TECHNOMIC
PUBLISHING CO., INC.

Biocompatible Polymers, Metals, and Composites

Edited by: M. Szycher, Ph.D.

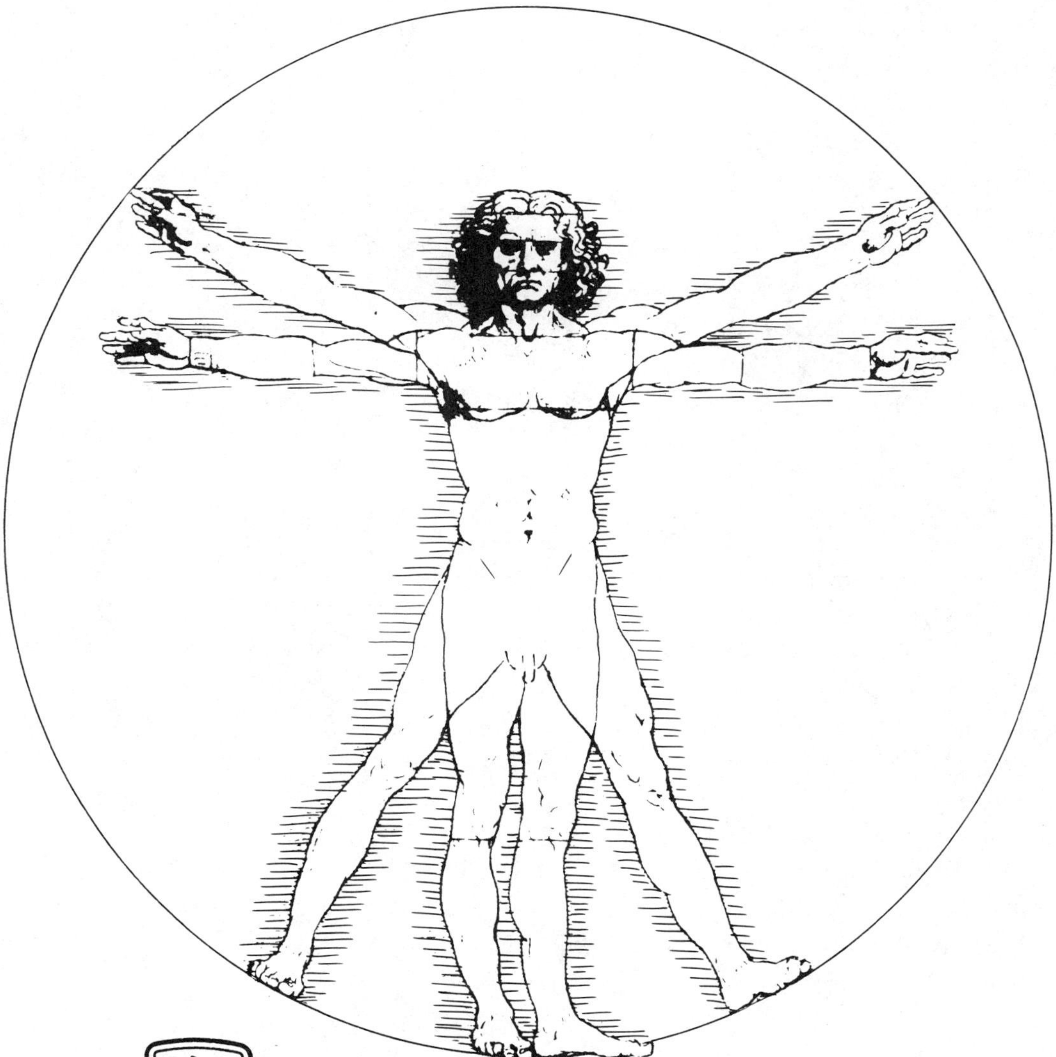

Sponsored by the SOCIETY OF PLASTICS ENGINEERS, INC.

851 New Holland Avenue
Box 3535
Lancaster, Pennsylvania 17604

Printed in U.S.A.
Library of Congress Card No. 82-74316
ISBN 87762-323-6

DEDICATION

This book is dedicated to my wife, Laurie, and to my sons, Mark and Scott, for their continued support and encouragement.

Foreword

Plastics in biomedical applications continue to be one of the most rapidly growing areas in plastics today. Certainly the technical challenge is one of the most demanding since polymer performance criteria are frequently confounded by polymer compatability with aggressive biological systems. Dr. Michael Szycher, the editor of this landmark volume on biocompatible polymers, metals and composites, is a recognized authority in this highly technical area. He has gathered together many of the leading technical people to contribute their ideas to this book. The book is thoughtfully formatted to allow for easy reader access and this care has been translated into the individual chapter construction. Dr. Szycher is one of the founders of the Medical Plastics Division of the Society of Plastics Engineers and is coeditor of the successful SPE-sponsored volume, "Synthetic Biomedical Polymers", also published by Technomic.

The Technical Volumes Committee of SPE has been charged with surveying and evaluating need for specific technical books since 1956. In that time, it has been the catalyst for publication of more than 50 books in important areas of the plastics industry that have not previously had definitive treatments. The committee works with authors and publishers, reviews and contents of manuscripts to determine their utility to SPE members, and most importantly, thoroughly reviews final manuscripts to ensure accuracy of the technical material.

This concern with technical accuracy and detail is typical of the way in which the Society deals with its other activities—education programs, conferences, periodicals, and meetings. Its greatest resource is its 26,000 practicing plastics engineers and technologists, a resource that has made SPE the largest and most respected organization of its type in plastics worldwide.

The Society of Plastics Engineers is pleased to sponsor and endorse this foundation volume edited by an outstanding SPE member and authored by many of the foremost technical people in the biomedical area today.

SOCIETY OF PLASTICS ENGINEERS, INC.
14 FAIRFIELD DRIVE, BROOKFIELD CENTER, CONNECTICUT 06805
TELEPHONE 203-775-0471

Contents

III
Current Topics in Biomaterials

IV
Emerging Technologies

V

Processing of Biocompatible Materials

Preface

Technologies have a life cycle of their own, similar in many ways to living organisms. An integral part of both the technological and organic life cycle is the maturation process. For any technical discipline, the maturation process involves greater rationalization; that is, the eventual replacement of the arts-practitioner, who relies heavily on experience and trial-and-error methods, by the professional who operates with prior understanding of fundamental concepts, and is thus capable of predicting, in advance, the expected behavior of a system based on scientifically defined principles.

The field of biomaterials is relatively new, and as such is in the process of undergoing a maturation process. It is apparent that biomaterials technology relies heavily on the classical sciences (chemistry, physics), but is also reinforced by basic engineering, anatomy, histology, hematology, and other disciplines too numerous to mention. A quick review of the biomaterials literature points out that there has indeed been a transition from the pragmatism or serendipity of early investigators, into a more controlled, scientifically based approach. Earlier attempts concentrated on selecting commercially available polymers, cleaning or purifying them as much as possible, and using them as a starting point in the fabrication of prototype prostheses. Lately, the tendency has been to specifically target the most suitable biomaterials to the intended application, biomaterials so specialized and expensive that they may never become commercially viable, except for their use in biomedical applications.

With these thoughts in mind, the intent of this book has been to emphasize, from a scientific viewpoint, the development, manufacture, and testing of those biomaterials most compatible with the human body. The result is that we have cut across disciplines, centers of medical research, and topics, in a deliberate effort to present the broadest view of the field. The contributors to this book represent many of the disciplines cited previously, and the topics originate from investigations conducted in the private, government, and academic sectors.

This book would not have been possible without the efforts of the contributors, who represent the vanguard of this young, emerging field. The sponsorship of the Society of Plastics Engineers, and the support of Thermo Electron Corporation have been invaluable. Specifically, I would like to acknowledge the interest and cooperation of those people who have been there on a daily basis: Victor L. Poirier, Manager of the Biomedical Group, Thermo Electron, for his unwavering support, Dorothy Lee Carchia for her heroic efforts in editing and proofreading, and Thomas L. Coyne for the design of the cover that graces this book.

Michael Szycher, Ph.D.
Director
Biomaterials Research
Thermo Electron Corporation

Waltham, Massachusetts
January 1982

I

Fundamental Concepts in Blood/Materials Interactions

Chapter 1

Thrombosis, Hemostasis, and Thrombolysis at Prosthetic Interfaces

Michael Szycher, Ph.D.
Thermo Electron Corporation
Biomedical Systems Division
101 First Avenue
P.O. Box 459
Waltham, MA 02254

I. ABSTRACT

Exposure of blood to artificial surfaces leads to adsorption of plasma proteins within a matter of seconds. Following this adsorption, there may be subsequent deposition of platelets and leukocytes, leading to blood coagulation on the surface of the biomaterial, a phenomenon known as mural thrombosis.

Blood coagulation results from the conversion of a soluble circulating plasma protein, fibrinogen, into insoluble fibrin. Though fibrinogen is soluble in plasma, it is suspended on the brink of insolubility and indeed can be readily polymerized into fibrin on the surface of artificial materials under a variety of conditions. The fibrin that is deposited on the walls quickly forms a meshwork of fibrils, the basis of a coagulum.

The formation of a coagulum may be preceded by platelet adhesion; these two phenomena occur more or less independently. It appears that in the latter stages of blood coagulation on a foreign surface, there is a mutual and cooperative interaction between the coagulation process and platelet aggregation. As it forms, the coagulum entraps other blood elements. Red blood cells appear to play primarily a passive role, adding only bulk. White blood cells are attracted by the thrombus, invade it, and concentrate there. Early in the process, through enzymatic release, leukocytes may contribute to fibrin formation and platelet recruitment; later, these leukocytes may take part in the digestion and resolution of the thrombus (thrombolysis).

II. INTRODUCTION

The increasing utilization of foreign materials in contact with blood has gained great importance in medical practice in recent years. In the past two decades there has been a virtual revolution in the development and clinical applications of blood-handling equipment.

To mention just a few examples, we can cite the now widespread utilization of hemodialysis equipment – better known to the lay public as artificial kidney machines. Hemodialysis machines accept blood from a patient suffering from a derangement in kidney function, purify the blood from certain toxic metabolites, and return the cleansed blood to the patient.

Another example is the worldwide use of cardiopulmonary bypass. This device has permitted the development of open-heart surgery. The instrument pumps blood through the patient, while the heart is stopped to allow for a surgical procedure to take place. At the same time, while the blood is circulating extracorporeally, the device also oxygenates the blood, thus performing the dual functions of both heart and lungs.

Other notable examples include angiographic catheters, chronic insulin monitors, and intraaortic balloon pumps. More recently, an artificial heart device has been developed. This temporary Left Ventricular Assist Device is now undergoing its third year of clinical trials at participating hospitals in the Boston area. This artificial heart is designed to help patients who cannot be weaned from cardiopulmonary bypass, or in patients whose myocardium is profoundly hypokinetic following cardiogenic shock.

The successful development of the Left Ventricular Assist Device, as well as cardiopulmonary bypass, are made possible only through the use of synthetic polymers that are chronically nonthrombogenic. That is, when these devices begin to pump blood, they do not cause blood to coagulate uncontrollably or to embolize, since this would immediately defeat the intended purpose.

This is a remarkable achievement, since normally blood coagulates rapidly upon mere contact with foreign substances. To be able to produce cardiovascular prostheses that are nonthrombogenic, we must first gain a thorough understanding of the basic mechanisms underlying blood coagulation. Only then can we hope to select the biomaterials and configurations most suitable for our purposes.

III. BACKGROUND

In normal arteries and veins, a continuous monolayer of cells, called the endothelium, forms a unique thromboresistant layer between circulating blood and potentially thrombogenic subendothelial tissues. The integrity of the endothelium is a fundamental requirement for maintenance of normal structure and function within the entire cardiovascular system.

Natural living endothelium is nature's premier nonthrombogenic blood interface. This remarkable hemocompatibility of living blood vessels is undoubtedly derived from the ability of the vessels to take an active role in their thromboresistance; vascular endothelium is a biochemically versatile tissue capable of many synthetic and metabolic functions. For example, endothelial cells produce prostaglandin PGI (prostacyclin), the most potent antiplatelet inhibitor known in biology; endothelial cells also synthesize a plasminogen activator which solubilizes mural fibrin; endothelial cells possess a surface enzyme capable of neutralizing adenosine diphosphate, thereby reducing platelet agglomeration; finally, normal endothelium has been shown to synthesize heparin — like anticoagulant substances. Thus, this thin cell, hardly visible in routine histologic sections, guarantees freedom from thrombosis and thromboembolism under normal circumstances.

However, what happens where we implant in the cardiovascular system a synthetic polymer that does not possess a living endothelium? Let us assume that we have synthesized an experimental biomaterial, and we wish to use it in chronic contact with blood. If we fashion this biomaterial in the form of an aortic graft, and implant it in the descending aorta, what physiological reactions can we expect? What would happen to the blood? What would happen to the blood-contacting surface of the biomaterial? To answer these questions, we must first examine the normal reactions of the blood, because it is precisely the normal reactions of the blood which will ultimately determine the success or failure of the implant.

IV. MURAL THROMBOSIS AND HEMOSTASIS

Under normal conditions, when a needle punctures a vessel wall, as depicted in Figure 1A, a series of responses is promptly elicited. As the needle is withdrawn from the vessel wall, as shown in Figure 1B, platelets adhere to the raw edges of the wound and then aggregate in an effort to plug the defect in the vessel wall, and thus prevent continuing hemorrhage; while this plug develops across the defect, a similar reaction takes place on the traumatized intimal surface to form an in situ mural thrombus. Platelets also adhere to the exposed connective tissue on the outside of the vessel, as shown in Figure 1C. Fibrin coagulation quickly follows platelet aggregation to further stabilize the mass. If not stabilized, surface fragments are apt to be dislodged by the blood, and carried away as emboli in the bloodstream.

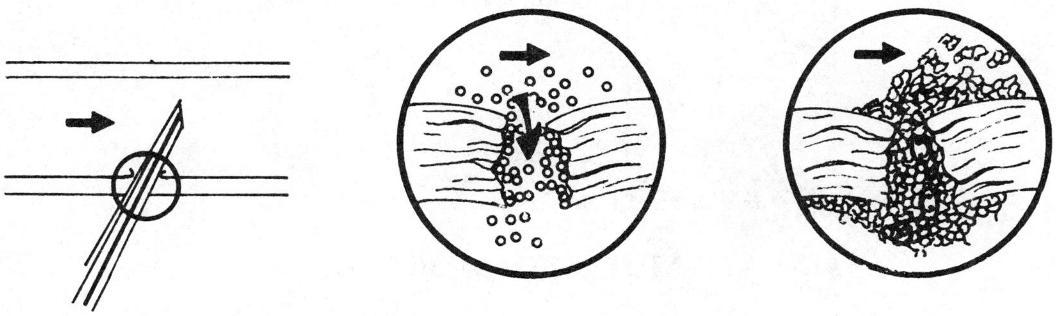

(A) (B) (C)

(A) Needle punctures a vessel wall; (B) Platelets adhere to wound; (C) Fibrin coagulation quickly follows, with occasional incorporation of leukocytes. If not stabilized, microemboli may be carried by bloodstream. Arrow = direction of blood flow.

Figure 1. Normal Hemostatic Mechanism.

This simple model exemplifies two basic concepts, thrombosis and hemostasis. Thrombosis is the manifestation of those functions of blood normally responsible for the formation of a clot. The principal mechanisms that have evolved in blood are platelet adhesion, platelet aggregation, and finally, fibrin coagulation (polymerization and crosslinking). Hemostasis refers to the combination of processes that account for the cessation of bleeding after surgery, or trauma to the vascular system; one process contributing to hemostasis involves the mechanism of thrombosis. Thus, hemostasis implies a return to normalcy, a restoration of equilibrium; therefore when we design and implant a cardiovascular prosthesis, we always strive to regain hemostasis as soon as possible.

Traditionally, blood coagulation was thought to be accomplished by the interaction of platelets and the formation of fibrin; in modern times the incredible complexity of blood coagulation is slowly being unraveled, dramatically illustrated by the many chapters in this book that deal specifically with the thrombogenicity of natural and synthetic blood interfaces.

Blood itself is composed of a liquid medium, plasma, and cellular elements, which constitute approximately 46 percent of the volume, shown diagrammatically in Figure 2. Cellular elements are subdivided into erythrocytes, leukocytes, and platelets, illustrated in Appendix A. Generally, erythrocytes do not form part of the coagulation process per se, although they are generally trapped within the sticky coagulum, giving rise to the familiar dark coloration we associate with a clot. By far the most important role is played by the platelets. Platelet adhesion and aggregation is one of the first steps in the formation of mural thrombi. An implanted biomaterial which is attractive to platelets can be expected to thrombose shortly thereafter.

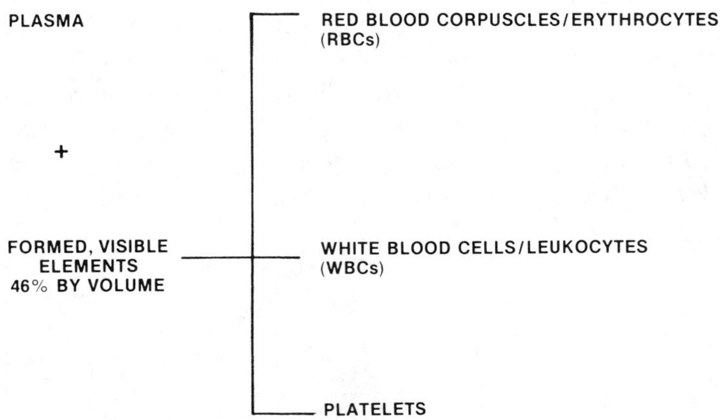

Figure 2. Human Blood Constituents.

V. PLATELETS (THROMBOCYTES)

As we have seen, hemostasis is one of the essential survival mechanisms; in man, hemostasis depends on the clotting of blood pumps, and on the aggregation of a particular type of circulating cell, the platelet. Platelets have only two well-established physiological functions: (1) to form hemostatic plugs in injured vessels, and (2) to provide a phospholipid material (platelet Factor 3) that greatly accelerates plasma coagulation.

Platelets are the smallest of the formed elements of the blood, averaging 1.5 μm in diameter and from 0.5 to 1 μm in thickness as determined by electron microscopy [1]. Normally, about $250 \times 10^3/mm^3$ (range 140 to $440 \times 10^3/mm^3$) are present in the circulation (range 140 to $440 \times 10^3/mm^3$ [2]. Microscopically, they appear as flat discs [3] and remain viable for 9 to 12 days in man, as estimated by in vitro whole population labeling with ^{51}Cr-chromate [4,5].

Ultrastructurally, the interior of the platelet is seen to contain a variety of granules, the least numerous being the mitochondria, comprising roughly 15 percent of the granule population. Two other intracellular storage granules are present: they are called, respectively, dense granules and α-granules. Interactions between platelets and certain substances (i.e., collagen, synthetic foreign surfaces) cause the release of granular material into the circulating blood; the specific release of granular material from the platelets in response to extracellular stimulation has been termed the platelet release reaction [6,7]. The term "platelet release reaction" is thus used to describe the specific extrusion to the platelet's environment of the content of platelet storage granules.

The platelet release reaction is of paramount importance in our understanding of mural thrombi on biomaterials, since the platelet granules represent individually functioning biological units capable of attracting more platelets, and also capable of initiating thrombosis. Platelets circulate in blood without adhering to each other or to normal endothelium. Their unique properties lie in changes that occur when the endothelium is broken, or when the platelets are exposed to a variety of foreign artificial surfaces.

Platelets adhere to biomaterials by means of pseudopodia; following this adhesion (the mechanisms of which are poorly understood), platelets undergo a variety of internal changes, known as the platelet release reaction, which results in their sticking to each other, a process known as platelet aggregation. This aggregation appears to be triggered by the release of adenosine diphosphate (ADP) which is present in high concentration within the platelets themselves. The ADP responsible for platelet aggregation is stored in electron-dense dark granules. ADP also causes the activation of a membrane phospholipase, which hydrolyzes membrane phospholipids to yield arachidonic acid. Arachidonic acid, in turn, is converted by a platelet enzyme called cyclooxygenase into a prostaglandin endoperoxide. This endoperoxide is then converted into a substance called thromboxane A_2, which is the most potent platelet aggregant known in medicine. Therefore platelets are self-sufficient laboratories, containing all the necessary ingredients needed for adhesion, aggregation, and the initiation of a mural thrombus.

The production of an irreversible aggregate of platelets is dependent on the platelet release reaction. ADP released from adherent platelets is sufficient to induce aggregation of a much larger number, so the release reaction may also be viewed as a biologic amplifier that rapidly converts a minimal stimulus into a massive response [8]. ADP extruded during the release reaction is only one of a number of pharmacologically active substances located within the platelet-dense bodies. Table 1 shows the contents of substances known to reside within the platelets.

To recapitulate, platelets respond to a variety of substrates, both natural and synthetic, by altering their shape, adhering to the materials to which they are exposed, and undergoing a release reaction. This release reaction involves a surprisingly rapid movement of subcellular granules to the surface of the platelet where they degranulate and contribute to the prolongation and amplification of mural thrombus.

This analysis of platelet function has emphasized its role to promote hemostasis and its participation in thrombogenesis. In addition, platelets are also important for other functional characteristics:

- Platelets and leukocytes tend to accumulate around each other; this interaction frequently leads to mural thrombosis.
- Adhesion of platelets nearly always occurs when blood contacts any artificial polymer, possibly leading to the activation of the intrinsic coagulation sequence.

Table 1. Substances Released During Platelet Release Reaction

Subcellular Localization	Constituent	Reference
Dense granules	5-Hydroxytryptamine (5-HT)	9
	Adenosine DiPhosphate (ADP)	10
	Adenosine TriPhosphate (ATP)	11
	Calcium	12
	Pyrophosphate	13
	Antiplasmin	14
α-granules	Acid hydrolases	15
	Potassium	16
	Fibrinogen	17
	Permeability factor	18
	Chemotactic factor	19
Unknown	Growth factor	20
	Bactericidal factor	21
	Platelet Factor 4	22

- Platelets recognize microscopic imperfections in the surface of "smooth" biomaterials, forming a microthrombus, which may embolize, and reform in a perpetual cycle.
- Platelet clumps form spontaneously in areas of blood stasis. These clumps are periodically carried downstream, resulting in a continuous shower of platelet microemboli.

The successful design of hemocompatible biomaterials demands detailed knowledge and understanding of platelet function and activity. Among the most important functions of platelets is their role in hemostasis; another crucial function is the participation of these elements in the coagulation sequence, particularly in the activation of the intrinsic pathway of coagulation, a subject to be discussed in detail subsequently.

VI. INTRINSIC COAGULATION SEQUENCE

We now turn our attention to blood plasma. The liquid phase of blood is composed of an aqueous medium, which normally contains a bewildering array of special substances. For the sake of simplicity, we will only discuss certain substances known to interact with implanted biomaterials, and which lead to the phenomenon of thrombosis. Of special interest are three families of proteins: the immunoglobulins, albumin, and the blood coagulation proteins. The blood coagulation proteins are a series of enzymes that work in a sequential fashion, with the final outcome being the polymerization of a blood-circulating monomer (fibrinogen) to form a crosslinked, stable biological macromolecule known as fibrin, depicted in Figure 3. Table 2 lists the individual coagulation factors according to the description established by the International Nomenclature Committee, which utilizes a roman numeral for each individual coagulation constituent. The numbers were assigned on a historical basis, with fibrinogen being the first factor purified and identified. Because of a mistake, Factor VI was assigned to a substance initially thought to be unique, but which later turned out to be merely an impure factor; since by that time Factor VII had already been discovered, it was decided to drop Factor VI from the list to avoid possible confusion. Arabic numbers 3 and 4 are assigned to mixtures of platelet membrane phospholipids, and a protein, that are known to contribute to the coagulation process; but to date the phospholipids have not been identified biochemically in a manner com-

Table 2. Nomenclature of Blood Coagulation Factors

Factor	Other Common Names
I	Fibrinogen
II	Prothrombin
III	Tissue Thromboplastin
IV	Calcium
V	Proaccelerin, Plasma Ac-globulin, Labile factor
-	Omitted
VII	Proconvertin, Stable factor, SPCA
VIII	Antihemophilic factor, AHF, antihemophilic globulin, AHG, Antihemophilic factor A
IX	Plasma thromboplastin component, PTC, Christmas factor, antihemophilic factor B
X	Stuart-Power factor
XI	Plasma thromboplastin antecedent, PTA
XII	Hageman factor, HF
XIII	Fibrin stabilizing factor, Fibrinase, Laki-Lorand factor
3	Platelet phospholipid clotting activity
4	Platelet antiheparin activity

Note: The coagulation factors are all proteins, with the exception of Factor IV (Ca^{++}). Factors VI, 1, and 2 are omitted since they were found to be impure macromolecules.

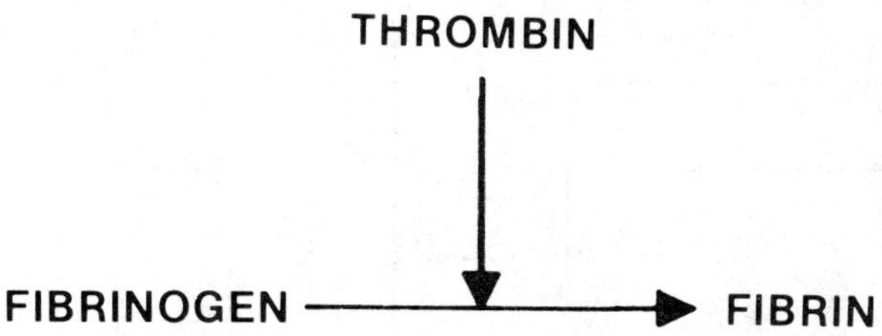

Figure 3. Formation of a fibrin meshwork by the proteolytic activity of thrombin on its substrate, fibrinogen. A fibrin meshwork is the final outcome of the coagulation cascade, and is an essential structural component of thrombus.

parable to other coagulation factors. Until they are identified in an unequivocal fashion, they are merely referred to as "phospholipids." A comprehensive glossary of known blood coagulation components is presented in Appendix B.

The coagulation of blood is mediated through a series of complex reactions involving the interaction of several enzymes, lipids, and ions. In the predominant reaction mechanism, an inactive circulating proenzyme is converted to an active proteolytic enzyme which has as its substrate another proenzyme. This principle is illustrated in Figure 4, which depicts the formation of fibrin monomer from its precursor fibrinogen, accomplished by the proteolytic proenzyme thrombin.

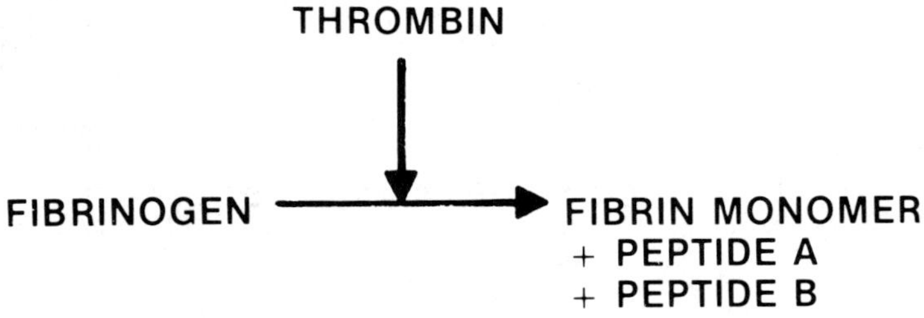

Figure 4. Formation of Fibrin Monomer by Cleavage of Peptides A and B.

Fibrinogen is a plasma protein that is synthesized in the liver parenchymal cells [23]. Its plasma concentration ranges between 200 and 400 mg/dl. Its biologic half-life is around 3 days. The fibrinogen molecule has a molecular weight of 330,000 Daltons, and consists of three pairs of disulfide-linked polypeptide chains designated $(A\alpha)_2$, $(B\beta)_2$, and γ_2 [24]. Since it circulates in dimerous form, [25] it is composed of a pair of alpha, beta, and gamma chains, shown in Figure 5. Peptides A and B represent the two fibrinopeptides cleaved from fibrinogen in the transformation of soluble fibrinogen into the spontaneously polymerizing fibrin monomer [26,27]. Covalent structure changes resulting from thrombin proteolysis reduce the molecular mass by an extremely small amount, approximately 6000 out of 340,000 mass units, but expose the polymerization sites of the fibrin monomer and permits gelation to occur.

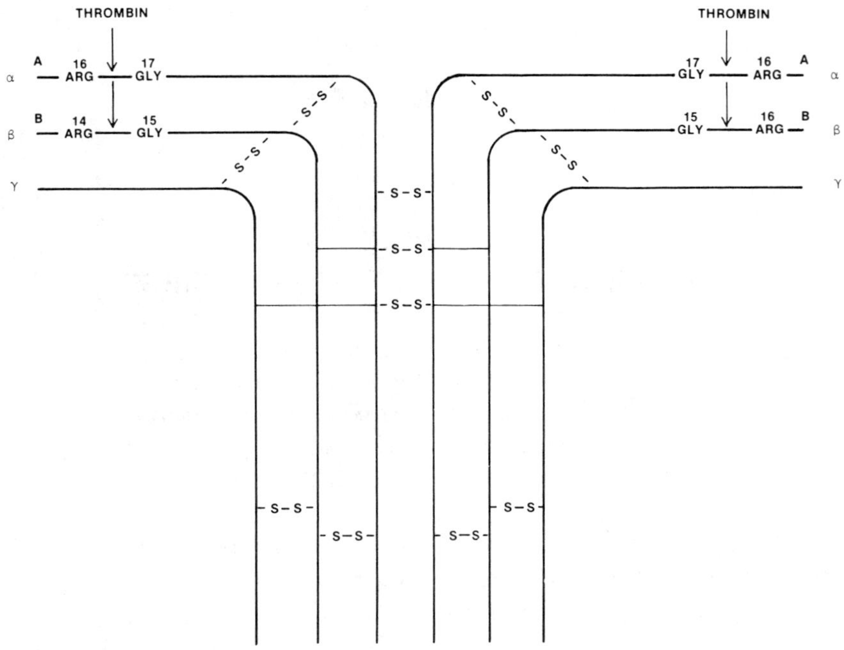

Figure 5. Molecular architecture of fibrinogen dimer. Peptides A and B are cleaved from the N-terminal portions of the α or β chain by the proteolytic action of thrombin.

The actual conversion of fibrinogen into fibrin can be divided into three phases:

(1) the proteolytic phase
(2) the polymerization phase
(3) the stabilization phase

(1) The proteolytic phase of fibrinogen conversion is heralded by the cleavage of two pairs of peptides from the fibrinogen molecule by the proteolytic enzyme thrombin [28,29]. One pair of peptides, called peptide A, is cleaved from the N-terminal end of the two alpha chains and one pair of peptides, called peptide B, is cleaved from the N-terminal end of the two beta chains. The gamma chains stay intact. The fibrinogen minus its peptides A and B is now called a fibrin monomer.

Although thrombin is a serine protease, it only splits Arg-Gly residues and thus is exquisitely specific as to its proteolytic action. One of these Arg-Gly bonds is located in the immediate vicinity of the N-terminal end of both the alpha and beta chains, thus cleaving the A peptide, which is 16 amino acids long, and the B peptide, which is 14 amino acids long.

(2) During the polymerization phase (Figure 6),which follows the proteolytic phase, the fibrin monomers aggregate or polymerize end-to-end, and side-to-side, thus forming a fibrin strand. The early polymerization phase is marked by primarily end-to-end association of the fibrin monomers, apparently reflecting the initial cleavage of the A peptides. Later coinciding with the release of the B peptide, the monomers polymerize side-to-side, thus reflecting the beta chain association.

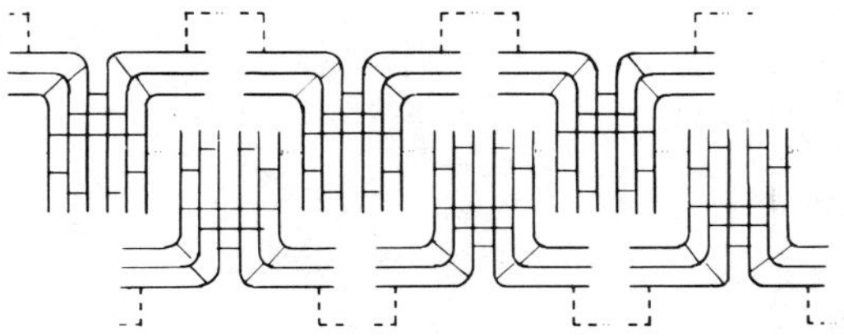

Figure 6. Polymerization Phase of Fibrin Formation.

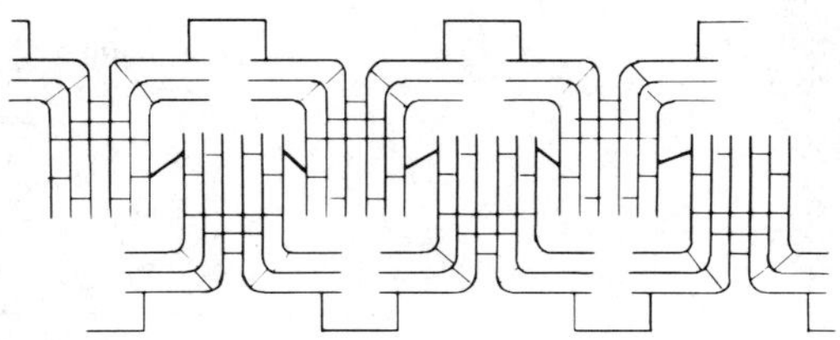

Figure 7. Stabilization Phase of Fibrin Formation (Crosslinking).

A fibrin strand, therefore, is composed of a large number of individual fibrin monomers, polymerized end-to-end and side-to-side. This polymerization sequence appears to be spontaneous, not requiring enzymatic intervention.

(3) The stabilization phase, shown in Figure 7, is characterized by the replacement of the initial hydrogen bonds between the individual monomers with covalent bonds, a crosslinking reaction. This covalent bond requires enzymatic mediation, and the enzyme facilitating this process is called Factor XIIIa, or "fibrin stabilizing factor." The covalent bond appears to occur between the epsilon amino groups of lysine and gamma carboxyl groups of aspartic acid.

The formation of fibrin is actually the last step in a complex series of reactions, which ultimately results in the formation of thrombus. The normal hemostatic process begins when a blood vessel is injured, and culminates in the formation of a fibrin-platelet meshwork that is a structural barrier to the further escape of blood, and the nidus for repair. When a biomaterial is implanted in the bloodstream, these basic mechanisms continue to operate, and may lead to undesirable or unexpected thrombosis.

So far, we have only discussed two aspects of the blood coagulation phenomenon, namely

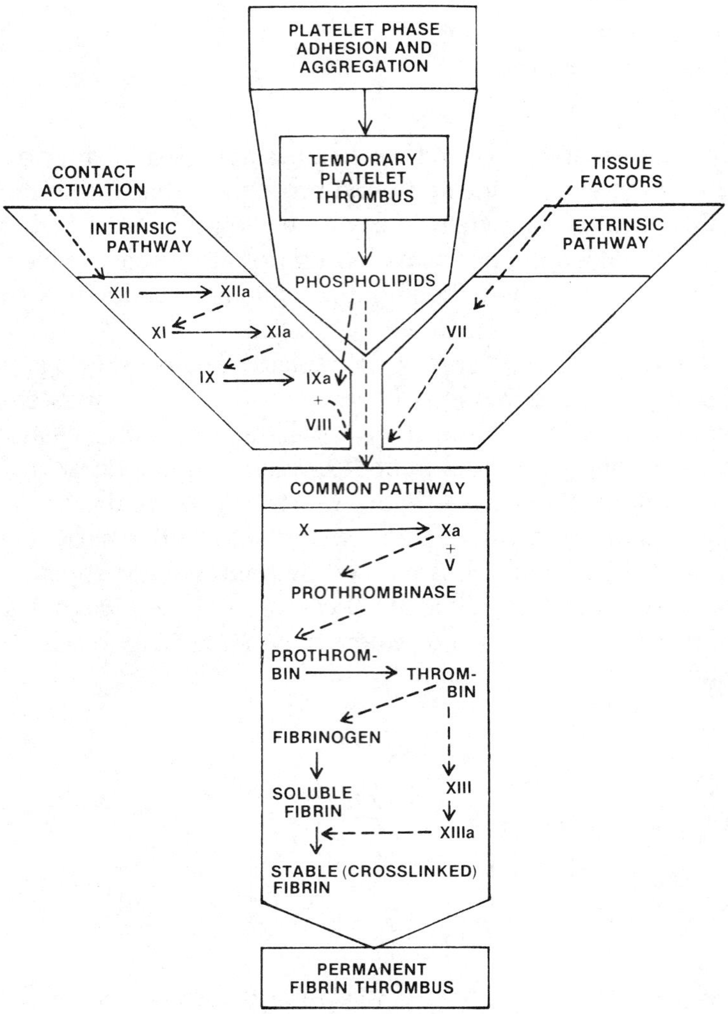

Figure 8. Blood Coagulation Cascade

the action of platelets and the formation of fibrin. In reality, fibrin is formed in response to a sequential system of reactions, as shown in Figure 8. As the figure indicates, fibrin can be formed in response to three independent mechanisms: the intrinsic pathway shown on the left, platelet activities shown in the middle, and the extrinsic pathway shown on the right.

The extrinsic pathway is activated by blood exposed to a variety of substances naturally found in tissues, known collectively as "tissue factors." Tissue factors include collagen, basement membrane constituents, lipids, and proteins. The generation of thrombus in blood exposed to tissue extracts occurs explosively in less than 10 seconds. There are no limiting steps, and the reaction proceeds rapidly to completion. The extrinsic pathway usually is not activated by the exposure to blood of a biomaterial, and is discussed here merely for the sake of completeness.

You may notice that starting at the top of the chart, the sequence is initiated by the activation of a single factor, either Factor VII of the extrinsic pathway, platelet adhesion with release of phospholipids, or the activation of Factor XII of the intrinsic pathway. This is shown diagrammatically by the addition of the small letter "a" following the factor. The activated factor then reacts with another factor; the second factor is then activated to act on a third factor, and so on, until the final step when thrombin acts on fibrinogen to form a fibrin meshwork. The sequence appears to follow a cascade, or waterfall effect, and for that reason, this chart is also known as the blood coagulation cascade.

In biomaterials work, it is the *intrinsic pathway* that is the most important. The exposure of blood to artificial surfaces leads in many cases to the adsorption of Factor XII upon the surface, with subsequent deposition of platelets and leukocytes. This adsorption of Factor XII may be of slight degree, or dependent on flow conditions. Factor XII may be activated, and the blood coagulation cascade will proceed to produce fibrin. During the polymerization of fibrinogen into fibrin, this mass is highly attractive to platelets, which may adhere to the thin layer of fibrin, agglomerate, release phospholipids, and amplify the speed of thrombus formation.

The intrinsic pathway, which may be provoked by exposure of blood to artificial surfaces, is initiated by conversion of Factor XII (Hageman Factor, a circulating protein present in normal plasma), into an active proteolytic enzyme whose natural substrate is Factor XI (Plasma Thromboplastin Antecedent), another circulating plasma protein proenzyme. It now appears that the initial activation step of Factor XII is not a simple direct consequence of surface adsorption and unfolding of the molecule; instead, present data indicate a complex activation step which involves interaction of at least four plasma proteins: Factor XII itself, Factor XI, prekallikrein, and high molecular weight kininogen (the precursor of the vasoactive substance bradykinin) [30,31]. Biochemical characteristics of prekallikrein and kininogen are presented in Appendix C.

These four proteins are collectively termed the "contact" system. The event that results in formation of the first active proteinase has not been established. There is evidence that adsorption of Factor XII on a surface alters its structure and increases its susceptibility to proteolysis by kallikrein. Meanwhile, another protein, high molecular weight kininogen, [32] apparently facilitates the adsorption of Factor XI on the surface, making it available to activated Factor XII which it serves as substrate.

As kallikrein converts Factor XII to Factor XIIa, Factor XIIa converts more prekallikrein to kallikrein (Figure 9), so a positive feedback mechanism seems to develop. Moreover, as kallikrein converts kininogen to kinin, the kinin converts more Factor XII to Factor XIIa, thus establishing another positive feedback system; this biological amplification system probably explains the explosive nature of the clotting process on artificial surfaces exposed to circulating blood.

A composite drawing of the entire mechanism of the contact activation system is presented in Figure 10. Note that platelet phospholipids as well as Ca^{++} ions intervene in the coagulation cascade in at least two steps (1) during formation of Factor XIa, phospholipids, and Ca^{++2} "complex" and (2) activation of prothrombin to thrombin, by formation of Factor Xa, Factor V, phospholipids, and Ca^{++} "complex." Thus platelet phospholipids, and presumably platelet Ca^{++} as well, are capable of triggering the coagulation cascade.

In summary, mural thrombus formation on the walls of an implanted biomaterial is, in effect, an exaggeration of the normal hemostatic mechanism. For instead of the formation of a hemostatic plug, which is designed simply to seal off a site of vascular injury, we find that the initiating events are the same, but the process may not stop until an abnormal mass is formed which may partially occlude the prosthesis, or embolize downstream. Like the hemostatic mechanism, mural thrombi on biomaterials involves the same two principal components, blood platelets and the various plasma proteins of the intrinsic coagulation sequence.

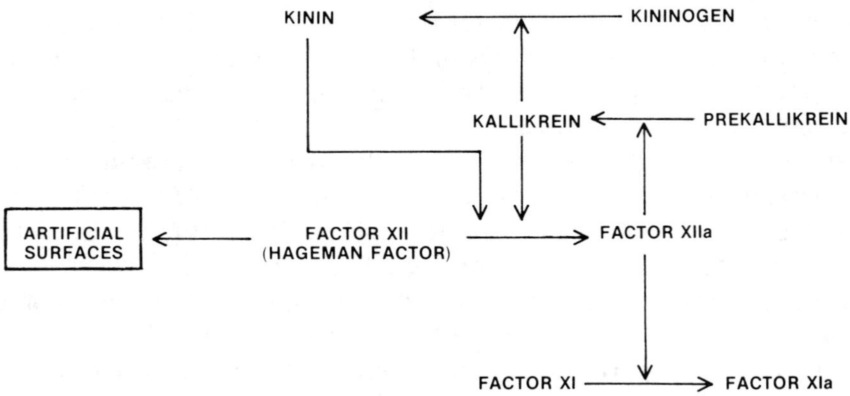

Figure 9. Positive feedback mechanism resulting in activation of factor XII, following exposure of artificial surfaces to circulating blood.

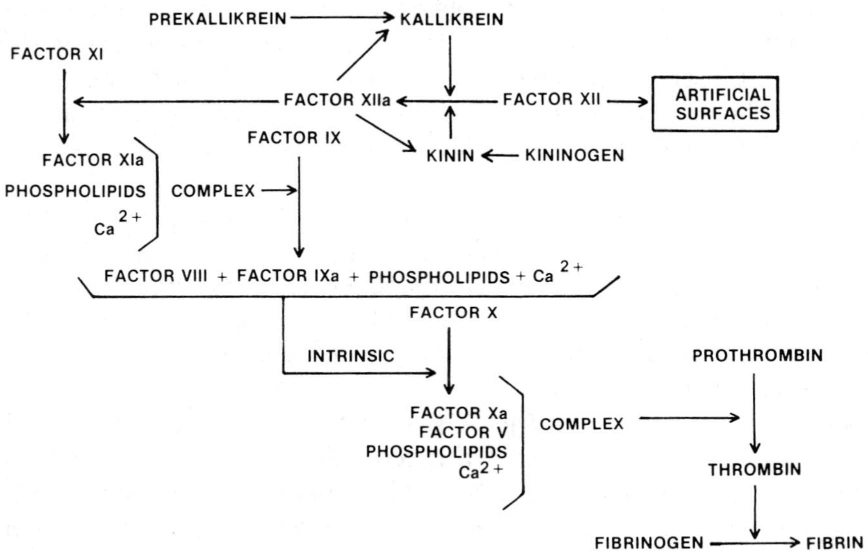

Figure 10. Composite mechanism of fibrin formation by contact activation on artificial surface.

VII. THROMBOLYSIS

The culmination of the coagulation sequence is the rapid transition of soluble fibrinogen into insoluble fibrin. The capacity of the fibrinolytic system to cause the dissolution of fibrin represents an essential defense or compensatory system reactive to uncontrolled activity of the coagulation sequence and critical for the preservation of the cardiovascular system [33]. Multimolecular systems intrinsic to the blood provide enzymatic effectors for controlled catabolism of fibrin and other proteins [34].

Components of the fibrinolytic systems present in plasma include: (a) fibrinolytic enzymes (proenzyme plasminogen and proteolytic agent plasmin), (b) activators of plasminogen, (c) inhibitors of fibrinolytic enzyme activators, (d) plasmin substrates, (e) catabolic degradation fragments of fibrinogen and fibrin, and (f) humoral antibodies to degradation fragments of fibrinogen and fibrin.

The proteolytic enzyme plasmin and its proenzyme plasminogen are the components of the major human fibrinolytic system. Plasminogen is a β-globulin composed of a single polypeptide chain, with a molecular weight estimated to range from 87,000 to 89,000 Daltons. In normal plasma it is present at a concentration of 200 to 495 μg/ml [35]. Plasminogen circulates in concert with fibrinogen and plasmin [36].

The conversion of plasminogen to plasmin is characterized by cleavage of the single-chain zymogen, resulting in a two-chain proteolytic enzyme structure interconnected covalently by a single disulfide bond. The chains are designated heavy (H chain: 55,000 Daltons) and light (L chain: 26,000 Daltons). Plasmin is capable of hydrolyzing arginyl and lysil bonds at neutral pH; this may explain the modest preference for fibrinogen and fibrin. However, a number of other plasma proteins, such as Factors V, VIII, and XII, are also subject to attack by plasmin. Thus, plasmin is a nonspecific proteolytic enzyme.

Recent evidence has shown that a major endogenous plasma activator system is Factor XIIa, depicted in Figure 11. In this system Factor XIIa directly activates plasminogen activator, and also converts prekallikrein to kallikrein. The latter amplifies the generation of more Factor XIIa; activated plasminogen proactivator then converts plasminogen to plasmin. Thus human plasma endogenously contains all proteins necessary for clot formation, as well as clot lysis (thrombolysis).

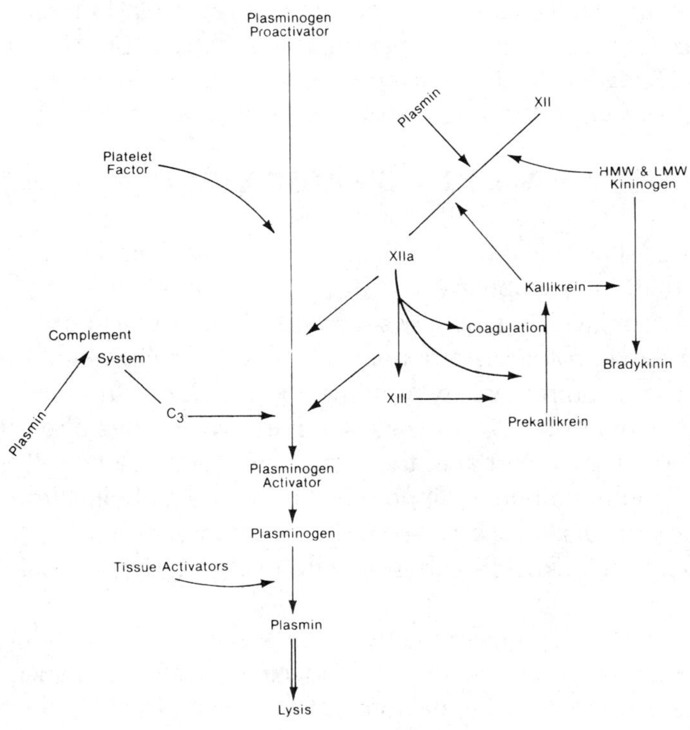

Figure 11. Activation of Plasminogen by Several Pathways.

Like other physiologic processes, the thrombolytic mechanism is controlled and governed by a number of inhibitory devices. To date, a total of nine naturally occurring components of the plasma have been demonstrated to inhibit the activity of the various fibrinolytic systems (Table 3) [37-45]. The inhibitory capacity is different for each inhibitor, and is variable, depending upon which protease in the pathway is complexed by the inhibitor.

Table 3. Naturally Occurring Plasma Components with Demonstrated Inhibitory Activity on Various Fibrinolytic Systems

Inhibitor	Molecular Weight	Concentration (mg/100 ml)	Reference Number
α_1-antitrypsin	55,000	200 - 400	37
α_2-macroglobulin	725,000	150 - 420	38
C1 esterase inhibitor	104,000	15 - 35	39
antithrombin III	65,000	17 - 30	40
inter-α-trypsin inhibitor	160,000	20 - 70	41
α_1-antichymotrypsin	69,000	30 - 60	42
α_2-antiplasmin (inter-α-antiplasmin)	67,000 - 80,000	unknown	43
antiactivator	50,000 - 80,000	unknown	44
α_1-antiplasmin	68,000	unknown	45

In essence, the activation of the intrinsic pathway is brought about by the surface activation of Factor XII, and the kallikrein-kinin system. As these proteases are activated to produce fibrin, an equal and opposite reaction may also take place to dissolve the formed fibrin, thus providing a coordinated and balanced hemeostatic integration between these antagonistic systems. Therefore, the activation of plasminogen by Factor XII represents a general mechanism for producing localized surface proteolysis; this mechanism may serve to limit and control the amount of mural thrombus formed on the walls of implanted prostheses.

VIII. PROTEIN ADSORPTION

When a biomaterial is initially placed in contact with blood, blood plasma proteins (albumin, fibrinogen/fibrin, γ-globulins) are immediately adsorbed onto the surface of the biomaterial. This protein layer is generally accepted to form almost immediately [46]. This initial adsorption of plasma proteins profoundly influences all subsequent events, and to a large extent determines the thrombogenicity/nonthrombogenicity of the implanted biomaterials.

In the first minutes of contact, it appears there are two modes of plasma protein adsorption at the blood/biomaterial interface: the first occurs as a result of the preferential, competitive adsorption of either albumin, fibrinogen/fibrin, or γ-globulins from the blood plasma, and the second mode occurs (following surface adsorption of proteins from the blood clotting sequence) as platelet and leukocyte adhesion, ultimately causing the polymerization of fibrin onto the surface.

A consensus is now developing among biomaterial scientists, that in those instances where albumin layering occurs in preference to fibrinogen, thromboresistance is favored [47-50]. Studies, which investigated the individual effects of albumin, fibrin, and γ-globulins on thrombosis, found that if albumin is preferentially adsorbed, there is little or no thrombus formation [51]. If, however, fibrinogen and γ-globulin are preferentially adsorbed, thrombosis may ensue, causing platelet adherence, aggregation, and release of platelet constituents. And as we have already discussed, platelet release products are known to activate the intrinsic cascade, and have also been shown [52] to activate Factor VII of the extrinsic pathway which then activates Factor X, and consequently cause fibrin polymerization.

Fibrinogen is thought to enhance platelet adhesion to glass and collagen fibrin; fibrinogen adsorption has also been implicated in the initial phases of the thrombogenic reactions [53-55]. Fibrinogen is also suspected of interacting with leukocytes [56] where, presumably, in those situations when fibrinogen is preferentially adsorbed and not stabilized by Factor XIII, the degree of platelet adherence and agglomeràtion is not solely mediated by the plasma proteins, such as albumin and γ-globulins, but rather by a complex series of interactions between fibrinogen, platelet, leukocytes, and other blood proteins.

Gamma globulins have not received as much attention as fibrinogen and albumin, but a careful study showed that γ-globulin coatings on an artificial surface not only enhanced platelet adhesion, but stimulated the platelet release reaction as well [57].

After the initial layer of plasma protein is adsorbed onto the biomaterials surface, a crosslinked fibrin network may develop over the next minutes to hours. It is within this fibrin network that the formed elements of the blood become entrapped, forming a mural thrombus. The rate of these simultaneous processes may be critical for the practicality of a material in a particular device. If the rate of thrombus formation is slow, the process of fibrinolysis may prevent gross thrombus formation. If controlled, a more permanent substrate develops which, with time (months) can become biologically reorganized or resolved into a defined type of pseudoneointimal lining [58-60].

This crucial interrelationship between adsorption of plasma proteins and the thrombogenicity of biomaterials has been extensively studied; the aim has been to better understand the interaction between blood and polymeric surfaces, to gain a fundamental knowledge about these phenomena. The goal is to contribute to the development of less thrombogenic artificial surfaces. Table 4 summarizes the concentrations of adsorbed plasma proteins on the surfaces of some important biomaterials.

An important observation that has been repeatedly made is that albumin minimizes platelet adhesion and thrombogenesis [63-65] and that albumin renders polymers less suscep-

Table 4. Surface Concentration of Adsorbed Plasma Proteins on Some Important Biomaterials

Polymer	Surface Distribution		Reference
	Albumin (%)	Fibrinogen and γ-Globulin (%)	
Polystyrene	17	83	61
Polyethylene	25	75	61
Silastic Rubber	32	68	61
Teflon FEP	37	63	61
Biomer Polyurethane	42	58	62
Tecoflex HR Polyurethane	37	63	62
Silicone-Urethane Copolymer	38	62	62

tible to cellular adhesion; Table 4 confirms these reported observations. We can see that as the percentage of albumin adsorbed on the surface increases, the polymers become less thrombogenic. Silicone rubbers, Teflon, and polyurethanes are among the best of the available hemocompatible materials.

IX. COMPLEMENT AND FIBRONECTINS

To this point we have discussed the interrelationship between (a) blood cells (platelets, leukocytes), (b) coagulation proteins (intrinsic and extrinsic pathways), and (c) plasma proteins (albumin, fibrinogen, γ-globulins). All of these components contribute significantly to the formation of mural thrombi on implanted biomaterials.

More recently, two other circulating plasma proteins have been shown to significantly affect the chronic hemocompatibility of implanted biomaterials, (1) complement and (2) fibronectins. Physiologically these proteins are unrelated, but when passively adsorbed onto biomaterials surfaces they appear to mediate the lysis and adhesion of blood cells to implanted prostheses.

Complement is a multimolecular, self-assembling biological system which constitutes the primary humural mediator of antigen-antibody reactions [66]. When the complement system is activated and acts against foreign cells it is called immunity. When the proteins of the complement system act against host cells, such reactions are called allergic or hypersensitive reactions. To date we know of 21 distinct proteins that are considered constituents of the complement system; 15 are considered components proper, 3 regulators, 1 enzyme inhibitor, and 2 inactivating enzymes.

Operationally, the complement system may be subdivided into two pathways, each comprising several functional units. The first, or classical pathway, is activated by IgG- and IgM-type complexes; its proteins have been divided into three functional units: (1) the recognition unit, (2) the activation unit, and (3) the membrane attack system. The characteristics of the proteins of the classical human complement system are presented in Table 5. The second pathway, called the alternative pathway, bypasses C1, C2, and C4 and acts on C5-9 in a manner analogous to that of the classical activation mechanism. It is the alternative pathway of complement activation that is the predominant system of complement activation in blood-materials interaction.

The alternative pathway can be activated by proteolytic enzymes (such as the blood-clotting enzymes). In some cases, these enzymes act by activating C3, as in the classical pathway. The proteins of the alternative pathway of complement activation are presented in Table 6. A schematic diagram of the interrelationship between the classical and alternative pathway mechanisms is shown in Figure 12.

Complement activation on a biomaterials surface is important for at least three reasons. (1) Activated complement mediates the chemotaxis and adhesion of leukocytes to foreign surfaces, [67] activation of the alternative pathway results in the release of soluble chemotactic factors (C3a and C5a) which attract polymorphonuclear leukocytes to the site; these leukocytes may also attract platelets, and help in the formation of mural thrombus. (2) Activated complement aggregates platelets, and encourages ADP release; denatured IgG fixes complement, aggregates platelets, and binds leukocytes [68]. (3) Polymorphonuclear leukocyte adhesion to artificial surfaces is a consistent finding in ex vivo stagnation point flow experiments. The clinical significance of this blood-foreign surface interaction is manifest on a

Table 5. Proteins of the Classical Human Complement System

Functional Unit	Protein	Surface Concentration (μg/ml)	Molecular Weight	Relative Electrophoretic Mobility
Recognition	Clq	180	400,000	γ_2
	Clr	---	180,000	β
	Cls	110	86,000	α
Activation	C2	25	117,000	β_1
	C3	1,600	180,000	β_2
	C4	640	206,000	β_1
Membrane Attack	C5	80	180,000	β_1
	C6	75	95,000	β_2
	C7	55	110,000	β_2
	C8	80	163,000	γ_1
	C9	230	79,000	α

Table 6. Proteins of the Alternative Pathway

Protein	Symbol	Serum Concentration (μg/ml)	Molecular Weight	Relative Electrophoretic Mobility
Nephritic Factor Analog	IF	---	150,000	γ_1
Properdin	P	25	184,000	γ_2
C3	C3	1,600	180,000	β_2
C3b	C3b	---	171,000	α_2
C3 Proactivator	C3PA or B	200	93,000	β
C3 Activator	C3A or $\bar{B}$	---	63,000	γ
C3 Proactivator Convertase	C3Pase or $\bar{D}$	---	24,000	α

widespread basis during cardiopulmonary bypass; leukocyte-platelet emboli are often found in the lungs of patients perfused in a CPB system not containing microaggregate filters [69].

The last of the circulating plasma proteins to be discussed are the fibronectins. The fibronectins [70,71] are a group of glycoproteins, variously known as CSP (cell surface protein) [72], FSA (fibroblast surface antigen) [73], LETS (large external transformation sensitive protein) [74], Galactoprotein [75], Z protein [76], and Clg (cold insoluble globulin) [77]. Fibronectins have been found on the surface of fibroblasts [78], smooth muscle cells [79], glial cells [80], epithelial cells [81], and endothelial cells [82].

Fibronectin (the name to be used in this chapter) is an α_2-glycoprotein with a molecular weight of 450,000 Daltons that consists of two nearly identical subunit polypeptides, held together by disulfide linkages. Native fibronectin appears as disulfide crosslinked dimers which occur mainly in two immunologically cross-reactive forms: on the surface of many cells (cellular fibronectin), and in the form of plasma fibronectin which circulates in human blood; the plasma form of fibronectin is commonly called cold insoluble globulin (Clg). Figure 13 shows the proposed primary structure of human Clg [83]. The dashed arrow indicates site of in vitro plasmic attack.

Cell surface fibronectin plays an important role in cell-cell interaction, as well as adherence

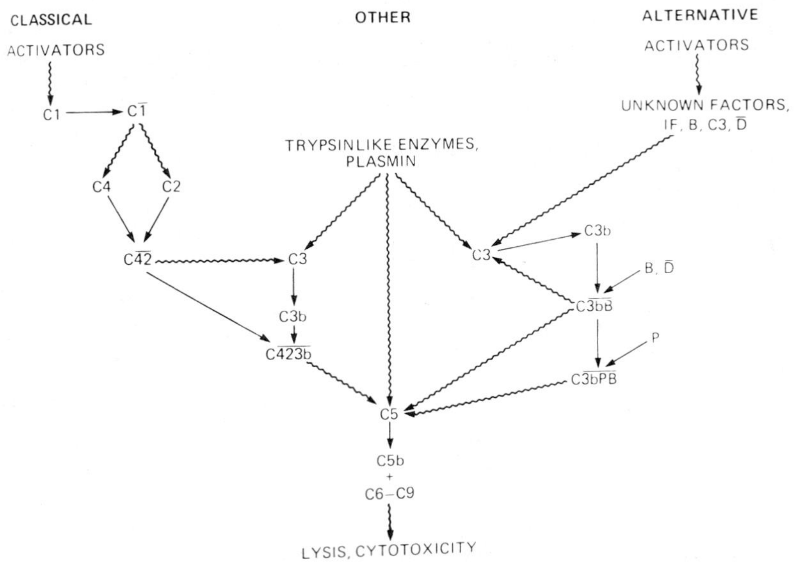

Figure 12. Schematic Diagram of the Mechanisms of Assembly of the Complement (C) System on the Surfaces of a Complement Activator.

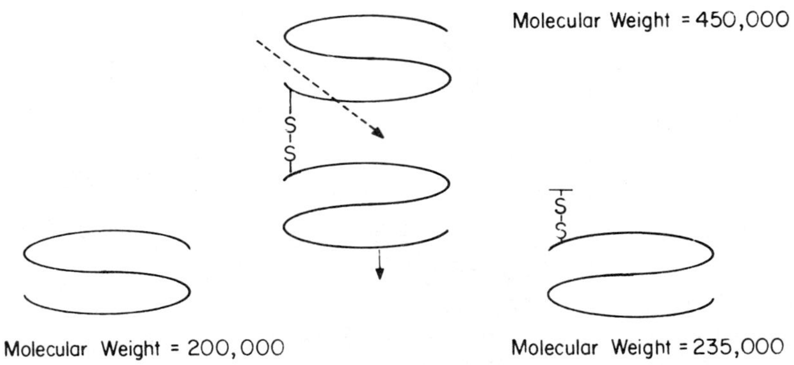

Figure 13. Primary Structure of Human Cold Insoluble Globulin.

of cultured cells to a substratum [84,85]. Cell surface fibronectin is antigenically related to plasma fibronectin, but subtle differences may exist [86]. Cell surface fibronectin may be the precursor of plasma fibronectin, and its release may be in response to low extracellular levels, or it may be nonspecifically released into the extracellular fluid as part of a normal pathway for its turnover. Plasma fibronectin promotes cell adhesion to tissue culture plastic and denatured collagen substrate [87,88] moreover, plasma fibronectin must be adsorbed on the substratum surface to obtain spreading of a variety of cell types on tissue culture plastic and attachment/spreading of cells on denatured collagen substrata [89,90]. The simplest unifying interpretation of these findings is that the fibronectins function as adhesive proteins that bind cells to other cells, and most importantly in the case of implanted polymers, it binds cells to artificial substrata.

The fibronectins appear to participate in the process of mural thrombosis by the following mechanisms:

(a) Plasma fibronectin, by virtue of its affinity for fibrin, is crosslinked to the α-chain of fibrin under physiologic conditions [91].

(b) Fibronectin binds to fibrinogen. This interaction is manifest in the coprecipitation of fibronectin with cryofibrinogen and other components in the cryoprecipitate that forms when plasma is kept at a low temperature (hence the name "cold insoluble globulin"). If blood is allowed to clot, a large fraction of fibronectin is incorporated into the fibrin clot [92].

(c) Fibronectin is present in platelet α-granules.

(d) Large External Transformation Sensitive (LETS) protein has been shown to promote red blood cell aggregation [93].

(e) Cold Insoluble Globulin (Clg) appears to be involved in the adhesion of platelets. The evidence [94] suggests the Clg is recruited from the plasma concomitant with binding of platelets to collagen. The presence of Clg appears to promote spreading of the platelets and platelet aggregation.

These observations are strongly indicative that fibronectins are an important component in the process of mural thrombosis. To date, these proteins have not received wide attention in regards to hemocompatible polymers; future research should focus on the fibronectins, to better elucidate how these proteins influence the thrombogenicity of implanted synthetic polymers.

X. INHIBITORS OF COAGULATION

Control of mural thrombosis on implanted biomaterials can be accomplished by the use of anticoagulants. Anticoagulants do not dissolve clots; in general, anticoagulants are used therapeutically to arrest an established thrombotic process or preoperatively to prevent a thrombus from developing. Their principal action is to prevent the formation of fibrin by inhibiting certain steps in the coagulation sequence.

Many anticoagulants have been described; anticoagulant drug therapy literature is extensive and clearly beyond the scope of this volume. We will discuss only four important anticoagulants: (1) Antithrombin III, (2) Heparin, (3) Dicumarol and Warfarin, and (4) Aspirin and Dipyridamole.

(1) **Antithrobin III.** This lipoprotein is believed to be the antithrombin with major physiologic significance [95-98]; antithrombin III appears to be synthesized in the liver [99], with a biologic half-life of 48 hours [100]. Antithrombin III is distributed widely in body fluids and apparently there is also a large extravascular reservoir of this material throughout the body [101].

Antithrombin III is the most potent controlling factor for the blood coagulation systems, since it is a strong inactivator of most of the activated enzymes that comprise the cascade sequence. Antithrombin III reacts with heparin, and the reaction of antithrombin III with heparin immobilized on a surface may explain, in part, the antithrombotic effect of such surfaces [102]. The mechanism of action of antithrombin III is not clear; it has been suggesgted that it acts as an enzyme that destroys thrombin, or that it inactivates thrombin by forming a complex [103.104]. Antithrombin III also inactivates other blood proteins such as plasmin [105], Factor VII [106], Factor Xa [107], and may inhibit Factor III [108].

(2) **Heparin.** Although heparin is considered a pharmaceutical agent it is actually a normal body constituent that is present in high concentrations in tissue mast cells, intestinal mucosa, and liver and lung parenchyma. Heparin is one of the complex carbohydrates known as

mucopolysaccharides or glycosaminoglycans. The presence of sulfate groups in the carbohydrate moiety gives heparin its highly negative charge, and has been shown to be essential for the drug's unique anticoagulant properties.

Heparin functions as an anticoagulant by binding to, and activating antithrombin. Heparin activation of antithrombin accelerates the rate at which this normal plasma globulin binds to a variety of activated coagulation factors such as thrombin; heparin is then released from the complex and rapidly binds to additional antithrombin molecules, continuing the process. The fact that heparin can recycle much like an enzyme and activates multiple antithrombin molecules, coupled with the fact that antithrombin inactivates coagulation proteins throughout the entire coagulation cascade (Figure 14), makes heparin a very potent and effective anticoagulant [109].

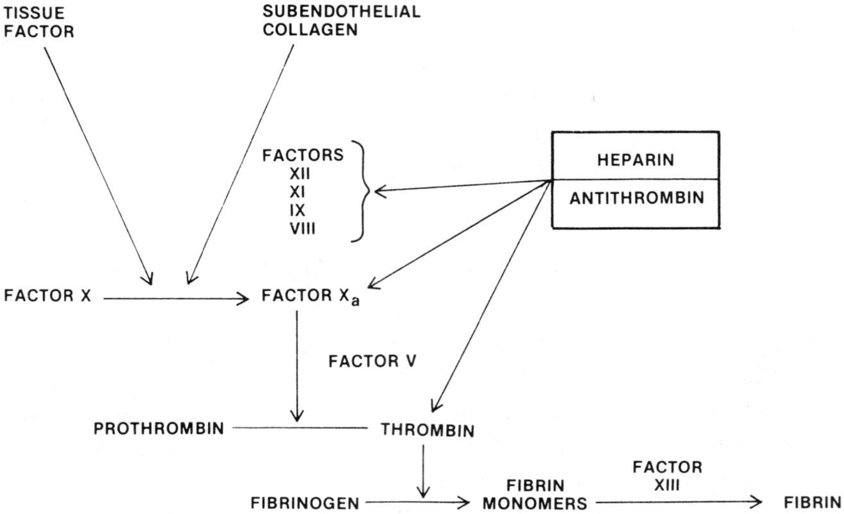

Schematic diagram shows how heparin interferes with the coagulation cascade initiated when injury causes blood to be exposed to subendothelial collagen or a released tissue factor. Heparin binds to antithrombin and forms a complex that neutralizes coagulation factors at three stages in the cascade. The complex prevents the activation of factor X into factor X_a through its effects on factors IX, XI, and XII early in the cascade. It also inhibits existing factor X_a. And it neutralizes previously formed thrombin, thus preventing the production of fibrin.

Figure 14. Sites of Heparin Action in Coagulation Cascade.

Heparin seems to act principally by binding to antithrombin III (cofactor), thereby greatly accelerating the enzyme neutralizing effect of this serine protease inhibitor. In the presence of heparin, the interaction of antithrombin with thrombin is virtually instantaneous. In addition to prothrombin, four other coagulation proteins are converted to active serine proteases (Factors XII, XI, IX, and X) and are therefore also neutralized by the heparin-antithrombin complex. Table 7 presents a summary of the known anticoagulant properties of heparin.

Table 7. Anticoagulant Properties of Heparin

1.	Inhibits activated Factors XII, XI, IX, X, and II.
2.	Inhibits the thrombin-mediated conversion of fibrinogen to fibrin.
3.	Inhibits the aggregation of platelets by thrombin.
4.	Inhibits activation of fibrin stabilizing enzyme.

(3) **Dicumarol and Warfarin.** Because of their widespread use, dicumarol and warfarin, the two most commonly employed oral anticoagulants, will be discussed together. Unlike heparin, these drugs have no direct effect on blood coagulation and their action is indirect, depending on properties that are manifest only in vivo.

The oral anticoagulants have only one major pharmacological effect – inhibition of blood-contacting mechanisms by interfering with the hepatic synthesis of the vitamin K-dependent clotting factors. This effect appears to be based on their antagonism to vitamin K by simple competitive inhibition [110,111]. As a result, the activity of the vitamin K-dependent clotting factors (II, VII, IX, and X) is reduced. The rate of decrease in the functional activities of the four coagulation factors involved is thought to be a function of the half-life of the factors; thus, after the administration of these oral anticoagulants, Factor VII activity falls first, followed sequentially by Factors IX, X, and II [112]. After stopping therapy, the activities of these factors return to normal in the reverse order.

Both of the extrinsic and intrinsic coagulation systems are affected. Factors VII and X are part of the extrinsic system and are required for the conversion of tissue thromboplastin of prothrombin to its active enzymatic form, thrombin. Factors IX and X are involved in the elaboration of blood thromboplastin. All four factors are considered of equal importance in hemostasis.

An indirect effect on platelets has been described, although it is by no means clear whether this is of any therapeutic value. Inhibition of platelet aggregation has been reported in a variety of in vivo test systems [113,114]. A therapeutic range of anticoagulation has been reported to be associated with a prolongation of platelet survival and with decreased platelet adhesiveness [115]. On the other hand, inadequate doses may have the opposite effect [116]. It is not likely that oral anticoagulants cause significant suppression of platelet-mediated thrombosis.

(4) **Aspirin and Dipyridamole.** The anticoagulants discussed so far have little or no discernible effect on platelet function when used in normal therapeutical dosage. However, since platelets play a primary role in the initiation of thrombus, particularly in the arterial system, we will review the effects of two agents (aspirin and dipyridamole) on the in vitro behavior of platelets. Platelets have been assigned a central role in hemostasis and thrombosis. They have turned out to be amazingly versatile structures: they adhere to sites of endothelial injury, aggregate to form platelet masses, release granules rich in a variety of secretory products, and synthesize, among other things, several types of prostaglandins. In normal hemostasis, platelets adhere to the severed margins of a vessel within seconds to a few minutes. It has been shown that platelets first stick by attachment of long pseudopods. Platelets, once attached, undergo a transformation to become relatively elongated cells, broadening the area of adhesion. Involved in this change in shape are the platelet contractile proteins actin and myosin and possibly their numerous microtubules. Seconds after adherence, the platelets release two types of granules: so-called alpha granules, having fibrinogen, beta thromboglobulin, cationic proteins, and platelet Factor 4 (a heparin-neutralizing protein), and dense bodies, rich in serotonin (5-hydroxytryptamine), ADP, ATP, and ionized calcium. The granule-release reaction is an energy-requiring process analogous to secretion in other cells systems. It is triggered by collagen, thrombin, trypsin, plasmin, antigen-antibody complexes, endotoxin, and fatty acids as well as a number of other compounds. It is believed that these stimuli to platelet activation inhibit membrane-bound adenyl cyclase, because decreased levels of cAMP are found in aggregated platelets. Simultaneously, there is an increased intraplatelet

concentration of calcium. Increase in this cation is a potent stimulus to platelet activation (contraction, aggregation, release). With platelet aggregation, a phospholipid (platelet Factor 3) becomes activated.

The initial platelet aggregation is an autocatalytic reaction which, once initiated, enters a logarithmic phase with the release of more ADP, serotonin, and ionized calcium. At this time, the clotting sequence leads to the formation of thrombin, which further augments platelet aggregation. But this initial platelet aggregation is temporary, and although the platelets are adherent, they have intact membranes. This temporary hemostatic plug is friable, and may readily be fragmented or dislocated in rapidly moving streams. Disaggregation of the platelets would soon follow, were it not for intercurrent events such as the generation of more thrombin and fibrin. Thrombin is the most powerful platelet aggregator identified to date, inducing generally larger, firmer, and more permanent aggregates. Under the influence of thrombin, platelets release all granules and lose their internal structure. While plasma membranes remain intact under the electron microscope, platelets appear hollow or ghostlike. In the past, this process of secondary or permanent aggregation has been called viscous metamorphosis. Secondary aggregation is energy-dependent; it depends on the metabolism of glucose by the platelets. In addition, recent studies show that certain of the prostaglandins now appear to be necessary as modulators of hemostasis [117].

Prostaglandins (PGs) are long-chain (20 carbon) hydroxyunsaturated fatty acids which are extremely potent physiologic and pharmacologic agents, active in microgram doses. A large number of PGs have now been identified, and each bears a letter designation, indicating the ring structure, and a number subscript, denoting the number of double bonds in the side chain, e.g., PGE_2, PGI_1 [118]. These are ubiquitous hormones produced locally in a variety of tissues and, for our purposes, in platelets and endothelial cells. They are all derived from arachidonic acid released from membrane phospholipid by activation of membrane phospholipase A. Arachidonic acid is rapidly transformed by cyclo-oxygenase into endoperoxides, which are then converted in PGs. The two most important of the PGs in blood clotting are PGI_2 and thromboxane A_2. Both are unstable compounds; the former is synthesized by prostacyclin synthetase in endothelial cells, while the latter is produced by thromboxane synthetase in platelets. PGI_2 and thromboxane A_2 have opposing effects on platelets and vascular smooth muscle, and thus appear to provide a local, finely balanced mechanism which may either favor or oppose platelet aggregation and blood clotting. PGI_2, formed in endothelial cells, prevents platelets from aggregating and initiating a clot. This action may be a main defense against unwanted platelet aggregation in normal blood flow [119]. Simultaneously, PGI_2 depresses normal muscular contractility of the vessel wall, thus inducing vasodilation and speeding blood flow, further militating against the buildup of platelet aggregates and clot formation. However, damage to blood vessel walls and loss of endothelial cells would create a local lack of PGI_2, and so this protective mechanism would be lost. At the same time, adherence of platelets would release thromboxane A_2, which induces both platelet aggregation and vasoconstriction [120]. Other prostaglandins such as PGE_2, $PGF_{2\alpha}$, and PGD_2 are less potent inhibitors of platelet aggregation in man. It is clear, then, that the PGs are major participants in the process of platelet aggregation.

Aspirin inhibits platelet aggregation by preventing the release of ADP, one of the substances that is important for platelet aggregation. Aspirin also inhibits the release of platelet ATP, serotonin, and other substances extruded from the cell during the release reaction. These findings suggested that aspirin inhibits the release reaction. The effects of a single dose of aspirin on platelets can be detected for 4 to 7 days after ingestion, at a time when salicylate is no longer detectable in the blood. The inhibitory actions of aspirin on platelets are due to its effect on the synthesis of platelet prostaglandins and thromboxane A_2, which are mediators of platelet release/aggregation. Platelets that have been stimulated to aggregate by various agonists synthesize PGH_2 (and then thromboxane A_2) from membrane-derived arachidonic acid. The enzyme responsible for the conversion of arachidonic acid to PGC_2 (the precursor of PGH_2) is known as cyclooxygenase (or prostaglandin synthetase). Aspirin acetylate inhibits this enzyme, irreversibly inactivates it, and thereby inhibits platelet aggregation and the release mechanism, as shown in Figure 15.

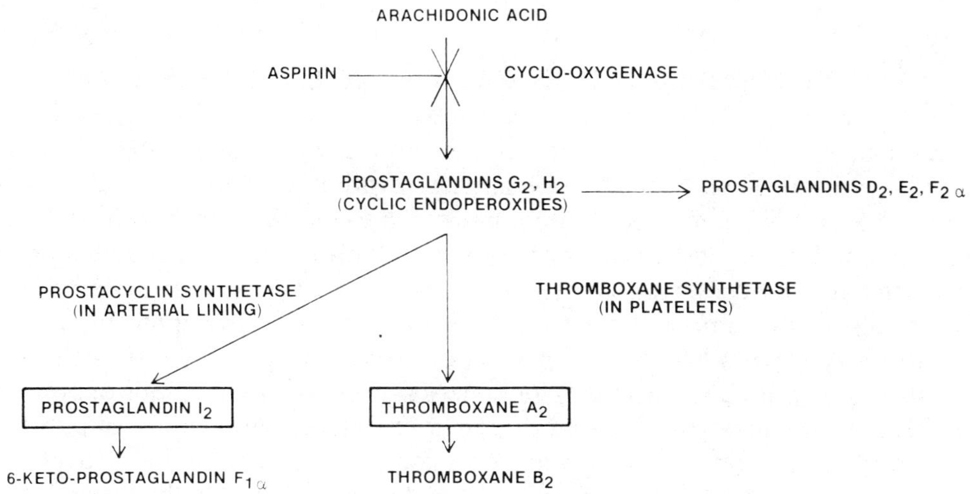

Figure 15. Inhibitory Effect of Aspirin on the Formation of Cyclic Endoperoxides.

Dipyridamole, a coronary vasodilator agent, also inhibits ADP-induced platelet aggregation. This drug is a pyrimidopyrimidine compound that was originally used to treat angina pectoris. Table 8 summarizes clinically significant effects of dipyridamole. Studies in 1965 showed that dipyridamole could inhibit platelet thromboembolism that ordinarily occurs after mechanical injury of the cerebral cortical blood vessel of rabbits. The antithrombotic properties of this drug were subsequently demonstrated in a variety of experimental and clinical situations. For example, administration of dipyridamole significantly reduced the incidence of thrombosis in rabbit cerebral or rat mesenteric arteries that had been injured by mechanical pinching, electric current, or ruby biolaser. It also prevented the development of arteriosclerosis in homocysteinemic baboons. In some experimental studies, however, no antithrombotic effect could be detected. In man, administration of dipyridamole in a daily divided dose of 400 mg together with crystalline warfarin sodium reduced the incidence of postoperative thromboembolism in patients undergoing cardiac valve replacement. Dipyridamole also prolongs platelet survival after cardiac valve surgery, suggesting that it may prevent the deposition of platelets on the prosthetic valves. Dipyridamole, administered together with anticoagulants, can also modifiy the vascular lesion that is associated with the rejection of renal allografts.

Table 8. Effect of Dipyridamole on Platelets

1.	Platelet thrombus formation (in vivo)	Inhibits
2.	Platelet aggregation (in vitro)	
	Collagen	No inhibition*
	ADP	No inhibition*
	Epinephrine	No inhibition*
3.	Platelet adhesion (glass beads)	Variable inhibition
4.	Platelet metabolism	Inhibits phosphodiesterase
5.	Platelet survival	Increases in some cases

*At clinically relevant concentrations

XI. SYNOPSIS OF BLOOD/MATERIAL INTERACTIONS

Normal vascular endothelium is the ideal nonthrombogenic surface, which is generally considered to be resistant to platelet adhesion and aggregation. On the other hand, a foreign surface devoid of endothelium may be thrombogenic due to platelet adhesion/agglomeration and the formation of a fibrin meshwork. Therefore, mural thrombosis and coagulation induced by blood/material interactions are a key concern in the area of medical prostheses.

It is now established that among the initial events that occur when synthetic materials contact blood is the very rapid adsorption of plasma proteins. This process seems to be completed in less than 3 seconds and effectively influences subsequent interactions of blood cells, especially platelets and leukocytes with the proteinated surfaces. Adsorption of plasma proteins can lead to the activation of the intrinsic blood coagulation cascade; this activation may be slight, or it may lead to the polymerization and crosslinking of fibrin on the blood interface.

To the best of our knowledge, the sequence of events appears to be the following: adsorption of plasma proteins, adhesion of platelets and leukocytes, activation of platelets followed by the release reaction, recruitment of nearby platelets by released products including ADP and thromboxane A_2, aggregation of recruited platelets upon the layer of adherent platelets with eventual formation of a mural thrombus. This mural thrombus frequently is associated with fibrin formation, and the presence of fibrin stabilizes the thrombus. Leukocytes contribute to activation of the blood coagulation sequence as well as to removal of fibrin and markedly altered platelets. This sequence is summarized below.

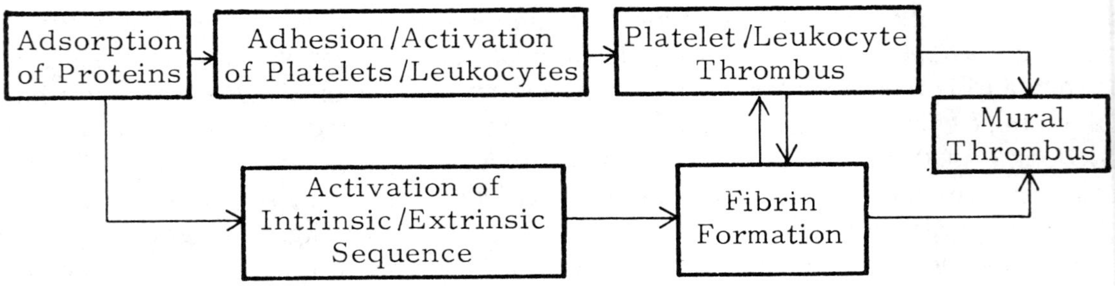

The formation of layers of adsorbed protein and adherent platelets and leukocytes upon artificial surfaces exposed to blood depends upon a number of factors. Among these are: the nature of the surface of the biomaterial, the specific types of plasma proteins adsorbed and the effect of this on activation of blood coagulation and complement and fibrinolytic systems, the type of anticoagulant that may be present in the blood, the flow properties of blood near the interface with the biomaterial, and possible low-grade activation of platelets and the blood coagulation system at points in the vascular system remote from the biomaterial. Some artificial surfaces appear to attract predominantly platelets, while other attract populations of neutrophils and macrophages. In either case, adherent platelets or leukocytes appear to contribute to activation of nearby platelets as well as the activation of the blood coagulation systems. These activated platelets and leukocytes appear to be capable of triggering both the intrinsic and extrinsic blood clotting systems; activation of these two systems reinforce each other.

The phases of fibrin formation are achieved through four major steps in the series of reactions which constitute the normal mechanism of coagulation. First, a substance which activates prothrombin is formed via two pathways: the intrinsic and extrinsic reactions. This substance is called prothrombin activator and all plasma factors except Factor XIII are necessary for its formation. The extrinsic pathway is a powerful activator of Factor X, producing large amounts of this factor. The mechanism, initiated by tissue thromboplastin, involves Factors VIII, X, and V. Thromboplastin activates prothrombin indirectly, not directly. Factor VII is unique to the extrinsic clotting mechanism. Intrinsic clotting occurs as a result of a series of reactions involving platelet Factor 3 and four factors unique to the intrinsic pathway (Factors XII and XI, the contact factors, and Factors IX and VIII, the factors missing in the two forms of hemophilia). Platelet Factor 3 is a lipid clotting factor made available by the platelets. It is the equivalent of the lipid portion of tissue thromboplatin and is referred to as partial thromboplastin. The extrinsic and intrinsic mechanisms merge at the point in the clotting process where Factor X is activated. Both systems produce a prothrombin activator through the interaction of activated Factor X(X_a), Factor V(V_a), calcium, and lipid. The intrinsic mechanisms receive lipid from platelet Factor 3, and extrinsic mechanisms from tissue thromboplastin.

The second major reaction in the coagulation process is the conversion of prothrombin to thrombin by the prothrombin activators. The first thrombin formed accelerates the further production of thrombin by activating Factors VIII and V, and by making platelet Factor 3 available. There is a sudden formation of large amounts of thrombin.

The third major reaction in clotting is the conversion of fibrinogen to fibrin by thrombin. Thrombin alters the fibrinogen molecule, forming a fibrin monomer, and subsequently allowing the formation of strands of fibrin.

The fourth and last step of coagulation involves stabilization of the fibrin clot. Factor XIII is used here to link the fibrin molecules together in a firm bond.

Lysis of a fibrin clot, part of the repair process is mediated by the plasminogen-plasmin system. Plasmin, a proteolytic enzyme, degrades fibrin to polypeptides of varying molecular weights known as fibrinogen degradation products. The reactions that lead to the generation of plasmin and fibrinolysis are as follows:

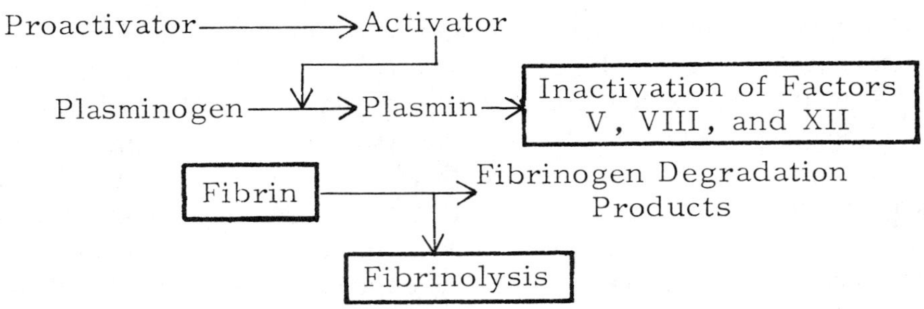

To control mural thrombosis, anticoagulants such as heparin are frequently used. Heparin acts on the intrinsic coagulation sequence by dramatically accelerating the rate of which antithrombin-heparin cofactor neutralizes the serial proteolytic enzymes in the cascade mechanism; however, heparin has no inhibitory effect on platelets. To control platelet-foreign surface reactions antiplatelet agents, such as aspirin and dipyridamole have been used successfully. Heparin, administered intravenously, may be used preoperatively but for chronic administration an oral anticoagulant, such as coumadin, is preferred.

The rationale in the development of thromboresistant materials as divided into two philosophies: smooth versus textured surfaces. The first approach is to prevent activation of the thrombogenic pathways by tailoring the physiochemical properties of the polymer surface to either minimize all blood interactions, or to selectively absorb a passivating albumin layer; in addition, pharmacologically active agents may be incorporated into the polymer via bulk dispersion, or by surface immobilization of the anticoagulants.

A second approach consists of using rough surfaces, such as velours, flocked or integrally textured surfaces, to encourage the formation of a living biological lining, derived from the blood itself. This pseudoneointimal lining, composed of collagen, fibrin, fibroblasts, and pseudoendothelial cells, has been used successfully for periods of 1 year in Left Ventricular Assist Devices (see chapter entitled "Hemocompatible Interfaces in Artificial Heart Devices").

In conclusion, we have made great strides in our efforts to produce cardiovascular devices that are chronically nonthrombogenic. Our success can be measured in terms of the many devices now in routine clinical use that would have been unthinkable just a few short years ago. By the judicious application of the highly specialized knowledge discussed in this book, we can look forward to the future development of safe and clinically reliable prostheses for the benefit of mankind.

REFERENCES

1. Hovig, T., "The Ultrastructure of Blood Platelets in Normal and Abnormal States," Series Haematol., 1:3 (1968).
2. Wintrobe, M. M., *Clinical Hematology,* Seventh Edition, Lea & Febiger, p. 388 (1974).
3. French, J. E., "Blood Platelets: Morphological Studies on Their Properties and Life Cycle," Brit. J. Haematol., 13:595 (1967).
4. Aster, R. H. and Jandl, J. H., "Platelet Sequestration in Man, I. Methods," J. Clin. Invest., 43:843 (1964).
5. Harker, L. A. and Finch, C. A., "Thrombokinetics in Man," J. Clin. Invests., 48:963 (1969).
6. Holmsen, H., Day, H. J., and Stormorken, J., "The Blood Platelet Release Reaction," Scand. J. Haematol., Supp. 8:1-26 (1969).

7. Grette, K., "Studies on the Mechanism of Thrombin-Catalyzed Haemostatic Mechanisms in Blood Platelets," Acta Physiol. Scand., 56, Suppl. 165 (1962).
8. Niewiarowski, S. and Thomas, D. P., "Platelet Release Reaction: The Effects on the Vessel Wall," Thromb. Diath. Haemorrh., Suppl. 40:199 (1970).
9. Davis, R. B. and White, J. G., "Localization of 5-HT in Blood Platelets: A Radiographic and Ultrastructural Study," Br. J. Haematol., 15:93-99 (1968).
10. Mill, D. C. B. and Thomas, D. P., "Blood Platelet Nucleotides in Man and Other Species," Nature (London) 195:715-729 (1969).
11. Baker, R. V., Blashko, H., and Born, G. V. R., "The Isolation of Blood Platelets of Particles Containing 5-HT and ATP," J. Physiol. (London) 149:55 (1959).
12. Martin, J. H., Carson, F. L., and Race, G. J., "Calcium Containing Platelet Granules," J. Cell Biol., 60:775-777 (1974).
13. Silcox, D. C., Jacobelli, S., and McCarty, D. J., "Identification of Inorganic Pyrophosphate in Human Platelets and its Release on Stimulation with Thrombin," J. Clin. Inves., 52:1595-1604 (1973).
14. Joist, J. H. et al., "Platelet Antiplasmin; Its Extrusion During the Release Reactions, Subcellular Localization, and Relation to Platelet Antiheparin," Thromb. Res. (in press).
15. Zucker, M. B., "Tests of Platelet Adhesion, Aggregation and Release," Thromb. Diath. Haemorrh., Suppl. 42:1 (1970).
16. Lages, B. et al., "Metal Ion Contents of Gel-Filtered Platelets from Patients with Storage Pool Disease," Blood, 46:119-130 (1975).
17. Castaldi, P. A. and Caen, J., "Platelet Fibrinogen," J. Clin. Pathol., 18:579 (1965).
18. Nachman, R., Weksler, B., and Ferris, B., "Increased Vascular Permeability Produced by Human Platelet Granule Cationic Extract," J. Clin. Invest., 49:274-281 (1970).
19. Weksler, B. B. and Coupal, C. E., "Platelet Dependent Generation of Chemotactic Activity in Serum," J. Exp. Med., 137:1419-1430 (1973).
20. Ross, R., et al., "A Platelet-Dependent Serum Factor Stimulates the Purification of Arterial Smooth Muscle Cells in Vitro," Proc. Nat. Acad. Sci., 71:1207-1210 (1974).
21. Weksler, B. B. and Nachman, R. L., "Rabbit Platelet Bactericidal Protein," J. Exp. Med., 134:1114-1130 (1971).
22. Weiss, H. J. and Rogers, S., "Platelet Factor 4 in Platelet Disorders – Storage Location and the Requirement of Endogenous ADP for its Release," Proc. Soc. Exp. Biol. Med., 142:30-35 (1973).
23. Barnhart, M. I. and Anderson, G. F., "Intracellular Localization of Fibrinogen," Proc. Soc. Exp. Bio. Med., 110:734 (1962).
24. Laki, K., *Fibrinogen,* N. Y., Marcel Dekker (1968).
25. Blomback, B., Henschen, A., et al., "N-Terminal Disulphide Knot of Human Fibrinogen," Nature, 218:130 (1968).
26. Doolittle, R. F., Horizons Biochem. Biophys., 3:164-191 (1977).
27. Doolittle, R. F., *The Plasma Proteins,* ed. F. W. Putnam, N.Y., Academic Press, 2:109-161 (1975).
28. Blomback, B., "Fibrinogen to Fibrin Transformation," *Blood Clotting Enzymology,* ed. Seeger, N.Y., Academic Press (1967).
29. Bailey, K., Lorand, L., and Middlebrook, W. R., "Action of Thrombin in the Clotting of Fibrinogen," Nature, 167:233 (1951).
30. Griffin, J. H. and Cochrane, C. G., "Recent Advances in the Understanding of Contact Activation Reactions," Sem. Thrombus. Hemostas., 5:254 (1979).
31. Nossel, H. L., "Interface-Induced Coagulation Reactions," *Vascular Grafts,* eds. Sawyer and Kaplitt, N.Y., Appleton-Century Crafts (1978).
32. Wiggins, R. C., Bouma, B. N., et al., Proc. Nat'l. Acad. Aci., USA, 74:4636-40 (1977).
33. Nemerson, Y., Silverberg, S. A., and Testy, T., "Self-Damping Mechanisms in Blood Coagulation," Thromb. Diath. Haemorrh., 32:57-64 (1974).
34. Robbin, K. C. and Summaria, L., "Biochemistry of Fibrinolysis," Thromb. Diath. Haemorrh., Suppl. 47:9-19 (1971).

35. Zoltan, R. P., Metz, E. T., and Russell, H. T., "Assay of Human Plasminogen in Plasmin by Affinity Chromatography," Clin. Chem., 18:654-657 (1972).
36. Alkjaersig, N., Sherry, S., and Fletcher, A., "The Mechanisms of Clot Dissolution by Plasmin," J. Clin. Invest., 38:1086 (1959).
37. Jacobsson, K., "Electrophoretic Demonstration of Two Trypsin Inhibitors in Human Serum," Scand. J. Clin. Lab. Invest., 5:97-98 (1953).
38. Todd, E. W., "Quantitative Studies on the Total Plasmin and the Trypsin Inhibitor of Human Blood Serum," J. Exp. Med., 89:309-324 (1949).
39. Ratnolf, O. D. and Lepow, K. H., "Some Properties of an Esterase Derived From Preparations of the First Component of Complement," J. Exp. Med., 106:327-343 (1957).
40. Abildgaard, V., "Purification of Two Progressive Antithrombins of Human Plasma," Scand. J. Clin. Lab. Invest., 19:190-195 (1967).
41. Steinbuch, M., "Isolation of an α_2 Globulin from Human Plasma," Nature, 192:1196 (1961).
42. Shulman, N. R., "Studies on the Inhibition of Proteolytic Enzymes by Serum," J. Exp. Med., 95:593-604 (1952).
43. Gallimore, M. J. and Shaw, J. T. B., "The Influence of Various Plasma Components on the Lysis of Dilute Human Blood Clots," Thromb. Diath. Haemorrh., 18:101-113 (1967).
44. Gallimore, M. J., "Inter-Antiplasmin: Its Distinction from Antiactivator," Thromb. Res., 12:687-692 (1978).
45. Bernick, M. B., "Inhibitor of Proteinases in Culture of Human Lung: A New Alpha 1-Antiplasmin?", Thromb. Res., 11:739-746 (1977).
46. Baier, R. E. and Dutton, R. C., "Initial Events in Interaction of Blood with a Foreign Surface," Am. Chem. Soc. Mts., Atlantic City, N.J., (1968).
47. Salzman, E. W. et al., "Protein Platelet Interaction on Heparinized Surfaces," J. Biomed. Nat. Res., 3:69 (1969).
48. Lyman, D. J. et al., "Platelet Interaction with Protein-Coated Surfaces," Throm. Diath. Hemorrh., Suppl. 42:109 (1971).
49. Zucker, M. B., and Vroman, L., "Platelet Adhesion Induced by Fibrinogen Adsorbed onto Glass," Proc. Soc. Exp. Biol. Med., 131:318-20 (1969).
50. Jenkins, C. S. et al., "Modification of Platelet Adherence to Protein-Coated Surfaces," J. Lab. Clin. Med., 81:280 (1973).
51. Packham, M. A. et al., "The Effect of Plasma Proteins on the Interaction of Platelets with Glass Surfaces," J. Lab. Clin. Med., 73:686-97 (1969).
52. Baumgartner, H. R. et al., "Platelet Adhesion, Release and Aggregation in Flowing Blood: Effect of Surface Properties and Platelet Function," Thromb. Haemoctas, 35(1): 124-138 (1976).
53. Dutton, R. C., et al., J. Biomed. Res., 3:13 (1969).
54. Vroman, L. and Adams, A. L., Thromb. Diath Haemorrh., 18:510 (1967).
55. Vroman, L. and Adams, A. L., J. Biomed. Mater. Res., 3:43 (1969).
56. Guest, M. M. et al., "A Possible Role of Leukocytes in Hemostasis," Bibl. Auct., 12:131-137 (1973).
57. Evans, G. T. and Mustard, J. F., "Platelet-Surface Reaction and Thrombosis," Surgery, 64:273-280 (1968).
58. Nose, Y., Kambic, H. E., et al., "In Vitro Test of Compatibility of Blood with Various Natural and Synthetic Surfaces," Thromb. Diath. Haemorrh., Suppl. 60:87-95 (1974).
59. Imai, Y., Tajima, K., and Nose, Y., "Biolized Materials for Cardiovascular Prosthesis," Trans. ASAIO, 17:6-9 (1971).
60. Szycher, M., Poirier, V., et al., "Biochemical, Histological, and Ultrastructural Assessments of Pseudoneointimal Lining Derived from Fibroblast-Seeded Integrally Textured Polymeric Surfaces," J. Biomed. Nat. Res., 15:247-265 (1981).
61. Brash. J. L. and Lyman, D. J., "Absorption of Plasma Proteins in Solution to Unchanged, Hydrophilic Polymer Surfaces," J. Biomed. Nat. Res., 3:175-189 (1969).

62. Szycher, M., Thermo Electron Corporation, unpublished data.
63. Mason, R. G. et al., "Effect of Certain Purified Plasma Proteins," Am. J. Patt., 73:183 (1973).
64. Gott, V. L. and Furuse, A., "Antithrombogenic Surfaces, Classification, and In Vivo Evaluation," Fed. Proc., 30:1679 (1971).
65. Salzman, E. W., "Nonthrombogenic Surfaces: Critical Review," Blood, 38:509 (1971).
66. Muller-Eberhard, H. J., "Complement," Ann. Rev. of Biochem., 44:697-724 (1975).
67. Ruddy, S., Gighi, I., and Austen, K., New Engl. J. Med. 287:489 (1972).
68. Ishizaka, T. and Ishizaka, K., Proc. Soc. Exp. Biol., 101:845 (1959).
69. Connell, R. S. et al., Ann. Thorac. Surg., 15:217 (1973).
70. Kuusela, P., Ruoslahti, E., Engvall, E., and Vaheri, A., "Immunological Interspecies Cross-Section of Fibroblasts Surface Antigen (Fibronectin)," Immunochemistry, 13:639-642 (1976).
71. Keski-Oja, J., Mosher, D. F., and Vaheri, A., "Cross Linking of a Major Fibroblast Surface-Associated Glycoprotein (Fibronectin) Catalyzed by Blood Coagulation Factor XIII," Cell, 9:29-35 (1976).
72. Yamada, K. M. and Weston, J. A., "Isolation of a Major Cell Surface Glycoprotein from Fibroblasts," Proc. Nat. Acad. Aci., USA, 71:3492-3496 (1974).
73. Ruoslahti, E., Vaheri, A., Kuusela, P., and Linder, E., "Fibroblast Surface Antigen: A New Serum Protein," Biochem. Biphys. Acta., 322:352-358 (1973).
74. Hynes, R. O., "Alteration of Cell-Surface Proteins by Viral Transformation and by Proteolysis," Proc. Nat. Acad. Sci., USA, 70:3170-3174 (1973).
75. Gahmberg, C. G. and Hakomori, S. I., "Surface Carbohydrates of Hamster Fibroblasts, II. Interaction of Hamster NIL Cell Surfaces with Ricinus Communis Lectin and Concanavalin A as Revealed by Surface Galactosyl Label," J. Bio. Chem., 250:2447-2451 (1975).
76. Blumberg, P. M. and Robbins, P. W., "Effect of Proteases on Activation of Resting Chick Embryo Fibroblasts and on Cell Surface Protein," Cell, 6:137-147 (1975).
77. Mosher, D. F., J. Biol. Chem., 250:6614-6621 (1975).
78. Wartiovaara, S. E., Linden, E., Ruoslahti, E., and Vaheri, A., "Distribution of Fibroblast Surface Antigen," J. Exp. Med., 140:1522-1533 (1974).
79. Bornstein, P. and Ash, J. F., "Cell-Surface Associated Structural Proteins in Connective Tissue Cells," Proc. Nat. Acad. Aci., USA, 74:2480-2484 (1977).
80. Vaheri, A., Ruoslahti, E., Westermark, B., and Ponten, J., "A Common Cell-Type Specific Surface Antigen in Cultured Human Glial Cells and Fibroblasts: Loss in Malignant Cells," J. Exp. Med., 143:64-72 (1976).
81. Chen, L. B., Mastland, N., et al., "Detection of the Large External Transformation Sensitive Protein on Some Epithelial Cells," Exp. Cell Res., 106:39-46 (1977).
82. Bornstein, P., Duksen, V., and Balian, G., "Organization of Extracellular Proteins in the Connective Tissue Cell Surface: Relevance to Cell-Matrix Interactions In Vitro and In Vivo," Ann. N.Y. Acad. Sci., USA 312:96 (1978).
83. Mosesson, M. W., "Structure of Human Plasma Cold-Insoluble Globulin and the Mechanism of its Precipitation in the Cold with Heparin or Fibrin-Fibrinogen Complexes," Ann. N.Y. Acad. Sci., 312:17 (1978).
84. Grinnel, F., "Cellular Adhesiveness and Extracellular Substrata," Int. Rev. Cyt., 53:65-244 (1978).
85. Yamada, K. M. and Olden, K., "Fibronectins: Adhesive Glycoproteins of Cell Surface and Blood," Nature, 275:179 (1978).
86. Yamada, K. M. and Kennedy, D. W., "Fibroblast Cellular and Plasma Fibronectin are Similar But Not Identical," S. Cell Bio., 80:492 (1979).
87. Klebe, R., "Isolation of a Collagen Dependent Attachment Factor," Nature, 250:248-251 (1974).
88. Kleinman, H. K., McGoodwin, E. B., and Klebe, R. J., "Localization of the Cell Attachment Region in Types I and +I Collagens," Biochem. Biophys. Res. Commun., 72:426-432 (1976).
89. Grinnell, F. and Hays, D. G., "Induction of Cell Spreading by Substratum Adsorbed Ligards Directed Against the Cell Surface," Exp. Cell Res., 116:275-284 (1978).

90. Grinnel, F. and Minter, D., "Attachment and Spreading of Baby Hamster Kidney Cells to Collagen Substrata: Effects of CIG," Proc. Nat. Acad. Sci., USA, 75:4408-4412 (1978).
91. Mosher, D. F., "Crosslinking of Plasma and Cellular Fibronectin by Plasma Transglutaminase," Proc. N.Y. Acad. Sci., 312:40 (1978).
92. Ruoslanti, E. and Vaheri, A., J. Exp. Med., 141:497-501 (1974).
93. Yamada, K. M., Yamada, S. S., and Pastan, I., "The Major Cell Surface Glycoprotein of Chick Embryo Fibroblasts in an Agglutinin," Proc. Nat. Acad. Sci., USA, 72:3158-3162 (1975).
94. Hynes, R. O. et al., "A Large Glycoprotein Lost from the Surfaces of Transformed Cells," Proc. N.Y. Acad. Sci., 312:337 (1978).
95. Verstraete, M., "Antithrombins," Thromb. Diath. Haemorrh., Suppl. 20:385 (1976).
96. Lewis, J. H., Walters, D., Didisheim, P., and Merchangt, W. R., "Application of Continuous Flow Electrophoresis to the Study of the Blood Coagulation Proteins and the Fibrinolytic Enzyme System, I. Normal Human Materials," J. Clin. Invest., 37:1323.
97. Abildgaard, U., "Inhibition of the Thrombin-Fibrinogen Reaction by)Antithrombin III Studied by N-Terminal Analysis," Scient. Clin. Lab. Invest., 20:207 (1967).
98. Abildgaard, U., "Inhibition of the Thrombin-Fibrinogen Reaction by α_2-Macroglobulin, Studied by N-Terminal Analysis,"Thromb. Diath. Haemorrh., 21:173 (1969).
99. Denny, G. P. and Minot, G. R., "The Origin of Antithrombin," Amer. J. Physiol., 38:233 (1951).
100. Hensen, A. and Loeliger, E. A., "Antithrombin III: Its Metabolism and its Function in Blood Coagulation," Thromb. Diath. Haemorrh., Suppl. 1, 9:1 (1963).
101. Monkhouse, F. C. and Milojevic, S., "Changes in Thrombin Generation and Antithrombin Titer Following Massive Bleeding and Transfusion in Dogs," Can. J. Biochem. Phys., 38:475 (1960).
102. Lindsay, R. M. et al., "Panel Conference Blood Surface Interactions," Trans. ASAIO, 26:603 (1980).
103. Abildgaard, U., "Inhibition of the Thrombin-Fibrinogen Reaction by α_2-Macroglobulin, Studied by N-Terminal Analysis," Thromb. Diath. Haemorrh., 21:173 (1969).
104. Abildgaard, U., "Binding of Thrombin to Antithrombin III," Scand. J. Clin. Lab. Invest., 24:23 (1969).
105. Abildgaard, U. and Egeberg, O., "Thrombin Inhibitory Activity of Fractions Obtained by Gel Filtration of Antithrombin III Deficient Plasma," Scand. J. Haemat., 5:155 (1968).
106. Seegers, W. H., Schroer, H., and Mitsuyasu, K., "Inactivation of Purified Autoprothrombin I with Antithrombin," Can. J. Biochem., 42:1425 (1964).
107. Biggs, R., Denson, K. W. E., Akman, N., Borett, R., and Hadden, M., "Antithrombin III, Antifactor Xa and Heparin," Brit. J. Haemat., 19:283 (1970).
108. Egeberg, O., "On the Natural Blood Coagulation Inhibitor System. Investigations of Inhibitor Factors Based on Antithrombin Deficient Blood," Thromb. Diath. Haemorrh., 14:473 (1965).
109. Rosenberg, R. D., "Heparin, Antithrombin and Abnormal Clotting," Ann. Res. Med., 29:367-378 (1978).
110. Lowenthal, J. and MacFarlane, J. A., "The Nature of the Antagonism Between Vitamin K and Indirect Anticoagulants," J. Pharmacol. Exp. Ther., 143:273 (1964).
111. Bell, R. G., Sadowski, J. A., and Matshciner, J. T., "Mechanism of Action of Warfarin, Warfarin Metabolism of Vitamin K," Biochemistry, 11:1959 (1972).
112. Kaxmier, F. J., Spittel, J. A., Jr., Thompson, J. J., Jr., et al., "Effect of Oral Anticoagulants on Factors VII, IX, X and II," Arch. Intern. Med., 115:667 (1965).
113. Cunningham, G. M., McNicol, G. P., and Douglas, A. S., "Effect of Anticoagulant Drugs on Platelet Aggregation in Chandler's Tube," Lancet, 1:729 (1965).
114. Poller, L., Thomson, J. M., and Priest, C. M., "Coumarin Therapy and Platelet Aggregation," Br. Med. J., 1:474 (1969).
115. Murphy, E. A., and Mustard, J. F., "Dicumarol and Platelet Turnover," Circ. Res., 9:402 (1961).
116. Horlick, L., "The Adhesive Index, A Measure of Platelet Stickiness. Its Response to Myocardial Injury and to Anticoagulant Treatment," *An International Symposium: Anticoagulants and Fibrinolysis,* eds., MacMillan, R. L., and Mustard, J. R., Philadelphia, Lea and Febiger, pp. 56-57 (1961).

117. Smith, J. B. et al., "Prostaglandins and Precursors in Platelet Function," In Symposium on Biochemistry and Pharmacology of Platelets, CIBA Foundation Symposium, p. 207 (1975).
118. Samuelsson, B. and Pauletti, R., *Advances in Prostaglandin, and Thromboxane Research,* New York, Raven Press (1976).
119. Bunting, S. et al., "Antithrombotic Properties of Vascular Endothelium," Lancet, 2:1075 (1977).
120. Editorial, "Prevention of Thrombosis," Lancet, 1:127 (1977).

APPENDIX A
MATURATION OF BLOOD CELLULAR ELEMENTS

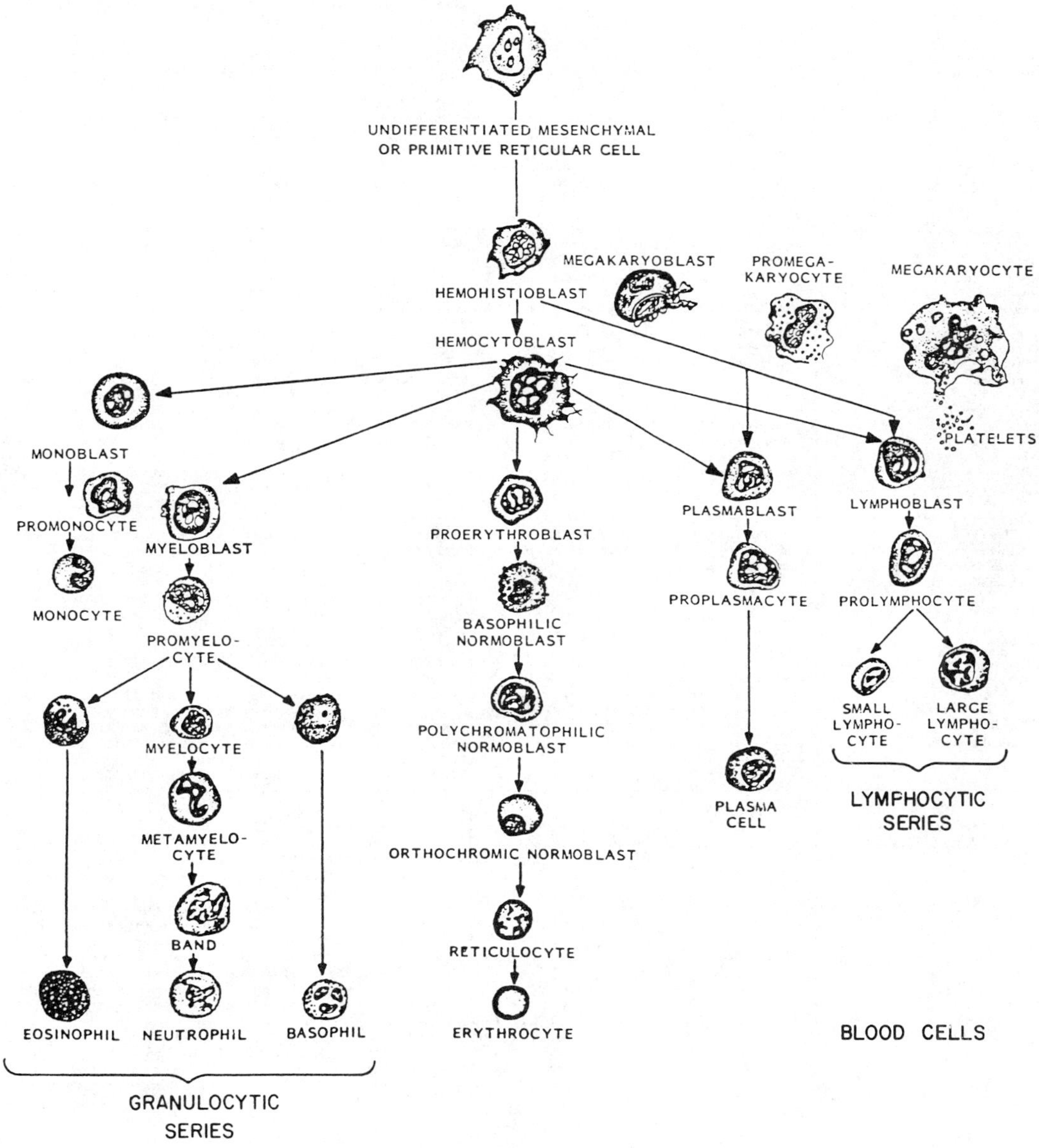

This diagram depicts the concept of a primitive, pluripotential cell precursor of all blood elements. This undifferentiated cell may give rise to red blood cells (erythrocytes), granulocytic, lymphocytic and plasma cell series (collectively known as leukocytes), and platelets.

APPENDIX B
GLOSSARY OF BLOOD COAGULATION COMPONENTS

Common Name and Synonyms	Function	Distinguishing Characteristics
Fibrinogen (I)	Soluble protein which after proteolysis by thrombin polymerizes to form the fibrin clot.	Mol wt 340,000; fibrous protein comprised of 6 disulfide-linked polypeptide chains, 2-Aα chains (mol wt 64,000), 2-Bβ chains (mol wt 55,000), and 2γ chains (mol wt 47,000). (See Fibrinogen)
Prothrombin (II) Factor II	Circulating precursor of the proteinase thrombin, converted to thrombin by the proteinase Factor Xa.	Mol wt 72,500, K-dependent single polypeptide chain glycoprotein (∿11% carbohydrate); contains 10γ -carboxyglutamic residues, thrombin forming half homologous with pancreatic serine proteinases thrombin mol wt 37,000. (See section on prothrombin conversion to thrombin.)
Thromboplastin (III) (sometimes tissue thromboplastin, or "tissue factor")	A homogenate of brain, lung, or other tissue which upon addition to blood plasma markedly shortens the time required for clot formation.	Thromboplastin preparations require the presence of a specific protein, tissue factor, and phospholipid for clot-promoting activity. (See section on activation of Factor X via the extrinsic system.)
Calcium Ion (IV)	1. Forms "bridges" between K-dependent proteins and acidic phospholipids of cell membranes; 2. Stabilizes Factor V, fibrinogen, and perhaps other proteins; 3. Involved in Factor XIII activation and subunit dissociation.	No distinguishing characteristics.
Factor V (V) Accelerator globulin Proaccelerin Labile factor	Accessory ("acceleration") protein which participates with the proteinase Factor Xa in prothrombin activation.	Mol wt ∿350,000; glycoprotein; may exist as oligomers of 350,000 in circulation; before its accelerating prothrombin proteolysis by Factor Xa it must be itself activated. (See section on activation processes in the blood coagulation system.)
Factor VII (VII) Proconvertin, Serum prothrombin conversion accelerator	Precursor of the proteinase that activates Factor X; first component of the "extrinsic" pathway of coagulation.	Mol wt 45,000-54,000; K-dependent single polypeptide chain; glyoprotein; undoubtedly contains γ-carboxyglutamic acid on the basis of its K dependence and its amino-terminal sequence homology with prothrombin and Factors IX and X. (See section on activation of Factor X via the extrinsic system.)
Factor VIII (VIII) Antihemophilic factor A (AHF); antihemophilic globulin (AHG) Platelet cofactor I	Controversial; accessory protein which participates with the proteinase Factor IXa in Factor X activation via intrinsic coagulation pathway.	Mol wt 100,000-2,000,000; ambiguity in molecular weight due to controversy about the particular species that participates directly in coagulation reactions versus other functions related to platelet physiology. (See sections on activation of Factor X via the intrinsic system and the relationship between Factor VIII and the von Willebrand Factor of hemostasis.)
Factor IX (IX) Christmas factor, antihemophilic factor B plasma thromboplastin component	Circulating precursor to proteinase which activates Factor X in the intrinsic pathway of coagulation.	Mol wt 55,400 (bovine) and 57,000 (human); K-dependent single polypeptide chain glycoprotein; carbohydrate - 25% (bovine) and 17% (human). Contains γ-carboxyglutamic acid; after proteolytic activation consists of two polypeptide chains - a heavy chain (mol wt 27,000), which is homologous to the pancreatic serine proteinases and a light chain, mol wt 16,000 which contains γ-carboxyglutamic acid residues. (See sections on activation of Factor X via the intrinsic system and contact activation system and activation of Factor IX.)
Factor X (X) Stuart-Prower factor, prothrombokinase Autoprothrombin III	Circulating precursor of the proteinase which converts prothrombin to thrombin.	Mol wt 54,500 (bovine) and 59,000 (human); K-dependent; two polypeptide chain glycoprotein; carbohydrate - 10% (bovine) and 15% (human). The heavy chain (mol wt 40,000) is homologous to the pancreatic serine proteinases, and the light chain (mol wt 15,000) contains 12 γ-carboxyglutamic acid residues. (See section on activation of Factor X.)
Factor XI (XI) Plasma thromboplastin antecedent (PTA)	Circulating precursor of enzyme Factor XIa which proteolytically converts Factor IX to Factor IXa.	Mol wt 124,000 (bovine) and 160,000 (human); both bovine and human Factor XI consist of two apparently equal molecular weight disulfide-linked polypeptide chains; proteolytic activation results in formation of 4 disulfide-linked polypeptide chains. (See sections on contact system of coagulation and activation of Factor IX.)
Factor XII (XII) Hageman factor	Circulating precursor to enzyme which proteolytically activates Factor XI.	Mol wt 74,000 (bovine) and 76,000 (human); single polypeptide chain glycoprotein; proteolytic cleavage forms a disulfide-linked two-chain molecule with a heavy chain (mol wt ∿50,000) and a diisopropylphosphorofluoridate-reactive serine containing light chain (mol wt 28,000). (See sections on contact system of coagulation and activation and activation of Factor IX.)
Factor XIII (XIII) Plasma transglutaminase (actually pro) Fibrin-stabilizing factor, (FSF) Fibrinoligane, Laki-Lorand factor	Circulating precursor of transglutaminase which covalently cross-links fibrin monomers in the fibrin polymer.	Mol wt 320,000 (plasma form, tetrameric); 160,000 (platelet form, dimeric). Molecule consists of two a subunits (plasma and platelet forms; mol wt 75,000) and two b subunits (plasma form only; mol wt 80,000). The a subunits are proteolytically cleaved to form the active transglutaminase, with the generation of a reactive cysteinyl thiol.

APPENDIX C

RELEVANT BIOCHEMICAL CHARACTERISTICS OF CONTACT SYSTEM PROTEINS

Common Name and Synonyms	Function	Distinguishing Characteristics
Prekallikrein (None) Fletcher factor	Precursor of proteinase kallikrein; cleaves Factor XII to form Factor XIIa and the high molecular weight kininogen to form bradykinin.	Mol wt 88,000 (bovine plasma) single polypeptide chain; kallikrein consists of a heavy chain, mol wt 52,000 and a light chain, mol wt 33,000-38,000; amino terminus of prekallikrein is homologous to the amino terminus of bovine Factor XI. (See sections on contact system of coagulation and activation of Factor IX.)
High-molecular-weight kininogen (None) Flaujeac, Fitzgerald, Williams factor (contact activation cofactor)	Source of bradykinin; accessory protein in activation of Factor XI by Factor XIIa and Factor XII kallikrein.	Mol wt 76,000 (bovine) and ∿150,000 (human); a single polypeptide chain glycoprotein, with ∿13% carbohydrate; cleavage by kallikrein releases bradykinin and a fragment that contains a large number of histidine residues. (See sections on contact activation system of coagulation and activation of Factor IX.)

Chapter 2

Mechanism of Adsorption of Proteins To Solid Surfaces and Its Relationship To Blood Compatibility

J. L. Brash
Departments of Chemical Engineering and Pathology
McMaster University
Hamilton, Ontario, Canada

ABSTRACT

A review of adsorption of proteins to solid surfaces is given. Fundamental aspects are first discussed including explanations of driving forces for adsorption, transport mechanisms and modes of binding of proteins to surfaces. Recent research in relation to the role of protein adsorption in the interactions between blood and solid surfaces is then described. Among the topics addressed are: rates of adsorption, quantities adsorbed, reversibility, competition aspects of adsorption and composition of the layer adsorbed from blood.

Supported by grants from Ontario Heart Foundation and Medical Research Council of Canada.

INTRODUCTION

Protein adsorption to solid surfaces is of interest for a volume on "Biomedical Materials" in several respects. Foremost among these is that it is an inevitable effect for any surface in contact with a protein-containing medium. This has been demonstrated for blood by Baier and Dutton [1] during direct observation of blood flow on a surface using reflected light microscopy. Brash and Lyman [2] also demonstrated, by infrared spectroscopy, the presence of proteins on a polyethylene surface after exposure to whole blood. The importance of protein adsorption in other areas of biomaterials application has also been recognized. For example fouling of insulin infusion devices due to insulin deposition on surfaces has been reported [3]. Also the impairment of contact lenses by protein adsorption from tear fluids represents a limitation to the longevity of these devices [4]. In blood contact situations adsorption is believed to be rapid. Thus Gendreau et al. [5] have found that proteins are present on a germanium surface within a few seconds of blood contact. Vroman et al. [6] have demonstrated the presence of fibrinogen on a number of surfaces within a few seconds of contact with plasma. Thus it is generally believed that protein adsorption is the first event occurring at the interface after blood contact. The arrival of cellular elements would be expected to be later because of their larger size and therefore smaller diffusion coefficients.

Events subsequent to protein adsorption are thus now known to occur through the intermediary of the adsorbed protein or "conditioning" layer as it has been called by Baier [7]. In this regard a number of studies have shown that the tendency of platelets to adhere and undergo secondary responses such as release is greatly influenced by the composition of the underlying protein layer. Packham et al. [8] showed an inhibitory effect of albumin and an enhancing effect of γ-globulin and fibrinogen in this regard. Work in our laboratory [9] has led to similar conclusions and has shown, moreover, that release from adherent platelets is relatively high when γ-globulin is adsorbed on the surface. Kim and coworkers [10-12] have proposed in this connection that platelet adhesion takes place via reaction between platelet enzymes (e.g., glycosyl transferase) and saccharide residues on adsorbed protein. Since albumin contains no sugar residues, such reactions cannot occur. The effect of proteins other than the common plasma proteins is effectively unknown. Recently [13] fibronectin has been suggested as a possible "adhesive" for platelet sticking.

In addition to the effects mentioned, foreign surface contact also triggers plasma coagulation and this clearly involves adsorption of the coagulation factor proteins as has been shown by several groups [14,15]. Indeed adsorption of Hageman factor to negatively charged surfaces (e.g., kaolin) is a recognized primary means of activation. All-in-all protein adsorption is a key event in blood surface interactions and must be understood more fully than at present if we wish, in turn, to understand the mechanisms of surface-induced thrombosis.

The material of this chapter is presented in two parts. In the first part a brief discussion of relevant fundamental principles is given. As a means of organizing this discussion, two questions are posed and answers are attempted: why do proteins adsorb, how do proteins adsorb? In the second part, recent research in relation to protein adsorption from blood is reviewed.

WHY DO PROTEINS ADSORB?

Adsorption of proteins at interfaces of all kinds is inevitable and virtually axiomatic; thus the question naturally arises why do proteins "like" interfaces. There are several answers to this question depending on the particular point of view. The thermodynamicist would say it is because adsorption results in a lowering of the system's free energy. The protein chemist might say it is because of the amphipathic character of the molecules with their polar nonpolar ambivalence. Others might say that adsorption is favored due to the macromolecular nature of proteins and to the associated limits on solubility. In fact all of these statements are valid and mutually compatible. We shall examine each of them briefly.

Any discussion of free energy change, ΔG, must consider its enthalpy and entropy components according to the definition:

$$\Delta G = \Delta H - T\Delta S$$

For a process to be spontaneous, as is protein adsorption, ΔG, from the point of view of the system must be negative. Thus either ΔH must be sufficiently negative or ΔS sufficiently positive to give a net negative result for ΔG. That is, adsorption must be sufficiently exothermic or have a sufficient associated gain of entropy. Enthalpy changes are available directly from calorimetric measurements [16,17] and even from the few data that have appeared it is clear that both enthalpically and entropically driven adsorptions can occur. Thus Norde and Lyklema [16] found ΔH for adsorption of albumin on negatively charged polystyrene ranged from positive to negative depending on the pH (Figure 1). In particular near the isoelectric point, where the protein is effectively uncharged, adsorption was endothermic and therefore driven by an increase in entropy. These observations may reflect the fact that hydrophobic interactions (see below) predominate under isoelectric conditions in this system. Nyilas et al. [17] found negative ΔH values for adsorption of γ-globulin on glass under neutral pH conditions where both surface and protein are charged.

It is clear that exothermic character can arise from the various interactions between protein and surface. These interactions can in principle involve covalent, electrostatic, and hydrogen bonding. Various nonbonding interactions are also possible. Entropy gain mechanisms, perhaps less obvious, result mainly from the disruption of structured water either near the protein or near the surface, i.e. from hydrophobic interactions.

The polypeptide chains of proteins consist of amino acids linked one to another by peptide bonds. The side chains of the amino acids contain, variously, negatively or positively charged groups, polar groups and hydrophobic groups. The ambivalent polar/nonpolar character of the protein as a whole clearly provides a driving force for concentration of the proteins at interfaces since differences in polarity will also exist across the interface. The process of adsorption viewed in this way can also be thought of as reducing the interfacial free energy or tension, a refinement on the overall thermodynamic description given above. Reduced interfacial tension is a driving force common to all adsorptions whether involving natural or synthetic materials, macromolecules or small molecules.

The interplay of molecular weight, solubility, and competition adsorption with other species including solvent molecules must also be considered when seeking an answer to the question: why do proteins adsorb? Absolute solubilities of proteins can be considered as low. Thus fibrinogen solubility ranges from about 3.0 to 0.4 mg ml^{-1} depending on pH and ionic strength [18]. For most proteins solubility rarely exceeds 1 percent by weight. Such low solubility might be thought of as a consequence of the high molecular weight and indeed solubilities tend to be higher for smaller proteins. Although other, more specific factors may determine the adsorption behavior in a particular system, nonetheless it is reasonable to view

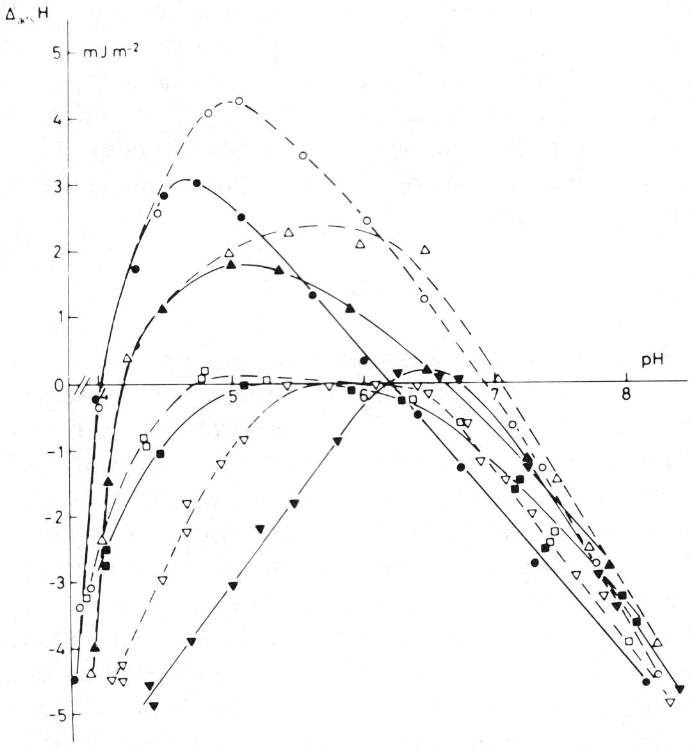

Figure 1. Enthalpy of adsorption of human plasma albumin on polystyrene latices. O, $\sigma_o = -15.5$ microcoulombs (μC) cm^{-2}; Δ, $\sigma_o = -6.3\ \mu C cm^{-2}$; □, $\sigma_o = -4.6\ \mu C\ cm^{-2}$; ∇, $\sigma_o = -2.3\ \mu C\ cm^{-2}$. T = 25°C. Open symbols, 0.01 M KNO_3; filled symbols, 0.05M KNO_3. (Reproduced with permission from reference 16).

adsorption as a consequence of limited solubility based on high molecular weight. Analogies with synthetic high polymer adsorption are perhaps illuminating in this regard. Thus it has been found that in polyisobutylene adsorption to carbon [19], the quantity adsorbed per unit surface area increases with increasing initial average MW. In addition there is a "fractionation" effect in that as the surface fills up, the average MW of the polymer remaining in solution decreases. For individual proteins which are of uniform MW, it is less easy to distinguish molecular weight effects. However it is likely that in mixtures of proteins, MW is a determining factor. Solubility and "goodness" or "poorness" of solvent are important in the adsorption of synthetic polymers. In general there is an increase in adsorption with decreasing solubility and with increasingly poor solvent as illustrated by adsorption of various polymers on glass [20]. Also Pefferkorn et al. [21] have shown for a water-soluble carboxylate-bearing copolymer, that increasing amounts are adsorbed with increase in MW and with decrease in solvent power (increasing NaCl concentration) at constant M.W. The extension of the adsorbed polymer into the solution (i.e. layer thickness) was shown to decrease with decreasing solvent power.

Analogous effects for proteins are illustrated by the fact that adsorption has frequently been found to be maximal at the isoelectric point [22,23] where solubility is a minimum. (This finding has also been explained in terms of a diminution in charge repulsion effects between adjacent protein molecules on the surface.) The concept of solvent power is strictly not applicable to proteins since it pertains to the change in average dimensions of the polymer coil as a function of solvent interactions. Protein molecules in the native state are of course not random coils and if they remain native do not significantly change dimensions. Solvent power, however, does have its protein analogy in the phenomena of salting in and salting out where an optimum range of salt concentration exists with respect to solubility.

In summary, it can be said that proteins adsorb because of their amphipathic character, their high MW and consequent limited solubility. The favorable free energy change associated with the adsorption process results primarily from the gain of entropy accompanying disruption of water structure, although many adsorptions are exothermic as well.

HOW DO PROTEINS ADSORB?

In considering this question we must address ourselves to three main topics: (a) how does the protein reach the surface, (b) how does it "react with" or "bind" to the surface, and (c) once adsorbed can the protein leave or desorb from the surface?

Transport

In most situations of practical interest, where a solution of protein is flowing past a solid surface, the protein reaches the surface by a combined diffusion-convection process. Having reached the surface the protein will bind by various mechanisms (see below). The binding process for any particular case will be governed by the intrinsic kinetics. Transport and binding are sequential elements of the adsorption process so that depending on their relative rates the adsorption rate may be controlled by one or the other or both. If transport is fast compared to binding then the rate of adsorption will be identical to the rate of binding. If binding is fast then transport will control.

Well-developed mathematical models are available to describe convective-diffusion and binding processes and with rate data of sufficient accuracy, the controlling step could be determined on the basis of fitting of data to the models. Such a procedure requires very precise measurements of initial adsorption rates. By "initial" is meant the stage of adsorption when most of the surface is still unoccupied. At the later stages when most of the surface is already occupied, the binding process will nearly always be rate-controlling since surface availability becomes the dominant factor. Also protein-protein interactions such as charge repulsion may become important. The initial stages of protein adsorption generally occur over a period of a few minutes and with available techniques, accurate rate data are difficult to obtain (most adsorption kinetics studies have been conducted over periods of several hours, well beyond initial conditions). Consequently little information is available regarding the question of transport versus binding control. However Robertson et al. [24] have recently shown by an in situ continuous measurement (total internal reflection fluorescence) that adsorption of both bovine serum albumin and fibrinogen to the surface of a silicone polymer are transport controlled under the concentration and flow conditions of their experiments. No general statement about rate control is ever likely to be possible since the situation will always depend on specific conditions.

With regard to transport in flowing blood as opposed to buffer solutions or plasma, the phenomenon of red cell-augmented diffusivities has frequently been discussed [25,26]. This augmentation results from the shear-induced lateral migrations [27] and rotations [28] of the RBC giving effects analogous to eddy diffusion. These phenomena are highly significant for transport of platelets and several papers [25,26,29] have reported platelet diffusivities greatly in excess of those predicted by Brownian motion. Whether RBC local motions can augment the diffusivity of proteins remains to be determined. We have found that the overall effect of RBC on adsorption is inhibitory [30], so that any effect on transport, if present, must be masked by the inhibition process.

In summary, then, it may be said that proteins move to a surface by molecular diffusion, which may be supplemented by convective transport in flow situations. No generalization can be made as to whether transport is rate limiting.

Modes of Interaction

In this section we consider only generalized binding and do not discuss specific covalent attachment via chemical reaction of protein with surface-localized functional groups. Such binding does not occur as a result of adsorption under biologic or quasi-biologic conditions and thus is irrelevant to the subject matter of this Volume.

Perhaps the most obvious means of binding protein to a surface is via electrostatic bond formation between charged groups on the protein and oppositely charged surface sites. This type of binding is exploited in the technology of ion exchange chromatography. The proteins in plasma are negatively charged at blood pH and thus would be expected to bind to cationic surfaces. The converse, namely that proteins should be repelled from negatively charged surfaces is not always true. Norde and Lyklema [16] have reported that the adsorption of negatively charged proteins on a negative polystyrene latex proceeds not only spontaneously, and thus with a decrease in free energy, but also exothermically. Possibly other interactions are involved in such cases. Also it is possible that attractive electrostatic bonds are formed with specific cationic sites on the protein, which will be present even though the net charge is negative. Electrostatic bonding undoubtedly plays a role in many protein adsorption systems and indeed has been used in schemes to fractionate plasma by manipulation of pH and ionic concentration and composition [31]. The sensitivity of electrostatic bonding to the ionic composition is of some significance for the adsorption of proteins from blood where almost certainly for protein bound in such a manner, adsorption would be reversible and subject to continuous exchange with other ions in the blood. Protein adsorption appears generally to be irreversible or at best partially and slowly reversible on many of the surfaces of interest for blood contact applications (see below for a more extensive discussion of reversibility). This is particularly true of hydrophobic polymer surfaces. In such cases electrostatic interactions are presumably of minor importance. By contrast we have recently found [32] that adsorption of fibrinogen to glass shows considerable reversibility and that desorption occurs in response to electrolytes. This, and other evidence [33] suggests the importance of electrostatic interactions in adsorption of proteins to glass.

Another possible protein-surface interaction, which depends very strongly on the surface chemical composition, is hydrogen bonding. This would be likely only for relatively polar substrates. For example undissociated silanol groups on glass may be envisaged as forming H-bonds with carbonyl groups of peptide bonds. Messing [33] has invoked such a mechanism to explain the effect of urea, a H-bond disrupting agent, on adsorption of proteins to glass.

H-bonding is of course an extremely important phenomenon in the internal structure of proteins, contributing strongly to the stability of the α-helical and β-sheet structures. Its role in binding to surfaces has not been thoroughly assessed.

Another feature of protein secondary structure that may be relevant to adsorption, are the β-turns. These have recently been extensively studied by Chou and Fasman [34] and have been defined by them as "regions of the protein involving four consecutive residues where the polypeptide chain folds back on itself by nearly 180°." The β-turns are stabilized in many instances by internal H-bonding between the first and fourth residues. In addition there appears to be a preference for certain amino acid residues to be incorporated in the turns, e.g. proline, glycine and asparagine. Interestingly hydrophobic residues have the smallest tendency to be incorporated. Again to quote Chou and Fasman [34], "it is the chain reversals that give a protein its globularity rather than linearity." Recently Loucheux [35] has argued that the β-turns occur in the surface regions of the protein and must therefore be involved in adsorption. This interesting suggestion remains for the moment tantalizing but unconfirmed.

Perhaps the most important general binding mechanism in the present context is that of hydrophobic interaction. Hydrophobic interaction may be defined as the interaction of nonpolar groups in aqueous media. Proteins are known to contain hydrophobic "patches" in their surface (Figure 2) [36] which would be available to interact with hydrophobic contacting surfaces, typified by organic polymers such as polyethylene or Teflon. The heat change involved in such interactions is small and the major thermodynamic driving force is believed to be the gain of entropy when structured water at the hydrophobic interface is transferred to the bulk. This concept is illustrated schematically in Figure 3 due to Ochoa [37]. It should be noted in passing that the globular structures of soluble proteins are believed to be in large measure determined and stabilized by internal hydrophobic bonding, a hypothesis first advanced by Kauzmann [38]. A recently-developed form of protein chromatography is based on hydrophobic interactions and has been reviewed by Yon [39] and by Ochoa [37]. The characteristics of this process may serve to illustrate the nature of hydrophobic interactions and the extent to which they are important in "blood-contact" protein adsorption. The effect of ionic strength is instructive. As the salt concentration is increased, the hydrophobic interactions intensify and the quantity adsorbed increases [40]. The converse is true for decreasing salt concentration. "Salting out" ions (e.g. NH_4^+, SO_4^{2-}) are more effective than chaotropic ions (e.g. SCN^-, I^-) in promoting adsorption [41]. This is of course the opposite of the effect of neutral salts on attractive electrostatic interactions. Addition of compounds such as ethanol or ethylene glycol has been used as a means of eluting proteins from hydrophobic supports [42]. This presumably results from the polarity-reducing effect of the additive. It is most likely via hydrophobic interaction that proteins bind to surfaces such as polyethylene, silicone and certain segmented polyurethanes. The available evidence suggests that such surfaces adsorb considerable quantities, corresponding to compact monolayers [43] and that there is no desorption and only slow, partial exchange between adsorbed and dissolved protein [44].

Clearly the degree to which any particular binding mode occurs depends to a large extent on the character of the surface, e.g. whether it is hydrophobic or hydrophilic, whether it is charged or neutral, whether it is polar or nonpolar. Systematic studies of adsorption from this point of view are lacking but a few data exist which perhaps give indications of a general nature. Work in our laboratory, for example, has dealt with adsorption of albumin and fibrinogen separately and in mixtures to a range of surfaces from hydrophobic to hydrophilic as shown in Table 1.

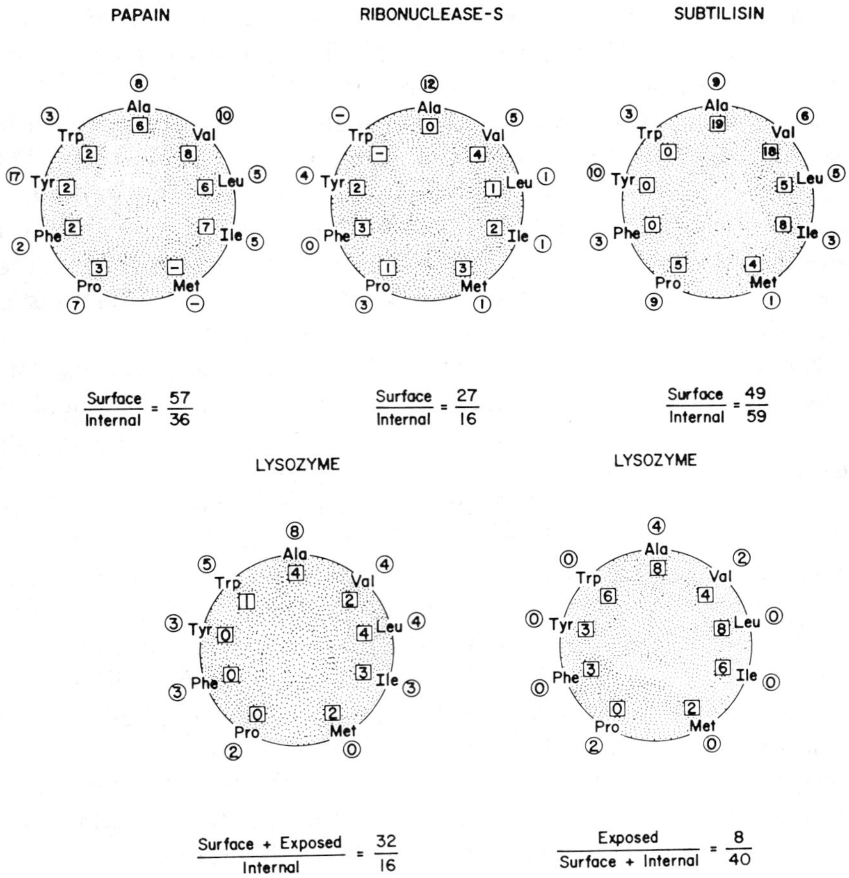

Figure 2. Top row: distribution of apolar groups between surface and interior of papain, ribonuclease, and subtilisin, respectively. Bottom row: two possible extreme representations for lysozyme; at left all side chains even partially accessible to solvent are classified as "surface"; on right, only side chains projecting fully into solvent are counted in circles outside envelope delineating the interior. (Reproduced with permission from reference 36.)

Quantities adsorbed are generally greater for hydrophobic substrates (bottom of Table), suggesting perhaps greater inherent binding capability or alternatively that adsorption to hydrophilic surfaces (whatever the binding mechanism) is subject to reversing influences such as desorption and ion exchange. Chuang et al. [45] have also observed greater affinity of plasma proteins for polyvinyl chloride, a hydrophobic surface, than for cuprophan dialysis membrane, a hydrophilic surface. Based on the influence of electrolytes, Mizutani [46] has argued that albumin is adsorbed to glass electrostatically and to siliconized glass by hydrophobic bonding. Waugh et al. [47, 48] have shown that thrombin binds more strongly to a poly(methyl methacrylate) surface than to glass. Similarly Chuang et al. [49] have found stronger binding of thrombin to polyvinyl chloride than to cuprophan.

The question of reversibility is also relevant to a consideration of the mechanism of adsorption. Reversibility is a somewhat controversial aspect of protein adsorption. Thus on solid surfaces adsorption has generally been found to be irreversible on any realistic time scale in the

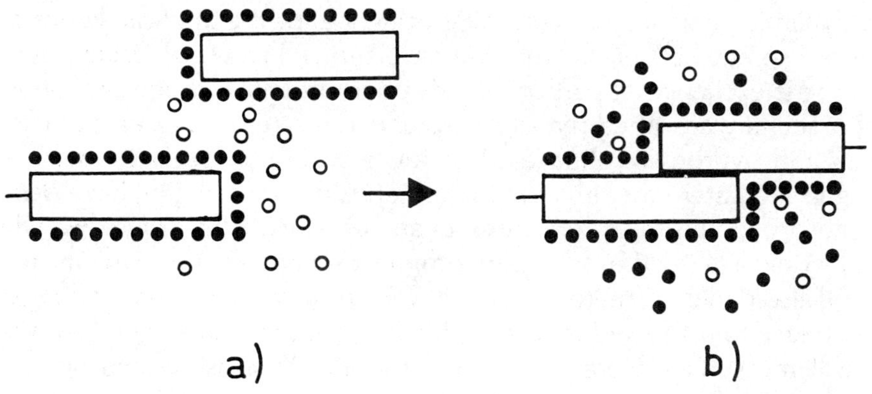

Figure 3. The mechanism of hydrophobic interaction. The water molecules around the hydrophobic "yard sticks" are dotted, for simplicity, in order to distinguish them from those in the bulk. Notice that the difference between a) and b) is only the improved degree of disorder (+ ΔS) of water molecules. (Reproduced with permission from reference 37).

Table 1. Adsorption of Albumin and Fibrinogen to Various Surfaces [43]

SURFACE	ALBUMIN* ($\mu g\ cm^{-2}$)	FIBRINOGEN* ($\mu g\ cm^{-2}$)
Polyurethane 1540 (Hydrophilic)	0.020 ± 0.009	0.034
Polyurethane 600 (Hydrophilic)	0.037	0.083
Collagen	0.086	0.615
Siliconized Glass	0.176	0.973
Polystyrene	0.196	1.051 ± 0.053
Polyurethane 1200 (Hydrophobic)	0.571	1.092

*Steady-state surface concentrations at 1 mg ml^{-1} (0.05 M tris, pH 7.35).

sense that no desorption occurs upon reduction of the bulk concentration to points lower on the isotherm. Such behavior is characteristic of a variety of systems but especially so of hydrophobic surfaces [2,50] while for hydrophilic surfaces both reversibility [43] and irreversibility [50] have been found. There is certainly no fundamental reason why desorption should not occur for proteins vis-a-vis other, simpler molecules, However the possibility of multiple contacts resulting in a very high activation energy for desorption could severely limit the rates of protein desorption.

Some systems [51,52] have shown reversibility in the sense that additional adsorption has been observed upon increasing the bulk concentration. Also, good agreement of adsorption data with a Langmuir model has frequently been found [2,45,53] thus implying reversibility in the sense of a dynamic equilibrium. Supporting evidence for the applicability of a Langmuir model, is however, somewhat sparse. Thus we have shown [32,44,54], using double isotope labeling, that there is exchange of part of the adsorbed protein with the protein in solution, even though the quantity adsorbed remains constant. The rates and extents of exchange are greater for glass and hydrophilic surfaces than for hydrophobic surfaces, again suggesting stronger binding in the latter case. In a similar fashion Chuang et al. [45] have demonstrated exchange of adsorbed proteins on cuprophan of the order of 40% whereas on polyvinylchloride only 6% of the adsorbed protein exchanged. Experiments reported by Kochwa et al. [55] also could be interpreted as showing turnover. They noted that exposure of a polyurethane surface to unlabeled protein "limited" subsequent uptake of the corresponding labeled protein. If the surface were saturated in the initial exposure, and no turnover occurred, then presumably no uptake of the labeled protein would take place.

Other work indicating a dynamic rather than a static character for adsorbed protein is that of Cuypers et al. [56] showing replacement of adsorbed fibrinogen by other proteins on exposure to serum. Also Vroman et al. [57] have recently shown that fibrinogen initially adsorbed from plasma to a "glass-like" surface is replaced within minutes by high molecular weight kininogen and factor XII. These studies suggest the importance of protein turnover for the blood-material interface problem in that it provides a mechanism whereby the composition of the adsorbed protein layer, known to be important for platelet-surface interactions [8], could change with time. Also it is possible, as pointed out previously [44], that "reflected" protein (i.e. protein that has been adsorbed, and then returned to the bulk) may be conformationally altered so that it can trigger some undesired response in the blood, e.g. coagulation. Evolution of the adsorbed layer with time is also suggested by recent work of Mizutani [58] and of Soderquist and Walton [51]. Mizutani has shown that various enzymes adsorbed to glass progressively lose activity over a period of several weeks and are dissociated to subunits. Soderquist and Walton found, similarly, that plasma proteins undergo a slow conformational change when adsorbed to copolypeptide and silicone surfaces.

RECENT RESEARCH ON PROTEIN ADSORPTION AS RELATED TO BLOOD INTERACTIONS

As stated in the introduction protein adsorption from blood to a foreign surface is the first event in a sequence leading to thrombus formation. A schematic representation of surface thrombogenesis, showing the initiating role of protein adsorption is shown in Figure 4. A considerable volume of research has been carried out in recent years relating to these phenomena. The following discussion of this work emphasizes the most recent contributions. Again the discussion will be divided into several subtopics, reflecting to some extent the questions which current research on protein adsorption is trying to answer. These are: (a) What is the time dependence of adsorption and what is the order of magnitude of the quantities adsorbed? (b) To what extent is the adsorbed protein "denatured" and how does this relate to blood interactions? (c) Given the fact that there are of the order of 100 individual protein species in plasma, what is the composition of the adsorbed layer? (d) Is there an influence of blood cells on adsorption?

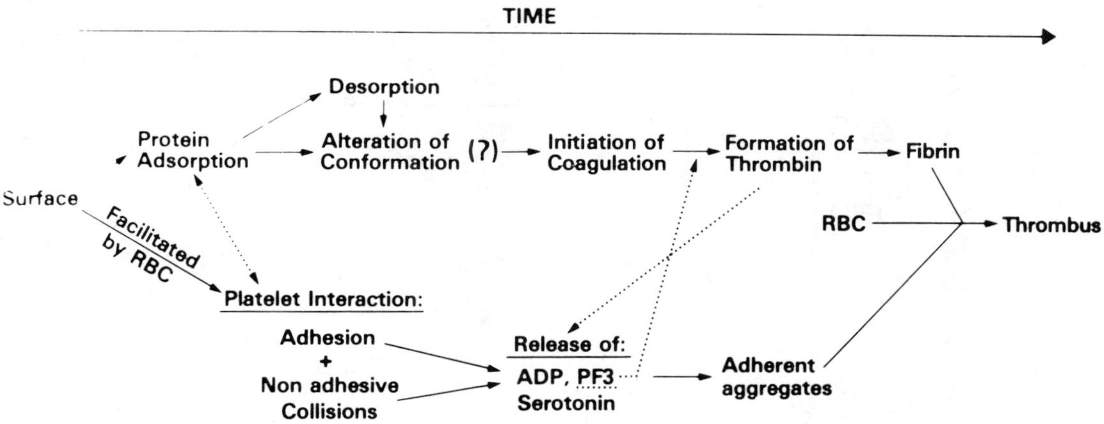

Figure 4. Sequence of events leading to thrombus formation on artificial surfaces. (Reproduced with permission from "Assisted circulation," F. Unger Ed., Springer-Verlag, New York, 1979).

(a) Kinetics of Adsorption, Quantities Adsorbed

As already discussed, detailed studies of adsorption kinetics with high time resolution have not been carried out. This is mainly because of the experimental difficulty of obtaining real time in situ kinetic data. Most experimental techniques such as radio-isotope labeling, require separation of the adsorbing surface from its "mother" solution before the measurement is made. Such techniques are thus not in real time and are subject to artefacts of the separation procedures (e.g. rinsing). Studies using such techniques with solutions of single proteins indicate that adsorption may be largely complete within a few minutes. For example Chan & Brash [32] found that fibrinogen adsorption to glass is 75% complete within 5 minutes under conditions where ultimate adsorption is of monomolecular layer proportions. Lee and Kim [53] reported adsorption times to equilibrium of the order of one hour. Real time studies have recently been reported by Robertson et al. [24] and by Van Wagenen et al. [59] using total internal reflection fluorescence, and by Gendreau et al. [5] using Fourier transform infrared attenuated reflection spectrocopy. Robertson's work indicates that adsorption of bovine serum albumin (BSA) and fibrinogen to silicone polymers can be diffusion controlled in the early stages under certain conditions of flow. Van Wagenen et al. showed that in adsorption to quartz from equimolar solutions of BSA and γ-globulin, BSA reached "equilibrium" in 8 seconds and γ-globulin in 40 minutes (in this case 75% of equilibrium was achieved in about 15 minutes).

With regard to amounts adsorbed, most protein-surface pairs exhibit a limiting surface concentration corresponding presumably to the capacity of the surface to accommodate protein. Thus adsorption isotherms, showing surface concentration as a function of solution concentration, usually approach a plateau beginning at moderate solution concentrations and extending to concentrations found in blood (e.g. Figure 5). The surface concentrations at these plateaux are of the order of 0.1 to 1.0 $\mu g\ cm^{-2}$. It can be deduced from the known geometry of protein molecules that such quantitites can be modeled as monomolecular layers. Only in a few instances have multimolecule layers been proposed [17,60].

Thus for adsorption from buffer solutions of single proteins, the available data suggest that proteins adsorb with rapid initial rates, approach a steady state concentration somewhat more slowly, and attain that steady state within perhaps an hour.

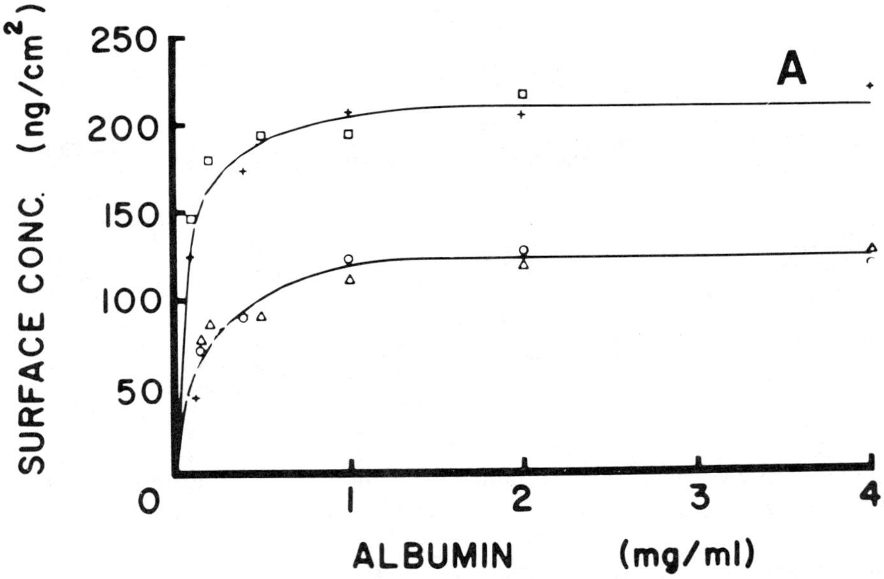

Figure 5. Adsorption isotherms of albumin and delipidated albumin onto Cuprophane and PVC. Results are averages of two to three determinations in each case. +—+, Albumin adsorption onto PVC; □—□, delipidated albumin adsorption onto PVC; o—o, albumin adsorption onto Cuprophane; Δ—Δ, delipidated albumin adsorption onto Cuprophane. (Reproduced with permission from reference 45).

In plasma, kinetics and "equilibria" are quite different and are not predictable from buffer solution data. As already indicated, Vroman et al. [6] have shown the presence of fibrinogen on various surfaces within seconds of plasma contact, but have also found that the fibrinogen disappears in the following few minutes [57]. Other groups have also shown transient adsorption of proteins from plasma or blood [55,61,62]. Additional discussion of plasma results is given below.

(b) Denaturation

In the blood context, the significance of denaturation relates to the possible activation of coagulation, to the effect on platelets of interacting with denatured proteins, and to the possible depletion of proteins by a rapid denaturation – desorption sequence.

One approach to the study of surface denaturation is to use data on quantity adsorbed in a "monolayer" (the usual configuration) to calculate average protein dimensions which can then be compared to known solution dimensions. Such an approach has usually led to the conclusion that gross dimensional alteration probably does not occur [2]. Perhaps the greatest weakness of this approach is that one is dealing with averages for a very large population of molecules and a small but significant subpopulation with altered dimensions would not be detected. In addition one assumes the surface distribution of protein to be uniform. There is some recent evidence [63-65] that such an assumption may not always be justified.

More recently various physical and biological techniques have been used for studying denaturation. The "bound fraction" measurements of Morrissey and Stromberg [66] based on infrared spectral shifts of protein amide I bands showed that albumin and prothrombin adsorbed on silica retain native conformation but γ-globulin may be altered at low surface coverage [67]. Chuang et al. [68] have made an extensive study of the biologic response of thrombin adsorbed on cuprophan and polyvinylchloride and have shown retention of several functions including reactivity with antithrombin III, with fibrinogen and with a specific antibody. Amidase activity was, however, lacking. Waugh et al. [47] similarly showed that thrombin adsorbed on glass retains its ability to clot fibrinogen. McMillin and Walton [69] showed using circular dichroism that fibrinogen is not conformationally altered on silica, whereas factor XII undergoes a major change. The same group has recently found [51] that proteins desorbed from synthetic polypeptide films show a loss of secondary structure (α – helix, or β – sheet). We have made similar observations for fibrinogen desorbed from glass [70]. Mizutani [58] has also recently shown that a number of enzymes adsorbed to glass gradually lose activity over a period of several weeks. All-in-all, the evidence on denaturation is somewhat varied and leads one to the conclusion that generalization should probably not be attempted; rather each system must be examined individually.

(c) Layer Composition in Plasma Contact

We turn next to the question of competitive adsorption and the composition of the layer adsorbed from plasma. In studies where simple mixtures of two or three components have been used [43,63,71-73] it has often been concluded that fibrinogen is preferentially adsorbed from mixtures with albumin or γ-globulin. These results could be taken as an indication that fibrinogen will predominate in the layers adsorbed from blood or plasma. We have observed [43] that the fibrinogen-to-albumin ratio correlates with platelet reactivity on various surfaces Horbett et al. [74] have drawn attention to the preferential adsorption of hemoglobin from plasma onto polyethylene and their results suggest that substantial adsorption of this protein might occur in blood. In this regard it should be noted that although hemoglobin is present in plasma only in trace amounts (~ 0.003 mg ml^{-1}), hemolysis occurring in the presence of a foreign surface may increase this value. In more recent work Horbett and Weathersby [75] have drawn attention to the differences in composition of the adsorbed protein layer as a function of the underlying surface composition in a series of copolymers of hydroxyethyl methacrylate and ethyl methacrylate. Compositional differences were also observed as a function of time.

Studies of quantities adsorbed from plasma in general show results considerably different from solutions of single proteins or simple mixtures. The work of Horbett et al. [74] as well as showing differences in composition between the adsorbed layer and plasma, also showed smaller values of surface concentration for plasma than for simple protein solutions of the same concentration. From this and other reported work it seems likely that the total surface concentration of the common plasma proteins (albumin, γ-globulin and fibrinogen) is less for plasma than for simple buffered solutions. This suggests that either there are trace proteins that are strongly surface active and are adsorbed in large quantities or that the plasma itself somehow restricts adsorption. In support of the latter hypothesis, Kochwa et al. [55], studying the adsorption of fibrinogen from plasma to a polyetherurethane, observed a maximum in the time course of adsorption at times of a few minutes. This was attributed to rapid initial adsorption followed by enzymatic removal of part of the fibrinogen, perhaps those molecules that had undergone a conformational change.

Recent work in our laboratory [61] using plasma has shown an early maximum in the adsorption of fibrinogen on polyethylene similar to that reported by Kochwa et al. [55]. However, other surfaces such as polystyrene showed kinetics similar to those in simple solution. Somewhat surprisingly, glass appeared not to adsorb fibrinogen for contact times between 2 minutes and 3 hours. This observation is in accord with the suggestion of Vroman et al. [57] that on activating surfaces, initially adsorbed fibrinogen is rapidly replaced (within minutes) by high molecular weight kininogen and factor XII. In agreement with Horbett et al., we found generally low surface concentration values of the abundant proteins, and again it is possible this is due to adsorption of unidentified trace proteins or to enzymatic action on initially adsorbed proteins.

Some investigators have found adsorption to be similar from plasma and simple solutions. Thus Kim et al. [76] reported on the adsorption of fibrinogen, γ-globulin, and albumin from plasma on various hydrophobic polymers including a segmented polyetherurethane. Their data indicated substantial adsorption to all surfaces with "normal" kinetics. Also Chiu et al. [77] found that surface concentrations of fibrinogen adsorbed from plasma to glass or carbon are about the same as or greater than from solution. Much work remains to be done to establish the exact composition of proteins adsorbed from plasma and blood, especially with respect to trace proteins. It does seem clear, however, that there is considerable surface specificity in this regard so that surface properties per se may be considered as determining the outcome of contact with blood.

(d) Red Cell Effects

Since red cells occupy approximately half the volume of blood it seems relevant to ask what effect they might have on protein adsorption. We have found [30,78] that in general the addition of RBC to protein solutions causes a reduction in the quantity of protein adsorbed, and in some cases the surface concentration passes through a transient maximum. Our most recent work [78] suggests that the effect derives partly from competitive adsorption of released hemoglobin. However the major effect is membrane- or particle-related since ghost cells are as effective as normal cells in reducing adsorption. With regard to surface-related thrombosis, it has usually been assumed that RBC exert their effect of augmenting platelet-adhesion via their hydrodynamic behavior. It now seems likely that at least part of the effect could be due to a reduction in the adsorption of platelet-protective proteins, or that red cells deposit an adhesive material on the surface.

CONCLUSIONS

It should be evident from the preceding discussion that a considerable body of information relative to protein adsorption from blood has accumulated in recent years, and that certain broad trends in behavior have emerged. Among these are that deposits are of monolayer proportions; that the layer forms rapidly but may "evolve" with time; that the composition of the layer varies with the surface, is different from that of blood and in some cases may be enriched in fibrinogen; that conformational change is probably not a general phenomenon though it occurs in some systems; and that red cells may play a role in restricting adsorption.

Looking to the future one might ask: what remains to be done? To this reviewer's mind, essential knowledge is still lacking concerning the composition of the layer adsorbing from blood. Thus we do not know in detail what proteins, and in what proportions, are adsorbed to different surfaces. This is particularly true of trace proteins. Immunological techniques such as used by Vroman [71] should be of value in this regard. In particular it seems important that we understand something of the way in which surface chemistry influences the composition of the layer. This could well be the key to development of thromboresistant surfaces since later blood response, e.g. platelet sticking, depends on the protein layer. More studies that permit "real-time," "in situ" observation are also required, so that events on the time scale of a few seconds can be resolved. Recent work using internal reflection fluorescence [24,59,60] and Fourier transform infrared internal reflection spectroscopy [5] seems promising from this point of view.

Finally it may be that a revival of past efforts to understand the surface-adsorption aspects of the initial or contact phase of blood coagulation would be useful. Considerable new biochemical knowledge of blood coagulation has been developed in recent years [15]. However an understanding of the role of surface, fundamentally a protein adsorption phenomenon, remains to be achieved.

REFERENCES

1. Baier, R. E. and Dutton, R. C. Initial events in interactions of blood with a foreign surface. *J. Biomed. Mater. Res.* 3, 191-206, 1969.
2. Brash, J. L. and Lyman, D. J. Adsorption of plasma proteins in solution to uncharged, hydrophobic polymer surfaces. *J. Biomed. Mater. Res.* 3, 175-189, 1969.
3. Sefton, M. V. Implantable micropump for insulin delivery. Amer. Chem. Soc. Adv. Chem. *199,* 511, 1982.
4. Royce, F. M., Ratner, B. D. and Horbett, T. A. Adsorption of proteins to copolymer contact lens materials from artificial tear solutions. Amer. Chem. Soc. Adv. Chem. *199,* 453-462, 1982.
5. Gendreau, R. M., Winters, S., Leininger, R. I., Fink, D., Hassler, C. R. and Jakobsen, R. J. Fourier transform infrared spectroscopy of protein adsorption from whole blood: ex vivo dog studies. Appl. Spectroscopy, *35,* 353-357, 1981.
6. Vroman, L., Adams, A. L., Klings, M., Fischer, G. C., Munoz, P. C. and Solensky, R. P. Reactions of formed elements of blood with plasma proteins at interfaces. *Ann. N.Y. Acad. Sci.* 283, 65-76, 1977.
7. Baier, R. E. The organization of blood components near interfaces. *Ann. N.Y. Acad. Sci.* 283, 17-36, 1977.
8. Packham, M. A., Evans, G., Glynn, M. F. and Mustard, J. F. The effect of plasma proteins on the interaction of platelets with glass surfaces. *J. Lab. Clin. Med.* 73, 686-697, 1969.
9. Whicher, S. J. and Brash, J. L. Platelet-foreign surface interactions: release of granule constituents from adherent platelets. *J. Biomed. Mater. Res.* 12, 181-201, 1978.
10. Lee, R. G. and Kim, S. W. The role of carbohydrate in platelet adhesion to foreign surfaces. *J. Biomed. Mater. Res.* 8, 393-398, 1974.
11. Lee, R. G. and Kim, S. W. Cyclic AMP and platelet adhesion to silastic surfaces. *Thromb. Res.* 4, 485-490, 1974.
12. Lee, E. S. and Kim, S. W. Adsorbed glycoproteins in platelet adhesion onto polymer surfaces: significance of terminal galactose units. *Trans. Amer. Soc. Artif. Int. Organs.* 25, 124-131, 1979.
13. Ihlenfeld, J. V., Mathis, T. R., Barber, T. A., Mosher, D. F., Riddle, L. M., Hart, A. P., Updike, S. J. and Cooper, S. L. Transient in vivo thrombus deposition onto polymeric biomaterials: role of fibronectin. *Trans. Amer. Soc. Artif. Int. Organs.* 24, 727-734, 1978.
14. Ratnoff, O. D. and Saito, H. Coagulation factors and the role of surface in their activation. *Ann. N.Y. Acad. Sci.* 283, 88-92, 1977.

15. Cochrane, C. G. and Griffin, J. H. Molecular assembly in the contact phase of the Hageman factor system. *Am. J. Med.* 67, 657-664, 1979.
16. Norde, W. and Lyklema, J. The adsorption of human plasma albumin and bovine pancreas ribonuclease at negatively charged polystyrene surfaces. V. Microcalorimetry. *J. Colloid Interface Sci.* 66, 295-302, 1978.
17. Nyilas, E., Chiu, T. H. and Herzlinger, G. A. Thermodynamics of native protein/foreign surface interactions. I. Calorimetry of the human γ-globulin/glass system. *Trans. Amer. Soc. Artif. Int. Organs.* 20, 480-490, 1974.
18. Leavis, P. C. and Rothstein, F. The solubility of fibrinogen in dilute salt solutions. *Arch. Biochem. Biophys.* 161, 671-682, 1974.
19. Gilliland, E. R. and Gutoff, E. B. Rubber-filler interactions: solution adsorption studies. *J. Appl. Polymer Sci.* 3, 26-42, 1960.
20. Rowland, F. W. and Eirich, F. R. Flow rates of polymer solutions through porous disks as a function of solute. II Thickness and structure of adsorbed polymer films. *J. Polymer Sci. A-1* 4, 2401-2421, 1966.
21. Pefferkorn, E., Dejardin, P. and Varoqui, R. Derivation by hydrodynamics of the structural characteristics of adsorbed polymers at liquid-solid interfaces. *J. Colloid Interface Sci.* 63, 353-361, 1978.
22. Bull, H. B. Adsorption of bovine serum albumin on glass. *Biochem. Biophys. Acta.* 19, 464-471, 1956.
23. Norde, W. and Lyklema, J. The adsorption of human plasma albumin and bovine pancreas ribonuclease at negatively charged polystyrene surfaces. I Adsorption isotherms. Effects of charge, ionic strength and temperature. *J. Colloid Interface Sci.* 66, 257-265, 1978.
24. Lok, B. K., Cheng, Y-I and Robertson, C. R., *J. Colloid Interface Sci.*, in press.
25. Feuerstein, I. A., Brophy, J. M. and Brash, J. L. Platelet transport and adhesion to reconstituted collagen and artificial surfaces. *Trans. Amer. Soc. Artif. Int. Organs.* 21, 427-434, 1975.
26. Turitto, V. Benis, A. M. and Leonard, E. F., Platelet diffusion in flowing blood. *Ind. Eng. Chem. Fundam.* 11, 216-223, 1972.
27. Goldsmith, H. L. Red cell motions and wall interaction in tube flow. *Fed. Proc.* 30, 1578-1588, 1971.
28. Keller, K. H. Effect of fluid shear on mass transport in blood. *Fed. Proc.* 30, 1591-1599, 1971.
29. Grabowski, E. F., Friedman, L. I. and Leonard, E. F. Effects of shear rate on the diffusion and adhesion of blood platelets to a foreign surface. *Ind. Eng. Chem. Fundam.* 11, 224-232, 1972.
30. Brash, J. L. and Uniyal, S. Adsorption of albumin and fibrinogen to polyethylene in presence of red cells. *Trans. Amer. Soc. Artif. Int. Organs.* 22, 253-259, 1976.
31. Curling, J. M., Berglof, J., Lindquist, L.-O. and Eriksson, S. A. Chromatographic procedure for the purification of human plasma albumin. *Vox Sang.* 33, 97-107, 1977.
32. Chan, B. M. C. and Brash, J. L. Adsorption of fibrinogen on glass: reversibility aspects. J. Colloid Interface Sci., *82*, 217-225 (1981).
33. Messing, R. A. Adsorption of proteins on glass surfaces and pertinent parameters for the immobilization of enzymes in the pores of inorganic carriers. *J. Non-Cryst. Solids.* 19, 277-283, 1975.
34. Chou, P. Y. and Fasman, G. D., β-turns in proteins. *J. Mol. Biol.* 115, 135-175, 1977.
35. Loucheux, C. Etude de l'interaction coude-β/interface. Paper presented at "Colloque des ATP Proteines aux interfaces et materiaux hemocompatibles." CNRS, Paris, 1978.
36. Klotz, I. M. Comparison of molecular structures of proteins: helix content, distribution of apolar residues. *Arch. Biochem. Biophys.* 138, 704-706, 1970.
37. Ochoa, J.-L. Hydrophobic (interaction) chromatography. *Biochimie* 60, 1-15, 1978.
38. Kauzmann, W. Some factors in the interpretation of protein denaturation. *Adv. Prot. Chem.* 14, 1-63, 1959.
39. Yon, R. J. Recent developments in protein chromatography involving hydrophobic interactions. *Int. J. Biochem.* 9, 373-379, 1978.

40. Porath, J., Sundberg, L., Fornstedt, L. and Olsson, I. Salting out in amphiphilic gels as a new approach to hydrophobic adsorption. *Nature* 245, 465-466, 1973.
41. Pahlmann, S., Rosengren, J., and Hjerten, S. Hydrophobic interaction chromatography on uncharged sepharose derivatives. Effects of neutral salts on the adsorption of proteins. *J. Chromatog.* 131, 99-108, 1977.
42. Laas, T. Agar derivatives for chromatography, electrophoresis and gel-bound enzymes. IV Benzylated dibromopropanol crosslinked sepharose as an amphiphilic gel for hydrophobic salting out chromatography of proteins with special emphasis on denaturing risks. *J. Chromatog.* 111, 373-387, 1975.
43. Brash, J. L. and Uniyal, S. Dependence of albumin-fibrinogen simple and competitive adsorption on surface properties of biomaterials. *J. Polymer Sci.* C66, 377-389, 1979.
44. Brash, J. L. and Samak, Q. M. Dynamics of interactions between human albumin and polyethylene surface. *J. Colloid Interface Sci.* 65, 495-504, 1978.
45. Chuang, H. Y. K., King, W. F. and Mason, R. G. Interaction of plasma proteins with artificial surfaces: protein adsorption isotherms. *J. Lab. Clin. Med.* 92, 483-496, 1978.
46. Mizutani, T. Use of silicone-coated porous glass for exclusion chromatography in an aqueous medium. *J. Chromatog.* 196, 485-488, 1980.
47. Waugh, D. F., Anthony, L. J. and NG, H. The interactions of thrombin with borosilicate glass surfaces. *J. Biomed. Mater. Res.* 9, 511-536, 1975.
48. Waugh, D. F., Lippe, J. A. and Freund, Y. R. Interactions of bovine thrombin and plasma albumin with low energy surfaces. *J. Biomed. Mater. Res.* 12, 599-625, 1978.
49. Chuang, H. Y. K., Crowther, P. E., Mohammad, S. F. and Mason, R. G. Interactions of thrombin and antithrombin III with artifical surfaces. *Thromb. Res.* 14, 273-282, 1979.
50. Macritchie, F. The adsorption of proteins at the solid-liquid interface. *J. Colloid Interface Sci.* 38, 484-488, 1972.
51. Soderquist, M. E. and Walton, A. G. Structural changes in proteins adsorbed on polymer surfaces. *J. Colloid Interface Sci.* 75, 386-397, 1980.
52. Norde, W. Adsorption of proteins at solid surfaces. In: *Adhesion and Adsorption of Polymers, Part B.* L. H. Lee (Ed.), New York: Plenum Publishing Corp., 1980, pp. 801-825.
53. Lee, R. G. and Kim, S. W. Adsorption of proteins onto hydrophobic polymer surfaces: adsorption isotherms and kinetics. *J. Biomed. Mater. Res.* 8, 251-259, 1974.
54. Brash, J. L., Uniyal, S. and Samak, Q. Exchange of albumin adsorbed on polymer surfaces. *Trans. Amer. Soc. Artif. Int. Organs.* 20, 69-76, 1974.
55. Kochwa, S., Litwak, R. S., Rosenfield, R. E. and Leonard, E. F. Blood elements at foreign surfaces: a biochemical approach to the study of the adsorption of plasma proteins. *Ann. N.Y. Acad. Sci.* 283, 37-49, 1977.
56. Cuypers, P. A., Hermens, W. T. and Hemker, H. C. Ellipsometric study of protein film on chromium. *Ann. N.Y. Acad. Sci.* 283, 77-85, 1977.
57. Vroman, L., Adams, A. L., Fischer, G. C. and Munoz, P. C. Interaction of high molecular weight kininogen, factor XII, and fibrinogen in plasma at interfaces. *Blood.* 55, 156-159, 1980.
58. Mizutani, T. Decreased activity of proteins adsorbed onto glass surfaces with porous glass as a reference. *J. Pharm. Sci.* 69, 279-282, 1980.
59. Van Wagenen, R. A., Rockhold, S. and Andrade, J. D. Probing protein adsorption II. Total internal reflection intrinsic fluorescence. *Amer. Chem. Soc. Adv. Chem., 199,* 351-370, 1982.
60. Burghardt, T. P., and Axelrod, D. Total internal reflection/fluorescence photobleaching recovery study of serum albumin adsorption dynamics. *Biophys. J.,* 33, 455-468, 1981.
61. Uniyal, S. and Brash, J. L. Patterns of adsorption of proteins from human plasma to solid surfaces. Thromb. Haemostas., in press.
62. Ihlenfeld, J. V. and Cooper, S. L. Transient in vivo protein adsorption onto polymeric biomaterials. *J. Biomed. Mater. Res.,* 13, 577, 1979.

63. Kochwa, S., Litwak, R. S., Rosenfield, R. E. and Leonard, E. F. Blood elements at foreign surfaces: in vitro evaluation of biomaterials in a spinning disc apparatus. *Ann. N.Y. Acad. Sci.* 283, 457-472, 1977.
64. Eberhart, R. C., Prokop, L. D., Wissenger, J. and Wolkow, M. A. Observation of albumin deposits on teflon surfaces. *Trans. Amer. Soc. Artif. Int. Organs.* 23, 134-139, 1977.
65. Ratner, B. D., Horbett, T. A., Shuttleworth, D. and Thomas, H. R., Analysis of the organization of protein films on solid surfaces by ESCA *J. Colloid Interface Sci.,* 83, 630-642, 1981.
66. Morrissey, B. W. and Stromberg, R. R. The conformation of adsorbed blood proteins by infrared bound fraction measurements. *J. Colloid Interface Sci.,* 46, 152-164, 1974.
67. Morrissey, B. W. and Fenstermaker, C. A. Conformation of adsorbed γ-globulin and β-lactoglobulin. Effect of surface concentration. *Trans. Amer. Soc. Artif. Int. Organs.* 22, 278-283, 1976.
68. Chuang, H. Y. K., Mohammad, S. F., Sharma, N. C. and Mason, R. G. Interaction of human α-thrombin with artificial surfaces and reactivity of adsorbed α-thrombin. *J. Biomed. Mater. Res.,* 14, 467-476, 1980.
69. McMillin, C. R. and Walton, A. G. A circular dichroism technique for the study of adsorbed protein structure. *J. Colloid Interface Sci.* 48, 345-349, 1974.
70. Chan, B. M. C. and Brash, J. L. Conformational change in fibrinogen desorbed from glass surface. *J. Colloid Interface Sci.,* 84, 263-265, 1981.
71. Vroman, L., Adams, A. L., Klings, M. and Fischer, G. Fibrinogen, globulins, albumin and plasma at interfaces. In: *Applied Chemistry at Protein Interfaces.* R. E. Baier (Ed.), Washington, D.C.: American Chemical Society, 1975, pp. 255-289.
72. Brash, J. L. and Davidson, V. J. Adsorption on glass and polyethylene from solutions of fibrinogen and albumin. *Thromb. Res.* 9, 249-259, 1976.
73. Horbett, T. A. and Hoffman, A. S. Bovine plasma protein adsorption onto radiation-grafted hydrogels based on hydroxyethyl methacrylate and N-vinylpyrrolidone. In: *Applied Chemistry at Protein Interfaces.* R. E. Baier (Ed.), Washington, D.C.: American Chemical Society, 1975, pp. 230-254.
74. Horbett, T. A., Weathersby, P. K. and Hoffman, A. S. The preferential adsorption of hemoglobin to polyethylene. *J. Bioeng.* 1, 61-67, 1977.
75. Horbett, T. A. and Weathersby, P.K. Adsorption of proteins from plasma to a series of hydrophilic-hydrophobic copolymers I. Analysis with the in situ radioiodination technique. *J. Biomed. Mater. Res.,* 15, 403-423, 1981.
76. Kim, S. W., Wisniewski, S.m Lee, E. S. and Winn, M. L. Role of protein and fatty acid adsorption on platelet adhesion and aggregation at the blood-polymer interface. *J. Biomed. Mater. Res. Symp.* 8, 23-31, 1977.
77. Chiu, T-H., Nyilas, E. and Turcotte, L. R. Microcalorimetric and electrophoretic studies of protein sorption from plasma. *Trans. Amer. Soc. Artif. Int. Organs.* 24, 389-402, 1978.
78. Uniyal, S. Brash., J. L. and Degterev, I. A. Influence of red blood cells and their components on protein adsorption. Amer. Chem. Soc. Adv. Chem., *199,* 277-292, 1982.

Chapter 3

Surface Thermodynamics of Protein Adsorption, Cell Adhesion and Cell Engulfment*

A.W. Neumann,[1,2,3] D.R. Absolom,[1,2,4] W. Zingg,[2,3,5] C.J. van Oss[4] and D.W. Francis[1,2]

ABSTRACT

A thermodynamic model provides qualitative and quantitative insight into attachment and detachment of cells and proteins to foreign surfaces. A correct prediction of the behavior of a system by the model suggests non-specificity; deviations are probably caused by specific interactions. Proteins and human blood cells were found to be relatively hydrophilic in their native state. The thermodynamic approach and the relevant methodology are described.

*Supported in part by the Natural Sciences and Engineering Research Council and the Medical Research Council of Canada.
[1]Department of Mechanical Engineering, University of Toronto, Toronto, Ontario, Canada M5S 1A4.
[2]Department of Surgery, Research Institute, Hospital for Sick Children, Toronto, Ontario, Canada M5G 1X8.
[3]Institute of Biomedical Engineering, University of Toronto, Toronto, Ontario, Canada M5S 1A4.
[4]Department of Microbiology, State University of New York at Buffalo, Buffalo, New York 14214.
[5]Institute of Medical Science, University of Toronto, Toronto, Ontario, Canada M5S 1A4.

I. INTRODUCTION

1. General

Exposing polymers, metals or ceramics to a biological environment by implanting a biomedical device elicits a number of reactions such as protein adsorption and cell adhesion to the surface of the device. These processes will invariably change the surface properties of the substrate and may cause, directly or indirectly, adverse reactions. Therefore it is generally agreed that the study of cell adhesion and protein adsorption is a necessity if we wish to analyze the performance of biomedical devices in contact with body fluids or tissues. It is further agreed that surface tension quantities are among the relevant quantities to investigate. Beyond this point, however, there is a bewildering array of postulates and approaches based on intuition and empiricism within a very limited range of observations. Such claims comprise statements to the effect that the critical surface tension of wetting γ_c of a biomaterial should have a certain value, say 25 ergs/cm^2, for that material to be thromboresistant. Another claim is that the interfacial tension between biomaterial and blood should be zero for good biocompatibility. More recently certain postulates have appeared with respect to "polarity" of the candidate biomaterials, in conjunction with an attempted division of interfacial tensions into "dispersion components" and "polar components" of surface tension.

Clearly, all such approaches are empirical, and while one should not object to empirical approaches that solve scientific problems and advance technology, little progress was brought about by these approaches up to now. As all of these make thermodynamic pretentions, by invoking interfacial quantities, it is appropriate to point out their intrinsic fallacies.

2. The Concept of "Critical Surface Tension"

With respect to the critical surface tension γ_c one must first of all state that its introduction by Zisman and his co-workers over thirty years ago presented one of the major advances in surface science [1]. One has to see this on the background of a general aversion and suspicion towards contact angles, which were believed to be best left alone due, in part, to the complicating phenomenon of contact angle hysteresis. Zisman showed that there were relations between surface tensions and contact angles, a fact which nobody before him was able to perceive. It all culminated in the introduction of his concept of γ_c, which proved very fruitful at the time. However, if we now take a critical view of the approach, we have to note that γ_c is defined operationally, but not thermodynamically. Thermodynamically, interfacial tensions are defined as partial derivatives of certain thermodynamic potentials with respect to surface area. The critical surface tension, γ_c, on the other hand is defined as a limiting value of a plot of the cosine function of the contact angle over the liquid surface tension. Thus this quality is not a thermodynamic parameter and definitely not a thermodynamic property and therefore precludes a thermodynamic analysis *ab initio*.

3. The Concept of "Zero Interfacial Tension"

Next, let us consider the postulate that thromboresistance necessitates a low or possibly zero interfacial tension. To be fair, it has to be pointed out that we ourselves introduced the concept long before it was introduced into the area of biomaterials. We did this in connection with the interpretation of the strength of adhesive joints [2]. It was found that under a given set of experimental conditions, there was indeed a correlation between the strength of adhesive joints and the interfacial tension such that maximum strength of the adhesive bond occurred at zero interfacial tension. This empirical argument was introduced after it became apparent that simple thermodynamic models did not correlate with the experimental observations. On this background it would be more reasonable to expect optimum thromboresistance for large values of interfacial tensions, i.e. the opposite of the present postulate.

The concept of "zero interfacial tension" may or may not have relevance to processes of cell and/or protein adhesion. However, the fact remains that if we merely consider individual interfacial tensions then we have left the domain of thermodynamics which requires that the net free energy change for the overall process be considered. Thermodynamics tells us that certain potentials are minimized in natural processes, and these potentials contain several interfacial tensions, so that we cannot expect a single interfacial tension to describe the observations. Unless it can be established that at least the crudest of thermodynamic models fails to predict cellular adhesion, protein adsorption or related processes in thrombus formation, there should be no room for postulates which are intuitive at best and arbitrary at the worst.

4. The Concept of "Polar and Dispersive Forces"

Finally, turning to questions of "polarity" and dispersion and polar components of surface tensions, it has to be realized that consideration of specific intermolecular forces does not arise in thermodynamic theory. The measurable thermodynamic parameters, such as surface tension, "integrate" over all the intermolecular interactions. Whether or not a division of interfacial tensions into dispersion and polar components is justified will be an open question until decisive tests will have been performed. The burden of proof is clearly on the proponents of the concept [3]. Surprisingly, nobody seems to have considered the necessity of such proof, in spite of the fact that the concept can be tested against independent phenomenological observations. One possible testing ground is the behavior of small particles, embedded in a melt, when encountered by the solidification front. A substantial body of such observations was published recently [4,5]. Clearly, in cases where the matrix material consists solely of C and H, the resulting interactions can only be due to dispersion forces, and the dispersion component of the surface tension, if it is a proper parameter at all, would reduce to the total surface tension, which could be considered within a proper thermodynamic free energy balance. The predictions of the particle interaction with the solidification fronts are in substantial conflict with the phenomenological observations, suggestion that the concept of dispersion components and polar components of interfacial tensions is not tenable. More details with respect to this problem will be presented elsewhere.

5. Basic Thermodynamic Considerations

Turning now to thermodynamics itself, we first have to consider what it might contribute to the problem of thromboresistance of biomaterials. One of the main uses of thermodynamics is that it provides an answer to the question of the directionality of natural processes. Thermodynamics tells us that a properly identified thermodynamic potential, in our case the free energy function, will be minimized at equilibrium. This implies that the process under consideration, e.g. platelet adhesion, will be favored if this process causes this function, pragmatically called the free energy F, to decrease. If F increases, the process is not possible.

6. The Thermodynamic Model

In order to make a quantitative prediction, we have to "model" the process. Consider a particle (P), e.g. a cell, initially suspended in a liquid (L), attaching to a solid (S) which is also immersed in this liquid (Figure 1). In the absence of gravity or any other external forces, as well as in the absence of any specific biochemical interactions, i.e. when we consider the cell simply as a deformable polymer particle, the change in the free energy ΔF^{adh} due to the process of cell adhesion is

$$\Delta F^{adh} = \gamma_{PS} - \gamma_{PL} - \gamma_{SL} \quad (1)$$

where γ_{PS} and γ_{PL} are the particle-solid and the particle-liquid interfacial tension, respectively, and γ_{SL} is the solid-liquid interfacial tension. The free energy is the maximum work obtainable from a process, here the adhesion of a cell, and the interfacial tensions are, by definition, the work required to generate the interfacial areas under consideration.

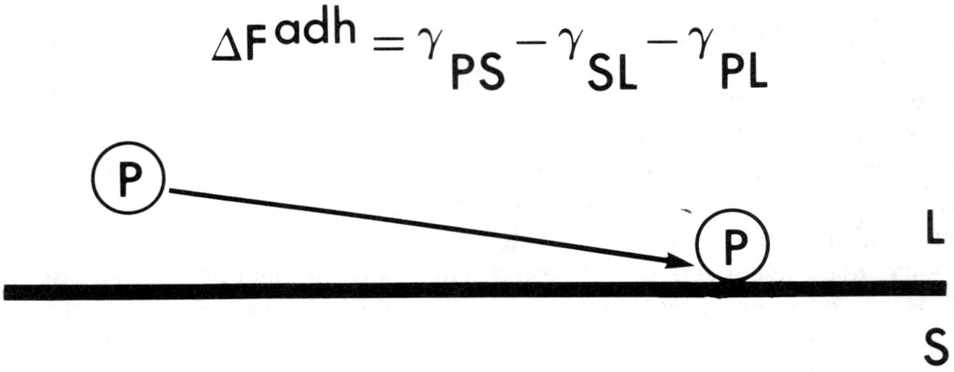

Figure 1. Schematic representation of the process of particle adhesion. P: particle; L: suspending liquid; S: substrate.

7. Critique of the Model

The introduction of this model and its quantitative prediction, *viz.*, eq. (1) is not a panacea. There are probably many reasons why this model might be inconclusive at best and misleading at the worst. Three possible causes for the breakdown of this model are:

1. The model may be an oversimplification geometrically; it considers, *prima facie*, no geometric or conformational changes of the species due to attachment.
2. The driving force for the attachment of the cell or the protein may not be primarily interfacial tensions, but e.g. specific biochemical interactions.
3. The evaluation of the interfacial tensions in equation (1) is not a matter free of controversy, cf. the above discussion.

Thus, there is a variety of reasons why such an approach might lead into difficulties. On the other hand, if we pursue this approach and find patterns of agreement between model predictions and observations which are broad enough to exclude statistical coincidence, we gain insight into the processes which might allow us to choose materials and design procedures which would help minimize or reduce undesired processes. Partial agreement and particularly the pattern in which the model breaks down may provide valuable information, e.g. on specific interactions in the system which are not contained in the model.

8. The Equation of State Approach

The crucial point in the actual application of the model is the problem of obtaining values for the interfacial tensions γ_{PS} and γ_{PL} in equation (1). We shall obtain these data from an equation of state approach [6], which allows the calculation of a surface tension γ_{SV} of a solid (S) in contact with a vapor (V), from a liquid surface tension γ_{LV} and a contact angle θ. The solid-liquid interfacial tension γ_{SL} can then also be calculated. These calculations may either be performed with the aid of computer programs [7] or from tables [8].

Already the simplest considerations of our simple model in conjunction with the equation of state relations predicts patterns of behavior far more complicated than the empirical postulates discussed above might suggest. As an illustration, we show in Figure 2 the free

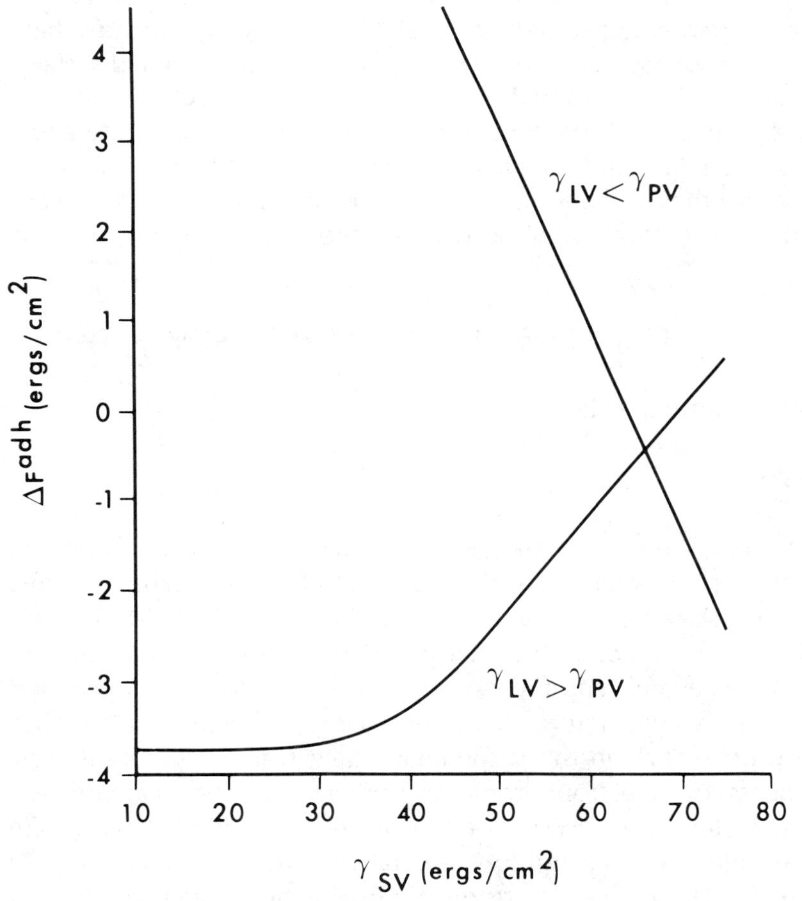

Figure 2. Dependence of the change in free energy on substrate surface tension (γ_{SV}).

energy of adhesion for a cellular species to surfaces of various surface tensions, for the two cases where the liquid surface tension is smaller and larger, respectively, than the surface tension of the cellular species. Obviously, the often asked important question whether cellular adhesion is expected to increase or to decrease with increasing surface tension (increasing hydrophilicity) of the substrate is an incomplete question.

9. Experimental Verification

Finally, we have to consider what type of experiment we shall perform and what features of the results shall be compared with the model. Basically, the latter tells us, through the positive or negative sign of ΔF^{adh}, whether or not adhesion is favored. Two patterns of behavior are conceivable in the case of a correspondence between prediction and observation. It might well be that the behavior of the system follows the thermodynamic prediction in an on-off mode, ie. positive values of ΔF^{adh} would result in the total absence of cellular adhesion and negative values of ΔF^{adh} would cause saturation of the solid surface with cellular species no matter how slightly or strongly negative this value would be. However, experience with such systems suggests that this pattern of behavior does not take place, probably because other unidentified forces are operative. We shall therefore focus our attention on the other alternative, i.e. the comparison of the extent of the reaction with the thermodynamic driving force, or, in other words, the extent of cellular adhesion in comparison to sign and magnitude of the free energy of adhesion ΔF^{adh}. Equation (1) indicates that cell adhesion and protein adsorption to a substrate depends on the suspending liquid surface tension (γ_{LV}), the substrate surface tension (γ_{SV}) and the surface tension of the cell or protein (γ_{PV}). In addition to these thermodynamic considerations, other factors, such as flow rate and electrical charges, may also be expected to affect cell and protein adhesion. For the moment, however, in order to gain insight into the mechanisms governing cell adhesion and protein adsorption, we shall focus our attention on those conditions where the thermodynamic principles are usually applicable.

II. CELL ADHESION AND PROTEIN ADSORPTION

1. Thermodynamic Aspects

a. Cell Adhesion

1. *Granulocytes.* We have investigated in detail the adhesion of human granulocytes to a range of polymer substrates such as polytetrafluoroethylene, nylon-6,6, low density polyethylene, polystyrene, acetal and sulfonated polystyrene [9,10]. Two critical points about these experiments should be noted. 1. The first is that the cells have been isolated and then resuspended, after several centrifugation washes, in a protein-free liquid medium. Thus we are assured that the polymer surfaces are *not* precoated with a protein layer before cell adhesion occurs. (The protein level in the suspending liquid was assayed both before and after the adhesion process by spectrophotometric and immunochemical means). 2. The isolated, washed granulocytes were resuspended in protein-free liquids having different surface tensions(γ_{LV}). The liquid surface tensions γ_{LV} ranged from approximately 73 ergs/cm² to 65 ergs/cm². The liquids used were mixtures of physiological saline with varying amounts of low

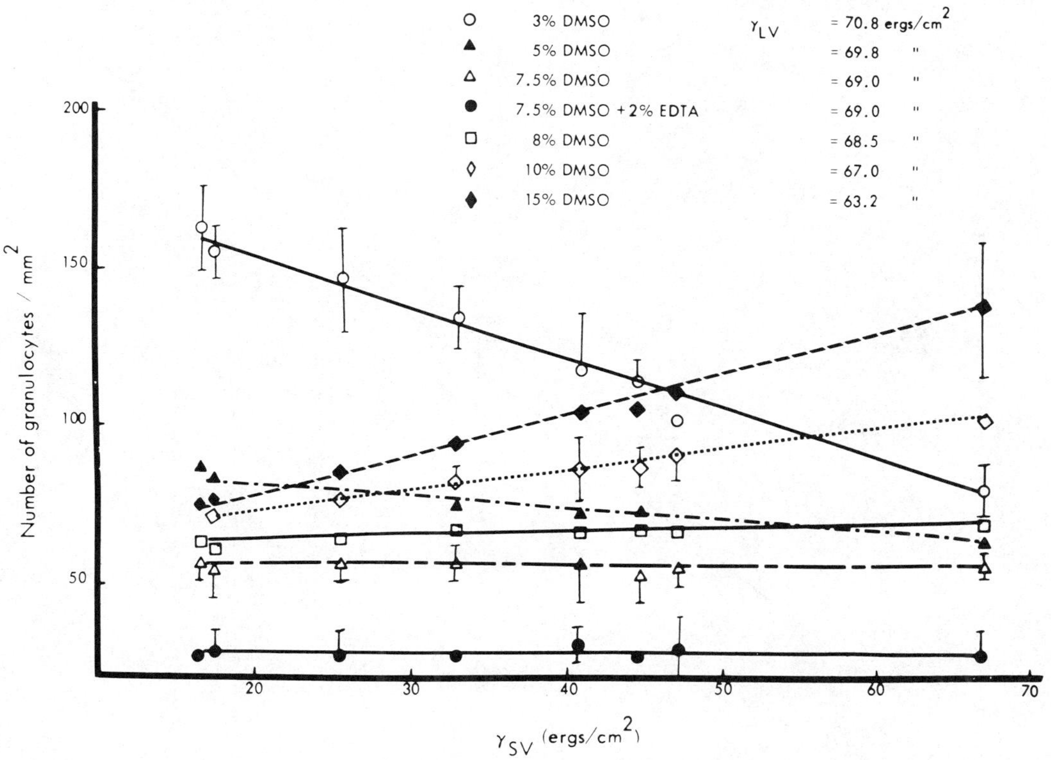

Figure 3. Granulocyte adhesion for the various liquid surface tensions; error limits are 95% confidence. (For graphical reasons, error limits are given only for some cases; the errors are similar in all cases.)

molecular weight substances such as dimethyl sulfoxide (DMSO). Typical results are given in Figure 3. We infer that the extent of granulocyte adhesion depends on the surface tension of the suspending liquid, in qualitative agreement with the predictions of the model, see Figure 2.

It was also shown that the extent of cell adhesion depends on the surface tension of the adhering particles. For this purpose blood cells of the same type *viz.* granulocytes, which had modified surface properties, were used. These physiologically defective cells were obtained from patients with juvenile peridontal disease [11]. In these cases the cell adhesion experiments resulted in plots similar to those shown in Figure 3. That the cell surface tension γ_{PV} for these physiologically deficient cells was different from that of normal granulocytes is easily seen from plots of the type given in Figure 3.

It is apparent from Figure 3 that the pattern of adhesion is different in three regions:

(1) $\gamma_{LV} > \gamma_{PV}$ where adhesion *decreases* with increasing γ_{SV}

(2) $\gamma_{LV} < \gamma_{PV}$ where adhesion *increases* with increasing γ_{SV}

(3) $\gamma_{LV} = \gamma_{PV}$ where the extent of adhesion is independent of γ_{SV}.

These observations are in qualitative accord with the theoretical predictions of the model as depicted in Figure 2.

2. *Platelets.* It is generally agreed that platelets are the first cellular elements which adhere onto a polymer material when contacted with blood. For this reason we have investigated the extent of platelet adhesion to various polymer materials. Platelet adhesion to various substrates was determined for short contact times, between substrate and platelet

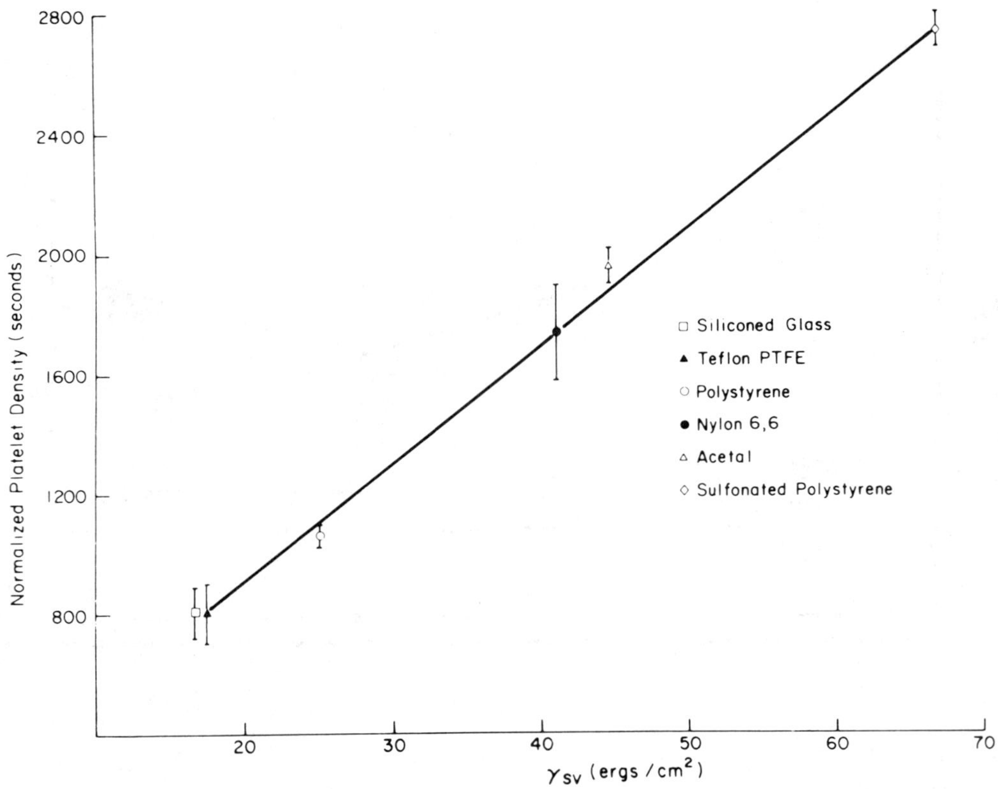

Figure 4. Platelet adhesion to various substrates as a function of γ_{SV}.

suspension, typically 4 minutes. These experiments indicate that the number of platelets adhering per unit surface area always *increases* with increasing surface tension of the substrates, cf. (Figure 4). During the course of these investigations [9-12] we were not able to obtain the analogous situation to granulocyte adhesion where cell adhesion *decreased* with increasing substrate surface tension at high values of γ_{LV}, i.e. in the absence of DMSO. Analysis of the suspending liquid of the platelet preparation revealed that it had a *lower* surface tension than that of the original suspending medium presumably due to the exudation of surface active agents by the adhering platelets. Therefore, in the case of platelets we are dealing *only* with the situation where $\gamma_{LV} < \gamma_{PV}$ and thus the experimentally observed pattern of adhesion is what would be expected from the thermodynamic model.

b. Protein Adsorption

During the course of these platelet adhesion studies we noted [12-14] the effect of various proteins in solution and preadsorbed onto polymer surfaces on platelet adhesion. Fibrinogen and immunoglobulin G promoted platelet adhesion whereas albumin resulted in decreased adhesion to the various polymer surfaces. These effects were presumably due to the prior adsorption of the proteins onto the polymers, thereby modifying the surface properties of the polymer substrates. These observations in conjunction with the generally accepted opinion that protein adsorption preceeds cell adhesion led us to investigate the role of interfacial tensions in determining the extent of adsorption of serum proteins onto various polymers. In particular we were interested in determining to what degree protein adsorption followed the pattern of cell adhesion and whether it could be described by the same thermodynamic principles.

For this purpose a similar strategy to that described for the granulocyte adhesion studies was adopted. Thus we investigated the role of substrate, suspending liquid and protein surface tension on the extent of protein adsorption. Human serum albumin, immunoglobulin G, immunoglobulin M and α_2-macroglobulin were studied [15]. The results of these experiments confirm quantitatively, in all cases, the predictions of the thermodynamic model. The surface tensions of the four serum proteins were determined from contact angle data [15,16] and are summarized in Table 1, from which we infer that the hydrophobicity increases from α_2M via albumin and IgM to IgG.

Table 1. Surface Tensions (γ_{PV} in ergs/cm²) for the Four Serum Proteins Found Via the Contact Angle and Via the Absorptivity Methods.

α_2M, α_2-macroglobulin; HSA, human serum albumin.

Protein	Contact angles in degrees ± S.E. (n = 30)	γ_{PV} derived from the contact angles	γ_{PV} derived from the adsorpitivities (Fig. 20)
α_2M	13.4° ± 0.5°	70.9	71.0
HSA	15.2° ± 0.3°	70.3	70.2
IgM	17.9° ± 0.2°	69.4	69.4
IgG	23.3° ± 0.6°	67.3	67.7

Adsorption isotherms of all four proteins on polytetrafluoroethylene are plotted in Figure 5. As the solvent in this case is a buffer without addition of DMSO, the liquid surface tension is γ_{LV} = 72.9 ergs/cm², i.e. the condition $\gamma_{LV} > \gamma_{PV}$ is satisfied in all cases. As expected from Figure 2, protein adsorption increases with decreasing surface tension of the protein. The adsorption isotherm of four serum proteins to various polymer substrates out of a single liquid surface tension (γ_{LV} = 72.9 ergs/cm²) is given in Figure 6. As expected from the thermodynamic model protein adsorption decreases with increasing substrate surface tension. The results of protein adsorption experiments for various surface tensions of the aqueous solvent as a function of substrate surface tension γ_{SV} are given for immunoglobulin G in Figure 7 and for human serum albumin in Figure 8. The substrates in these experiments are polytetrafluoroethylene, polystyrene, low density polyethylene, acetal, poly(ethyleneterephthalate) and sulfonated polystyrene. The bulk protein concentration was sufficiently high to assure adsorption saturation, i.e. to reach the plateau values of Figure 5.

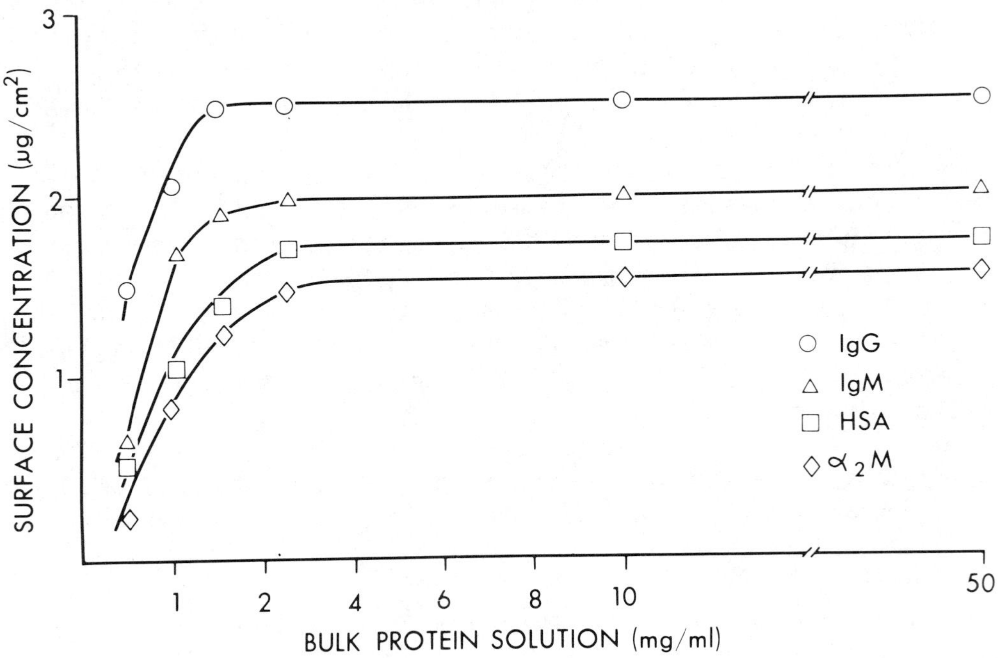

Figure 5. Adsorption isotherm of four serum proteins on poly(tetrafluoroethylene). Proteins were dissolved in a phosphate saline buffer, γ_{LV} = 72.9 ergs/cm²; pH 7.3; ionic strength = 0.15.

The curves in Figures 7 and 8 have a striking similarity with the curves for granulocyte adhesion, cf. Figure 3. It is apparent from Table 1 and these figures that for $\gamma_{LV} > \gamma_{PV}$, and a single γ_{LV}, adsorption of the protein species decreases with increasing substrate surface tension. When $\gamma_{LV} < \gamma_{PV}$, the opposite is true, and when $\gamma_{LV} = \gamma_{PV}$, protein adsorption is independent of γ_{SV}. Thus the extent of adsorption for a single protein species is, as described above, dependent on both γ_{LV} and γ_{SV}, in accord with the thermodynamic model. This is illustrated in Figure 8, where the adsorption of albumin to a range of polymer surfaces under conditions of varying γ_{LV} is depicted.

2. Other Factors

Under physiologically relevant conditions the adhesion/adsorption process is considerably more complex and several additional factors have to be taken into consideration, e.g. electrical interactions and protein-protein displacement.

1. **Electrostatic Interactions.** In any system consisting of condensed phases there are basically two kinds of interactions, i.e. van der Waals and electrical interactions. There is a close correlation between the van der Waals interactions and the thermodynamic free energies as discussed here [17]. Electrostatic interactions, however, may be expected to influence the adhesion phenomena discussed so far. While it is not the purpose of this chapter to treat electrical phenomena in depth, we wish to illustrate how electrical interactions can modify the type of phenomena considered here.

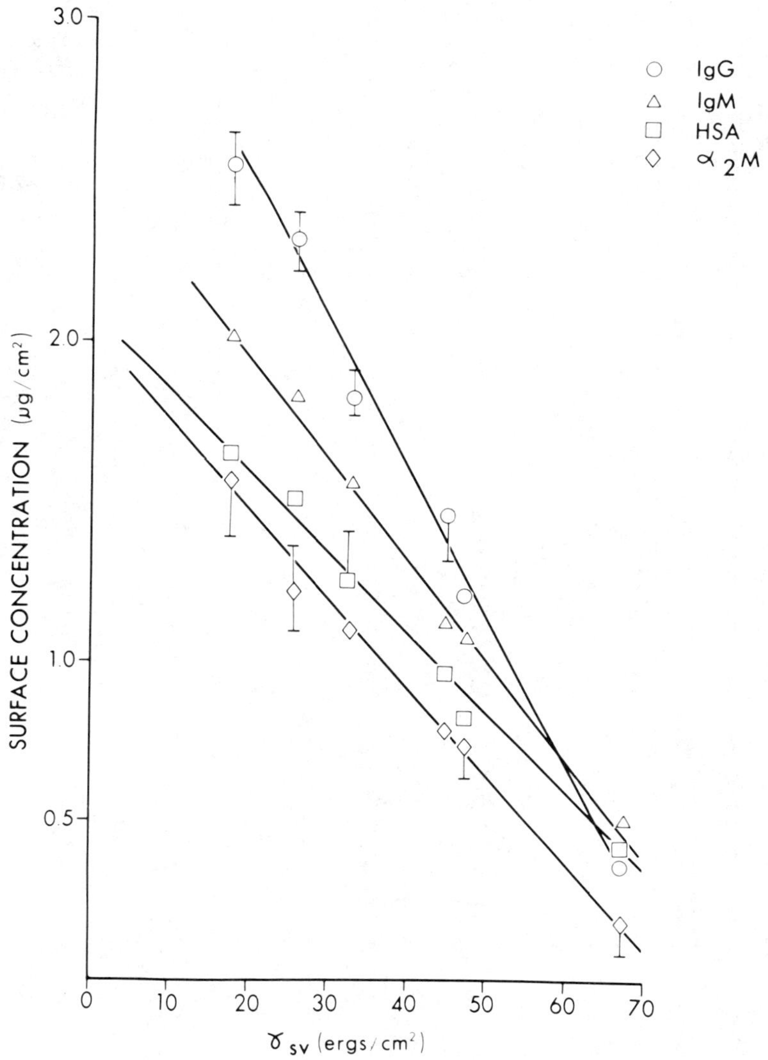

Figure 6. Adsorption of the four serum proteins to the various polymer substrates at a single liquid surface tension (γ_{LV} = 72.9 ergs/cm²).

It can be shown from Equation (1) that when

$\gamma_{LV} = \gamma_{PV}$,

$\Delta F^{adh} = 0$ since $\gamma_{PL} = 0$ and $\gamma_{PS} = \gamma_{SL}$

From Figures 3 and 7 it is apparent that under these conditions a comparatively small but nevertheless positive and constant level of adhesion/adsorption still could be measured. The extent of this adhesion/adsorption is independent of the substrate surface tension γ_{SV} and cannot be ascribed to a van der Waals attraction. In order to clarify whether this level of cell adhesion may be due to electrostatic interactions, we have investigated the effect of ionic strength and plurivalent cationic bridging between the cells and the polymer substrates [11]. The results are summarized in Figure 9. Lowering the ionic strength of the suspending medium (in which $\gamma_{LV} = \gamma_{PV}$, $\Delta F^{adh} = 0$) results in a considerable reduction in the extent of cell adhesion

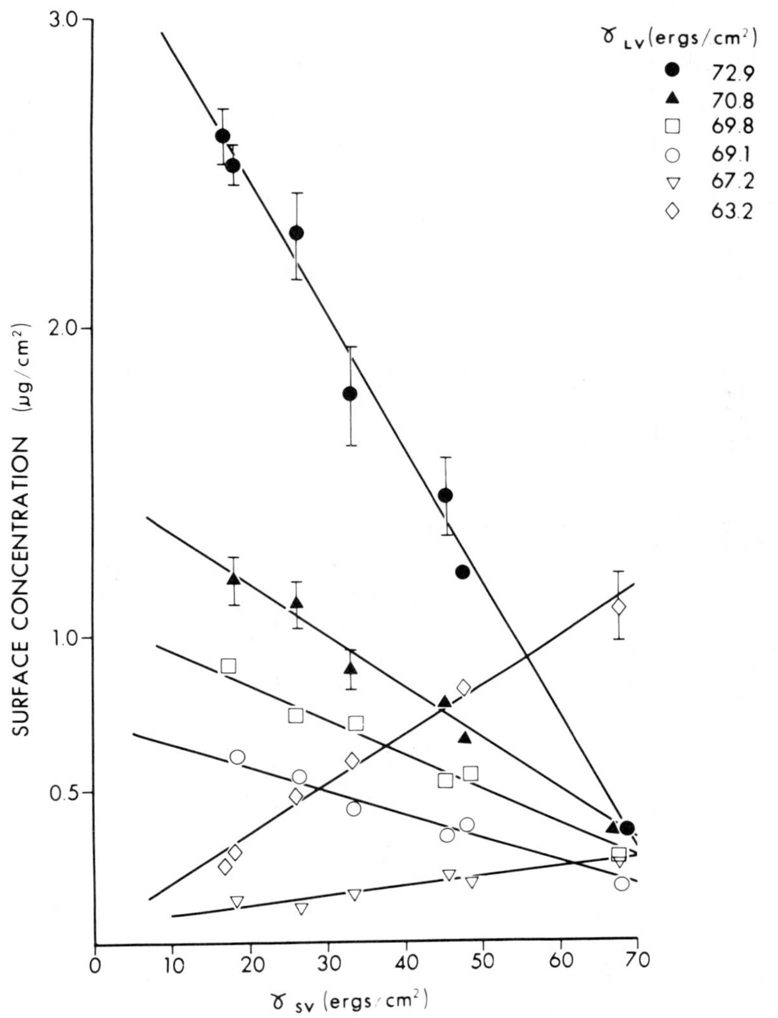

Figure 7. Immunoglobulin G adsorption for the various liquid surface tensions; error limits, 95% confidence.

which may be partially explained in terms of the familiar electrokinetic phenomenon of increasing ζ-potential accompanying a decrease in ionic strength. Thus, at a lower ionic strength, and therefore at a higher ζ-potential, a stronger electrostatic repulsion between the cells and the various surfaces should prevail, which then would indeed give rise to decreased cell attraction and thus less cell adhesion. At the same time further dilution with H_2O not only lowers the overall ionic strength (while increasing the ζ-potential), but also decreases the concentration of plurivalent cations available for ion-bridging, which also leads to a decrease in cell adhesion. It is apparent from Figure 9 that even under conditions of very low ionic strength ($\mu \cong 0$) and $\Delta F^{adh} = 0$, a small and constant number of cells still attach to the various low ζ-potential surfaces. In order to test whether the remaining level of cell adhesion is due to bridging by plurivalent cations, a chelating agent, sodium ethylene diamine tetra-acetic

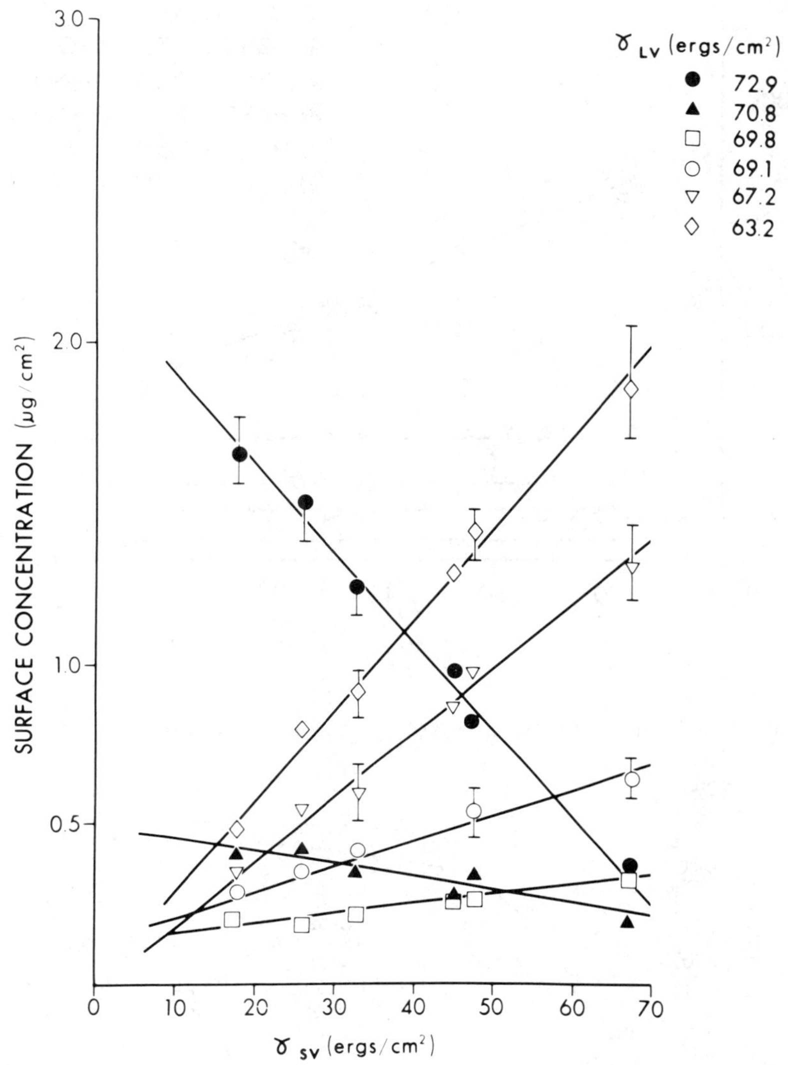

Figure 8. Human serum albumin adsorption for the various liquid surface tensions; error limits 95% confidence.

acid was added to the low ionic strength buffer, again under conditions where $\Delta F = 0$. This effectively reduced the residual cell adhesion to an almost negligible level (Figure 9). Thus it is clear that electrostatic interactions can indeed play a significant role in determining cell adhesion. However when the substrates used are polymer surfaces, the extent of the ionic contribution to cell adhesion tends to be constant for all of the surfaces, resulting in a constant level of adhesion to all of the surfaces.

2. **Kinetics of Platelet Adhesion.** The question of the kinetics of adhesion and adsorption was discussed so far only briefly, in connection with protein adsorption, see Figure 5. The granulocyte and platelet adhesion data discussed so far represent the level of adhesion at more or less arbitrarily chosen times of contact between suspension and substrate. From the

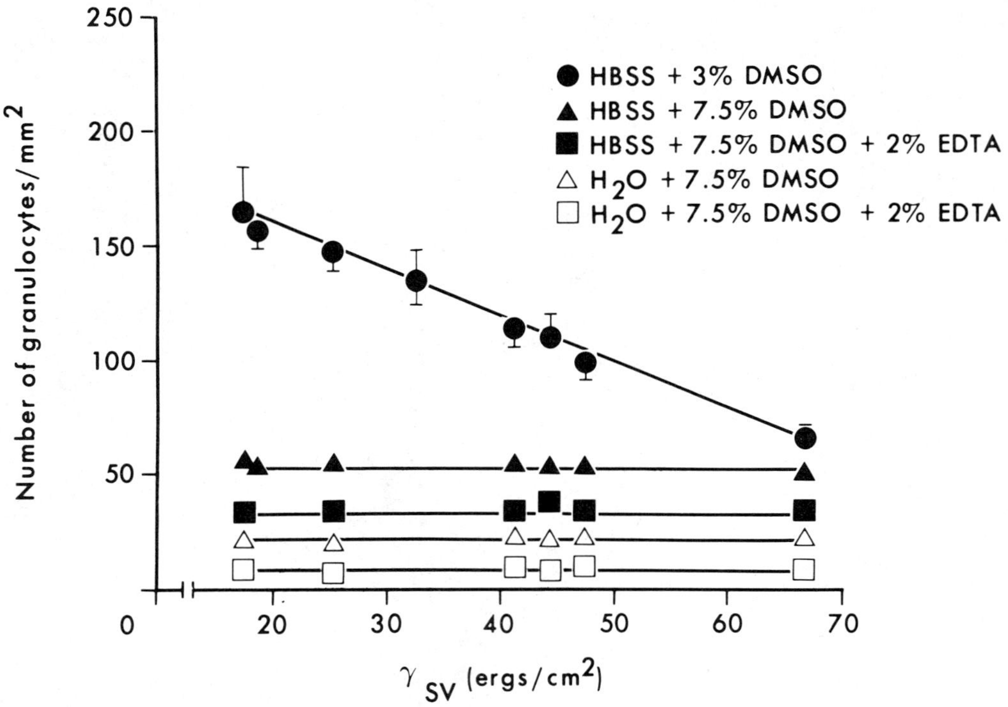

Figure 9. Granulocyte adhesion to various polymer substrates as a function of the liquid composition.

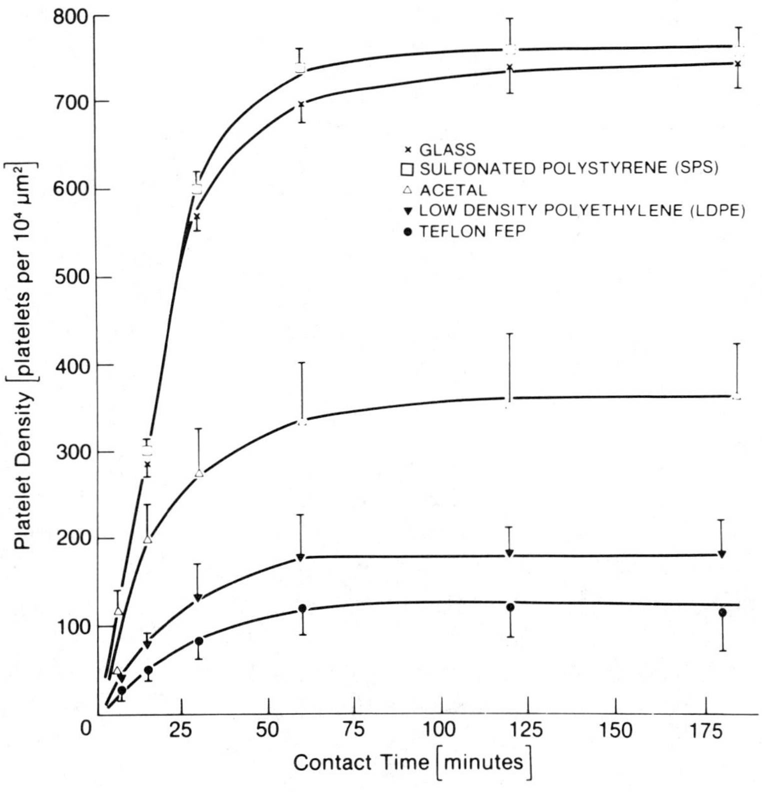

Figure 10. Kinetics of platelet adhesion to various solid substrates. Platelet preparation by gel filtration. Error limits: 95% confidence. Substrates as indicated.

point of view of the thermodynamic model it would be more desirable to compare ΔF^{adh}, i.e. the driving force for the process of cell adhesion, with the equilibrium or saturation level of adhesion. Therefore, kinetics of platelet adhesion was studied [18]. Two types of suspensions of pig platelets were used, one prepared according to Tangen et al. [19] and the other according to Mustard et al. [20]. The results obtained with the preparation according to Tangen et al. are given in Figure 10. The results with the preparation according to Mustard et al. show the same features, except that the saturation levels for glass and sulfonated polystyrene are markedly lower, near 500 platelets per $10^4\ \mu m^2$. It is to be noted that platelet adhesion reaches saturation after approximately one hour and that platelet adhesion increases with increasing surface tension of the substrate.

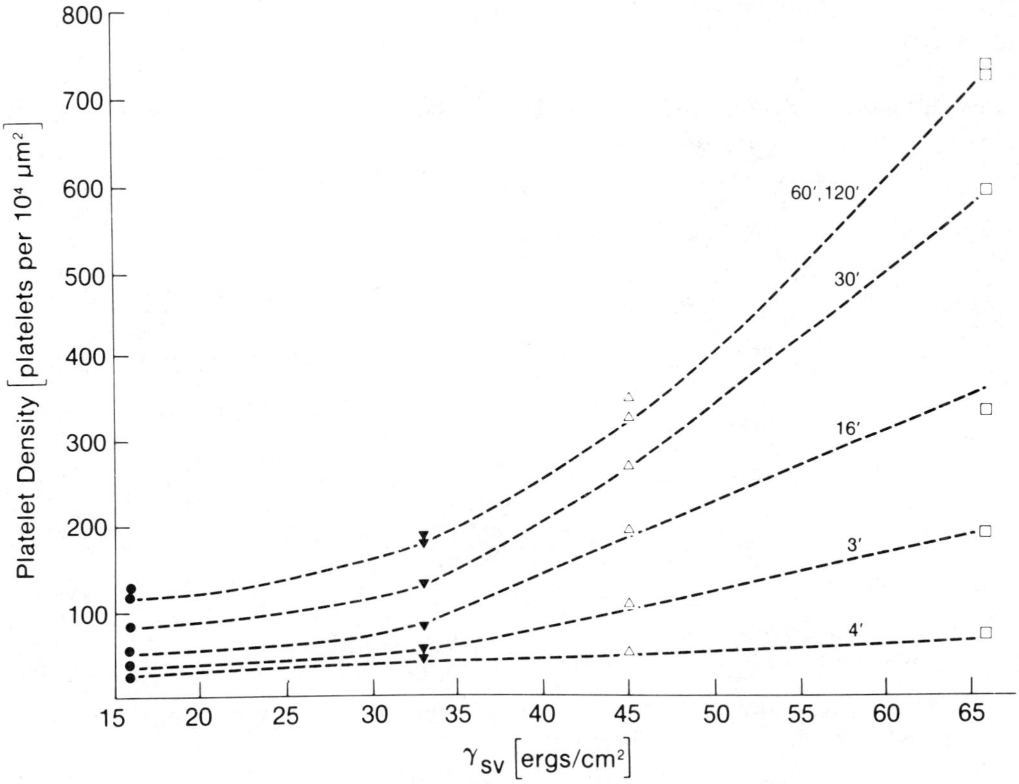

Figure 11. Platelet adhesion as a function of substrate surface tension γ_{SV} for various contact times. Platelet preparation by gel filtration. Symbols as in Figure 10.

Comparing platelet adhesion after 4 minutes as plotted in Figure 4 with the thermodynamic prediction of Figure 2 for $\gamma_{LV} < \gamma_{PV}$, we note that the curvature at low γ_{SV} drawn in Figure 2 is absent in Figure 4. In order to test whether this lack of quantitative agreement between model and experiment may be due to the kinetics of platelet adhesion, the data of Figure 10 were used to replot in Figure 11 platelet adhesion over γ_{SV}, for a number of contact times between platelet suspension and substrate. It is interesting to note that at contact times of 4 minutes the resulting curve is again virtually straight, whereas the curves corresponding to the plateau of Figure 10 show a curvature compatible with the model (Figure 2).

3. **The Effect of Substrate Topography on Cell Adhesion.** An effect of surface roughness on platelet adhesion has been suspected for a long time [21]. In order to test whether these findings imply that platelets adhere more readily to rough than to smooth substrates, standard static adhesion tests were performed with smooth and roughened glass, both in the natural hydrophilic state and after siliconizing [22]. The results show that there is no difference in platelet adhesion between smooth and rough surfaces, neither in the hydrophilic nor the hydrophobic state. In a flow system surface topography plays an important role in cell adhesion [22,23]. This effect is dependent on the nature of the substrate material. In the case of hydrophilic surfaces (high energy surfaces) e.g. sulphonated polystyrene, surface roughness does not influence cell adhesion. In the case of hydrophobic, or low energy surfaces, the effect of surface roughness on cell adhesion under flow conditions is marked [23]. Results relating to the effect of surface topography are summarized in Table 2. The marked effect observed on rough hydrophobic surfaces may be due to the entrapment of air pockets as has been suggested by Ward et al. [21].

Table 2. Platelet Adhesion from Suspension in Laminar Flow Test (Number of Platelets adhering)/(10^4 μm^2 Surface Area).

	a Smooth glass	b Rough glass	c Smooth silane	d Rough silane
Mean	15.4	3.3	8.1	14.9
Number of Tests*	4	4	4	4
Standard Deviation	± 4.9	± 1.8	± 2.9	± 4.1
Significance of difference between T	a and b	a and c	b and c	c and d
	> 99%	> 95%	> 99.8%	> 95%

Concentration: 200,000 Pig Platelets/mm^3; Flow rate: 6ml/min; Duration of flow: 4min.

* In each test, each type of surface was investigated in triplicate; on each individual slide 10 microscopic fields were evaluated.

T The reported statistical confidence level values were determined by performing a comparison test with the means of the various samples. It was assumed that all the data points are independent, normally distributed variables with unknown but equal variances.

III. APPLICATION TO BIOTECHNOLOGICAL PROBLEMS

1. Hydrophobic Chromatography

The thermodynamic model may be applied to preparative procedures for the procurement of large quantities of granulocytes and serum proteins. These procedures require that we initially maximize cell or protein adhesion to a single substrate and subsequently achieve selective desorption of the particles of interest from the matrix material. We have previously described in detail the conditions under which such a desorption can be achieved [24,25]. In brief, what is required is that the surface tension of the suspending buffer is lowered to a surface tension intermediate between that of the protein or cell of interest and the polymeric carrier. Under such conditions the free energy of adhesion will be positive and the van der Waals interactions between the cells/protein and the polymer are rendered repulsive [26]. If at the same time a chelating agent is added to the eluting buffer so as to obviate the effect of electrostatic interactions due to plurivalent cationic bridging then complete desorption of large quantities of proteins or cells from the polymer material ensues. This procedure has been applied to protein purification by means of hydrophobic chromatography [27,28] and to granulocyte elution from nylon fibers [29] as illustrated in Figure 12. This figure indicates the

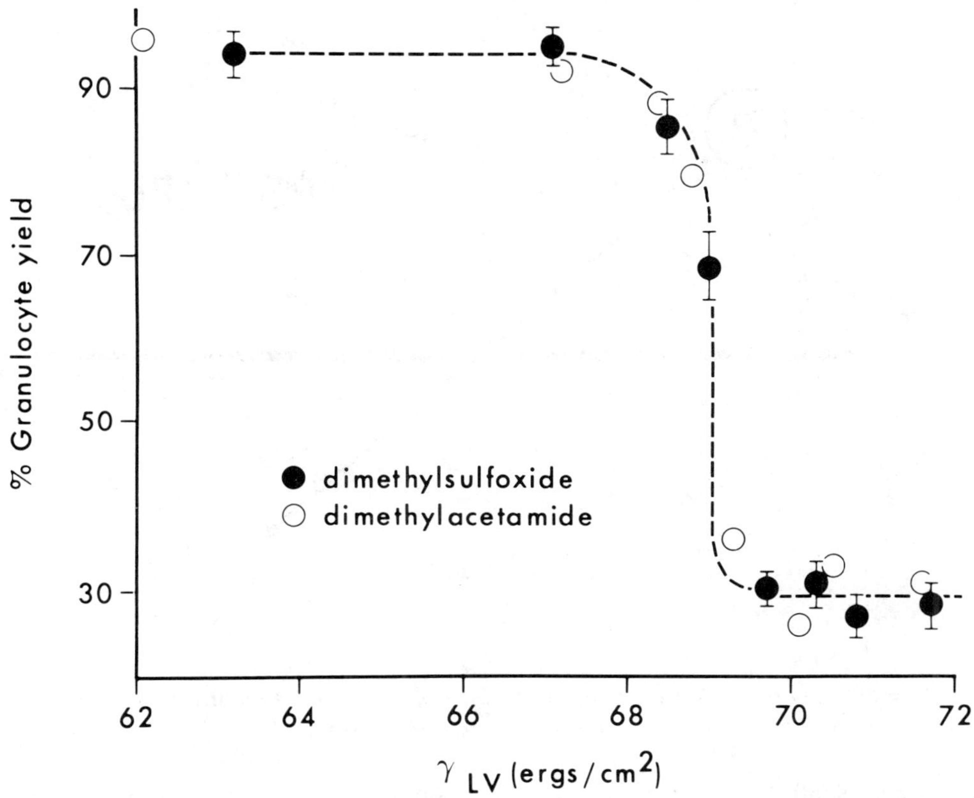

Figure 12. Granulocyte elution from nylon fibers as a function of the surface tension of the eluting buffer.

role of both electrical and van der Waals interactions in determining the overall cell adhesion to a polymer surface. When the electrical interactions between the cell and nylon matrix are overcome (through the incorporation of a chelating agent into the buffer) a cell yield ≅ 30% is achieved. When however the attractive van der Waals interaction is rendered repulsive, through the lowering of the surface tension of the buffer to a value intermediate between that of the adhering cells and the nylon, a three-fold increase in cell yield is achieved. This enhanced yield is reflected by the sharp inflection point in Figure 11 which occurs at the point where $\gamma_{LV} = \gamma_{PV}$.

Complete dissociation of antigen-antibody complexes [30-33] and elution in affinity chromatography [31,34] can also be achieved by the same procedure, with an appropriate increase in pH (instead of chelation) to effect a reversal in electrostatic attraction.

2. Phagocytic Engulfment

The preceding sections suggest that even if one is primarily interested in thromboresistance of biomaterials, it may be of interest not to concentrate on only platelet adhesion and protein adsorption, but to take a wider view and consider, say attachment and detachment of granulocytes as well. Extending this reasoning one step further it may be expected that consideration of the process of ingestion of small particles (e.g. bacteria) by white cells may provide further clues for the understanding of the behavior of platelets [16,35].

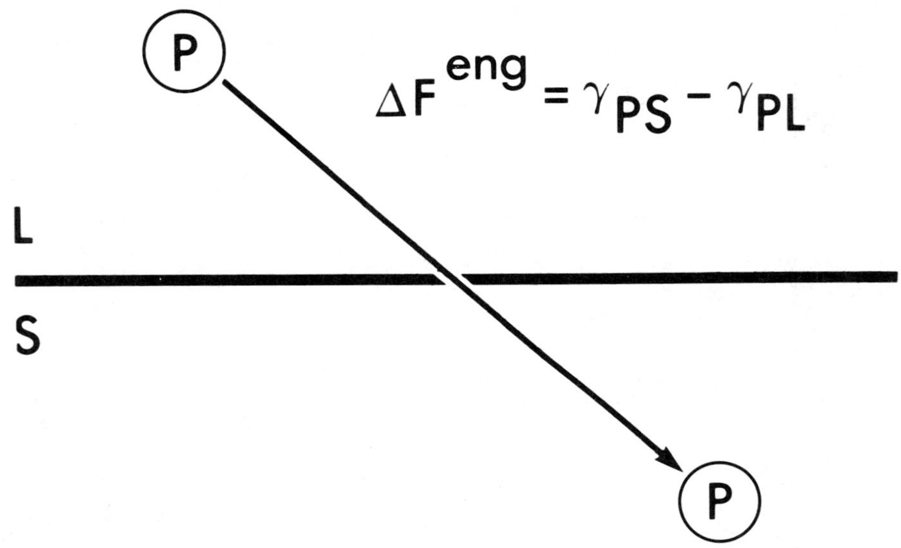

Figure 13. Schematic representation of the process of cell engulfment; P: particle, S: cell membrane, L: suspending liquid.

Thermodynamically the process of ingestion is similar to that of adhesion, see Figure 13. In the process of ingestion, particle-liquid interfacial area is replaced by particle-solid (cell) interfacial tension, and the free energy change for the process is:

$$\Delta F^{adh} = \gamma_{CP} - \gamma_{PL}, \tag{2}$$

where γ_{CP} and γ_{PL} represent cell-particle and particle-liquid interfacial tension, respectively.

This model for particle ingestion corresponds completely to the model of particle adhesion as depicted in Figure 1. The correspondence between adhesion and phagocytic ingestion was recognized as early as 1922 by Fenn [36], who suggested that cell adhesion was simply a case of frustrated phagocytosis. During the course of these studies we have concentrated on the analysis of ingestion mechanism by two kinds of cells, *viz.* granulocytes [37,38] and platelets [39,40]. The particles which were to be ingested consisted of several strains of bacteria having a range of surface tensions. In direct analogy to the cell adhesion and protein adsorption studies described earlier in this chapter, we have investigated the relationship between the extent of particle ingestion and particle surface tension on the one hand and the influence of liquid surface tension on the other hand.

The phagocytic cells (granulocytes or platelets) were obtained following standard isolation procedures. The particles to be ingested comprised of five strains of well characterized bacteria. These bacteria were used either as is or after coating with non-specific antibodies. This opsonization was achieved by incubating the bacteria with a 1% (w/v) solution of human γ-globulin (Cohn's Fraction II) [16]. The bacteria and phagocytic cells, at fixed standard concentrations, were then suspended in buffered liquids having different surface tensions prepared through the admixture of varying amounts of dimethylsulfoxide. Fixed proportions of the cells and bacteria were then mixed and incubated for a standard period, after which the extent of bacterial ingestion was quantitated.

a. Non-specific Ingestion

Engulfment is dependent on the operative interfacial tensions as in cell adhesion and protein adsorption (cf. Figures 3 and 7) and is described by two regimes as is shown in Figure 14:

(1) $\gamma_{LV} > \gamma_{CV}$. Under this condition the more hydrophobic bacteria are ingested to a larger extent than the more hydrophilic ones, i.e. ingestion *decreases* with increasing bacterial surface tension.

(2) $\gamma_{LV} < \gamma_{CV}$. Under this condition the more hydrophilic bacteria are ingested to a greater extent, i.e. ingestion *increases* with increasing bacterial surface tension.

b. Specific Interactions

If however, the bacteria are precoated with antibodies (i.e. opsonized) as described earlier, then a specific receptor-ligand interaction occurs between the opsonized bacteria and the granulocyte membrane. This promotes a specific ingestion process which is essentially independent of the surface tension of the suspending liquid (Figure 15). The extent or level of engulfment of the *opsonized* bacteria increases with increased bacterial hydrophobicity. This however is not due to the surface properties of the opsonized bacteria (all species of opsonized bacteria investigated have a surface tension of $\cong 60 - 70$ ergs/cm^2) but reflects the increased non-specific adsorption of γ-globulin onto the more hydrophobic bacteria during the opsonization procedure [37,41]. Consequently, there will be an increased number of receptor-ligand interactions between the granulocyte membrane and the more hydrophobic bacteria, resulting in an increased ingestion. Conversely, there is a lesser extent of interaction between the granulocyte membrane and the hydrophilic bacteria, to which fewer antibody molecules attach. Interestingly, a quantitative assessment of opsonization indicates that this process follows an identical pattern to protein adsorption onto polymer surfaces described earlier and may be described by the same thermodynamic parameters. Thus granulocyte engulfment of bacteria can be shown to have both specific as well as non-specific components [37,38].

Platelet ingestion of small particles, on the other hand, appears to be entirely non-specific in character and is dependent on the surface tension of interacting components *viz.* bacteria

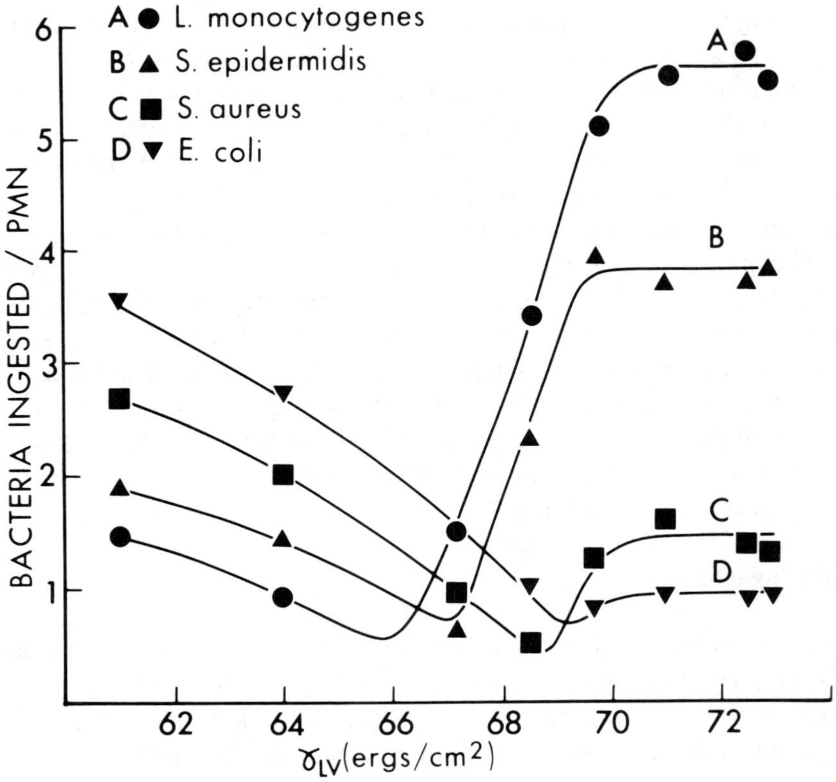

Figure 14. Experimentally determined extent of bacterial ingestion by human granulocytes as a function of the surface tension of the suspending aqueous media.

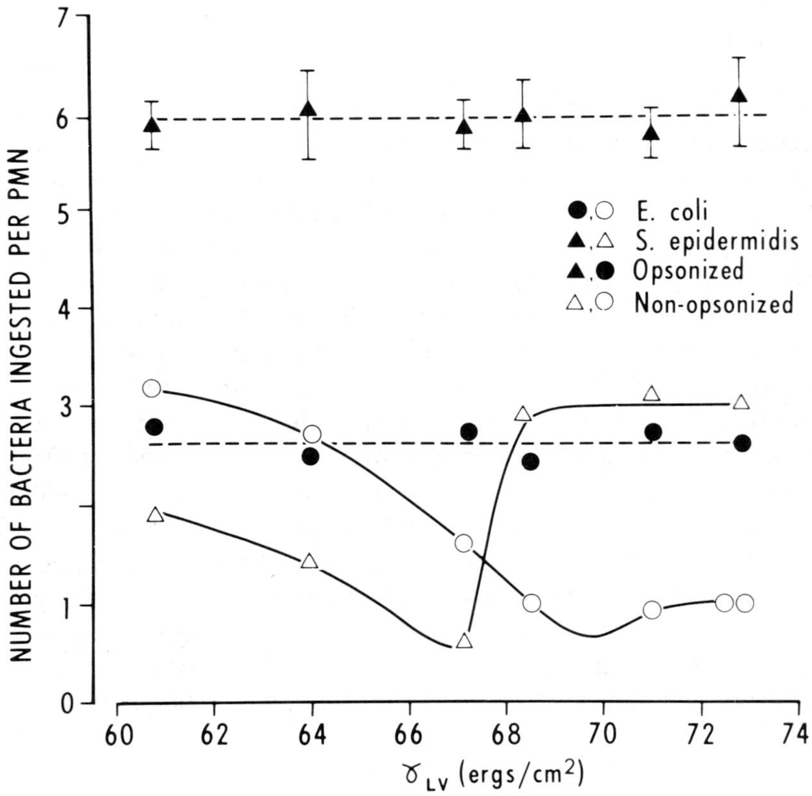

Figure 15. Effect of opsonization of bacteria on ingestion by human granulocytes.

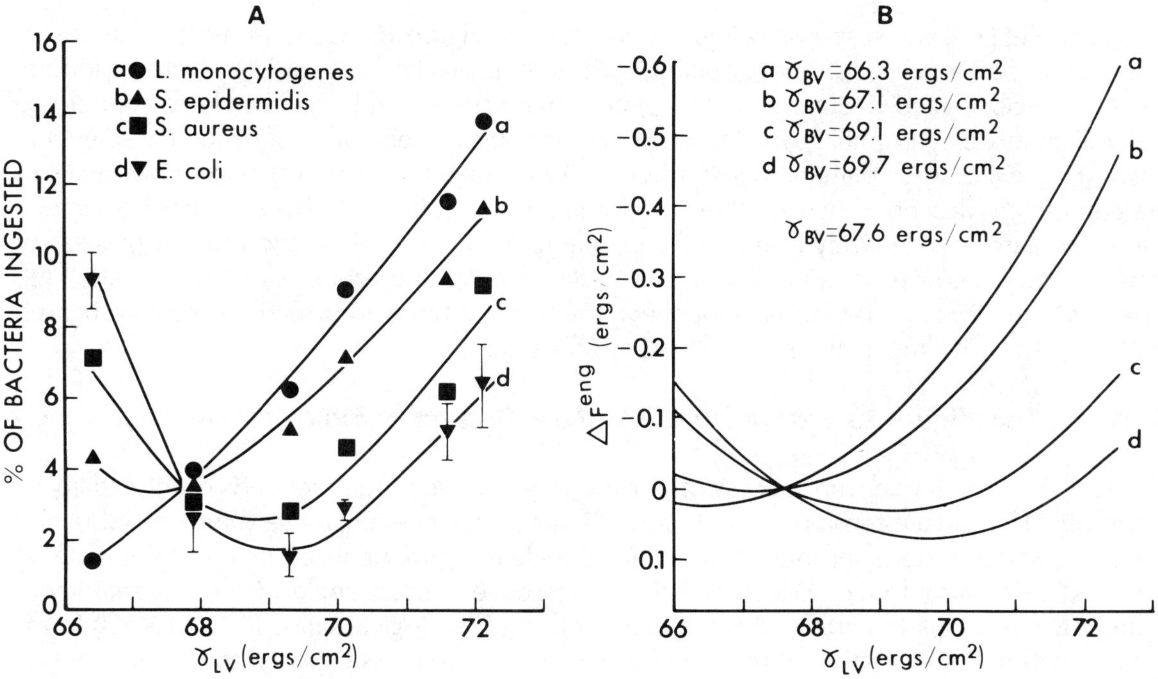

Figure 16. Free energy of engulfment as a function of the surface tension of the suspending aqueous media for the four species of non-opsonized bacteria (B) and the experimentally determined extent of the same bacteria ingested by pig platelets in the same aqueous media (A). Errors are 95% confidence limits.

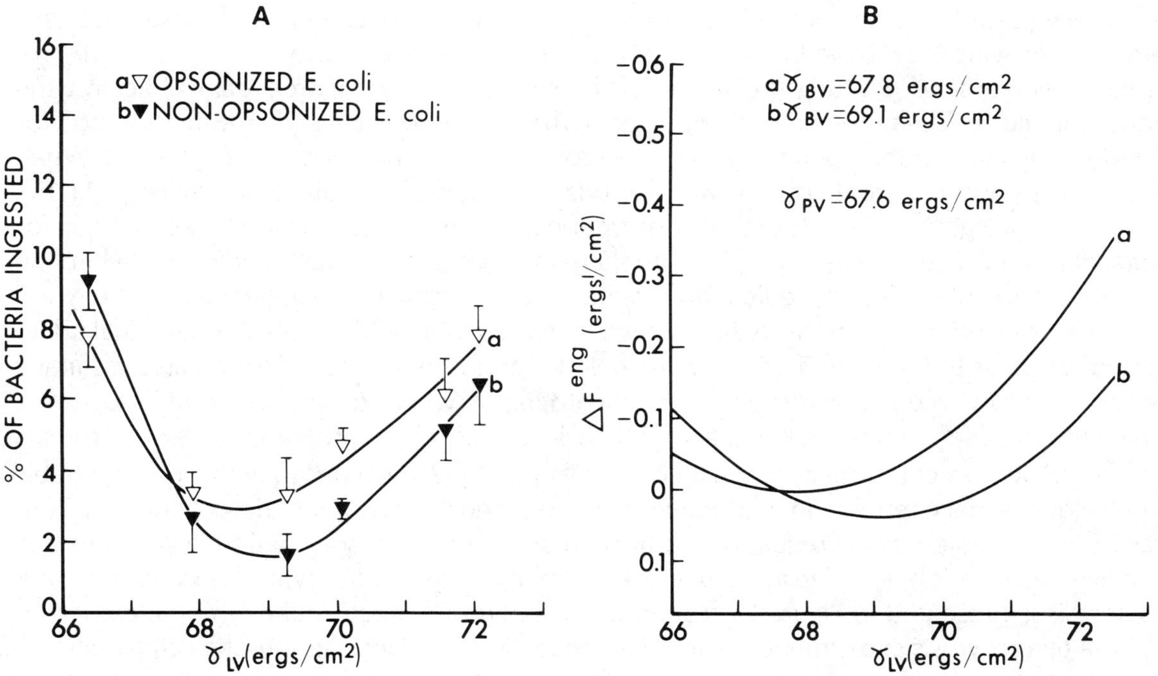

Figure 17. Comparison of the extent of ingestion of opsonized and non-opsonized E. coli. A – experimental, B – theoretical.

(γ_{BV}), platelet (γ_{PV}) and suspending liquid medium (γ_{LV}). (Figure 16). Opsonization (i.e. antibody coating) of the particles does not appear to promote a specific receptor-ligand interaction between the opsonized bacteria and the platelet membrane, and serves only to render the somewhat more hydrophilic particles more hydrophobic thereby promoting increased engulfment (Figure 17). Thus platelet ingestion of both opsonized and non-opsonized bacteria can be completely described by one thermodynamic model [39]; the process of particle engulfment by platelets is entirely non-specific in character, in contradistinction to the process of granulocyte phagocytosis, which has both specific as well as non-specific components [37-39]. The consequences of this difference between the two cell types is currently being investigated with respect to its implications for cell adhesion studies.

3. Novel Techniques to Determine the Surface Tension of Biological Material

As mentioned earlier the success of our thermodynamic model depends on the ability to determine the surface tension of the biological material. Generally these values are obtained *via* an equation of state approach from contact angle measurements on layers of the material exposed to an air interface [15,16,37,39]. The effective contact angle of the material is obtained by measuring the angle which a 10 μl drop of physiological saline (0.15 M NaCl) forms on the material as a function of the time for which the material is exposed to the air. Contact angles of fresh drops of saline are measured at five minute intervals over a period of approximately 1 hr. Initially the contact angle measured is close to zero but then rapidly increases to a plateau value which is generally constant for between 10 and 40 minutes and tends to be characteristic for the material being measured (Figure 18).

The cell adhesion and protein adsorption as well as the studies of bacterial ingestion by granulocytes and platelets not only provide insights into the mechanisms of these processes but also provide novel methods for determining the surface tensions of cellular or proteinaceous materials. Plotting the slopes of the straight lines in Figures 3 and 7 against the various liquid surface tensions (γ_{LV}) employed in these experiments yields another method for the determination of the operative surface tension of the adhering particles. (Figure 19). When the slope is equal to zero then $\gamma_{LV} = \gamma_{PV}$, the surface tension of the adhering particles [9-11,15].

A study of Figure 12 reveals that the desorption method can serve as another technique for obtaining cellular surface tensions [29]. The sharp increase in eluted cell yield occurs when the surface tension of the liquid medium equals the surface tension of the adhering cells, i.e. $\gamma_{LV} = \gamma_{CV}$. The desorption step in these experiments occurred within 30 minutes of the initial adhesion of the cells to the nylon fibers. This technique cannot be employed to obtain the surface tension of proteins e.g. in hydrophobic chromatography where desorption from an octyl- or phenyl-sepharose® matrix takes place [27] or in affinity chromatography [31,34]. Proteins tend to undergo a conformational change on adsorption [42] and consequently a considerably lower liquid surface tension (increased energy) is required to bring about desorption [43]. Thus considerably less energy is required to prevent association (or adsorption) than is required to achieve dissociation (or desorption) [30,44]. An interesting and typical example of this hysteresis is presented in Figure 21 for the dissociation of antigen-antibody complexes.

The phagocytosis experiments, in addition to yielding novel insights into the cell-particle interaction, also provide a means for determining the surface tension of the small ingested particles [37-39]. Consideration of Figures 13 and 16 reveals that in each case a certain minimum ingestion occurs which is characteristic for each of the bacterial species employed. This

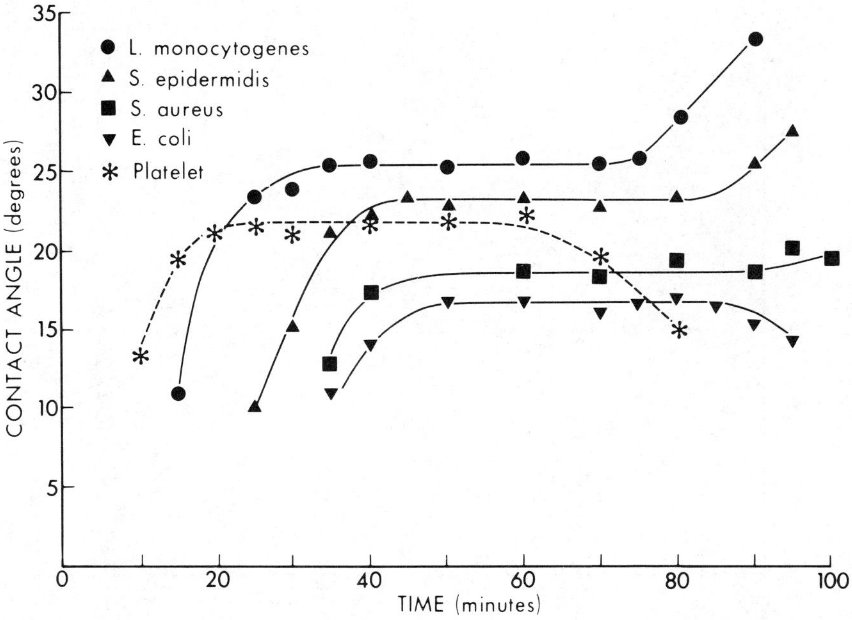

Figure 18. Contact angles of saline of non-opsonized bacteria and platelets as a function of water evaporation from the wet biological substrate, measured in terms of time. Each symbol is the average of ten individual contact angle readings on each of four different drops, at approximately the same time, on one and the same substrate.

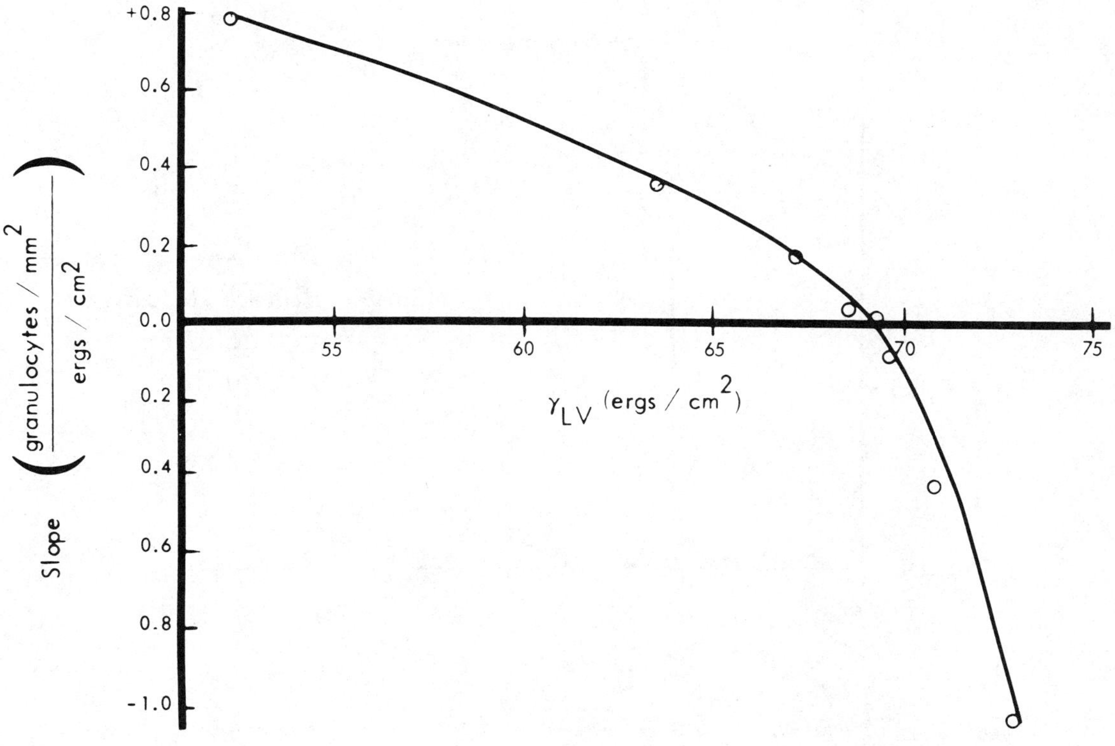

Figure 19. Slopes of the straight line data of Figure 3 versus γ_{LV}. *Slope is zero for* $\gamma_{LV} = \gamma_{PV} = 69.0$ *ergs/cm². The points are computer curve fitted to a second order polynomial and the intercepts taken from that curve fit.*

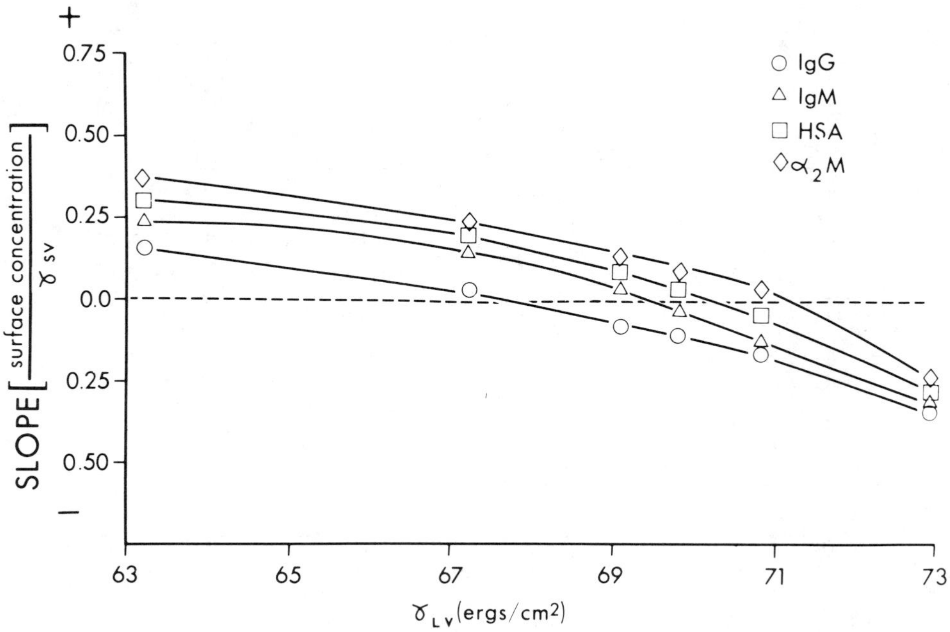

Figure 20. Slopes of straight line data of the type illustrated in Figure 7. The slope is zero for $\gamma_{LV} = \gamma_{PV}$ for each of the four proteins investigated. The points are computer curve fitted to a second order polynomial and intercepts taken from that curve fit.

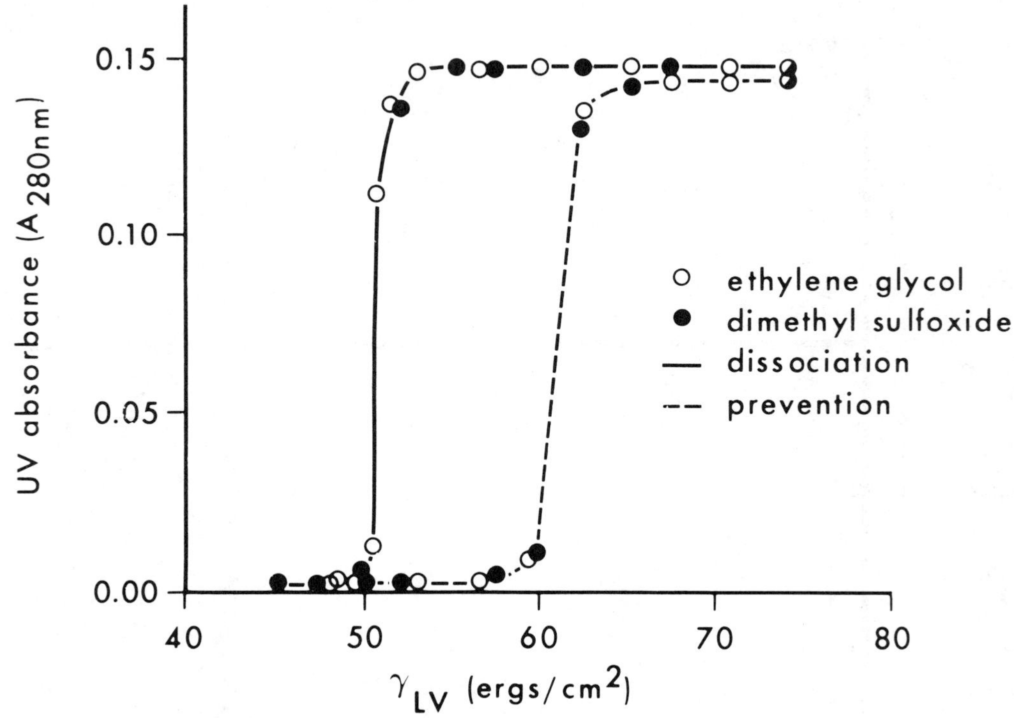

Figure 21. Dissociation and prevention of formation of antigen-antibody (Ag-Ab) precipitates in liquid media of various surface tensions. The Ag-Ab precipitate dissociation curve is indicated by a full line; the curve indicating the prevention of Ag-Ab precipitate formation is drawn as a broken line.

minimum corresponds to a certain liquid surface tension which is equal to the surface tension of the bacteria, i.e. minimum ingestion occurs where $\gamma_{LV} = \gamma_{PV}$. In the case of an entirely non-specific process such as platelet phagocytosis (Figure 16) it is also possible to obtain the surface tension of the phagocytic cells. This is obtained from that point where all the curves have a common intersection which corresponds to a certain liquid surface tension, i.e. the common intersection occurs where $\gamma_{LV} = \gamma_{CV}$. This technique for determining the surface tension of the phagocytic cells cannot be used when the ingestion process has both specific as well as non-specific interactions [37]. Under such circumstances no common point of intersection occurs, cf. Figure 14.

The theoretical concepts of these techniques for obtaining cell and protein surface tensions will be discussed elsewhere together with a description of the freezing front technique [4,5,45] as well as the method involving the determination of the maximum stability of suspensions for obtaining cellular surface tensions [46,47].

IV. CONCLUSIONS

1. The thermodynamic model proposed provides qualitative and quantitative insight into attachment and detachment of cells and proteins to foreign surfaces. Crucial phenomena, such as the reversal of the dependence of cell adhesion when γ_{LV} changes from $\gamma_{LV} > \gamma_{CV}$ to $\gamma_{LV} < \gamma_{CV}$, or the correct prediction of the minimum in bacterial ingestion by platelets as well as granulocytes when $\gamma_{LV} = \gamma_{BV}$ are convincing evidence that the thermodynamic model is a good starting point for the study of such phenomena. This point is further reinforced by the fact that protein adsorption follows the same patterns as cell adhesion.

2. It is quite clear that not all the processes considered follow the prediction of the thermodynamic model. The most striking exception to the general pattern is phagocytic ingestion of opsonized bacteria by granulocytes, which proves to be independent of the surface tension γ_{LV} of the suspending liquid. However, this observation is linked to the known specific antibody-cell membrane receptor interactions. Thus we see that the thermodynamic model may also be used to decide questions of specificity vs non-specificity. As long as the model predicts correctly the behavior of the system, one may conclude that the interactions are probably non-specific.

The question whether *all* deviations from the thermodynamic model are due to specificities is difficult as yet to resolve completely; it will be dealt with in detail elsewhere. There are some indications that certain deviations from the model are not due to specificity but to limitations of the model.

3. Proteins and human blood cells are relatively hydrophilic in their native state. Typically they have surface tensions in the range from 60-70 ergs/cm^2 at room temperature. To our knowledge the only human tissue that is extremely hydrophobic is cartilage [48]. To measure contact angles in air on proteins, cells and tissue with liquids of relatively low surface tension such as methylene iodide, alcohols and various hydrocarbons is virtually meaningless, not only because of physiological reservations, but for thermodynamic reasons as well. Since Zisman's work it has been well known that liquids with surface tensions lower than that of a solid may well form finite contact angles on this solid (autophobicity) [1]. It is attributed to the interaction of liquid molecules with the solid, such as orientation, resulting in a solid surface with a surface tension which is smaller than that of the liquid. But even if it were correct that the response of biological substances to low surface tension liquids were more complicated,

say, in that the finite contact angle reflected properties of lower levels of the membrane, this would still be largely irrelevant because most biological processes occur in aqueous media and not in hydrocarbons.

4. While there may be limitations to the thermodynamic model, no serious shortcomings of the equation of state for interfacial tensions could be found in all the investigations described here. Indeed, it would be difficult to perceive of serious problems with the approach if we consider that, e.g. contact angle measurements on a layer of granulocytes, granulocyte adhesion to various polymeric substrates and granulocyte elution from Nylon fibers all yield the same value of the surface tension of granulocytes. However, as questions of the possibilities and modalities of surface tension determination on biological substances transcend the scope of this article, they will be dealt with in detail elsewhere.

V. ACKNOWLEDGEMENTS

This work was supported in part by the Medical Research Council of Canada (#MT 5462) and the Natural Sciences and Engineering Research Council of Canada (#A 8278). Two of the authors (AWN and DRA) acknowledge support of the Ontario Heart Foundation through fellowships.

REFERENCES

1. Zisman, W.A. Contact angles, wettability and adhesion. Adv. Chem. Ser. *43*, 1-51 (1964).
2. Wolf, K.L., Driedger, O., Neumann, A.W., and Sell, P.J. On adhesion, contact angles and interfacial tension. DECHEMA Monographs *51*, 31-44 (1964).
3. Fowkes, F.M. Introductory lecture: Attractive forces at solid-liquid interfaces. In: *Wetting*. Soc. Chem. Industry (U.K.) Monograph *25*, 3-30 (1967).
4. Omenyi, S.N., Neumann, A.W., and van Oss, C.J. Attraction and repulsion by solidification fronts. I. Thermodynamic effects. J. Appl. Phys. *52*, 789-795 (1981).
5. Omenyi, S.N., Smith, R.P., and Neumann, A.W. Determination of solid/melt interfacial tensions and of contact angles of small particles from the critical velocity of engulfing. J. Colloid Interface Sci. *75*, 117-125 (1980).
6. Neumann, A.W., Good, R.J., Hope, C.J., and Sejpal, M. An equation of state approach to determine surface tensions of low energy solids from contact angles. J. Colloid Interface Sci. *49*, 291-304 (1974).
7. Omenyi, S.N. Attraction and repulsion of particles by solidifying melts. Ph.D. Thesis, University of Toronto, 1978.
8. Neumann, A.W., Absolom, D.R., Francis, D.W., and van Oss, C.J. Conversion tables of contact angles to surface tensions. Separ. Purif. Methods *9*, 69-163 (1980).
9. Absolom, D.R., Neumann, A.W., Zingg, W., and van Oss, C.J. Thermodynamic studies of cellular adhesion. ASAIO Trans. *25*, 152-156 (1979).
10. Neumann, A.W., Absolom, D.R., Zingg, W., and van Oss, C.J. Surface thermodynamics of leukocyte and platelet adhesion to polymer surfaces. Cell Biophysics *1*, 79-92 (1979).
11. Absolom, D.R., van Oss, C.J., Genco, R.J., Francis, D.W., and Neumann, A.W. Surface thermodynamics of normal and pathological human granulocytes. Cell Biophysics *2*, 113-126 (1980).
12. Neumann, A.W., Moscarello, M.A., Zingg, W., Hum, O.S., and Chang, S.K. Platelet adhesion from human blood to bare and protein coated polymer surfaces. J. Polymer Sci. Polym. Symp. *66*, 391-398 (1979).
13. Newmann, A.W., Zingg, W., and Hum, O.S. Adhesion of platelets to smooth solid surfaces. Biomed. Tech. *20*, 57-59 (1975).

14. Hum, O.S., Neumann, A.W., and Zingg, W. Platelet interaction with smooth solid substrates determined by an open static method. Thromb. Res. *7*, 461-470 (1975).
15. van Oss, C.J., Absolom, D.R., Neumann, A.W., and Zingg, W. Determination of the surface tension of proteins. I. Surface tension of native serum proteins in aqueous media. Biochim. Biophys. Acta *670*, 64-73 (1981).
16. van Oss, C.J., Gillman, C.F., and Neumann, A.W. *Phagocytic Engulfment and Cell Adhesiveness.* Marcel Dekker, N.Y. (1975).
17. Neumann, A.W., van Oss, C.J., and Zingg, W. Thermodynamic aspects of phagocytosis and thrombosis. Klin. Wochenschr. *53*, 1021-1027 (1975).
18. Neumann, A.W., Hum, O.S., Francis, D.W., Zingg, W., and van Oss, C.J. Kinetic and thermodynamic aspects of platelet adhesion from suspension to various substrates. J. Biomed. Mater. Res. *14*, 499-509 (1980).
19. Tangen, O., and Berman, H.J. Gel filtration of blood platelets. A methodological report. Adv. Exp. Med. Biol. *34*, 235-243 (1972).
20. Mustard, J.F., Perry, D.W., Ardlie, N.G., and Packham, M.A. Preparation of suspensions of washed platelets from humans. Brit. J. Haematol. *22*, 193-204 (1972).
21. Ward, C.A., Ruegsegger, B., Stanga, D., Zingg, W., and Herbert, M.A. Relation of proteins, platelets and gas nuclei in adhesion to a synthetic material. Am. J. Physiol. *233*, 100-105 (1977).
22. Zingg, W., Neumann, A.W., Strong, A.B., Hum, O.S., and Absolom, D.R. Platelet adhesion to smooth and rough hydrophobic and hydrophilic surfaces under conditions of static exposure and laminar flow. Biomaterials *2*, 156-158 (1981).
23. Strong, A.B., Absolom, D.R., and Zingg, W. A new flow cell for platelet adhesion studies. Annals Biomed. Eng. (In press).
24. van Oss, C.J., Absolom, D.R., and Neumann, A.W. Applications of net repulsive van der Waals forces between different particles, macromolecules or cells in liquid. Colloids and Surfaces *1*, 45-56 (1980).
25. Neumann, A.W., Omenyi, S.N., and van Oss, C.J. Attraction and repulsion of solid particles by solidification fronts. III. van der Waals interactions. J. Phys. Chem. *86*, 1267-1270, (1982).
26. van Oss, C.J., Neumann, A.W., Good, R.J., and Absolom, D.R. The influence of extremely small attractive as well as repulsive van der Waals forces on cell interactions. Adv. Chem. Ser. *188*, 107-114 (1980).
27. van Oss, C.J., Absolom, D.R., and Neumann, A.W. Repulsive van der Waals forces. II. The mechanisms of hydrophobic chromatography. Separ. Sci. Technol. *14*, 305-317 (1979).
28. van Oss, C.J., Neumann, A.W., Omenyi, S.N., and Absolom, D.R. Repulsive van der Waals interactions: Their role in various separation methods. Separ. Purif. Meth. *7*, 245-271 (1979).
29. Absolom, D.R., van Oss, C.J., and Neumann, A.W. Elution of human granulocytes from nylon fibers by means of repulsive van der Waals forces. Transfusion *21*, 642-657 (1981).
30. van Oss, C.J., Absolom, D.R., Grossberg, A.L., and Neumann, A.W. Repulsive van der Waals forces. I. Complete dissociation of antigen-antibody complexes by means of negative van der Waals forces. Imm. Comm. *8*, 11-29 (1979).
31. Absolom, D.R. Affinity chromatography. Separ. Purif. Methods *10*, 239-286 (1981).
32. van Oss, C.J., Beckers, D., Engelfriet, C.P., Absolom, D.R., and Neumann, A.W. Elution of blood group antibodies. I. Red cell antibodies. Vox Sanguis *40*, 367-371 (1981).
33. Hovanec, D.L., Absolom, D.R., van Oss, C.J., and Gorzynski, E.A. The relationship to coagglutination of immunoglobulin class dissociated from *E. coli*- antibody complexes. J. Clin. Microbiol. *12*, 608-610 (1980).
34. van Oss, C.J., Absolom, D.R., and Neumann, A.W. Role of attractive and repulsive van der Waals forces in affinity and hydrophobic chromatography. In: *Affinity Chromatography and Related Methods.* T.B. Gribnau, J. Visser and R.J. Nirvard (Eds.), Elsevier, Amsterdam, 1982.

35. Zingg, W., Absolom, D.R., Francis, D.W., van Oss, C.J., and Neumann, A.W. Platelet phagocytosis as a model for platelet adhesion. Proc. 2nd European Conference on Biomaterials, Goteberg, Sweden (1981).
36. Fenn, W.O. The adhesiveness of leukocytes to solid surfaces. J. Gen. Physiol. *5,* 143-148 (1922).
37. Absolom, D.R., van Oss, C.J., Zingg, W., and Neumann, A.W. Phagocytosis as a surface phenomenon. VI. Opsonization by a specific adsorption of IgG as a function of bacterial hydrophobicity. J. Reticuloendothelial Soc. *31,* 59-70 (1982).
38. Neumann, A.W., Absolom, D.R., Zingg, W., Francis, D.W., and van Oss, C.J. Thermodynamic aspects of granulocyte phagocytosis. (Submitted for publication).
39. Absolom, D.R., Francis, D.W., Zingg, W., van Oss, C.J., and Neumann, A.W. Platelet phagocytosis of bacteria: Surface thermodynamic aspects. J. Colloid Interface Sci. *85,* 168-177 (1982).
40. Zingg, W., Absolom, D.R., Francis, D.W., van Oss, C.J., and Neumann, A.W. Platelet phagocytosis of bacteria. (Submitted for publication).
41. van Oss, C.J., Absolom, D.R., and Neumann, A.W. Phagocytosis as a surface phenomenon. In: *the Reticuloendothelial System.* Eds. H. Friedman, M.R. Escobar and S.M. Reichert. Plenum Press, N.Y. Vol. 4 (in press).
42. Absolom, D.R., van Oss, C.J., Zingg, W., and Neumann, A.W. Determination of surface tensions of proteins. II: Surface tension of serum albumin, altered at the protein-air interface. Biochim. Biophys. Acta. *670,* 74-78, 1981.
43. de Bruin, H.G., van Oss, C.J., and Absolom, D.R. Desorption of protein from polystyrene latex particles. J. Colloid Interface Sci. *76,* 254-255 (1980).
44. Absolom, D.R., van Oss, C.J., and Neumann, A.W. Repulsive van der Waals forces. III. Complete dissociation of dextran-antidextran immune complexes. (In preparation).
45. Spelt, J.K., Absolom, D.R., Zingg, W., van Oss, C.J., and Neumann, A.W. Surface tension determination of biological cells by means of the freezing front technique. Cell Biophysics. (In press).
46. Omenyi, S.N., Snyder, R.S., van Oss, C.J. Absolom, D.R., and Neumann, A.W. Effects of zero van der Waals and zero electrostatic forces on droplet sedimentation. J. Colloid Interface Sci. *81,* 402-409 (1981).
47. Omenyi, S.N., Snyder, R.S., Absolom, D.R., van Oss, C.J., and Neumann, A.W. Enhanced erythrocyte suspension layer stability achieved by surface tension lowering additives. J. Dispersion Sci. and Technol. (In press).
48. Chappuis, J., Sherman, I., and Neumann, A.W. (Submitted for publication).

Chapter 4

Protein/Surface Interaction

Leo Vroman, Ph.D.
Interface Laboratory
Veterans Administration Medical Center
Brooklyn, New York 11209

ABSTRACT

On many materials, rapid adsorption of specific plasma proteins out of blood is followed by activation of enzymes and further interactions with proteins at or near the surface. On surfaces that activate clotting, plasma deposits fibrinogen and replaces it with factors that initiate coagulation; in blood, platelets adhere preferentially where they still find fibrinogen. Similar interactions involving globulins may govern the deposition of certain white blood cells. Events are found to be affected by narrow spaces and by flow.

If we live in a world of causal relationships, then the very first events that occur when blood touches a new surface must be the cause – or at least part of the causes – of all later events. Biologically oriented scientists may conveniently believe that man-made materials have a very limited repertoire of causes to affect blood with, while engineers may prefer to think that the blood has a very limited repertoire of responses to a great variety of surface effects. This latter error is at present the one that concerns me most. If we continue the evaluation of vascular implants in terms of a single value: the amount of thrombus produced by the device, then we regard all thrombi identical but for size. Such blurred vision ignores that no two thrombi are alike, and that preventing the formation of one thrombus may not be like preventing any other thrombus, no two being provoked by exactly the same pattern of events in space and time. Even a device produced with a perfectly homogeneous surface must go through an unpredictable landscape of adventures during and immediately after its implantation in the bloodstream. On dry material, the air/blood/material interface wil advance at a finite speed and create a gradient of events, or deposit a protein film formed at the interface, onto the solid wherever it is hydrophobic.

It is generally agreed now that adsorption of specific proteins has specific consequences. Progressing from a description of early molecular events to later visible ones, our understanding should be able to grow proportionally. In an effort to do so [1], large gaps became clearly noticeable in our knowledge of areas between a) material surface properties and protein adsorption (perhaps in part because it is preceded by adsorption of ions), b) adsorption of protein and adhesion of platelets (perhaps because specific receptors on the platelets for the adsorbed protein are only now beginning to be studied), c) protein adsorption and granulocyte adhesion (a process at least as complex as that of platelet adhesion), d) protein adhesion and fibrin formation. The latter relationship has proved to be quite involved only because it has been studied more, and it has been studied because it seems deceptively simple to the beginner: plasma forms fibrin in man-made containers and not in our circulation. Also, nature has provided us with patients who congenitally lack various clotting factors. Many of these factors would not have been discovered if they had not been totally absent in, e.g., hemophiliacs. The ability of normal plasma, and more recently, of purified proteins prepared from normal plasma, to correct specific deficiencies has led to a sharpened image of molecular events that lead to clotting. It has become clear to us [2-4] as well as to others [5,6], however, that the behavior of any protein species present in plasma cannot be predicted from the behavior of the purified protein. For example, by observing the adsorption of matter out of normal intact plasma onto oxidized silicon crystal slices in the ellipsometer [3], and identifying the adsorbed material by subsequent exposure to various antisera, we found that the plasma will first deposit fibrinogen and then remove it again. In undiluted normal plasma this process may take less than one minute on the oxidized silicon surface [2], and somewhat longer on glass [7]. The removal of fibrinogen probably does not involve true proteolysis [4] but removability of purified proteins in general [5] and of fibrinogen specifically [6] may well be affected by the nature of the substrate. We found that it is mainly High Molecular Weight Kininogen (HMWK) that replaces the adsorbed fibrinogen: a patient lacking kininogens deposited fibrinogen rapidly but removed it quite slowly from glass [7] and, in the ellipsometer, from oxidized silicon slices.

The timing of fibrinogen deposition, and especially of its removal from man-made surfaces by the blood may be clinically crucial: in vitro at least, human platelets adhere preferentially where fibrinogen is adsorbed [17,18], for example on many hydrophobic solids. On many of these, fibrinogen is deposited and remains for platelets to adhere to. Platelets suspended in fibrinogen-free medium will adhere to glass that had been exposed to intact plasma for no more than a few seconds; they will not adhere where plasma had resided on the glass for several minutes [6,17].

The deposition of HMWK onto a surface is part of the process of activation of clotting; HMWK acts as a carrier of clotting factor XI and of prekallikrein, transporting them to the surface [8] where they react with factor XII. The light chain of HMWK is involved in this transport [9]; the molecule must be intact to function [10] and is needed to render prekallikrein active in the intrinsic clotting system [11]. The interaction of adsorbed factor XII, with factor XI and prekallikrein (perhaps taken specifically to factor XII by their carrier HMWK) may be further complicated by the ability of factor XII to activate itself at the interface [12,13]. The preferential adsorption of HMWK onto at least certain surfaces [14] may in itself suffice to remove preadsorbed fibrinogen; if so, activation of plasminogen to proteolytically active plasmin by surface activation of factor XII [15,16] and/or by its autoactivation may not be involved in this removal of fibrinogen film.

Possibly, factor XII displaces fibrinogen on activating surfaces. When factor XII is activated by its contact with a solid, some of its molecules will merely change their shape but will remain adsorbed in the active state. Often referred to as α-HF$_a$, the adhering form is able to activate factor XI and to cleave prekallikrein yielding kallikrein. Other molecules of adsorbed factor XII will release an active fragment, β-HF$_a$, which will not be able to activate factor XI but will split prekallikrein [19]. Kallikrein is also released into the bulk plasma and it in turn will cleave HMWK [20]. Probably, where activation is a result of enzymatic cleavage this process may continue and destroy the activity it has created. If so, we must expect some consumption of clotting factors involved in this early phase of coagulation. We did indeed find that activated plasma deposits fibrinogen but has lost its ability to remove fibrinogen from activating substrates [3,4]. On glass, platelets resuspended in their original intact versus activated plasma will adhere more to glass by several orders of magnitude if suspended in the activated plasma aliquot.

The finding that thrombosis rather than intravascular clotting is enhanced by activation of the intrinsic system [21] may be explained on this basis. Any resemblance between in vitro and in vivo effects must always be suspected however: it may be coincidental. Whether or not it is true that a grossly averaged property of the endothelium – such as it wettability [22] or its surface charge [23] – under certain conditions parallels it non-thrombogenicity, the blood nearsightedly viewing only the minute surface detail that it is touching, may be blind to the crude statistical mean that is all we see of these details.

On the other hand, I do believe that certain physical conditions may affect in vitro phenomena similarly on a relatively wide range of materials, allowing us to suspect that these conditions may have a similar influence on the mosaic of properties presented to the blood by the endothelium in vivo.

There are two such physical conditions that have concerned us recently: the presence of narrow spaces, and that of flow. Thus far, our most recent data can be summarized as follows. On glass (as well as on oxidized silicon and on anodized tantalum), wherever spaces are between about 0.6 and 20 micrometers wide, the plasma penetrating such areas will contain enough fibrinogen to coat the surrounding glass, but will not contain enough HMWK to remove this fibrinogen deposit. Within this narrow "residual fibrinogen" zone, platelets entering wherever space allows them,will adhere to this residual fibrinogen film. We demonstrated these phenomena by allowing plasma, platelet-rich plasma or whole blood to enter a space left between a glass slide and a convex lens of known curvature resting on that slide. Within a space of less than .6 microns wide, plasma was unable to deposit fibrinogen, and under certain conditions deposited albumin instead [24]. In effect then, a narrow space may act like a diluent, allowing a protein with higher concentration but lower affinity for the surface, to be adsorbed. When plasma was diluted with a buffer solution, it did indeed leave a larger circle of fibrinogen with an increasing central "hole," and when the height of the plasma at the outer edge of the fibrinogen ring was computed and then plotted against plasma dilution, a straight line resulted with an extrapolated intercept at 0 layer height and 0 dilution (infinitely high concentration).

Whole heparinized blood left a larger ring of platelets between lens and slide, than did its red cell-poor platelet-rich supernatant; and red cells added to intact plasma caused it to leave a larger ring of fibrinogen [24]. The enhancing effect of red cells upon platelet retention may therefore act neither via a substance released by the cells [25] nor via a simple and direct influence on flow [26]: the red cells may act as a diluent of the plasma so that less HMWK is available and fibrinogen will remain in relatively wider spaces of about 40 microns, easily reached by platelets that will then adhere.

Effects of flow on the pattern of adhesion of platelets to surfaces that are potentially clot-promoting, may be indirect as well. We found that in a stagnation point flow chamber [27], flow beyond the 4 support points of the test surface (a glass coverslip) is disturbed, forming a line of reduced flow from support point to chamber periphery. On these lines, removal of fibrinogen from the glass by flowing plasma was delayed, and deposition of platelets was markedly enhanced [28].

The following very general rule may be applied: where plasma will deposit fibrinogen, and where circumstances allow this fibrinogen to remain (e.g. on many hydrophobic solids, but on negatively charged, clot-promoting ones only where texture or geometry creates narrow spaces or where flow is reduced, and where the blood plasma is diluted), platelets will adhere. The rule does not imply that deposition of a single layer of platelets must lead to thrombus formation; the opposite may be true.

There are indications that many paths lead to white cell adhesion. Kallikrein [29] formation, and complement activation such as formation of C5a [30] and its effect on the solubility and availability of antibody/antigen complexes [31] can be expected to link the process of surface activated clotting to that of immune adhesion. The distortion suffered by gamma globulin upon adhering to a rigid substrate may resemble its modification by complexing with antibodies, and lead to interactions with the complement system. IgG exposed to various hydrophobic interfaces will bind complement, while its exposure to un-siliconized (and therefore wettable) glass does not [32]. We found [33] that granulocytes in whole heparinized blood adhere to gamma globulin films that had been deposited onto a hydrophobic rather than onto a hydrophilic substrate. Ellipsometry recordings showed that normal intact plasma deposits matter on gamma globulin films, but then removes even more than it deposited if the substrate was wettable [34]. It is tempting to combine the findings of this paragraph into a few rather simple conclusions: IgG is adsorbed onto certain non-wettable surfaces in such a position or conformational change that it irreversibly binds one or several complement components, thus localizing chemotactic activity at its surface and causing granulocyte adhesion (and spreading). On wettable, clot-promoting surfaces such as glass, binding of complement is reversible, perhaps because activation of factor XI at the interface causes plasmin generation

[35]. Our experiments with the ellipsometer did indicate that factor XII in intact state was needed at the interface or in solution to cause removal of the matter deposited by plasma onto an IgG film on the clot-activating substrate [34].

Plasma fibronectin, though probably not involved in platelet adhesion and aggregation [36,37], may be adsorbed out of plasma onto various surfaces under certain conditions [38]; possibly, it plays a role in white cell adhesion.

The study of chemotactic agents and their development in the course of clotting, complement activation, fibrinolysis and other physiological events that allow themselves to be observed in vitro, is expanding too rapidly to allow a fair report here. Within each of these systems, and probably beyond in reactions that link the systems together, various dormant enzymes are both activated and destroyed by other enzymes. Activation itself is often a prelude to destruction, so that any material surface introduced to the blood will be populated by a sequence of proteins acting and interacting within seconds, each at its own rate, with or without attracting the relatively large formed elements floating above them (Figure 1).

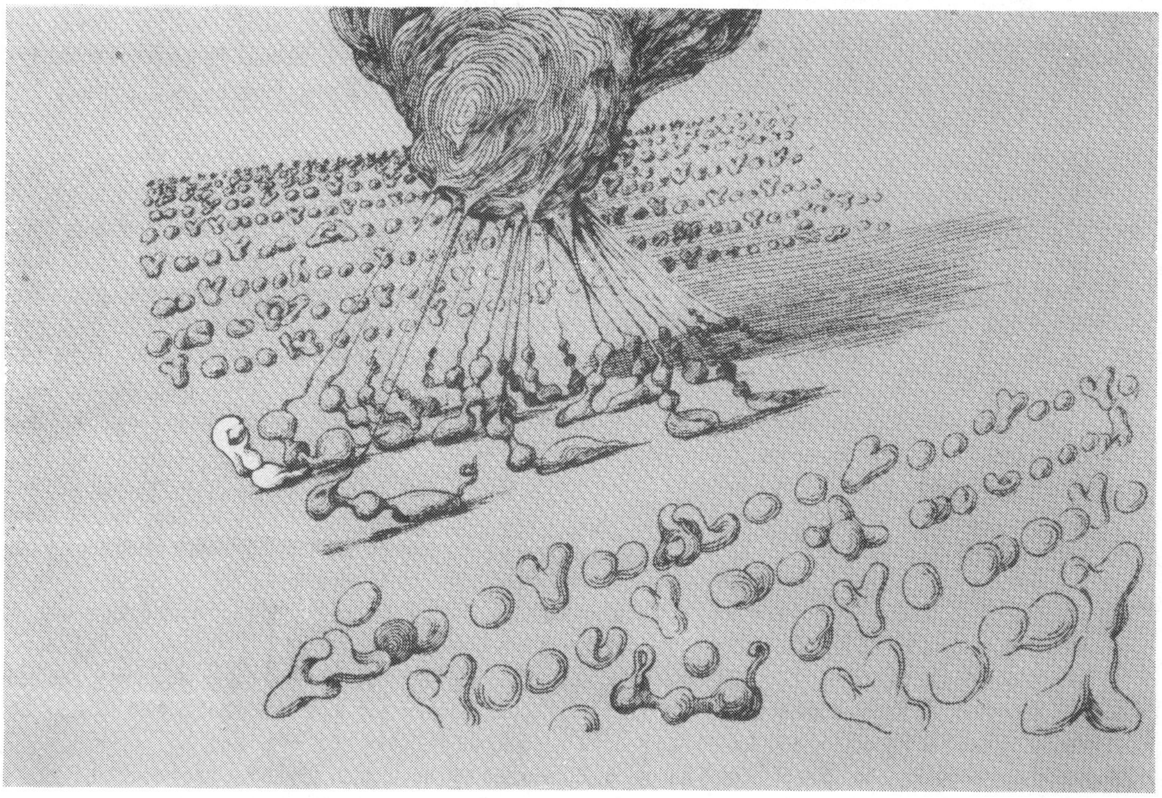

Figure 1. Concentrations and activities of plasma proteins related to platelet adhesion. An audience of 500 albumin molecules and 250 globulin molecules watches passively as 25 molecules of adsorbed fibrinogen (shown as rather flexible players, each consisting of 3 spheres on a rod) attract a platelet (the balloon floating above them), while a single high-molecular-weight kininogen molecule (white, carrying a molecule of factor XI) disengages one fibrinogen molecule from the glass-like field. The proportions of albumin:globulins:fibrinogen:HMWK are approximately 500:250:25:1.

With its proteins and even with its ions, the plasma probes the substrates it touches, sensing its details within a scale of Ångstroms. Visible fibrin formation and the adhesion of platelets and white blood cells are, in turn, probes of the pattern in the substrate of proteins carpeting whatever material we introduce. But these visible probes are relatively huge and therefore poor indicators of this underlying pattern. Obviously then, we will not understand it and its essential ultrafine details, unless we first try to understand events that occur in plasma when it touches large uniform areas of man-made materials. Even there, we will find a host of interacting reactions whose distribution in time and space will reflect the delicate web of interrelations within the plasma itself. For example, we have not even touched upon the many inhibitors affecting these reactions at interfaces. Until now, the literature contains no sharply distinguishing criteria by which to separate specific from non-specific effects: many proteins, for example, interfere with the adsorption (and subsequent activation) of clotting factors merely by being adsorbed themselves. Substrate materials can inhibit non-specificially as well, e.g. by adsorbing a clotting factor in such a position that its active site will remain hidden. Specific inhibitors of activation, chemotaxis or proteolysis may hide behind any change of activity found in an adsorbed enzyme: an enzyme may become active when the activity of its inhibitor is inhibited by another activator. On a heterogeneous surface, such events may occur side by side. In effect, flow, changes of geometry and temperature are forces gross enough to be compared with a storm causing an ocean of wind chimes to sing briefly as it breaks.

REFERENCES

1. *The Behavior of Blood and its Components at Interfaces.* L. Vroman and E. F. Leonard, eds. Ann. New York Acad. Sci. 283, 1977.
2. Vroman, L. and Adams, A. L. Findings with the recording ellipsometer suggesting rapid exchange of specific plasma proteins at liquid/solid interfaces. Surface Sci. 16:438, 1969.
3. Vroman, L. and Adams, A. L. Peculiar behavior of blood at solid interfaces. J. Polymer Sci. 34:159, 1971.
4. Vroman, L. and Adams, A. L. Possible involvement of fibrinogen and proteolysis in surface activation. Thromb. Diath. Haemorrh. 18:510, 1967.
5. Brash, J. L. and Uniyal, S. Adsorption of albumin, fibrinogen and IgG from human plasma onto solid surfaces. Plast. Med. Surg. 3:29, 1979.
6. Helmus, M. N., Malhotra, O. P. and Gibbons, D. F. Plasma interaction on block copolymers as determined by platelet adhesion. Adv. Chem. Series 199: 1981 (in press).
7. Vroman, L., Adams, A. L., Fischer, G. C. and Munoz, P. C. Interaction of high molecular weight kininogen, factor XII and fibrinogen in plasma at interfaces. Blood 55:156, 1980.
8. Wiggins, R. C., Bouma, B. N., Cochrane, C. G. and Griffin, J. H. Role of high-molecular-weight-kininogen in surface-binding and activation of coagulation Factor XI and prekallikrein. Proc. Natl. Acad. Sci. USA 74:4636, 1977.
9. Thompson, R. E., Mandle, R. and Kaplan, A. P. Studies of binding of prekallikrein and Factor XI to high molecular weight kininogen and its light chain. Biochemistry 76:4862, 1979.
10. Chan, J. Y. C., Movat, H. Z., and Burrows, C. E. High molecular weight kininogen: its ability to correct the clotting of kininogen-deficient plasma after cleavage of bradykinin by plasma kallikrein, plasmin or trypsin. Thromb. Res. 14:817, 1979.
11. Scott, C. F. and Colman, R. W. Function and immunochemistry of prekallikrein-high-molecular-weight-kininogen complex in plasma. J. Clin. Invest. 65:413, 1980.
12. Wiggins, R. C. and Cochrane, C. G. The autoactivation of rabbit Hageman Factor. J. Exp. Med. 150:1122, 1979.

13. Silverberg, M., Dunn, J. T., Garen, L. and Kaplan, A. P. Autoactivation of human Hageman Factor, J. Biol. Chem. 255:7281, 1980.
14. Ratnoff, O. D. The relative amidolytic activity of Hageman factor and its fragments. The effect of high-molecular-weight-kininogen and kaolin. J. Lab. Clin. Med. 96:267, 1980.
15. Mandle, R. J. Jr. and Kaplan, A. P. Hageman-factor-dependent fibrinolysis: Generation of fibrinolytic activity by the interaction of human activated factor XI and plasminogen. Blood 54:850, 1979.
16. Goldsmith, G. H., Saito, H. and Ratnoff, O. D. Activation of plasminogen by Hageman factor (factor XII) and Hageman factor fragments. J. Clin. Invest. 62:54, 1978.
17. Zucker, M. B. and Vroman, L. Platelet adhesion induced by fibrinogen adsorbed onto glass. Proc. Soc. Exp. Biol. Med. 131:318, 1969.
18. Mason, R. G., Shermer, R. W. and Zucker, W. H. Effects of certain purified plasma proteins on the compatibility of glass with blood. Am. J. Pathol. 73:183, 1973.
19. Revak, S. D., Cochrane, C. G., Bouma, B. N. and Griffin, J. H. Surface and fluid phase activities of two forms of activated Hageman factor produced during contact activation of plasma. J. Exper. Med. 147:719, 1978.
20. Schiffman, S., Mannhalter, C. and Tyner, K. D. Human high molecular weight kininogen. Effects of cleavage by kallikrein on protein structure and procoagulant activity. J. Biol. Chem. 255:6433, 1980.
21. Gurewich, V., Nunn, T. and Lipinski, B. Activation of intrinsic or extrinsic blood coagulation in experimental venous thrombosis and disseminated intravascular coagulation: pathogenetic differences. Thromb. Res. 14:931, 1979.
22. Baier, R. E. The role of surface energy in thrombogenesis. Bull. New York Acad. Med. 48:257, 1972.
23. Sawyer, P. N. and Srinivasan, S. The role of electrochemical surface properties in thrombosis at vascular interfaces: cumulative experience of studies in animals and man. Bull. New York Acad. Med. 48:235, 1972.
24. Vroman, L., Adams, A. L., Fischer, G. C., Munoz, P. C. and Stanford, M. Proteins, plasma and blood in narrow spaces of clot-promoting surfaces. Adv. Chem. Series 199:, 1982 (in press).
25. Hellem, A. J. The adhesiveness of human blood platelets in vitro. Scand. J. Clin. Lab. Invest. 12 (Suppl.) 1960.
26. Goldsmith, H. L. Red cell motions and wall interactions in tube flow. Fed. Proc. 30:1578, 1971.
27. Morton, W. A. and Cumming R. D. A technique for the elucidation of Virchow's triad. Ann. New York Acad. Sci. 283:477, 1977.
28. Stanford, M. Effects of flow on the activation of the intrinsic clotting system. Ph.D. thesis, in preparation.
29. Schachter, M. Kallikreins: a group of serine proteases with bioregulatory actions. Pharm. Rev. 31:1, 1979.
30. Craddock, P. R., Hammerschmidt, D., White, J. G., Dalmasso, A. P. and Jacob, H. S. Complement (C5a)-induced granulocyte aggregation in vivo. A possible mechanism of complement-mediated leukostasis and leukopenia. J. Clin. Invest. 60:260, 1977.
31. Miller, G. W. and Nussenzweig, V. Complement as a regulator of interactions between immune complexes and cell membranes. J. Immunol. 113:464, 1974.
32. Miekka, S. I. and Gozze, I. Anticomplementary activity of human immunoglobulin G. I. Mechanism of the artefactual increase in anticomplementary activity of IgG during the assay. Vox Sang. 29:101, 1975.
33. Vroman, L., Adams, A., L., Klings, M., Fischer, G. C., Munoz, P. C. and Solensky, R. P. Reactions of formed elements of blood with plasma proteins at interfaces. Ann. New York Acad. Sci. 283:65, 1977.
34. Vroman, L., Adams, A. L., Klings, M. and Fischer, G. Fibrinogen, globulins, albumin and plasma at interfaces. Adv. Chem. Series 145:255, 1975.

35. Saito, H. The participation of plasma thromboplastin antecedent (Factor XI) in contact-activated fibrinolysis. Proc. Soc. Exper. Biol. Med. 164:153, 1980.
36. Harfenist, E. J., Izzotti, M. J., Packham, M. A. and Mustard, J. F. Plasma fibronectin is not involved in ADP-induced aggregation of rabbit platelets. Thromb. & Haem. 44:108, 1980.
37. Sochynsky, R. A., Boughton, B. J., Burns, J., Sykes, B. C., McGee, L. O., Fabian, I. and Aronson. M. The effect of human fibronectin on platelet collagen adhesion. Thromb. Res. 18:521, 1980.
38. Grinnell, F. and Feld. M, K. Adsorption characteristics of plasma fibronectin in relationship to biological activity. J. Biomed. Mater. Res. 15:363, 1981.

Chapter 5

Activation of Complement by Polymers in Contact with Blood

George A. Herzlinger
Belmont Instrument Corporation
Belmont, MA 02178

ABSTRACT

Complement activation is well known to mediate cellular response to foreign materials in the context of inflammation, but has only recently gained attention in relation to biomaterials. In this review we consider a) the extent to which materials in contact with blood activate complement components and b) the role of complement activation in mediating cell adhesion to blood contact surfaces.

Complement activation by diverse materials has been investigated. Nylon 6,6, cellophane, polymethyl methacrylate, asbestos fibers, urate crystals, and even oxygen bubbles have all been shown by various investigators to activate the complement cascade when in contact with blood or whole serum. Nylon has been found to be an especially potent activator, and has been studied by several investigators. Nylon-induced activation proceeds rapidly within the first few minutes of blood contact at biological temperature. It is highly temperature dependent, requires Ca^{++} ions, and involves a pathway originating with Cl. By contrast, cellophane membranes activate complement by the alternative pathway which is independent of Ca^{++}. No general mechanism for surface induced complement activation has been established. The diversity of material for which activation is seen, suggests complement mediation of cellular effects at a variety of blood contact surfaces.

Cellular effects due to complement activation by blood-contact materials have been documented. Activation of complement by nylon or cellophane extracorporeal blood circuits has been shown to produce sequestration of leukocytes in the pulmonary vasculature when blood from these circuits reenters the body. This phenomenon has been established in several different clinical situations including hemodialysis, cardiopulmonary bypass, and leukapheresis filtration. Parallel phenomena have been observed in vitro: plasma containing activated complement induces granulocyte aggregation and enhances granulocyte adhesiveness to surfaces.

The role of complement in mediating cell adhesion at blood-contact surfaces has been studied by the effect of in vivo depletion of C3 on white cell and platelet adhesion to polymer surfaces in a canine ex vivo blood flow experiment. Cell adhesion to smooth polymer surfaces was studied after profound reduction of C3 levels with cobra venom factor (CVF). CVF administration had little effect on cell counts, coagulation times or ADP levels required to to produce platelet aggregation in vitro, while both platelet and leukocyte adhesion to smooth polymer surfaces were sharply reduced in the CUF experiments relative to identical experiments with normal dogs. Nylon surfaces which normally would be covered with a dense layer of platelets and leukocytes were nearly free of adherent cells. Reduction in the number of adherent leukocytes and platelets to polymethyl methacrylate, the other polymer studied, was also observed. Complement activation would seem to play a major role in mediating short term leukocyte and platelet adhesion to smooth polymer blood contact surfaces.

*Work supported in part by N.I.H. Contract #N01-HV-9-2901, while the author was at Avco Everett Research Lab., Inc., Everett, MA 02149.

1. RATIONALE: WHY STUDY COMPLEMENT ACTIVATION BY BIOMATERIALS?

Introduction of a foreign substance into the body generally results in an inflammatory type of response culminating in the mobilization of white blood cells, especially polymorphonuclear leukocytes (PMNS) at the invasion site. In the case of particulate substances, cellular engulfment and ingestion (phagocytosis) may also result.

In studies of blood flow on smooth polymer surfaces deposition of large numbers of white blood cells, especially PMNS, is generally observed during the first few minutes of blood/surface contact, provided the fluid shear forces of the flow are not too large [1,2]. PMN attachment to explanted devices is also seen [3].

A natural question in connection with these phenomena is: To what extent do synthetic materials in contact with blood elicit an inflammatory-like response? Do white blood cells adhere to synthetic surfaces in a process which parallels preparation for phagocytosis? Answers to these questions require study of the substances in blood responsible for PMN mobilization and adhesion: the complement system of proteins. The structure and function of these important enzymatic proteins has been elucidated in the last 20 years. Detailed descriptions of the complement system may be found in textbooks and reviews [4,5,6,7]. Some of the basic properties are discussed in Section 2 below.

2. THE COMPLEMENT SYSTEM

The complement system consists of a series of enzymes with activation of early components inducing activation of later components in a cascading sequence. The nine primary complement components are denoted Cl through C9. The most abundant component in serum, and the pivotal component in the cascade is C3. Its concentration in human plasma is approximately 1.6 mg/ml, comparable to that of fibrinogen. It is common to all known activation pathways, as discussed below, and its split products have potent biological activity including induction of chemotaxis, and the ability to bind neutrophils and other phagocytes. The C3 activation step involves a feedback mechanism, in which activated (cleaved) C3 molecules promote further C3 activation. Activated C3 also produces activation of the later components of the cascade.

Discussion of the mechanism of complement activation is primarily that of the mechanism by which cleavage of the C3 molecule is initiated. Two primary pathways are known. In the classical pathway, antigen-antibody complexes provide a site for binding and cleavage of the first complement component Cl in the presence of Ca^{++} ions. The site of the antibody (IgG) molecule responsible for Cl binding can also be exposed by heat aggregating the IgG molecules. Once activated, Cl promotes activation of components C4 and C2. These form a complex Cl42 which constitutes a primary activator of C3.

Alternative pathway activation of C3 involves substances which can bind C3 and "serum factors" directly without involvement of earlier complement components. The primary serum factors, known as factor B, factor D, and properdin are involved in an amplification step in which C3 split products regenerate additional C3 activation. The amplification process is prevented from continuing identifinitely by control (inactivating) proteins. Complete discussion of the details of both the classical and alternative pathways are given in the reviews [6,7]. The known alternative pathway activators are primarily polysaccharides. Two such activators of interest are zymosan, yeast cell wall particles, often used as a reference activator in the laboratory, and endotoxin, a lipopolysaccharide found in the cell walls of bacteria. A third activator, cobra venom factor (CVF), a purified component of cobra venom, has the unusual property of forming a C3 activator (convertase) with serum, which is not affected by the inactivating control proteins. Animals treated with CVF in the laboratory have nearly depleted serum levels of C3. Finally, it should be noted that alternative pathway activation, unlike that of the classical (Cl) pathway, does not require Ca^{++} for initiation of the process.

No matter which activation process triggers the complement cascade, the C3 activation step involves both amplification, and production of split products with potent biological activity. C3a, the smaller fragment, promotes histamine release from mast cells and induces chemotaxis of leukocytes. C3b, the large antigen-bearing fragment, binds to many types of cells, including PMNs, B-lymphocytes, monocytes, and red blood cells (primates) [8]. C3 binding to platelets has also been determined [9]. Activated C3 produces activation of the later components in cascading fashion. C5a a split product of C5 activation strongly influences white blood cell (PMNs) adhesion and chemotaxis. Components C6 through C9 form a complex capable of direct lysis of cell membranes. In the case of bacteria, endotoxin-mediated activation results in bacterial destruction. The complement system is thus a direct non-cellular source of immunological protection.

Cell lysis, as the final stage of complement activation, is often used to quantify complement activity. Sheep erythrocytes are incubated with antiserum to the sheep rbc membranes in the presence of varying dilutions of test serum. The curve of hemolysis versus serum dilution determines the complement activity of the serum, with the dilution level at 50% hemolysis, or "CH50", often used as a quantitative measure of complement activity [10].

In considering complement activation by biomaterials, two questions must be answered:

a) To what extent do synthetic blood-contact materials activate complement components? (and by what mechanism?)

b) What are the cellular effects due to this activation?

Investigation into these questions are discussed in Sections 3 and 4 respectively.

3. COMPLEMENT ACTIVATION BY POLYMERS IN CONTACT WITH BLOOD

Although complement activation by synthetic ("foreign") materials has been studied for years in the context of immunology, it has only recently received attention by those studying biomaterials used in prosthetic devices. Initial studies focused on explaining clinical symptoms associated with blood-surface interaction in various extracorporeal devices. Thus Craddock and coworkers studied pulmonary complications and systemic leukopenia experienced by hemodialysis patients [11]. These syndromes were found to be due to pulmonary sequestration of leukocytes consequent to complement activation by cellophane dialysis membrane. It was also shown that cellophane activates plasma complement *in vitro* and that activated plasma produces granulocyte aggregation as measured by an *in vitro* nephelometric aggregation assay. The assay was similar to standard platelet aggregometry and utilized granulocytes which had been separated from blood by density gradient centrifugation methods. The stirred granulocyte suspension, when monitored in the aggregometer showed biphasic aggregation upon adding activated plasma [12]. Further study showed that incubation of plasma with dialysis membrane or with laboratory polysaccharides produces a transient increase in granulocyte adhesiveness [13]. Immunoelectrophoresis showed the offending complement component to be split product of C5, C5a. A clinical syndrome (pulmonary edema, leukopenia) was thus related to a specific complement subcomponent.

In terms of known activation mechanisms, cellophane-induced activation is not inconsistent with other alternative pathway activation observed in the laboratory, since cellophane, like zymosan, inulin and other laboratory alternate pathway activators, is a polysaccharide. However, soon after the dialysis membrane investigation, a parallel phenomenon was observed in connection with nylon fiber leukapheresis filtration [14,15]. In this procedure, drawn blood is pumped over a nylon fiber filter to which granulocytes adhere preferentially, with the bulk of the blood returned to the donor. Human donors were found to experience sharp leukopenia early in the procedure. Plasma extracted from the blood return line was found to have granulocyte aggregating activity, C5a (activated C5) and Factor B activity (Hammerschmidt, *et al.*) [14]. Parallel studies by a second investigating group (Nusbacher, *et al.*) demonstrated directly that complement components were consumed in the nylon filtration process, including substantial reductions in C1, C4, C2, C3, and C5, with total hemolytic complement (CH50) also reduced [15]. Involvement of Cl implies a process akin to the classical pathway.

Nylon, as a polyamide, contains numerous NHC=0 groups analogous to the peptide groups of proteins. It is obviously quite different chemically from known alternative and classical pathway activators. Strong nylon induced complement activation is surprising.

Recently we studied the details of the nylon 6,6 activation process and examined activation due to a second polymer as well, polymethyl methacrylate (PMMA) [16]. Our investigation was motivated by the observation of surface binding of large numbers of white blood cells to a variety of polymer test surfaces (more than 30 different materials) evaluated in a canine *ex vivo* blood flow experiment at Avco Everett Research Laboratory [2]. Dog serum was used in the investigation because most biomaterials used in prosthetic devices are tested in dogs, and because cell adhesion to the same polymers could be evaluated in the *ex vivo* blood flow preparation. Polymer to be tested for complement activating ability was first converted to microspheres, vastly increasing the surface available for polymer-serum contact to greater than 100,000 sq cm of material. The particle formation process is applicable to a wide variety of polymers, and involves no surfactant or other surface active agent. See [16] for details.

By utilizing a very large serum-polymer interface, the surface-induced reaction could potentially involve a sizeable fraction of total complement protein. In addition, the use of a dispersed microparticulate ensured rapid diffusion of proteins to the polymer surface with diffusion times very small fractions of a second. The microparticle methods enabled quantitative measurement of complement activity with reaction rates not artificially prolonged by diffusion.

In an experiment, serum was exposed to a fixed amount of polymer suspension, usually on the order of 1-2 mg/ml, at biological temperature for a fixed period of time. The reaction was then quenched by cooling to 0°C and the particles removed by centrifugation. The serum was then assayed for C3 level and C3 split products using Laurell "rocket" immunoelectrophoresis, and antigen-antibody cross immunoelectrophoresis (XAA) [17, 18]. The latter method directly yields a plot of quantity of C3 versus electrophoretic mobility, with split products of the C3 molecule showing increased mobility.

Both nylon and PMMA rapidly activated C3 within a few minutes of serum contact. Nylon activity was much greater and was studied in detail. Nylon activation increased with increasing surface area up to a saturation level of 20% of the total C3 in serum. Saturation was reached at 350 square cm/ml, equivalent to activation of 0.05% of the total C3 in 1 ml of serum for each square cm of nylon surface.

The time course of the reaction was studied in detail: during the first 2 minutes there is little activity, after which the reaction rapidly develops. The bulk of the reaction is complete in less than 10 minutes, with no further development. The nylon-serum reaction is completely inhibited by removal of Ca^{++} with chelating agent, Mg EGTA, and was highly temperature dependent. Activity at 30°C was reduced by at least a factor of 5 relative to that at canine biological temperature, 39°C.

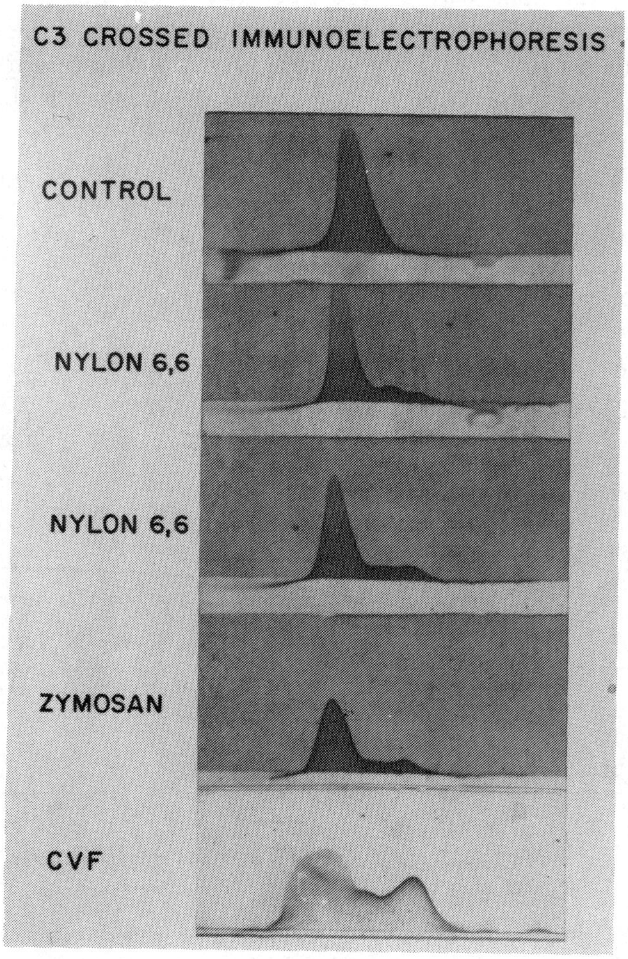

Figure 1. Laurell XAA curves showing C3 conversion in canine serum at 39°C.

A) Control held at 39°C for 50 minutes with no added polymer.
B,C) Sera exposed to 6 mg/ml nylon 6,6 for 20 and 50 minutes respectively (saturation conditions).
D) Serum exposed to 6 mg/ml zymosan for 20 minutes. The curve is identical in appearance to curves B), C).
E) Much larger amount of conversion induced by 2 U/ml CVF in 10 minutes. Converstion peaks appear at the same mobilities as for nylon and zymosan.

Figure 1 shows several Laurell XAA plates. Each crossed immunoelectrophoresis run produces a plot of antigenic C3 concentration (y-axis) versus mobility (x-axis). The control serum plate shows a single peak at the C3 mobility, while the plates run with nylon and zymosan particles show additional peaks at higher mobility indicating the presence of C3 split products. From the area under the conversion peaks the relative amount of converted (activated) C3 was calculated. Both the zymosan and nylon plates involve sera exposed under saturation conditions, with 20% maximum attainable conversion. In contrast, the plate run with CVF (bottom) shows more than twice as much conversion for the same time period. CVF will, in time, convert nearly all available C3. Note that XAA plates from nylon and zymosan are nearly identical, despite the fact that the nylon conversion was shown to be Ca^{++} dependent unlike that of zymosan, an alternative pathway activator. C3 activation was the primary phenomenon observed in the experiments. C3 binding was not observed. Total C3 serum levels were not affected by exposure to polymer — no antigenic C3 remained bound to the polymer surface. The quantitative relationship between surface area and activation is shown in Figure 2.

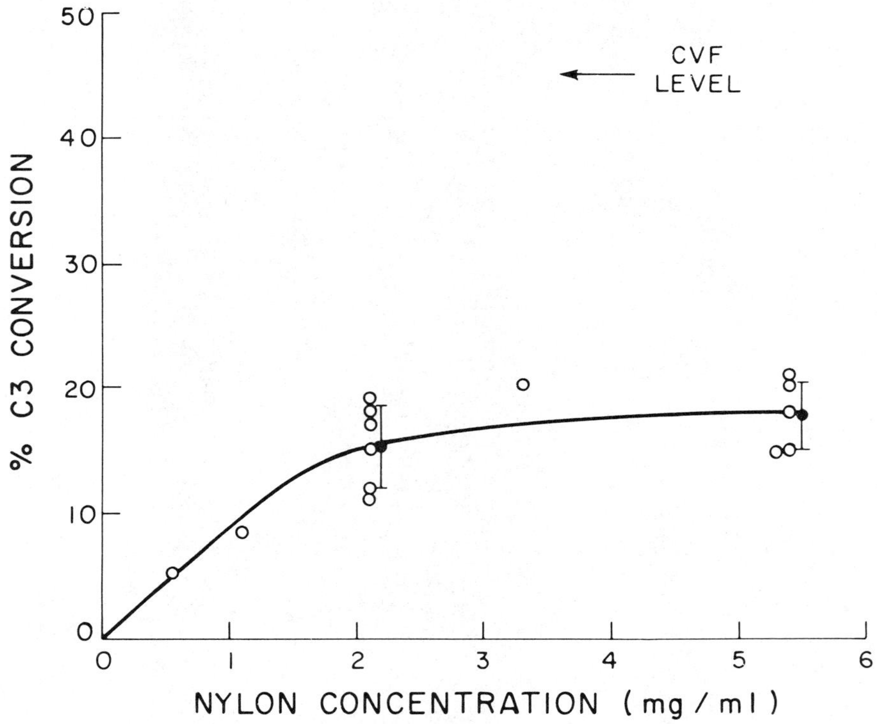

Figure 2. Dose-response curve for nylon-induced C3 conversion. Percent of converted C3 is shown vs. nylon concentration for 10 minute, 39°C polymer/serum incubations. Also shown is the level of C3 converstion induced by 2 U/ml CVF under identical conditions. Brackets indicate standard deviations computed from the data.

Nylon induced activation has recently been studied in other clinical situations, and, in fact, a variety of other man made materials have also been found to activate complement. Substantial C3 activation during cardiopulmonary bypass has been demonstrated in which a nylon mesh bubble oxygenator lining was utilized (Chenoweth, *et al.*) [19]. Incubation of the mesh with plasma produced rapid C3 activation *in vitro. In vitro* activation was also demonstrated to a lesser extent by bubbling oxygen through heparinized whole blood: the bubble oxygenation process itself produced increased C3 split product levels over that observed in control (no oxygenation) situations. This result indicates the possibility of complement activation occurring at many types of surfaces.

Indeed other substances have been shown to activate complement. These include, for example, urate crystals which initiate the painful inflammation of gout (Giclas), and asbestos fibers (Hasselbacher) [20,21]. Urate-induced activation was shown to involve both C1 and C4, but was apparently independent of IgG [20].

In summary, studies to date have documented potent, and rapid C3 activation by nylon, as well as activation by a variety of other materials including cellophane, PMMA, an oxygen interface, asbestos, etc. These situations have in common an adsorption interface where plasma protein reorientation or denaturation can take place. It is known that heat denatured IgG will activate C1 in much the same way as immune complexes. It is not known whether adsorption-induced denaturation of plasma protein, results in a parallel effect. Most of the surface activation studies do indicate the involvement of C1 either through demonstration of Ca^{++} dependence or through direct measurement of Cl depletion, suggesting a process akin to the classical pathway. However, the mechanism of surface-induced activation is not established, nor is it known why nylon 6,6 is such a potent activator. Whatever the mechanism, the diversity of materials shown to activate complement components suggests the possibility of complement mediation of cellular effects in blood/surface phenomena.

4. CELLULAR EFFECTS MEDIATED BY COMPLEMENT IN BLOOD-SURFACE INTERACTION

Studies of the cellular consequences of complement activation by blood contact synthetic materials have centered primarily on three types of phenomena:

a) the effect of complement activation on cellular adhesiveness and aggregation as measured *in vitro*.

b) the effect of complement activation by extracorporeal circuits on increased cellular adhesiveness and sequestration upon re-entering a vascular bed.

c) observation of cell adhesion and aggregation to blood contact surfaces in animals in whom one or more complement components have been depleted by pharmacological agents.

An example of an *in vitro* assay is the white blood cell (PMN) aggregation assay of Craddock, *et al.* which has already been discussed. In our studies of activation by nylon particles we investigated the direct action of nylon particles on canine platelets, in citrated plasma, using a standard platelet aggregometer to monitor optical density. We observed platelet aggregation in response to both zymosan and nylon particles. An initial increase in optical density occurs as particulate is added to the stirred platelet suspension. This is followed by a slow decrease in optical density as platelet aggregates are formed. Aggregation induced by nylon was inhibited by complete removal of Ca^{++} by Mg EGTA, while that due to zymosan persisted. The Ca^{++} dependence corresponds directly to that observed for C3 activation by the 2 materials and is consistent with complement involvement in the aggregation process. (Note that particle aggregation alone without platelets would not produce the observed effect in the aggregometer. This and other details of the platelet aggregation experiments are described in [16]).

The phenomena of increased cellular adhesiveness induced by complement activation in extracorporeal blood circuits has been discussed already in connection with: a) hemodialysis, b) cardiopulmonary bypass and c) leukapheresis filtration. In each case, formation of complement split products C3a or C5a in the extracorporeal circuit was documented and related to sequestration of leukocytes *in vivo*.

The third type of investigation involves observation of cellular adhesion and surface aggregation on blood contact surfaces in animals whose C3 level had been depleted by a pharmacological agent. We carried out this type of investigation using CVF to sharply reduce the C3 level of experimental animals *in vivo,* and compared cellular adhesion to polymer surfaces from this group to that of untreated animals [22]. We utilized an *ex vivo* blood flow preparation which enabled direct real-time microscopic observation of test surfaces.

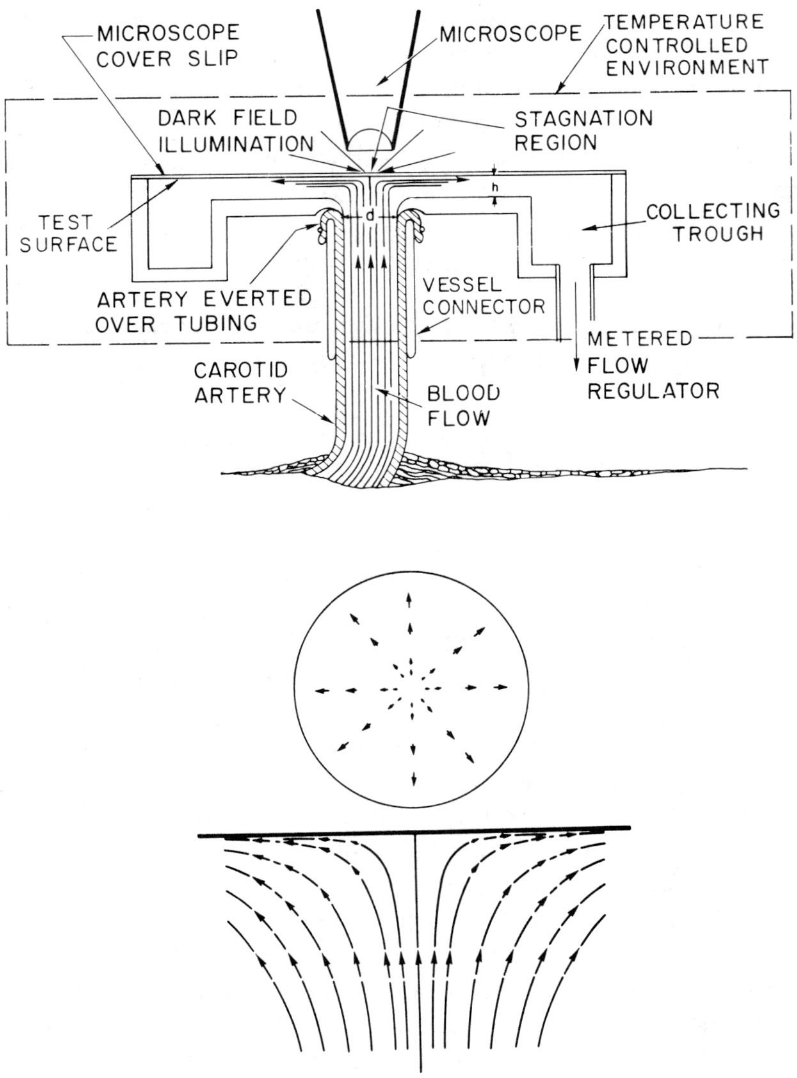

Figure 3. Stagnation point flow apparatus (Top) and flow pattern (Bottom).

In the experiment, arterial blood from an anesthetized dog impinges directly upon a test surface in stagnation point flow configuration (Figure 3). The Stagnation Point Flow Preparation has been described in detail elsewhere [1,2]. The flow pattern in the preparation is cylindrically symmetric, with surface shear rate increasing linearly with radius from a central stagnation point (Figure 3). Only blood originating near center streamlines reaches the test surface so that prior blood/surface contact is eliminated. The blood flow preparation, originated by Petschek and Kantrowitz, [1] and developed as a controlled experiment by Cumming, [2] had been used for a number of years to document blood/surface phenomena for a wide variety of materials. A general set of phenomena was observed for all materials tested [2]. On smooth surfaces, platelet adhesion is observed during the first few minutes of blood flow with rapid formation of a platelet monolayer. Somewhat slower adhesion of white blood cells, especially PMNs, also occurs with a dense layer of white cells forming within a shear limited circular region after about 10 minutes of flow. Adhesion of platelets and PMNs to a wide variety of surfaces is the dominant short term blood/surface effect observed with smooth surfaces. The universal involvement of PMNs suggests a role for complement in mediating this short-term cell adhesion. Thus cell adhesion from CVF-decomplemented dogs was compared with that observed with normal dogs under otherwise identical conditions [22].

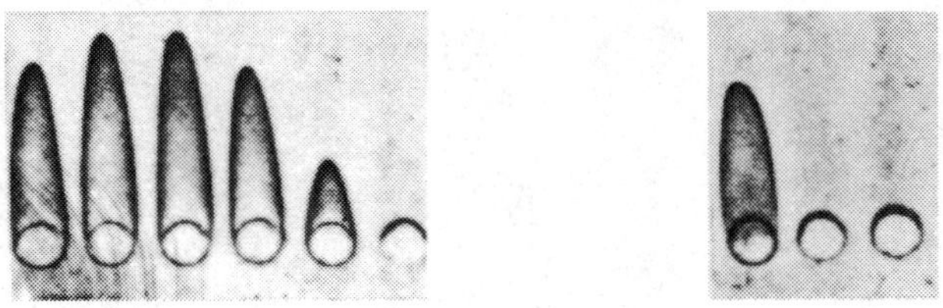

1 2 3 4 5 6

DILUTION 1 : 8

5 6 7

DILUTION 1 : 4

1	PRE CVF
2	+ 10 MIN
3	+ 30 MIN
4	+ 1 HR
5	+ 4 HR
6	+ 20 HR
7	+ 44 HR

Figure 4. Time evolution of in vivo response to CVF. Area under each rocket shaped curve is proportional to the C3 level. At 4 hours the C3 is depleted by about 2/3 while at 1 day only about 2% of the original level remains.

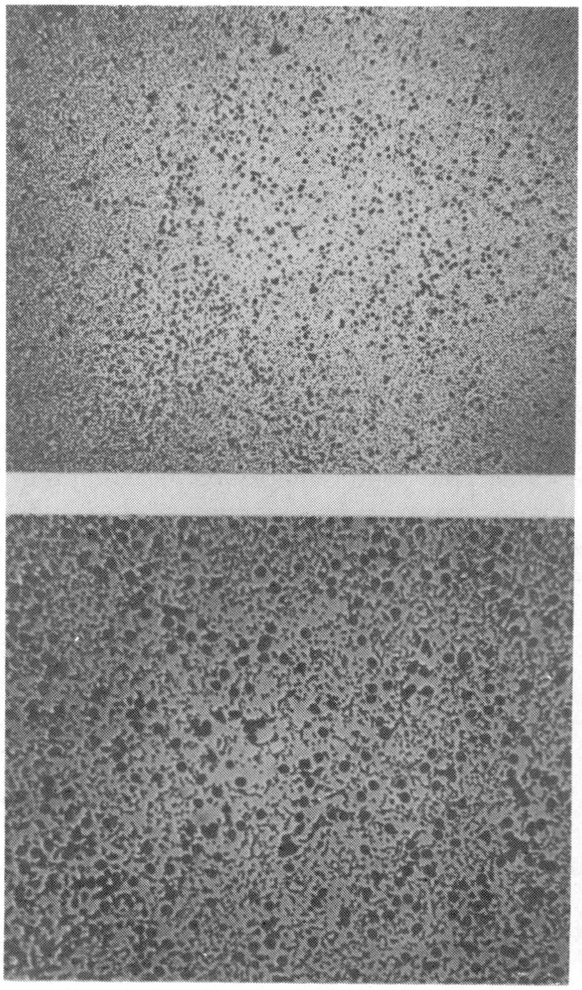

Figure 5. Post-test micrograph of nylon 6,6 surface after 10 minute blood/surface exposure at 39°C – control experiment. Upper photo, field approximately 1250μ × 950μ, lower photo, field approximately 625μ × 475μ.

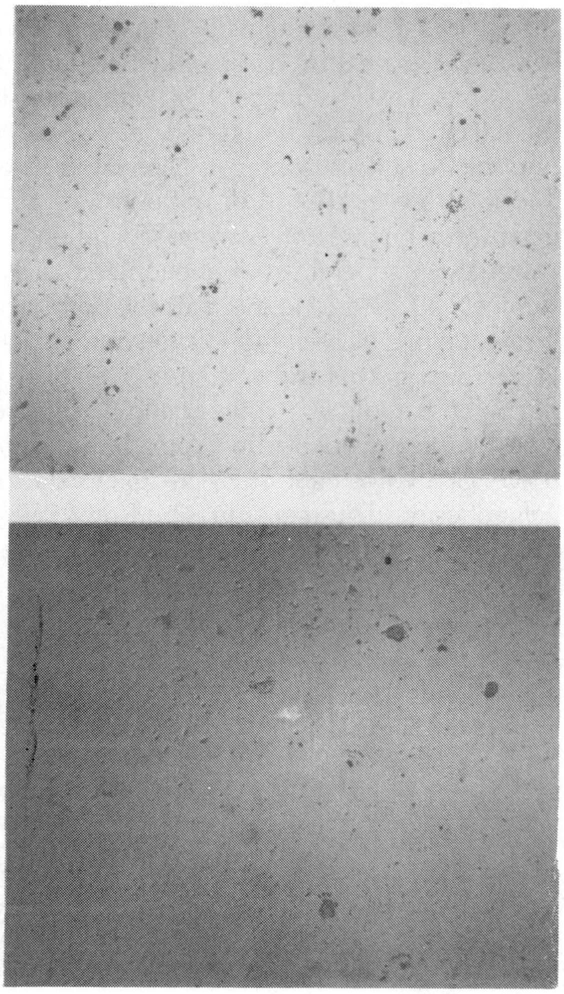

Figure 6. Post-test micrographs of nylon 6,6 surfaces, after 10 minute blood/surface exposure at 39°C – CVF experiments. Field shown for each surface, 1250μ × 950μ.

CVF, administered a day prior to the flow experiment sharply reduced antigenic C3 while not affecting white blood cell count, platelet count, coagulation times (PT and PTT times), or platelet aggregation induced by ADP (a non-complement dependent process). Transient neutropenia/neutrophilia reported by others in other animal models, was not observed, perhaps due to use of *Naja Haje* CVF (which preactivates only C3 directly; *Naja Naja,* the other form, directly activates both C3 and C5) [23].

CVF reduced antigenic C3 by about a factor of 50 while leaving nearly all hematological parameters intact. Figure 4 shows Laurell rocket immunoelectrophoresis plates which document the dramatic drop in C3 level. In some experiments CH50 was measured, rather than C3. CVF reduced CH50 by only about a factor of 10 from the control level. The larger fraction of hemolytic activity indicates that serum C3 is normally present in excess over that needed to

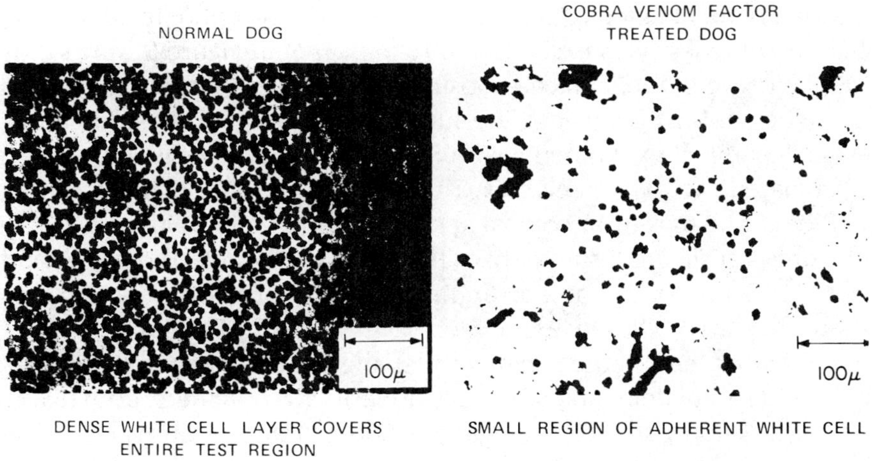

Figure 7. Comparison of control and CVF experiments for PMMA surfaces exposed to flowing blood for 10 minutes at 39°C.

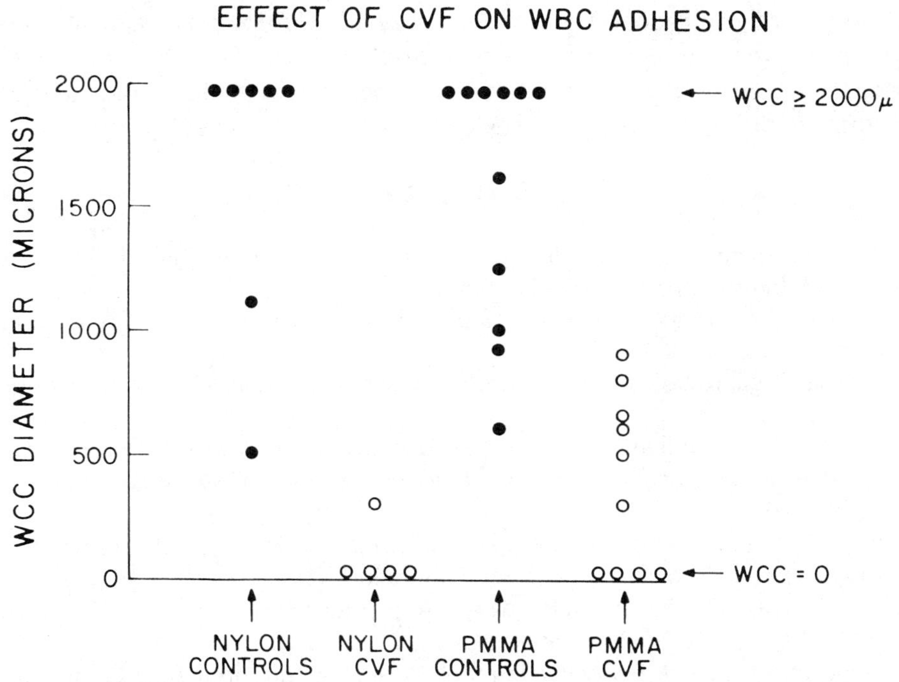

Figure 8. Summary of data showing effect of CVF on leukocyte adhesion to PMMA and nylon 6,6 surfaces. Shown are data for the diameter of the region of adherent leukocytes or white cell circle (WCC) for both CVF and control experiments, for both nylon and PMMA surfaces.

functionally limit the complement cascade, and that nearly all C3 must be depleted in order to inactivate the complement system.

Although complete functional decomplementation could not be achieved, a substantial effect on cell adhesion was observed. Results of the experiments are summarized in Figures

5,6,7,8. Figure 5 shows a nylon 6,6 surface after 10 minutes of blood/surface contact for a control (no CVF) experiment. Platelet aggregates are seen over the entire test region, while the circular area of adherent leukocytes exceeds 1100 μ in diameter. Figure 6 shows 2 nylon 6,6 surfaces after 10 minutes of blood/surface exposure for a CVF experiment run two days prior to that of Figure 6. The contrast is striking. The surfaces from the CVF experiments show little or no cell adhesion. Nearly all experiments with nylon surfaces show similar effect: the CVF administration eliminated the "white cell circle" and sharply reduced platelet adhesion. Figure 7 shows typical PMMA surfaces from control and CVF experiments, with again, a significant difference in cell adhesion. Figure 8 summarizes the white cell adhesion data for both polymers. The effect for nylon surfaces is dramatic and clear cut, the PMMA data show more scatter, with a significant ($p < .001$) difference between control and CVF groups.

We conclude that, at least in the canine model, there is evidence that complement activation mediates short term platelet and white cell adhesion to polymers: Both nylon and PMMA activate C3 *in vitro.* Nylon particles aggregate canine platelets. Removal of C3 by preactivation with CVF and subsequent clearance of split products, results in reduced short-term cell adhesion to smooth nylon and PMMA surfaces. It should be noted that thromboembolic events may still occur in C3 depleted animals, platelet response to non-complement stimuli is still intact, and indeed thrombus formation on roughened polymer surfaces was observed in the stagnation Point Flow preparation for CVF animals. Complement activation is only one mechanism which can be triggered at the blood/polymer interface, but one which available evidence indicates is especially important in mediating white blood cell and platelet adhesion to smooth surfaces during the early phases of blood/surface contact.

REFERENCES

1. Petschek, H.E., Adamis, D., Kantrowitz, A.R., "Stagnation Point Flow Thrombus Formation," Trans. Am. Soc. Artif. Intern. Organs, 14:256, 1968.
2. Cumming, R.D., "Important Factors Affecting Initial Blood Material Interactions," Trans. Am. Soc. Artif. Intern. Organs, 26:304, 1980.
3. Baier, R., "The Organization of Blood Components Near Interfaces," Ann. NY Acad. Sci. 283:17, 1977.
4. Cooper, N.R., "The Complement System," in Fundenberg, H. W., Sites, D. P., Caldwell, J.L., and Wells, J.V. (eds.), *Basic and Clinical Immunology,* Los Altos, CA., Lange Medical Publications (1976), Chapter 6.
5. Lachmann, P.J., "The Immunochemistry of Complement," in Hobart, M.J. and McConnell, I. (eds), *The Immunosystem,* Oxford, Blackwell Sci. Publications (1975).
6. Ruddy, S., Gigli, I., and Austen, K.F., "The Complement System of Man," New Eng. J. Med., 287:489-495, 545-549, 592-596, 642-646, 1972.
7. Fearon, D.T., and Austen, K.F., "Activation Mechanisms of The Alternative Complement Pathway and Amplification Step," in Bing, D.H. (ed), *The Chemistry and Physiology Of The Human Plasma Proteins,* New York, Pergamon Press, (1979), p. 229.
8. Henson, P.M., "The Adherence of Leukocytes and Platelets Induced by Fixed IgG Antibody or Complement," Immunology. 16:107, 1969.
9. Hauch, T.W., and Rosse, W.F., "Platelet Bound Complement C3 in Immune Thrombocytopenia," Blood 50:1129, 1977.
10. Mayer, M., "Complement and Complement Fixation," in Kabat, E., Mayer, M., *Experimental Immunochemistry,* Springfield, Ill., Charles C. Thomas, (1961).

11. Craddock, P.R., Fehr, J., Dalmasso, A.P., Brigham, K.L., Jacob, H.S., "Hemodialysis Leukopenia. Pulmonary Vascular Leukostasis from Complement Activation by Dialyzer Cellophane Membranes," J. Clin. Invest. 59:879, 1977.
12. Craddock, P.R., Hammerschmidt, D.E., White, J.G., Dalmasso, A.P., and Jacob, H.S., "Complement C5a Induced Granulocyte Activation *In Vitro:* A Possible Mechanism of Complement-Mediated Leukostasis and Leukopenia," J. Clin. Invest., 60:201, 1977.
13. O'Flaherty, J.T., Craddock, P.R., and Jacob, H.S., "Effect of Intravascular Complement Activation on Granulocyte Adhesiveness and Distribution," Blood, 51:731, 1978.
14. Hammerschmidt, D., Craddock, P., McCullough, J., Kronenbrug, R., Dalmasso, A., Jacob, H., "Complement Activation and Pulmonary Leukostasis During Nylon Fiber Filtration Leukapheresis," Blood, 51:721, 1978.
15. Nusbacher, J., Rosenfeld, S., MacPherson, J., Thiem, P., Leddy, J., "Nylon Fiber Leukapheresis: Associated Complement Component Changes and Granulocytopenia," Blood, 51:359, 1978.
16. Herzlinger, G.A., Bing, D.H., Stein, R., and Cumming, R., "Quantitative Measurement of C3 Activation at Polymer Surfaces," Blood, 57:764, 1981.
17. Laurell, C.B., "Quantitative Estimation of Proteins by Electrophoresis in Agarose Gel Containing Antibodies," Anal. Biochem., 15:45, 1966.
18. Laurell, C.B., "Antigen-antibody Crossed Electrophoresis," Anal., Biochem., 10:358, 1965.
19. Chenoweth, D.E., Cooper, S.W., Hugli, T.E., Stewart, R.W., Blackstone, E.W. and Kirklin, J.W., "Complement Activation During Cardiopulmonary Bypass: Evidence For Generation of C3a and C5a Anaphylatoxins," New Eng. J. Med. 304:497, 1981.
20. Giclas, P.C., Ginsberg, M.H. and Cooper, N.R., "Immunoglobulin G Independent Activation of The Classical Complement Pathway by Monosodium Urate Crystals," J. Clin. Inves., 63:759, 1979.
21. Hasselbacher, P., "Binding of Immunoglobulin and Activation of Complement by Asbestos Fibers," J. Allergy and Clin. Immun., 64:294, 1979.
22. Herzlinger, G.A., Cumming, R.D., "Role of Complement Activation In Cell Adhesion To Polymer Blood Contact Surfaces," Trans. Am. Soc. Artif. Intern. Organs, 26:165, 1980.
23. Vogt, W., vonZabern, J., Hinsch, B., Przyklenk, H., Schmidt, G., "Differences Between Cobra Venom Factor (CVF) from Naja Naja and Naja Haje: Binding Capacity and Support of C5 Cleavage by Factor B." (Abstract), J. Immunol. 124:544, 1980,

II

Strategies for Hemocompatibility

Chapter 6

Hemocompatible Interfaces in Artificial Heart Devices

Michael Szycher, Ph.D.
Director, Biomaterials Research
Thermo Electron Corporation
Waltham, Mass.

AND

William F. Bernhard, M.D.
Professor of Surgery
Cardiovascular Surgical Research Laboratories
Children's Hospital Medical Center
Boston, Mass.

ABSTRACT

A new technique has been developed for producing Model 11S Biomer bladders with Integrally Textured (IT) hemocompatible interfaces. For the past four years we have been routinely fabricating IT polymeric blood-contacting sufaces from negative-replica silicone molds, which are a high-fidelity topographical facsimile of conventionally flocked bladders. Our objectives are threefold: (1) to develop hemocompatible interfaces that promote the formation of stable pseudoneointimal linings, (2) to investigate means of accelerating replacement of initial fibrin coagulum by a collagenous, cellular lining, and (3) to characterize the resultant pseudoneointimal lining biochemically, histologically and ultrastructurally.

Systematic in vivo studies were undertaken to evaluate the newly developed polymeric surface in terms of its ability to form a thin, stable biologic lining. Control experiments were carried out to compare results with previous experience utilizing polyester fibril conventionally flocked surfaces. Additional studies were conducted to define the effects of cell seeding of integrally textured surfaces. A total of 28 experients have been conducted to date; 16 bladders were seeded with allogeneic fetal cells prior to implantation, and 12 bladders were unseeded, to serve as controls. In vivo trials of seeded surfaces have resulted in the formation of strong, cellular, and highly collagenous linings, with collagen contents varying between 31 and 65 percent. These lining contain viable cells and thus exhibit high cellular activity, as evidenced by postexplant cell culture techniques. This indicates that a living, viable pseudoneointima has been generated. On the other hand, control (nonseeded) linings do not produce significant amounts of collagen in their linings.

In addition to investigating means of integrally texturing the surfaces of Biomer bladders, we have also been studying alternative methods of integrally texturing the nonflexing, rigid metal surfaces of our blood pumps. Our studies have identified an unusually promising method, known as powder metallurgy (PM) surfaces, now in its sixth year of in vivo trials. The PM method involves sintering titanium spheres which are metallically bonded to titanium component substrates without the use of adhesives; this IT porous metal coating develops a thin, semitransparent, smooth biologic lining when implanted in experimental animals.

I. BACKGROUND

The National Heart, Lung, and Blood Institute (NHLBI) of the Department of Health, Education, and Welfare, established a program for the development of an artificial heart and related circulatory assist devices in 1964. An organized effort was initiated to develop implantable artificial heart devices to meet discrete clinical needs. Contracts were awarded to several contractors to conduct studies basic to artificial heart research and development. Targeted activities were multidisciplinary, combining the talents of surgeons, physicians, engineers, and chemists. The ultimate goal was to integrate developments in these areas in order to achieve a fully implantable, internally powered, temporary assist system that would have clinical application.

Such expectation has a sound physiological basis; of all major organs of the body, the heart performs only one function – pumping of blood. All other major organs perform a variety of metabolic and endocrine activities. By contrast, the heart can be viewed as strictly a fluid-moving device. Conceptually, an impaired natural heart could be replaced by a totally artificial device, if some major problems could be overcome.

Among the problems to be resolved were the manufacture of devices small enough to fit the anatomical constraints of the human thorax, the development of control consoles capable of anticipating cardiac cycle, and the manufacture of a prosthesis that is not only reliable and durable, but is also capable of overcoming the body's immunologic response mechanism and tendency to clot blood at the mere surface contact with any substance deemed alien to itself.

Thermo Electron was one of the original contractors selected by NHLBI to conduct artificial heart research, and has remained a leader in this field. After extensive testing involving laboratory animals, major advances in hardware design and a breakthrough in the development of blood-compatible surfaces culminated in the approval of Thermo Electron's Left Ventricular Assist Device (LVAD) for clinical use. Major impetus for these clinical trials came from statistics compiled by the American Heart Association, which show that more than 500,000 Americans die each year of heart disease, 180,000 under the age of 65.

A substantial fraction succumbs because of inadequate cardiac function. Many of these individuals have otherwise intact organ systems and cannot be helped by current or projected methods of conventional medical and surgical treatment. A portion of these patients could be saved by mechanical intervention; it is for this patient population that circulatory assist and artificial heart devices are intended. Because death and disability from heart disease are most commonly due to the pumping inadequacy of an infarcted left ventricle with the remainder of the heart providing sufficient function, an effective LVAD was considered a major priority at Thermo Electron. Other research groups, both in America and abroad, have focused their attention on total heart replacement.

For a left ventricular device, the period of intended application may be expected to range from just a few hours up to permanent implantation. For some patients, the vicious cycle of cardiac inadequacy (i.e., failure of the heart to nourish itself leading to myocardial infarction). might be reversed in a matter of hours or days, and only temporary or short-term circulatory systems would be needed. In other cases, where heart disease may be so advanced and extensive that adequate myocardial healing proves impossible, a permanently implantable device might be used.

This investigation was specifically designed to develop blood interfaces suitable for long-term (>2 years), or permanently implanted, LVADs. One of the most challenging problems in the biomaterials field is to devise a surface that overcomes or accommodates the tendency of blood to clot upon mere physical contact with a foreign surface. Clearly, if a device is intended to pump blood, it must somehow bypass or minimize the phenomenon of thrombogenicity.

Polyurethanes can be made nonthrombogenic, if their surface is devoid of microscopic imperfections. Imperfections on the order of 1 to 2 microns are recognized by platelets, thus triggering the coagulation cascade. The difficulties involved in the manufacture of totally defect-free surfaces led Thermo Electron to a new approach: flocking all blood-contacting surfaces with precision-cut polyester fibrils that would encourage the formation of a biological lining.

Although the precise mechanism of pseudointima formation is not totally understood, a large body of knowledge has been accumulated over the years, which allows some explanation of kinetic events. There is general agreement that certain plasma proteins coat the surface of any substance exposed to blood. This conditioning monomolecular layer is deposited within seconds, and greatly influences subsequent occurrences.

The plasma proteins found to absorb on the surface of polyurethanes are gamma globulins, fibrinogen, and albumin. In some cases, where albumin is preferentially adsorbed, the surface undergoes a passivation process, remaining in a state of dynamic equilibrium. In other cases, where fibrinogen is adsorbed, it undergoes polymerization to fibrin, attracting platelets, which leads to thrombus formation. Adsorption of plasma proteins onto polymeric surfaces is currently an area of intense scientific investigation.

When a flocked surface is exposed to blood, there is little doubt that plasma proteins are adsorbed onto each polyester fibril. Within several minutes, platelets adhere and agglomerate in the interstices of the flocked matrix. Shortly thereafter, a sticky network of fibrin is deposited between the platelets, attracting and retaining circulating erythrocytes and leukocytes. This process continues until all the exposed fibrils are covered. This initial thrombus is capable of flexing for several weeks, and since it was derived from the blood itself it is nonthrombogenic. After two or three months, fibroblasts spontaneously penetrate the lining, colonize, and begin to synthesize collagen. With the passage of time, collagen slowly replaces fibrin; this maturation and organization results in a more stable pseudoneointimal lining.

II. INTRODUCTION

Blood compatible materials are essential to circulatory support devices; many of the crucial requirements for a material to be considered satisfactory have been discussed in a number of review publications [1,2,3,4]. Numerous materials have been considered for use in prosthetic devices. These have been classified into five broad categories: (1) synthetic materials, such as ionic, polarized, or neutral polymers and pyrolytic carbons; (2) synthetic materials with additives, such as heparin and biolized surfaces; (3) hydrogels; (4) textured surfaces, such as flock, velour, and microfiber scaffold; and (5) composite-based, or combinations of the above.

In our early work (1968) with assist pumps, flexible bladders were fabricated with molded smooth silicone rubber with no surface treatment. Five animal pump experiments were conducted with this type of surface; and within three to five days, the surface was covered with a progressively thickening layer of thrombus (despite anticoagulation) [5]. These discouraging results prompted investigations of surfaces that promote formation of a biological interface.

The previous efforts of Liotta, DeBakey, and coworkers, who utilized velour cloth to promote growth of an organized fibrin layer, provided a basis for our initial work [6,7,8]. Our approach consisted of lining the integral blood-contacting surfaces of the pump with precision-cut polyester fibrils to promote the formation and adhesion of a thin fibrinous coagulum.

Pump bladders, flocked with polyester fibrils, demonstrated impressive performance in eliciting a stable biological lining that provides the desired biocompatibility. The fibrin coagulum that initially covers the polyester fibrils gradually organizes and is eventually covered, in part, with a cellular layer. However, flocked bladders are not without inherent limitations; during pumping, the bladder undergoes constant flexing and subjects the adhesively bonded fibril matrix to continual distortion forces. It is logical to anticipate possible failure of this bond in long-term chronic applications. To circumvent this problem, it was felt that textured surfaces integral to the bladder material would allow a matrix bed for biologic deposition and avoid separation by having a surface with the same modulus as the base material.

The concept of an IT surface promises to overcome the limitations of adhesively bonded flocked bladders, while retaining the fundamental advantages of the conventional flocked surface. We recognize that other textures may be equal to, or better than, the flock replica topography; however, the flocked surface concept represents a known quantity that has consistently proven successful and, in addition, provides a well-characterized reference control for measuring the suitability of a newly developed blood interface. During the past four years we have pursued the development and refinement of Model 11 Biomer bladders with IT surfaces; the effort has been quite successful and we are routinely fabricating prototype IT Biomer bladders from negative-replica silicone rubber mandrels.

Studies conducted over the past ten years have shown that pseudoneointimal lining develop on both the static and flexing surfaces of implantable vascular prostheses [9,10]. The deposition of circulating blood elements is seen initially. Early in the maturation process, an organized fibrin layer develops. After a few weeks, occasional areas of spontaneous cellular proliferation and in situ collagen synthesis may be observed. However, this process proceeds at a slow and unpredictable pace. In an effort to accelerate development of a thin, collagenous, organized cellular interface, we have conducted a series of experiments seeding Model 11 IT Biomer bladders with cultured bovine fetal cells. These allogeneic cells were selected not only because of their rapid reproduction in vitro, but also because their primitive nature apparently does not provoke an adverse immunologic response in recipient animals. When implanted, cell-seeded Biomer bladders form thin, strong, highly collagenous, biologic linings. We consider the formation of pseudoneointimal linings composed largely of native collagen to be a highly desirable event, since it represents an end stage in the intravascular healing process.

A similar sequence of events takes place when a PM surface is implanted in the blood stream. Sintered PM surface is utilized on all rigid blood interfaces of the artificial heart; i.e., the apical inlet tube, and both inlet and outlet conduits. Immediately post-implantation, a thin layer of thrombus forms within the porous structure of the PM surface and, after several weeks organization, collagenization and pseudoendothelialization progressively transform the fibrin thrombus into a living biologic lining closely resembling the inner surfaces of natural blood vessels.

Thus, the concept of a porous hemocompatible interface is used in both flexible and rigid components. For applications requiring flexibility, such as the polyurethane bladder, polymeric interdigitating fibrils compose the interface; for rigid pump applications, a sintered porous titanium composes the preferred blood surface. Since no adhesives are utilized in the fabrication of these two topographies, and since the entire cross section is composed of the same material, we call these interfaces integrally textured (IT) surfaces.

Table 1 presents a list of materials used in the fabrication of IT bladders and PM surfaces.

Table 1. Materials

- Biomer - A linear, segmented polyether-based polyurethane; Ethicone, Inc., Somerville, N.J. The polymer is used as recieved, with no further chemical modifications.
- DiMethyl Acetamide - Solvent for Biomer; used to dilute incoming Biomer solution to usable viscosity; spectrophotometric grade; Aldrich Chemical Co., Milwaukee, WI.
- Silastic J RTV - Two-component silicone rubber; Dow Corning Corp., Midland, MI.
- Methylene Chloride-Phenol - 30 percent solution, reagent grade; used as solvent for nylon monofilaments; Anachemia Ltd., Montreal, Canada
- Nylon Monofilaments - 3 denier, specially finished for electrostatic flocking; C-Labs, Inc., Somerville, Mass.
- Ti-6%Al-4%V spheres - Nuclear Metals Inc., Concord, Mass.
- Hydroxyethyl Cellulose (Hec) WP-09-L Union Carbide Corp., Needham Heights, Mass.
- Acationox - nonionic metal free detergent, Scientific Products, Cat #SP-101.
- Sodium Sulfate, anhydrous - Fisher Scientific Co., Fair Lawn, N.J.
- Aluminum Potassium Sulfate - Fisher Scientific Co., Fair Lawn, N.J.
- Sodium Carbonate - Fisher Scientific Co., Fair Lawn, N.J.
- Leomin KP Type F - Fatty acid amide quarternized with dimethyl sulfate; American Hoeschst Coventry, R.I.

III. FABRICATION OF FLEXIBLE INTEGRALLY TEXTURED (IT) SURFACES

A. Integral Textures on Planar Surfaces

We have pursued the development of aortic grafts and bladders possessing an IT surface, which is a high-fidelity facsimile of the present flocked surface. We first developed the technique to produce a flock-like texture on a planar surface, and then addressed the considerably more difficult problem of duplicating this texture on the inside of a curved surface, which is necessary to produce a bladder master mold. The effort has been quite successful and we have been able to produce flock replicas from silicone molds with IT surfaces.

In order to develop an appropriate process for the manufacture of IT surfaces, a chronological approach was undertaken. The effort was divided into three sequential steps: flat sheet production, straight cylinders for aortic graft production, and complex bladder shapes. The manufacturing process is shown diagrammatically in Figure 1.

Initial efforts used randomly flocked surfaces as masters from which transfers were made, and these produced rather poor quality IT surfaces. These masters produced a rough surface, but it was almost devoid of fibrils. This was understandable, as the random fiber orientation did not lend itself well to demolding. Using transfer molds made from electrostatically flocked

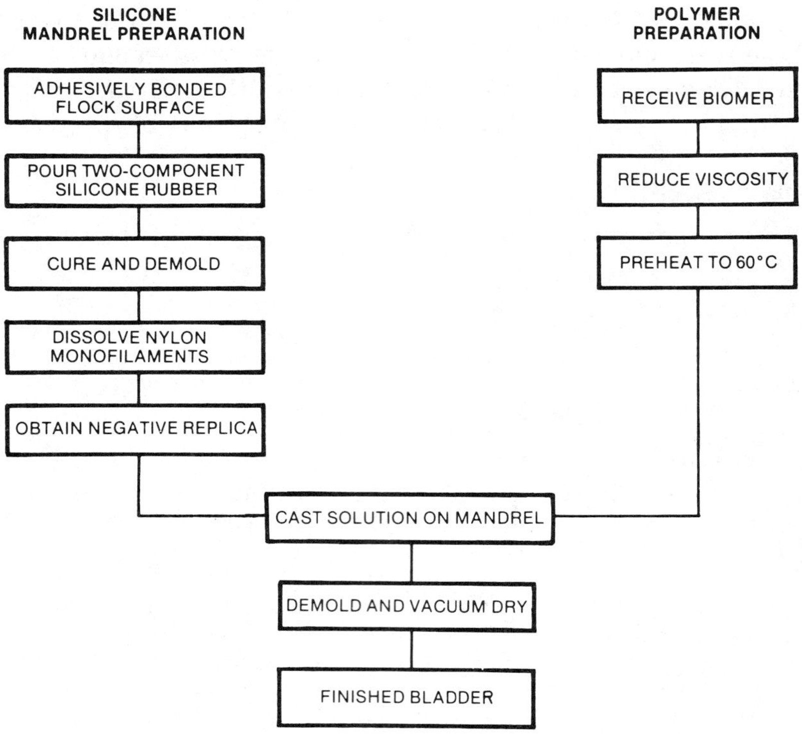

Figure 1. Diagram of fabrication process for producing integrally textured surfaces.

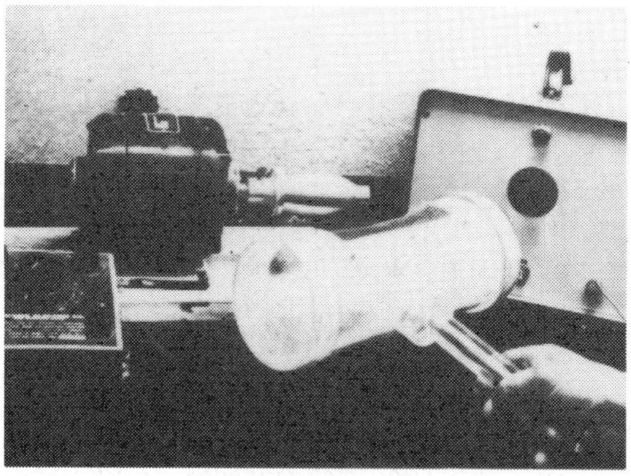

Figure 2. Electrostatic flock applicator for planar surfaces.

surfaces gave significantly improved results. Figure 2 depicts the apparatus used for electrostatically flocking planar surfaces; shown are the flock applicator and the variable high-voltage control module.

Using this apparatus, an electrostatically flocked flat sheet master was manufactured. Silicone rubber was poured onto this surface and allowed to cure for 24 hours. The parts were separated, and the silicone transfer mold was immersed in a 50-percent solution of phenol in methylene chloride to dissolve any residual, embedded, polyester fibrils. Such a test sheet is shown in Figure 3. The surface characteristics of this flat sheet are illustrated in Figures 4 and 5, with the negative-replica topography plainly visible. The deep holes represent the spaces previously occupied by the fibrils before being dissolved.

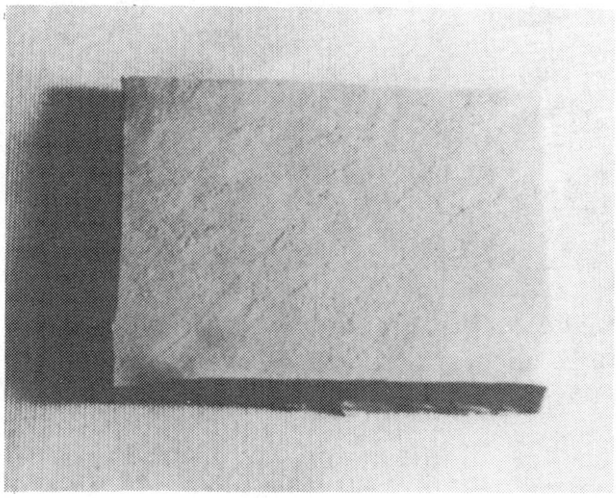

Figure 3. Flat silicone rubber transfer mold obtained from an electrostatically flocked master sheet.

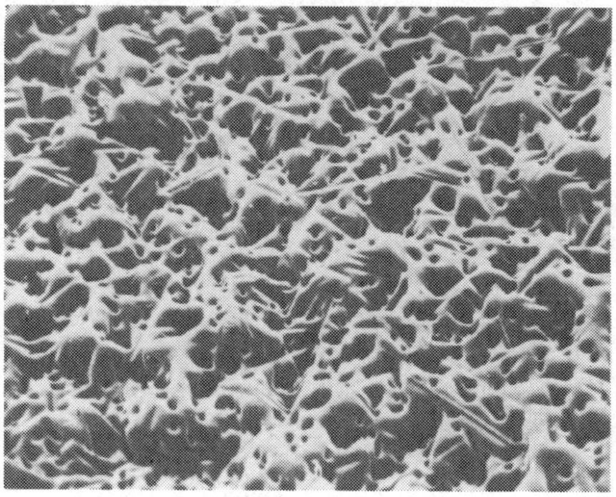

Figure 4. Surface morphology of flat silicone rubber transfer mold.

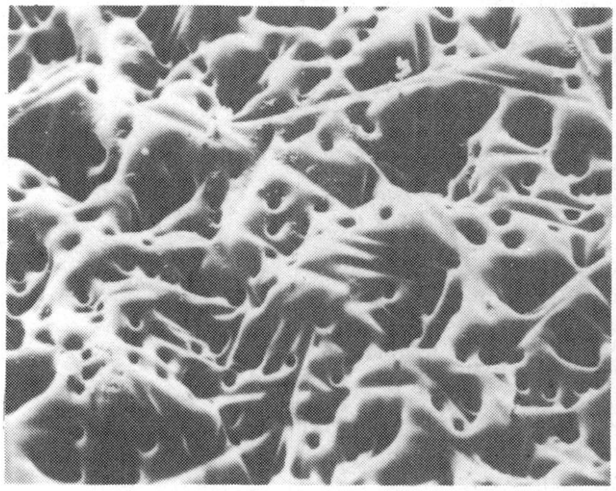

Figure 5. Surface morphology of flat transfer mold.

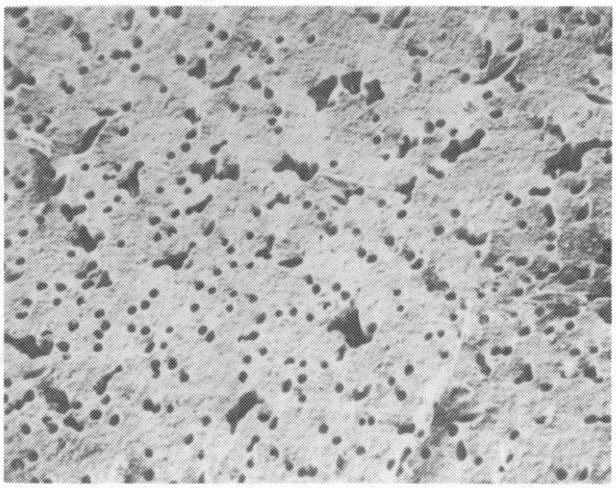

Figure 6. Section of flat transfer mold showing perpendicular aspect of fiber orientation.

One of the most desirable characteristics being sought in electrostatically flocked masters is the ability of the electrical field to orient fibers perpendicular to the surface. To ascertain if this property was indeed being met, part of the surface was cut away, exposing the underlying matrix. Figure 6 clearly shows the parallelism of the pores. This condition mirrors the original alignment of the electrostatically flocked fibrils.

One last question that remained to be answered at this juncture was whether the phenol solution would completely dissolve the embedded fibril. Figure 7 demonstrates the thorough

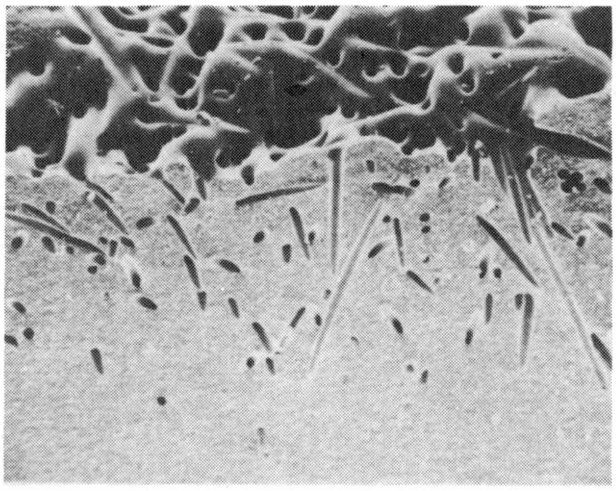

Figure 7. Section of flat transfer mold showing complete solvation of residual polyester fibrils within mold. Note that there are no traces of polyester to the extreme depths of the pores.

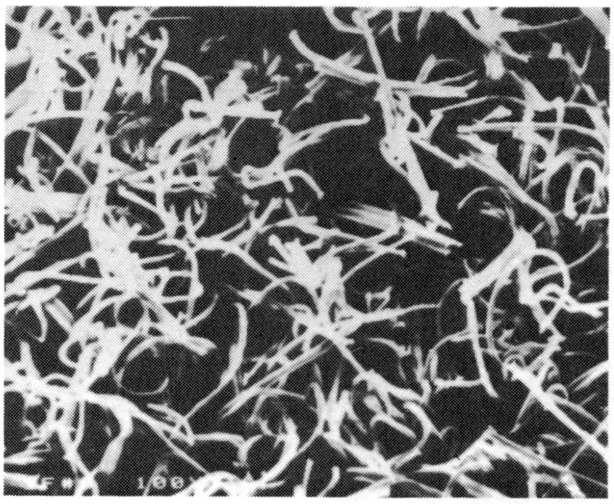

Figure 8. The topography of an integrally textured surface, showing the interlocking fibrillar network similar to conventionally flocked surfaces.

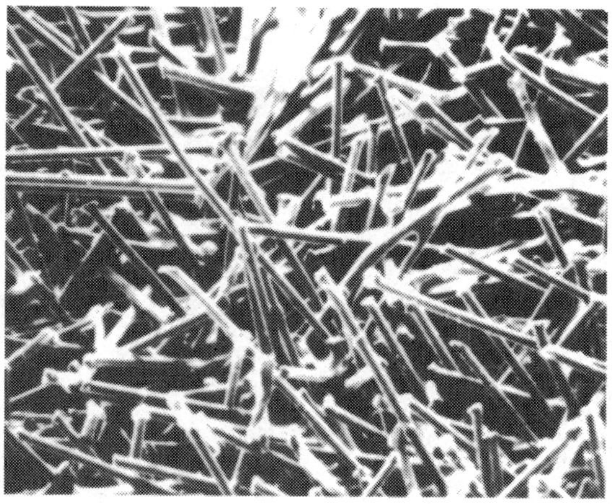

Figure 9. Characteristic photomicrograph of a conventionally flocked surface.

solvation and removal of the polyester fibril to the innermost depths of the pores. No trace of fibril is discernible in the photomicrograph.

IT surfaces obtained from this flat transfer mold were highly encouraging. A typical result is shown in Figure 8. As shown, the resultant surface topography assumes an interlocking fibril network similar to conventionally flocked bladder surfaces. For comparison purposes, Figure 9 presents a characteristic photomicrograph of a conventional bladder. The structural analogy between these two surfaces is readily apparent.

B. Integral Textures on Straight Cylinders

Having been successful in reproducing flock-like textured surfaces on flat sheets, we next proceeded to develop a technique suitable for electrostatically flocking the inner surface of straight cylinders. Application of fibers by electrostatic methods to cylinders presents some problems not encountered with flat surfaces. The diameter of the cylinder limits the distance between electrodes, which is an important control parameter normally used in electrostatic coatings.

Efforts were directed at the production of masters with controlled flock density and perpendicular fiber orientation relative to the material surface. To accomplish these goals, an innovative electrostatic method was evolved. The process consisted of machining a split brass housing in the desired configuration. The housing is secured on a lathe and the unflocked surfaces masked prior to application of an epoxy adhesive.

The epoxy adhesive was specifically designed to exhibit good adhesive qualities to the polyester fibrils, while maintaining a long, open tack. The solid contents are adjusted to 8 percent nonvolatiles, ensuring a mixture of sprayable viscosity, approximately 400 cp. As it is turned on the lathe, the adhesive is lightly sprayed inside the housing, using an airbrush. Flock is next applied to the interior of the housing using a specially designed applicator, in a high-voltage field. The entire apparatus is shown in Figure 10. This method proved eminently satisfactory, yielding high reproducible results from trial to trial.

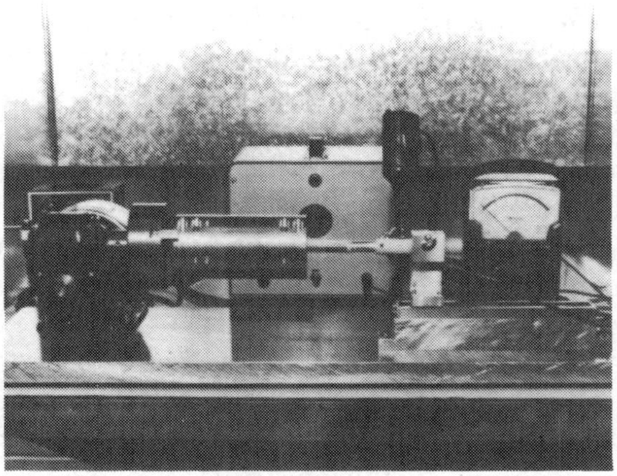

Figure 10. Electrostatic flocking apparatus for cylindrical molds.

Another question centered on the correct flock finish. Flock suitable for electrostatic flocking must meet certain critical requirements to ensure a suitable surface. Precision-cut monofilaments must be surface treated with antistatic agents to maintain their surface conductivity within narrow limits; empirical determinations showed that a resistivity of between 10^8 and 10^9 ohm-cm was necessary. In addition, a proper finish is also required to enhance siftability and to prevent agglomeration during processing.

Commercially available monofilaments used in flock production are invariably surface coated with a complex mixture of fatty acids and silicones designed to provide lubrication during stitching and looming. This finish must be completely removed and a new finish applied so the flock will "fly" correctly within the electrostatic field. Failure to obtain a suitable finish results in an unsuitable master mold, since the monofilaments will be randomly oriented.

The stripping procedure consists of adding 120 grams of precision-cut flock to 2 liters of boiling wter, maintained at a pH of 10 with sodium carbonate; proper wetting and dispersion of the monofilaments is ensured by continuous mixing, and the addition of 0.5 milliliter of a surfactant such as acationox. The slurry is stirred for 40 minutes.

The slurry is next allowed to decant for 15 minutes without stirring, with the turbid supernatant decanted. One liter of deionized water is added, the slurry resuspended by stirring, and again allowed to decant. The operation is repeated several times until the supernatant fluid is clear; finally, the flock suspension is filtered through a Buchner vacuum funnel using Whatman No. 31 low ash filter paper. At this point the flock is free of incoming surface finish.

The electrostatic-grade finish is applied to the monofilaments by immersing the stripped flock in a bath consisting of 2 liters deionized water, 10 grams of fatty acid amide quarternized with dimethyl sulfate, 40 grams of sodium sulfate, and 3 grams of aluminum potassium sulfate. As in the previous operation, the bath is maintained at a pH of 10 and a temperature of 50°C, with continuous stirring for 30 minutes. The flock is then filtered on the Buchner funnel to remove most of the solution without washing. The wet flock is dried in an oven for 14 hours at 65°C and sifted on a U.S. Standard No. 30 sieve (28 mesh), to loosen agglomerated fibers.

At this point, a brief explanation of electrostatic flocking is in order. Electrostatic flocking is a process designed to electrically charge fibrils and make them adhere in a vertical position on a coating of adhesive, thereby producing an artificial suede effect.

In practice, the machine is fed with either a.c. or d.c. current. The current initially energizes the fibrous flock so that it forces the individual fibrils to orient in a vertical direction, along the lines of force of the electrostatic field between the operating electrodes.

At this point, a strong electrostatic field exists, having been obtained by flowing current between two parallel plates, with the force lines perpendicular to the adhesive layer. Under the influence of this electrostatic field, the precharged fibrils are driven vertically into the adhesive surfaces producing the desired suede effect.

Most of the successful electrostatic flocking methods now in use produce suede-like effects on flat surfaces. For our purposes, a technique had to be devised for electrostatically flocking the inner surfaces of bladder-shaped cylinders.

This seemingly simple requirement severely complicates the procedure. In this case, the bladder-shaped cylinder is one of the electrodes; the second electrode, traversing the entire centerline, must be machined at close tolerances to the same contour as the cylinder. That is, the gap between the inner electrode and the inner surfaces of the cylinder must be identical at all points.

First, the basic law of electrostatics known as Coulomb's Law must be obeyed. It states that the intensity of the field is inversely proportional to the square of the distance between the electrodes. True application of Coulomb's Law implies that a uniform force field is attainable only if the electrodes are parallel.

Second, since the flock is secured by an adhesive base, it assumes the thickness of the adhesive to be evenly distributed across the entire inner surface of the cylinder. Too little adhesive allows the fibrils to fall, whereas too much adhesive tends to orient the fibrils in a semivertical position, probably due to formation of a meniscus caused by surface tension.

A third, and probably most important factor, is the conductivity of the flock, necessary for electrostatic movement. Electrically charged fibrils lose their conductivity factor due to a loss of humidity in the discharging process. Therefore, it is essential that adequate moisture be maintained during the process. The humidity can be regulated by carefully formulating a suitable flock finish, and by storing the flock inside an environmental chamber.

Lastly, two general types of electrostatic machines can be used: alternating current (a.c.) and direct current (d.c.). With a.c. electrostatic fields, the fibers are oriented so that they stand on end, perpendicular to the adhesive. On the other hand, d.c. fields not only orient the fibers, but also accelerate them towards the adhesive to improve penetration. For this reason, a fibril finish specifically tailored for d.c. electrostatic flocking, was developed.

Another notable achievement was reached in the development of an acceptable demolding process. Having obtained a highly satisfactory electrostatically flocked master, we attempted to fabricate metal transfer molds. The molds were to be made by pouring molten Cerrocast alloy inside the master, demolding, and subsequently dissolving the polyester fibril; if accomplished, this method would result in a negative-replica metal transfer mold, with its attendant high dimensional stability, excellent heat transfer properties, and long serviceability.

Demolding thin polyurethane films from metal transfer molds proved unyieldingly difficult. The intricate topography of the negative-replica surface provided a high degree of mechanical interlocking. In addition, the urethane tends to be a natural adhesive to the metal surface. Metal molds, desirable for their dimensional stability and serviceability, proved unsuccessful. All attempts to demold thin polyurethane films from metal mandrels failed, even with the aid of parting agents. A good solution to this problem was found by switching to silicone-based masters. The silicone rubber transfer molds provided inherent release mechanisms because of their surface properties and ability to deform; consequently, the urethane film was able to be demolded with relative ease. Figure 11 shows a typical, cylindrical, silicone rubber mandrel obtained from an electrostatically flocked master mold.

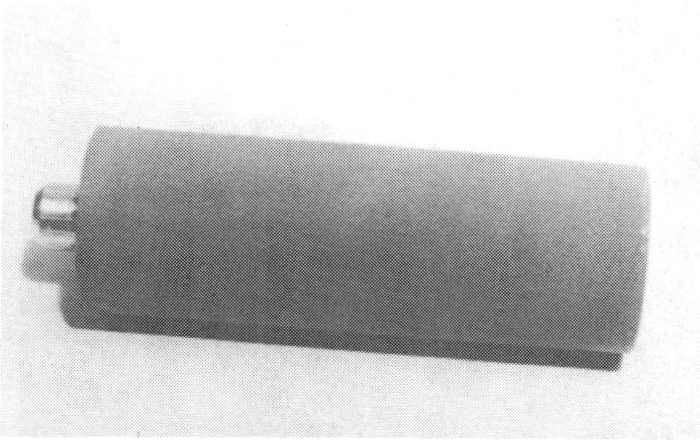

Figure 11. Cylindrical silicone rubber transfer mandrel.

C. Integral Textures on Bladder Shapes

Inner surfaces of split aluminum master molds were specially machined to match the complex shape of Model 11 axisymmetric bladders. Because the inner diameter of such master molds varies longitudinally, a special modification to the electrostatic coater had to be designed. The distance between electrode and mold profoundly influences flock density; the closer the distance, the higher the fibril density. To be useful, the inner surface of the flock master mold must exhibit a uniform flock density.

To accommodate this crucial requirement, a singular flock applicator was fabricated. Its length was such that it protruded beyond either end of the brass housing. A longitudinal window was machined and covered with a 20-mesh fiberglass screen. This allows for uniform flock release and reduction of clumps of flock. One end is equipped with a nonconductive acrylic holding fixture that was designed to be held in the tailstock of the lathe; this end houses one high-voltage terminal. The other end of the applicator allows for flock loading.

After loading the applicator with flock, the housing is rotated on the lathe at 30 rpm. A 5-kilovolt charge is applied. The applicator is then positioned within the housing orifice so that it projects from both ends symmetrically, with the window facing downward. The voltage is increased to 10 kilovolts, or just below arcing potential. Flock is continually released to the housing by activating an electric vibrator. The housing is periodically tapped manually with an acrylic rod in order to allow loose flock to fall back to the applicator and become repolarized. To better ensure even flock distribution, the applicator is manually moved in a reciprocating motion along its longitudinal axis. Once flocking has been completed, the housing and applicator are removed from the lathe.

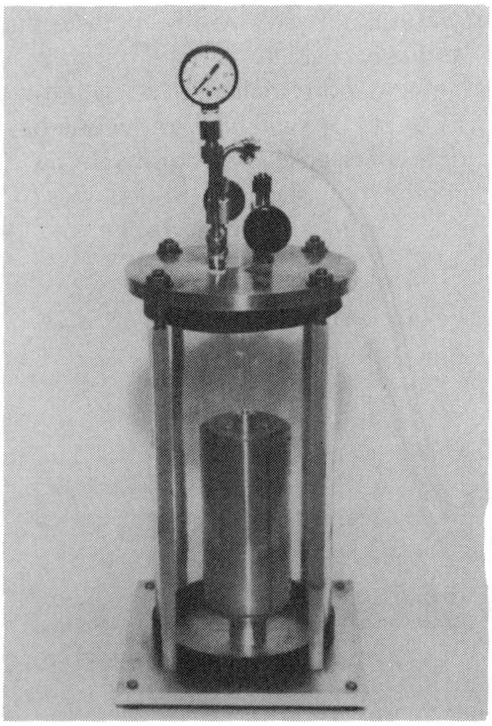

Figure 12. Vacuum chamber used for deaerating transfer molds.

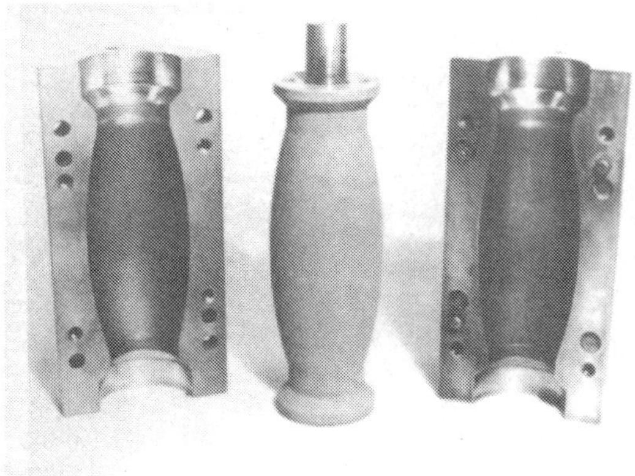

Figure 13. Silicone rubber transfer mandrel flanked by open halves of the brass master molds.

The electrostatically flocked housing is then ready for use in casting the room temperature vulcanizing (RTV) silicone rubber mandrel. The entire composite is deaerated simultaneously, ensuring complete penetration of the silicone between fibrils, as well as releasing any entrained air pockets in the liquid matrix. Figure 12 shows the vacuum chamber used for this purpose. Following cure of the silicone rubber, the mandrel is demolded. The remainder of flock

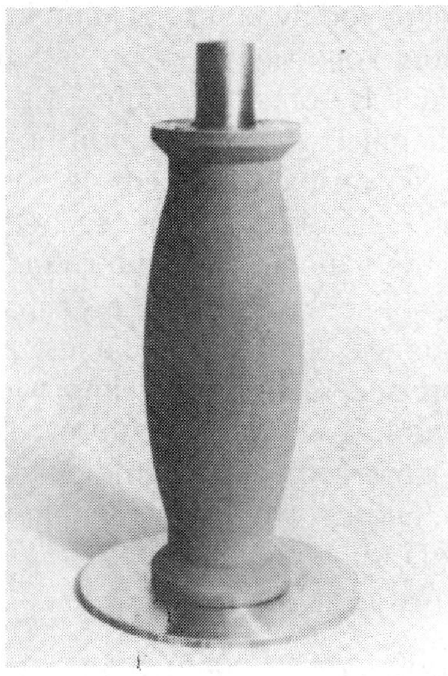

Figure 14. Closeup view of bladder-shaped transfer mandrel.

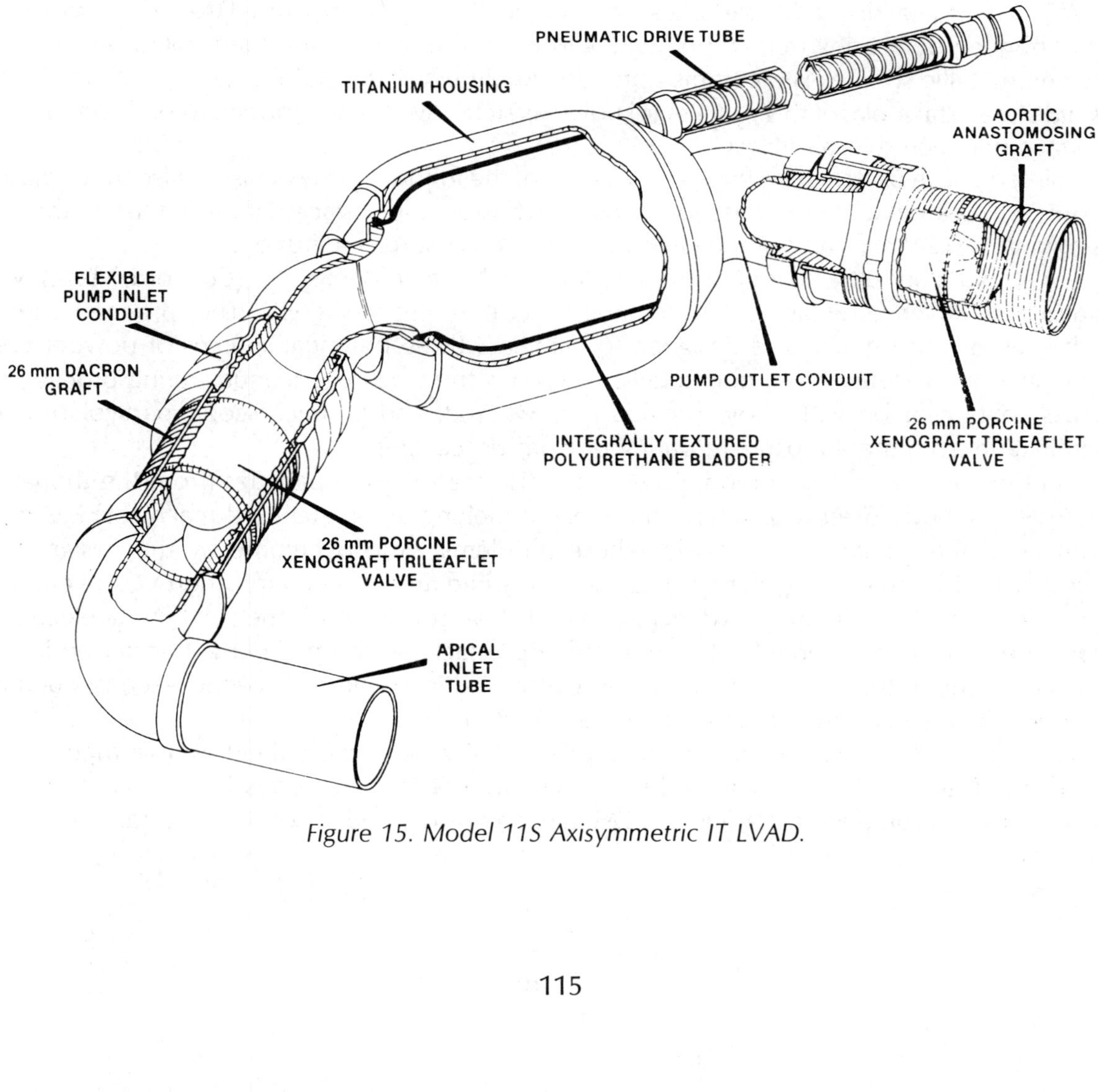

Figure 15. Model 11S Axisymmetric IT LVAD.

fibrils and epoxy adhesive are removed by ultrasonication in a 50-percent solution of phenol in methylene chloride for 48 hours. Following these procedures, a mandrel bearing a negative replica of the electrostatic flocking is obtained. Figure 13 presents an exploded view of the demolded mandrel, with the open halves of the master mold. Figure 14 is a closeup view of the silicone mandrel, ready for dip casting to obtain the desired shape and surface.

At this stage, the last experimental obstacle was reached. Although silicone rubber mandrels afforded easy demolding, the material proved too fragile to serve as a mandrel in continuous use. The mandrel is reusable only as long as it is capable of withstanding the abuse of rolling a tight bladder over its surface. Some of the earliest silicone mandrels had a tendency to tear during the demolding process. Considerable improvement was realized by switching to Dow Corning Type J silicone rubber, which possesses excellent physical properties. Silastic J mandrels have now withstood more than 50 demoldings without encountering a single failure. These silicone rubber mandrels are now routinely utilized in the fabrication of the Model 11S axisymmetric IT LVAD, shown in Figure 15.

IV. FABRICATION OF RIGID IT SURFACES

A. Powder Metallurgy (PM)

A Powder Metallurgy (PM) part is a shaped object that has been formed from metal powders and bonded by heating below the melting point of the major constituents [11]. Bonding between metallic spheres is a complex process during which several reactions – mostly in the solid state – take place; this process is known as sintering [12] (the formation of a common interface between two particles).

Sintering can be achieved by a combination of the following mechanisms: viscous or plastic flow, evaporation and condensation, volume diffusion and surface diffusion. Our method of sintering Ti-6%Al-4%V alloys appears to take place via surface diffusion.

We obtain our ultraclear titanium powder from Nuclear Metals, Inc. (Concord, Mass.) who utilize an advanced plasma arc rotating electrode process (REP). This process, shown schematically in Figure 16, is designed to eliminate three potential sources of powder contamination: (1) metallic and nonmetallic inclusions from powder manufacturing process, (2) cross contamination with alloys previously powdered, and (3) microscopic particulate contamination from the atmosphere during powder processing.

In the past, metallic inclusion, particularly discrete tungsten particles (from the thoriated tungsten cathode used to establish the electric melting arc in standard machines) has contaminated the titanium REP powder; these problems were overcome by the design of a specialized REP chamber (Figure 17); another possible area of contamination was overcome by processing the titanium powders in Class 10 clean rooms. After the solid metal electrode rods are converted to powder in the plasma REP machine, the powder is transferred into a sealed vessel; further processing is always conducted in an inert atmosphere; consequently, the powders never come in contact with ambient air.

Excellent sphericity, uniformity and reproducibility can be obtained by this method, as shown in Figure 17A. Sphericity and uniformity are critical parameters in titanium powders, since many properties of the finished PM surface are dependent on these parameters (i.e., porosity, density, strength).

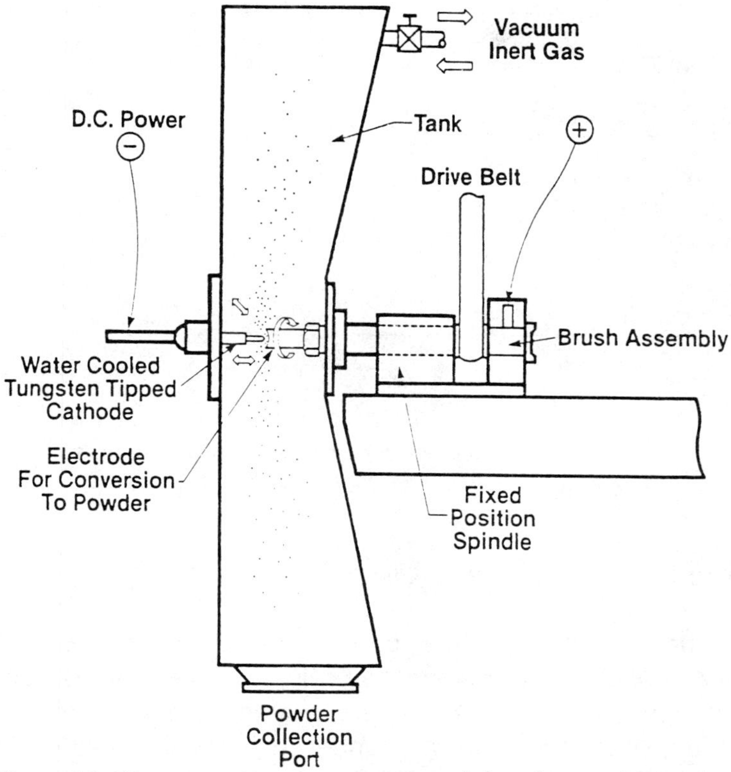

Figure 16. Diagrammatic representation of the plasma-arc rotating electron process. (Courtesy, Nuclear Metals, Inc.).

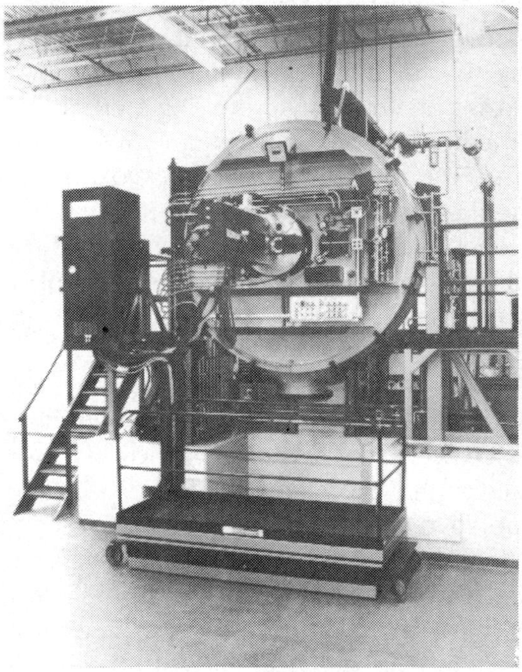

Figure 17. Specialized chamber for the production of titanium spheres. (Photo courtesy, Nuclear Metals, Inc.).

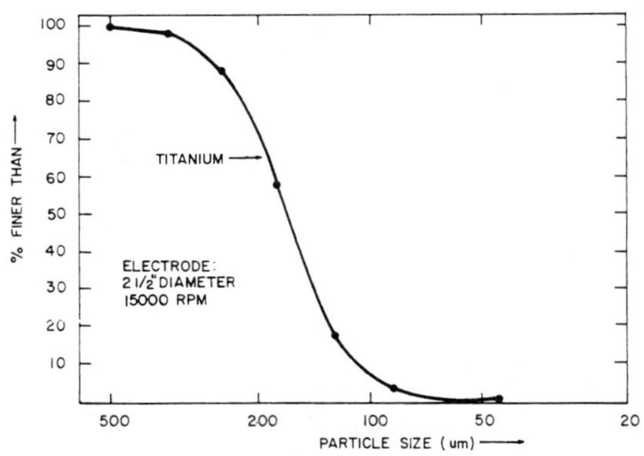

Figure 17A. Size distribution of REP Ti alloy powders.

B. Texturing of Rigid Metallic Surfaces Using PM Technology

Flocked surfaces have traditionally been used at Thermo Electron as a means of obtaining blood compatibility through the formation of a thin, fibrin-cellular coagulum. Identical surfaces have been employed as the blood-containing interface of both flexible members (bladders) and nonflexible components (housing, connecting conduits) of our LVADs. Until recently, preparation of conventionally flocked surfaces required the use of reactive adhesives to bond the polyester fibrils to the substrates.

In addition to investigating a means of texturing the surfaces of Biomer bladders, we have also been studying alternative methods of texturing the nonflexing (metal) surfaces of our blood pumps. Concerning the texturing of nonflexing (metal) pump components, our investigations have been utilizing an unusually promising method, known as PM, now in its sixth year of in vivo trials. The method involves use of titanium spheres which are consistently and reliably bonded to titanium components without the use of adhesives (PM interfacing). Our involvement with PM surfaces began in 1976, when laboratory studies were conducted in an effort to reproduce the excellent results reported by McGregor [13] and Brest [14]. McGregor indicated that porous metal coatings permitted the development of a pseudoneointima when exposed to flowing blood in canines. A thin, semitransparent, smooth, continuous fibrous lining was routinely obtained.

Metal inlet and outlet conduits of the Model 11 LVAD were sent for PM preparation to the Ontario Research Foundation, the laboratory that developed the PM coating process used by McGregor. The assist device with the PM-coated elbows was subsequently implanted by Children's Hospital Medical Center (CHMC) on December 14, 1976 (Calf No. 528). The animal had an uneventful postoperative course, and was maintained on assisted circulation for 2½ months at a flow of 4.5 L/min. Elective sacrifice of the calf occurred on February 23, 1977. Anticoagulation with Coumadin (sodium warfarin) was maintained throughout the study (prothrombin time maintained between 20 and 26 seconds). Autopsy examination revealed no gross evidence of thromboembolic organ damage (thrombocytopenia) produced by the pump or PM surface. These encouraging results were reported by Poirier, Szycher, and Bernhard in 1978 [15].

The adhesion of individual particles to the underlying titanium substrate and to each other was satisfactory. The sintering process used in the fabrication of PM surfaces produces solid phase diffusion at the points of contact, and results in a three-dimensional, interconnected, honeycombed structure, with a luminal blood-contacting surface composed of titanium spheres (Figure 18). It is important to note that this surface is obtained without the use of adhesives, and is therefore integral with the substrate.

PM surfaces are envisioned as an ideal substitute for conventional Dacron flock on all metal surfaces. This interconnecting structure provides a strong mechanical interlock for the biologic lining; the structure can be expected to reliably withstand years of implantation, since only permanent metallic bonds are obtained.

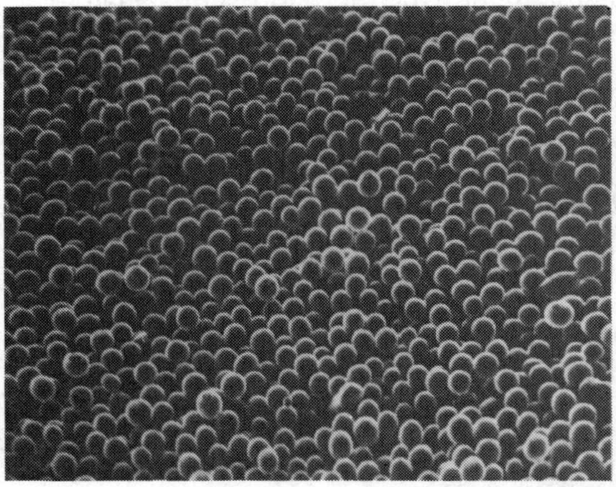

Figure 18. View of powder metallurgy surface integrally formed with sintered titanium spheres.

C. Fabrication of Prototype Pumps with PM Surfaces

To pursue the development of porous metal surfaces further, we have developed techniques for applying these coatings to the blood-contacting surfaces of the blood pump itself. In the standard PM process, fine granular powder is compacted under high pressure (60,000 psi) to obtain a desired shape. The compacted part is demolded as a semirigid component and, subsequently, heated to approximately 80 percent of its melting point. This heating cycle promotes crystal agglomeration (sintering) of the powder, and results in a fused solid structure. Modifications of this process are routinely used to fabricate commercially porous metal components. By careful selection of powder size and compaction pressures, porous components can be produced with varying densities for use as filters, mufflers, thermal insulating materials, and hydraulic dampening devices.

We have additionally modified this process to achieve a uniform porous coating on blood-contacting surfaces of rigid metal components. Spherical powdered metal is sieved to achieve the desired porosity, as predicted by the following expressions:

$$\text{Minimum Porosity} = 0.172\ r^2$$

$$\text{Maximum Porosity} = 4.172\ r^2$$

where:

porosity = void area
r = sphere radius.

The process developed at Thermo Electron results in a multilayered coating and a sintering operation in a single high-temperature cycle. Surface preparation proceeds as follows: the surface to be coated is prepared with a high-viscosity (>5000 cp) solution of hydroxyethylcellulose in dimethyl acetamide. Sieved titanium powder (Ti-6%Al-4%V) is dusted on the wet surfaces in a manner similar to the preparation of conventionally flocked surfaces, with excess powder removed by blowing dry nitrogen gas over the surface. Next, the composite is placed inside a furnace, and heated to 1250°C for 2 hours under a vacuum of 5×10^{-5} torr. This heating cycle completely vaporizes the hydroxyethylcellulose binder, and at the same time bonds the spheres at the points of contact by a sintering process.

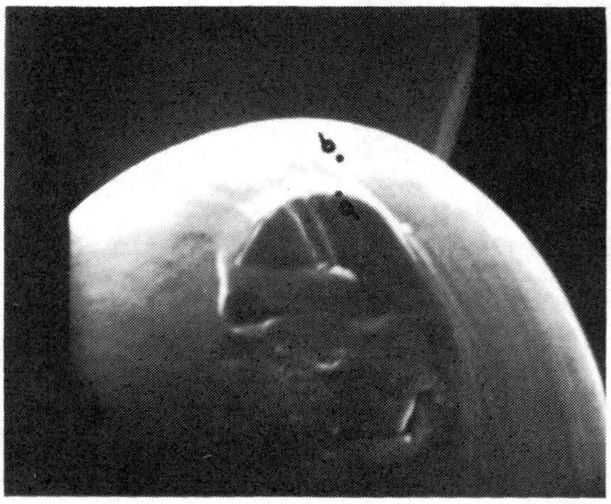

Figure 19A. Microprobe analysis of representative sphere. Point (a) – Fracture surface; Point (b) Sphere surface.

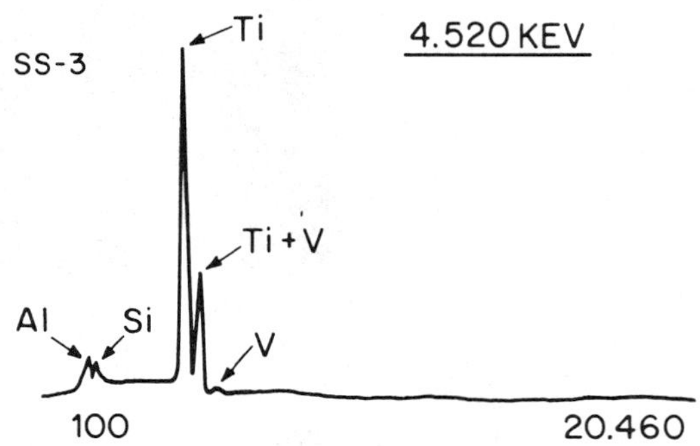

Figure 19B. Microprobe fingerprint of point (b), sphere surface showing characteristic. Titanium, aluminum, and vanadium peaks, as well as surface silicone contamination.

To verify that a true sintering process was indeed taking place, a section of PM surface was selected at random, and interstitial attachment between spheres and substrate was assayed by electron microprobe analysis. To accomplish this aim, spheres were forcibly detached from the underlying substrate, and the bonding material was analyzed using an SEM probe; the spheres themselves were analyzed at the same time, by probing a point adjacent to the bonded material. Results are shown in Figures 19 and 20, which indicate that the bonding material is composed primary of titanium and aluminum, with a reduction in vanadium content. The surface of the spheres, which in this case serves as a control, is composed of titanium aluminum, and vanadium, with some ubiquitous silicone contamination. From these results, we conclude that a true sintering process is occurring, and we are obtaining true metal-to-metal bonds within our honeycomb. A scanning micrograph of this bond is shown in Figure 21.

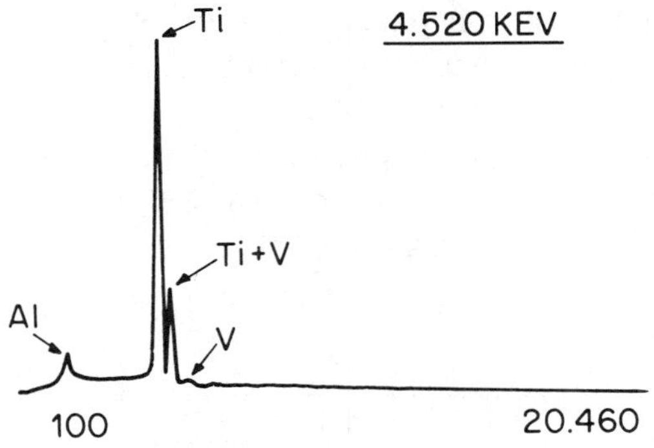

Figure 20. Microprobe fingerprint at point (a), fracture surface, showing an increase in aluminum concentration, and a small decrease in vanadium. This spectra clearly shows that a metallic bond exists between spheres, albeit at a slightly different composition than the surface alloy.

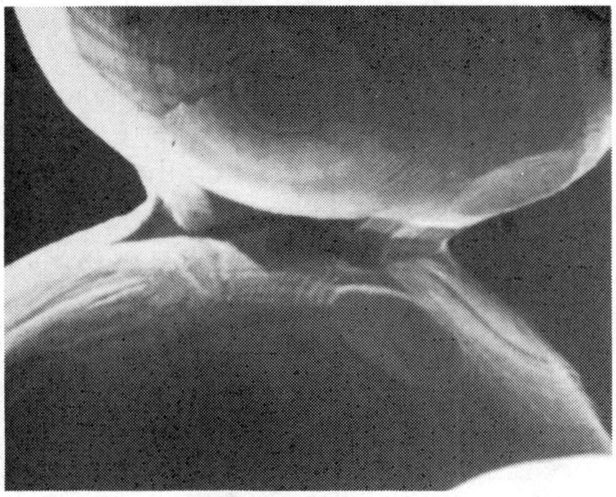

Figure 21.

D. In vivo Investigations Employing PM Surfaces

Encouraged by these results, a systematic evaluation of PM surfaces was initiated by fabricating titanium cylindrical conduits textured with PM blood-contacting surfaces for use as thoracic aortic grafts in calves. The basic design of the prosthesis is shown in Figure 22; the conduit was coated with a PM finish in two sphere sizes ranging from 44 to 74 μm. The interstitial matrices formed with the smaller particles exhibited equivalent pore diameters in the 10- to 85-μm-diameter range, whereas the larger spheres resulted in 35- to 180-μm-diameter pores.

Eight conduits were implanted in the descending thoracic aorta of calves by the surgical team of the CHMC Cardiovascular Laboratory. Four conduits were implanted in anticoagulated

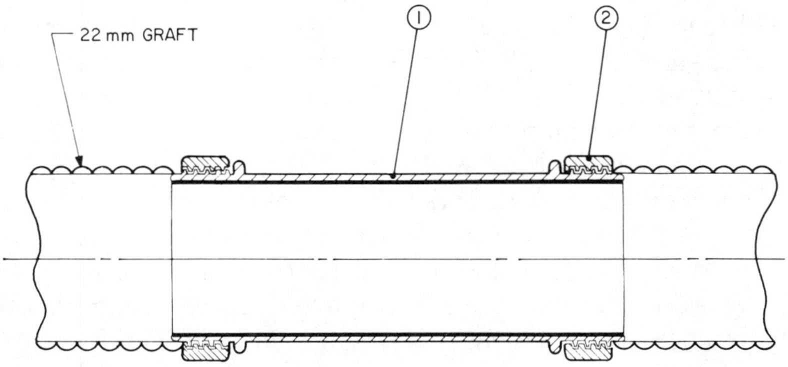

Figure 22. Cross section of aortic graft segment with PM-coated surface.

animals (sodium warfarin) and the remaining four were not anticoagulated (controls). Each subset was broken down into two sphere sizes with varying implantation periods. The results, shown in Table 2, confirmed our preliminary findings, indicating that PM surfaces provided a satisfactory anchoring for the PNI layer. All conduits remained patent throughout the experiments, and demonstrated that the PM coating did not damage the cellular blood components (platelets and erythrocytes) nor result in systemic embolization of fibrin segments.

Table 2. PM-Coated Conduits

Powder Size (μm)	Anticoagulated			Not Anticoagulated		
	Calf No.	Bond Strength (g/cm)	Duration (Day)	Calf No.	Bond Strength (g/cm)	Duration (Day)
44 - 74	T3	3 → 15	44	T15	5 → 22	51
44 - 74	T4	*	96	T16	*	116
149 - 420	T13	3 → 6	46	T7	12 → 38	37
149 - 420	T14	—	105	T8	8 → 35	119

*T4 was not evaluated because the bond was considered to be less than what was required to install the test sample into the tensile testing apparatus.

More recently, Whalen and Nose [16] presented an extension of these studies conducted at the Cleveland Clinic. In this report, the blood-contacting inner surfaces of the Model 12A PVAD were coated with a sintered titanium PM surface and implanted in a series of nine calves for short periods (10 to 56 days).

These surfaces were fabricated using 45 to 75, 75 to 150, and 150 to 225-μm-diameter spheres. In each experiment, the pump diaphragm employed was coated with a polyester fibril textured surface, which served as a control. The PM-surface PVADs were implanted in 90-kg calves, and pumped in a synchronous counterpulsation mode for the duration of the study. No postoperative anticoagulants were used, and three experiments were performed with each surface.

A comparison of the PM and polyester fibril surfaces is presented in Figure 23. The polyester fibril surfaces are randomly oriented, 75-μm-diameter fibrils of 320-μm average length, at a density of 100 to 150 fibrils/mm^2. The effective "mat thickness" of this surface is in the range of 200 μm.

Study of the PM surface has shown that there are several layers of spheres in the sintering coating, as shown in Figures 24 thru 27. The effective mat thickness of the PM surface obviously depends on the particle size; thus, it ranged from an effective thickness comparable to the fibril surface (in the case of the largest particle size surface, 150 to 225 μm to considerably finer for the 45- to 75-μm surface).

In the nine experiments that were undertaken, there was a relationship between PNI thickness and surface particle size. In order of increasing particle size range, the measured PNI thicknesses were: 70 to 220 μm, 70 to 400 μm, and 190 to 600 μm. Thus, as one might expect, the coarser the surface and the larger the effective mat thickness, the thicker the PNI deposition. The raw PNI thickness measurement data are given in Table 3. The raw data do not consider technical problems encountered, such as an obstructed inflow cannula, and the data spread within each sphere size is accountable if particular experiments are analyzed in detail.

While PNI deposition was minimal using the finest particle size surface, there was evidence

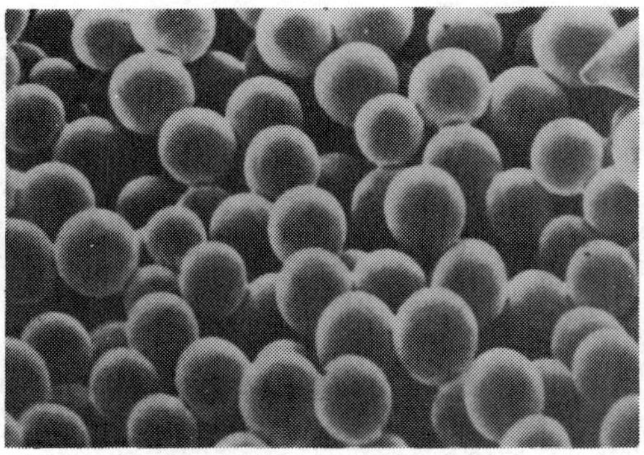

(a) PM surface as applied to housing.

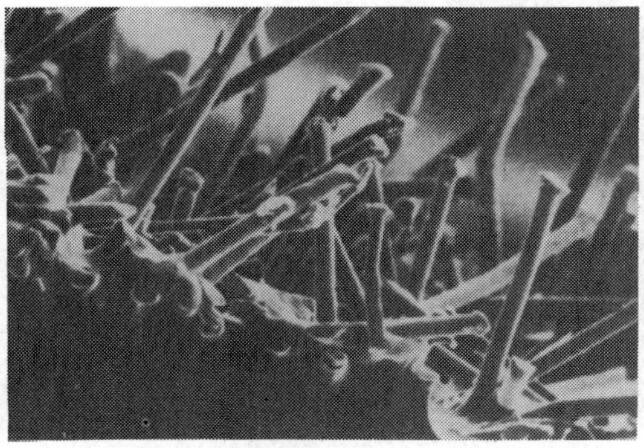

(b) Flock surface as applied to diaphragm.

Figure 23. An SEM comparison of the powder metal (PM) surface with a conventionally flocked surface prior to implantation.

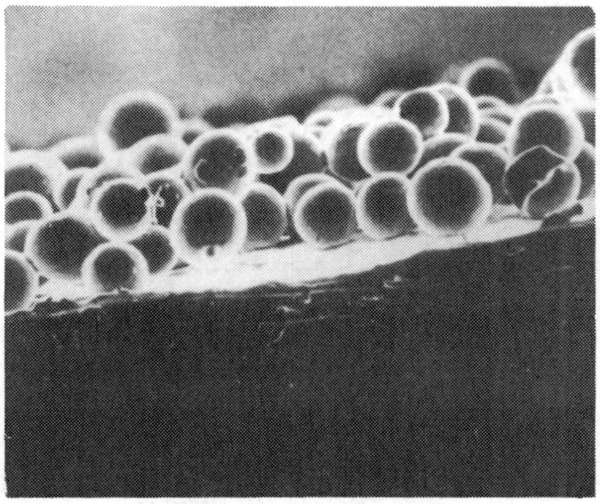

Figure 24.

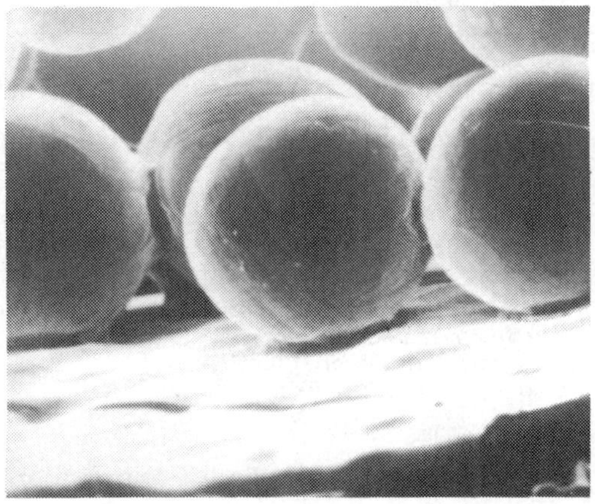

Figure 25.

of PNI detachment in two of the three studies with that surface. In addition, the PNI qualitatively was more easily detached from the PM surface with the smallest (45 to 75 μm) sphere size/surface than for the larger particle size surface. Accordingly, for application in a blood pump, the 45- to 75-μm sphere size surface does not appear suitable. On the basis of these results, the 75- to 150-μm sphere size surface was selected as the optimum choice among the size ranges evaluated, since it yielded satisfactory PNI attachment and produced a thinner lining than the surface composed of the largest spheres (150 to 225 μm).

It is apparent that PNI organization on the PM surface is different from that observed on conventional polyester fibril surfaces. It appears that the early fibrin coagulum on the PM surface entraps fewer red cells compared to the flocked fibril surface. This leads to a diminished

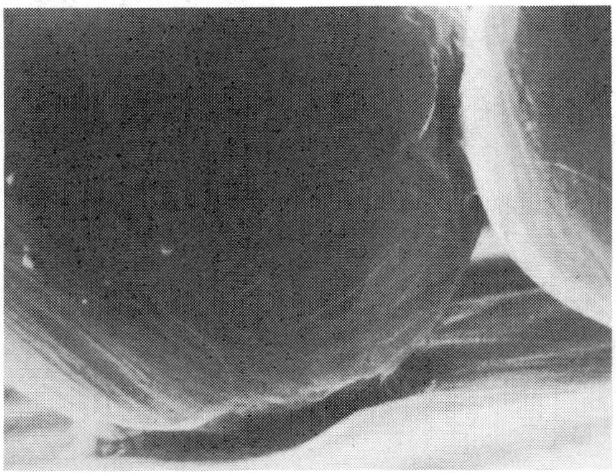

Figure 26.

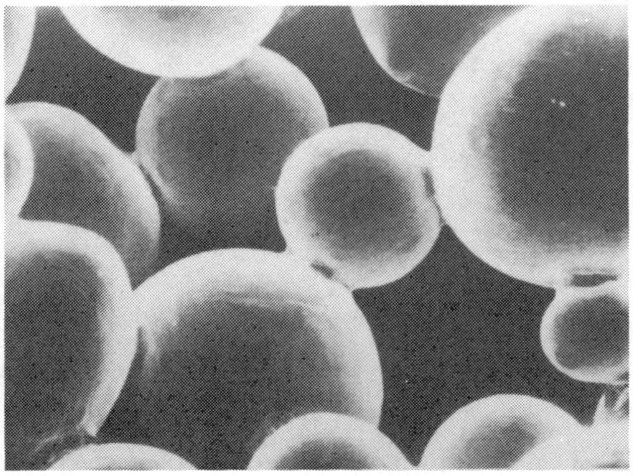

Figure 27.

Table 3. PNI Thickness Measurements

Particle Size	S: 45-75 μm			I: 75-150 μm			L: 150-225 μm		
Exp. Number (Time in days)	78295 (13)	78303 (23)	78313†† (41)	78304 (10)	78276 (37)	78260† (54)	78273 (7)	78292 (28)	78314†† (56)
PNI Thickness Housing	150**	70-220	70-240 (900)*	60-200	70-400	40-370	40**	196-600	50-250

*Fresh red blood cell deposition
**Only few measuring points
†80% inflow cannula obstruction
††Pump off >3 hrs, in first week of study

leukocyte reaction at the PNI/PM surface interface, since early organization of the PNI includes lysis or phagocytosis of damaged cells and debris. The result is that organization proceeds more rapidly, because initial cellular accumulation on the PM surface is less [17]. In this series of experiments, large mesenchymal cells appeared on the PM surface within 10 days, and areas containing fibroblasts and collagen synthesis were noted after 23 days.

With time, fibroblasts increase in number, and much of the original fibrin matrix is replaced by collagen. Eventually, the cell layer at the surface, morphologically, begins to resemble endothelial cells. These experiments emphasize that a stable, thin, and well-adhered pseudoneointimal lining is obtained by use of PM surfaces as blood-contacting interfaces.

E. Conclusions

In vivo experiments performed at CHMC and Cleveland Clinic Foundation of Artificial Organs are strongly supportive of the view that PM surfaces are a suitable interface for blood pump metallic components. The multiple bonds between individual spheres, and between spheres and substrate, result in metallic meniscus formation, producing a type of IT surface not subject to adhesive bond failure.

Thus, the concept of IT surfaces is being universally utilized in both flexible and rigid applications. Flexible applications include all Biomer components where the polymeric fibrils, as well as the underlying bladder wall, are made of one material: polyurethane. Rigid applications include titanium inlet and outlet conduits, titanium housings and, lately, we have also been using PM-surfaced apical tubes in all our heart assist pumps.

These studies indicate that PM surfaces exhibit excellent blood compatibility, resulting in the formation of thin pseudoneointimal linings on the nonmoving, metallic parts of blood pumps. This is not only due to its good blood compatibility, but also to the exceptional mechanical strength and durability of PM surfaces. Because of its inertness, desirable mechanical properties and good blood compatibility, titanium PM surfaces seem to be very promising materials for chronic blood pumps.

V. IN VIVO STUDIES

A total of 28 LVAD experiments have been conducted to date. The studies have been purposely divided into nonseeded (control) implantations and seeded experiments. Of these, 12 were nonseeded controls and 16 were seeded preoperatively with cultured fetal fibroblasts.

A. Surgical Procedures

Thermo Electron's Model 11S LVADs were implanted in calves weighing 80 to 90 kg. Preoperative medication consisted of atropine sulfate (0.6 mg) and morphine sulfate (8.0 mg), with anesthesia induced with sodium thiopental (Pentothal), and maintained with 1 percent halothane by means of a mechanical ventilator. Pump implantations were carried out through a left lateral thoracotomy incision in the sixth intercostal space, with placement of the device in series between the left ventricular apex and the descending thoracic aorta. The devices were pulsed asynchronously (70 bpm) throughout the experiments by means of an extracorporeal actuating system and stroke volume limiter to prevent overcollapse of the Biomer bladder.

Holstein calf recipients were initially anticoagulated with intravenous heparin (activated clotting time increased to a mean of 300 seconds) for three days, and subsequently maintained with oral sodium warfarin (Coumadin). Prothrombin times were prolonged to approximately twice the control time (22 to 28 seconds) and followed daily. Routine hematology and blood chemistry studies include hematocrit, white blood count and differential, serum sodium, potassium and chloride, blood urea nitrogen, serum creatinine, total bilirubin, platelet count, plasma hemoglobin, and mechanical fragility.

B. Cell Culture Techniques

Fresh Holstein fetuses of two to four months' gestation with the placental membranes intact were obtained from a local abbatoir. The material was prepared and draped in the operating room and the fetus was exposed through a short incision. Multiple connective tissue specimens were obtained, including sections of fascia overlying the chest wall musculature and a segment of ligamentum nuchae. Tissues were cleansed in Hanks balanced salt solution (HBSS) (Grand Island Biological Co., Grand Island, N.Y.), minced into specimens weighing approximately 1 gram, and plated in 10 percent bovine calf serum and Sevoian's medium.

Incubation at 37°C, in a humidified atmosphere at 5 percent CO_2, resulted in cell attachment within 24 to 48 hours. When a uniform monolayer developed, the cells from the primary culture were harvested and divided. For subculture, monolayers were washed with HBSS (without calcium and magnesium ions) to raise the monolayer pH to 8.0. Loosening of the layer was effected with a trypsin-ethylenediaminetetraacetate (EDTA) solution, which was then decanted. Sevoian's medium was added to the residual film to inactivate the trypsin and prevent cell lysis. The harvested cells were divided, replanted in the complete medium (5×10^5 cells/60 mm plate), and incubated. Doubling time in subculture was 24 hours.

C. Long-Term Storage of Cultured Fibroblasts

For long-term storage of cells, liquid nitrogen was utilized. Fetal fibroblasts obtained by the previously described procedures were pelleted out of trypsin-EDTA and suspended (at a concentration of 5×10^6 cells/ml) in F-10 medium supplemented with 10 percent dimethylsulfoxide and 20 percent calf serum. Cell aliquots (1.5 ml) sealed in glass ampules were frozen in a Linde BF4-1 controlled-temperature unit at a rate programmed to decrease the temperature of the freezing medium 1°C/min (from ambient 22°C to −65°C, followed by a rapid drop in temperature to −190°C). After freezing, the ampules were transferred in liquid nitrogen vapor and stored in a Linde Nitrogen repository at −195°C.

D. Fibroblast Seeding of IT Surfaces

Approximately 30-million cultured fibroblasts (from a single Holstein fetus) were pooled and suspended in 50 ml medium. A cell count was done on the suspension for an exact concentration figure and the suspension was transferred into the sterile polyurethane pumping chamber of an assist device. The chamber, assembled within a tightly sealed titanium housing, was rotated in a mechanical device for 3 hours at 6 to 8 revolutions per hour. Following rotation, the cell-seeded surface remained in the rotational device at room temperature (25°C) under sterile conditions until ready for implantation. At that time the culture medium supernate was drained away and collected to determine cell retention (cell count). A cell retention of over 60 percent provided a distribution of 360 cells/mm^2 and was considered optimum. Viability of the cells following rotation within the pumping chamber was checked by plating the residual cells returned and observing the growth pattern of subsequent passages.

E. Summary of Implantations

Tables 4 and 5 present a summary of experiments conducted to date. The following paragraphs describe the in vivo studies.

Calf No. 541

LVAD implantation in Calf No. 541 was carried out on May 26, 1977 without difficulty. The animal did well postoperatively for 32 days when it suddenly expired in the presence of a surgical technician who was cleaning the animal's stall. Autopsy examination did not reveal any evidence of thromboembolic damage to the parenchymatous organs. However, the animal was found to have an extensive bronchopneumonia that had not been apparent

Table 4. Nonseeded (Control) Implantations

Calf No.	Days Bypass	Reason for Experiment Termination	Gross Appearance	Histological/Ultrastructural Assessment
552	21	Scheduled sacrifice	Thin, grayish-white lining	Mostly fibrin, interspersed with trapped blood cells
553	23	Elective sacrifice	Thin, smooth, grayish-white lining	Fibrinous coagulum, with enmeshed cellular elements
584	30	Scheduled sacrifice	Reddish membrane (2- to 3-mm thick), thinnest is middle portion	Loose fibrin, with entrapped erythrocyte and leukocyte
589	31	Scheduled sacrifice	Lining loose and thick (2 to 3 mm), maximum thickness at inflow/outflow annulus	Multiple layer of loose fibrin, with trapped round cells; abundant erythrocytes
590	31	Scheduled sacrifice	Reddish membrane; few foci of calcification	Fibrous lining consisting of up to 4 layers of different densities of fibrin
541	32	Thromboembolism	Bladder covered with thin (1 to 2 mm) lining	Layered fibrinous lining; highly edematous
564	38	Elective sacrifice	Thin, glistening layer; well attached	Highly cellular lining, composed of fibrin and collagen
585	39	Scheduled sacrifice	Lining loose and thin; some areas of bladder not covered with intima - spontaneous detachment	Layered, loose fibrin, weak foreign body - giant cell reaction. Edematous fluid throughout.
578	44	Scheduled sacrifice	Gray-brown membrane, thicker in outflow region; 3 flexion creases containing fibrin ridges (2 to 3 mm)	Fibrin deposition, diffuse calcification and moderate giant cell formation; focal infiltration at inflammatory cells
566	60	Elective sacrifice	Reddish-gray membrane covering surface (1- to 4-mm thick); two patches of gray-white tissue (1 cm) well adhered to bladder; some calcified nodules	Meshwork at mature fibrin, acellular; giant cell reaction at base; few elongated cells in a matrix of collagen (section from grayish-white patch)
576	61	Poor pump filling	Thickened layer of fibrin; areas of spontaneous pseudoendothelium	Multiple layers of dense fibrin meshwork; surface rough with multiple red cells and occasional round cells. Abundant material staining (+) for collagen, underneath white areas
567	69	Twisted outflow conduit with partial pump obstruction	Reddish-brown layer thickest in inflow and outflow area (2 to 4 mm), thinnest in central zone (1 to 2 mm)	Three layers noted: acellular basal zone; middle layer, fibrin; luminal zone cellular (monocytes, lymphocytes embedded in fibrin)

clinically. This pneumonitis and an acute glomerulonephritis were the causes of death in this case. Examination of the blood pump indicated that the bladder surface was covered with a layer of fibrin that varied between 1 and 2 mm in thickness. There were occasional ridges and irregularities present, but no definite flexion creases were observed. There was no evidence of pseudoendothelial formation. The inflow and outflow xenograft valves appeared to be in satisfactory condition, and the metal elbows were intact and free of gross thrombus. In summary, this animal died unexpectedly and suddenly; autopsy examination confirmed the presence of a severe pneumonia and kidney infection.

Calf No. 552

Pump implantation in Calf No. 552 was undertaken on November 2, 1977 and the animal was sacrificed after 21 days of satisfactory circulatory support. Autopsy examination revealed no evidence of infection or embolic organ damage. The pump bladder contained a thin, well-attached fibrin lining, and the inflow and outflow valves were free of thrombus and calcification. Microscopic examinations of the brain, kidneys, heart, adrenal glands, pancreas, liver, spleen, and lungs were within normal limits.

Table 5. Cell-Seeded Integrally Textured Surfaces

Calf No.	Days Bypass	Reason for Experiment Termination	Gross Appearance	Histological/Ultrastructural Assessment
571	36	Elective sacrifice	60 percent of surface covered with thin (0.9 to 1.2 mm) layer of gray-white tissue, fibrin comprising remainder	Three layers present: fibrin at base with some cellularity, comprised of fibroblasts, multinucleated giant cell; middle: collagen, acellular; luminal layer: cellular with flattened cells
605	47	Elective sacrifice	Thin (0.9 to 1.5 mm) lining, apparently well attached; smooth surfaced	Dense collagenous lining, containing many fibroblastic cells, predominantly oriented in a longitudinal fashion
604	54	Elective sacrifice	Thin (0.5 to 1.0 mm) lining; smooth surfaced	Collagenous lining, of unusually high fibroblastic cell density. A thin layer of fibrin covers the blood-contacting surface.
613	61	Elective - loss of bladder compliance	Surface lined with very thin lining	Large amounts of fibrin covering a collagenous underlining at the outflow end
582	74	Obstruction of inflow conduit (kinked Dacron graft)	Surface lined with white, strong tissue (1- to 1.5-mm thick); occasional foci of calcification	High fibroblastic activity with dense collagen deposition; giant cell reaction surrounding polymeric fibrils. Occasional acute and chronic inflammation
569	78	Air embolus due to flange separation	Lining thickened (2 to 3 mm) due to inflow valve obstruction	Thin collagenous lining near bladder; loose, layered fibrin on top (thrombus)
597	85	Poor pump filling; unsatisfactory blood flow through LVAD	Lining lifted from underlying bladder. Lumpy, irregular surface. Thick, poorly attached lining.	Very thick (6 mm) in some portions. Necrotic cells surrounded by dystrophic calcification.
587	111	Elective sacrifice	Biologic lining thin, smooth, and well attached, inflow and outflow valves calcified.	Three layers present: cellularity at base, round cells, fibroblasts and some ingrowth of collagen around polymeric fibrils; middle layer - loose collagenous network; luminal layer - multiple spindle-shaped cells oriented circumferentially.
558	123	Broken struts supporting inflow conduit	Thin, well-attached layer of grayish-white tissue	Three layers present, as above; collagen stain intensely positive, particularly near luminal surface. Good collagen infiltration around polymeric fibrils.
594	149	Elective - inflow obstruction	Thin collagen lining. Well attached.	Highly collagenous lining. On some thick areas (2 to 4.0 mm) evidence of dystrophic calcification.
591	150	Poor and irregular pump filling. Outflow valve calcified.	Thin (0.5 to 1.0 mm), but poorly attached lining. Scattered calcified areas.	Both ends (inflow and outflow) separated from bladder. Space filled with fibrin, platelets, red cells, edematous fluid and debris. Collagen near bladder, covered with fibrinous lining.
583	163	Wound infection	Surface covered with thin, white, glistening membrane (0.5- to 1.0-mm thick) throughout	Fibrous tissue with fibroblast-like cells at basal layer; occasional giant cells at middle and base - one calcific zone
579	240	Elective sacrifice	Surface covered with thin, grayish-white, strong, glistening lining throughout	Cellular collagenous tissue with spindle-shaped cells; excellent collagen infiltration around polymeric fibrils
586	270	Elective sacrifice	Bladder surface covered with thin, well-adhered, grayish-white tissue	Highly collagenous lining, interspersed with spindle cells, giant cells towards base
581	338	Elective sacrifice	Well-adhered, strong, glistening, thin lining (0.5- to 1.0-mm thick)	Highly collagenous lining; good collagen infiltration around polymeric fibrils. Luminal layer composed of multiple, spindle-shaped, flattened cells.
603	367	Elective sacrifice	Strong, glistening, thin lining (0.3- to 0.6-mm thick)	Collagenous lining; luminal layer composed of many elongated, flattened cells (pseudoendothelium)

Calf No. 553

The third implantation, Calf No. 553, was undertaken on November 7, 1977. This experiment was terminated after 23 days of pumping because of the development of an air leak at the inflow flange of the pump housing. The animal was in excellent condition at the time of sacrifice. Autopsy examination revealed no evidence of thromboembolic damage, and the pump bladder was covered with a thin, smooth layer of fibrin. The xenograft valves were entirely normal in appearance and there was no evidence of free thrombus within the metal elbows of the device. In summary, the experiment was terminated after 23 days due to a mechanical failure at the inflow flange of the pump housing.

Calf No. 558

A Model 11 pump was implanted in this animal on December 28, 1977. The textured surface had a mat thickness of 430 microns. This experiment was terminated after 124 days due to a mechanical failure. The supporting cage of the valved conduit separated at its welded points, causing obstruction of the inflow valve and inflow conduit. Examination of the pump bladder surface revealed a thin layer of grayish-white membrane which was well attached to the underlying textured surface. There was no loose thrombus on the bladder surface. The inflow valve conduit was kinked; this occurred when the protected cage separated at its welded points. The outflow valved conduit was satisfactory.

In summary, Calf No. 558 received a fibroblast cell-seeded pump bladder which was removed after 124 days of partial left ventricular bypass. A smooth, thin, fibrous membrane was well attached to the underlying textured surface.

Calf No. 564

Control pump implantations to evaluate the textured Biomer surface were initiated on September 12, 1978 in Calf No. 564. A Model 11 pump with inflow and outflow Dacron conduits containing xenograft valves was implanted in the left pleural space, and was pumped at rates of 60 to 70 bpm for 38 days (flows of 3.5 to 4.5 L/min). The experiment was interrupted because of a fracture of one of the protective struts on the inflow conduit. Kinking of the Dacron inflow graft occurred, which severely limited pump filling.

Autopsy examination revealed no evidence of infection or thromboembolic damage associated with pump implantation. Microscopic examination of specimens obtained from parenchymatous organs revealed only focal alveolar collapse in the left lung and interstitial inflammatory cell infiltrates in both kidneys.

Examination of the xenograft valves and the metal elbows containing flocked polyester fibrils was unremarkable. The valves were completely intact and the flocked elbows contained patchy areas of thin, adherent fibrin. The pump bladder was covered with a thin, adherent layer of reddish-gray material, and was sectioned for biochemical analysis and microscopic pathologic examination. To our surprise, amino acid analysis revealed that approximately 30 percent of the surface contained hydroxyproline, and the rest consisted of fibrin and blood cell derivatives. There was no elastin present.

Microscopic examination of the pump bladder lining revealed relatively dense bundles of collagen in the middle layer of what appeared to be a three-layer pseudoendothelium. The inner layer adjacent to the polyurethane fibrils contained a few giant cells in the region of the fibrils and a loose architecture of cellular debris and fibrin. No red cells were present in this area. The middle collagenous layer contained spindle-shaped cells that resembled fibroblasts or modified smooth muscle cells. The luminal surface of the pseudoendothelium revealed adherent white cells, predominantly monocytes.

Total thickness of the pseudoendothelial layer in the inflow section ranged from 500 to 550 microns; in the central section, from 320 to 500 microns; and, in the outflow section, from 800 to 920 microns.

This pump bladder specimen was superior in appearance to many other specimens we have seen in the past, even though the experiment was of relatively short duration. The unexpected finding of approximately 30 percent of the surface containing collagen was of considerable interest and may have been the result of spontaneous implantation of histiocytes from the blood circulating through the pump. In addition, connective tissue cells from the apical inflow area of the left ventrical may also have accumulated in the pump bladder at the time of pump implantation.

Calf No. 566

A second control pump implantation was carried out on September 22, 1978 in Calf No. 566. This animal was pumped for a period of 60 days, at which time it was subjected to elective sacrifice for blood interface examination. Autopsy examination revealed no evidence of infection or thromboembolytic organ damage. Microscopic examination of sections from parenchymatous organs was unremarkable. The xenograft valves and metal elbows of the pump were completely free from any thrombus accumulation.

Ninety percent of this bladder surface consisted of fibrin, with only a few small patches of spontaneously forming pseudoendothelium. The fibrin was mature in form and intermixed with small amounts of cellular debris, possibly derived from platelets.

The white patch from the control bladder lining contained elongated cells, with fibroblast-like morphology, embedded in a matrix of mature collagen fibrils.

In summary, this control bladder lining consisted of over 90 percent fibrin and cellular debris, with one small patch of pseudoendothelium. The thickness of the bladder varied from 1.0 to 4.0 mm in the central areas and was thicker in the inflow and outflow ends of the bladder. There were folds of thrombus on both the inflow and outflow ends and, in these areas, the thickness increased to approximately 5.0 to 7.0 mm.

This was a more typical control bladder interface consisting predominantly of smooth, relatively thick fibrin and one spontaneously formed patch of pseudoendothelium measuring approximately 1.0 cm in diameter.

Calf No. 567

A control pump was implanted in Calf No. 567 on September 22, 1978. This animal was maintained with Coumadin anticoagulation (as are all animals undergoing pump implantation), and was sacrificed on December 5, 1978 because of difficulty with pump ejection. A mechanical problem developed because of a twisted Dacron outflow graft, but the change in pump output was detected immediately after it occurred, permitting elective termination of the experiment before any interface damage could occur.

Autopsy examination revealed no evidence of infection or thromboembolic organ damage. The xenograft valves and pump elbows were in satisfactory condition, with no evidence of thrombus accumulation. Microscopic examination of the parenchymatous organs was unremarkable.

Gross examination of the pump bladder revealed a generally thickened fibrin layer over the polyurethane textured surface, with one (1.0 cm) whitish area of the bladder.

Histologic examination of the bladder surface was carried out in several areas to include the white patch of pseudoendothelium, and the more generalized area of fibrin covering the major portion (95 percent) of the bladder surface. The thickest part of the lining was found in the outflow area (4.5 mm), which consisted of fibrin and necrotic debris, with no organization by collagen fibrils. Special stain showed a few areas of calcification of the bladder here as well as in the inflow region. The thinnest portion of the fibrin lining was noted in the center (where the patch of pseudoendothelium was located), and this contained collagen fibers in addition to fibrin.

Pump Calf No. 569

Pump Calf No. 569 had a fetal fibroblast-seeded pump bladder. This animal was sacrificed on December 19, 1978 after sustaining a massive air embolus secondary to acute separation of the bladder flange for a distance of approximately 3.0 cm. Autopsy examination also revealed two fractured inflow struts protecting the xenograft valve, which kinked the Dacron graft and obstructed the inflow valve. This obstruction had existed for an undetermined period of time, probably extending over many days. Although autopsy examination did not disclose any thromboembolic organ damage, the pump bladder was filled with thrombus extending up to 1.0 cm in thickness.

Pump Calf No. 571

Pump Calf No. 571 received a Mode 11 device seeded with fetal fibroblasts. The animal was sacrificed because of poor pump filling after 38 days (pump flows of 3.5 to 4.5 L/min) on December 15, 1978. Although no definite point of obstruction was found in the pump system at the time of autopsy examination, the problem related to angulation of the inflow tube toward the ventricular septum. Of interest was the presence of a separation of the bladder flange in this device for a distance of 1 cm, a factor that would have abruptly terminated the experiment in another few days because of massive air embolization (as occurred in Calf No. 569).

Careful autopsy examination did not disclose any evidence of infection or thromboembolic organ damage in this calf. Microscopic sections of parenchymatous organs revealed only focal interstitial lymphocytic infiltration in the kidneys. Gross examination of the pump bladder disclosed large areas of thin, grayish-white tissue attached to the polyurethane fibrils, in addition to patchy areas of thin fibrin. Approximately two-thirds of the pump bladder consisted of the grayish-white lining material, and one-third of a reddish-brown fibrin layer.

Histologic examination of the specimen was carried out, and three layers were observed within the pseudoendothelium, with the part adjacent to the polyurethane fibrils consisting of both fibrin and loose collagen fibers. There were also occasional giant cells present. The middle layer consisted of very dense collagen fibers, with occasional spindle-shaped fibroblast-like cells. The innermost luminal area was extremely cellular, showing spindle-shaped fibroblast cells as well as multiple round cells. The cellular lining toward the luminum was discontinuous and showed occasional patches of very thin fibrin. The total thickness of the biological lining ranged from 0.9 to 1.2 mm and was slightly thicker in the inflow area (2.0-mm thick).

This cell-seeded pump bladder specimen, removed after 38 days of partial left ventricular bypass, revealed a great deal more collagen than in the previous control specimens (which consisted mostly of fibrin). Collagenous material was firmly attached to the polyurethane fibrils to provide satisfactory adherence of the developing pseudoendothelial layer.

Calf No. 576

Calf No. 576 received a control Model 11 pump on February 8, 1979. The bladder flange and inflow struts of the device were modified to prevent strut fracture and flange separation which proved troublesome in previous pump experiments. This experiment was terminated after 61 days. Examination of the pump bladder revealed a somewhat thickened (3.5 mm) fibrin layer which was lingular and not well attached to the underlying textured surface. There were no areas of calcification and the inflow and outflow elbows were free of loose thrombus. The inflow valve was not remarkable, but the outflow valve contained one cusp which was not flexible. No definite calcification was noted. Examination of the brain, liver, heart, lungs, and kidneys was not remarkable; there was no evidence of thromboembolic damage.

Calf No. 578

LVAD implantation was carried out on February 26, 1979 and was a control study (no cells). The experiment was terminated after 44 days because of inadequate pump filling. Autopsy examination disclosed a kinked outflow Dacron graft which partially blocked ejection of blood from the device. A surgical error was responsible for the problem because the graft had been longer than necessary to bridge the space between the outflow end of the LVAD and the side of the descending thoracic aorta.

Examination of the pump surface revealed a moderately thick, irregular layer of fibrin with several small grayish-white patches of pseudoendothelium. There was no evidence of calcification. The inflow and outflow elbows were free of loose thrombus, and the xenograft valves were unremarkable. Examination of the brain, kidneys, lung, adrenal glands, and other organs was also unremarkable.

In summary, this control experiment was terminated after 44 days due to an outflow graft obstruction.

Calf No. 579

LVAD implantation was carried out on March 12, 1979 and consisted of a Model 11 LVAD seeded with bovine fetal fibroblasts. This experiment was continued for a total 283 days and was terminated because of a superficial infection around the percutaneous lead. The animal's health was excellent throughout the study, and partial left ventricular bypass (flow of 4.0 L/minute) was maintained throughout. The textured surface in this bladder had a mat thickness of 430 microns.

The bladder surface was covered with a very thin layer of grayish-white tissue consistent with pseudoendothelium. Replacement of the original fibrin surface was almost complete. The lining appeared to be well attached to the underlying textured fibrils. Examination of the xenograft valves disclosed moderate cusp calcification with a fracture of an outflow cusp in a region of calcification. There was no evidence of thrombus on the valves or in the pump elbows. Pathologic examination of the brain, kidneys, heart, and lungs was unremarkable. There was no evidence of thromboembolic organ damage.

In summary, this fibroblast-seeded textured surface had developed a thin collagenous lining which was well attached to the underlying fibrillar surface.

Calf No. 581

A Model 11 pump was implanted in this animal on March 20, 1979. The textured surface of the bladder had a mat thickness of 430 microns. This experiment was terminated after 338 days due to the presence of a rising white blood count secondary to an infection in the region of the percutaneous lead.

Examination of the pump bladder surface revealed a thin, grayish-white membrane which was well attached to the underlying textured surface. There was no loose thrombus on the bladder surface. The outflow xenograft valve was moderately calcified, the inflow valve contained calcification in discrete areas and remained flexible. The pump elbows were free of thrombus accumulation.

Autopsy examination revealed pneumonitis which probably resulted in the leukocytosis. Examination of the brain, kidneys, liver, and spleen was not remarkable.

In summary, Calf No. 581 received a fibroblast cell-seeded pump bladder which was removed after 338 days of satisfactory partial left ventricular bypass. A smooth, thin, fibrous membrane was well attached to the underlying textured surface.

Calf No. 582

LVAD implantation was carried out on March 26, 1979. The pump consisted of a Model 11 device with a textured surface having a mat thickness of 430 microns. The animal was sacrified after 74 days because of poor pump function. It was discovered at autopsy examination that the outflow valve was occluded with thrombus and heavily calcified. The pump bladder, which was seeded with bovine fetal fibroblasts, was covered with a thin, glistening layer of fibrous tissue despite the presence of almost complete pump obstruction. The inflow valve was not calcified and there was no loose thrombus within the pump elbows or on the pump bladder. Examination of the brain, lungs, spleen, liver, and kidneys did not reveal any thromboembolic damage.

In summary, Calf No. 582, who received a fibroblast-seeded Model 11 device, was sacrificed because of pump outflow obstruction. The cause of the problem was a severely calcified outflow valve. Despite this fact, the pump bladder contained a well-developed, thin fibrous membrane.

Calf No. 583

LVAD implantation was carried out on April 3, 1979 employing a Model 11 device and a textured bladder surface with a mat thickness of 430 microns. The experiment was continued for 163 days employing Coumadin anticoagulation. Termination of the experiment at this time was carried out to permit examination of the pump bladder surface.

There was no loose thrombus present. The lining measured 0.5-1.0 mm in thickness throughout. There was mild calcification of the outflow xenograft valve and no calcification of the inflow valve. There was no obstruction of the device or pump bladder by loose thrombus. Examination of the brain, kidneys, lungs, and heart was unremarkable.

Examination of the textured bladder surface revealed the presence of a uniform, thin, grayish-white membrane which was well attached to the polyurethane fibrils. There was no evidence of loose thrombus on the bladder surface. Examination of the xenograft valves revealed a few areas of calcification on the three inflow cusps but the valve remained flexible. The pump elbows and outflow valve were free of loose thrombus and there was no calcification present. Examination of the brain, kidneys, and lungs was unremarkable. There was no evidence of embolic damage.

In summary, this experiment, which continued for 163 days, revealed the presence of a thin, fibrous lining attached to the textured bladder surface.

Calf No. 584

Pump implantation was undertaken on April 12, 1979 without complication. This was a control experiment (no cells) with the animal maintained on Coumadin until the time of sacrifice. The experiment was continued for 33 days without difficulty, and sacrifice was undertaken at that time according to the experimental protocol.

Examination of the pump bladder revealed a somewhat thickened (3.0 mm) fibrin layer which was irregular and not well attached to the underlying textured surface. There were no areas of calcification and the inflow and outflow elbows were free of loose thrombus. The inflow valve was not remarkable but the outflow valve contained one cusp which was not flexible. This cusp was the septal leaflet with muscle fragments at the base. No definite calcification was noted. Examination of the brain, liver, heart, lungs, and kidneys was not remarkable. There was no evidence of thromboembolic damage.

Calf No. 585

LVAD implantation in this animal was carried out on April 26, 1979 without complication. This was a control experiment (no cells) with a textured surface of different dimensions than those used previously. The fibrils were 18 microns in diameter, 380 microns in length with a mat thickness of 310 microns. This experiment was scheduled for a period of approximately one month, and the animal was sacrificed after 38 days of partial left ventricular bypass. Coumadin anticoagulation was maintained throughout the study.

Examination of the pump bladder surface revealed a thin layer of fibrin which was poorly attached to the underlying textured fibrils. The valved conduits and pump elbows were unremarkable. There was no valve obstruction but a small area of calcification was noted in the muscular cusp of the outflow valve. Examination of the heart, liver, adrenals, kidneys, and lungs was not remarkable. There was no evidence of embolic damage present.

In summary, a control experiment with a textured surface having a mat thickness of 310 microns revealed poor attachment of the thin fibrin lining underlying polyurethane fibrils.

Calf No. 586

A Model 11 pump was implanted in this animal on May 7, 1979. The textured surface of the bladder had a mat thickness of 430 microns. This experiment was terminated after 270 days due to the presence of a rising white blood count secondary to an infection in the region of the percutaneous lead.

Examination of the pump bladder surface revealed a thin, grayish-white membrane which was well attached to the underlying textured surface. There was no loose thrombus on the bladder surface. The outflow xenograft valve was moderately calcified and stiff but the inflow valve (also containing calcification in areas) remained flexible. The pump elbows were free of thrombus accumulation.

Autopsy examination revealed a diffuse pneumonitis which probably resulted in the leukocytosis. Examination of the brain, kidneys, liver, and spleen was not remarkable. There was no thromboembolic organ damage present.

In summary, Calf No. 586 received a fibroblast cell-seeded pump bladder which was removed after 270 days of satisfactory partial left ventricular bypass. A smooth, thin, fibrous membrane was well attached to the underlying textured surface.

Calf No. 587

LVAD implantation in this animal was undertaken on June 5, 1979. The pump bladder contained a textured surface with a mat thickness of 430 microns. The bladder was seeded with bovine fetal fibroblasts prior to implantation and the calf was electively sacrificed after 111 days. At that time, a thin, grayish-white membrane was well attached to the underlying textured surface. There was no loose thrombus present on the lining.

The outflow xenograft valve was heavily calcified and there was moderate calcification of the inflow valve as well. Autopsy examination revealed no evidence of embolic damage to the parenchymatous organs examined.

In summary, Calf No. 587 contained a cell-seeded pump bladder which formed a fibrous lining on the textured surface.

Calf No. 589

A Model 11 LVAD was implanted in this animal on June 18, 1979 containing a textured surface with fibrils measuring 18 microns in diameter, 230 microns in length and a mat thickness of 200 microns. This experiment was terminated after 30 days, as scheduled. Examination of the pump bladder lining revealed it to be relatively thick (3.0 mm) and not well attached to the underlying surface. There were scattered areas of calcification sent. The inflow and outflow elbows and xenograft valves were not remarkable. Examination of the brain, pancreas, heart, lungs, liver, and kidneys showed each of these organs to be within normal limits in appearance. Microscopic examination was also not remarkable.

In summary, this control experiment revealed relatively poor attachment of the fibrin lining to the underlying textured surface with some areas of calcification present.

Calf No. 590

LVAD implantation was carried out on June 19, 1979 without difficulty. This control experiment (no cells) was scheduled for a period of one month and the animal was sacrified after 31 days. Coumadin anticoagulation was maintained throughout the study.

Examination of the pump bladder surface revealed a thin fibrin lining which seemed to be well attached to the underlying textured surface (mat thickness 200 microns). A few scattered areas of calcification were noted. The pump elbows and xenograft valves were normal in appearance. Examination of the brain, kidneys, lungs, myocardium, and liver was not remarkable.

In summary, this one-month control experiment with a textured surface (mat thickness 200 microns) was well attached to the underlying fibril surface in contrast to other similar experiments.

Calf No. 591

An LVAD was implanted in this animal on July 30, 1979. The experiment continued for five months (150 days) and was terminated because of inadequate pump filling.

Examination of the pump bladder revealed a grayish-white, thin membrane which was not well attached to the underlying textured surface. This lining had detached in several areas and caused intermittent pump obstruction during ejection of blood from the device. The textured surface in this case had a reduced mat thickness of 310 microns.

Examination of the xenograft valves revealed them to be flexible, but moderate calcification was present on one cusp of the outflow valve. There was no loose thrombus on the pump bladder surface or within the pump elbows.

In summary, this fibroblast-seeded pump bladder developed a thin, fibrous membrane but it was not well attached to the textured surface of reduced mat thickness (310 microns).

Calf No. 594

LVAD implantation was carried out on September 10, 1979 employing a Model 11 pump with a textured fibril surface (mat thickness 430 microns). Elective sacrifice of the calf was necessary on February 6, 1980 (149 days) because of an inflow obstruction.

Examination of the pump bladder at autopsy revealed large areas of thin (less than 1.0 mm) areas of pseudoendothelium at the inflow area, middle segment, and just proximal to the outflow region of the bladder. There were scattered areas of calcification, the present measuring 2.0 to 4.0 mm in diameter. Also present were areas of fibrin which were thin (1.0 to 2.0 mm), which appeared to be involved in the collagenous development. It was apparent that if the experiment had lasted 8 to 12 months, the entire pump bladder might well have been covered with a thin layer of collagen. There was no separation of the biologic layer from the underlying textured surface. There appeared to be somewhat more calcification in this fibroblast-seeded specimen than in others examined during the current program.

The cause for the inflow obstruction was a separation of polyester flock from the inflow metal elbow which resulted in occlusion of this structure with thrombus, which limited flow to approximately 10 to 20 percent of normal.

Separation of flock from the metal portions of the device is an unusual complication not found in any other pump during the current three-year program. Examination of the heart, liver, adrenals, kidneys, lungs, and GI tract was unremarkable. There were no abnormalities at microscopic examination of the various organs. There was no evidence of thromboembolic organ damage noted.

Calf No. 597

LVAD implantation was carried out on October 2, 1979 without complication. The device was a Model 11 pump with a textured surface (mat thickness 200 microns).

The experiment continued uneventfully for 85 days when poor pump function was noted. The animal was sacrified at this time, and examination of the bladder lining revealed that a tissue layer had completely lifted away from the underlying polyurethane fibril matrix. This loose membrane was responsible for pump obstruction and the rapid onset of poor LVAD function.

Examination of the xenograft valves revealed a small area of calcification in one cusp of the outflow valve. There was no valve obstruction and the pump elbows were free of thrombus buildup. Autopsy examination was unremarkable.

In summary, this cell-seeded Model 11 LVAD developed a thin, fibrous lining which completely separated from the underlying textured surface. This bladder had a mat thickness of 200 microns.

Calf No. 603

This animal was implanted with a Model 11 LVAD on December 3, 1979. The integrally textured bladder was seeded with bovine fetal fibroblasts prior to implantation. The experiment was continued for 367 days to permit inspection of the pseudoneointimal lining.

Upon gross examination, the biological lining appeared exceptionally thin, smooth and glistening. A small focus (2 mm in diameter) of calcification was noticed on the inflow annulus; the rest of the lining was free of calcific plaque. The lining was noticeably free of trapped red blood cells or hemosiderin, displaying a white pearlescent appearance.

Calf No. 604

Model 11 pump implantation in this animal was undertaken on January 16, 1980. The textured pump bladder with a mat thickness of 200 microns was seeded with bovine fetal fibroblasts prior to implantation. The experiment was terminated after 54 days to permit inspection of the textured bladder surface. The polyurethane fibrils were covered with a thin, grayish-white membrane which was well attached to the underlying surface.

In summary, Calf No. 604 received a Model 11 cell-seeded pump bladder (mat thickness 200 microns) which developed a thin fibrous lining which was well attached to the underlying polyurethane surface.

Calf No. 605

A Model 11 LVAD with a textured bladder (380-micron mat thickness) was implanted on January 23, 1980. The experiment was continued during Coumadin anticoagulation for a period of 87 days. The animal was sacrificed to permit examination of the bladder surface.

At this time, a thin, grayish-white membrane appeared to be well attached to the underlying polyurethane fibrils. The xenograft valves were not calcified and the entire pump was free of loose thrombus. Pathologic examination of the heart, lungs, kidneys, and brain was unremarkable.

In summary, Calf No. 605 with a bladder containing a mat thickness of 380 microns demonstrated a developing pseudoendothelial lining after 47 days. The lining was well attached.

Calf No. 613

Pump implantation in this animal was undertaken on May 22, 1980 and consisted of a Model 11 LVAD containing a textured surface with a mat thickness of 230 microns. Sacrifice of this animal was carried out on July 23, 1980 and was prompted by a difficulty in flexion of the pump bladder.

At the time of autopsy examination, the bladder showed a marked buildup of fibrin with a rugal appearance in the outflow end of the device. This was laminated thrombus measuring up to 5.0 and 8.0 mm in thickness. The inflow end of the bladder revealed a very thin (approximately 200 to 400 microns) layer of collagen which was glistening and well attached to the underlying fibril matrix. There did not appear to be any gross calcification present. The thick layer of thrombus at the outflow end of the bladder also partially obstructed the outflow elbow, resulting in difficulty in compression of the pump bladder.

There was no evidence of embolic damage to parenchymatous organs and examination of the heart, liver, adrenals, brain, kidneys, and lungs was not remarkable. Microscopic examinations of these organs were also within normal limits. In summary, there was a marked increase in thickness of the fibrin layer covering the textured fibrils in the outflow half of the pump bladder. This extremely thick layer was in striking contrast to the very thin collagenous tissue found in the inflow portion of the same bladder. The reason for this discrepancy was not apparent at autopsy examination.

VI. CHARACTERIZATION OF BIOLOGIC LININGS

A. Glycosaminoglycans (GAGs)

1. Structure and Function of GAGs

Glycosaminoglycans are polysaccharides that are found in practically all tissues, usually in covalent association with protein. Seven types are commonly recognized; six of these are structurally related, with a carbohydrate backbone consisting of alternating uronic acid (L-iduronic acid and/or D-glucuronic acid) and hexosamine (D-glucosamine or D-galactosamine) residues. All except one, hyaluronate, are sulfated. These polysaccharide types are distinguished by their monomer composition, by the position and configuration of their glycosidic linkages, and by the amount and location of their sulfate substituents. The hyaluronate and chondroitin sulfate species have rather simple structures whereas other (such as the dermatan sulfate, heparan sulfate and heparin species) may contain a larger number of different disaccharide units, arranged either in block structures or in less well-ordered, complex sequences. These structures are established during biosynthesis, by polymer-modification reactions that appear to be coordinated in a specific manner, yet operate by a partly random selection mechanism.

A large number of macromolecules may bind to GAGs. The majority of ligands are proteins or protein conjugates; however, GAGs capable of interchain binding have also been implicated. In addition, a number of as yet unidentified components; for example, on cell surfaces, are believed to mediate certain observed biological effects of GAGs. Binding between GAGs and other macromolecules has been postulated in highly diverse functional contexts, such as the structural organization of the extracellular matrix in connective tissues, the control of hemostasis, the specific binding of plasma proteins to the blood vessel wall, and the regulation of cell behavior and metabolism.

Our interest in GAGs stems from the fact that GAGs are thought to be synthesized by fibroblasts prior to collagen fibrogenesis, thus providing an extracellular matrix for collagen fibril formation and maturation. The synthesis and analysis of GAGs in our biologic linings represent a crucial first step in the in situ formation of a highly collagenous autologous pseudoneointimal lining, closely resembling normal arterial walls. In addition, normal arterial walls contain hyaluronate, proteoglycans of chrondroitin 4- and 8-sulfates, dermatan sulfate, and heparan sulfate, with most of these substances identical in the arterial intima.

2. Chemical Structure

Chains consist of alternating sugars of hexosamine (glucosamine or galactosamine) and another sugar (glucuronic acid, iduronic acid or galactose).

Most compounds can be represented as repeating disaccharide units.

HYALURONIC ACID

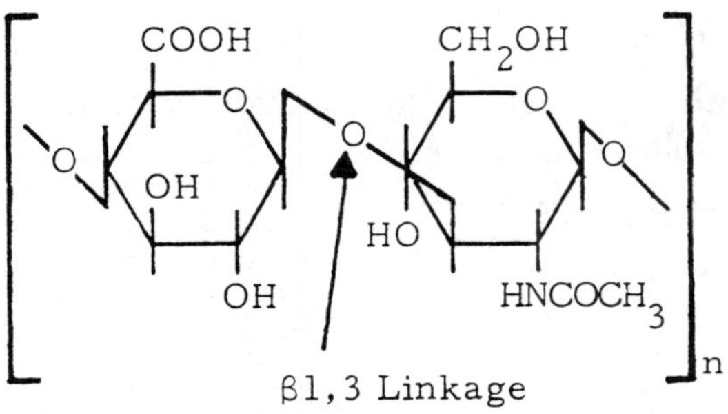

N-acetylglucosamine
glucuronic acid
no sulfate
5×10^5 MW

DERMATAN SULFATE
(Chondroitin Sulfate B)

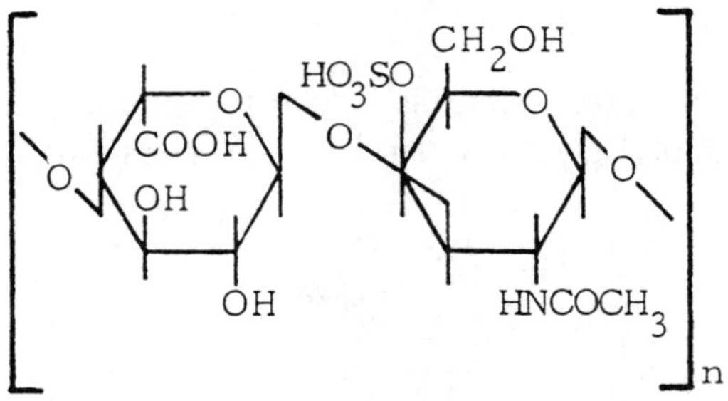

N-acetylgalactosamine (4 sulfated)
iduronic acid (occasionally 2 sulfated)
$2\text{-}5 \times 10^4$ MW

CHONDROITIN 6-SULFATE
(Chondroitin Sulfate C)

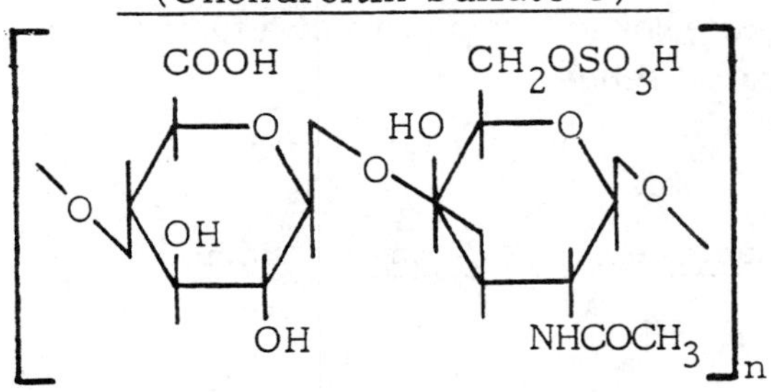

N-acetylgalactosamine (6 sulfated)
(can also be 4 sulfated)
glucuronic acid
$2\text{-}5 \times 10^4$ MW

KERATAN SULFATE

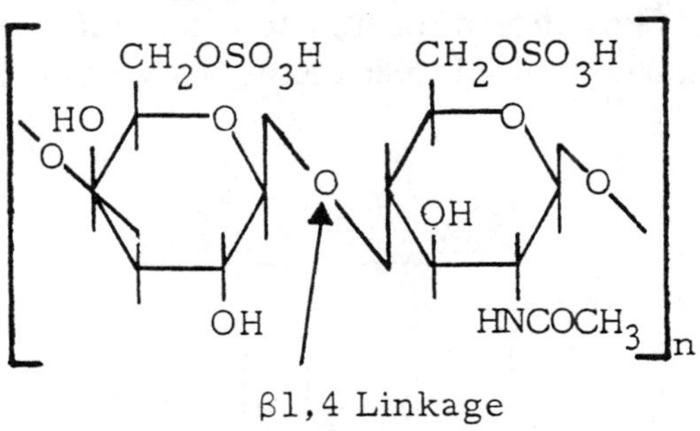

N-acetylglucosamine (6 sulfated)
galactose (6 sulfated)
$5\text{-}20 \times 10^3$ MW

Heparin has more variations in sulfate and uronic acid content.

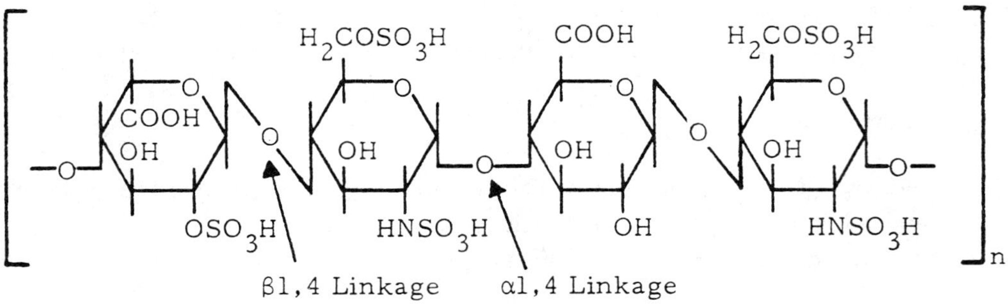

glucosamine (6 sulfated)
glucuronic acid
iduronic acid (2 sulfated)
$1\text{-}3 \times 10^4$ MW

Heparan sulfate is similar to heparin but with less sulfate. It has variations in N-sulfate and N-acetyl groups while heparin is essentially N-sulfated.

HEPARAN (Heparitin) SULFATE

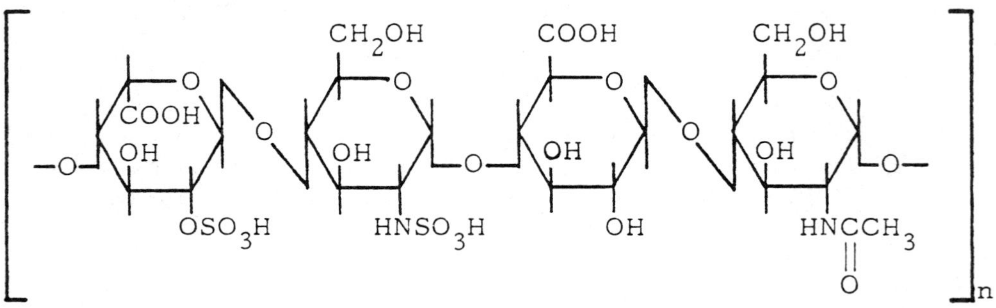

glucosamine N-sulfated
N-acetylglucosamine (sometimes 6 sulfated)
glucuronic acid
iduronic acid (sometimes 2 sulfated)

Chrondroitin sulfate and most other GAGs are linked to a protein by a tetrasaccharide, as shown below. The linkage is a glycosidic bond to serine.

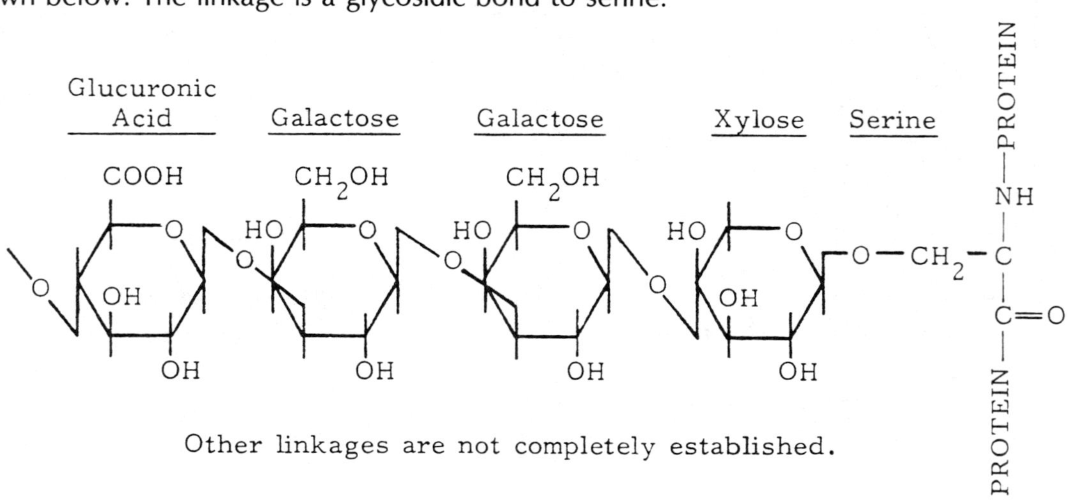

Other linkages are not completely established.

Hyaluronic acid is the only GAG that is not certainly linked covalently to proteins and it does *not* contain sulfate.

Definition of GAGs

- Mucopolysaccharides is the original term used to describe a group of polysaccharides that are viscous or mucinous. This group of compounds was chemically heterogeneous.
- At present, mucopolysaccharide is still viewed as a general term. However, these compounds are now usually called proteoglycans and glycosaminoglycans.
- GAGs are extremely large (10^4 to 10^6 molecular weight units), unbranched heteropolysaccharides containing hexosamines. The GAGs are generally attached to a protein core. The intact molecule is called a proteoglycan.

The different types of GAGs commonly distinguished in vertebrate tissues are shown in Table 6. They are all polyanions that have acidic sulfate and/or carboxyl groups, and many of their functional properties have been attributed to their polyelectrolyte nature. Generally, the GAGs do not occur as free polysaccharide chains in vivo, but as proteoglycans in which several chains are covalently linked, at the reducing terminal sugar, to a polypeptide core.

Table 6. Occurrence and Properties of Glycosaminoglycans

Polysaccharide	Mol. Wt. ($\times 10^{-3}$)	Repeating Period Monosaccharides	Sulfate per Disaccharide Unit	Other Sugar Components[a]	Examples of Occurrence In Mammalian Tissues
Hyaluronate	4-8000	D-glucuronic acid D-glucosamine	0	b	Various connective tissues, skin, vitreous humor, synovial fluid, umbilical cord, cartilage
Chondroitin 4- and 6-sulfates	5-50	D-glucuronic acid D-galactosamine	0.1-1.3	D-galactose D-xylose	Cartilage, cornea, bone, skin, arterial wall
Dermatan sulfate	15-40	D-glucuronic acid L-iduronic acid D-galactosamine	1.0-3	D-galactose D-xylose	Skin, heart valve, tendon, arterial wall
Heparan sulfate	—	D-glucuronic acid L-iduronic acid D-glucosamine	0.4-2	D-galactose D-xylose	Lung, arterial wall, ubiquitous on cell surfaces (?)
Heparin	6-25	D-Glucuronic acid L-iduronic acid D-glucosamine	1.6-3	D-galactose D-xylose	Lung, liver, skin, intestinal mucosa (mast cells)
Keratan sulfate	4-19	D-galactose D-glucosamine	0.9-1.8	D-galactosamine D-mannose L-fucose sialic acid	Cartilage, cornea, intervertebral disc

a. Including the sugar components of the polysaccharide-protein linkage region.
b. The occurrence in hyaluronate of arabinose has been suggested but not conclusively verified.

3. Interaction of GAGs with Collagen

There is now general agreement that most of the GAGs occur in the native state covalently bound to protein [18,19,20,21]. The GAGs of connective tissues (most of which occur as proteoglycans) form, along with fibrous proteins, collagen, and elastin, the major macromolecular elements of the tissues. The relationship that these components bear to each other, and to the water and microions of the intercellular matrix [22], presumably accounts for the physical properties of the tissue; therefore, binding between the macromolecules has far-reaching physiological implications.

All GAGs, except hyaluronate, which lacks sulfate groups, and keratan sulfate, which lacks carboxyl groups, bind to collagen by electrostatic interaction at physiological pH and ionic strength; GAGs of higher charge density and larger molecular size bind with higher affinity; and, finally, the presence of L-iduronic acid residues appears to promote the binding process. The interaction is thus akin to the cooperative electrostatic binding of GAGs to a number of other proteins. The number of polysaccharide chains bound to each collagen monomer varies, depending on the type of polysaccharide, between two and five; however, a dermatan sulfate of high molecular weight (41,000) could bind as many as five molecules of collagen per chain.

Thus we see that proteoglycan-collagen interaction influences the deposition of collagen fibrils, as well as the final organization of the fibril. For these reasons, we analyzed selected biologic linings, in an effort to determine in a quantitative manner the presence of GAGs within our pseudoneointimal linings. The experimental protocol and results are discussed in the next section.

4. GAGs in LVAD Autologous Linings

The tissue from the bladders was digested with papain and Pronase, centrifuged, and concentrated to a small volume (200 μl). Much of the collagen and elastin was present in the pellet. An appropriate number of aliquots (5 to 20) were subjected to the mentioned electrophoretic analysis. In order to obtain reliable data, we analyzed each sample at least five times. A large aliquot of the digest was used to measure the low content of hyaluronic acid, and a small aliquot was necessary for the determination of those GAGs present in high concentrations. After the two-dimensional electrophoresis was completed, the resulting cellulose acetate plates were stained with Alcian blue, the resulting spots were cut out, and the dye was eluted and quantitated.

This method circumvented many disadvantages of previously used techniques. The advantages of this procedure are threefold:

- It simultaneoulsy resolves seven standard GAGs (chondroitin sulfates A, G, and C, heparan sulfate, hyaluronic acid, and keratan sulfate).
- The GAGs can be quantitated on microgram levels (10 mg of dry, defatted tissue are sufficient for this purpose; the sensitivity of the procedure lies between 1 and 5 μg of a GAG; the reproducibilty of the results is ±5 percent).
- The proteolytic digest of the tissue can be applied directly without fractionation to the cellulose acetate plate used for this type of electrophoretic analysis.

Results of our analysis are presented below:

Glycosaminoglycan Distribution in Neointimal Lining of LVAD Bladder 558 Expressed in Relative Percentage

Sample No.	Hyaluronic Acid (%)	Heparan Sulfate (%)	Dermatan Sulfate (%)	Chondroitin Sulfate C (%)
1	6	2	55	37
2	12	Trace	70	18

B. Collagen

The macromolecular structure of blood vessels consists primarily of elastin and collagen fibrils lying in a "ground substance matrix" or glycosaminoglycan-proteoglycan mixture. Therefore, a basic understanding of the nature of collagen, and its role in autologous biologic pseudoneointimal linings seems indispensable if the objective is to construct cardiac prostheses capable of continuous, reliable operation for periods of at least two years. The following sections describe our efforts to elicit, characterize, and evaluate the in situ synthesis of collagen, by the pre-seeding of our bladders with allogeneic fetal fibroblasts.

1. Nomenclature

Several genetically distinct types of collagen have now been described in the literature. The most abundant type of collagen, Type I, consists of two α_1 and one α_2 chain [23,24,25]. A Type II collagen, isolated from cartilage, consists of three α_1 (II) chains, which are distinct from the alpha chains of Type I [26-30]. A Type III collagen has been isolated from fetal tissue [31,32]; a fourth classification has now been described as Type IV collagen found in basement membrane, and Descemet's membrane [33]. Corneal stromal collagen has been identified as Type I [34]. It has been reported that Type II collagen has been localized by antibody studies in the anterior stroma and Bowman's and Descemet's membrane [35,36]. Type III collagen has traditionally been associated with the cardiovascular system. More recently, a corneal collagen (Type V) has been identified, although there is no universal agreement on this.

A summary of collagen types and tissue distribution follows.

Types of Collagen

Organ	Source	Collagen Type*				
		I $(\alpha 1)_2\alpha 2$	II $(\alpha 1)3$	III $(\alpha 1)3$	IV $(\alpha 1)3$	V(?) $(\alpha 1)3$
Dermis	Adult	+++	-	+	*	
	Embryo	++	-	++	*	
Tendon		++++	-	-	-	
Bone		++++	-	-	-	
Lung	Alveoli	++++	-	-	*	
	Bronchi	-	++	-	-	
Dentin		+++	-	+	-	
Eye	Lens	-	-	-	*	++++
	Cornea	++++	-	-	*	
	Vitreous body	-	-	-	-	++++
	Fibrous sclera	+++	-	-.	-	
	Cartilaginous sclera	+	+++	-	-	
Cartilage		+	+++	-	-	
Cardiovascular System		+	-	+++	*	
Basement Membrane		-	-	-	++++	

* ++++: only detected molecular species
+++: predominant molecular species
++: abundant
+: traces
-: undetermined or absent, basement membrane(s) not included.

2. Biosynthesis and Fibrogenesis

The formation of a collagen fiber is complicated owing to the nature of the collagen molecule. The biosynthetic process of soluble collagen formation includes not only the usual DNA-RNA-ribosomal systems but also requires the following post-translational biochemical events:

- The hydroxylation of key prolyl and lysyl residues to form hydroxyproline and hydroxylysine. These reactions are catalyzed by the enzymes prolyl hydroxylase and lysyl hydroxylase, respectively.
- Certain of the hydroxylysyl residues are glycosylated with either the disaccharide unit, glucosylgalactosyl-, or by galactosyl- alone. Glycosylating enzymes are required for this event to occur, and each saccharide unit, glucose or galactose, is incorporated via its UDP derivative.
- The three-stranded helical structure is formed by the interaction of an extra register peptide on the individual chains, which causes the three alpha chains to join and form a triple helix. These register peptides contain cysteine residues which are probably involved in bringing the chains together. An enzyme, procollagen peptidase, then cleaves the register peptide portions of the three-stranded collagen. Many laboratories are currently investigating the nature of this step in the biogenesis of collagen fibers.
- The extrusion of collagen molecules from the cell that synthesized it is also being studied in several laboratories, but little definitive data are presently available about the exact nature of this step.
- The formation of 640 A spacing native fibers is the next requirement in the sequence. Little is known of the nature of this step.
- The crosslinking of lysine and hydroxylysine residues occurs, resulting in aldol condensates, Schiff bases, and histidinohydroxymerodesmosine.

The biosynthesis and fibrogenesis of collagen is summarized in Figures 28 and 29 respectively. As these figures indicate, collagen is unique among proteins. The molecular properties are strongly influenced by a number of postribosomal modifications which include:

- Enzymatic Cleavage of a Procollagen Precursor
- Hydroxylation of Proline and Lysine
- Extracellular Formation of Collagen Fiber
- Intermolecular Crosslinking Process

In our studies, we are interested in obtaining highly collagenous linings, since the in situ synthesis and maturation of collagen represents an end stage in the intravascular healing process. In addition, we have also found that collagenous pseudoneointimal linings exhibit better overall adhesion to IT Biomer bladders.

3. Collagen in LVAD Autologous Linings

The main feature of all collagens is the consistent proportion of glycine in the helical region (33 percent of the total residues present, or every third residue), and the presence of hydroxyproline and hydroxylysine. Glycine, alanine, proline, and hydroxyproline constitute two-thirds of the total residues.

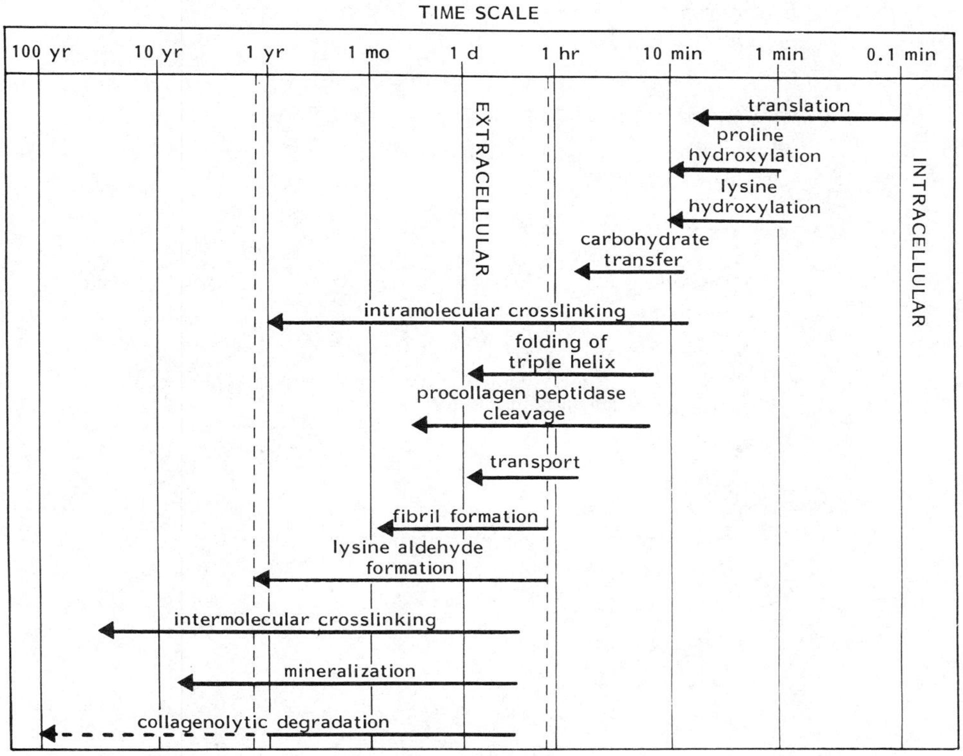

Figure 28. Temporal sequence in collagen biosynthesis.

Collagen is also unique in its hydroxyproline content. In fact, the presence of hydroxyproline is diagnostic of collagen. Furthermore, hydroxyproline uniformly represents 100 amino acid residues for each 1000 residues of amino acids in the protein backbone. It is this consistency which conveniently allows the accurate quantitation of collagen.

For instance, if a tissue contains an unknown mixture of collagen and other proteins, the amount of hydroxyproline is directly indicative of the percent collagen present. Thus, if the amino acid analysis of a tissue contains 50 residues of hydroxyproline per 1000 residues, we can safely conclude that collagen represents 50 percent of the protein mixture, since pure collagen would contain 100 residues of hydroxyproline per 1000 amino acid residues. In our investigations, we take full advantage of this fact, when analyzing the collagen contents of pseudoneointimal linings emanating from both seeded and nonseeded bladders experiments.

In our protocol, amino acid analysis is performed by cutting a strip approximately 0.5 × 7.0 cm from the pump lining. Adhering tissue is manually removed from the polyurethane and homogenized in H_2O. An aliquot of the homogenate is hydrolyzed, in vacuo, in 6N HCl at 110°C for 20 hours.The hydrolysates are analyzed on a Beckman Amino Acid Analyzer, Model 119CL.

The percentages of collagen from the amino acid analyses of pump linings maintained for various periods of time, both cell seeded and unseeded (controls), are given in Tables 7 and 8. These percentages are based on the assumption that pure collagen would contain 100 hydroxyproline residues per 1000 amino acids. As expected from previous studies, the tissue derived from cell-seeded bladders contained considerably more collagen than that from control linings, as judged by hydroxyproline content.

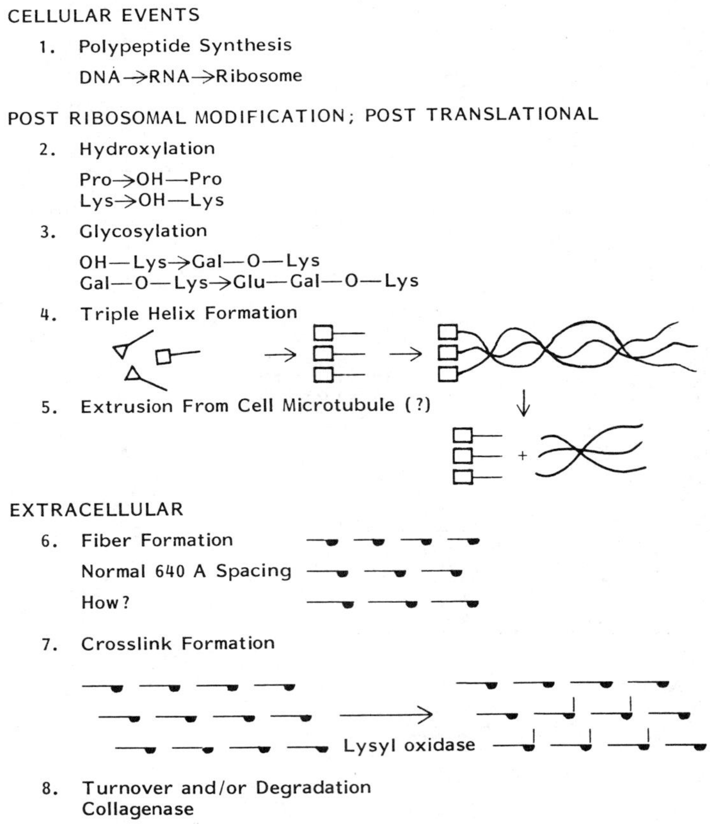

Figure 29. Fibrogenesis.

Table 7. Amino Acid Composition of Neointimal Linings (Nonseeded Controls)

Amino Acid	LVAD 584 30 Days	LVAD 589 31 Days	LVAD 590 31 Days	LVAD 564 38 Days	LVAD 585 39 Days	LVAD 578 44 Days	LVAD 566 60 Days	LVAD 576 61 Days	LVAD 567 69 Days	Purified Calf Aortic Collagen
Hydroxyproline	1.1	0.4	0.5	34.6	Trace	1.1	None	1.7	2.9	91.9
Aspartic	119.1	109.8	106.3	87.1	112.8	119.1	121.4	117.4	114.7	48.1
Threonine	63.9	70.7	70.6	46.4	66.6	63.9	64.6	64.0	66.2	19.2
Serine	67.4	74.5	86.2	65.4	71.1	67.4	78.9	69.4	88.5	34.2
Glutamic Acid	107.2	109.5	106.4	100.9	115.4	107.2	113.5	118.3	108.8	72.2
Proline	55.6	67.3	86.9	89.6	53.5	55.6	57.1	60.7	69.6	106.7
Glycine	87.0	87.5	84.8	171.5	87.8	87.0	89.6	90.1	100.0	316.7
Alanine	67.8	59.5	65.7	91.9	56.1	62.8	58.0	56.3	71.0	120.0
Valine	60.0	64.4	53.3	54.1	61.9	60.0	47.6	57.8	55.6	34.9
Isoleucine	34.9	44.6	34.6	27.1	45.1	34.9	33.7	37.3	35.9	17.9
Leucine	80.4	72.1	70.8	66.9	73.7	80.4	70.8	73.4	78.7	34.0
Tyrosine	36.8	36.9	36.8	24.8	36.0	36.4	36.4	37.2	38.7	5.1
Phenylalanine	39.2	35.3	34.8	28.5	34.9	39.2	33.5	35.4	39.0	15.7
Lysine	72.9	53.1	51.6	41.7	63.4	72.9	69.0	68.4	68.0	25.0
Histidine	23.2	21.2	19.2	20.1	20.1	23.2	22.4	18.9	25.2	5.5
Arginine	51.1	53.9	50.9	54.1	54.1	51.1	53.0	51.9	ND	46.5
Cysteine	16.1	20.4	21.7	11.9	27.3	16.1	21.5	21.7	27.3	ND
Methionine	21.1	18.3	19.0		27.3	21.1	26.9	20.2	ND	ND

ND = Not Determined

Table 8. Amino Acid Composition of Neointimal Linings (Seeded Bladders)

Amino Acid	LVAD 511 36 Days	LVAD 605 47 Days	LVAD 604 54 Days	LVAD 582 77 Days	LVAD 558 123 Days	LVAD 583 163 Days	LVAD 579 240 Days	LVAD 586 270 Days	LVAD 581 338 Days	LVAD 603 367 Days
Hydroxyproline	31.1	52.2	54.5	47.1	65.9	32.9	49.6	49.3	65.3	46.0
Aspartic	98.6	84.6	81.1	75.4	74.8	88.0	77.7	82.6	68.4	95.3
Threonine	69.9	47.8	45.9	44.1	43.3	50.1	39.0	42.2	36.6	47.6
Serine	55.0	54.0	52.7	59.3	51.0	53.0	52.1	54.0	49.6	56.6
Glutamic Acid	114.1	96.8	96.0	93.7	96.8	100.9	94.8	93.1	86.1	104.8
Proline	79.3	93.6	94.2	88.8	57.4	73.1	91.9	98.6	101.3	88.2
Glycine	159.5	135.3	139.8	190.2	203.9	169.4	203.4	205.6	234.3	165.9
Alanine	87.3	86.2	89.8	84.5	69.6	84.3	85.0	88.6	90.4	88.3
Valine	20.9	52.6	52.1	48.8	12.3	50.8	42.5	39.2	38.2	54.7
Isoleucine	32.6	28.9	30.6	24.9	24.9	36.7	25.5	19.2	20.4	32.7
Leucine	73.4	58.2	59.0	57.1	58.4	58.9	54.8	48.4	48.1	59.0
Tyrosine	29.1	21.9	21.0	20.5	24.0	26.9	20.2	21.0	16.2	25.3
Phenylalanine	33.7	28.4	28.2	25.6	22.2	27.7	22.5	23.9	20.4	26.7
Lysine	50.7	44.6	46.1	42.6	55.6	45.7	39.6	43.6	34.3	1.0
Histidine	18.0	15.0	14.5	13.1	17.3	15.4	12.8	12.4	10.0	12.8
Arginine	56.1	59.1	59.0	48.0	58.9	51.8	51.3	49.7	50.0	56.3
Cysteine	ND	16.1	13.7	16.7	27.3	15.8	16.3	14.7	10.5	ND
Methionine	16.2	14.7	11.9	11.5	41.3	14.2	13.4	13.7	11.4	15.5

ND = Not Determined

4. Explanting for Cell Growth

A strip of approximately 1.5 × 7.0 cm is cut lengthwise from the pump lining and washed three times with the Dulbecco's Medium with antibiotics. The pseudoneointimal tissue is removed manually from the polyurethane and washed twice more with the same medium. The strip of tissue is cut into 1-mm^3 pieces, and the explants are transferred to a 75-cm^2 tissue culture flask. The flask is allowed to stand 10 minutes with the cap end up to drain most of the medium from the explants in order to promote adherence. The medium is removed and the loosely capped flask is placed upright again in a humidified 5% CO_2/95% air incubator at 37 °C for 30 minutes. Dulbecco's Medium, supplemented with 10-percent fetal bovine serum and containing 3.7 grams sodium bicarbonate per liter, penicillin (100 units/ml), and streptomycin (100 μg/ml), is added to the flask to cover the explants (10 ml). The loosely capped flask is incubated undisturbed for a week. After this time, the medium is changed twice weekly with 20 ml of fresh medium. The cells which grew out from the explants after a total of 15 days are detached with a 0.5% trypsin/0.2% EDTA solution (GIBCO) in Modified Puck's Saline A solution, centrifuged, resuspended in medium, and seeded into new flasks (first passage). In some cases, the cells are trypsinized after one week in first passage and subcultured (second passage). When there is a sufficient number, cells are pulsed with ^{14}C-proline, except that 10 ml of medium containing 10 μCi^{14}-proline is used.

All tissues pulsed with ^{14}C-proline were capable of synthesizing collagen, as seen by the presence of nondialyzable ^{14}C-hydroxyproline (summarized below) in both the medium (soluble proteins) and tissue fractions. However, the pulsed, cell-seeded pump linings were capable of synthesizing more collagen in proportion to other proteins than the control linings, as exhibited by the higher percentage of the total radioactivity in hydroxyproline.

^{14}C-Proline Pulse of Pump Linings (Percent cpm In Hydroxyproline)

Pump Lining	Calf No.	Days of Bypass	% Hydroxyproline* (cpm)	
			Tissue	Medium
Nonseeded	584	30	0.6	2.6
	589	31	---	2.3
	590	31	7.3	3.9
	585	39	1.1	0.6
	578	44	3.3	8.7
	566	60	---	3.1
	576	61	0.9	2.5
	567	69	---	Trace
Seeded	571	36	11.4	13.0
	605	47	2.6	6.0
	604	54	5.4	5.2
	582	77	12.7	9.8
	587	111	11.7	8.7
	583	163	14.9	12.8
	579	240	8.1	7.2

$$*\% \text{ Hydroxyproline} = \frac{\text{cpm hydroxyproline}}{\text{cpm hydroxyproline} + \text{cpm proline}} \times 100$$

5. ^{14}C-Proline Incorporation by Tissue

Tissue adhering to the polyurethane is forcibly stripped with forceps from a 1.5- × 7.0-cm section of pump lining, and placed in a petri dish with medium devoid of fetal bovine serum, or proline. Added to the medium are 50 μg/ml of sodium ascorbate; after two washes of 5 ml each, the tissue is incubated for 24 hours in 5 ml of the same media containing 10 μCi ^{14}C-proline (specific activity 260 μCi/mole, Schwartz-Mann). The medium is removed, the tissue is washed three times with 1-ml aliquot of 0.9% NaCl and the washes are added to the supernate fraction. This fraction is centriguted, and dialyzed exhaustively against water. The tissue is suspended in 3 ml of H_2O and also dialyzed. Both dialyzed media and tissue are lyophilized and then hydrolyzed in 6NHCl at 110°C for 20 hours. The hydrolysates are subsequently placed on an amino acid analyzer equipped with a split-stream arrangement to analyze for ^{14}C-hydroxyproline and ^{14}C-proline.

Results are summarized on the following page.

Some of the control pump linings, as well as some of the cell-seeded pump linings, exhibited cell outgrowth. Although there appeared to be more cell outgrowth from the explants derived from cell-seeded linings, the actual number of cells may not be significant since prior handling may affect tissue viability. However, one must bear in mind that cell outgrowth from the control linings suggests cell infiltration. ^{14}C-proline pulse studies were performed on cells grown from one control and from one seeded pump lining and the percent hydroxylation on a radioactive basis is also given in the table. The amount of collagen synthesized by cells from the one control lining was comparable to the amount of collagen synthesized by the seeded lining. It should be pointed out that the percent hydroxylation expresses the percen-

Pump Lining	Calf No.	Days of Bypass	Number of Cells	% Hydroxylation* (cpm)	
				Media	Tissue
Nonseeded	584	30	1.15×10^{6}	-	-
	589	31	Minimal	-	-
	590	31	Minimal	-	-
	585	39	None	-	-
	578	44	1.12×10^{6}	39.0	8.9
Seeded	582	77	5.30×10^{6}	36.8	3.4
	587	111	4.30×10^{6}	-	-
	583	163	Minimal	-	-

$$^{*}\%\ \text{Hydroxylation} = \frac{\text{cpm hydroxyproline}}{\text{cpm hydroxyproline} + \text{cpm proline}} \times 100$$

tage of the total radioactivity in hydroxyproline. Since collagen contains approximately equal amounts of hydroxyproline and proline, the percentage of the radioactivity in the collagen would be twice that found in the hydroxyproline.

C. Histological Assessments

1. Introduction

Specimens of untouched linings are immersed in buffered glutaraldehyde fixative immediately after animal sacrifice. The specimens are analyzed by light microscopy, transmission electron microscopy, and scanning electron microscopy. Pertinent protocols used in these analyses are described in the following sections.

2. Light Microscopy

Specimens of biological linings are dehydrated (through the use of graded alcohol solutions) and embedded in paraffin. Hematoxylin and Eosin (H&E) staining is performed for overall morphology, Periodic Acid Schiff (PAS) for polysaccharides, Masson Trichrome for connective tissue and collagen, Elastica Van Giesson for elastin, and Alcian Blue for acid polysaccharides.

3. Transmission Electron Microscopy (TEM)

After fixation in cacodylate-buffered glutaraldehyde, the specimens are washed in 0.1 M cacodylate containing 7 percent sucrose (pH 7.2). Postfixation is accomplished with 1 percent aqueous osmium tetroxide for 1 hour at room temperature. Specimens are then stained with 0.1 percent aqueous uranyl acetate and dehydrated through graded alcohols and propylene oxide. Subsequently, samples are embedded in Epon 812 for sectioning and examined on a Philips EM 300 high-resolution electron microscope at 80 kV acceleration voltage. Special attention is given to the identification of cells lining the blood-contacting pseudoneointimal surface, the ultrastructure of all cells beneath the surface, as well as the relationships of these tissue components to the polymeric substrate.

4. Scanning Electron Microscopy (SEM)

Following fixation in cacodylate-buffered glutaraldehyde, specimens are dehydrated through graded alcohols and Freon-13. The specimens are dried by the critical point drying method and coated with gold by the sputter-coating method. Special attention is given to cells forming the blood-pseudoneointimal interface, and their ability to form a continuous lining.

SEM findings are compared with TEM and light microscopy data, and the results correlated with biochemical findings.

5. Nonseeded (Control) Studies — Results

Although there are variations among bladders, in general, the linings from nonseeded bladders are typically quite thick (2.0 to 4.0 mm), and have an edematous, spongy appearance. Adhesion of the biologic lining to the Biomer fibrils is poor, and only a few tips of the fibrils are integrated into the biologic lining. The polymeric fibrils are usually surrounded by large, empty-appearing spaces, with occasional clusters of cellular material, cauliflower-like in appearance, which probably represent multinucleated giant cells. The empty-looking spaces may represent artifacts of fixation, but also reflect poor adherence to the biologic lining to the bladder wall.

The luminal surface of the biologic lining shows a complex fibrin meshwork with ellipsoid cavities, up to 10 μm in diameter. Multiple round to elongated cells, with partially ruffled surfaces are quite common. In addition, a few round cells and red blood cells are found. Platelets are sparse, and in most cases do not spread.

Deeper into the lining, it consists almost exclusively of multiple layers of fibrin meshwork with occasional trapped red cells, and foci of polymorphonuclear leukocytes. Sparse, randomly distributed, round cells are located in holes of the fibrin meshwork throughout the specimen. Abundant platelet ghosts and cellular debris are found throughout this layer.

Occasionally, a collagenous, cellular area is found within the middle layer. This represents spontaneous in situ synthesis of collagen by fibroblastic-like cells. Surrounding this collagenous area are spindle cells appearing like fibroblasts. The spindly cells are oriented predominantly ina longitudinal direction, although some cells are also oriented circumferentially. Abundant material, staining positive for mucopolysaccharides and collagen is located between these cells.

The innermost layer, located adjacent to the polymeric fibrils, shows patches of loosely organized fibrin, sparse round cells, a few giant cells, and a small foci of calcification. With increasing longevity of implant; i.e., over 60 days, the calcific plaques become more prevalent, with some amalgamation of crystals. Large, empty areas surround the polymeric fibrils. Abundant cellular debris is found in most areas.

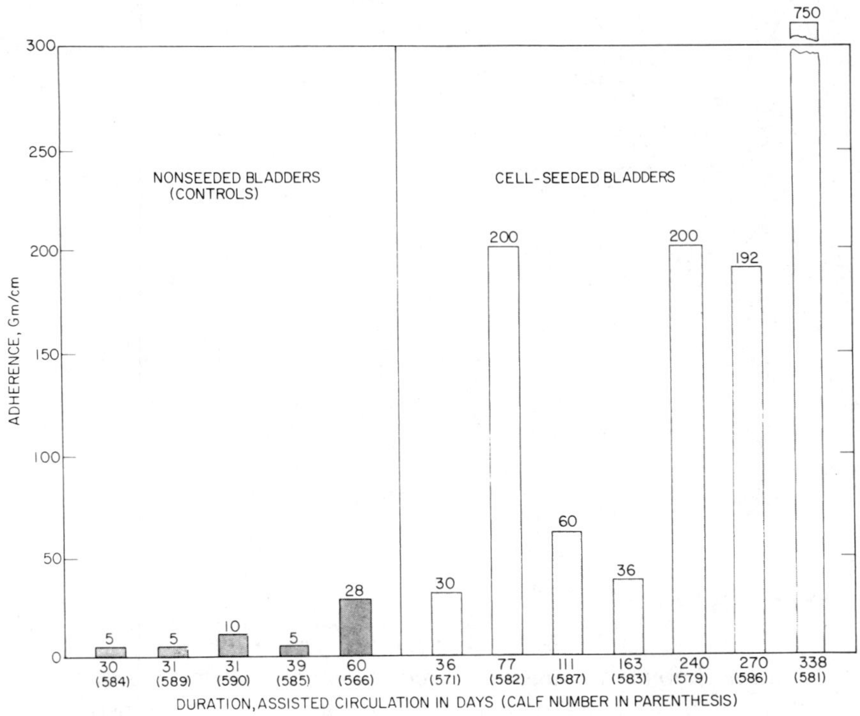

Figure 30. Attachment of Pseudoneointimal Linings to Biomer Bladders. Nonseeded (control) bladders, display poorer adhesion due to the presence of fibrin at the PNI/bladder interface. In contrast, the highly collagenous linings of seeded experiments are much better attached.

6. Seeded Studies – Results

The appearance of the pseudoneointimal linings of the fibroblast-seeded studies was strikingly different from the controls. In most of the studies, which ranged in duration from 36 to 367 days, the linings were thin, smooth, and well-adhered, seldom exceeding 1.5 mm in thickness. Semi-quantitative gross observations revealed linings with substantially less calcification, despite longer implant duration, and in many cases no calcific plaque at all.

Typically, pseudoneointimal linings derived from fibroblast-seeded bladders show three distinct layers: (1) a peripheral, rather cellular layer, containing the polymeric fibrils, (2) a medial layer with fibroblastic cells surrounded by parallel layers of collagen fibrils, and (3) a luminal layer, also collagenous, but with a thin covering of precipitated plasma proteins as the blood interface. The luminal surface is mostly noncellular, very smooth, and apparently devoid of endothelial cells.

Collagen content increases with implantation time, as expected. The collagen density is most apparent in the peripheral (basal) and middle layers as shown by collagen and PA' stains.

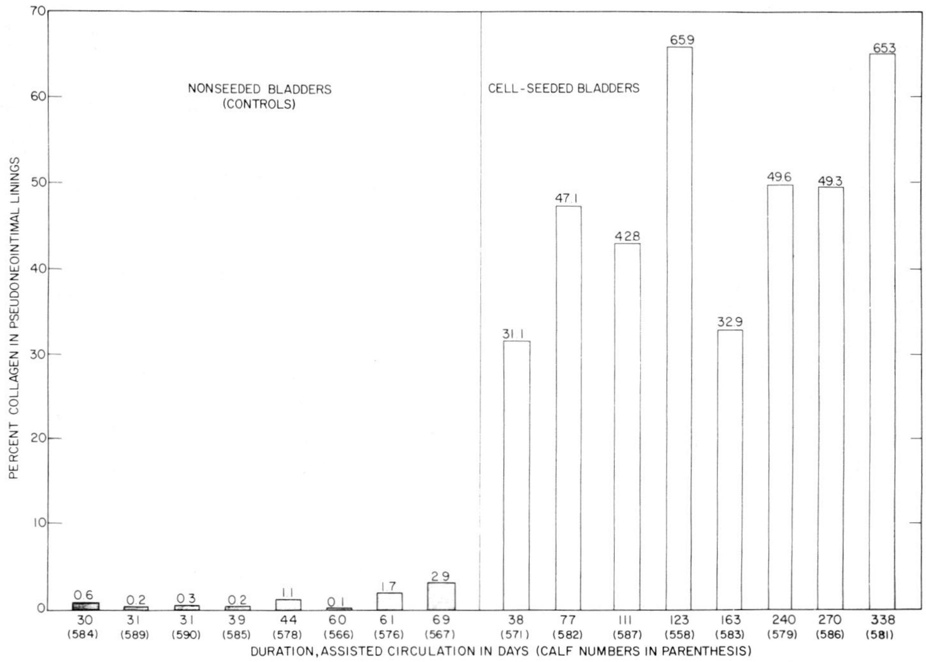

Figure 31. Concentration of Collagen in Pseudoneointimal Linings. It is quite evident that pseudoneointimal linings derived from cell-seeded experiments contain significantly higher amounts of collagen, and are thus much stronger than fibrin-based linings.

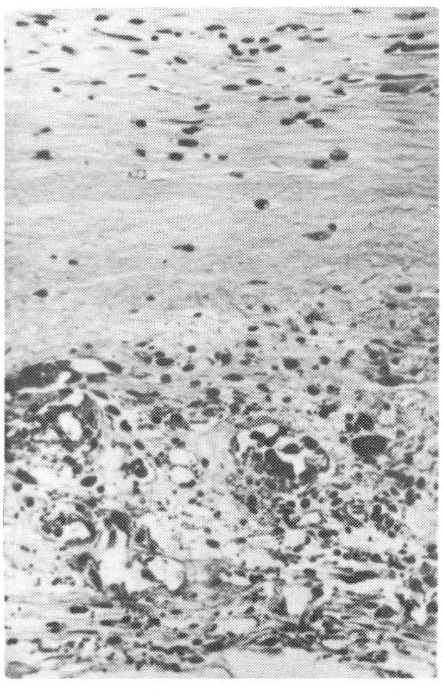

Figure 32. Cross Section of a Fibroblast-Seeded Bological Lining. This photograph, from LVAD Calf No. 558, shows a typical tri-layered structure with extensive collagen in the middle and lumenal layers. (320x).

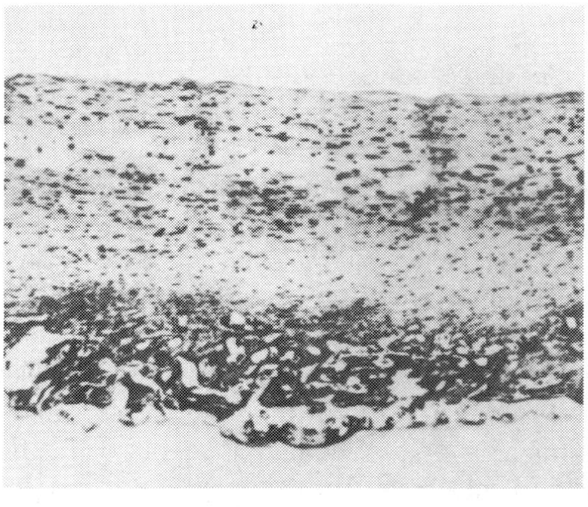

Figure 33. Lower magnification (50x) of lining from LVAD Calf No. 558, clearly demonstrating the trilaminar layers of the Neointima.

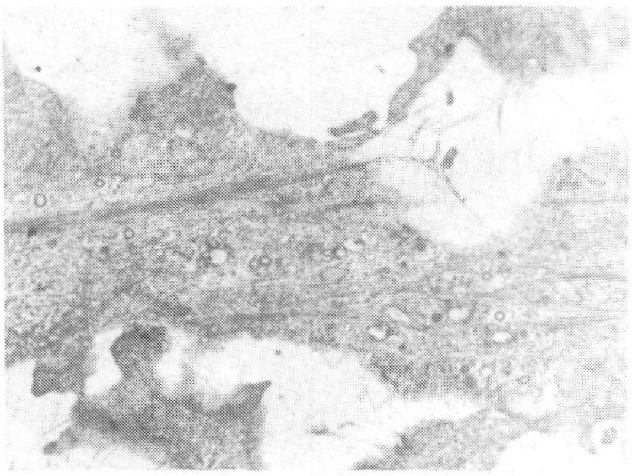

Figure 34. Transmission Micrograph of Cell Used for Seeding Bladder. The cell at the center has been sectioned in a plane parallel to the cell culture flask growing surface. The cell is elongated, containing bundles of microfilaments, which lie parallel to the long axis of the cell. Microtubules and ribosomes are also present. Note extracellular fibrillar material which has a structure consisten with that of collagen when observed in cell culture (27,500x).

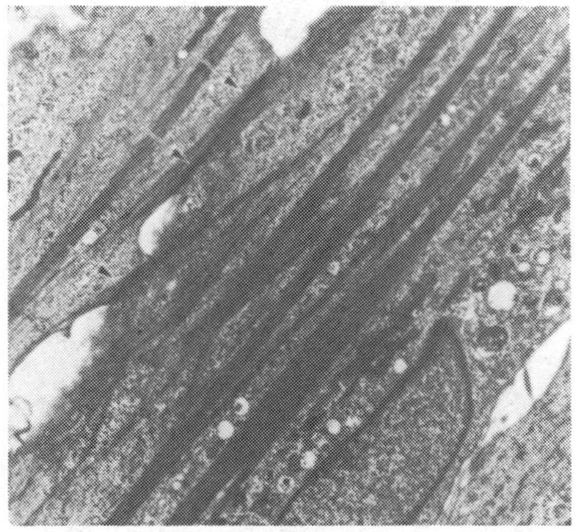

Figure 35. Cells Used for Seeding Bladder (in culture). This transmission micrograph shows two fibroblast-like cells with two areas of close association, occurring at desmosomes (arrows). Note bundles of microfilaments (stress fibers) and associated dense bodies; the microfilaments terminate at the desmosomes. (9240x).

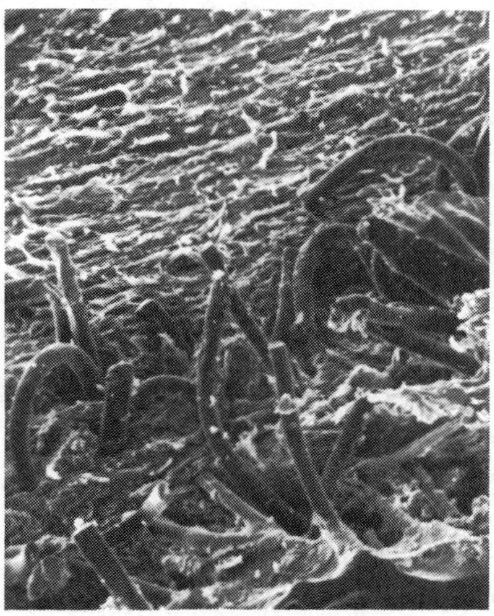

Figure 36. Calf No. 568, Scanning Electron Micrograph (SEM). This cut surface shows the polymeric fibrils, which are quite tightly interwoven with fibrillar and some cellular elements. The remainder of the biological lining shows a densely packed fibrillar layer in intimate contact with the polymeric fibrils (200x).

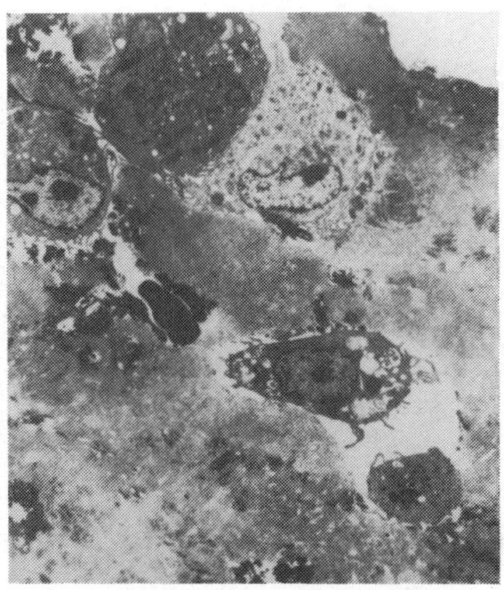

Figure 37. Calf No. 553 (23 Days Implantation) Nonseeded Control. Transmission electron photomicrograph representative of the surface of the biologica material. The blood-contacting surface is composed of white blood cells, fibrin, trapped erythrocytes, and platelet debris. White blood cells are seen at various levels within the lining (8000x).

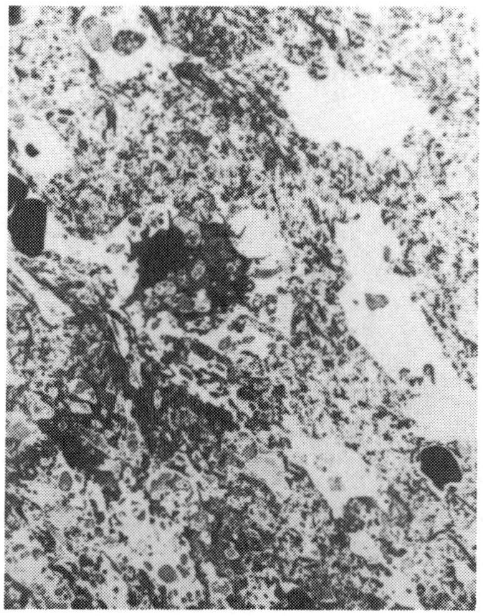

Figure 38. Calf No. 553 (23 Days Implantation) Nonseeded Control. Transmission electron micrograph of the middle layer of the biologic material. A loosely organized, highly edematous, fibrinous layer typifies the linings of nonseeded cells. In this micrograph, a white blood cell and three red blood cells (showing as electron dense elliptical portions) are visible. (8000x).

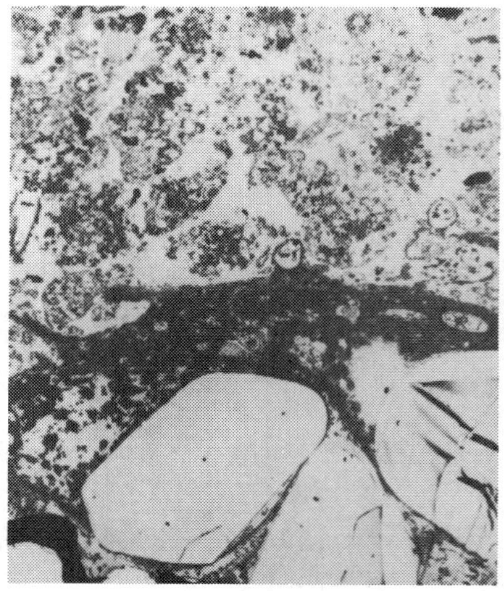

Figure 39. Calf No. 553 (23 Days Implantation) Nonseeded Control. Transmission electron photomicrograph of the basal area of the biologic material that formed on the LVAD. The basal portion is composed of fibrin and platelet profiles. This layer provides the continuity between the biologic material and the LVAD substrate. Portions of the spaces previously occupied by the Biomer fibrils are visible at the bottom of the micrograph. The fibrils are surrounded by a thin, edematous layer of fibrin. (8000x).

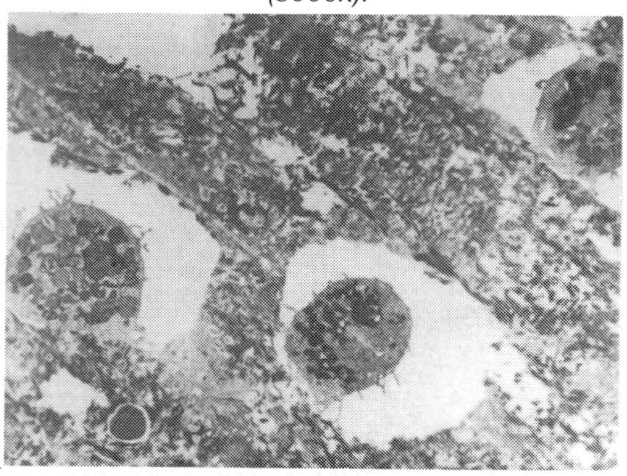

Figure 40. Calf No. 566 (60 Days Implantation) Nonseeded Control. Specimen No. 1, fibrinous portion of the lining. Dense meshwork of mature fibrin and precipitated serum proteins. In free spaces are three round cells showing microvilli and granules typical of monocytes. These cells also show larger phagocytic vacuoles containing structures of various electron densities. One cell has an eccentric nucleus with a chromatin pattern usually seen in monocytes. There is also a red cell surrounded by a small empty space. This micrograph is representative of all nonseeded (control) linings (8000x).

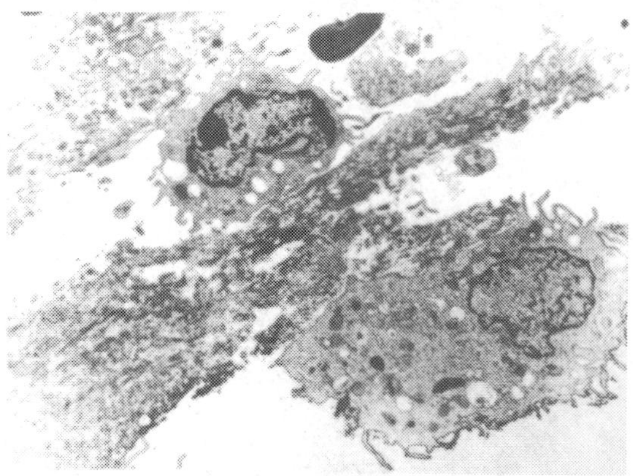

Figure 41. Calf No. 568, Nonseeded Control, Transmission Electron Microscopy (TEM). Electromicrographs from the apparent lumenal surface of the lining showing a monocytic cell that is rounded and shows abundant cytoplasmic villi. The cytoplasm shows the typical granules of a monocyte. The adherence is relatively firm to a material that appears to be fibrin. Particularly dense interstitial material with a relatively rough surface is present on the rest of the lumenal surface. There is also a red cell and a similar cell embedded in between the interstitial material. (8000x).

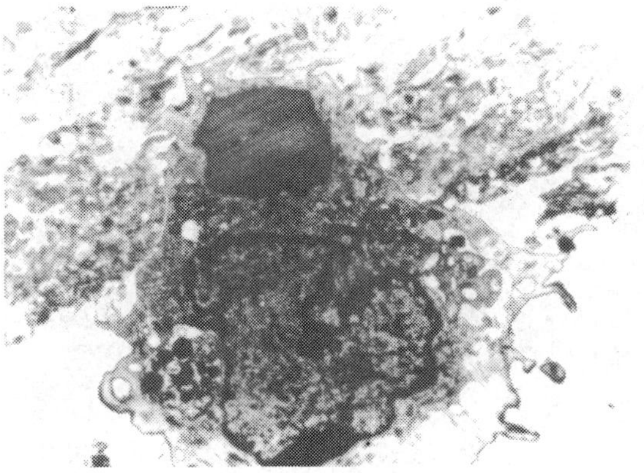

Figure 42. Calf No. 568, Nonseeded Control, TEM. A cell found adhering to and partially embedded in the luminal surface of the lining, this cell is definitely phagocytic and shows a typical phagocytic vacuole with droplets and granular material and probably also a partially phagocytosed red cell. Most of the excess cellular material consists of fibrin of variable density (12,420x)..

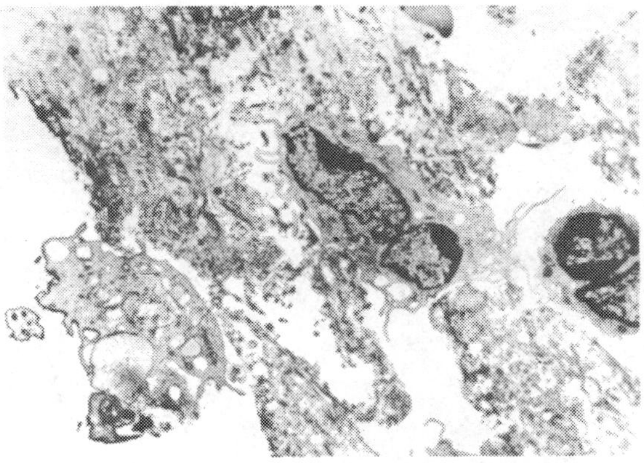

Figure 43. Calf No. 568, Nonseeded, TEM. A low-power view of a cell attached to the lumenal surface of the lining. This cell also is phagocytic and has the characteristics of a monocyte. Two more cells are embedded in a relatively dense fibrillar interstitium consisting mostly of fibrin (6,095x).

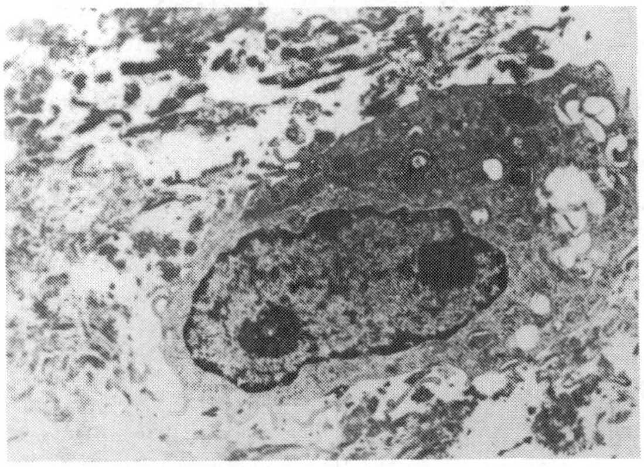

Figure 44. Calf No. 568, Nonseeded, TEM. A monocytic cell with typical granules and a few vacuoles embedded predominantly in fibrin that is loosely arranged. This cell is also located just underneath the surface and does not show the typical features of the fibroblasts. It lacks the very active rough endoplasmatic reticulum that was seen in other cells (12,420x).

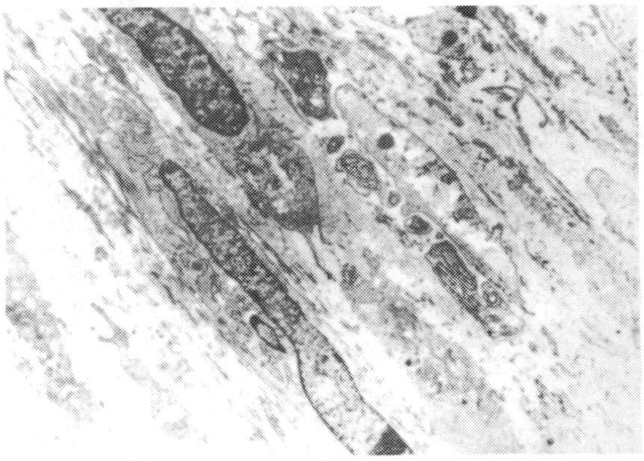

Figure 45. Calf No. 568, Nonseeded, TEM.Deeper in the lining there are parallel spindle-shaped cells resembling fibroblasts, with relatively active rough endoplasmic reticulum. The interstitial material looks somewhat more organized and is essentially fibrillar (12,420x).

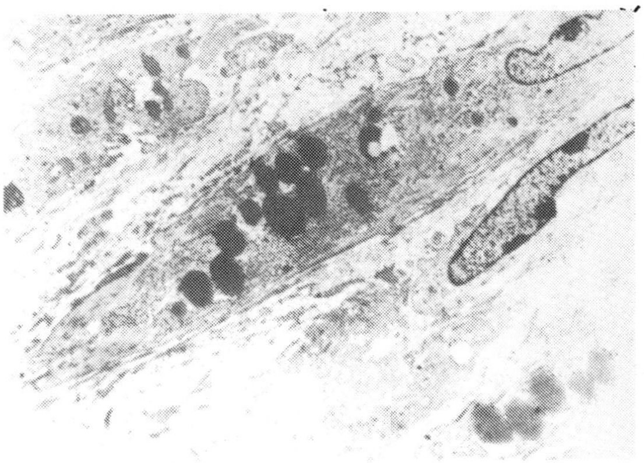

Figure 46. Calf No. 568, TEM. Somewhat deeper in the lining there are spindle-shaped cells relatively densely packed that show the morphology of fibroblasts and a relatively active, although not much dilated, rough endoplasmic reticulum. There are some peripheral areas showing actin filaments with dense bodies. Two of the cells contain quite prominent lipid droplets. The interstitial material is somewhat more organized than in the surface and appears to be young collagen (12,420x).

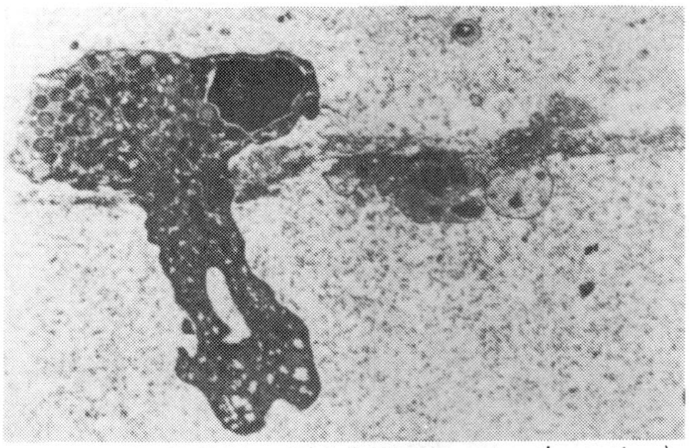

Figure 47. Calf No. 586 (270 Days Implantation), Fibroblast Seeded. Transmission electron micrograph taken at the blood-contacting surface shows cores of flocculant material and the luminal surface. A somewhat more organized, but still amorphous, floccular material comprises the biological lining. A very fine dense structure separates the two areas; however, this structure is definitely not collagenous. Extensions of cells with granules resembling those of polymorphonuclear leukocytes are adherent to the blood interface. One cell clearly identifiable as a polymorphonuclear leukocyte is seen penetrating through the very thin boundary layer. (12,420x).

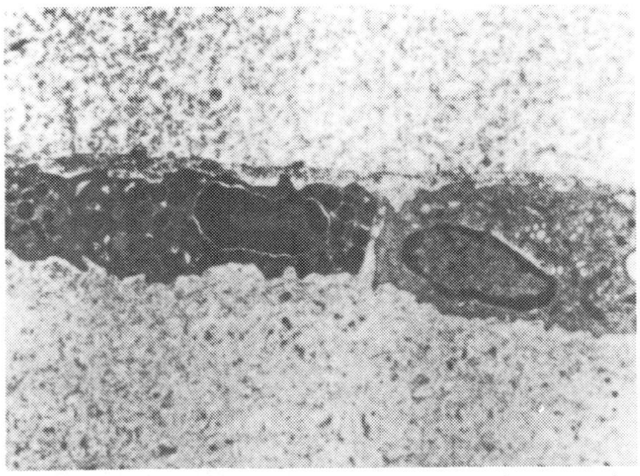

Figure 48. Calf No. 581 (338 Days Implantation), Fibroblast Seeded. Transmission electron micrograph taken from the surface of the biologic lining shows a very loose architecture with floccular and amorphous material both inside and outside of the borderline. This material resembles precipitated plasma proteins. Two cells are visible within the lining. One is a polymorphonuclear leukocyte with typical granules and the other resembles a monocyte. (12,420x).

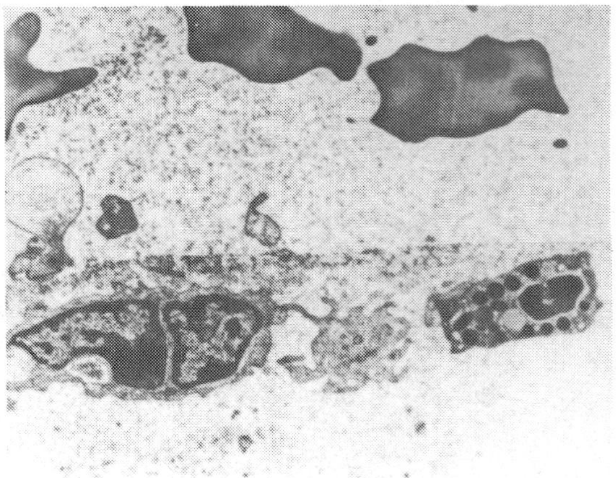

Figure 49. Calf No. 586 (270 Days Implantation), Fibroblast Seeded. Transmission electron micrograph at the blood interface. The biologic lining is at the bottom of the photograph, containing white blood cells. The top of the photograph shows postmortem thrombus, with three enmeshed red blood cells. Although the pseudoneointimal lining is highly collagenous, the actual blood interface is composed of precipitated plasma proteins and cells. This may help explain why our collagenous linings are nonthrombogenic, since collagen is not in direct contact with blood. (12,420x).

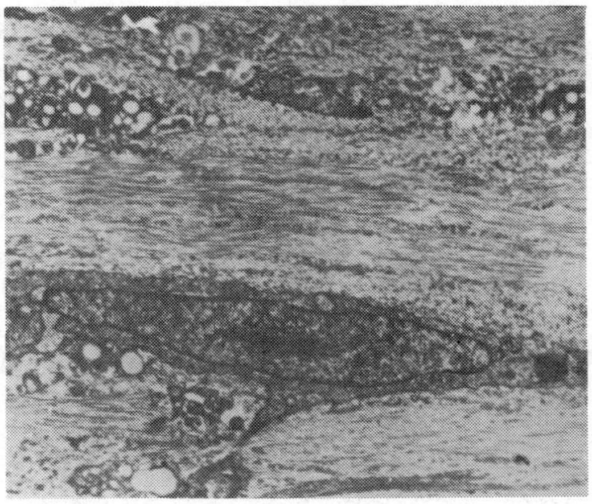

Figure 50. Calf No. 581 (338 Days Implantation), Fibroblast Seeded. Transmission electron micrograph of a portion of the bladder lining taken from the collagenous-dense center, showing a viable fibroblast, surrounded by bundles of mature collagen fibers. The collagen fibers can be seen arranged in longitudinal as well as cross-sectional bundles. In some layers within the collagen bundle, there are portions of necrotic cells and cellular debris. (12,420x).

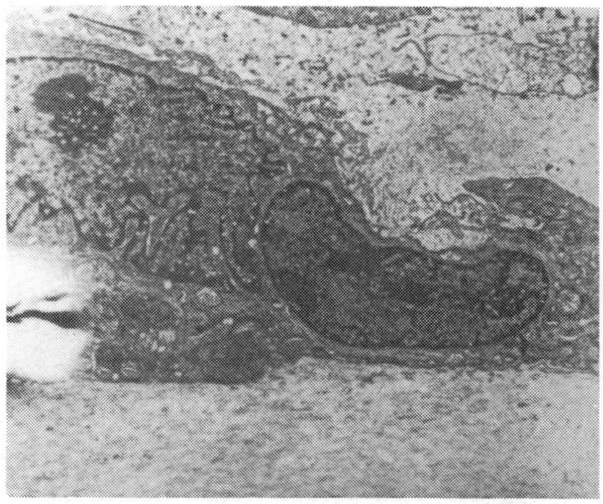

Figure 51. Calf No. 594 (149 Days Implantation), Fibroblast Seeded. Transmission electron micrograph taken in the region of the bladder shows a large multinucleated giant cell partially in direct contact with the Biomer fibril. The giant cell is surrounded by mature collagen fibers positioned longitudinally as well as in cross section (12,420x).

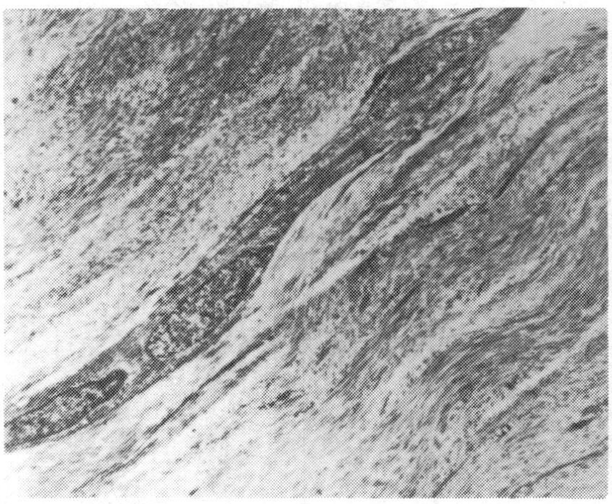

Figure 52. Calf No. 586 (270 Implantation), Fibroblast Seeded. Transmission electron micrograph showing densely packed, highly organized layer of collagen with elongated fibroblastic cells which appear to be less active than cells seen in other specimens. (8,170x).

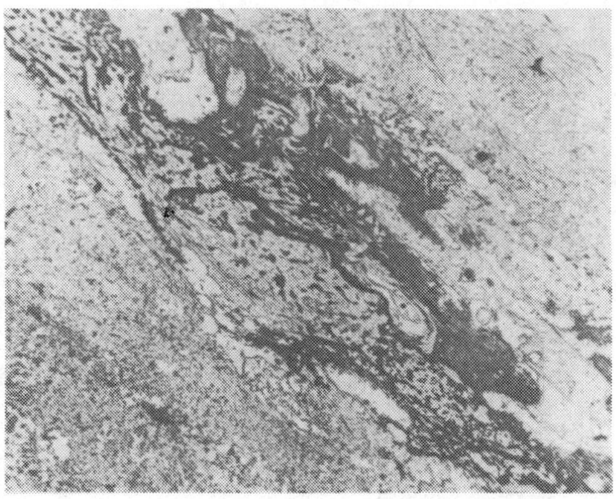

Figure 53. Calf No. 581 (338 Days Implantation), Fibroblast Seeded. Transmission electron micrograph taken adjacent to the bladder interface. The Biomer fibrils are not visible. There are three layers, two peripheral ones with collagen and loose amorphous material and a central one with rather densely packed fibron. This entire area is virtually acellular, except for a few very thin cytoplasmic extensions of fibroblastic cells. (9,740x).

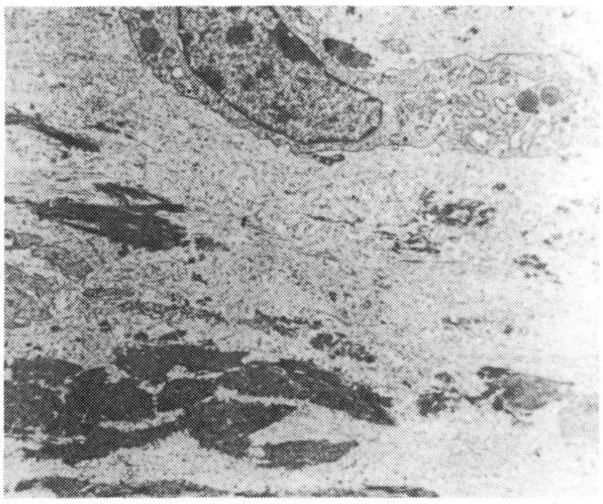

Figure 54. Calf No. 586 (270 Days Implantation), Fibroblast Seeded. Representative area from the center of the biologic lining showing organized fibrin and collagen intermixed in various directions. A viable fibroblast shows good preservation and abundant cytoplasmic detail. (8,740x).

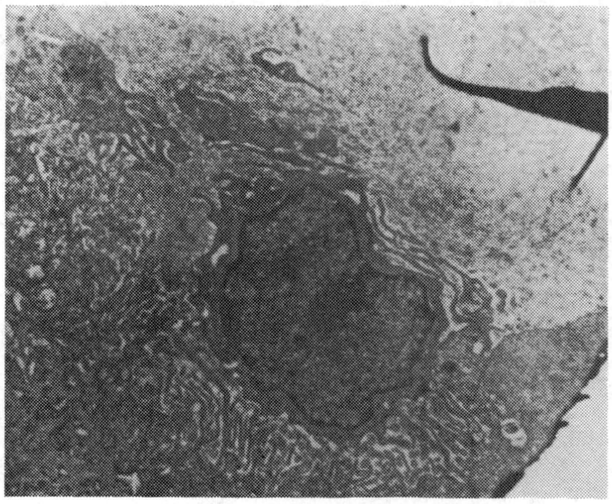

Figure 55. Calf No. 594 (149 Days Implantation), Fibroblast Seeded. Transmission electron micrograph adjacent to the polymeric fibrils which appears as a white area in the corner. Remains of the polyurethane appear as condensed electrondense patches. A similar dark patch is overlaying a large area of collagen. This is an artifact representing polymeric materials smeared onto the biological material. The cells shown are fibroblastic in nature and show bizarre interdigitating cytoplasmic extensions. The cytoplasm of a second cell is located adjacent to a portion of the fibril. However, such close contacts are rather exceptional. (12,420x).

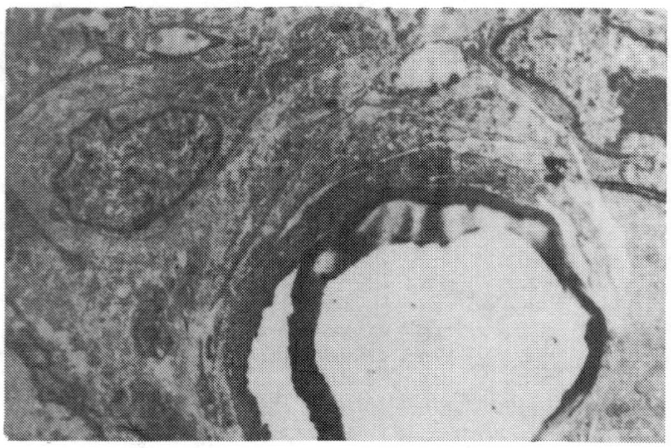

Figure 56. Polymeric Fibril/Cellular Interface. Intimate contact between cellular extension and Biomer fibril is clearly seen. All cells in this region of Calf No. 582 are fibroblastic in nature and concentrically arranged; no fibrin is seen in this section, explaining the good adherence between biologic lining and bladder.

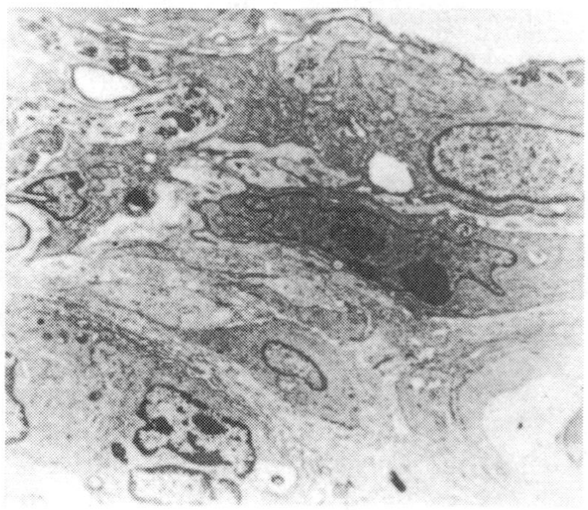

Figure 57. Calf No. 586 (270 Days Implantation), Fibroblast Seeded. Highly cellular area in the region of the polymeric fibrils. The cells show a variety of shapes and sizes as well as variable nuclear density and chromatin patterns. These cells appear viable and show a rather active cytoplasm. Between the cells we find mostly amorphous material and some debris. (8,740x).

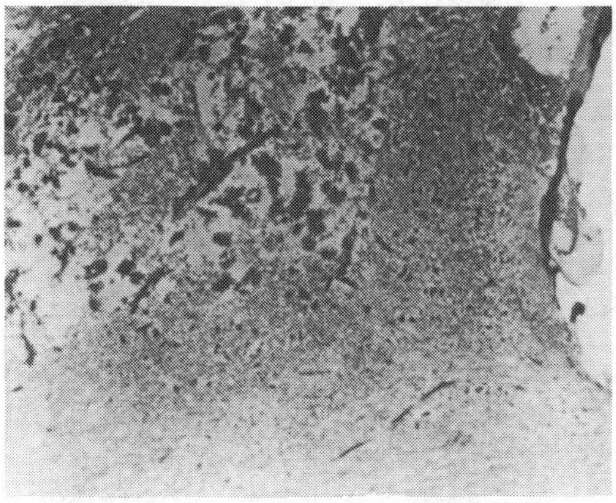

Figure 58. Calf No. 581 (338 Days Implantation), Fibroblast Seeded. Micrograph taken from an area surrounding the Biomer fibrils. The fibril location is partially visible at the edge of the photograph, showing up as the white area with a dark periphery. This particular fibril is not in contact with a viable cell. It is surrounded, instead, by grey, amorphous material. Some mature collagen fibers and dark-appearing bundles of fibrin are seen opposite the Biomer fibril. At the opposite end of the photograph, an extension of a viable fibroblast is located at a considerable distance from the Biomer fibril. (8,740x).

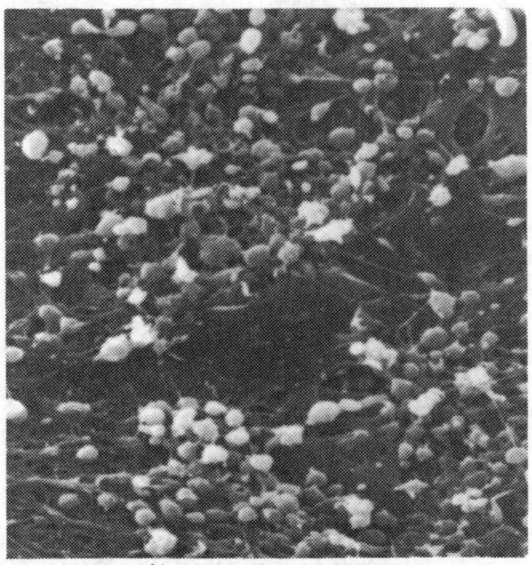

Figure 60. Calf No. 568, SEM. Representative area showing several cells which have become flattened, and retain only slight evidence of surface ruffles. Predominant are disc-shaped platelets and flat, structureless cells located on a fibrillar meshwork. Note that platelets are virtually absent on the surface of flattened cells. It is also interesting that most platelets appear as individual cells not forming larger aggregates. Some of the fibrillar-appearing background actually represents pseudopods of spreading platelets. (2000x).

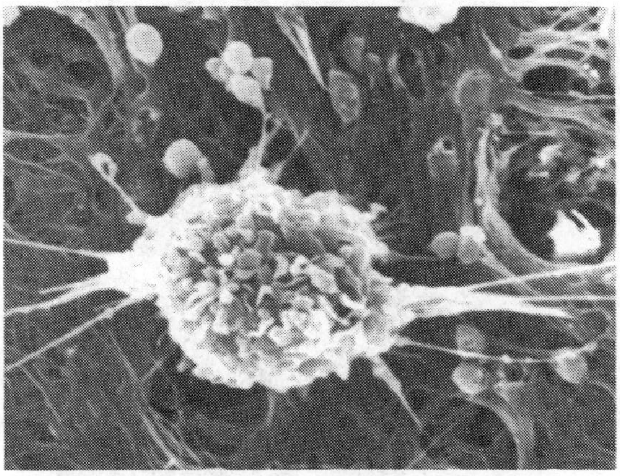

Figure 59. Calf No. 568, SEM. Close-up electron micrograph of a round cell with delicate cytoplasmic extensions and a ruffled cytoplasmic surface adhering to a fibrillar meshwork. The small, disc-shaped elements surrounding this cell represent platelets. Only a few platelets show some spreading; most of the others retain their discoid shape. Our observations are strongly suggestive that ruffled-surface monocytic cells attach themselves to the biologic lining, lose their surface ruffles and eventually become flattened cells, with many ultrastructural characteristics at endothelid cells. This process will be shown in the next series of scanning micrographs. (4000x).

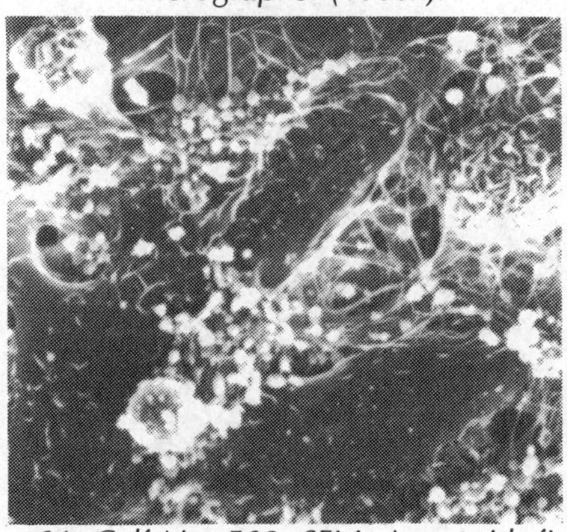

Figure 61. Calf No. 568, SEM. Area with five flat cells, multiple platelets in various stages of shape change, and pseudopod formation; also present are a small round cell with a fine granular surface and two round cells with ruffled cytoplasmic surfaces. One of these is flattening out and shows small portions of the cytoplasm without ruffled surface. Although some fibrillar structures, possibly extensions of platelets of fibrin strands, are occasionally seen covering the flat cells, most of the surface of these cells is empty and smooth. (1500x).

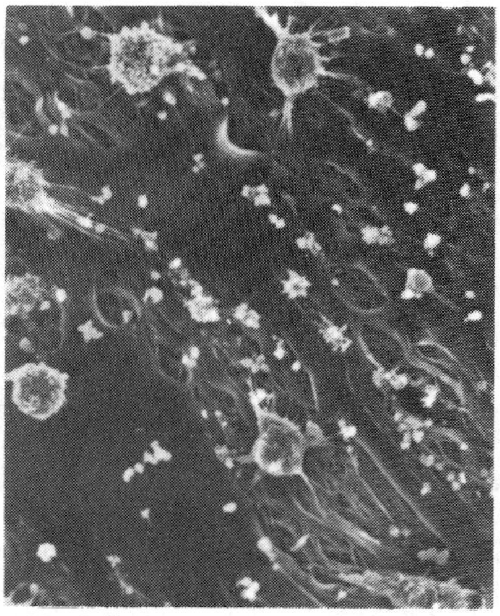

Figure 62. Calf No. 568, SEM. A rare area where the flat, superficial cells are predominant. The super-imposed round cells, with the ruffling surface, extend delicate multiple cytoplasmic extensions to the surface of these flat cells as well as to the underlying fibrillar meshwork. The smallest formed elements most likely represent platelets that have spread only a little, and some debris. It is noteworthy that large area of the surfaces of the flat cells do not show any adhering material. (1000x).

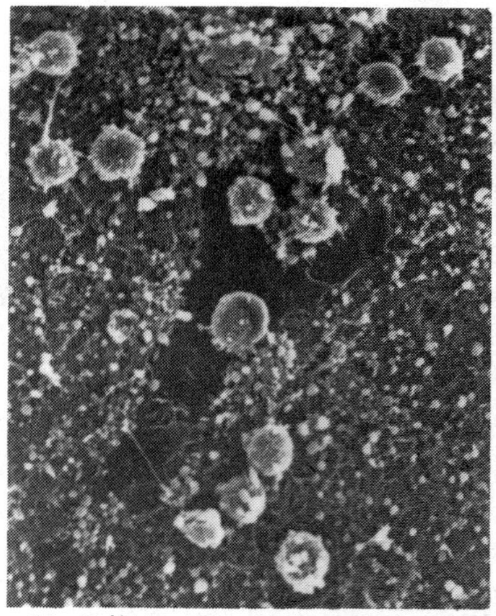

Figure 63. Calf No. 571, Cell-Seeded, SEM. In this experiment, we can observe another group of extremely flat cells together with multiple, relatively uniform, round cells. The round cells obviously adhere to the fibrillar meshwork as well as to the smooth surface of the flat cell. Platelets, in contrast, adhere to the round cells and to the fibrillar meshwork but not to the flat, smooth cell. (1200x).

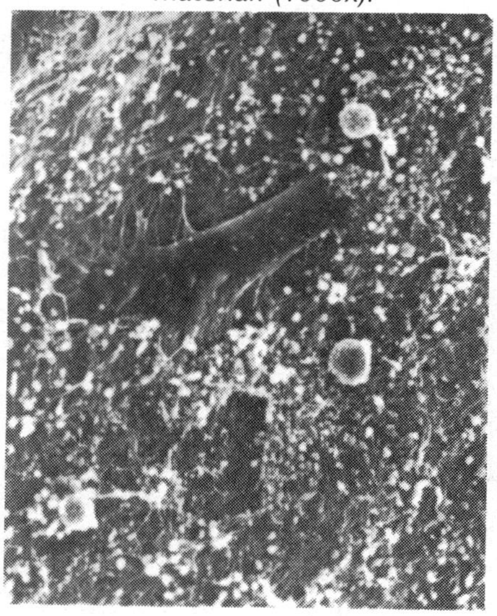

Figure 64. Calf No. 571, Cell-Seeded, SEM. One flat cell with an extremely smooth surface and delicate cytoplasmic extensions is surrounded by three round cells with a fine granular surface showing no cytoplasmic extensions. The rest of the surface shows a relatively dense meshwork of fibrillar material, multiple discrete platelets with occasional pseudopods, and few, barely recognizable, spread platelets. (1000x).

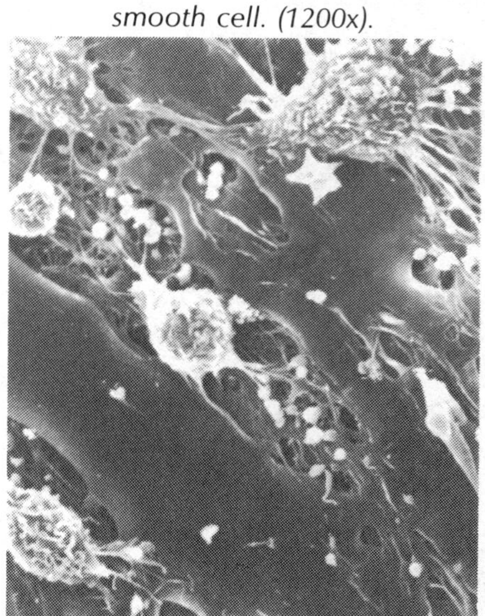

Figure 65. Calf No. 571, Cell-Seeded, SEM. Similar area showing an incomplete covering of the fibrillar meshwork with extremely flat cells, showing a very smooth surface. Five individual cells with ruffled surfaces are found in different stages of spreading; the largest one especially shows multiple, delicate, cytoplasmic extensions but also a relatively flat cytoplasmic extension lacks surface ruffling. The few platelets present show only short pseudopods, if any, and appear to adhere predominantly to the fibrillar meshwork. (1500x).

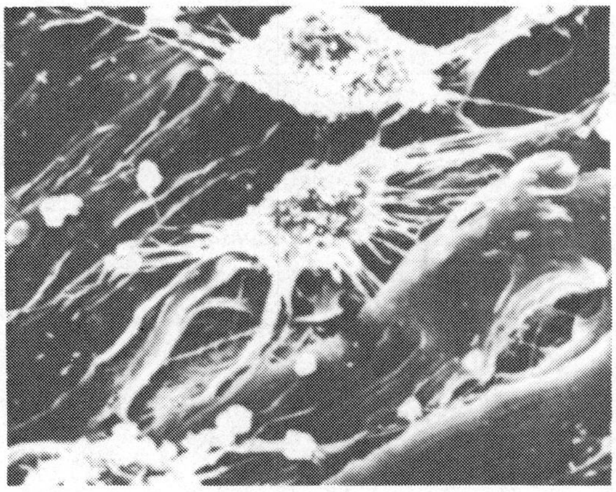

Figure 66. Calf No. 571, Cell-Seeded, SEM. Close-up of an area with multiple, smooth-surfaces, superficial cells covered by three round cells with ruffled surface and multiple, delicate, long cytoplasmic extensions to the surface of the smooth cells as well as to the underlying fibrillar meshwork. Only occasional platelets are present, apparently adhering to the round cells or to defects in the smooth cell layer. The three round cells with ruffled surfaces will eventually cover the spaces between the flattened cells. When this happens, the true blood-contacting surface of the PNI lining is composed of a cellular monolayer reminescent of normal endothelium. (2000x).

7. Preliminary Conclusions

We have successfully developed a method for obtaining highly collagenous pseudoneointimal linings (ranging from 30 to 69 percent collagen) by preoperatively seeding bladders with allogeneic fetal cells. A total of 12 in vivo experiments, ranging from 1 month to over 11 months duration, show cellular linings composed largely of newly synthesized collagen, in a GAG matrix composed of dermatan sulfate, chondroitin sulfate C, hyaluronic acid, and heparan sulfate.

Integrally textured surfaces have been specifically designed to encourage the formation of a biologic lining consisting of proteins derived entirely from the host. Our experiments to date have shown that a continuous lining is formed within a relatively short period of time.

A comprehensive assessment of resultant pseudoneointimal linings requiring a fundamental understanding of the nature of biologic materials that have accumulated during in vivo experiments. An understanding of the biochemical moieties present in the lining is crucial, since these constituents ultimately decide the suitability and integrity of the lining in long-term implants. We have studied the temporal events occurring in an intimal lining by mechanical, biochemical, histological, and ultrastructural methods.

Systematic in vivo studies have been conducted comparing nonseeded (control) bladders with fibroblast-seeded bladders. Histological and biochemical analyses confirm, on a quantitative basis, that much more collagen accumulated on cell-seeded lining than on control linings. Radioactive pulse experiments indicate that the tissue from the fibroblast-seeded pump linings synthesize more collagen, in vitro, than the tissue from the control linings. Cell outgrowth from explants of both control and seeded linings are also shown to possess high degrees of biosynthetic activity in vitro.

Substantial differences exist between nonseeded (control) and seeded linings; these differences are illustrated in Figures 30 through 66. A summary of our conclusions follows on the next page:

MODE	DISADVANTAGES	ADVANTAGES
Nonseeded	1. Thick, uncontrolled linings	1. No handling prior to surgery
	2. Loose fibrin adhesion to bladder	2. Satisfactory for short implantation periods
	3. Ectopic calcification	
Fibroblast Seeded	1. Need to study immunologic response (if any)	1. Thin, collagenous linings
	2. Requires a storage bank for harvested fibroblasts	2. Smooth, nonthrombogenic blood interface
	3. Requires seeding time (4 hrs) prior to surgical implantation	3. Excellent adhesion to bladder
		4. Substantially less calcification even after 11 months implantation

ACKNOWLEDGEMENT

The authors acknowledge the invaluable help of Dr. Carl Franzblau of Boston University School of Medicine for his measurement of pseudointimal collagen content, and Dr. Christian Haudenschild of Mallory Institute of Pathology for his pathological assessments of retrieved prostheses.

REFERENCES

1. Stoffey, D. G. et al., "A Review of Nonthrombogenic Materials," J. Macromol. Sci. Chem., *A3:*119-131 (1969).
2. Bruck, S. C., "Biomaterials, Medical Devices, and Artificial Organs," *1:*79 (1973).
3. Leininger, R. L., "Critical Reviews in Bioengineering," *1:*3, 333 (1972).
4. Szycher, M., "An Integrated Approach to Hemocompatible Polymers: A Test Protocol," Chapter 1 in *Synthetic Bomedical Polymers,* Technomic Publishing Co. (1980).
5. Bernhard, W. F., "An Improved Blood-Pump Interface for Left Ventricular Bypass," Annals of Surgery, *168:*750 (1968),
6. Liotta, D. et al., Cardiovascular Res. Bull., *4:*69 (1966).
7. Hall, C. W. et al., J. Biomed. Mat. Res., *1:*179 (1967).
8. DeBakey, M. E. et al., Nat. Acad. Sci., National Research Council, Washington, D.C., Chapter 18 (1966).
9. Bernhard, W. F., Colo, N. A., Wesolowski, J. S., Szycher, M., Fishbein, M. C., Parkman, R., Franzblau, C., and Haudenschild, C. C., "Development of Collagenous Linings on Impermeable Prosthetic Surfaces," J. Thorac. Cardiovasc. Surg., *79:*552-564 (1980).
10. Bernhard, W. F., Colo, N. A., Szycher, M., Wesolowski, J. S., Haudenschild, C. C., Franzblau, C., Parkman, R., and Liss, R., "Development of a Nonthrombogenic Collagenous Blood-Prosthetic Interface," Ann. Surg., *192:*369-381 (1980).
11. *ASTM Annual Book of Standards,* Part 9, American Society for Testing and Materials, Philadelphia, Pa., p. 63 (1978).

12. *Sintering and Related Phenomena,* Ed. Gordon and Breech, Science Publishers, N.Y., London (1967).
13. McGregor, D. C. et al., "Porous Metal Surfaces: A Radical New Concept in Heart Valve Design," Trans. ASAIO, *22*:646 (1976).
14. Brest, A. N., *Heart Substitutes, Mechanical and Transplant,* Charles C. Thomas, Pub., p. 47 (1966).
15. Keiser, J., Bernhard, W., Poirier, V., Gernes, D., Szycher, M., and Robinson, W., "Development and Evaluation of Unilateral and Bilateral Cardiac Assist Devices," Annual Technical Report NO1-HV-4-2910-4, NTIS (January 1978).
16. Whalen, R. L., and Nose, Y., "Development of a Left Heart Assist Blood Pump," Annual Technical Report NO1-HV-7-2934-2, NTIS (June 1979).
17. Harasaki, H., Snow, J., Gerrity, R., Whalen, R., Ozana, K., Kiraly, R., and Nose, Y., "Powdered Metal Surface for Blood Pumps," ASAIO Proceedings, Vol. 25 (In Press).
18. Mathews, M. B., "Connective Tissue," Macromolecular Structure and Evolution, Springer, Berlin/Heidelberg/New York (1975).
19. Comper, W. D. and Laurent, T. C., *Physiol. Rev.* (1978).
20. Silbert, J. E. and Reppuci, A. C., J. Biol. Chemn., *251*:3942-47 (1976).
21. Lindahl, U. and Roden, L., *Glycoproteins, Their Composition, Structure and Function,* Ed. A. Gottschalk, pp. 491-517, Amsterdam: Elsevier, p. 1378, 2nd Ed. (1972).
22. Rees, D. A., Int. Rev. Sci. Biochem., *5*:1-41 (1975).
23. Piez, K. A., Weiss, E., and Lewis, M. S., "The Separation and Characterization of the α- and β-Components of Calf Skin Collagen," J. Biol. Chem., *235*:1987 (1960).
24. Miller, E. J., Martin, G. R., Piez, K. A., and Powers, M. R., "Characterization of Chick Bone Collagen and Compositional Changes Associated with Maturation," J. Biol. Chem., *242*:5481 (1967).
25. Kang, A., Piez, K. A., and Gross, J., "Characterization of the α Chains of Chick Skin Collagen and The Nature of the NH_2-terminal Cross-Link Region," Biochem., *8*:3648 (1969).
26. Miller, E. J. and Matukas, U. J., "Chick Cartilage Collagen: A New Type of $\alpha 1$ Chain Not Present in Bone or Skin of the Species," Proc. Nat. Acad. Sci., *64*:1264 (1969).
27. Trelstad, R. L., Kang, A., Igarashi, S., and Gross, J., "Isolation of Two Distinct Collagens from Chick Cartilage," Biochem., *9*:4993 (1970).
28. Miller, E. J., "Isolation and Characterization of a Collagen from Chick Cartilage Containing Three Identical α Chains," Biochem., *10*:1652 (1971).
29. Strawich, E. and Nimni, M. E., "Properties of a Collagen Molecule Containing Three Identical Components Extracted from Bovine Articular Cartilage," Biochem., *10*:3905 (1971).
30. Toole, B. P., Kang, A., Trelstad, R., and Gross, J., "Collagen Heterogenity Within Growth Regions of Long Bones of Rachitic and Nonrachitic Chicks," Biochem. J., *127*:715 (1972).
31. Miller, E. J., Epstein, E. H., and Piez, K. A., "Identification of Three Genetically Distinct Collagens by Cyanogen Bromide Cleavage of Insoluble Human Skin and Cartilage Collagen," Biochem. Biophys. Res. Comm., *42*:1024 (1971).
32. Miller, E. J., "Structural Studies in Cartilage Collagen Employing Limited Cleavage and Solubilization with Pepsin," Biochem., *11*:4903 (1972).
33. Kefalides, N. A., "Isolation of a Collagen from Basement Membranes Containing Three Identical α Chains," Biochem. Biophys. Res. Comm., *45*:226 (1971).
34. Trelstad, R. and Kang, A., "Collagen Heterogeneity on the Avian Eye: Lens, Vitroeus Body, Cornea, and Sclera," Experiment Eye Research, *18*:395-406 (1974).
35. Linsenmayer, T. F., Smith, G. N., and Hay, E. D., "Synthesis of Two Collagen Types in Embryonic Chick Corneal Epithelium In Vitro," Proc. Natl. Acad. Sci., *74*:(1):39-43 (1977).
36. VonDerMark, K., VonDerMark, H., Tripl, R., and Trelstad, R., "Immunofluorescent Localization of Collagen Types I, II, and III in the Embryonic Chick Eye," Dev. Biol., *59*:75-85 (1977).

Chapter 7

The Development of Cellular Linings in Artificial Vascular Prostheses

William E. Burkel, Ph.D.
Department of Anatomy
University of Michigan

ABSTRACT

Cells and tissue fragments have been seeded into artificial vascular prostheses in order to provide a blood compatible surface for many years. While early experiments involved microfiber-lined polyurethane devices, more recent experiments have used standard vascular grafts. Specific methods for lining grafts with cells vary, but three general methods have been used. After harvesting cells or tissue fragments they have been: a) immediately seeded into grafts and the grafts implanted, b) cultivated in vitro, *seeded into grafts and implanted and c) seeded into grafts, the grafts cultivated* in vitro *and then implanted. Recent studies using methods a and b to seed endothelium into standard 6mm ID Dacron and Teflon thoracoabdominal prostheses have shown that these grafts are 60% covered with endothelium at 2 weeks and over 80% covered at 1 month with total healing of the grafts between 1 and 4 months, while controls remain thrombogenic for over a year. Similarly, 4mm ID externally supported Dacron iliofemoral grafts heal as rapidly as the 6mm grafts and have significantly higher patency rates than unseeded controls.*

Funded by National Heart Lung and Blood Institute Contract NO1-HV-2054 and Grant HL23345.

Since the modern era of vascular grafting began in 1952 when Voorhees and colleagues [1] implanted an artificial vessel fabricated from parachute cloth, surgeons have appreciated the need for a stable, nonthrombogenic flow surface in artificial vascular grafts. To accomplish this end two major approaches have been pursued. One was to develop nonthrombogenic vessels, either because of their physical-chemical structure, or due to the addition of clot inhibiting additives such as heparin. The second and more common approach has been to take materials, which though thrombogenic, provide a conduit which from the mechanical-surgical point of view make good grafts and fabricate them in such a way that the normal healing processes of the body provide a nonthrombogenic, or at least acceptably passive, flow surface.

The biologic surface which ultimately develops in nearly all currently available grafts, called a neointima (if it is covered with true endothelium) or a pseudointima (if the surface is not endothelium), arises from, or is formed from the seeding out of blood elements, (e.g. platelets, cells and fibrin), from perigraft tissue ingrowth and from pannus ingrowth longitudinally from the host vessel. This surface may be passivated to flowing blood, but unless covered by endothelium is unstable and thrombogenic. If flow is compromised in nonendothelial lined conduits, even momentarily, catastrophic events may occur leading to complete occlusion of the graft. Ideally, a graft becomes totally healed (i.e. be completely incorporated in perigraft tissue and lined by endothelium) as shown in Figure 1.

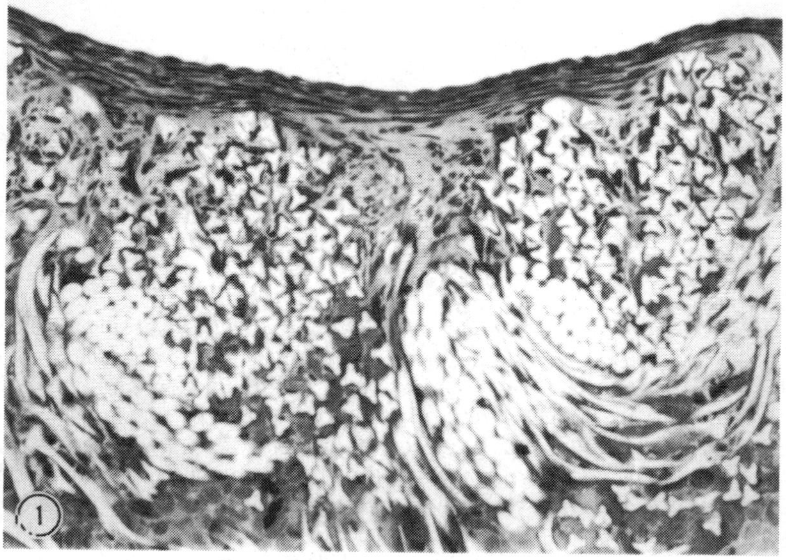

Figure 1. Longitudinal section through a Dacron double velour vascular graft showing complete healing and incorporation into perigraft tissue. Although this graft had been seeded with endothelial cells and only implanted for 2 weeks in a dog, it demonstrates the desired result in an artificial graft. The luminal surface (above) is completely covered by true endothelium. The underlying subendothelial tissue is cellular and thin (30-60μm), being composed of spindle-shaped smooth muscle cells superficially, and more pleomorphic fibroblasts and collagenous fibers closer to the graft fibers. The graft interstices are completely infiltrated with cells and connective tissue. The Dacron fibers in the lower half of the graft (external surface) are infiltrated with large multinucleated foreign body giant cells characteristic of this type of graft. LM ×120.

As is clear from the wide variety of vascular substitutes currently in use and under development, both biologic and artificial, the ideal prosthesis has not yet been found and the autologous vein graft is still the standard to which all others are compared. Indeed as Baier, et al. have remarked, the vascular substitutes presently in use are at best "physiologically tolerable" [2] and useful only in diameters greater than 6mm ID or in special high flow situations.

The one feature which clearly distinguishes natural vessels from their artificial counterparts is the presence of the cellular endothelial lining. A lining which, in addition to being truly nonthrombogenic, is capable of repair and renewal. Since such a lining develops in grafts slowly in man, if at all [3,4], investigators have seeded a variety of cells and tissue fragments [5] into artificial devices *in vitro* to provide a pseudo or neointima. Alternatively, others have tried to enhance the body's normal healing reactions and neo or pseudointimal development by optimizing the physical characteristics of the graft itself [6-9].

Much of the early work with seeded prostheses was done on diaphragms and bladders of artificial hearts and heart devices [10-15]. These devices were necessarily nonporous and generally composed of microfiber or flocked surfaces embedded into or glued to polyurethane bladders or diaphragms (Figures 2 and 3). To produce these pseudointimas, suspensions of cultured cells or tissue fragments were centrifuged into, or left to settle on, the microfabric after which the device was placed in a tissue culture chamber to allow the cells to attach and form a confluent surface (Figures 4-7).

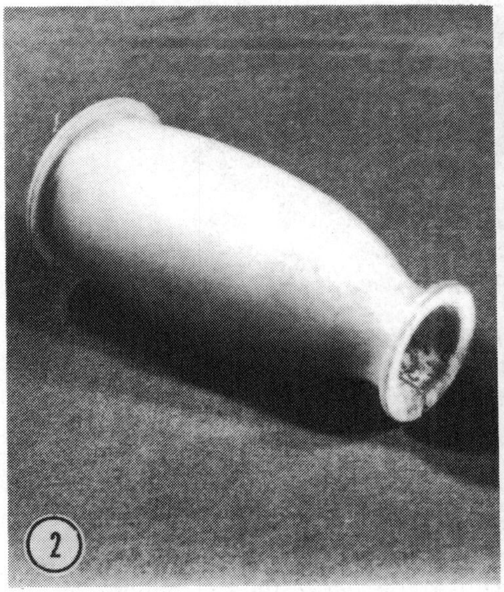

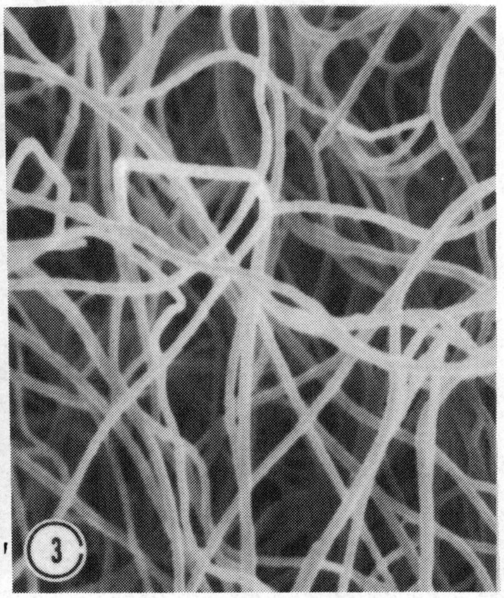

Figure 2. A bladder from a Thermoelectron (TECO) left ventricular assist device (LVAD). It is composed of a flexible, but nonporous, outer wall of polyurethane lined with a nonwoven polypropylene microfiber fabric (see Figure 3). × 0.6.

Figure 3. Scanning electron micrograph of a nonwoven polypropylene microfiber scaffold, manufactured by Union Carbide, such as used to line artificial vessels and LVADs. The small diameter fibers, which are coated with Parylene C and microwave discharge treated, form an ideal substrate for the growth of cultured cells. (see Figures 4-6). SEM ×1100.

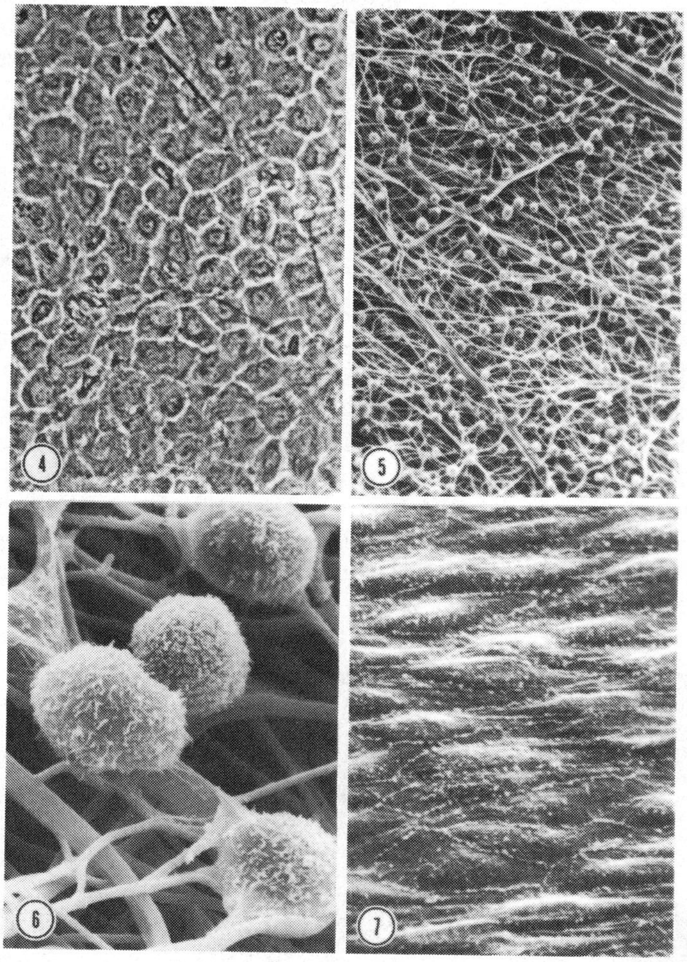

Figure 4. Human epidermal cells in tissue culture. These cells have been isolated from human skin by trypsinization and cultivated for periods of up to one year. Similar cells (Figure 7) have been used to produce pseudointimas in dogs. Phase contrast LM ×350.

Figure 5. Scanning electron micrograph of a polypropylene microfiber scaffold similar to Figure 3 seeded with human epidermal cells. The evenly distributed cells have just attached to the microfibers (see Figure 6). SEM ×140.

Figure 6. Scanning electron micrograph of same specimen as Figure 5 showing details of cellular morphology and beginning attachment of cells to the microfiber scaffold. When in suspension the cells are spherical and covered with microvilli which upon seeding attach to the microfibers. The cells then spread out by sending small processes along the fibers (center). SEM ×1500.

Figure 7. Scanning electron micrograph of the luminal surface of a polypropylene microfiber lined graft seeded with autologous epidermal cells cultivated in vitro for 2 weeks (see figure 8 method C) and implanted in a dog for 4 months. The morphological appearance of the surface is identical to that of normal endothelium. SEM ×850.

While this method has potential and was successfully used [10-16] it has several drawbacks. First, the microfabric-lined devices while good for cell growth, were extremely thrombogenic if not covered with cells and consequently could not be used in a tubular form unless they had a large bore. The microfiber lined devices sometimes varied from batch to batch and the cells and pseudointima did not always develop uniformly over the whole surface. Since methods to evaluate the cellular surface while keeping it intact and alive were not available, a complete cellular surface could not be assured upon implantation. The tissue culture step always posed a potential for microbial contamination which would preclude pseudointimal development and implantation. Lastly, even if a complete lining did develop *in vitro*, one could not be certain that the surgical procedure or handling might not damage the cellular surface leading to eventual thrombosis.

At about the time interest in cell-lined prostheses began to wane somewhat because of the problems mentioned above, Herring and his colleagues [17] found that the normal healing process in standard Dacron artificial vascular grafts could be considerably improved by adding scrapings from the inner surface of veins to the blood used to preclot grafts. While neither the use of venous tissue, nor seeding in blood were in themselves unique, the combination and the use of standard Dacron grafts produced dramatic results. Since we had considerable experience in isolating endothelial cells [18] and growing them in culture, we used enzymatically harvested endothelial cells [19-21] to seed grafts using the method described by Herring, et al.

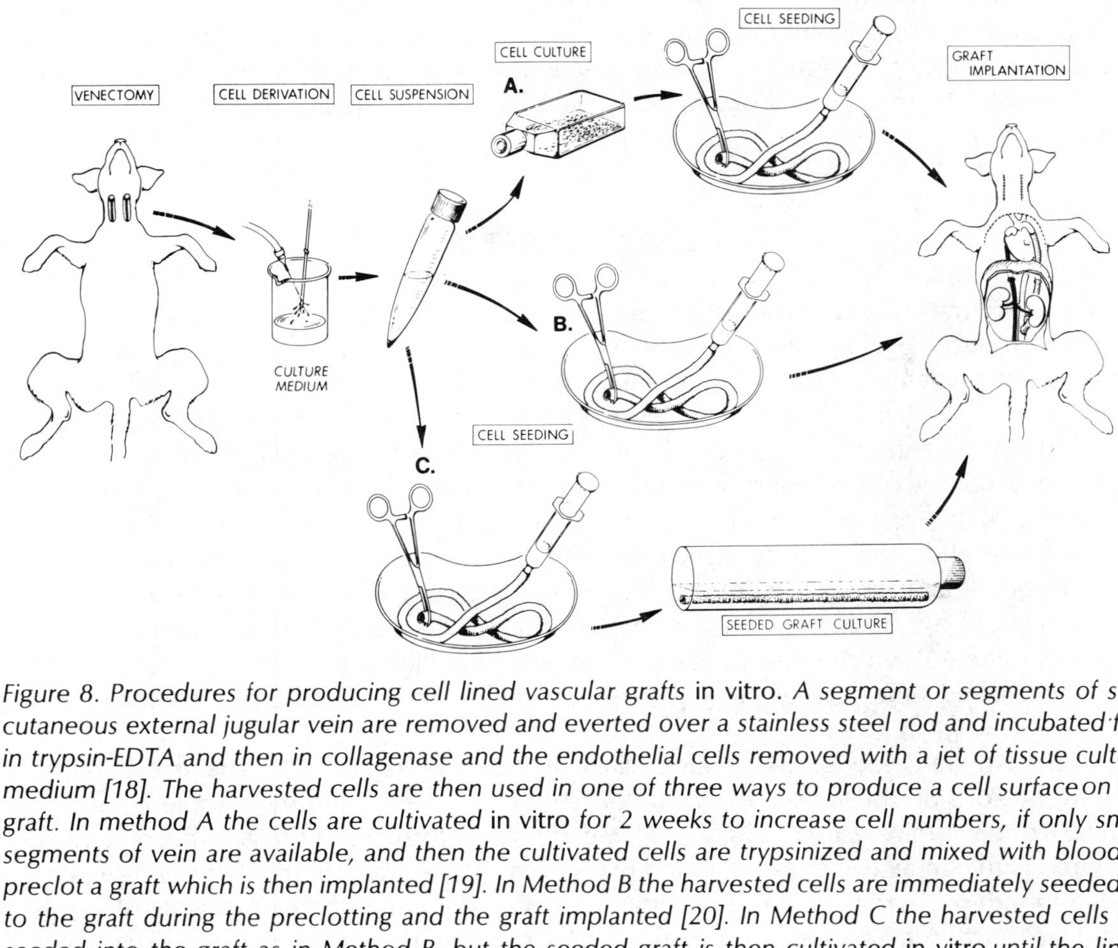

Figure 8. Procedures for producing cell lined vascular grafts in vitro. *A segment or segments of subcutaneous external jugular vein are removed and everted over a stainless steel rod and incubated first in trypsin-EDTA and then in collagenase and the endothelial cells removed with a jet of tissue culture medium [18]. The harvested cells are then used in one of three ways to produce a cell surface on the graft. In method A the cells are cultivated* in vitro *for 2 weeks to increase cell numbers, if only small segments of vein are available, and then the cultivated cells are trypsinized and mixed with blood to preclot a graft which is then implanted [19]. In Method B the harvested cells are immediately seeded into the graft during the preclotting and the graft implanted [20]. In Method C the harvested cells are seeded into the graft as in Method B, but the seeded graft is then cultivated* in vitro *until the lining develops, after which the cell-lined graft is implanted as shown in Figures 4-7.*

The method used in our experiments is summarized in Figure 8. The procedure involves 4 basic steps which may be modified for different types of neointima production. The first step is to remove the jugular vein or veins from the dog. Secondly, the veins are everted over a stainless steel rod, rinsed and incubated in first trypsin-EDTA and then collagenase and the cells washed from the vessel. Thirdly, the resultant cell suspension is used to produce an endothelial lining (Figure 8A, B, C). In variation A the cells may be cultivated *in vitro* to increase the cell number. After a suitable period of time, the culture is trypsinized to get a cell suspension, which is seeded into a graft during preclotting. In variation B the cells isolated from the veins are immediately seeded into the graft. In variation C the whole graft is cultured after seeding with cells and only implanted after an endothelial lining has developed *in vitro*. In the last step the graft (seeded with cultured cells, cells immediately after isolation or the cultivated graft) is implanted. Methods A and B produce equal results [19, 20] with B to be preferred because of its simplicity if enough cells are available. Variation C is the most complex, but may be useful for small vessels or in vessels with low flow (e.g. venous replacements) if care is taken not to damage the cell surface during implantation. This method was used routinely in the past and occasionally produced good results (Figures 2-7). A simpler alternative to step C however, in small diameter grafts or low flow situations (to be described later) is method B with systemic drug therapy to prevent thrombosis until the lining has developed *in vivo*. Using methods A and B and the alternative to C above, grafts have been implanted as thoracoabdominal bypasses and iliofemoral interposition grafts in dogs and the Dacron prostheses studied at periods of 18 hours to 1 year. Seeded polytetrafluoroethylene (PTFE, Gore Tex) grafts have also been used as thoracoabdominal bypasses and studied at 2 and 4 weeks post-implantation.

DACRON GRAFTS

The incorporation and healing in unseeded grafts was classically described by MacKenzie and Loewenthal in 1960 [22] and needs only be summarized in reference to the grafts we have used. When implanted, 6mm ID grafts (Figure 9) are initially infiltrated with blood cells, platelets and fibrin (Figure 10), but by two days are relatively clean internally, being covered only with platelets and fibrin (Figures 11 and 12). The "clean-looking" platelet-fibrin coagulum begins to become covered with fresh thrombus thereafter, however, reaching a maximum (about 80% of the surface covered by thrombus) at 2 weeks (Figure 13). During this time connective tissue and foreign body giant cells infiltrate the graft interstices and pannus tissue (smooth muscle and endothelium) begin to grow into the graft at the anastomotic line. As time progresses the fresh thrombus on the luminal surface is replaced by a fibrin coagulum (Figures 15 and 16) which over a period of months becomes organized and finally covered with endothelium, the rate of healing varying with the species and type of graft involved [23,4].

In contrast, grafts seeded with endothelial cells heal very rapidly [21]. The first endothelial cells are obvious on the surface of the graft at 4 days (Figure 17) and by 2 weeks cover more than 60% of the luminal surface (Figures 14 and 18). The interstices of the graft become rapidly infiltrated with connective tissue cells and many areas of the graft are totally healed (Figure 1). By one month more than 80% of the surface is covered by endothelium which is still only a monolayer in thickness and the incorporation of the graft seen in Figure 1 continues to

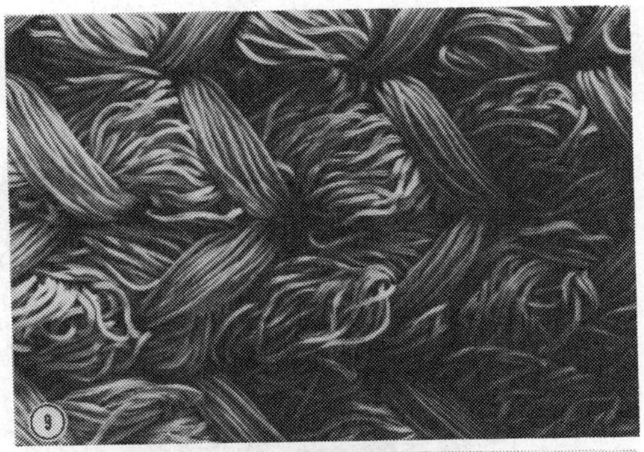

Figure 9. Luminal surface of a 6mm ID Dacron double velour warp knitted vascular graft (Meadox) used for thoracoabdominal bypasses. The larger irregular fiber bundles are composed of triangular fibrils and give the surface its velour character. (See Figure 1 for its sectioned appearance). SEM ×35.

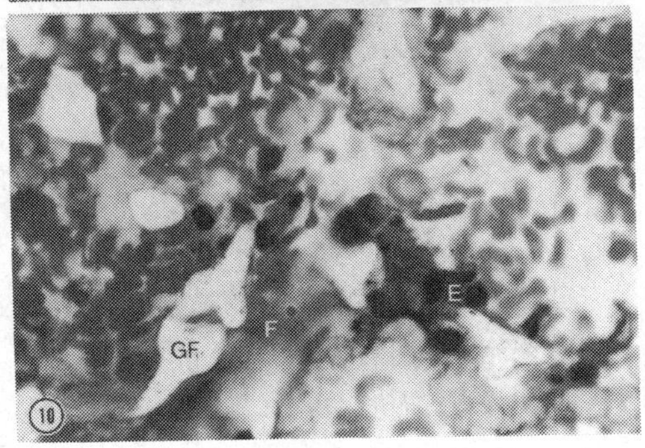

Figure 10. Cross section of a Dacron graft immediately after preclotting. The interstices of the graft are filled predominately with RBCs enmeshed in fibrin (F). Occasionally clumps of endothelial cells (E) are visible among graft fibers (GF). Endothelial cells are rarely found on the luminal surface immediately after seeding, but reach it by migrating. LM ×500.

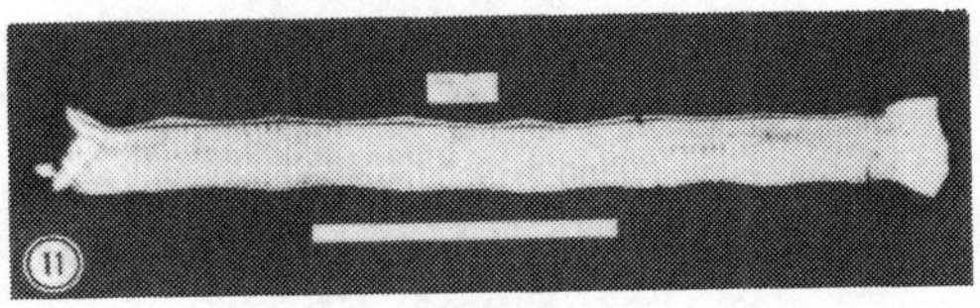

Figure 11. Gross photograph of a thoracoabdominal bypass removed from a dog 2 days after implantation. The surface is almost entirely free of thrombus and covered with platelets, fibrin and WBCs (see Figures 13 and 14). ×0.2.

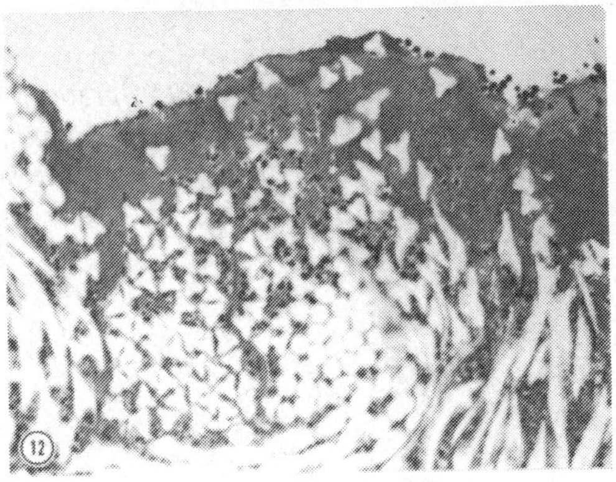

Figure 12. Micrograph of a cross section of a Dacron graft 2 days after implantation. The luminal surface is covered primarily with a thin layer of fibrin, platelets and WBCs. The zone immediately deep to the surface is almost exclusively fibrin. LM ×150.

progress. Between 1 and 4 months seeded grafts are totally healed and lined with endothelium whereas in unseeded grafts the fibrin-platelet coagulum and fresh thrombus may persist for more than a year (Figure 19). The histological picture of seeded grafts is similar to earlier times, but with a more well developed subendothelial tissue composed of mature collagen and smooth muscle (Figures 20 and 21).

The results with Dacron grafts are essentially the same whether cells are seeded into the grafts immediately (Figure 8A) or if they are cultivated for 2 weeks prior to seeding and implantation (Figure 8B) if comparable numbers of cells are used.

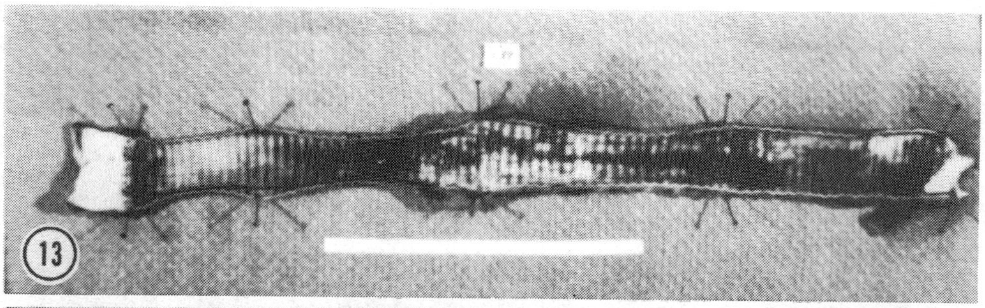

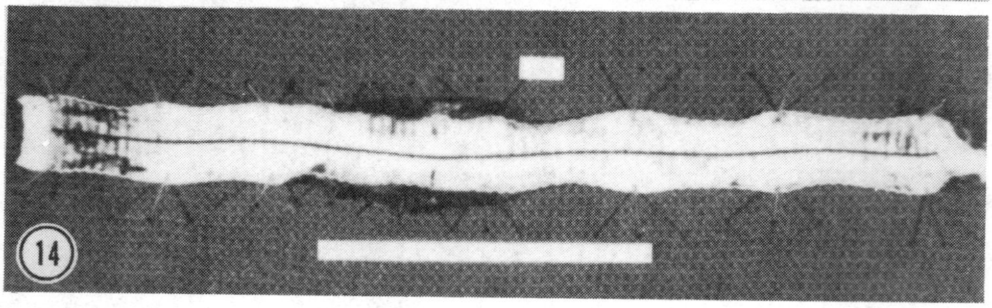

Figure 13. Gross photograph of a thoracoabdominal bypass graft 2 weeks after implantation. The control unseeded grafts are about 80% covered with thrombus, 5% endothelium and 15% fibrin. ×0.4.

Figure 14. Experimental, seeded graft. These grafts are about 15% covered with thrombus and about 60% true endothelium with the remainder fibrin at 2 weeks. ×0.4.

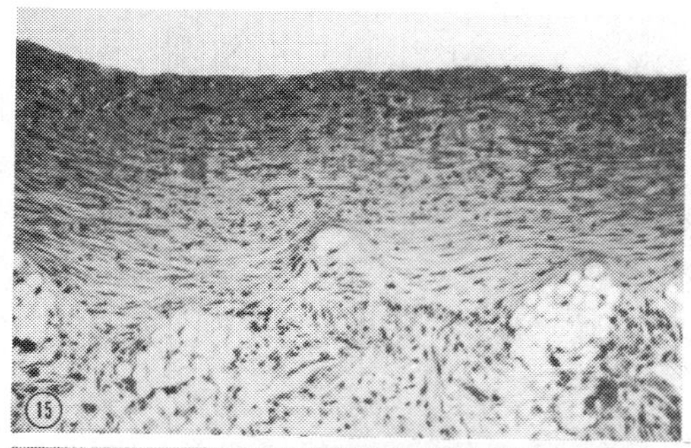

Figure 15. Section of an unseeded bypass graft 1 month after implantation. The bulk of the graft (80%) is covered by a fibrin coagulum several hundred microns thick in most places. The interstices of the graft are filled with connective tissue and foreign body giant cells, but the surface is unstable and potentially thrombogenic. LM ×50.

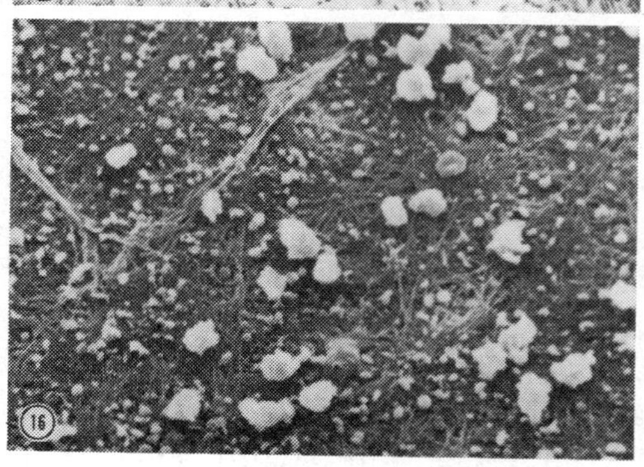

Figure 16. Surface of 1 month unseeded graft. The thrombus has been replaced by a fibrin coagulum with numerous platelets and WBCs on the surface. SEM ×700.

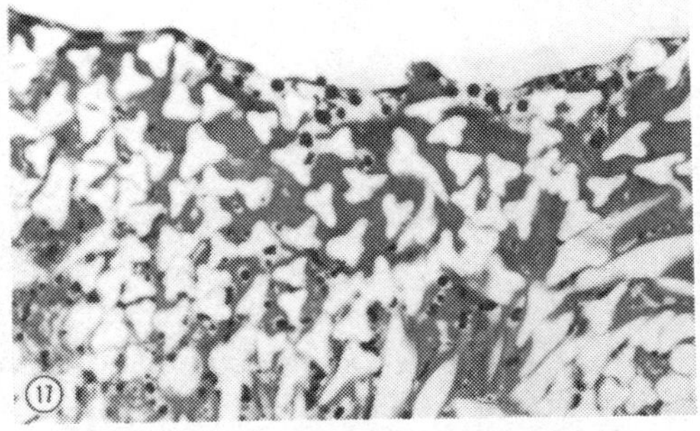

Figure 17. Cross section of a Dacron thoracoabdominal bypass graft 4 days after seeding with endothelium. The interstices of the graft are filled with fibrin above and WBCs below, but areas of endothelium are clearly visible on the surface. LM ×125.

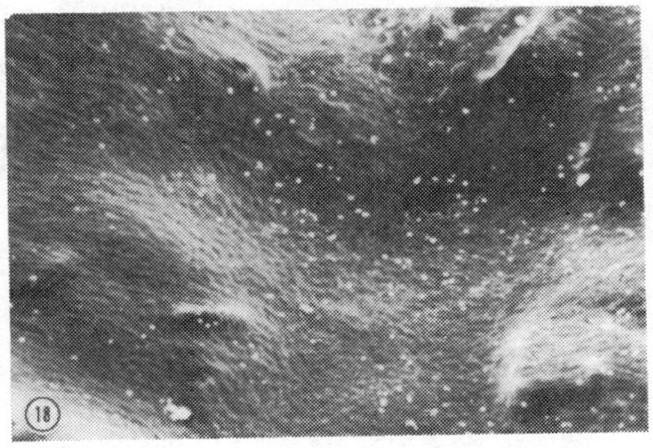

Figure 18. Scanning electron micrograph of a 14 day Dacron thoracoabdominal bypass graft. The surface is completely covered with a monolayer of endothelium. The rounded projections are endothelial cell nuclei, the white dots WBCs. The hill-valley contour is due to crimps of the graft (see Figure 1). SEM ×70.

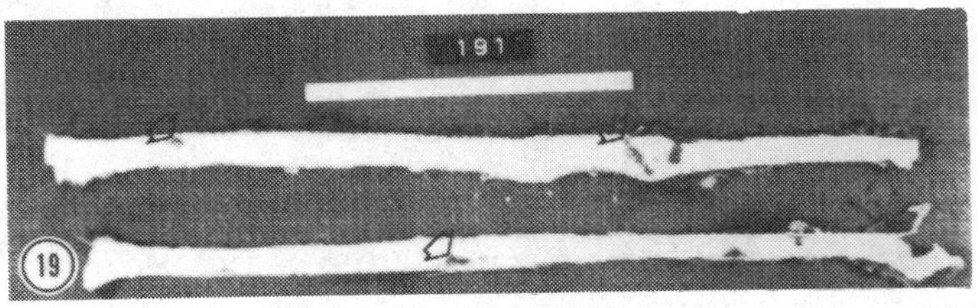

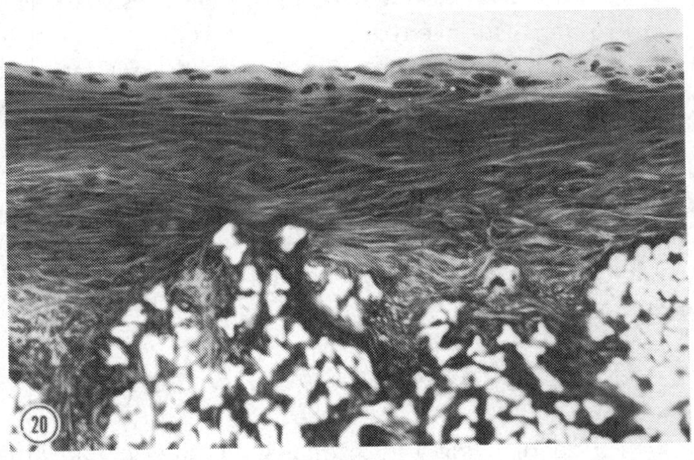

Figure 19. Gross photograph of a unseeded control graft implanted for 1 year in the thoracoabdominal position. While most of the surface is endothelial, numerous areas of thrombus are still visible (arrows). Seeded grafts in contrast are completely surfaced with endothelium by 4 months. ×0.28.

Figure 20. Cross section of a 1 year seeded Dacron implant. The graft is totally incorporated and covered with mature endothelium. The subdothelial tissue is composed of smooth muscle near the surface and fibroblasts closer to the graft fibers, with collagenous fibers throughout. LM ×150.

Figure 21. Transmission electron micrograph of a seeded graft removed 1 year after implantation. The internal surface is composed of typical endothelium with interdigitating cell junctions. The underlying tissue is composed of a layer of dense basal lamina-like material and several layers of typical smooth muscle cells (below). Compare to Figure 19. TEM ×5,000.

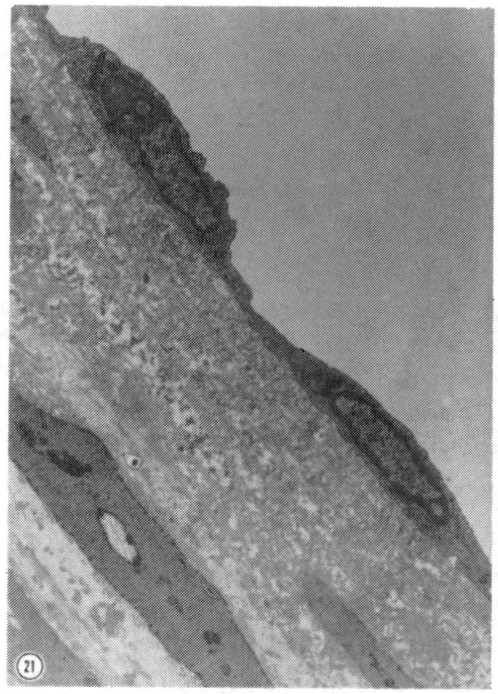

POLYTETRAFLUOROETHYLENE GRAFTS

PTFE Grafts present a problem to the seeding method since they are nonporous to blood except at high pressures and are not normally preclotted before use (Figure 22). Consequently fewer cells are trapped in the graft during seeding procedures than with Dacron. The cells which are seeded on the luminal surface readily cover it (Figures 23 and 24) with endothelium at about the same rate as in the Dacron grafts, (i.e. more than 60% coverage at 2 weeks, more than 90% coverage at 4 weeks) [24]. The similar coverage in Teflon grafts to that of Dacron when fewer cells are present is no doubt attributable to the fact that the cells are all on the flow surface and do not need to migrate to the lumen as they do in the porous grafts. In contrast to Dacron, however, PTFE grafts are essentially nonporous from the exterior and consequently the lining consists of a monolayer of seeded endothelium with the underlying blood cells, platelets and macrophages coming from the lumen (Figures 23 and 24). Control grafts are covered with a thin layer of fibrin and platelets (Figure 25) except for pannus ingrowth.

SMALL DIAMETER DACRON GRAFTS

The development of a cellular lining in arterial grafts larger than 8mm ID, while advantageous in terms of lessening chances in thrombosis and consumption of blood elements [25, 26] is not essential in man if flow through the conduit is adequate. Grafts smaller than 8mm ID are only used reluctantly in a clinical setting, however. Since the only adequate small diameter vessel substitute currently in use is the autologous saphenous vein, the availability of a small graft would be welcome.

When grafts of 6mm and smaller ID are used in peripheral arterial reconstruction they

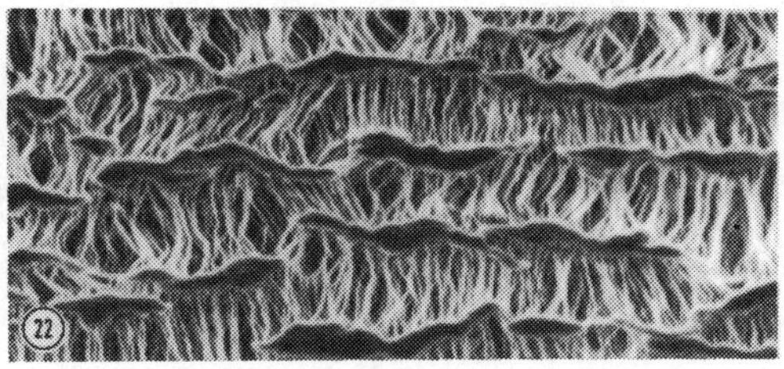

Figure 22. Surface view of PTFE Graft. The luminal surface is composed of nodes and connecting fibrils. The pore size and hydrophobicity of the graft make it nonporous to blood. SEM ×325.

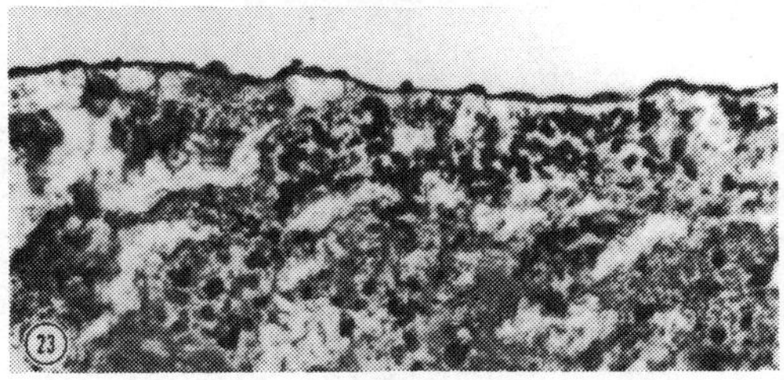

Figure 23. Section of a seeded PTFE thoracoabdominal bypass graft 1 month after implantation. The luminal surface consists of a monolayer of endothelium. Since these grafts are essentially impermeable to cells from the exterior, the bulk of the graft wall is filled with fibrin. Dark pleomorphic macrophages are characteristically found beneath the endothelial lining in the seeded grafts but usually not in the bare areas. LM ×220.

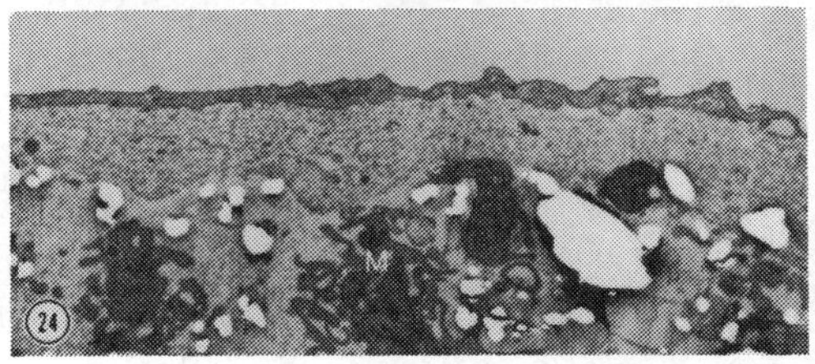

Figure 24. Transmission electron micrograph of a PTFE graft 1 month after implantation. The luminal surface is covered by an attenuated layer of endothelium overlying a layer of basal lamina-like material. The fine fibrils of Teflon have pulled out of the tissue block during sectioning and leave negative (i.e. white) images. The interstices between fibrils are filled with fluid, fibrin and macrophages (M). TEM ×4200.

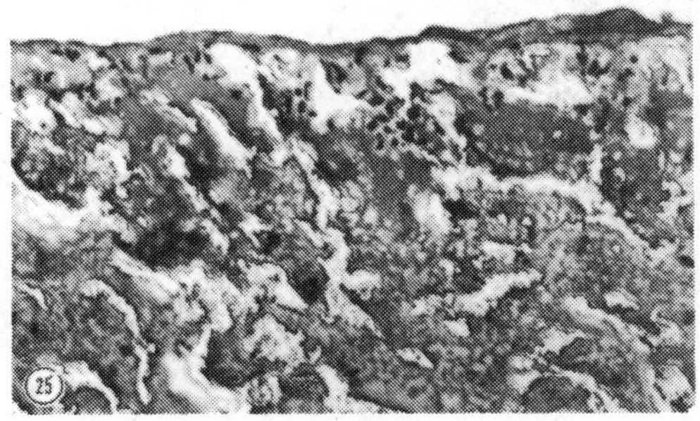

Figure 25. Section of an unseeded control PTFE graft at 1 month post implantation. Endothelium is only found at the anastomotic lines in these grafts. The remainder of the surface is covered by a thin layer of fibrin and platelets overlying the whitish PTFE nodes and fibrils. LM ×180.

are frequently subject to occlusion because of the thrombogenic nature of the surface, reduced flow from poor runoff or kinking of the conduit. As a test for the endothelial seeding method in small grafts (4mm ID), conduits have been placed between the iliac and femoral arteries in the dog. To preclude the effects of kinking of the graft as it passes under the inguinal ligament, externally supported, noncollapsible grafts were used (Figures 26 and 27).

Our initial attempts at producing endothelial linings in these grafts, implanted immediately after seeding of cells, were disappointing as half of both seeded and unseeded grafts were thrombosed between 1-10 days. It was apparent that most of the failures occurred acutely – sometimes before the dog left the surgery suite – and that the endothelial cells were not sufficiently established to be able to prevent thrombosis in the early postoperative stages. It had been shown that treatment of dogs with aspirin and dipyridamole prior to and after implantation of grafts [27] considerably reduced thrombotic sequelae. Therefore in a second experiment dogs were treated with dipyridamole (50mg, bid) for 4 days preoperatively and aspirin (5 gr qd) 1 day preoperatively and the regimen continued until grafts were removed after one week. With this pharmacological intervention all grafts remained patent.

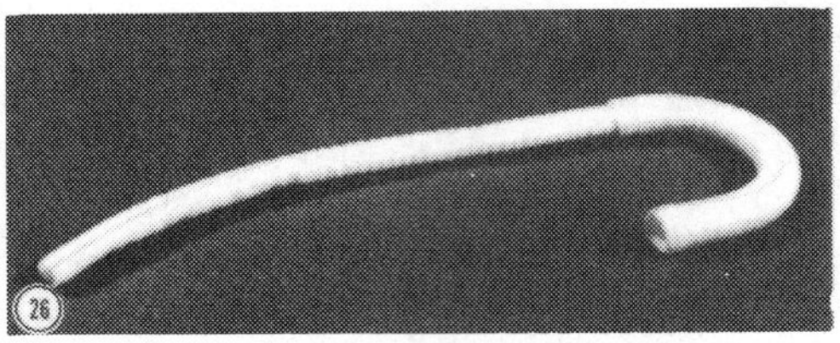

Figure 26. USCI externally supported Dacron graft, 4mm ID. The main portion of the graft is supported by a non-collapsible coil of polyethylene. The proximal end has a crimped sewing cuff while the distal end is uncrimped. ×0.5

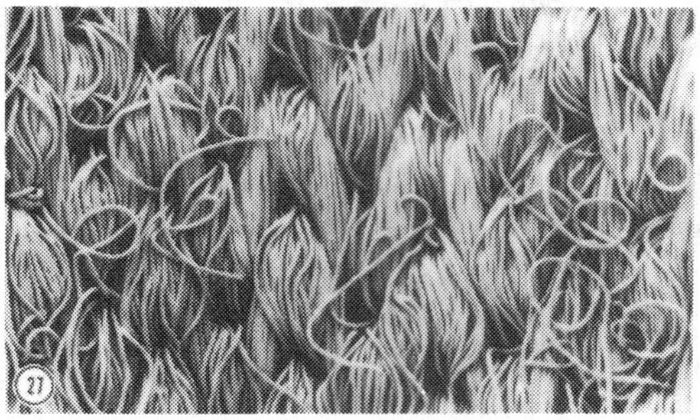

Figure 27. Surface of USCI graft is shown in Figure 26. SEM ×35.

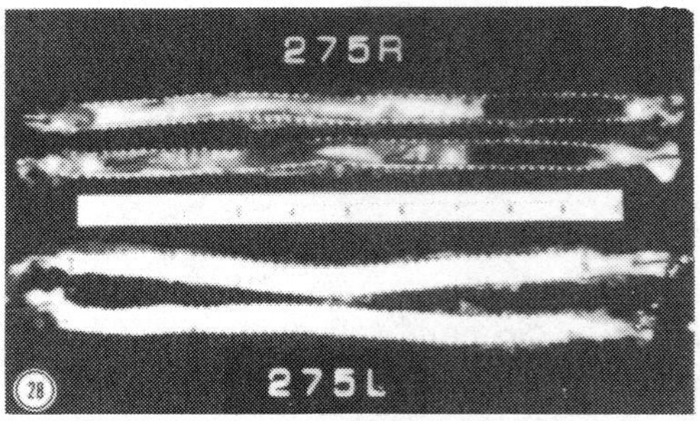

Figure 28. Gross photograph of 2 externally supported 4mm ID USCI grafts 8 weeks after implantation in the iliofemoral position. The seeded graft below is lined with endothelium while the unseeded graft has been occluded with thrombus for a considerable period. The white polyethylene support coil is apparent at the edges of the grafts ×0.5.

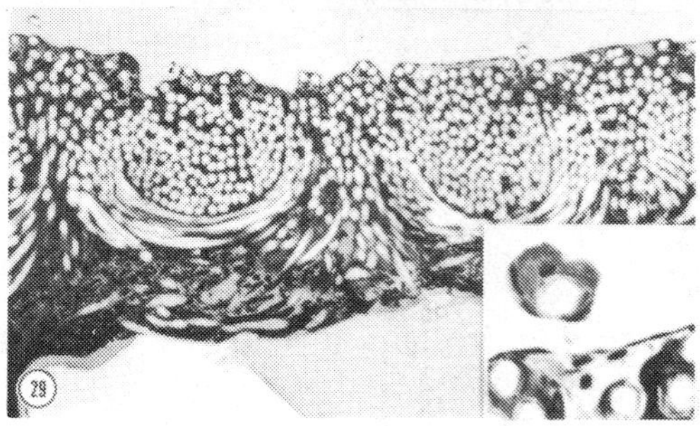

Figure 29. Section of a 4mm ID seeded graft 2 weeks after implantation showing the thin endothelial lining on the surface as well as fibers projecting into the lumen of the vessel. The graft is completely healed. The grayish structure at the bottom of the picture is a portion of the supporting coil of polyethylene. LM ×70. Inset: Isolated graft fiber projecting into the lumen is covered with endothelial cells. LM ×250.

In a third experiment the dogs were pretreated with aspirin and dipyridamole as above and then one iliofemoral graft was seeded with endothelium while the contralateral graft was not. The aspirin and dipyridamole were discontinued two weeks after implantation. In these experiments all the control grafts were patent at 2 weeks, half were occluded at four weeks and all were occluded at 8 weeks (Figure 28). In contrast only 2 of 12 seeded grafts were occluded, one at 2 weeks (anastomotic failure) and 1 at 8 weeks post implantation. The endothelial lining, while like that in Dacron grafts, was much thinner because of the uncrimped configuration of the graft (Figure 29).

From morphological and immunological data [19] it is clear that the surface of seeded grafts is true endothelium. The question arises however as to whether the lining is functioning as an endothelium. It was shown by Harker, et al. [25] that platelet survival could be directly related to the amount of endothelial surface in baboon grafts. Recently, Clagett, et al. [26] have shown that platelet survival in dogs with woven Dacron thoracoabdominal bypasses was still below normal 18 months after implantation. In addition, both 5-hydroxy tryptamine (5HT, serotonin) uptake and content in platelets were still abnormal 16 months after graft implantation.

In order to ascertain the effectiveness of the seeded grafts from a functional point of view we repeated the thoracoabdominal bypass experiment in collaboration with Clagett and his colleagues. In these experiments base-line blood and platelet data (clotting times, Beta thromboglobulin, 5HT content and uptake, and platelet survival) were accumulated on dogs, then seeded or unseeded grafts implanted and the blood and platelet values followed from 2-12 weeks postoperatively. Data accumulated to date, while not complete, indicate that blood values in dogs with seeded grafts have returned to normal by 8 weeks and that the surface does produce prostacycline (PGI_2), while unseeded grafts lag significantly behind.

It is clear from our data that the methods described above dramatically improve the rate of graft healing in dogs, providing a complete endothelial lining between 1 and 4 months, while control grafts still have thrombus at 1 year. In addition it has been shown that the lining which develops is morphologically endothelium and that it functions as a true intima metabolically.

REFERENCES

1. Voorhees, A.B., Jr.; Jaretzki, A., III; Blakemore, A.H. The use of tubes constructed from Vinyon "N" cloth in bridging arterial defects. Ann. Surg. 135(3):332-336, 1952.
2. Baier, R.E.; Akers, C.; Perlmutter, S.; Gott, V.L.; O'Riordan, J. Interfacial biophysics of materials in contract with blood. Annual Report, 1976. Contract No. NO-1-HV-3-2953, National Heart and Lung Institute, National Institutes of Health, Bethesda, Maryland 20014. Available from National Technical Information Service. Springfield, VA.
3. Berger, K.; Sauvage, L.R.; Rao, A.M.; Wood, S.J. Healing of arterial prostheses in man: its incompleteness. Ann. Surg., 175:118-127, 1972.
4. Sauvage, L.R.; Berger, K.; Wood, S.J.; Yates, S.G.; Smith, J.C.; Mansfield, P.B. Interspecies healing of porous arterial prostheses: observations, 1960-1974. Arch. Surg. 109:698-703, 1974.
5. Burkel, W.E.; Kahn, R.H. Cell-lined, nonwoven microfiber scaffolds as a blood interface. Ann. N.Y. Acad. Sci. 283:419-442, 1977.
6. Wesolowski, S.A.; Fries, C.C.; Karlson, K.E.; DeBakey, M.; Sawyer, P.N. Porosity: primary determinant of ultimate fate of synthetic vascular grafts. Surg. 50:91-96, 1961.
7. Fry, W. J.; DeWeese, M.S.; Kraft, R.O.; Ernst, C.B. Importance of porosity in arterial prostheses. Arch. Surg. 88:836-842, 1964.
8. Wesolowski, S.A.; Fries, C.C.; McMahon, J.D.; Martinez, A. Evaluation of a new vascular prosthesis with optimal specifications. Surg. 59:40-56,1966.
9. Sauvage, L.R.; Berger, K.; Wood, S.J.; Sameh, A.A.; Wesolowski, A.S.; Golaski, W.M.; Demonenico, M.; Hartmann, J.R. A very thin, porous knitted arterial prosthesis; experimental data and early clinical assessment. Surg. 65:78-88,1969.
10. Liotta, D.; Hall, C.W.; Villanueva, A.; O'Neal, R.M.; DeBakey, M.E. A permanent autologous lining for implantable blood pumps: a pseudoendocardium. Cardiov. Res. Cent. Bull. 4:69-80,1966.
11. Ghidoni, J.J.; Liotta, D.; Hall, C.W.; O'Neal, R.M.; DeBakey, M.E. *In Vivo* culture of tissue fragments which produce viable cellular linings covered by endothelium (neointimas) in impermeable, velour-lined arterial prostheses, bypass pumps, and valvular prostheses. Trans. Am. Soc. Artif. Int. Organs 14:69-72, 1968.
12. Bernhard, W.F.; Hussain, M.; George, J.B.; Curtis, G.W. Fetal fibroblasts as a substratum for pseudoendothelial development on prosthetic surfaces. Surg. 66:284-290, 1969.

13. Adachi, M.; Suzuki, M.; Kennedy, J.H. Preoperative coating of velour-lined circulatory assist devices with fibrin coagulum membrane (FCM). Trans. Am. Soc. Artif. Int. Organs 16:7-11,1970.
14. Mansfield, P.B.; Wechezak, A. Tissue cultured cells as an endothelial lining of prosthetic materials. In: Organ Perfusion & Preservation, J.C. Norman, Ed.; New York, N.Y., Appleton-Century-Crofts, 189-201, 1968.
15. Schultz, L.; Bull, B.S. Braunwald, N.S. Use of tissue culture techniques to evaluate new materials developed to serve as artificial heart linings. Surg. 69:557-562, 1971.
16. Kahn, R.H.; Burkel, W.E. Propagation of pseudo-intimal linings of vascular prostheses. In Vitro 8:451-458, 1973.
17. Herring, M.B.; Dilley, R.; Jersild, R.A., Jr.; Boxer, L.; Gardner, A.; Glover, J. Seeding arterial prostheses with vascular endothelium. The nature of lining. Ann. Surg. 190(1):84-90, 1979.
18. Ford, J.W.; Burkel, W.E.; Kahn, R.H. Isolation of adult canine venous endothelium for tissue culture. In Vitro 17(1):44-50, 1981.
19. Graham, L.M.; Vinter, D.W.; Ford, J.W.; Kahn, R.H.; Burkel, W.E.; Stanley, J.C. Endothelial cell seeding of prosthetic vascular grafts: early experimental studies with cultured autologous canine endothelium. Arch. Surg. 115:929-933, 1980.
20. Graham, L.M.; Burkel, W.E.; Ford, J.W.; Vinter, D.W.; Kahn, R.H.; Stanley, J.C. Immediate seeding of enzymatically derived endothelium in Dacron vascular grafts: early experimental studies with autologous canine cells. Arch. Surg. 115:1289-1294, 1980.
21. Burkel, W.E.; Vinter, D.W.; Ford, J.W.; Kahn, R.H.; Graham, L.M.; Stanley, J.C. Sequential studies of healing in endothelial seeded vascular prostheses: histologic and ultrastructure characteristics of graft incorporation. J. Surg. Res. 30:305-324, 1981.
22. MacKenzie, D.C.; Lowenthal, J. Endothelial growth in nylon vascular grafts. Br. J. Surg. 48:212-217, 1960.
23. Wesolowski, S.A. Performance of materials as prosthetic blood vessels. Bull. N.Y. Acad. Med. 48(2):331-356, 1972.
24. Graham, L.M.; Burkel, W.E.; Ford, J.W.; Vinter, D.W.; Kahn, R.H.; Stanley, J.C. Expanded polytetrafluoroethylene vascular prostheses seeded with enzymatically derived and cultured canine endothelial cells. Surg. 91:550-559, 1982.
25. Harker, L.A.; Slichter, S.J.; Sauvage, L.R. Platelet consumption by arterial prostheses: the effects of endothelialization and pharmacologic inhibition of platelet function. Ann. Surg. 186(5):594-601, 1977.
26. Clagett, G.P.; Russo, M.; Hufnagel, H. Platelet changes after placement of aortic prostheses in dogs. I. Biochemical and functional alterations. J. Lab. Cl. Med. 97(3):345-359, 1981.
27. Oblath, R.W.; Buckley, F.O.; Green, R.M.; Schwartz, S.I.; DeWeese, J.A. Prevention of platelet aggregation and adherence to prosthetic vascular grafts by aspirin and dipyridamole. Surg. 84(1):37-44, 1978.

Chapter 8

Biolized Surfaces as Chronic Blood Compatible Interfaces

Helen E. Kambic, M.S., Shun Murabayashi, Ph.D., and Yikihiko Nosé, M.D., Ph.D.
Department of Artificial Organs
Cleveland Clinic Foundation
Cleveland, Ohio

ABSTRACT

Various means have been employed to enhance or increase the level of blood compatibility of polymers. For example, one can reduce blood materials interactions by manipulation of the dose, route and sequence of anticoagulant administration. Physical and chemical alterations of the polymer surface can decrease the body's response. Thus, the blood compatibility may be enhanced by variations of the specific surface groups, the surface charge, the chemical reactivity and through the use of proteins and natural tissue derived materials. The blood compatibility of any material depends upon the ability of the contact surface to interact with plasma proteins and yet demonstrate the capacity to remain free of thrombus. The term "biocompatibility" is the response of a material to a series of complex reactions and interactions with blood leading to a high degree of specificity. Many materials remain foreign to the body and are rejected outright; others, may cause damage with prolonged contact and still others remain accepted by the body for years. It becomes apparent that such remarkable phenomena must have some surface-cellular basis.

Our laboratory has accumulated considerable experimental evidence in recent years regarding the specific biological characteristics of "biolized materials" and their properties which determine the extent of their blood compatibility. This chapter will examine the historical development of biolized materials and their specific application in blood pump development.

This work was supported in part by NIH Contracts NO1-HB-3-2914, NO1-HV-4-2960, and NIH Grant HL-17435.

INTRODUCTION

Biolization

Our experience in the past has shown that polymers have unique properties that can be enhanced by protein addition. Since that time technological advances have aided in the determination of specific factors influential in the development of "biolized surfaces." We have established that: a) protein additives alone will not enhance the blood compatibility of a material, but only when reacted with aldehydes; b) protein concentrations of 5-7% are essential for surface coatings or polyblends (mixtures of protein and polymer); c) glutaraldehyde concentrations of 0.45% are sufficient for crosslinking reactions involving the reactive groups within the protein; d) natural tissue materials such as the aorta, aortic valve and pericardium show excellent blood compatibility once aldehyde treated; e) aldehyde treated materials must remain hydrated and f) complete aldehyde removal is essential before implantation.

The term "Biolization" was conceived in the laboratories of the Department of Artificial Organs of the Cleveland Clinic Foundation in 1971 [1,2]. Since then the term has been used to refer to either the chemical or thermal treatment of natural tissue or to the chemically or thermally treated protein (natural tissue derivatives) either coated or blended with other polymers. The hypothesis states that the following two step process would increase the blood compatibility of virtually any material: 1) biological activation by a biological agent, such as protein or polysaccharide and 2) biological inactivation by aldehyde, heat or other treatments. The biological inactivation of protein has become the basis of our philosophy concerning blood compatibility.

Contact between blood and a polymeric material produces reactions of extreme complexity. Both the surface and physical characteristics control the sequence and extent of clotting. Current research into these reactions by others has shown that the initial event after blood contact is the adsorption of protein [3,4]. The deposition of the protein layer is hypothesized as the precursor to the adhesion of platelets and the activation of clotting mechanisms resulting in thrombus formation [5,6]. Many workers now agree that one of the first significant proteins is fibrinogen [7]. Despite the type of protein adsorbed, the nature of the protein will affect the behavior of the surface in contact with blood. In order to achieve a truly antithrombogenic surface, one approach would be the attachment of a benign layer that does not initiate blood coagulation or damage blood elements [8]. With this approach in mind, our attempt to "fool Mother Nature," was to evaluate the most readily available source of natural protein material, which was natural tissue.

Natural tissue is fundamentally protein. Nosé [1,9] and others have demonstrated the effective utilization of aldehyde treated natural tissue in functional cardiac prosthesis. Such materials are currently widely accepted for use as valve and arterial substitutes [10]. Nose has shown that cardiac prostheses used for the second time showed better blood compatibility than after the first use. The re-use of hemodialyzers has been demonstrated by others [11] and resulted in minimal platelet and blood cell adhesion on the dialysis membranes. In each case, the devices were sterilized with formaldehyde after initial use. As mentioned before, materials once implanted in the body will be coated with plasma proteins immediately. But in these cases, the blood contacting surfaces of the reused devices were coated with biological protein and then treated with formaldehyde. The materials used in these early prosthetic heart pumps and dialyzers were dramatically different, and the biological components deposited on

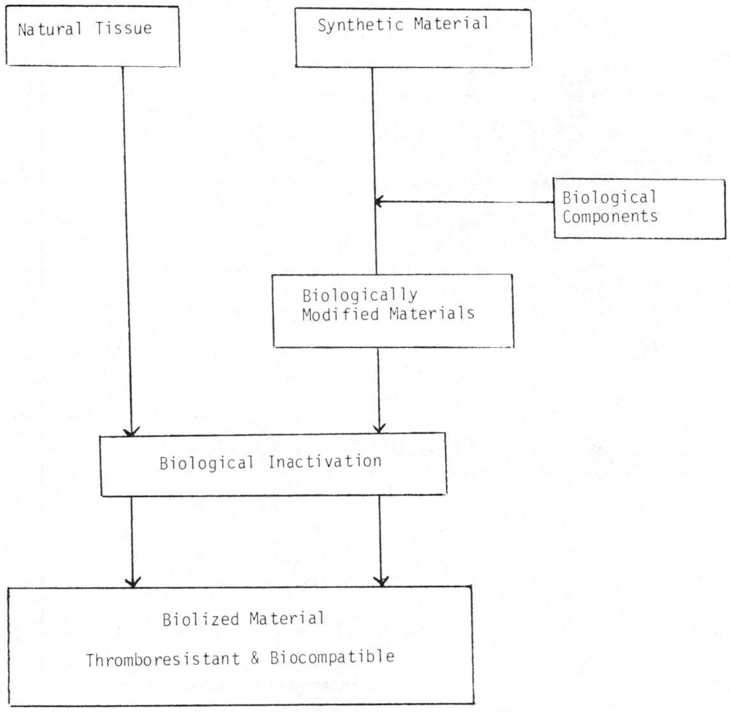

Figure 1. Hypothetical process of biolization.

their surface also differed. However, with formaldehyde treatment, both surfaces showed improved blood compatibility. Formaldehyde played an important role in the improved results. Further in vitro studies revealed that the presence of these biological components (protein) on a surface alone did not always enhance blood compatibility. Once treated by aldehyde, heat, etc., surfaces now became quite blood compatible. These treatments made biological materials nonspecific and insoluble due to the denaturation or the chemical reactions involved in crosslinking. The kind of process that was actually occurring was not completely understood at the time, and the term "Biolization" was introduced to describe the process. Together with the term, the hypothetical process for the production of biocompatible and blood compatible materials was also proposed as shown in Figure 1. The materials to be used for this process could be either natural or artificial in origin, but they must contain protein, polysaccharide or other biological components. Synthetic polymers could be subjected to this condition either by mixing biological components or by coating them (Biological activation). Our laboratory has hypothesized that the general thromboresistance of natural tissue is due to the protein or other biological components in their inactivated form. When a surface is treated with heat or aldehyde it becomes "biologically inactivated". Biological inactivation means the denaturation, insolubilization, or cross linking of biological components. From these observations, it was conceived that by extracting proteins or other biological components from natural tissue and blending them with synthetic polymers, the blood compatibility of the polymer would improve. This concept then allows the versatility of selecting polymers based on their physical properties for a given application, rather than being restricted to the use of only natural tissue or to a narrow range of available medical polymers. The "biologically activated polymer" is aldehyde treated in a solid state to produce a biolized polymer.

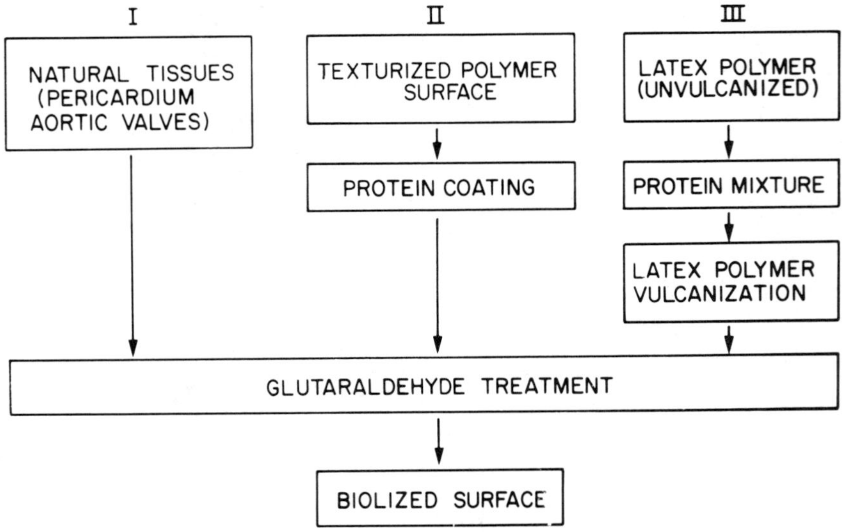

Figure 2. Three difference processes applied to generate biolized surfaces.

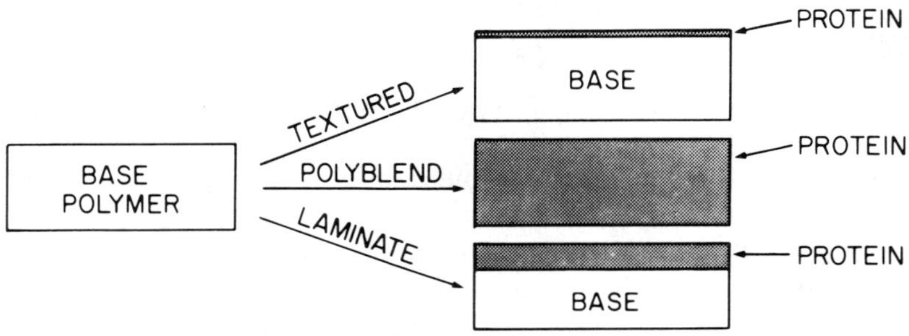

Figure 3. Three methods of adding protein to synthetic base polymers. 1) Protein impregnation into a thin porous or textured polymer surface, 2) mixtures of protein and polymer forming polyblends, 3) laminates of polyblends (2) with pure base polymer.

The direction of our biolized material development was then oriented to the design of protein coatings and polyblends. Three different processes to generate biolized materials have been developed to include the aldehyde treatment of a) natural tissue; b) polyblends, mixtures of proteins and polymers and c) protein coatings applied to high flex elastomers shown in Figure 2. In order to establish a good biolized synthetic surface synthetic polymers require the addition of protein to the base polymer (biological activation) prior to the aldehyde treatment. Figure 3 demonstrates three means of protein addition to polymers. In the first case, the cast polymer contains a thin porous or textured surface onto which the protein is impregnated. In the second case, the protein is mechanically blended with the polymer solution prior to casting. The third case represents a laminate of the polyblend and the unaltered base polymer. These three methods have been developed using various polymer systems and with successful modifications have been incorporated into the current biolized prostheses.

Historical Review

As early as 1970 the demand for strong elastic materials for the new artificial (wave pulsating heart) pump was evident [12]. Natural rubber alone was unsuitable, but with removal or water soluble protein components from the rubber and their replacement with albumin or heparin, the strength of the polymer was retained. The original rubber protein was replaced with polymeric material of homologous origin. A further expansion of this idea was the utilization of homologous or heterologous aortic natural tissue surfaces for incorporation into the blood pump systems.

Modified natural rubber was prepared by the addition of modifiers, Pluronic F-68, dog albumin, heparin, and heparin-benzalkonium chloride complex emulsions and then treated with formaldehyde. In vivo durability tests for up to 3 months showed no alteration in the mechanical properties of the modified and unmodified rubbers. In the case of natural rubber and additives, all modified rubber showed an initial decrease in in vitro clotting tests. The exception was natural rubber-albumin treated with 3% formaldehyde solution. Formaldehyde treatment greatly improved the blood compatibility and these results were in good agreement with those obtained with biological materials. Alcohol preserved aorta also showed remarkable blood compatibility over the untreated natural tissues.

In order to incorporate these findings, an artificial heart pump was constructed utilizing formaldehyde preserved heterologous calf valves; the remaining inside surface was coated with polyester fabric and the connector between the pump and body was a woven dacron graft shown in Figure 4 (partially biolized heart). In a series of implantations in sheep for 43 hours and 6 days revealed no clot formation of the valve fabric interface. Heterologous aortic graft for valves and alcohol or formaldehyde treated natural component surfaces were then established as candidate materials for the construction of artificial hearts [1].

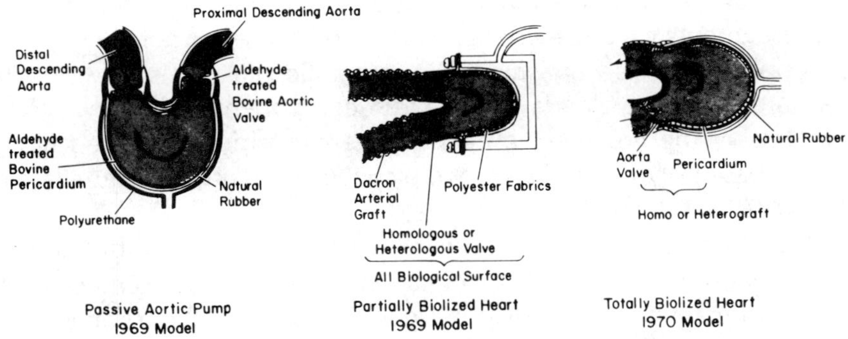

Figure 4. Historical development of biolized cardiac prostheses developed at the Cleveland Clinic.

Based on these concepts, 2 variations of an artificial heart device were made incorporating the combined use of biological and polymeric materials. The strength of the biological material could be augmented by reinforcement or lamination with the polymeric form. In one device, the partially biolized heart used for intraaortic implantation was fabricated from bovine pericardium, and used a dacron fabric inner pump and aortic valves all formaldehyde preserved. This passive aortic pump is shown in Figure 4.

In September 1976, we elected to sacrifice an animal implanted with the passive biolized pump in the aorta 5 years previously [13]. The single ventricular device had an outside polyurethane case. No provision for actually pumping the device was included, but the configuration was such that it could have functioned as an assist pump. The device was interposed in the aorta so that all the cardiac output to the descending aorta went through the pump in Figure 4. At autopsy the device was patent with no thrombus, although some calcium deposition was noted in certain areas of the pump. The valves leaflets were hypotrophic due to inactivity. This remarkable experiment demonstrated the compatibility of stationary biolized materials for cardiac prosthesis.

The totally biolized artificial heart, utilized 4% formaldehyde preserved pericardium and aortic valve with the calf aortic valve with aorta sutured together. The biological tissue sac thus formed was dipped in specially treated natural rubber latex so the latex coated the outside surface of the tissue. In using pericardial tissue, the endothelium faced the blood side. After curing, the natural rubber latex and tissue material formed a one sheet tissue rubber laminated material to provide improved mechanical properties. The totally biolized heart is described in Figure 4. The first sac type TAH driven by a pneumatic power source used this concept combined with a polyurethane housing that provided overall rigidity for the device. In 1973 a world record was established for a TAH implant with a survival of 17 days [14]. Although the results were very encouraging, limitations of the pericardium and natural rubber laminate were evident and the search continued for more durable flexing materials for total artificial heart (TAH) use.

Biolized Polyblends

Polyester and polyether urethanes were evaluated to further test the biolization hypothesis and confirm their use as coatings for blood contact applications. The latex urethanes were the next logical step after using the natural rubber latex system in studying the effects of protein additives. The method of polymer preparation and general composition of the hard and soft segments for these urethanes are reported elsewhere [15]. The commercially available latex polyurethanes were studied as unmodified cast films, as well as homogenous biolized protein urethane polyblends. The protein component, gelatin, was insolubilized in the polymer matrix by the crosslinking agent, glutaraldehyde. Laminated films were composed of a layer of base polymer and a second biolized layer forming a laminate or polyblend approximately 0.010-0.20″ thick.

The mechanical properties of laminated films were not comprised by the addition of the gelatin protein, in that both base and biolized laminated films showed mechanical properties on the same order of magnitude as shown in Figure 5. Although the gelatin modified the surface morphology of both polyester and polyether films, optimal conditions of the processing procedures produced films with good mechanical strength and hydrolytic stability. Proper fusion of the latex particles and a low rate of solvent evaporation established good molecular realignment of the polymer spheres; good fusion was evident between the laminated layers.

The results from the in vivo implantations for histocompatibility analysis indicated that the latex urethanes after 30 days implantation in rats were as histologically compatible as the control material, Biomer. The addition of gelatin to polymer did not significantly alter tissue responses, compared to the polymer alone. In contrast, when polymers with gelatin were aldehyde treated, the overall cell response was reduced. The aldehyde treatment may mask the sites for interaction of the cells with gelatin or they may control the rate of removal in the

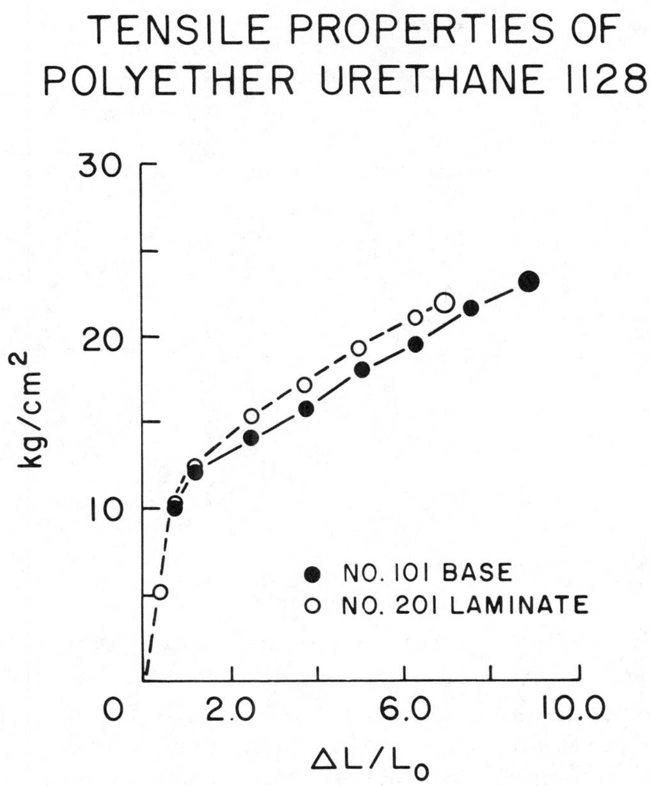

Figure 5. Stress strain curves for Sample 101 base polymer and Sample 201 biolized laminated urethane polymers.

case of phagocytosis [16]. Capsule density and cell response for all polymers tested indicated that the urethane was the major influence on tissue response.

The biolization of the urethanes showed an improved blood compatibility over that of the base polymers alone. This was supported by results from the Kinetic Clotting test [17] which showed predominantly white thrombus formation with a reduction in platelet attachment on these surfaces. This work with the urethanes extended our concept of biolization to include the mixing of protein additives to improve the blood compatibility of selected polymers. These favorable results led us to further developments whereby protein coatings could now be incorporated into the porous surface layers of materials selected for their excellent mechanical properties, specially, those properties pertinent to the development of an artificial heart pump.

Textured Surfaces

The search for improved diaphragm materials for blood pumps which could be biolized led to the development of a high flex polyolefin rubber, called Hexsyn. The Goodyear Tire and Rubber Co (Akron, Ohio) supplied a compression molded rubber which could be formed into a hemispherical blood pump diaphragm. Pneumatically driven active cardiac prostheses, i.e., the total artificial heart (TAH) and the left ventricular assist device (LVAD) were constructed of biolized materials. The first in a series of blood pumps used a 5% gelatin coated velour fabric

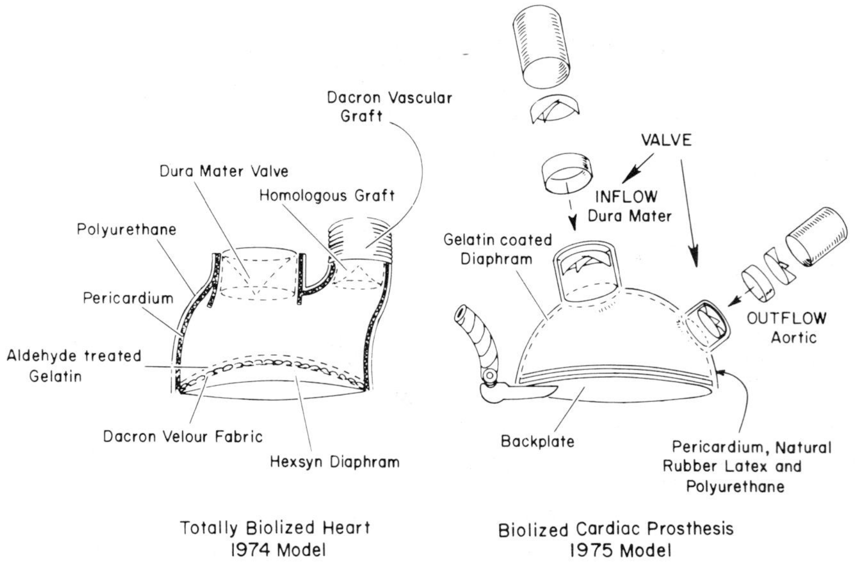

Figure 6. Biolized cardiac prosthesis development 1974–1975.

laminated to the flexible rubber diaphragm treated with 0.45% glutaraldehyde solution [18] as shown in Figure 6. Animal survivals were as long as 24 days for the TAH and 27 days for the LVAD. The dacron velour covered diaphragm used in these prostheses frequently ruptured due to voids in the rubber during molding. The PNI (pseudoneointima) formed on the velour surface was over one mm thick, furthermore, the diaphragm became stiffer as the PNI developed.

Due to the problems experienced with the fabric covered hemispherical diaphragms, the fabric was eliminated and a textured polyolefin rubber diaphragm was developed with a porous surface having 50-80μ diameter pores.

In order to mechanically anchor the protein coating on both the pump housing and diaphragm surface must be textured. The diaphragm surface was integrally textured using a salt casting technique after compression molding [19]. The pump housing surface is coated with a textured layer of Avcomat 610 using a similar technique. The resulting surface texture is nominally 100 microns thick with open pores nominally 20 microns in diameter. After final assembly, biolization of the pump is done by dipping the entire pump in a gelatin solution using vacuum to fill the pores in the textured surfaces and then crosslinking the gelatin coating in place with glutaraldehyde. By coating the pump after assembly, the entire blood contact surface is seamless with no discontinuities. With gelatin impregnated into the pores, additional coatings provided a smooth surface for blood contact. Figure 7 shows the surface coatings after using various concentrations of gelatin. This biolized surface combined with the natural tissue valves fabricated from human dura mater eliminated the need for anticoagulants in these types of blood pumps. This gelatin coated diaphragm was used with a pericardium lined blood pump housing for both TAH and LVAD devices until 1978 and produced a 145 day TAH implant and a 10.5 month LVAD implant [20]. A schematic of this biolized 1975 model is shown in Figure 6. Both of these devices were actuated pneumatically with air pressure acting directly on the pump diaphragm. One of the major problems with this type of actuation is that control of the pneumatic drive pressure is critical to prevent overdistention of the diaphragm with possible cracking of the gelatin layer occurring. Also the diaphragm type of pump did not

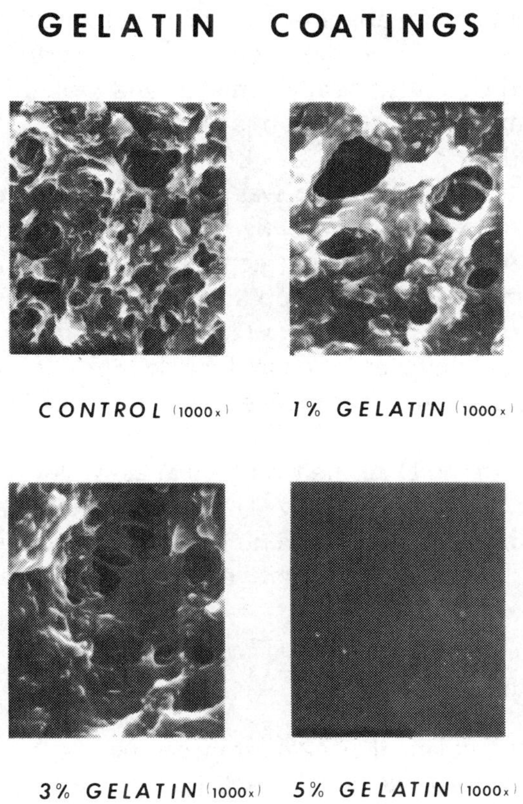

Figure 7. A scanning electron micrograph of the control textured polyolefin rubber (1000×). Pore size range 40-100μm. The surface appearance after coating with 1%, 3% and 5% gelatin solutions is compared. Using 1% and 3% gelatin solutions, the surface remains rough with unfilled pores (1000×), whereas with the 5% gelatin solution, the rough porous structure is filled and covered with a smooth gelatin layer.

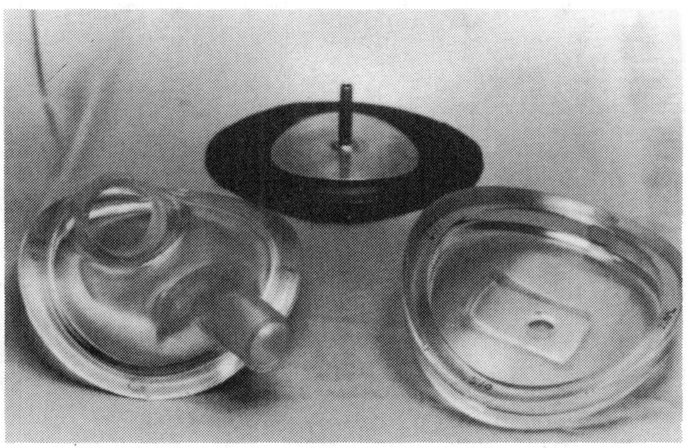

Figure 8. A compression molded and texturized flat (5″) diaphragm is shown with the inner and outer pump housings for pusher plate assist blood pumps.

lend itself to coupling with implantable mechanical actuators being developed by other contractors. For these reasons, in 1977 development was initiated on a biolized pusher plate type blood pump which could be mechanically actuated and would have controlled diaphragm movement to prevent damage to the gelatin layer [21].

The diaphragm molding process was also improved. After 1.0% gelatin and 0.4% glutaraldehyde treatments, the diaphragm was mounted on the elliptical backplate and attached to the housing shown in Figure 8. The entire prosthesis was stored in 0.4% glutaraldehyde-buffered solution with the exception of the dura mater valves. Bovine aortic valves (24 mm) were reinforced with dacron, aldehyde-treated and sutured to the outflow position of the device [22]. Dura mater valves (28 mm) were fabricated in house according to the method of Zerbini [23]. They were used in the inflow position and directly sutured to the natural atrium. Prior to implantation, the device was pumped in 7 liters of saline for 2 hours to remove excess aldehyde.

The basic construction of the LVAD (left ventricular assist device) is essentially the same as that for the total cardiac prosthesis. The LVAD connector tube lined with aldehyde treated pericardium is inserted into the natural left ventricle with a circular knife. The lining of the connector was originally jugular vein however, fabrication difficulties led to the subsequent use of pericardium.

Gelatin

The protein component, gelatin, has no existence in nature, but is derived from the parent protein, collagen. The collagen-to-gelatin transition is a process whereby the highly organized water-insoluble collagen is transformed from an assymetric network of linked tropocollagen fibers to a system of water soluble independent molecues [24]. The dissociation of the polypeptide chains by thermal or chemical processes leads to a class of products termed gelatins outlined in Figure 9. The nature of the gelatin product after collagen fiber degradation

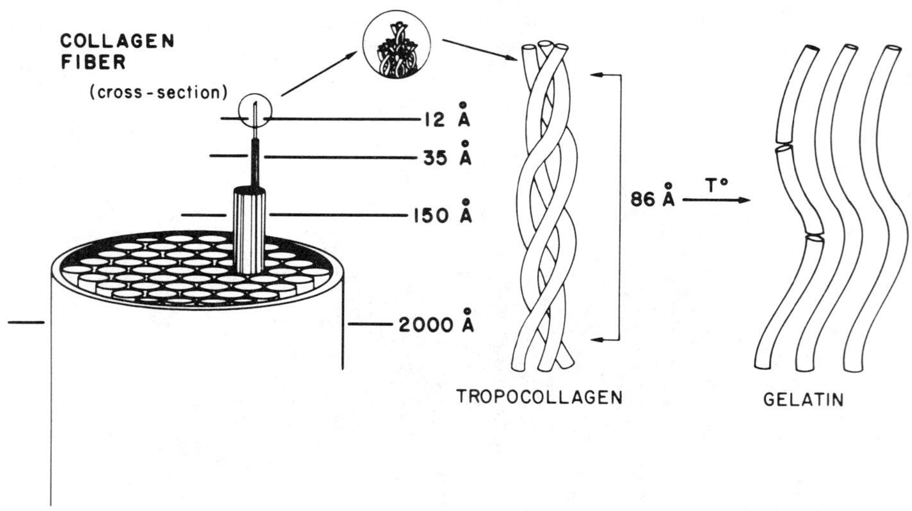

Figure 9. A schematic representation of the orientation of the tropocollagen fibers in collagen and the different levels of collagen organization. The dissociation of the polypeptide chains by thermal or chemical processes separates the chains and breaks them into segments. An assortment of gelatin molecules with different lengths and molecular weights are produced.

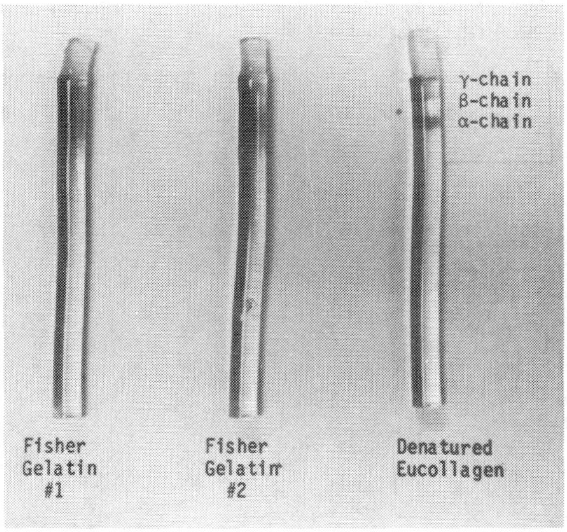

Figure 10. Polyacrylamide gel electrophoresis of Fisher gelatin A (Lot #776351), Fisher gelatin B (Lot #793029) and the purified eucollagen showing the characteristic α, β and γ polypeptide chains. Proteins migrated from the top (anode) to the bottom. Gelatin solutions were diluted to a 5 mg/7 ml solution and samples (0.2ml) were prepared and run at 2-3 m amps/gel for 2 hours.

depends on the amino acid composition of the chains, which determines the phase transition parameters, the degree of polymerization and in particular the order of hydrolysis of the main peptide bonds. The GPC (gel permeation chromatography) of the Fisher gelatin on agarose showed a predominance of these randomly coiled peptide chains with the largest chain components appearing as the α-chain with an M_w of approximately 96,000. The heterogeneity of the gelatin molecules is clearly more evident in the polyacrylamide gel electrophoresis as shown in Figure 10. The three chains designated α, β, γ vary in molecular weight. A large proportion of the high molecular weight contaminant material is presumed to be by products of the commercial alkaline preparation of gelatin. Figure 11 represents the major amino acid components found in the hydrolysates from the multiple 3 chain gelatin. The high content of Glycine (GLY) and Alanine (ALA) correlates well with results obtained from others [25,26] and is consistent with the fact that Glycine occurs at every third residue of the collagen chain.

Gelatin can be classified as a type of natural hydrogel. Once aldehyde treated, the nature and form of the crosslinked gelatin was found to have a very strong influence on the final mechanical and blood compatibility properties on the textured rubber substrate material. Two gelatins were fully characterized as to their stability, mechanical properties and aldehyde crosslinking. The properties of these gelatins are outlined in Table 1. Table 2 describes the steps involved in the Biolization procedure using gelatin. The mechanical properties of the gelatins were measured by preparing 5% gels. The stress strain curves for each of the gelatins and their corresponding bloom strength is shown in Figure 12. A 5% Fisher gelatin showed the greatest elasticity and flexibility when compared to all other gelatins tested. However, by altering and or raising the temperature for gelatin, elastic gels could be produced with longer gelation times. The tensile curves for gels crosslinked with glutaraldehyde concentrations from 0.2-2.0% showed relatively little change in mechanical properties.

Table 1. Properties of Calfskin Gelatins.

	Eastman Kodak (1099)*	Fisher (G-7)**
Gel Strength	348 Blood	108 Bloom
Ash	0.08%	<2.0%
Moisture	9.5%	9.8%
Gelation Temperature	21° - $17^{o}C$	20° - $16.5^{o}C$
Albumin	190 parts per million	-
$M_w^{\dagger}$	200,000	90,000
$M_n^{\dagger}$	70,000	-
Molecular Weight Distribution	15,000-200,000	15,000-95,000
pH	4.9	5.6

*Eastman Kodak, Rochester, New York, USA

**Fisher Scientific, Fair Lawn, New Jersey, USA

$M_w^{\dagger}$ - weight average molecular weight

$M_n^{\dagger}$ - number average molecular weight

Table 2. Pump Biolization Procedure.

Assemble pump housing, diaphragm and actuator.
↓
Dip the assembly in 5% gelatin solution.
↓
Reduce pressure for 30 min.
↓
Return to 1 atm for 5 min.
↓
Reduce pressure for 5 min.
↓
Return to 1 atm for 5 min.
↓
Return to 1 atm.
↓
Place the assembly in high humidity chamber at 4°C for 15 min.
↓
Dip in gelatin solution at 30°C for few seconds.
↑↓
Place in high humidity chamber at 4°C for 15 min.
↓
Submerge in 0.45% Glutaraldehyde solution at 4°C for 10 hrs.
↓
Store in 4% Formaldehyde solution at room temp until used.

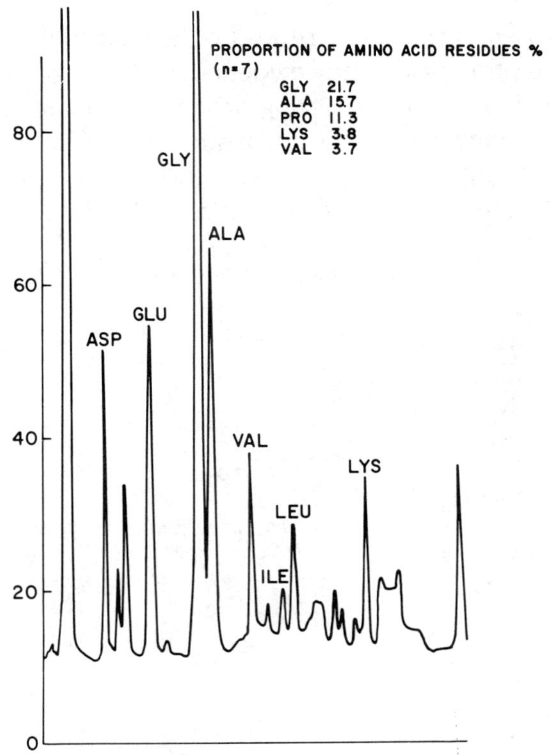

Figure 11. Elution pattern of the hydrolysates of Fisher gelatin using the Glenco Amino acid analyzer. The major residues are identified on the chromatogram and expressed as the percentage of total residues obtained. Hydrolysates were prepared using 12N HCL: proprionic acid (1:1) in shaded tubes under N_2 for 2 hours at 155°C.

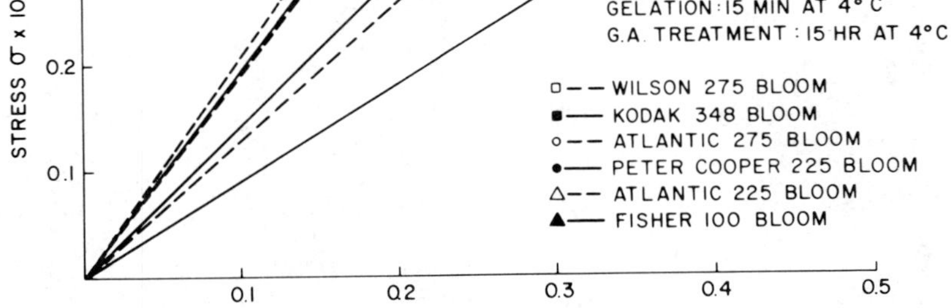

Figure 12. The characteristic stress strain curves obtained for 5% gelatin solutions allowed to gel and crosslinked by glutaraldehyde. The gel strength for each gelatin is also included.

The stress strain measurements of the textured polyolefin rubber gelatin composite were performed with special attention paid to any evidence of cracking to the gelatin surface on the rubber, since in some previous pumps, cracking of the gelatin surface and or detachment of the gelatin was observed in a few cases. The stress strain curves of the gelatin coated samples and the uncoated textured rubber samples are shown in Figure 13. As expected the gelatin coating had not altered the stress strain characteristics of the base polyolefin rubber material.

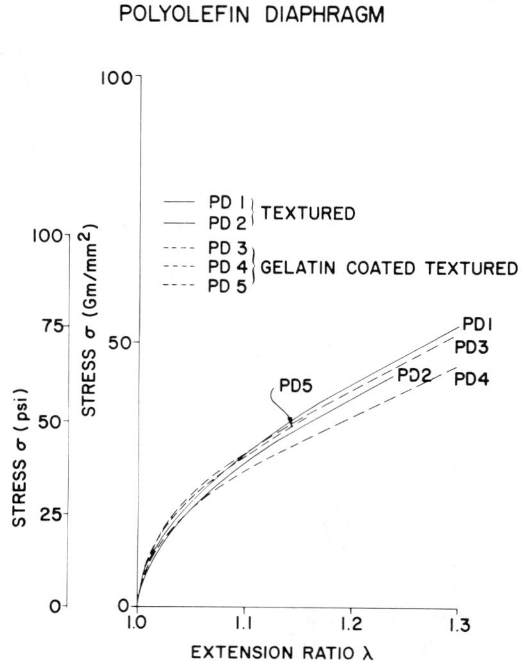

Figure 13. A comparison of the stress strain characteristics of textured polyolefin rubber with and without the gelatin coatings.

Table 3. Toxicity Results.

Material	Test	Result
Polyolefin Rubber	Tissue culture agar overlay rabbit muscle implant hemolysis test	nontoxic
Dacron Thread	Rabbit muscle implant	nontoxic
Gelatin Coated Dacron Thread	Rabbit muscle implant	nontoxic

Materials Science Toxicology Laboratories, University of Tennessee

Table 4. Glutaraldehyde.

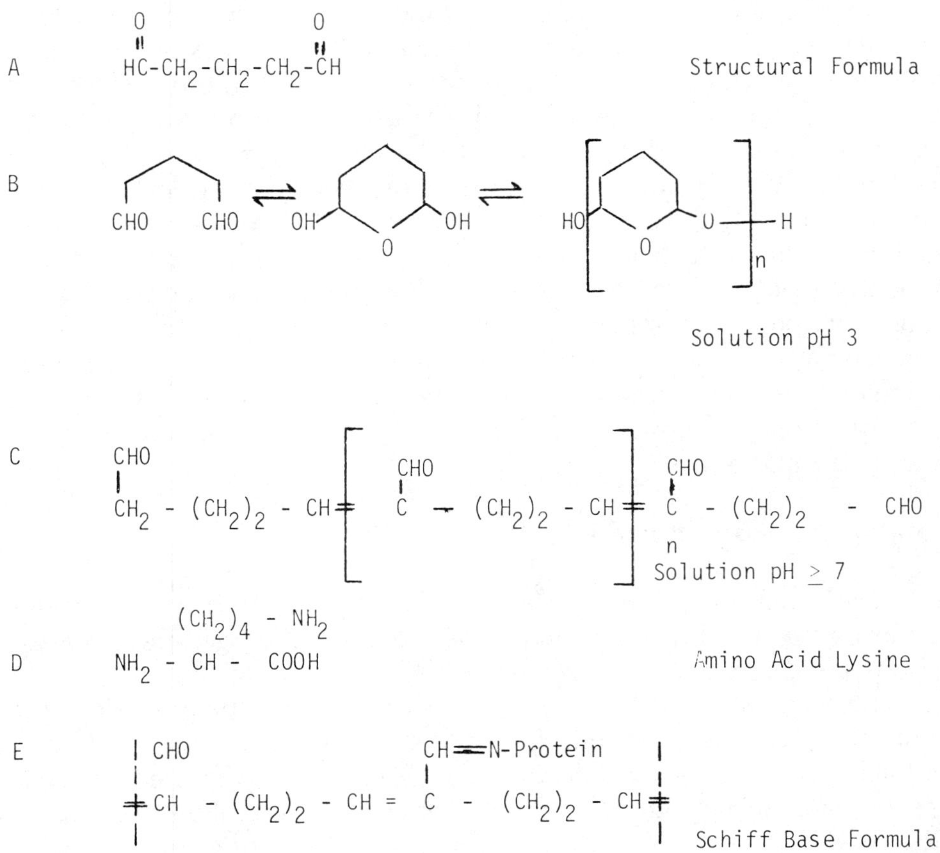

Glutaraldehyde structure and reactions with protein: A) structure of glutaraldehyde, B) commercial solution at pH 3, C) crosslinking solution at pH ≥ 7, D) structure of the amino acid lysine, E) reaction of protein and Schiff base formation between (C) and the amino acid lysine (D).

Gelatin coated samples were also subjected to cyclic endurance tests and run at 100 cycles/min and at extension ratios of 15-60%. No deformations of cracking were found over this range of extensibility, with gelatin surfaces remaining intact and well anchored to the rubber substrate. The ultimate extension ratio of the cross-linked gelatin alone was in the range of 45%. When composites were tested no cracking was observed at extension ratios of 60%. Currently used pusher plate pumps diaphragms have a maximum extension ratio of 15% and therefore current techniques for gel coatings are satisfactory for these types of diaphragms.

Toxicity evaluation of the gelatin was performed by subcutaneous muscle implantation of 5% gelatin coated onto dacron thread and uncoated dacron thread used as control. All materials were classified as nontoxic with the results as indicated in Table 3.

Glutaraldehyde

For many years, glutaraldehyde has been the most effective crosslinking agent among the difunctional reagents due to its interaction with the reactive groups of proteins, particularly the ε-amino group of Lysine. On the other hand, the crosslinks introduced by formaldehyde have been demonstrated to be unstable [28]. The use of formaldehyde for blood pumps is recommended and used only for maintaining sterility after preliminary protein polymerization by glutaraldehyde. When the pH of commercial glutaraldehyde is raised to pH $\geqslant 7$ at which crosslinking is carried out, the dialdehyde undergoes aldol condensation with itself followed by dehydration to generate α, β unsaturated polymers [29]. The reaction results in a Schiff base that forms with the aldehyde is in conjugation with a double bond. Glutaraldehyde structure and reactions with protein are outlined in Table 4. The use of glutaraldehyde as an effective crosslinking agent for proteins depends upon the concentration, pH, and temperature of the protein complex. The insolubilization of the soluble proteins at pH 7.4 satisfies the conditions required for the composite formation. 0.45% glutaraldehyde solutions are buffered with 0.1M Na_2HPO_4 and NaH_2PO_4 at pH 7.4.

Current Status of Biolized Prosthesis

It is now acceptable that pneumatically actuated total artificial heart can maintain normal physiology in experimental animals for several months requiring extracorporeal actuation systems and pneumatic actuation lines through the skin.

Now potential clinical applications to be considered involve the possibility of developing totally implantable cardiac prosthesis functioning for up to 2 years. Our group at the Cleveland Clinic has initiated the development of a mechanically actuated total artificial heart system capable of coupling with either thermal or electrical actuation systems.

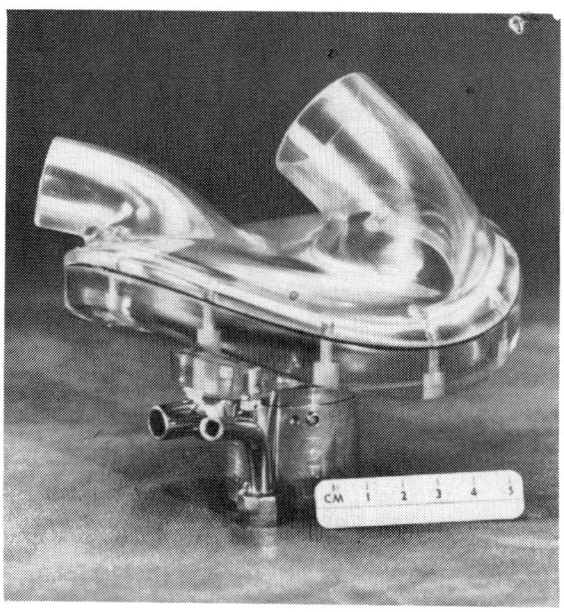

Figure 14. Cast epoxy developmental left ventricular assist device.

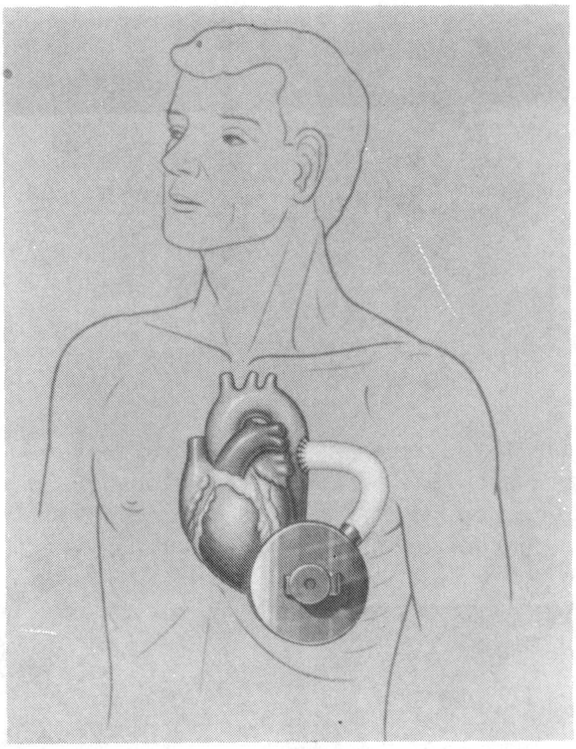

Figure 15. Anatomical location of the left ventricular assist pump.

The current left ventricular assist pump was designed from the beginning specifically for human implantation. This pusher plate type pump was designed for use with a mechanical actuation sytem. The pump is 11 cm in diameter and 3 cm thick providing a net stroke volume of 83 ml through a pusher plate displacement of 1.5 cm and is shown in Figure 14. It is capable of pumping up to 9.6 L/min at 120 beats/min with 15 mmHg inlet pressure. Major consideration in the design was given to the exact location of the pump in the human patient. It was decided to locate the pump intrathoracically and the actuator parathoracically for several reasons. The most reliable component, the pump, would be located intrathoracically and the actuator parathoracically for best conformance to anatomical constraints. In addition, the ribs would protect all the blood and vascular connections. The pump would be in close proximity to the natural heart to provide maximum efficiency and effectiveness, and minimum orientation effects on filling. Blood is obtained from the left ventricular apex and returned to the descending thoracic aorta. The pump geometry and placement inside the chest were arrived at by detailed anatomy studies using computerized axial tomography on living individuals. It was designed to fit the curvature of the left lateral thoracic wall to minimize lung displacement and avoid compression of the major vessels and pulmonary hilus. Space for the actuator is created by removal of the 6th or 7th rib to allow use of the rib space together with the subcutaneous location as in Figure 15. Five implants were done to evaluate long term biocompatibility and performance. The experiments in this series ranged in duration from one to seven months. Results of these implants revealed that the biolized pumps were all generally clean as shown in Figure 16, even in the presence of infection. Minor localized deposition was seen in all of the pumps at two locations on the diaphragm-housing junction. This area was later identified as having higher than design strain levels due to shrinkage of the diaphragm

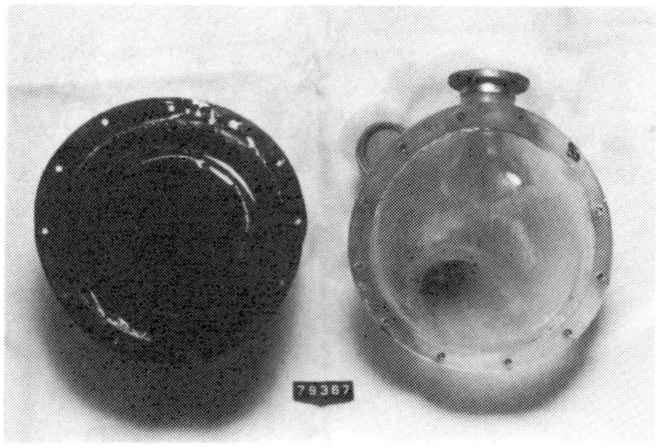

Figure 16. A compression molded and texturized flat diaphragm is shown with the inner and outer pump housings for a pusher-plate assist blood pump after implantation for four months without anticoagulants.

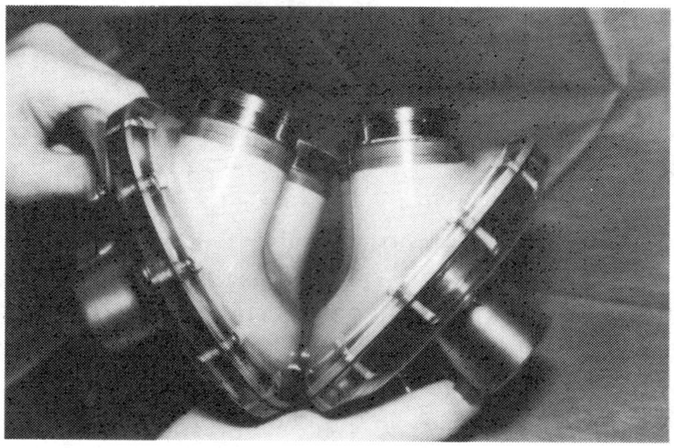

Figure 17. Total artificial heart pumps with pneumatic actuators.

during manufacture. Minor design changes to the diaphragm mold to compensate for the shrinkage have since eliminated this problem.

Total Artificial Heart Development

The pusher plate type blood pump has also been utilized for a Total Artificial Heart. The design of the pump has followed directly from the LVAD pump. In the TAH, two pusher plate pumps are utilized to replace the right and left ventricles of the natural heart. The dimensions of the pumps are similar to those of the LVAD, however the TAH pumps are in a flat rather than curved configuration and the blood ports have been changed to accommodate the arterial and atrial connections (Figure 17). Actuation of the pumps is provided by the same pneumatic actuators as used on the TLVAD system. Although this does not represent a finalized human configuration, it allows developmental testing of the device and various control methods to be performed. Implants of this device have been performed for durations of 45 and 108 days in calves during which various control methods were evaluated [30,31]. The Hall effect pusher plate position signal from each pump is used to control pumping. Utilizing this signal for control of the pump gives it good sensitivity to both preload and afterload. Preliminary results with this system indicate that it can provide more physiological hemodynamics than previous types of pumps. Further development will consolidate the components in an arrangement suitable for human implantation and will include an implantable actuation system.

ACKNOWLEDGEMENT

The authors wish to thank Miss Jan Kodish for typing this manuscript.

REFERENCES

1. Nosé, Y., Tajima, K., Imai, Y., Klain, M., Krava, G., Schriber, K., Urbanek, K., and Ogawa, H. Artificial heart constructed with biological material. Trans. Am. Soc. Artif. Intern. Organs, 17:482, 1971.
2. Imai, Y., Tajima, K., Nosé, Y. Biolized materials for cardiovascular prosthesis. Trans. Am. Soc. Artif. Intern. Organs, 17:6, 1971.
3. Vroman, L., Adams, A., Klings, M., Fischer, G., Munoz, P., and Solensky, R. Reactions of formed elements of blood with plasma proteins at interfaces. Ann. N.Y. Acad. Sci., 283:65, 1977.
4. Lyman, D.J., Metcalf, L.C., Albo, D., Jr., Richards, K.F., and Lamb, J. The effect of chemical structure and surface properties of synthetic polymers on the coagulation of blood. 111. In vivo adsorption of proteins on polymer surfaces. Trans. Am. Soc. Artif. Intern. Organs, 20B:474, 1974.
5. Macfarlane, R.G. The theory of blood coagulation. Chapter 1 in *Human Blood Coagulation Haemostasis and Thrombosis* (Ed. R. Biggs), Blackwell, London, 1972.
6. Lyman, D.J., Knutson, K., McNeil, B., and Shibatani, K. The effects of chemical structure and surface properties of synthetic polymers on the coagulation of blood. IV. The relation between polymer morphology and protein adsorption. Trans. Am. Soc. Artif. Intern. Organs, 21:49, 1975.
7. Baier, R.E. Blood compatibility of synthetic polymers perspective and problems. Chapter in *Polymers in Medicine and Surgery,* Vol. 8 (Eds. R.L. Kronenthal, Zale Oser, and E. Martin), Plenum Press, New York, 1975.
8. Falb, R.D. and Grode, G.A. Convalent Bonding of proteins to solid surfaces. Fed. Prod., 30:1688, 1971.
9. Kambic, H., Picha, G., Kiraly, R., Koshino, I., and Nosé, Y. Application of aldehyde treatments to cardiovascular devices. Trans. Am. Soc. Artif. Intern. Organs, 22:664, 1976.
10. Ionescu, M.I., Ross, D.N., Wooler, G.H., (Eds.) *Biological Tissue in Heart Valve Replacement.* London, Butterworths 1972.
11. Wing, A.J., Brunner, F.P., Brynger, H.O.A., Chantler, C., Donckerwolcke, R.A., Gurland, H.J., Jacobs, C., and Selwood, N.H. Mortality and morbidity of reusing dialyzers. Br. Med. J. 2:853, 1978.
12. Imai, Y., Von Bally, K., and Nosé, Y. New elastic materials for the artificial heart. Trans. Am. Soc. Artif. Intern. Organs, 16:17, 1970.
13. Harasaki, H., Kiraly, R., and Nosé, Y. Endothelialization in blood pumps. Trans. Am. Soc. Artif. Intern. Organs 24:415, 1978.
14. Nakazono, M., Koiso, K., Kamai, T. Agishi, T., Urzua, J., Kiraly, R., Kambic, H., Surovy, R., Carse, C., and Nosé, Y. A case report of 17 days survival with an implanted artificial heart in a calf. Japanese Heart Journal, 15:485, 1974.
15. Kambic, H., Barenburg, S., Harasaki, H., Gibbons, D., Kiraly, R., Nosé, Y. Glutaraldehyde protein complexes as blood compatible coatings. Trans. Am. Soc. Artif. Intern. Organs, 24:426, 1978.

16. White, M.J., Kohno, I., Rubin, A.L., Stenzel, K.H., and Miyata, T. Collagen films: Effect of crosslinking on physical and biological properties. Biomater. Med. Devices Artif. Organs, 1(4):703, 1973.
17. Kambic, H., Kiraly, R.J., and Nosé, Y. A Simple in vitro screening test for blood incompatibility of materials. J. Biomed. Mater. Res. (Symp. number 7), 10(4):561, 1976.
18. Nose, Y., Urzua, J., Jacobs, G., Arancibia, C., Nakiri, K., Picha, G., Kambic, H., Morinaga, N., Mitamura, Y., and Washizu, T. Development and evaluation of cardiac prosthesis 1st. Annual report contract No. NO1-HV-4-2960-1 May, 1975.
19. Kiraly, R.J., Arconti, R., Hillegass, D., Harasaki, H., and Nosé, Y. High flex rubber for blood pump diaphragms. Trans. Am. Soc. Artif. Intern. Organs, 23:127, 1977.
20. Tsushima, N., Kasai, S., Koshino, I., Jacobs, G., Morinaga, N., Washizu, T., Kiraly, R.J., and Nosé, Y. 145 days survival of calf with calf with total artificial heart (TAH) Trans. Am. Soc. Artif. Intern. Organs, 23:526, 1977.
21. Nose, Y. Principal investigator, Development and Evaluation of Cardiac Prosthesis. NIH Annual Report NO1-HV-4-2060-6, April 1979.
22. Harasaki, H., Snow, J., Jacobs, G., Kiraly, R.J., and Nosé, Y. Biological tissue valves in cardiac prosthesis. Trans. Am. Soc. Artif. Intern. Organs 24:332, 1978.
23. Nakiri, K., Jacobs, G., Pennza, P., Aranciba, C., Kiraly, R.J., and Nosé, Y. Dura mater valve for cardiac prostheses. Trans. Am. Soc. Artif. Intern. Organs 21:573, 1975.
24. Veis, A. *The Macromolecular Chemistry of Gelatin.* Academic Press, New York, 1964.
25. Traub, W., and Piez, K.A. Chemistry and structure of collagen. Adv. Protein Chem. 25:243, 1971.
26. Bensusan, H., An investigation of the products of an enzymatic hydrolysis of collagen. Biochemistry 8(12):4716, 1969.
27. Kambic, H., Murabayashi, S., Harasaki, H., Suwa, S., Pepoy, M., Hayashi, K., Hillegas, D., Kiraly, R., and Nosé, Y. Composite polymeric materials: Evaluation of crosslinked gel protein surfaces. Proc. 2nd Mtg. Int. Soc. Art. Organs 3 (Suppl):203, 1979.
28. Cater, C.W. The evaluation of aldehydes and other difunctional compounds as crosslinking agents for collagen. J. Soc. Leath. Trades Chem. 47:259, 1963.
29. Peter, K., and Richards, F.M. Chemical crosslinking reagents and problems in studies of membrane structure. In: *Annu. Rev. Biochem.* E.E. Snell, ed. Annual Reviews Inc. Palo Alto, CA 1977.
30. Harasaki, H., Takatani, S., Suwa, S., Jacobs, G., Snow, J., Kiraly, R.J., and Nosé, Y. Hemodynamic regulation in total artificial heart recipients. Artif. Organs 5:38, 1981.
31. Takatani, S., Harasaki, H., Suwa, S., Murabayashi, S., Sukalac, R., Jacobs, G., Kiraly, R.J., and Nosé, Y. Pusher-plate type TAH system operated in the left and right free running variable rate mode. Artificial Organs, 5(2):132, 1981.

Chapter 9

Blood-Blood Pump Surface Interaction

Hiroaki Harasaki, M.D., Ph.D., Raymond J. Kiraly, M.S.M.E. and Yukihiko Nose, M.D., Ph.D.
Department of Artificial Organs
Cleveland Clinic Foundation
Cleveland, Ohio

ABSTRACT

Total artificial hearts and left ventricular assist devices using various blood contacting surfaces were implanted and evaluated in calves without anticoagulants for up to 5 months and 10 months, respectively. The surfaces included biologically derived, chemically treated materials, such as glutaraldehyde-treated bovine pericardium and glutaraldehyde treated gelatin, and rough, synthetic surfaces, i.e., polyester flock and powdered metal surfaces. The glutaraldehyde-treated pericardium, polyester flock and powdered metal acted as "pseudoneointima (PNI) generating surfaces," and varying degrees of collagenation and endothelialization were observed. These processes occurred rather slowly in an insular manner on the surface having no direct connection to the natural tissue, and progressed with time. Calcification was observed in the PNI along the diaphragm-housing junction and of the flexing area of the diaphragm after 13 days of implantation. Mechanical stress and resultant thick PNI formation were the possible factors in promoting the calcification process. The smooth gelatin surface, in contrast, did not elicit PNI formation and behaved as a PNI non-generating surface. In an animal study of up to 7 months, the gelatin surface showed excellent blood compatibilty without any sign of biodegradation. Based upon these experiences, the smooth gelatin surface is now being used in TAH's and LVAD's fabricated and tested at the Cleveland Clinic.

This work was supported in part by NIH Contracts NO1-HV-4-2960, NO1-HV-3-2934, and NIH Grants HL-17435, and HL-24286.

INTRODUCTION

The development of cardiac assist and replacement devices has been hampered mainly because of a lack of satisfactory blood-contacting materials. Efforts were begun two decades ago and work has been carried out to identify or synthesize new artificial surfaces which interact with blood in favorable ways. Although the ultimate goal of such endeavors is to develop artificial surfaces whose interfacial phenomena are similar to those with the natural endothelial lining, none have been shown to meet this goal. Although the state of art of biomaterials having contact with blood is such, significant progress has been achieved in the past decade. Various types of total artificial hearts (TAHs) and left ventricular assist devices (LVADs) have been successfully tested in animals for up to 10 months. Various blood contacting materials have been used based upon different concepts. These include synthetic polymers, metals, carbons, natural macromolecules, modified tissue and various living cellular linings. The concepts behind these materials may be categorized into two major approaches. One is the surface which elicits the pseudoneointima (PNI) formation, and the other intends minimal cellular and/or protein reaction at the interface. The former is usually referred to as a rough surface, and the latter as a smooth surface [1], although no precise definition has been established on the surface roughness or smoothness.

In this chapter the blood contacting materials currently used in the cardiac assist or replacement devices and their in vivo performance will be reviewed with a special emphasis on the biolized surfaces [2], textured synthetic and metal surfaces, which have been tested at the Cleveland Clinic Foundation using the same animal model and the same pre-, intra- and post-operative management.

Chemically Treated Natural Tissues

In the history of the development of biological tissue valves, various chemicals have been introduced and tested to treat the natural tissues in an effort to minimize immunological reactions and to preserve the tissue integrity. It was in 1969 when Carpentier and his colleague [3] introduced glutaraldehyde for this purpose and coined a term of "bioprosthesis" to denote a tissue valve preserved with glutaraldehyde. It was not long until the glutaraldehyde-treated porcine aortic valve and the pericardial valve had begun to be utilized widely in clinical medicine, where superiority of this preservation method over other methods was clearly shown in terms of the blood compatibilty and durability. It was almost the same time when glutaraldehyde-treated natural tissues or proteins were introduced by our group to line the blood contacting surface of the artificial hearts [2]. The freshly obtained bovine pericardium was washed thoroughly with water and treated in 0.45% glutaraldehyde in 0.1M phosphate buffer at pH 7.4 for several days at room temperature. After cross-linking the pericardium was mounted on a silastic mold, sutured and fabricated in a pump configuration. The outer surface was then backed with natural rubber and segmented polyurethane (Figure 1). In the early developmental stage, the passive pumps lined with this glutaraldehyde-treated pericardium (biolized pump) were interposed into the calve's descending aorta in an end-to-end fashion to characterize its interaction with circulating blood. It was shown that without usage of anticoagulant, this "biolized surface" reacted favorably with blood, and five and a half years later almost the entire surface was lined with a layer of endothelial cells (Figure 2 and 3) which is the best known interfacial surface. Because of this satisfactory result, glutaraldehyde-treated

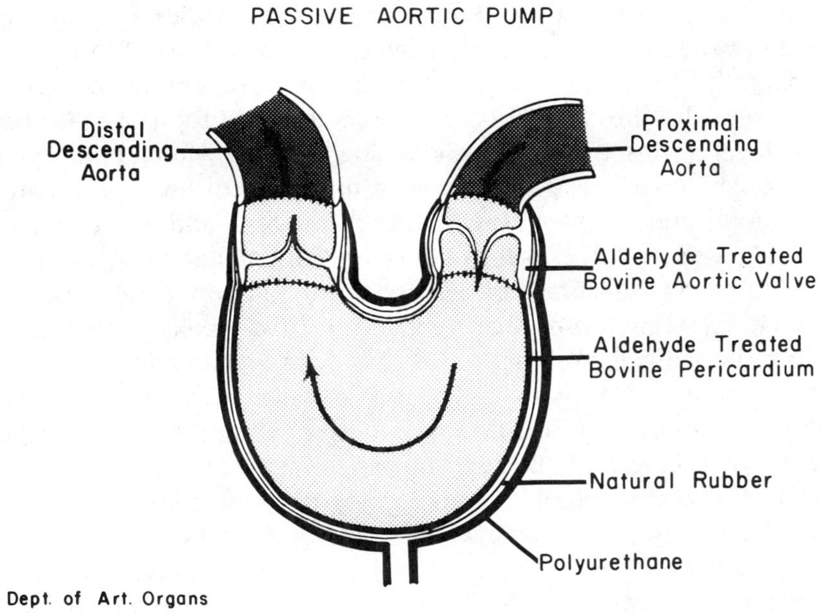

Figure 1. A schematic illustration of a "biolized" blood pump. The entire blood contacting surfaces were made of biologically derived, chemically treated materials.

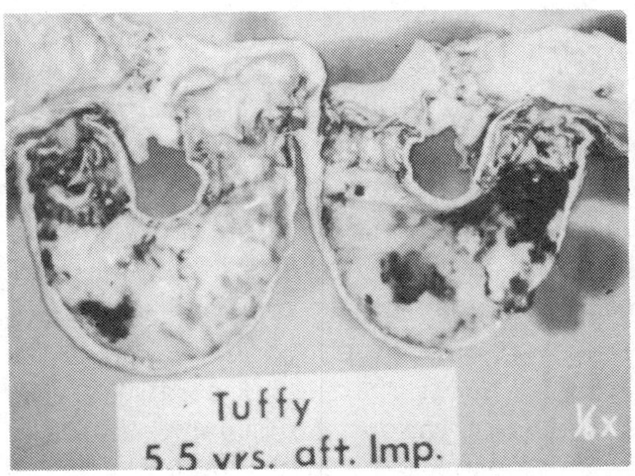

Figure 2. A passive aortic pump lined with a biolized surface. The device was implanted in the discending thoracic aorta of a calf for five and a half years without anticoagulant. Almost entire surface is covered by a glistening, thin pseudoneointima. The dark area shows insudation of blood underneath the PNI.

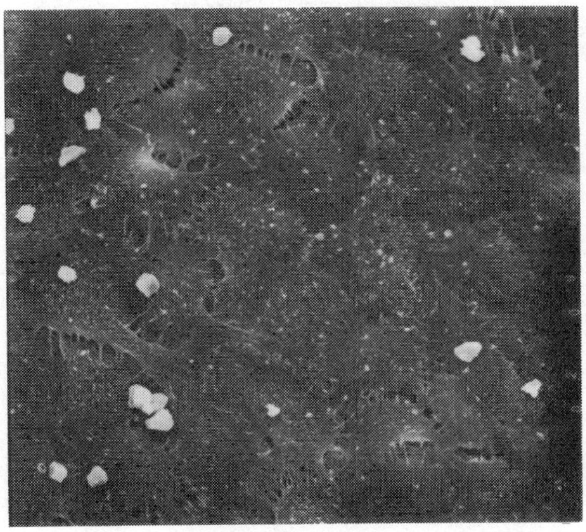

Figure 3. A scanning electron microscopic surface appearance of the pseudoneointima formed on the glutaraldehyde-treated pericardium. Flattened cells coalesce each other. However, occasionally the cell boundaries still do not show a typical structure of marginal fold of the natural endothelial layer.

pericardium was incorporated into functioning blood pumps, i.e., total artificial hearts (TAH) and left ventricular assist devices (LVAD) and tested in calves without anticoagulation. Eighteen TAH's and 19 LVAD's were evaluated in calves for up to 5 and 10 months, respectively.

The pericardium thus treated is a macroscopically smooth, but microscopically rough surface. After treatment, the mesothelial layer is denuded, and the sub-mesothelial fine fibrils and/or collagen layer forms the blood contacting surface. After contact with blood this microscopically rough surface was covered by a thin layer of fibrin and platelet matrix [4]. Within 2 weeks, fibrin underwent a polymerization process, and was compacted causing a resultant decrease in the total thickness of the layer. Concomitantly polymorpho- and mononuclear cells appeared on the surface of this polymerizing fibrin-platelet matrix, and invaded into this layer phagocytosing the cellular debris. After two weeks, flattened endothelial-like cells appeared on the surface, and by the sixth week of implantation, coalescence of these cells was observed in an insular manner. The area covered with an endothelial cell layer, as confirmed by the presence of Weibel-Palade bodies, increased with time. Figure 4 shows a pump housing of a LVAD used for 78 days. The pericaridum surface is covered by a very thin, semitranslucent PNI with a geographic pattern in the outflow region. By the fifth month, approximately one third of the surface area was covered by endothelial cells. The remaining surface was not endothelialized. However, the tightly packaged fibrin layer was also shown to be thrombo-resistant, since occasional platelets seen on this fibron surface retained the discoid shape or showed slightly deformed, contact or spread type of transformation [5].

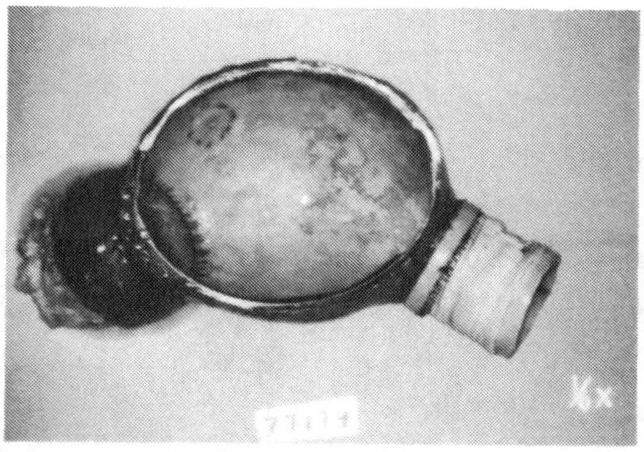

Figure 4. A LVAD pump housing used for 78 days in a calf without anticoagulant. The PNI is so thin that sutures of the air removal port and the valve housing are still recognized. No thrombi or calcified foci are seen.

The endothelialization in the blood pump takes place rather slowly and in an unreliable way. In the healing process of porous vascular grafts, it is well known that the porosity of the material [6] and the migration of fibroblasts, myofibroblasts, or smooth muscle cells through the lattice from the perivascular tissue plays a critical role, and in animals, endothelialization can occur relatively quickly on the collagenized pseudoneointima. The slow process of endothelialization seen in blood pumps may be attributed to the lack of porosity of the material, and, in addition, to complex fluid dynamics in the pump. The origin of the endothelial cell is a subject of controversy. In the studies of various vascular prostheses, it has been postulated that the endothelial cell lining starts at the host-graft junction directly and continuously from the host endothelial lining [7], from the endothelial cell of the capillaries which penetrate the interstices of the graft [8], from the "multipotential cells" in the circulating blood [9,10], or in the tissue itself [11]. Since the endothelialized areas occur discretely and in an insular fashion in the impervious blood pump, the origin of the endothelial cell is "blood born" and the multi-potential cell, possibly monocyte, and/or endothelial cell detached from the upstream surface of the natural cardiovascular system could be the precursor to the pump endothelialization. Nevertheless the glutaraldehyde-treated pericardium, which is macroscopically smooth but electron microscopically rough, exposing submesothelial fibrils less than 0.1 μm in diameter, is ultimately covered by an endothelial layer. The difference of PNI formed on this surface, when compared to the macroscopically rough surface as mentioned in the next sections, is that the thickness of the initially formed fibrin-platelet matrix is thinner than those on the macroscopic rough surfaces possibly due to the difference in surface roughness and other physico-chemical surface properties.

Although the application of this material is limited to a non-moving part of the blood pump, i.e., the pump housing, its blood compatibility and durability are promising even without usage of anticoagulants.

Chemically Treated Protein Coatings

It is known that any artificial surface is covered instantaneously by plasma proteins on contact with blood. The subsequent blood surface interactions (triggering the intrinsic coagulation process and platelet adhesion), are believed to be dependent upon the nature and amount of this initial protein coating formed on the artificial surface, which is governed mainly by the physico-chemical properties of the surface [12]. The precise mechanisms of this initial blood-surface interaction remain the subject of controversy. A hypothesis was raised by Nose et al. in 1971 [2], in that proteins cross-linked and immobilized with aldehyde treatment was expected to react with blood in a favorable way by alleviating its physico-chemical activities and antigenicity. The term "biolized surface" was coined to refer to the chemically and/or thermally treated biologically derived materials (proteins) either coated on or blended into a synthetic base material. This approach was thought to be practical in light of the fact that any synthetic material can hardly meet two fundamental requirements for blood pump application, namely high flex life and substantial blood compatibility. Gelatin (denatured collagen) has been used for this purpose because of availability and ease of processing. A gelatin layer was impregnated into the textured polyolefin rubber, which was shown to have sufficiently high flex life for use as a pump diaphragm [13]. Here the degree of surface smoothness is controllable by changing the concentration of the gelatin solution and the size of the surface texture of the base polyolefin rubber [14].

Studies were conducted on the effects of the gelatin solution concentration on blood compatibility. Either 1% or 5% gelatin-in-water solution was used. The gelatin layer coated on the textured polyolefin rubber diaphragm was gelated in a chamber at 4°C and then cross-linked with 0.45% glutaraldehyde in 0.1M phosphate buffer overnight at 4°C. The coating with 1% gelatin solution was incomplete, and the rough textured surface, having 10 to 50 μm pore size, was partially exposed. This gelatin coated rough surface acted as a PNI generating surface and rather thick PNI was formed (up to 3 mm) in the diaphragm-housing (D-H) junctional region within one month. Another problem encountered was that the 1% gelatin coated hemispherical diaphragm showed extensive calcification after 316 days of pumping in the calf. Histological and electron microscopical analyses of this surface disclosed that the gelatin layer had been detached from the base polyolefin diaphragm and the resultant deposition of blood elements underwent the calcification process. In contrast, the 5% gelatin coated diaphragm showed a microscopically smooth, and complete covering of the textured surface. After contact with blood, the 5% gelatin coated surface was covered by only a thin layer of proteinaceous material (Figure 5), and was essentially free of cellular and fibrin deposition. Spread or contact type platelets (Figure 6) and flattened cells were occasionally observed, however, platelet aggregation or PNI was not formed unless detachment of the gelatin layer occurred in the stress concentration areas, especially along the perimeter of the hemispherical diaphragm.

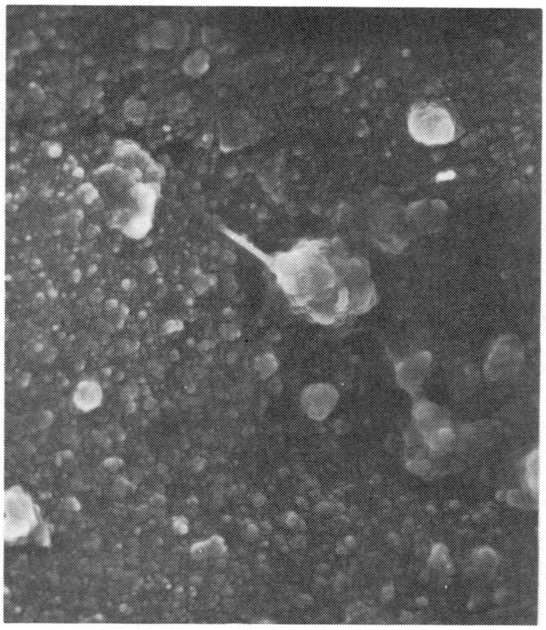

Figure 5. A scanning electron micrograph of 5% gelatin surface after contact with blood. The surface is covered with granular proteinaceous materials. In the center, a degraded platelet is seen (10,000x).

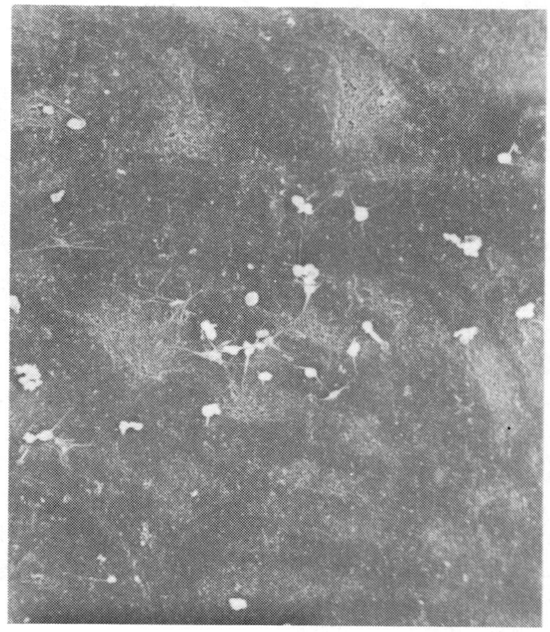

Figure 6. The 5% gelatin surface appears quite blood compatible. Occasional platelets seen after 3 months pumping are of contact and/or spread type, and no fibrin network or platelet aggregation is observed (3,000x).

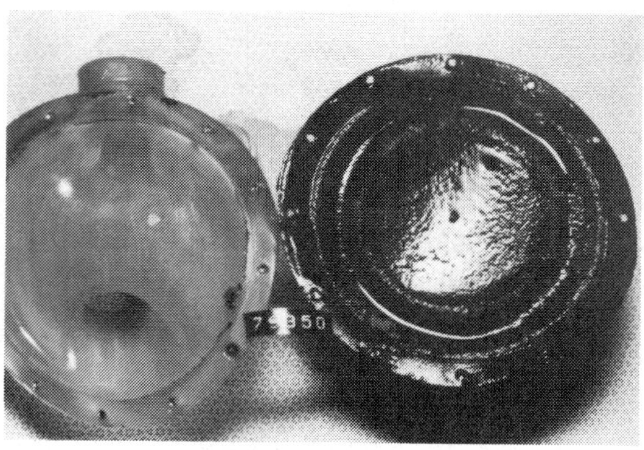

Figure 7. A pusher-plate type LVAD coated with 5% gelatin. The blood contacting surface of both housing and diaphragm is clear without thrombus.

This latter problem has been solved by employing a pusher-plate type diaphragm, where the maximum strain in the flexing region of the diaphragm was designed not to exceed 15%. Figure 7 shows a 5% gelatin coated, pusher-plate type LVAD used for 7 months in a calf without anticoagulants. The housing of this pump was also coated with 5% gelatin on textured Avcomat 610^{R}. The blood contacting surface of both diaphragm and housing was clean, without PNI formation. Thus, it is shown that the blood-material interaction occurs in different ways depending upon surface roughness, even though the surface is composed of the same material. The smooth gelatin surface has been tested in 22 pusher plate type TAH's [15] and LVAD's [16] for 1 to 7 months in calves without anticoagulants. The blood compatibility of this surface was shown to be excellent and no evidence of biodegradation or detachment of the gelatin layer, which is mechanically held in the pores of the textured base material, has been observed.

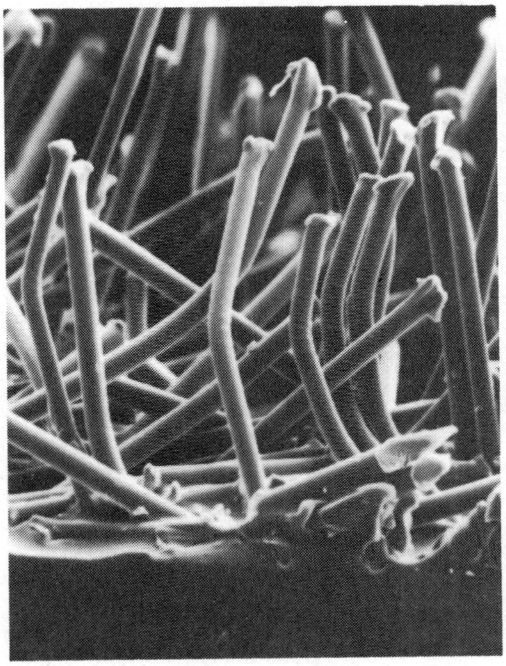

Figure 8. A cross section of a polyester flock surface. Polyester fibrils (300 μm long) are bonded to the base Biomer and forming a quite rough surface (300x).

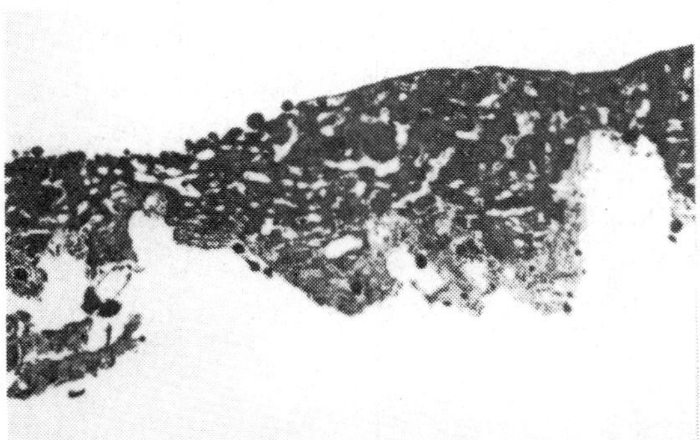

Figure 9. A pseudoneointima formed on a polyester flock surface after 2 months of implantation. In the right one half of the picture, the PNI is covered by a single layer, i.e., endothelial layer (PTAH, 160x).

Textured Polymer Surface

The first circulatory assist pump used by DeBakey [17] in 1961 was lined with Dacron velour to enhance PNI formation. The subsequent animal studies using this material, however, showed thrombus accumulation and scattered areas of calcification, which were caused by the thick pile depth of the velour. To ameliorate these problems, polyester fibril-flocked surface was introduced. Polyester fibrils, 300 μm long and 17 μm wide, are randomly bonded using adhesive to the base polymer. After curing and rinsing, overcoating with a diluted solution of urethane adhesive was added to fill any voids and improve the bonding of the fibrils. Figure 8 shows a SEM photograph of this material. This rough, synthetic textured surface has been extensively studied in several institutes including ours as a blood contacting surface of the LVADS [18,19,20]. The initially formed platelet-fibrin matrix was shown to be replaced with fibroblasts and collagen bundles, and endothelialization was ultimately observed after months of implantation (Figure 9). Although this desirable healing process of the PNI takes place in the non-deforming parts of the blood pump, such as the housing and the pusher-plate supported region of the diaphragm, the flexing region of the diaphragm showed a progressive increase in PNI thickness (Figure 10) with resultant calcification (Figure 11). The role of stress in the calcification process was analyzed and has been reported elsewhere [21,22]. In brief, when this type of surface is used in the deforming part of the blood pump (i.e., flexing area of the diaphragm), strain exerted during the pumping cycle creates fibril movement. The mutual orientation of fibrils changes according to the diaphragm position. The implication is that any PNI formed on and around the fibrils is mechanically disrupted, causing surface irregularity and resultant new deposition formation on this disrupted PNI surface. Invasion of fibroblasts or covering by an endothelial layer is rarely seen in the flexing area of the diaphragm. Figure 12 shows a x-ray photograph of the diaphragm used for 79 days. It is clearly shown that calcification is confined in the flexing

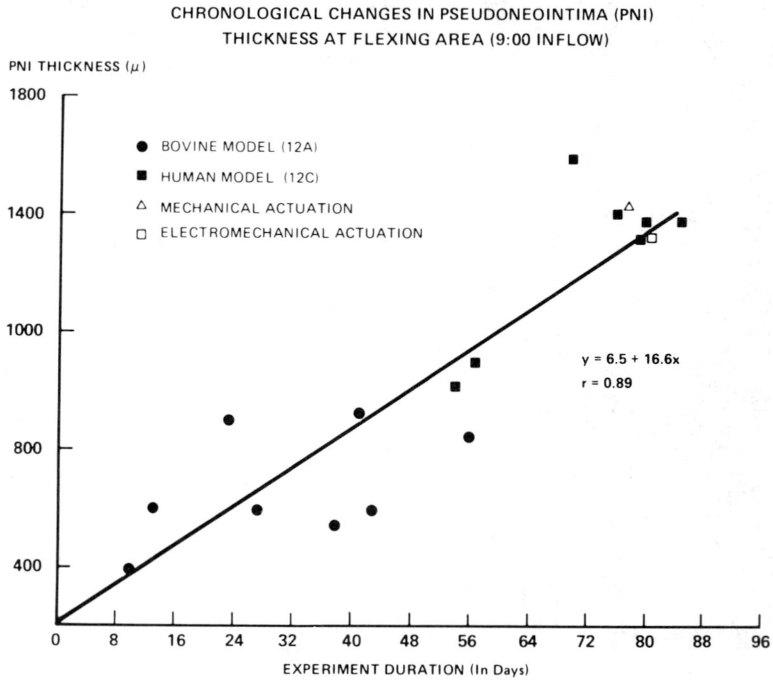

Figure 10. PNI thickness at the flexing area of the polyester flock coated diaphragm. Regardless of the type of pumps and actuation methods, the thickness increased with time, reaching more than 1.4 mm after 2 months of implantation. Closed circle and square denote a pneumatic actuation.

area of the diaphragm especially along the perimeter of the pusher plate, which has the most deformation. Transformation of amorphous calcium phosphate to crystalline, hydroxyapatite seems to take place within 2 weeks as revealed by TEM, energy dispersive x-ray microanalysis and x-ray diffraction analysis showing a typical apatite diffraction patter with a major peak at a 2θ angle of 32.5° (Figure 13).

Although it is known that vulnerability to calcification differs among the animal species and with age, no evidence has been shown in that this complication would not take place in humans. Further studies are necessitated to optimize the surface characteristics of this type of surface and to elucidate the pathogenesis of calcification, which may lead to device malfunction and/or systemic embolism.

Szycher and his colleague [23] introduced an integral-flock surface, where the flock fibrils and the base substrate are of the same material and are continuous in nature. Seeding of fetal calf fibroblasts on this improved textured surface before implantation was shown to enhance the healing of the PNI with rapid collagenation of the layer. Dystrophic calcification seldom occurs in the living tissue. This new approach with quick PNI healing will certainly minimize calcification in blood pump, especially in the the flexing region where tissue healing is always delayed.

Textured Metal Surface

Porous metals have been used successfuly in the fabrication of various endoprostheses.

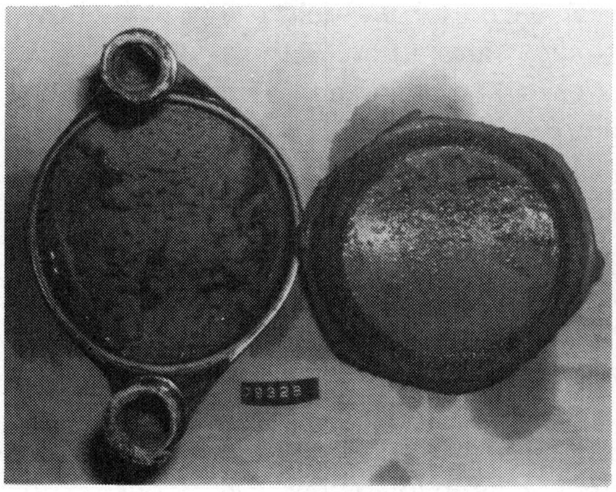

Figure 11. A pusher-plate type LVAD lined with a polyester flock surface used for 43 days. The diaphragm is centrally supported by a pusher plate. The peripheral flexing area of the diaphragm shows a diffuse and extensive calcification.

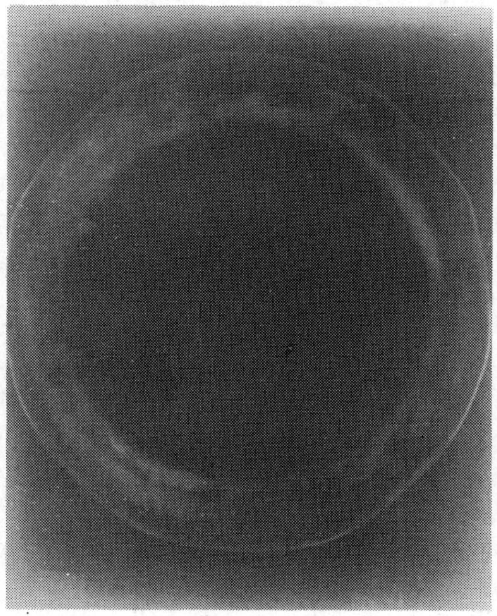

Figure 12. A x-ray picture of the diaphragm. The distribution of calcification is confined to the peripheral flexing area.

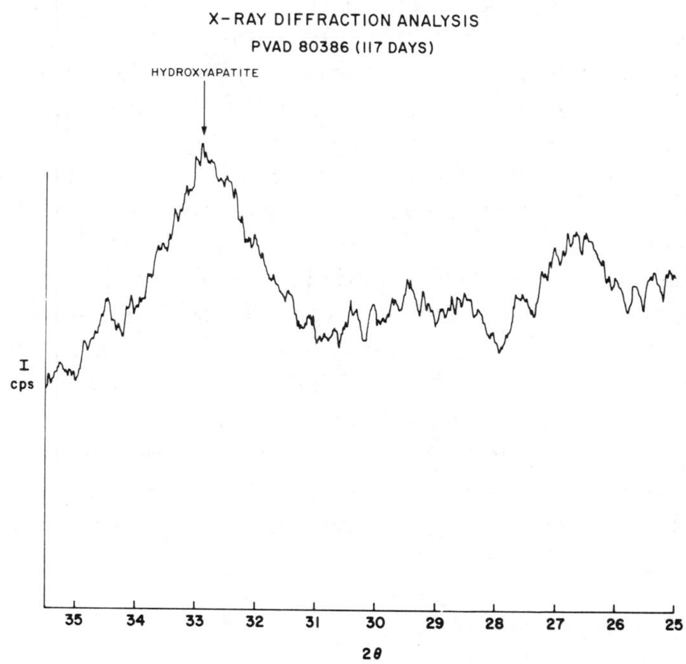

Figure 13. A x-ray diffraction analysis of calcified area of the diaphragm used for 117 days. It is shown that calcium phosphate is of crystalline form having a typical peak at a 2θ angle of 32.5°

These surfaces can be biologically fixed by allowing tissue ingrowth into their pores. In the cardiovascular application, MacGregor and his coworkers [24] introduced in 1976 a porous metal surface, made of a cobalt-base alloy, to cover the valve cages. Endothelialization was shown to occur quite quickly. Porous pure titanium and its alloys also attracted the attention for endoprosthetic use because of its inertness within the human body and a rather low density and elastic modulus, when compared with traditional cobalt alloys [25,26]. Encouraged by these previous works, powdered titanium alloy (Ti: 90%, Al: 6%, V: 4%) was applied as a blood contacting surface, in the housing of the LVADs by our group [27]. The titanium alloy spheres were prepared in an inert atmosphere by a sputtering process. Three different sizes of spheres were prepared by sifting through screens; small 45-75 μm, intermediate 75-150 μm, and large 150-225 μm. Each size of spheres were coated on the titanium housing with a sintering process by heating to 1300°C for 3-4 hrs. Nine LVADs, three of each particle size, were implanted in calves without anticoagulants for 7 to 56 days. As observed on the polyester flock surface, the rough, powdered titanium surface after contact with blood was covered with a platelet-fibrin matrix with a variable degree of erhtyrocyte and leukocyte involvement. By 2 weeks of implantation, polymorphonuclear and mononuclear cells appeared on the surface, some of them invading the PNI from the surface showing a "tunnel" formation. By the fifth week, discrete, insular areas of collagenation and endothelialization were observed. At the PNI-metal interface polymorphonuclear cells and/or mononuclear cell reaction was minimal, suggesting the good tissue compatibility of this material. No significant difference in histological reactions or in PNI thickness was observed among the pumps coated with different sized particles. The PNI thickness ranged from 40 to 600 μm, and appeared almost translucent macroscopically. Figure 14 shows a close up view of such PNI formed on the small particle size porous metal surface after 13 days. Even after 37 days, the PNI was so thin that the surface texture of the underlying metal surface was still observable (Figure 15). Although the basic cellular constituents and thickness of the PNI did not differ among the three particle sizes, there were differences in adherence of the PNI to the surface depending on the particle size. The thin, membraneous PNI formed on the small size (45-75 μm) was anchored poorly, and was partially detached from the powdered metal surface after 23 and 41 days of implantation, accompanied by relatively fresh red thrombi. Because of this, the small particle size of 45 to 75 μm range is not thought to be suitable for blood pump application. In contrast, the PNI on the intermediate (75-150 μm) and large (150-225 μm) particle sizes were securely anchored on the pm surface without signs of detachment. A textured titanium surface was also tested in dogs as a blood contacting surface of a vascular conduit implanted in the abdominal aorta, showing a similar PNI formation pattern as observed in the blood pump.

Although the experience with this new blood contacting surface is limited, because of its inertness, desirable mechanical properties, and good tissue and blood compatibility, the textured metal surface seems to be a very promising material for the non-moving components of the blood pump.

Smooth Synthetic Polymer Surface

Smooth polymer surfaces are currently used widely in various cardiac assist and replacement devices. The usage of this type of blood contacting surface is based on the intention that no activation of blood coagulation takes place at the interface.

Silicone-based elstomers are among the most widely used biomedical materials and are

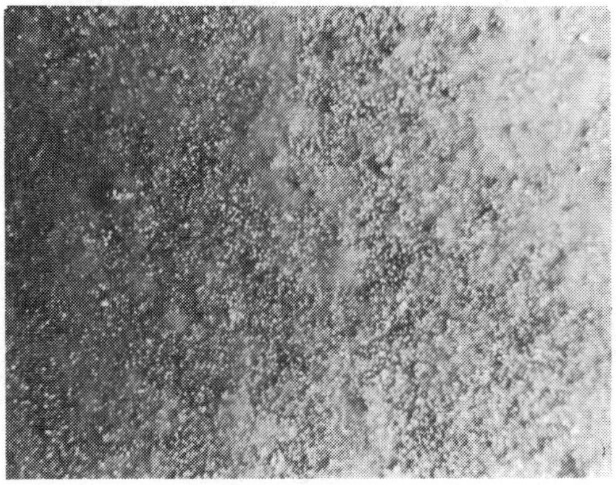

Figure 14. A close-up view of the PNI formed on the textured metal surface. The PNI is very thin and semi-transulucent. The PNI surface appears quite smooth.

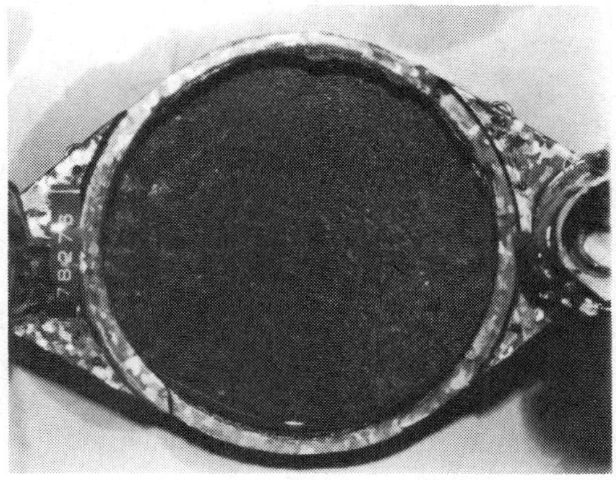

Figure 15. A pump housing used for 37 days. The textured metal surface (particle size: 150-225 μm) is still recognized, and the PNI formed on top is scarcely seen with this magnification. No sign of secondary thrombus formation is noted.

generally regarded as among the most stable and blood compatible materials. Application of silicone rubber to artificial hearts is not new and the total artifical hearts made in the initial stage by Akutsu et al. [28] was lined by this material. The prerequisites for cardiovascular application of this type of surface are the purity and smoothness of the surface in addition to the satisfactory mechanical properties. The surface should be microscopically smooth without discontinuity and be devoid of any foreign particles such as dust or surface inclusions derived during fabrication. These surface irregularities can serve as nidi for localized thrombi. It is also stressed that the design of the device should avoid any stagnation points or sizable step formations, such as a sharp diaphragm-housing junction or any junction between components. Frequent and rather massive thrombus formation has been reported to occur at the valve-pump junction. In the past several years the inertness and durability of silicone elastomers in the biological environment has come under question. Biodegradation, possibly due to lipid adsorption, caused the failure of silicone heart valve poppets. The failure is also known to be quite sensitive to the simultaneous presence of both stress and biologically active fluid such as blood. An occasional pump rupture was reported in the early stages of pump development using silicone rubber. The presence of filler in the silicone elastomers, although they increase the tensile strength, was shown to adversely affect the blood compatibility. Silcone rubber free of silica filler was introduced to improve the blood compatibility [29].

Polyether urethane has been extensively used in blood pumps since its introduction as a biomedical material in 1967 [30-32]. A compound made of polyurethane and siloxane (Avcothane 51) has also been used [33]. Although these rather new synthetic polymers have shown good blood compatibility, complete freedom from thromboembolism has not yet been achieved. To minimize thrombus formation, the surface should be pure and microscopically smooth, avoiding any contamination of dust particles or surface imperfections caused during fabrication [34].

Recent progress in long-term animal implantation of blood pumps in several institutes has disclosed a previously unexpected problem occurring on the blood contacting surface of these smooth synthetic materials. Calcification in the blood pumps using these materials is now recognized as a frequent and serious complication regardless of the type of blood pump, species of experimental animals used, and their age. The pathogenesis of calcification has not been studied in detail. Whether it occurs with the same mechanism as seen on the PNI-generating surfaces is not answered yet. It was reported that calcified deposits are preferentially seen in stress concentration areas of the moving diaphragm. It was also noted that the location of calcified depositions coincide with the loci of surface imperfection or surface defects [35]. It is possible that any surface defects caused during fabrication or created after usage in the stressed areas of the material behave as nidi for localized thrombi, the cellular components of which subsequently are degraded and become the site of nucleation of calcium phosphate. The other possibility, however, of direct deposition of calcium phosphate on these smooth synthetic surfaces still remains. Further studies are warranted to answer these questions.

CONCLUSION

In this chapter, we reviewed briefly the blood-material interfacial phenoma, which occur in the various blood pumps. The interactions of the materials to the circulating blood are affected by many factors, such as fluid dynamics in the pump, permiability of the surface, coagulability of blood passing through the pump, and physicochemical properties of the material. This fact makes it difficult to compare different materials used in different types of blood pumps, and tested in different animals species with or without anticoagulation. For the same reasons, there has been difficulty in establishing reliable and reproducible in vitro screening test method to predict the occurrance in blood pumps. Many approaches have been taken to develop materials which simultaneously possess good blood compatibility and mechanical properties to fulfill the requirements as blood pump materials. Any material, however, has it own advantages and disadvantages, and as yet, no material has been developed which is truely comparable to the endothelial lining of the cardiovascular system. The PNI generating surface is not recognized by blood as a foreign surface once the surface is covered by the PNI, the components of which derive from blood itself. The unpredictability of PNI formation, and calcification in the moving parts appear to be the major problems in long term implantation. Regarding the smooth surface approach, the degree of smoothness seems to play an important role. At present stability of surface smoothness after long term usage in a blood pump in vivo is not known. Nevertheless, the majority of the researchers in this field now agree that any of these materials is safely usable for short-term human applications, and the clinical studies in LVADs have been conducted under the auspices of National Heart, Lung and Blood Institute since 1975. We are now at the stage to expand this modality toward various chronic heart diseases on the long-term or even permanent basis. To accomplish this purpose, and to meet the pressing need, further studies and developments of materials are mandatory unifying the efforts of polymer chemists, surface chemists, fluid mechanical engineers, biologists and medical workers.

ACKNOWLEDGMENT

The authors are grateful to Miss Abbie Fields and Miss Jan Kodish for their invaluable help in preparation of this manuscript.

REFERENCES

1. Nose, Y., Arancibia, C., Koiso, K., Urzua, J., and Kiraly, R. J. *In:* Platelets, Thrombosis and Inhibitors, Didishein,P., Shimamoto, T., and Yamazaki, H., Eds., F. K. Schattauer Verlag, Stuttgart-New York, 67-77, 1974.
2. Nose, Y., Imai, Y., Tajima, K., Ogawa, H., Klain, M., von Bally, K., and Effler, D. B. Cardiac prosthesis utilizing biological material. J. Thorac. Cardiovasc. Surg., 62:714-724, 1971.
3. Carpentier, A., Lemaigre, G., Robert, L., Carpentier, S., and Dubost, C. Biological factors affecting long-term results of valvular heterografts. J. Thorac. Cardiovasc. Surg., 58:467-483, 1969.
4. Nose, Y., Kiraly, R. J., and Picha, G. Surface characteristics of cardiac prostheses in vivo. J. Biomed. Mater. Res. Symposium, 8:85-100, 1977.
5. Harasaki, H. Kiraly, R., and Nose, Y. Endothelialization in blood pumps. Trans. Am. Soc. Artif. Intern. Organs, 24:415-424, 1978.
6. Wesolowski, S. A., Fries, C. C., Karlson, K. E., DeBakey, M. E., and Sawyer, P. N. Porosity: Primary determinant of ultimate fate of synthetic vascular grafts. Surgery, 50:91-96, 1961.
7. MacKenzie, D. C., and Lowenthal, J. Endothelial growth in nylon vascular grafts. Br. J. Surg., 48:212-217, 1960.
8. Poole, J. C. F., Sabiston, D. C., Jr., Florey, H. W., and Allison, P. R. Growth of endothelium in arterial prosthetic grafts and following endarterectomy. Surg. Forum, 21:225-227, 1962.
9. Harker, L. A., Slichter, S. J., and Sauvage, L. R. Platelet consumption by arterial prostheses: The effects of endothelialization and pharmacologic inhibition of platelet function. Ann. Surg., 186:594-601, 1977.
10. MacKenzie, J. R., Hackett, M., Topuzlu, C., and Tibbs, D. J. Origin of arterial prosthesis lining from circulating blood cells. Arch. Surg., 97:879-885, 1968.
11. Bull, B., Fuchs, J. C. A., Braunwald, N. S. Mechanism of formation of tissue layers on the fabric lattice covering intravascular prosthetic devices. Surgery, 65:640-648, 1969.
12. Feijen, J., Bengeling, T., Bantjes, A., and Sibinga, C. T. S. Biomaterials and interfacial phenomena. Adv. Cardiovasc. Phys. 3:100-132, 1979.
13. Kiraly, R. J., and Hillegass, D. V. Polyolefin blood pump components. In: Synthetic biomedical polymers. Concepts and applications. Szycher, M., and Robinson, W. J., (eds.). Technomic Publishing Co., Westport, CT, p. 59-71, 1980.
14. Harasaki, H., Kiraly, R., Murabayashi, S., Pepoy, M., Fields, A., Kambic, H., Hillegass, D., and Nose, Y. Cross-linked gelatin as a blood contacting surface. Artif. Organs, 3(S):216-221, 1979.
15. Harasaki, H., Takatani, S., Suwa, S., Jacobs, G., Snow, J., Kiraly, R., and Nose, Y. Hemodynamic regulation in total artificial heart (TAH) recipients. Artif. Organs, 5:38-45, 1981.
16. Nose, Y., Kiraly, R., Ozawa, K., Sukalac, R., Przybycz, J., Murakami, T., Snow, J., Harasaki, H., Jacobs, G., Murabayashi, S., Golding, L., Castle, C., and Hillegass, D. Development and evaluation of cardiac prosthesis. Annual Report No. NO1-HV-2-2960-5, Cleveland Clinic Foundation, Cleveland, OH (April, 1979).
17. DeBakey, M. E. Left ventricular bypass pump for cardiac assistance. Clinical experience. Am. J. Cardiol. 27:3-11, 1971.
18. Poirier, V. Fabrication and testing of flocked blood pump bladders. In: Synthetic biomedical polymers. Concepts and applications. Szycher, M., and Robinson, W. J. (eds). Technomic Publishing Co., Westport, CT, 73-115, 1980.
19. Turner, S. A., Milton, L. T., Poirier, V. L., and Norman, J. C. Sequential studies of pseudoneointimae with long-term THIE-type ALVAD's thickness, calcification and compositional analyses. Artif. Organs, 5:18-25, 1981.
20. Harasaki, H., Kambic, H., Whalen, R., Murray, J., Snow, J., Murabayashi, S., Hillegass, D., Ozawa, K., Kiraly, R., and Nose, Y. Comparative study of flocked vs. biolized surface for long-term assist

pumps. Trans. Am. Soc. Artif. Intern. Organs, 26:470-474, 1980.

21. Nose, Y., Harasaki, H., and Murray, J. Calcification of artificial surfaces that contact blood. Trans. Am. Soc. Artif. Intern. Organs, *in press.*
22. Harasaki, H., Gerrity, R., Kiraly, R., and Nose, Y. Calcification in blood pumps. Trans. Am. Soc. Artif. Intern. Organs 25:305-309, 1979.
23. Szycher, M., Bernhard, W., Franzblau, C., and Handenshild, C. Integrally textured polymeric surface for cardiac assist devices. In: Artificial Organs, proceedings of the Second Meeting of the International Society for Artificial Organs. International Society for Artificial Organs, Cleveland, 210-215, 1980.
24. MacGregor, D. C., Pilliar, R. M., Wilson, G. J., Goldstein, W., Rubis, L. J., Blackwell, R., Lixfeld, W., Scully, H. E., and Silver, M. D. Porous metal surface: A radical new concept in prosthetic heart valve design. Trans. Am. Soc. Artif. Intern. Organs, 22:646-653, 1976.
25. Hirschhorn, J. S., McBeath, A. A., and Dustoor, M. R. Porous titanium surgical implant materials. J. Biomed. Mater. Res. Symposium, 2:49-67, 1971.
26. Nilles, J. L., Karagianes, M. T., and Wheeler, K. R. Porous titanium alloy for fixation of Kee prostheses. J. Biomed. Mater. Res. Symposium, 5:319-328, 1974.
27. Harasaki, H., Snow, J., Gerrity, R., Whalen, R., Ozawa, K., Kiraly, R., and Nose, Y. Powdered metal surface for blood pump. Trans. Am. Soc. Artif. Intern. Organs, 25:225-230, 1979.
28. Akutsu, T., Mirkovitch, V., Topaz, S. R., and Kolff, W. J. Silastic sac type of artificial heart and its use in calves. Trans. Am. Soc. Artif. Intern. Organs, 9:281-285, 1963.
29. Kolobow, T., Stool, E. W., Weathersby, P. K., Pierce, J., Hayano, F., and Suaudeau, J. Superior blood compatibility of silicone rubber free of silica filler in the membrane lung. Trans. Am. Soc. Artif. Int. Organs, 20:269-276, 1974.
30. Boretos, J. W. Pierce, W. S., Baier, R. E., Leroy, A. F., Donachy, H. J. Surface and bulk characteristics of a polyether urethane for artificial hearts. J. Biomed. Mater. Res. 9:327-340, 1975.
31. Pierce, W. S., Brighton, J. A., Donachy, J. H., Landis, D. L., Rosenberg, G., Prophet, G. A., White, W. J., and Waldenhausen, J. A. The artificial heart. Progress and promise. Arch. Surg., 112:1430-1438, 1977.
32. Rennenkamp, F., Affeld, K. Clevert, H. D., Frnak, J., Gerlach, K., Grosse-Siestrup, Ch., Henning, E., Kleibach, H., Krautzberger, W., Kuhlmann, F., Lemm, W., Monhaupt, A., Unger, V., Weidemann, H., Zartnack, F., and Bucherl, E. S. Long time results with seamless blood pumps out of polyurethanes for the replacement of the heart. Proc. ESAO, 4:94-98, 1979.
33. Lederman, D. M., Singh, P. I., Russell, F. B., Morgan, R. A., Cumming, R. D., Levine, F. H., Austen, W. G. and Buckley, M. J. Discontinuity-free integrally valved left heart blood pump. Proc. ESAO, 4:74-78, 1979.
34. Coleman, D., Lawson, J., and Kolff, W. J. Scanning electron microscopic evaluation of the surfaces of artificial hearts. Artif. Organs, 2:166-172, 1978.
35. Coleman, D. L., Lim, D., Kessler, T., Andrade, J. D. Calcification of non-textured implantable blood pumps. Trans. Am. Soc. Artif. Intern. Organs, *in press.*

Chapter 10

Pseudoneointimal Analyses of Chronically-Implanted Textured Blood Pumps

Stephen A. Turner[1], B.S., Mattie I. Bossart[2], Ph.D., Warren C. Clay[3], B.S.M.E., and O. Howard Frazier[4], M.D.

ABSTRACT

Texturing of internal blood pump surfaces provides a substrate for the deposition of a biologic pseudoneointimal lining derived from the circulating blood. Pseudoneointimal (PNI) analyses were performed following 27 chronic in vivo *evaluations, ranging from two days to greater than one year in the calf. These analyses included radiographic, histologic, and ultrastructural evaluations. From the studies described herein, a general trend in PNI accretion and maturation has been formulated. This can be summarized generally: (< 14 days) fibrin and platelet deposition; (14-30 days) fibrin compaction with infiltration of leukocytes; (40-60 days) formation of white fibrous (collagen, fibrin, fibroblasts) plaques in addition to the accellular fibrin matrix; (≥ 60 days) plaques increase in number and area with a maturation of fibroblasts to myofibroblasts occurring within a collagen matrix. Endothelialization occurred at the surface of the plaques separating the collagen matrix from the circulating blood. The remaining portion of the pump is covered by a thin (< 50 microns), adherent, thromboresistant, fibrin matrix. Ultrastructural studies verify morphologically the existence of an upper continuous endothelium, and indicate that a variety of cell types are present within the fibrous plaques. Though limited to the flexing portion of the pump diaphragm, calcification of the PNI did occur. These studies indicate that the textured surface utilized in the THI blood pump is a suitable blood interface for chronic mechanical circulatory support in the calf.*

This work was supported in part by National Heart, Lung, and Blood Institute, Devices and Technology Branch, Contracts NO1-HV-7-2936, and NO1-HV-0-2915.
[1]Research Associate, Cardiovascular Surgical Research Laboratories, The Texas Heart Institute, Houston, Texas.
[2]Director, Electron Microscopy, Department of Pathology, St. Luke's Episcopal Hospital, Houston, Texas.
[3]Program Manager, Thermo Electron Corporation, Waltham, Massachusetts.
[4]Director, Cardiovascular Surgical Research Laboratories, The Texas Heart Institute, Houston, Texas.

INTRODUCTION

Over the past decade, considerable progress has been made in the development of long-term circulatory assist (left ventricular assist devices) and replacement (total artificial heart) devices. The eventual goal is that of tether-free, totally implantable, electrically-actuated systems for use in man. To meet these objectives, demonstration of blood compatibility at the blood material interface is essential. Two basic approaches have evolved to meet this requirement.

One approach relies on a smooth, nonthrombogenic surface usually fabricated from polyurethane or its derivatives [1-3]. The other utilizes a textured biomaterial and is either pretreated with autologous or cultured cells [4], impregnated and coated with glutaraldehyde cross-linked gelatin [5] or simply left untreated to allow the formation of a biologic lining from the circulating blood [6]. All of these surfaces have shown satisfactory blood compatibility in short and intermediate-term ($\leqslant$ 3 months) experimental studies in animals. Controversy persists, however, regarding the use of textured or smooth surfaces for chronically implanted blood pumps. A variety of blood-contacting surfaces are currently being utilized in long-term blood pump evaluations (Table 1). The purpose of this section is to describe and summarize experience with the THI blood pump utilizing a textured blood-contacting surface in the calf.

More specifically this section will 1) describe briefly the THI blood pump and blood-contacting surface; 2) summarize the methods employed to analyze the explanted blood pumps; 3) describe, in detail, the development, ultrastructure, and calcification of the biologically-derived pseudoneointimal linings formed within THI blood pumps during 27 chronic, bovine experiments; 4) discuss the results, potentials, and problems of textured blood-contacting surfaces and; 5) present a review and discussion of the nature and possible etiology of blood pump calcification, a problem common to both textured and smooth surfaces.

THI BLOOD PUMP

The THI blood pump is a single-chambered, pusher-plate blood pump designed for transverse abdominal placement between the left ventricular apex and the infrarenal abdominal aorta (Figure 1). During in-vitro and in-vivo testing, it has been found to meet and exceed the National Heart, Lung and Blood Institute's (NHLBI) long-term blood pump criteria for providing flow rates $\geqslant$ 10 L/min at pumping rates $\leqslant$ 120 B/min into mean arterial pressures $\geqslant$ 120 mm Hg, with a mean filling pressure $\leqslant$ 15 mm Hg.

The blood pump is fabricated at Thermo Electron Corporation and has four major components: a rigid outer housing with inlet and outlet ports, a pusher-plate diaphragm, valved inlet and outlet conduits and a pusher-plate displacement transducer. The maximum stroke volume is 90 ml with a pusher-plate excursion of 1.52 cm. The pump housing and all external metallic components are fabricated from a titanium alloy (Ti6A14V). This alloy satisfies the requirements of fabricability, chemical and mechanical stability, biocompatibility, corrosion resistance, strength and weight. The pump diaphragm has a thickness of 0.08 cm and is fabricated from Biomer, a linear-segmented polyether polyurethane. This elastomer was selected on the basis of fabricability, chemical and mechanical stability, biocompatibility and durability [7].

Previoiusly, all blood-contacting surfaces except the valves and vascular grafts were

Table 1. Experimental Long-term (> 2 yr) LVADs and TAHs.

Institution	Device	Geometric Description	Blood-Contacting Surfaces
Avco-Everett Research Laboratories Everett, Massachusetts	AVCO LVAD	Diaphragm-Type Pump	Smooth, Avcothane
Andros, Incorporated Berkeley, California	Andros Model IIA Solenoid Actuated LVAS	Dual Pusher-Plate/ Diaphragm Type Pump	Smooth, Polyurethane
Chirurgishe Universitats-Klinik Berlin	Berlin TAH	Ellipsoid	Smooth, Segmented Polyurethane
Chirurgische Universitats-Klinik Innsbruck, Austria	Ellipsoid Heart	Ellipsoid	Smooth, Segmented Polyurethane
Cleveland Clinic Foundation Cleveland, Ohio	Cleveland Clinic LVAD	Pusher-Plate/ Diaphragm Type Pump	Smooth, Aldehyde-treated, Gelatin Coated Polyolefin
Cleveland Clinic Foundation Cleveland, Ohio	Cleveland Clinic Biventricular Assist Device	Pusher-Plate/ Diaphragm Type Pump	Smooth, Aldehyde-treated, Gelatin Coated Polyolefin
Institute of Transplantation of Organs and Tissues Moscow, USSR	USSR TAH Nr1 and Nr2	Sac-type/ Diaphragm Type Pump	Smooth, Silastic and Polyurethane
Pennsylvania State University Hershey, Pennsylvania	Pennsylvania State University Artificial Heart	Angle Port Pump Diaphragm Type	Smooth, Segmented Polyurethane
Texas Heart Institute Houston, Texas	THI E-type ALVAD	Pusher-plate/ Diaphragm Type Pump	Textured, Powdered Metal with Polyurethane Diaphragm
Texas Heart Institute Houston, Texas	Akutsu III TAH	Diaphragm Type Pump	Smooth, Segmented Polyurethane
Thermo Electron Waltham, Massachusetts	Model IX E-ALVAD	Pusher-plate/ Diaphragm Type Pump	Textured, Powdered Metal with Polyurethane Diaphragm
Thoratec Laboratories Berkeley, California	Thoratec Model U1-C LVAD	Pusher-plate/ Diaphragm Type Pump	Textured, Microporous Polyurethane, Tissue Interface
University of Tokyo Tokyo, Japan	Paracorporeal TAH	Sac-Type Pump	Smooth, Polyvinyl Chloride Paste
University of Utah Salt Lake City, Utah	Jarvik-5 Jarvik-7	Diaphragm-Type Pump	Smooth, Segmented Polyurethane

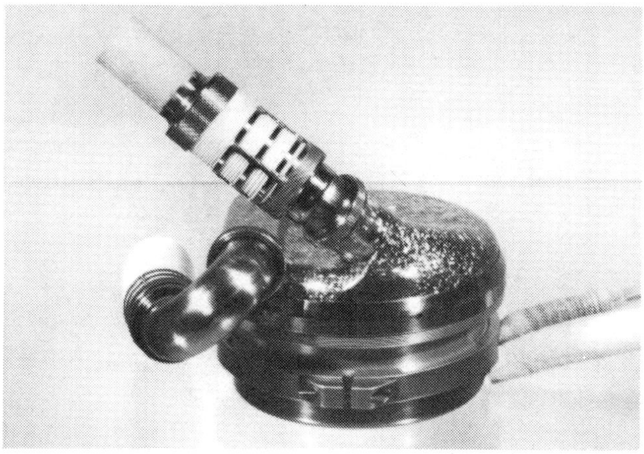

Figure 1. Integrated THI/Gould left ventricular assist system (LVAS) with flexible inlet and outlet conduits.

textured with polyester fibrils (17 microns in diameter, 320 microns in length and surface density of 150 fibrils/mm^2) to promote the deposition of a stable, adherent, biologically-derived pseudoneointima (PNI) from the circulating blood. Although these conventionally-textured surfaces performed well during in-vivo evaluations with durations exceeding one year, degradation of the polyurethane adhesive bonds between the fibrils and substrate represented a potential failure mode.

To prevent this potential problem, textured powder metallurgy (PM) techniques have been developed and incorporated in the fabrication of the metallic blood-contacting surfaces of the pump. This texturing method involves the use of titanium spheres which are reliably bonded (by sintering) to all titanium blood-contacting components, resulting in a multi-layered, interconnected, porous substrate [8]. In addition, a method of fabricating flexing pump diaphragms without the use of adhesives has been developed by Szycher et al [4]. The process involves production of a transfer mold which has been cast against a flocked master mandrel. The result is an integrally-textured Biomer diaphragm – an analogue of conventionally-flocked surfaces.

MATERIALS AND METHODS

Twenty-seven THI blood pump flexing diaphragms and rigid upper pump housings were analyzed following in-vivo studies ranging from 2 to 393 days in calves. In all except 3 of the 27 animals, postoperative anticoagulation consisted of daily Coumadin (2.5-7.5 mg to maintain prothrombin times at 2 to 2½ times normal), Persantine (400 mg) and Ascriptin (1 to 2 gm). In 15 studies, pump actuation was EKG synchronous; 12 systems were actuated asynchronously. In 13 studies, an electrical energy converter provided actuation, while 14 studies were pneumatically driven.

Calves used in these studies were 3-5 months of age and weighed between 75-100 kg. Complete blood counts and coagulation profiles were obtained routinely to assess continuing biocompatibility.

Immediately following pump explantation, the diaphragms with overlying pseudoneointima were removed for gross characterization. Following visual examinations of the PNI for homogeneity, color, texture and thickness, the diaphragms and opposing upper pump housings were photographed and placed in cold lactated Ringer's solution. Representative PNI sections from both the flexing and rigid portions of the diaphragm and the metal pump housing were placed in 10% formalin for light microscopy. Histologic examinations of hematoxylin-eosin or Gomori's (for collagen) stained PNI sections were performed.

For ultrastructural studies, samples of PNI plaques formed on rigid and flexing portions of the diaphragm were placed in 3% glutaraldehyde and examined by routine transmission electron microscopy methods. Respentative samples from these areas were also "en Bloc" stained with tannic acid to identify elastin. Samples from heavily calcified flexing portions of the diaphragm were decalcified using 3% glutaraldehyde – 0.1M EDTA solution. Thin sections from these preparations were post-stained with uranal acetate and lead citrate. Ultrastructural examinations were performed using a Siemens 101 electron microscope.

A modified radiographic technique (Kodak Min-R film exposed at 15 mas, 56 KV/for 1/12 second at 12 inches) was employed to demonstrate the location and relative density of radiopaque calcium-bearing material on the diaphragm. The radiographic and histologic data were then correlated. Based on the percent of calcification per total diaphragm surface area, numerical valves were assigned to each diaphragm: trace, 1+; slight, 2+; moderate, 3+; severe, 4+. Additional characterization of calcium-bearing deposits was performed using transmission and scanning electron microscopy and elemental spectral analyses.

Based on cross-sectional PNI measurements using a micrometer correlated with radiographs, thickness maps were constructed for each diaphragm. This information allowed correlations to be made relating PNI thickness to calcification and to determine areas of increased PNI deposition.

Experimental Results

Pseudoneointimae formed within THI blood pumps were evaluated in 27 calves using the methods described. Taken serially, these studies provide a means of studying the sequence of events involved in PNI deposition and stabilization. Blood compatibility appeared excellent as hematocrits and platelet counts stabilized, and plasma hemoglobins were within normal limits 24 hours following device implantation.

PNI Development

Within 48 hours of initial blood contact, the diaphragm surface was completely covered with a smooth biologically-derived PNI lining. Initially the PNI consisted of fibrin, platelets and a few trapped red blood cells (Figure 2). This fibrin matrix increased in thickness ($\geqslant$ 200 microns) during the first month of pumping and was composed of a trilaminar fibrin lining consisting of a loosely arranged upper layer overlying a compacted and, generally acellular basilar layer. Polymorphonuclear and morphonuclear cells were distributed within the upper fibrin layer.

After approximately one month of pumping, the majority of the PNI decreased in thickness ($\leqslant$ 75 microns) as compaction of the fibrin matrix occurred. At this time, the lines of layer demarcation were less identifiable and the PNI was primarily acellular as the leukocytes along the upper portion of the matrix decreased in number. Scanning electron micrographs showed only occasional erythrocytes and platelets on the well-organized fibrin surface, indicating that the substrate was thromboresistant.

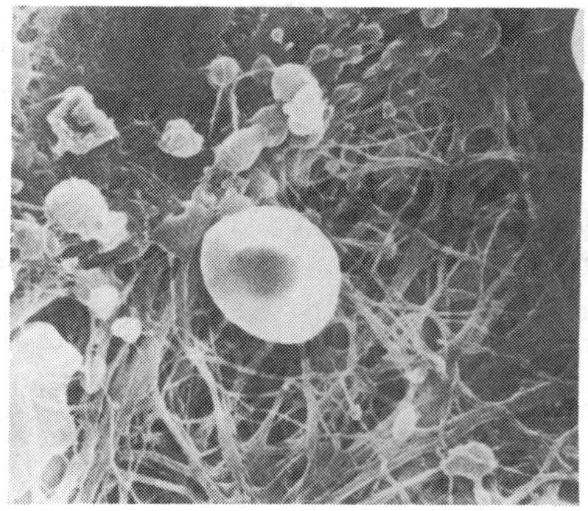

Figure 2. Scanning electron micrograph of the pseudoneointima formed after two days in the anticoagulated calf. This section from the diaphragm surface shows a fibrin matrix with several platelets, and an erythrocyte adhered to the surface. (× 6000).

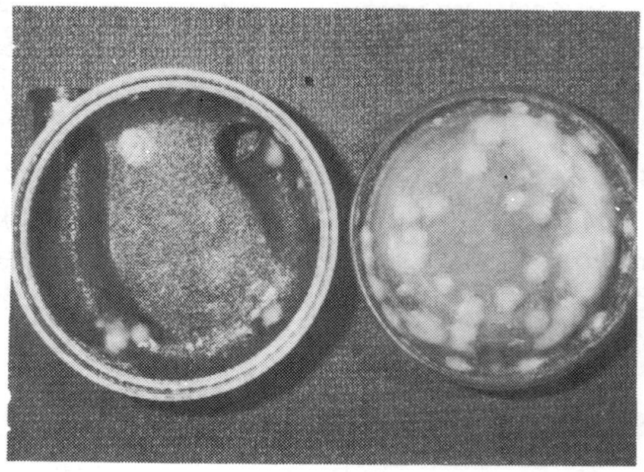

Figure 3. Photograph of the THI E-type upper pump housing (left) and opposing Biomer diaphragm (right), after 48 days of pumping in the calf. The white areas are composed of fibrin, collagen, and fibroblasts. The remaining areas of the pump are composed of a thin fibrin matrix, approximately 50-75 microns in thickness.

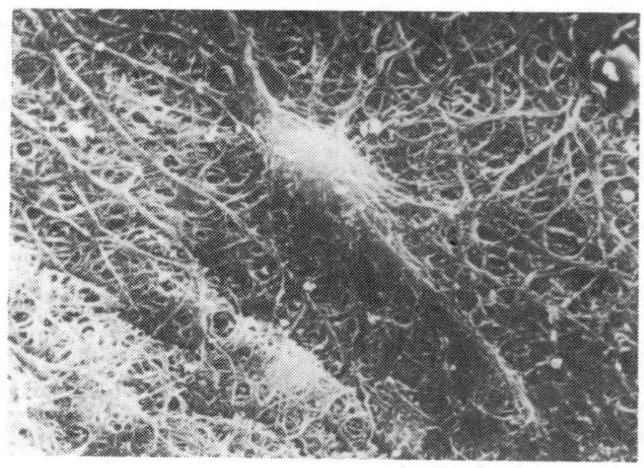

Figure 4. Scanning electron micrograph of the pseudoneointimal lining after 45 days of in-vivo pumping in the calf. This section shows a fibroblast (center), within a well organized fibrin matrix. (× 2100).

At six weeks, two distinctive types of PNI were identified. In addition to the fibrin lining, scattered white plaques appeared along the diaphragm and housing surfaces (Figure 3). The white areas measured approximately 150-500 microns in thickness and were firmly adherent to the blood-contacting surface. (Scanning electron micrographs showed evidence of fibroblast infiltration on the surface of these areas (Figure 4). In cross-section, these areas were composed mainly of fibrin, fibroblasts, collagen and a few macrophages.) The matrix was well organized and appeared to be overlapping with apparent tunnel formation. An overlying fibrin layer separated the collagen/fibroblast matrix from the circulating blood.

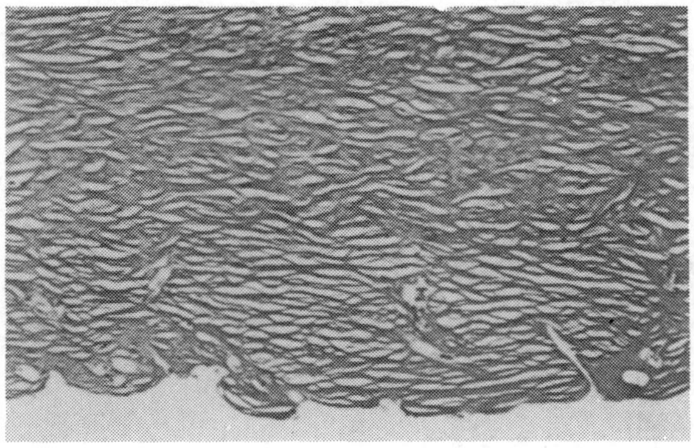

Figure 5. Photomicrograph of the PNI plaque formed after 150 days of pumping in the anticoagulated calf. Along the upper surface, a continuous endothelial lining overlies the collagen-fibroblast matrix. The basilar PNI demonstrates the points of biomaterial/biologic lining surface. (×175).

After approximately two months, the upper pump housings and diaphragms were covered by a thin fibrin lining (50-60% of the entire pumping surface) as well as numerous plaques of white, adherent PNI (40-50%). Relatively few changes with regard to the fibrin matrix occurred after this time. Grossly, the fibrin matrix showed no evidence of thrombogenicity and the lining was usually less than 50 microns in thickness. Microscopically, the fibrin matrix was mostly acellular and very well organized. The white plaques along the pumping surfaces were composed primarily of fibroblasts within a collagen matrix underlying an endothelial lining (Figure 5). The plaques were very adherent to the prosthetic interface and measured approximately 500-1000 microns in thickness. No thrombus was observed on the surface of this type of PNI. Further characterization of the cellular and extracellular components of these plaques from longer-term studies (> 100 days) was performed using transmission electron microscopy.

PNI Ultrastructure

Following fixation in 3% glutaraldehyde, the layer of PNI was easily removed from the underlying pump diaphragm. Cross-sections of the plaque-like material were oriented so that the diaphragm and blood-contacting surfaces could be identified. Figure 6 shows the tissue-like appearance of the PNI with its overlying endothelium. Plaques could be classified into two groups based on the ultrastructural characteristics of the cells and the location of the PNI on the diaphragm.

Within plaques from the non-flexing portion of the diaphragm, the majority of cells had the appearance of fibroblasts (Figure 7) and myofibroblasts (Figure 8). These cells formed layers parallel to the underlying diaphragm. The central area of the cells was characterized by elongated nuclei with large nucleoli and peripheral chromatin. The nuclei were irregular peripherally. In general, the cytoplasm of the elongated cells contained abundant Golgi, dilated endoplasmic reticulum, and moderate numbers of mitochondria. Progressing from the endothelial layer to the diaphragm surface, a successive maturation of fibroblasts to myofibroblasts was observed. The cells became more attenuated with the terminal ends becoming adjacent and frequently overlapping; however, no cell junctions were formed. Myofilaments with dense bodies which characterize myofibroblasts were more abundant in cells associated with the abluminal areas of plaques. In these cells, filamentous material traversed the cell cortices into the surrounding matrix (Figure 9). In addition, fewer profiles of endoplasmic reticulum were present in these cells. The cisternae were markedly dilated and proteinaceous material occupied the cytoplasm. No basal lamina invested these cells.

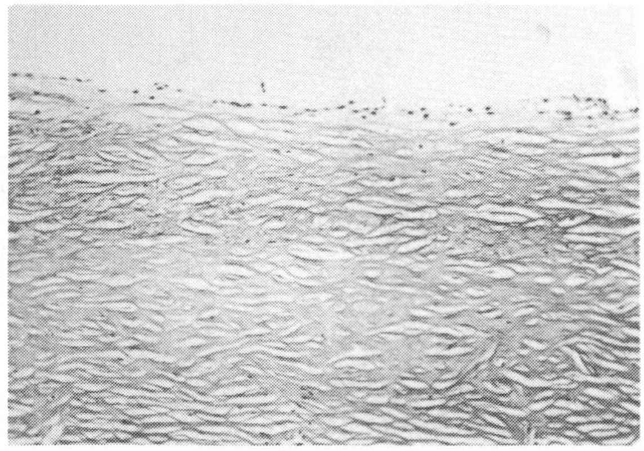

Figure 6. Higher magnification of the endothelial lining associated with the plaque-like PNI. A continuous layer of cells separates the collagen-fibroblast matrix from the circulating blood. (× 440).

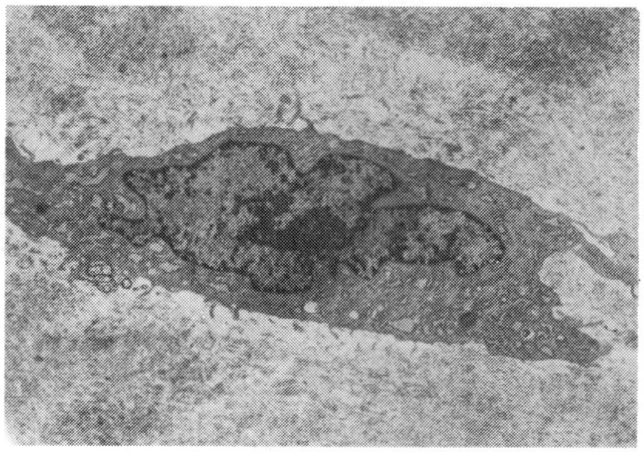

Figure 7. Transmission electron micrograph of a cell, with ultrastructural characteristics of a fibroblast, inside the collagen and proteinaceous matrix of the plaque. (× 8200).

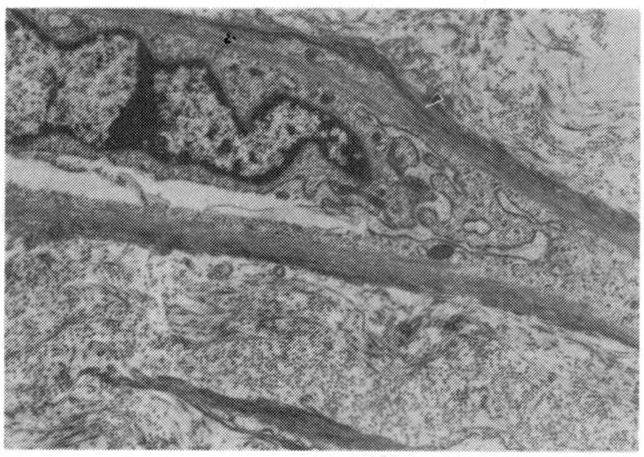

Figure 8. A myofibroblast with its surrounding collagen matrix. The arrow indicates peripheral myofilaments with associated dense bodies. (× 15000).

Collagen appeared to be the primary extracellular constituent in these plaques. In tissue directly underlying the endothelial cells, the collagen was sparce. The collagen was more compact and longitudinally oriented between the more basally attenuated myofibroblasts. Periodicity of collagen fibrils measured 600 nm in diameter. In cross-section the collagen was irregular peripherally with electron-dense attachments extending from angular points. These structures measured 500 nm and could be seen attached at sites in longitudinal sections of collagen.

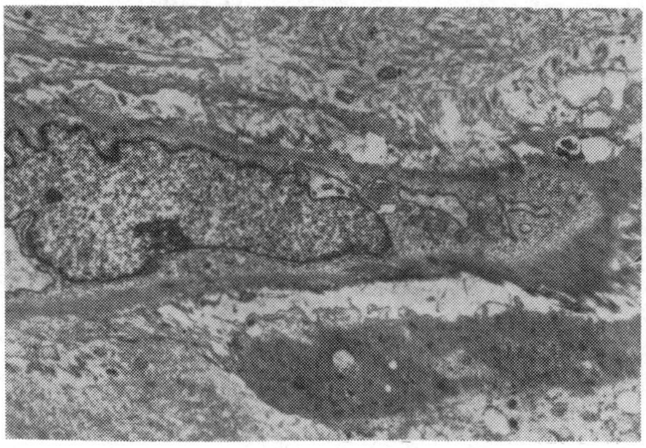

Figure 9. A mature myofibroblast, showing filaments extending into the matrix (arrow). (× 15000).

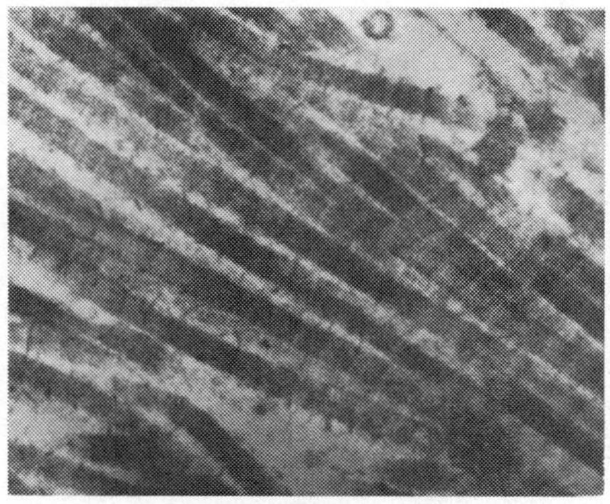

Figure 10a. Transmission electron micrograph of longitudinally cut collagen.

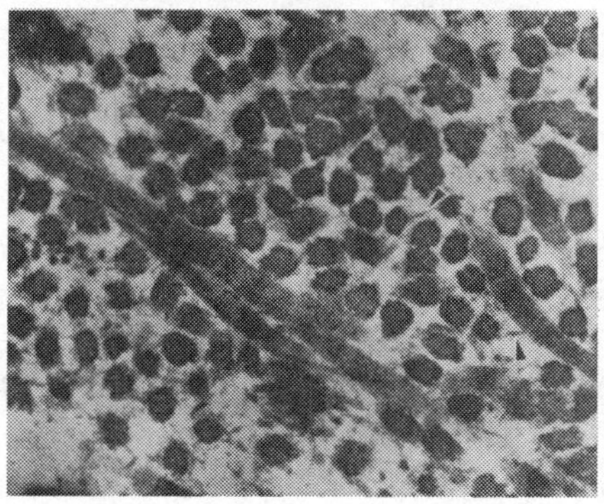

Figure 10b. Collagen cut in cross-section. The appendages seen in longitudinally sectioned collagen, are also seen in cross-sectioned collagen (arrow). (× 90000).

In addition to collagen, the extracellular matrix incorporated varying amounts of electron dense amorphous material (characteristic of mucopolysaccharide) containing a ground substance. Admixed with these materials were filaments appearing hollow and measuring 150 nm in diameter (Figure 10). No elastin was present within the plaques.

Plaques from the flexing portion of the diaphragm had a layering pattern similar to the linings seen in the non-flexing areas. The matrix was composed of short fibrils and amorphous proteinaceous non-filamentous material, interspersed with scattered collagen fibrils. Unlike the plaques described previously, the types of cells were different and more varied in these samples. The population of cells included obvious lymphocytes, monocytes, macrophages (Figure 11) and multinucleated giant cells (Figure 12), as well as fibroblasts and myofibroblasts.

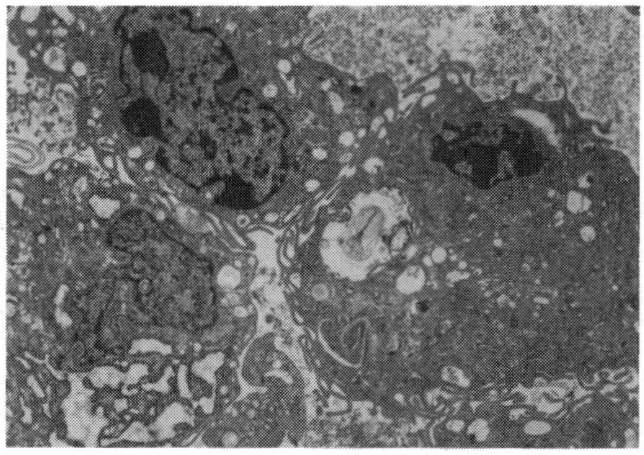

Figure 11. Macrophages from flexing portion of PNI plaque. (× 9000).

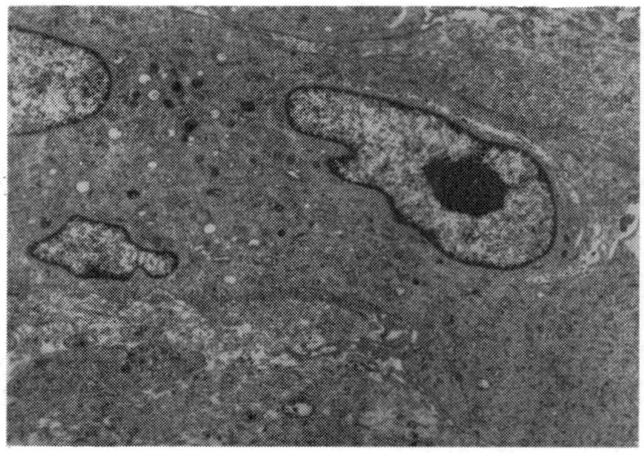

Figure 12. Multinucleated giant cell, from flexing portion of PNI plaque. (× 6000).

It is interesting to note that many cells appeared to be intermediates between these various cells (Figure 13 a,b,c). As in the other plaques, a loosely anchored layer separated the matrix from the circulating blood. Myofibroblasts formed layers parallel to the base of the plaque. An occasional cell could be seen randomly oriented within the plaque. These cells had characteristics of either lymphocytes, monocytes or macrophages. In addition, the cells showed a spectrum of appearances and were considered to be mobile, based on the presence of pseudopods. Occasionally a fibroblastic-like cell was found to contain cytolysosomes (Figure 14). Additionally, multinucleated giant cells were seen with myofilaments having dense bodies (Figure 15).

A loosely anchored confluent cell layer covered the plaques, from both the flexing and non-flexing portions of the diaphragm, separating the underlying tissue from circulating blood and forming an interface (Figure 16). These flatened cells formed a single layer, were underlined by an incomplete basal lamina, and had junctions characteristic of endothelial cells (Figure 17). Centrally located nuclei were often oriented toward the base of the cell. Varying amounts of peripheral chromatin nucleoli were present.

Organelles within the cytoplasm were sparse. The predominant organelle was a short profile of dilated rough endoplasmic reticulum. In addition, small clusters of polyribosomes, round to oval mitochondria, and fine filaments occupied the cytoplasm. Occasionally, bundles of myofilaments were located near the apical and basal sides of the endothelial cells. Pincytotic vesicles were present on both upper and lower sides of the cell, but were not prominent. In a few instances, isolated groups of endothelial cells were seen underlying the

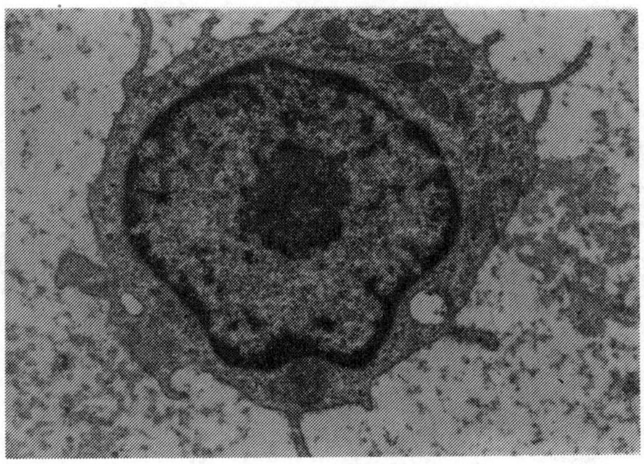

Figure 13a. Small cell from plaque, having no definite differentiation characteristics. (× 16000).

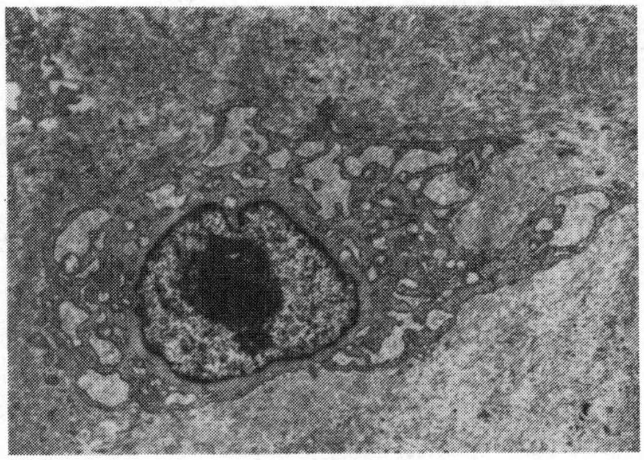

Figure 13b. Small cell showing some fibroblastic characteristics. (× 8000).

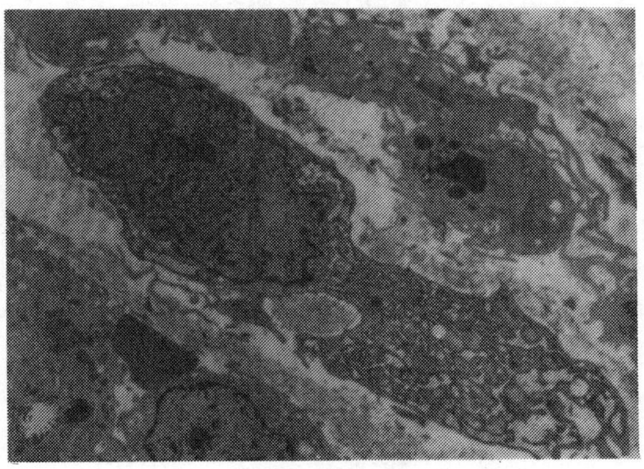

Figure 13c. Cell in the center appears to be a fibroblast. The surrounding cells are macrophages (× 5200).

external layer. These groups always occurred adjacent to the blood-contacting surface of the PNI. A discussion of these ultrastructural findings is presented on page 229. The predominant type of PNI from the flexing portion of the PNI was calcified and subsequently had to be decalcified prior to examination. The ultrastructure of these samples will be reviewed in the following section.

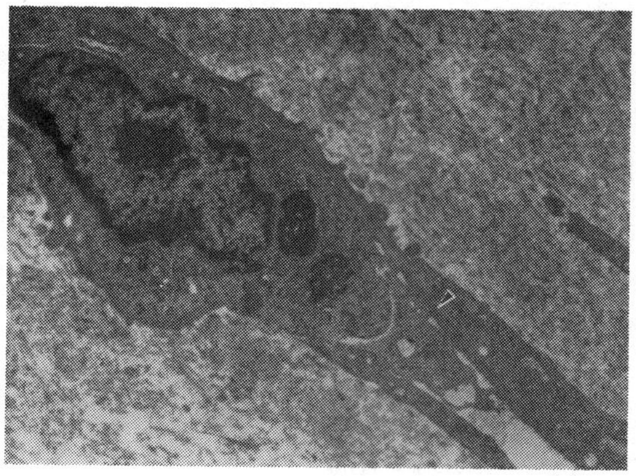

Figure 14. Transmission electron micrograph of a cell, that has some fibroblastic characteristics, but contains phagocytized material. The arrow indicates myofilaments in the adjacent cell. (× 8000).

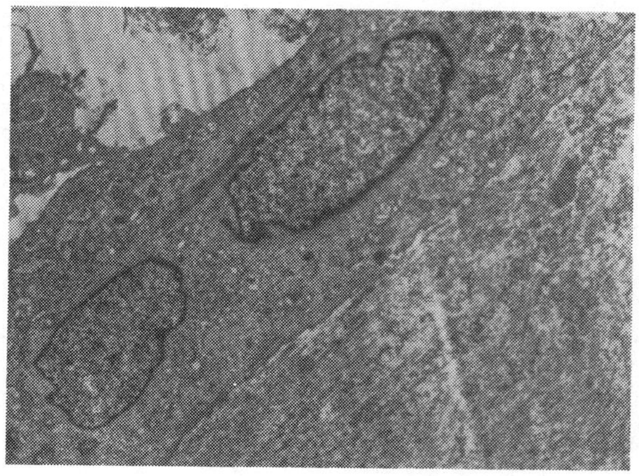

Figure 15. Myofilaments with dense bodies are shown within the cytoplasm of a multinucleated giant cell. (× 6000).

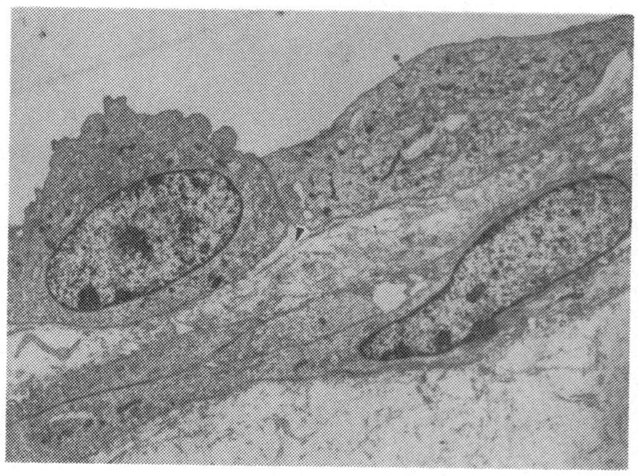

Figure 16. Portions of two endothelial cells overlying an internal cluster of the same cells. Arrow indicates basal lamina material. (× 7800).

PNI Calcification

With the advent of longer pumping durations, the problem of calcification and increased PNI thickness along the flexing periphery of the pump diaphragm has become more apparent. Figure 18 shows the flex pattern of the THI blood pump diaphragm and a PNI thickness map constructed following micrometer measurements and radiographic analyses. Although this portion of the blood-contacting surface comprises less than 15% of the total prosthetic interface,

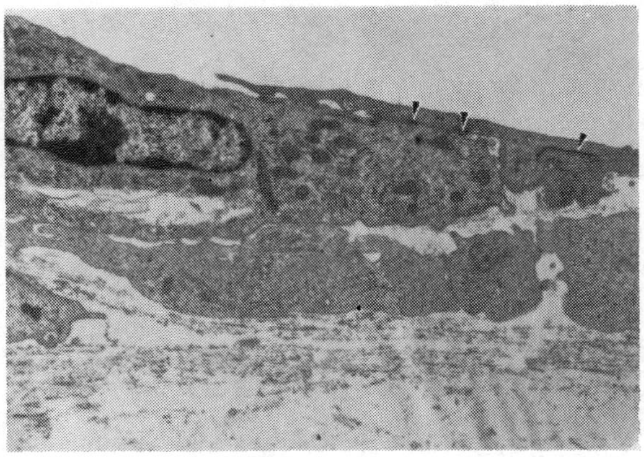

Figure 17. Endothelial layer showing cell junction (arrows. (× 10000).

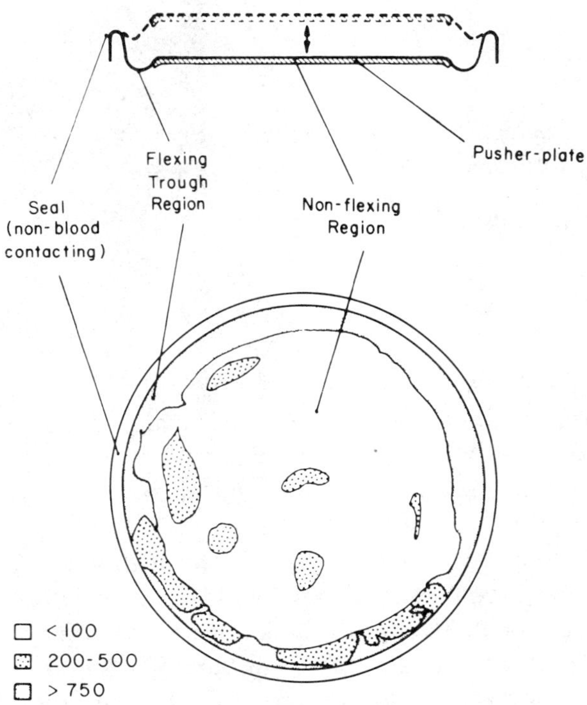

Figure 18. Illustration of the flex (roll) pattern of the THI blood pump diaphragm (upper) and a representative PNI thickness map, from a 108-day in-vivo evaluation. The flexing portion of the diaphragm is characterized by increased PNI thickness.

it continues to pose a potential problem in long-term studies. Based on our series of chronic THI blood pump implantations, several observations and conclusions concerning PNI calcification are noteworthy. On radiographic and histologic examination, PNI calcification occurred consistently at the flexing circumference of the pump diaphragm (Figures 19-20). In a few instances where smooth, adherent, connective tissue (fibrin and collagen) covered the flexing area,

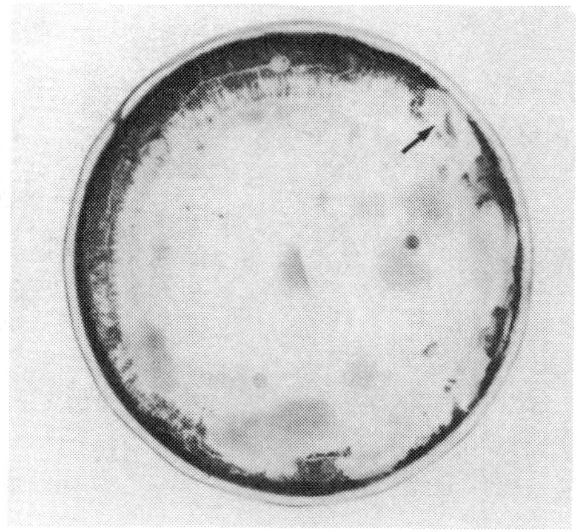

Figure 19. Xeroradiograph of a pump diaphragm following 108 days of electrical actuation in the anticoagulated calf. The darkened areas around the diaphragm periphery demonstrate PNI calcification. Along the top of the diaphragm, several cracks in the PNI lining are apparent; these cracks were limited to the biologic lining and did not involve the biomaterial. It is interesting to note, that only mild calcification is detectable in areas where collagenous plaque formation occurred (arrow).

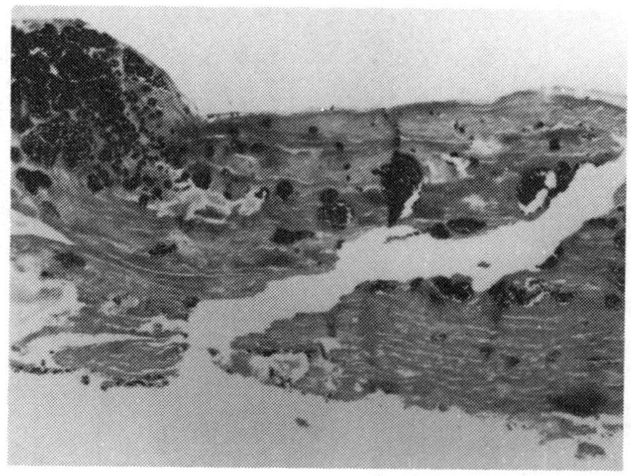

Figure 20. Photomicrograph of the calcified (darkened areas) PNI, from the flexing portion of the diaphragm.

calcification was minimal. It appears that the autogenous formation of a stable biologic lining precludes the occurrence of calcification. No calcification occurred on the rigid upper pump housing or on the pusher-plate backed (non-flexing) portion of the pump diaphragm. These findings implicate further the effects of mechanical tissue injury or flexure as major determinants of PNI calcification.

Light microscopic analyses indicated that PNI calcification was greatest when the thickness of the biologic layer exceeded 500 microns. In addition, calcific deposits were most predominant in the basal layers of the PNI at the level of the Dacron fibrils. Inflammatory cells and platelet aggregates were observed primarily in the PNI from flexing regions.

Transmission electron microscopy indicated that the calcified samples were quite different from the plaque samples described previously in that no collagen was present. The framework of the PNI in these areas was composed of long fibrin strands. Cellular elements included numerous red cells, mononuclear cells from peripheral blood, and macrophages, which were often multi-nucleated (Figure 21). The macrophages showed extensive phagocytic activity. No organized endothelium was found overlying these tissue-calcified areas. The decalcified areas had the appearance of psammoma bodies and the nucleation site for calcification could not be identified.

Scanning electron microscopy revealed a well organized fibrin lattice on all non-flexing portions of the pump. In mechanically stressed regions, the fibrin strands were disrupted (Figure 22). The calcific nuclei appeared to originate from surfaces of the individual fibrin strands. The flex area was less thromboresistant as numerous red cells and platelets were present.

Figure 21. Multinucleated macrophage superimposed on Dacron fibril (asterisk). Red cells and a portion of fibrin strand are seen in the PNI from this area which is partially calcified. (× 9000).

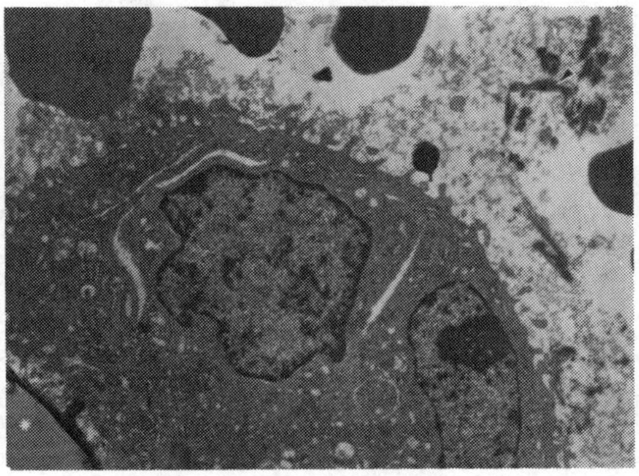

Figure 22. Scanning electron micrograph of the PNI from the flexing portion of an E-type diaphragm. The fibrin fibrils are disrupted and loosely organized. A platelet is present in the upper right corner of the micrograph. (× 8500).

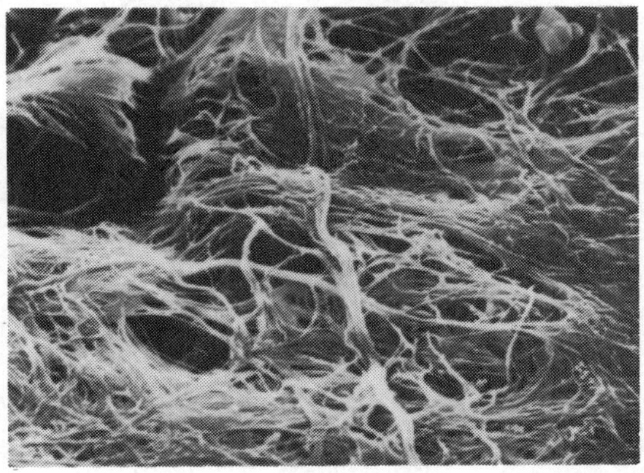

Examination of the calcific material with both transmission and scanning electron microscopy indicated that the deposits consisted of microcrystals which produced a powder diffraction pattern. X-ray spectral analyses indicated the presence of calcium and phosphorus. Calcium spectra were the strongest in intensity, indicating a higher concentration of this element. From reference data, the diffraction pattern and elemental composition of the deposits were consistent with calcium orthophosphate hydrate, $Ca_3(PO_4)_2 \cdot nH_2O$.

In a limited study comparing the pump diaphragms from non-anticoagulated calves after 79, 88 and 155-day durations with continuously anticoagulated (control) calves of 70, 95 and 150-day durations, no significant differences in PNI calcification were observed. Calcification was limited to the flexing periphery of both groups, although it occurred to a lesser degree in the control group.

In our series of studies, calcification was restricted to the biologic lining and did not involve the pumping diaphragm (except in the 393-day study); loss of compliance of the diaphragm was observed in only one instance. The degree of PNI calcification was variable in progression as there were no identifiable correlations in studies of $\leqslant$ 6 months duration (Table 2). Additionally, no significant differences in PNI composition, thickness, distribution, or calcification were noted with regard to synchronous versus asynchronous actuation modes.

Table 2. Summary of Calcification Analyses of the THI E-Type ALVAD.

Calf No.	Duration (Days)	Pumping Mode	Calcium Content Diaphragm Periphery
H-351	2	Async.	0
H-470	10	Sync.	0
H-500	11	Sync.	0
H-411	12	Async.	1+
H-454	14	Async.	0
H-437	25	Async.	1+
H-435	26	Sync.	4+
H-465	30	Async.	2+
H-415	32	Async.	3+
H-442	40	Async.	2+
H-453	44	Sync.	2+
H-490	44	Sync.	2+
H-439	45	Async.	1+
H-502	48	Sync.	2+
H-404	50	Async.	4+
H-468	70	Sync.	4+
*H-479	79	Sync.	3+
*H-480	88	Sync.	3+
H-452	95	Sync.	3+
H-492	108	Sync.	4+
H-462	112	Async.	3+
H-497	131	Sync.	3+
H-449	137	Async.	2+
H-440	150	Sync.	3+
*H-456	155	Sync.	4+
H-451	181	Sync.	1+
H-446	393	Async.	4++

* No postoperative anticoagulation.

DISCUSSION

The interpretation of data obtained from sequential pseudoneointimal analyses in experimental animals is difficult. It has been suggested that the hematological differences between experimental animals and man are so significant that valid scientific conclusions regarding blood compatibility of biomaterials cannot be made in experiments of this type [9]. Still, characterization of the PNI formed within chronically-implanted, textured blood pumps remains the best mechanism available for assessing the biocompatibility of blood-contacting materials.

The textured interface utilized in THI blood pump *in-vivo* evaluations was designed to promote the deposition of a controlled, adherent, biologically-derived PNI from the circulating blood. Until recently, preparation of these surfaces required the use of reactive adhesives to bond polyester fibers to underlying substrates. The long-term integrity of such a design has, however, been questioned [10].

While endurance testing conducted at Thermo Electron Corporation has demonstrated excellent integrity and adherence of the fibril matrix to the surface of the pump diaphragm, it is recognized that adhesively-bonded surfaces represent a potential failure mode. Consequently, alternative techniques of fabricating textured flexing and non-flexing blood-contacting surfaces have been developed. Encouraging results have been reported by Poirier and Szycher [11], and Whalen and Nosé [12] using powdered metal (PM) texturing for metal non-flexing pump components. Our initial results using powdered metal surfaces in a limited number of studies have shown excellent PNI adherence and integrity. Thus far, no deleterious effects attributable to the PM-textured surface have been noted.

A method of fabricating flexing pump diaphragms which eliminates the need for adhesives has been developed by Szycher [13]. The process involves production of a transfer mold which has been cast against a flocked master mandrel. The result is an integrally textured Biomer diaphragm. The use of both the PM surface and the integrally textured Biomer diaphragm overcomes the limitations associated with adhesively bonded flock texturing, with retention of the fundamental advantages of textured surfaces.

The positioning of a pumping interface and its accessory conduits within the circulatory system of a vertebrate animal creates an environment in which the intravascular fluid dynamics differ from those established by the normal evolutionary development of the animal. The normal physiologic interactions and adaptations of both formed blood elements and endothelial linings to shear forces and flow patterns are disturbed by the implantation of these devices. Ultrastructural analyses of the cellular reactions within these areas and at the pumping interface help elucidate adaptations in the organism to changes created by chronic circulatory assist.

The finding of plaques composed of cellular elements interspersed with collagen and covered by an endothelium was startling. It is tempting to suggest that these plaques are the *in-vivo* counterparts of *in-vitro* plaques established from hematopoetic cell cultures [14-20]. They also have an internal structure and cell composition similar to granulation tissue in which myofibroblasts are established [21-22]. These plaques also have the cellular progression of immature fibroblast-like cells to mature and degenerating myofibroblasts as seen in granulation tissue. Presently, the origin of the fibroblastic cell responsible for differentiating into myofibroblasts is proposed to be a multipotential cell present in blood or adventitia of small blood vessels, having ultrastructural characteristics similar to the cells observed in our evaluations [21] (Figure 13 a,b,c).

Numerous human pathological entities support the theory that such a cell exists. Myofibroblasts appear in the stroma of malignant neoplasms, quasineoplastic proliferative conditions and as a response to injury [23]. They are also found in aortic intimal thickenings, cirrhosis of the liver [21], and proliferative myositis and myositis ossificans in which calcification occurs [24]. In all of these instances, collagen production is associated with the occurrence of myofibroblasts and elastin is absent. This finding correlates well with the sections in our studies.

In the present study, fibrous plaques were separated from the circulating blood by a layer of cells having ultrastructural characteristics specific for endothelial cells [25]. The cells formed a continuous attenuated layer and rested on an underlying electron dense lamina. The organelles were sparce and pinocytotic vesicles were present on both sides of the cells. No Wiebel-Palade bodies, organelles specific for endothelial cells, were observed. Although these structures have been reported in bovine carotid endothelium [26], they are lacking in bovine aortic endothelial cells [27]. Endothelial cells are reported to migrate along the long axis of the aorta in response to injury [28], and to divide following toxic injury or mechanical desquamation [29]. However, there is no experimental model in which the movement of endothelium occurs across a barrier. The present study documents the finding of endothelium in sites remote from native endothelium.

In previous studies, we hypothesized that the intrinsic fibrinolytic system was responsible for the decrease in PNI thickness [6]. In other studies when endothelial cells were seeded on grafts treated with blood, the fibrin underlayer decreased and disappeared [30]. This was an effect of fibrinolysis produced by the seeded cells. In addition, clonal growth of bovine endothelial cells has been reported to increase in dishes coated with fibrin [31]. In this experimental setting, the cells had a high level of plasminogen activator and exhibited anchorage independent growth. Confluent cultures from bovine aortic endothelial cells exhibit "sprouting" [32], an infolding of small cell clusters. As shown in Figure 16, this was observed in our studies in the endothelium layer but was not observed in deeper areas of collagen and myofibroblasts.

These studies indicate that endothelialization may be possible in chronically-implanted blood pumps. Similarities of plaques and endothelium produced on the pumping surfaces to those reported in *in-vitro* studies is not surprising, since blood plasma supplies all the necessary nutrients and growth factors in infinite supply. Endothelialization in our studies appeared to be random in distribution usually covering less than 50% of the pumping diaphragm. Complete endothelialization may not be necessary, however, since the remaining portions of the pump are covered by a thin fibrin layer which appears to be sufficiently nonthrombogenic.

These ultrastructural studies in conjunction with histologic evaluations indicated that the textured surface utilized in the THI blood pump is a suitable blood interface for chronic mechanical circulatory support in the calf. Hemocompatibility was excellent as hematocrits, platelet counts, and plasma hemoglobins stabilized 24 hours post-implantation. The textured surface promoted a stable, adherent, thin PNI lining and has been shown to be thromboresistant. The 27 experimental studies described herein demonstrate a general trend in PNI accretion and maturation which can be summarized chronologically:

< 14 days – Fibrin and platelets completely cover all pumping surfaces. Infiltration of polymorphonuclear and mononuclear cells occurs within the fibrin matrix.

14-30 days – Continued deposition of fibrin and infiltration of polymorphonuclear cells along the upper portions of the PNI. Compaction of the fibrin matrix occurs, starting in the underlying acellular basilar layers. Disruption and calcification of the PNI begins at the flexing periphery of the diaphragm.

30-40 days – Continued compaction and subsequent thickness reduction of the fibrin matrix occurs. The leukocytes associated with the upper fibrin matrix decrease in number as the lining becomes generally acellular. Calcification along the flexing periphery continues.

40-60 days – Few changes within the acellular fibrin matrix occur; however, white plaques of fibrous tissue appear randomly distributed on the blood-contacting surfaces. These white areas are composed primarily of fibrin, collagen and fibroblasts. A loosely held confluent cell layer covers these plaques separating the underlying collagen matrix from circulating blood.

> 60 days – No significant changes occur within the thin (and now acellular) fibrin matrix. The white fibrous plaques increase in number and in area. These islands show a maturation of fibroblasts to myofibroblasts within a collagen matrix as well as an upper endothelial layer immediately in contact with the circulating blood.

Although these results are encouraging, a major concern regarding chronically implanted blood-pumps is the propensity for calcification to occur, particularly in mechanically flexed areas of the diaphragm. Depending on the degree of calcification one or more of the following may occur: 1) systemic embolization of calcific deposits; 2) perforation or abrasion of biosynthetic pumping surfaces; and 3) loss of compliance of flexing pump diaphragms resulting in compromised system performance. Although calcification has been reported on all surface types currently utilized in long-term *in-vivo* studies, controversy persists regarding its incidence, extent and etiology. Presented is a review and discussion regarding the nature and possible etiology of blood pump calcification.

General Mechanisms of Calcification

Pathologic calcification is a common reaction of tissue to injury. The process is initiated and perpetuated by a positive balance (and subsequent accumulation) of calcium and phosphate ions from the body fluids toward the affected tissue. When the accumulation is localized and no generalized abnormality in physiologic calcium metabolism exists, the calcification is termed dystrophic.

In dystrophic calcification, initiator complexes appear in extracellular substances upon tissue injury or death. Immediately afterwards, protein-calcium-phosphate complexes appear which form nucleation sites for calcification. This is followed by the formation of nucleation centers and secondary crystal growth of apatite at ion concentrations of normal extracellular fluid.

The mechanisms involved in the deposition of calcium salts under physiological conditions are still poorly understood. However in recent years, *in-vivo* evaluations of chronically implanted blood pumps in experimental animals have provided a means of studying calcification. A summary of factors which may induce, promote or contribute to calcification in chronically implanted blood pumps is presented in Table 3. A brief discussion of some of the factors is presented below.

Table 3. Factors Which May Promote, Induce or Contribute to Calcification In Chronically-Implanted Blood Pumps.

Factor	Relationship*	Reference
Flex (Mechanical Injury)	+	5,6,33,34,35,36,37
Thickness	+	5,6,33,35
Anticoagulation Regimen	+/-	39,40,41
Surface Imperfections/Defects	+	38,42,43
Species/Animal Model	+/-	33,37,42,43,44
Diffusion/Permeation	-	47
Pumping Duration	+/-	6
Pumping Mode (Async vs Sync)	-	6,33
Calcium Binding Proteins	+	45
Localized Lipid Absorption	+	42,46
Local Changes in Surface pH	+/-	42
Local Changes in Surface Temp.	+/-	42
Actuation (Pneumatic vs Electrical)	+/-	48

* + related
- unrelated
+/- possibly related or varying reports

Flex (Mechanical Injury)

Currently, the most accepted contributing factor to blood pump calcification is mechanical flexure of the biosynthetic pumping surfaces. As shown in Figure 19, the pump diaphragm of the THI blood pump is fixed to the housing at its outer diameter and to a pusher-plate located concentric with its center. The flexing portion of the diaphragm (the roll) spans the gap between the pusher-plate and outer diameter. As the pusher-plate translates axially, the shape of the roll must continuously change to accommodate the changing relationship between the inner and outer points of attachment. This is commonly referred to as diaphragm flexure. It occurs in all pusher-plate type assist devices, currently under development.

Our studies [6,33,35] and others [5,34,36,37,38] have shown that calcification is predominant in the flexing areas of the pump diaphragm (c.f., Figure 20). However, calcification has been minimal or absent in the rigid (non-flexing) upper housing and in the portions of the diaphragm that are backed by the pusher-plate. Whalen and associates [34] showed that calcification was induced in the PNI as a result of high cyclic strain which caused disruption and degeneration of the PNI lining. Microscopically, we have found that the PNI is firmly adhered to the flock fibrils in rigid (non-flexed) areas, but less adherent and poorly organized in flexing portions of the diaphragm. The unstable nature of the PNI in the flexing area is attributable to continuous fibril movement at the PNI/diaphragm interface. This particular phenomenon is unique to textured diaphragms, since smooth surfaces do not promote a PNI lining. Smooth surfaces do, however, calcify, although the cause appears to be related to cracks resulting from prolonged mechanical strain or fabrication defects [38,42,43]. Thrombus attaches at these sites and subsequently calcifies with time. Recently, Nosé and co-workers [5] have reported encouraging results using a biolized surface (gelatin). Except for small amounts of calcification associated with areas of detachment of the gelatin layer, no calcification was observed in the flexing portion of the diaphragm for periods up to four months. We have found that when an autogenous collagenous PNI matrix is formed on the flexing periphery of the diaphragm, calcification is minimal. To achieve a similar effect, Szycher and co-workers [4] are seeding pump diaphragms with allogenic fetal fibroblasts, in an effort to create a stable biologic lining. A stable lining on the flexible areas of the diaphragm may prevent or at least minimize calcification.

Thickness

Calcification due to increased PNI thickness applies only to textured surfaces. Our studies have shown that PNI calcification is increased in areas greater than 500 microns in thickness, except when collagen is present [6,33,34]. Since areas of increased PNI thickness occur predominantly in high flex regions of the diaphragm, it is difficult to assess which is more of a contributing factor to calcification. It is hypothesized, however, that a critical thickness is reached where complete washing of PNI is precluded, and, therefore, oxygen and substrate diffusion are inadequate. In a previous study, the earliest calcified lesion was seen in the deepest portion of the PNI [36]. A possible sequence of events occurring in the basilar PNI, as a consequence of mechanical injury, inadequate oxygen and substrate diffusion, is presented in Figure 23.

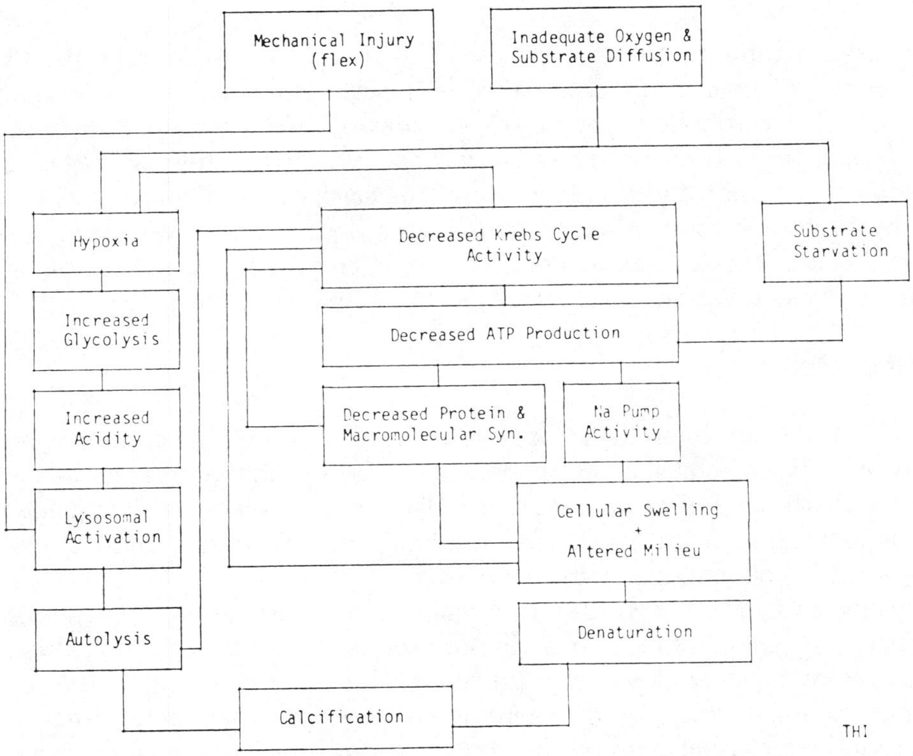

Figure 23. A possible sequence of events occurring in basilar PNI as a consequence of mechanical injury, inadequate oxygen, and substrate diffusion.

Anticoagulation Regimen

Early in our initial investigations utilizing textured surfaces, we considered the effects (if any) of anticoagulation on PNI calcification. As described previously, we use a regimen of Coumadin, Persantine and Ascriptin to maintain the prothrombin time at 2 to 2½ times normal (30 to 45 seconds). In a limited number of studies, we have seen no significant differences in PNI calcification in anticoagulated and non-anticoagulated calves following pumping durations up to 150 days using textured diaphragms. Our studies do not conform to those of Pierce et al [39] which showed that anticoagulation with sodium warfarin (Coumadin) inhibited blood pump calcification, possibly by blocking the formation of λ-carboxyglutamic acid containing proteins. Since λ-carboxyglutamic acid (GLA) is a vitamin K dependent, Ca^{++} binding protein, it is postulated that vitamin K antagonism (via warfarin or its analogues) would result in inhibition of GLA synthesis, and, therefore, loss of calcium binding potential. It should be emphasized that in this study a smooth, collapsible diaphragm was used. Another group using a similar smooth pumping surface and flex pattern found no apparent relationship between the anticoagulation regimen and calcification [41]. It is unlikely that therapeutic levels of Coumadin given systematically for anticoagulation are sufficient to inhibit totally, the synthesis of GLA proteins. However, localized distribution or binding of the drug at biomaterial sites prone to calcification may have potential.

Surface Imperfections/Defects

The problem of surface defects as contributing factors to PNI calcification have been observed predominantly in smooth surfaces [38, 42, 43]. It has been reported that surface defects can occur on moving surfaces as a result of cyclic mechanical strain. Similarly, fabrication imperfections, microbubbles, and discontinuities of the diaphragm have a tendency to develop calcification. In both instances, calcification penetrates the diaphragm surface and may cause further abrasion and eventual failure. The calcification of these defects is probably preceded by thrombus formation and subsequent degeneration. We have seen surface defects associated with calcification in only one instance (393 days). In this case, it appeared that the surface defect was an effect of calcification rather than a cause.

Species/Animal Model

For a number of years, it has been suggested that blood pump calcification is enhanced in young, growing experimental animals (sheep, goats, calves) and that the problem may not be as severe in man. This hypothesis is based on 1) differences in serum calcium (and phosphate) levels in man and experimental animals, and 2) the propensity toward calcification (xenograft valves) observed in children, but not seen in adults.

In the first instance, it has been suggested that serum calcium levels are significantly higher in calves or growing animals than in man. In our experience, we have found calcium levels of Hereford calves to be very close to those reported in man (9.45 mg/100 ml in calves vs 8.5-10.5 mg/100 ml in man) [49]. There is, however, considerable variability among laboratories, and we have also found differences among various breeds of calves.

In the latter instance, studies have shown that children develop xenograph valve calcification more rapidly and to a greater extent than adults [50]. Thus, it has been suggested that the adult sheep or goat may be a viable alternative to the growing calf as an animal model for chronic blood pump studies. Recent reports of *in-vitro* evaluations have suggested that adult human sera as well as adult bovine and, to a lesser degree, sheep sera, may cause sera calcification of certain materials [43]. The same study showed calcification of a non-textured blood pump after 77 days in the adult sheep. Therefore, it appears that differences exist among man and experimental animals regarding calcium metabolism; however, this does not necessarily eliminate human sera from involvement in calcium phosphate deposition on biomaterials.

Water Diffusion/Permeation

To test the possibility that calcification is related to diffusion/permeation of water from the circulating blood into and through the pump diaphragm, a series of studies were conducted in our laboratories utilizing a modified pusher-plate [47]. The pusher-plate was fabricated with small perforations in the central portion to allow water diffusion/permeation to occur at non-flexing areas of the diaphragm. Histologic and radiographic analyses revealed no calcification of the diaphragm associated with the perforated areas. As in previous studies, calcification was limited to the flexing region of the diaphragm. From these studies, it appears that water diffusion/permeation does not contribute significantly to the etiology of PNI calcification.

Pumping Duration/Mode

In our series of chronic THI blood pump implantations, there has been considerable variability with regard to PNI calcification and pumping duration [6]. While it would seem that

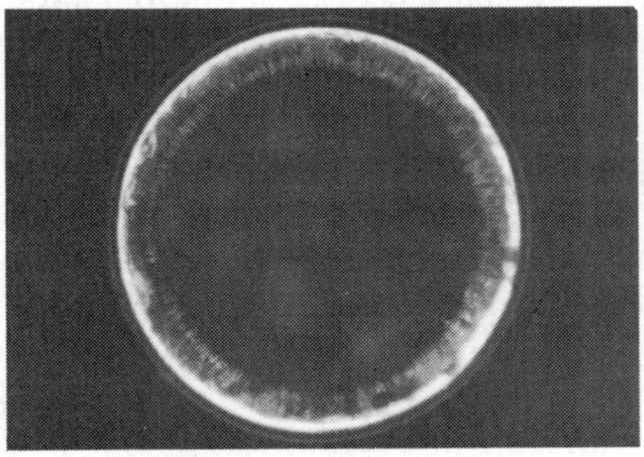

a. Radiograph of a THI E-type diaphragm following three months of electrical actuation in the calf. The diaphragm periphery is concentrated with radiopaque material.

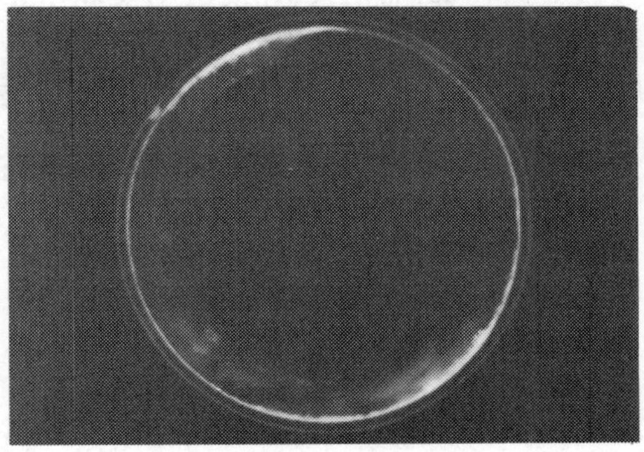

b. Radiograph of a THI E-type diaphragm, following six months of electrical actuation in the calf. Only trace amounts of radiopaque material are seen in the flexing periphery.

calcification should increase with time, we have found the progression of PNI calcification of textured surfaces to be variable in studies of $\leqslant$ 6 months duration. However, in our 393-day study, calcification was extensive. Figures 24a and 24b show a radiographic comparison of diaphragms explanted from calves following 3 and 6-month pumping durations. No infection or other disease processes were apparent in either case. Both animals were females approximately four months old at the time of implantation. The animals were anticoagulated with Coumadin and pumped synchronously. As shown in the figure, the 6-month diaphragm was significantly less calcified than the 3-month diaphragm. A possible explanation may be that the 6-month diaphragm embolized portions of its PNI/calcium matrix from the flex area. However, no symptoms related to embolization were observed during the implantation period, and post-mortem examination revealed no evidence of calcium emboli. (There is also the possibility of calcium resorption in the calf.) Table 2 compares the relative PNI calcification along the flex area following studies with durations from 2 to 39 days. Thus far, we have found no significant differences regarding pumping mode (EKG synchronous or asynchronous). Table 2 lists the pumping modes for the 27 THI blood pump implantations with associated calcification and pumping durations.

Localized Absorption and Binding

As described previously, the presence of the vitamin K dependent, calcium binding protein λ-carboxyglutamic acid (GLA) has been associated with calcium deposits (c.f., Anticoagulation). Lian and associates [45] have found GLA in both normal bone mineralization and pathologically calcified tissues. GLA has the specialized function of binding protein to promote protein-phospholipid interactions and has been isolated in calcified atherosclerotic plaques and calcified heart valves. Lian et al. have hypothesized that calcium binding proteins may play an important role in pathologic calcification, and, perhaps, pharmacologic intervention might inhibit the calcium process. Studies of this nature are continuing.

Additional hypotheses have been formulated by others, specifically, the role of lipids as precursors to diaphragm calcification. *In-vivo* and *in-vitro* studies of smooth and textured

LVAD diaphragms following bovine implantation, indicate the presence of calcium complexed long-chain fatty acids (LCFA) [42,46]. This group theorizes that precursor anchoring sites provided by sorbed biologic species facilitate and initiate calcification.

CONCLUSIONS

Taken together, our studies indicate that the textured surface used in the THI blood pump is a satisfactory blood interface for chronic mechanical circulatory support in the calf. A viable, adherent, thromboresistant PNI lining was formed on all blood-contacting surfaces and hemocompatibility was excellent. Calcification of the PNI lining occurred in the flexing portion of the pump diaphragm, but was greatly reduced when autologous plaque formation occurred in this area. This finding suggests that preoperative cell seeding or culturing to achieve fibrous plaque formation, especially in the flexing portion of the diaphragm, may help in limiting PNI calcification. Endothelialization occurred and was associated with the fibrous plaques. The finding of endothelium and fibroblasts in sites remote from native endothelium suggests that precursor or multipotential cells may exist in the circulating blood. The occurrence of intermediate cell types in the deeper PNI matrix, although a preliminary finding, also supports such a hypothesis.

ACKNOWLEDGEMENTS

The authors gratefully acknowledge the engineering and technical support of John Fuqua, Stephen Igo, Michael McGee, and Ruben Trono of the Texas Heart Institute; and Donald Dempsey, David Gernes, Victor Poirier, and Michael Szycher of Thermo Electron Corporation. Additionally, we would like to thank Karen Brandt, Marianne Kneipp, Evelyn Lawrence, and Rebecca Teaff for their editorial assistance in the preparation of this manuscript. Finally, special thanks goes to Ken Hoge for providing excellent photographic work.

REFERENCES

1. Pierce, W.S., Myers, J.L., Donachy, J.H., Rosenberg, G., Landis, D.L., Prophet, G.A., Snyder, A.J.: Approaches to the artificial heart. Surgery 90(2):137-148, 1981.
2. Kolff, W.J., Stellwag, F.: Blood at artificial organ surfaces: Progress to date as stepping stones for the future. Ann NY Acad Sci 283:443, 1977.
3. Oyer, P.E., Stinson, E.B., Portner, P.M., Ream, A.K., Shumway, N.E.: Development of a totally implantable, electrically-actuated left ventricular assist system. Am. J. Surg. 140:17, 1980.
4. Szycher, M., Poirier, V., Bernhard, W.F., Franzblau, C., Haudenschild, C.C., Toselli, P.: Integrally textured polymeric surfaces for permanently implantable cardiac assist devices. Trans. Am. Soc. Artif. Intern. Organs. 25:493-499, 1980.
5. Harasaki, H., Kambic, H., Whalen, R., Murray, J., Snow, J., Murabayashi, S., Hillegass, D., Ozawa, K., Kiraly, R., Nosé, Y.: Comparative study of flocked vs. biolized surface for long-term assist pumps. Trans. Am. Soc. Artif. Intern. Organs. 25:470-474, 1980.
6. Turner, S.A., Milton, L.T., Poirier, V.L., Norman, J.C.: Sequential studies of pseudoneointimae within long-term THI E-type ALVAD's: Thickness, calcification, and compositional analyses. Artif. Organs 5:18, 1981.
7. Szycher, M., Poirier, V., Keiser, J.: Selection of materials for ventricular assist pump development and fabrication. Trans. Am. Soc. Artif. Intern. Organs. 23:116, 1977.

8. Harasaki, H., Snow, J., Gerrity, R., Whalen, R., Ozawa, K., Kiraly, R., Nosé, Y.: Powdered metal surface for blood pumps. Trans. Am. Soc. Artif. Intern. Organs. 25:225, 1979.
9. Bruck, S.D.: Considerations of species-related hematological differences in the evaluation of biomaterials, Biomater. Med. Devices Artif. Organs. 5:97, 1977.
10. Olsen, D.B., Razecca, K., Jarvik, R., Kessler, R.T., Pons, L., Kolff, W.J.: Hemocompatibility of Polyurethanes for Heart Replacement. In, *Advances in Biomaterials,* Chichester, England, John Wiley and Sons (in press), 1981.
11. Keiser, J., Bernhard, W., Poirier, V., Gernes, D., Szycher, M., Robinson, W.: Development and Evaluation of Unilateral and Bilateral Cardiac Assist Devices. Annual Technical Report to NHLBI NO1-HV-4-2910-4, NTIS, Jan. 1978.
12. Whalen, R.L., Nose, Y.: Development of a Left Heart Assist Blood Pump. Annual Technical Report to NHLBI NO1-HV—7-2934-2, NTIS, June 1979.
13. Szycher, M., Bernhard, W.F., Franzblau, C., Haudenschild, C.C.: Integrally textured polymeric surfaces for cardiac assist devices: Artif. Organs. 4:210, 1980.
14. Van Slyck, E.J., Weiss, L., Dully, M.: Chromosomal evidence for the secondary role of fibroblastic proliferation in acute myelofibrosis. Blood 36:729-735, 1970.
15. Jacobson, R.J., Salo, A., Fialkow, P.J.: Agnogenic myeloid metaplasia: A clonal proliferation of hematopoietic stem cells with secondary myelofibrosis. Blood 51(2):189-194, 1978.
16. Friedenstein, A.J., Chailakhjan, R.K., Lalykina, K.S.: The development of fibroblast colonies in monolayer cultures of guinea-pig bone marrow and spleen cells. Cell Tissue Kinet 3:393-403, 1970.
17. Golde, D.W., Gocking, W.G., Quan, S.G., Sparkes, R.S., Gale, R.P: Origin of human bone marrow fibroblasts. Br. J. Haematol. 44:183-187, 1980.
18. Wilson, F.D., O'Grady, L., McNeill, C.J., Munn, S.L.: The formation of bone marrow derived fibroblastic plaques *in vitro:* Preliminary results contrasting these populations to CFU-C. Exp. Hematol. 2:343-354, 1974.
19. Greenberg, B.R., Wilson, F.D., Woo, L., Jenks, H.M.: Cytogenetics of fibroblastic colonies in PH^{1}-positive chronic myelogenous leukemia. Blood 51:1039-1044, 1978.
20. Hentel, J., Hirschhorn, K.: The origin of some bone marrow fibroblasts. Blood 38(1):81-86, 1971.
21. Ryan, G.B., Cliff, W.J., Gabbiani, G., Irle, C., Montandon, D., Stakov, P.R., Majno, G.: Myofibroblasts in human granulation tissue. Hum. Pathol. 5:55-67, 1974.
22. Gabbiani, G., Hirschel, B.J., Ryan, G.B.: Granulation tissue as a contractile organ. A study of structure and function. J. Exp. Med. 135:719-734, 1972.
23. Seemayer, T.A., Schurch, W., Lagace, R.: Myofibroblasts in human pathology. Hum. Pathol. 12(6): 491-492, 1981.
24. Gokel, J.M., Meister, P., Hubner, G.: Proliferative myositis. A case report with fine structural analysis. Virchows Arch (Pathol Anat) 367:345-352, 1975.
25. Mason, R.G., Mohammad, S.F., Saba, H.I., Chuang, G.Y.K., Lee, E.L., Balis, J.U.: Functions of endothelium. Pathol. Annu. 9:1-48, 1979.
26. Folkman, J., Haudenschild, C.: Angiogenesis *in vitro.* Nature 288:551-556, 1980.
27. Wechezak, A.R., Holbrook, D.A., Way, S.A., Mansfield, P.B.: Platelet adherence in endothelial cell cultures. Blood Vessels 16:35-42, 1979.
28. Schwartz, S.M., Haudenschild, C.C., Eddy, E.M.: Endothelial regeneration. Quantitative analysis of initial stages of endothelial regeneration in rat aortic intima. Lab Invest 38(5):568-579, 1978.
29. Sholley, M.M., Gimbrome, M.A. Jr., Cotran, R.S.: Cellular migration and replication in endothelial regeneration. A study using irradiated endothelial cultures. Lab Invest. 38(1):18-24, 1977.
30. Graham, L.M., Burkel, W.E., Ford, J.W., Vinter, D.W., Kahn, R.H., Stanley, J.C.: Immediate seeding of enzymatically derived endothelium in Dacron vascular grafts. Early experimental studies with autologous canine cells. Arch. Surg. 115:1289-1293, 1980.

31. Laug, W.E., Tokes, Z.A., Benedict, W.F., Sorgente, N.: Anchorage independent growth and plasminogen activator production by bovine endothelial cells. J. Cell. Biol. 84:281-293, 1980.
32. Cotta-Pereira, G., Sage, H., Bornstein, P., Ross, R., Schwartz, S.: Studies of morphologically atypical ("sprouting") cultures of bovine aortic endothelial cells. Growth characteristics and connective tissue protein synthesis. J. Cell. Physiol. 102:183-191, 1980.
33. Turner, S.A., Trono, R., Anderson, H.J., Ugorji, C.C., Norman, J.C.: Factors affecting pseudoneointimal (PNI) calcification in chronically implanted blood pumps. Abstracts, Am. Soc. Artif. Intern. Organs. 9:25, 1980.
34. Whalen, R.L., Snow, J.L., Harasaki, H., Nosé, Y.: Mechanical strain and calcification in blood pumps. Trans. Am. Soc. Artif. Intern. Organs. 26:487, 1980.
35. Turner, S.A., Trono, R., Milton, L.T., Norman, J.C.: Further observations on the etiology and effects of calcification within long-term (>2 year) implantable prosthetic blood pumps. Abstracts, Clin. Res. 28(4):716A, 1980.
36. Harasaki, H., Kiraly, R., Nosé, Y.: Calcification in blood pumps. Trans. Am. Soc. Artif. Intern. Organs. 25:305, 1979.
37. Harasaki, H., Murray, J.D., Whalen, R., Nose, Y.: Calcification at blood material interface. Abstracts, Am. Soc. Artif. Intern. Organs. 10:27, 1981.
38. Hennig, E., Keilbach, H., Bohme-Schmokel, D., Bucherl E.S.: Calcification of artificial heart valves and artificial hearts. Abstracts, Am. Soc. Artif. Intern. Organs. 10:27, 1981.
39. Pierce, W.S., Donachy, H.J., Rosenberg, R., Baier, R.: Calcification inside artificial hearts: Inhibition by warfarin sodium. Science 208:601, 1980.
40. Turner, S.A., Sterling, R., Fuhrman, T.M., Norman, J.C.: Necessity for anticoagulation in long-term LVAD's: Experimental studies with the THI E-type ALVAD. Abstracts, Am. Soc. Artif. Intern. Organs. 10:31, 1981.
41. Hastings, W.L., Aaron, J.L., Deneris, J., Kessler, T.R., Pons, A.B., Razecca, K., Olsen, D.B., Kolff, W.J.: A retrospective study of eight calves surviving five months on the pneumatic total artificial heart. Abstracts, Am. Soc. Artif. Intern. Organs. 10:5, 1981.
42. Coleman, D.L., Andrade, J.D., Kolff, W.J.: Calcification of long-term artificial heart implants. Abstracts Am. Soc. Artif. Intern. Organs. 8:23, 1979.
43. Coleman, D.L., Lim, D., Kessler, T., Andrade, J.D.: Calcification of non-textured implantable blood pumps. Abstracts, Am. Soc. Artif. Intern. Organs. 10:3, 1981.
44. Litwak, P., Hill, J.D., Rodvien, R., Robinson, J., Ward, R.S., Buck, K.E.: The goat: A model to meet changing needs in device evaluation. Abstracts, Am. Soc. Artif. Intern. Organs. 9:9, 1980.
45. Lian, J., Bernhard, W., Levy, R.J., Szycher, M.: Blood material interaction. Proc., National Heart, Lung and Blood Institute, Devices and Technology Branch Contractors' Meeting, 1980, p. 112.
46. Owen, D.R., Zone, R.: Analysis of a possible mechanism of surface calcification of biomedical elastomer. Abstracts, Am. Soc. Artif. Intern. Organs. 10:29, 1981.
47. Turner, S.A., Holub, D.A., Poirier, V.L., Fuqua, J.M., Norman, J.C.: Initial studies on calcification of the pseudoneointima formed within chronic blood pumps: Mechanical flex vs. diffusion/permeation of water. Abstracts, Clin. Res. 28(4):716A, 1980.
48. Milton, L.T., Fuqua, J.M., McGee, M.G., Norman, J.C.: Pseudoneointimal calcification in long-term THI E-type ALVAD's: Pneumatic vs. electrical actuation. Abstracts, Am. Soc. Artif. Intern. Organs. 10:22, 1981.
49. Wallach, J.: Interpretation of Diagnostic Tests (Second Edition). Little, Brown and Company, Boston, 1974, p. 8.
50. Kutsche, L.M., Oyer, P., Shumway, N.E., Baum, D.: An important complication of Hancock mitral valve replacement in children. Circulation 60 (Suppl I): 98, 1979.

Chapter 11

Carbons in Heart Valve Prostheses: Foundations and Clinical Performance

Frederick J. Schoen, M.D., Ph.D.
Pathologist, Brigham and Women's Hospital
Assistant Professor of Pathology
Harvard Medical School
75 Francis Street
Boston, MA 02115

ABSTRACT

Carbons are widely used clinically in prosthetic heart valves, as a result of their favorable mechanical and biological properties. Pyrolytic carbons, deposited in a fluidized bed, have high strength, and high fatigue and wear resistance. Compatibility with blood and soft tissue are good. After a brief summary of the materials science and biocompatibility of biomedical carbons, we review the clinical performance of substitute heart valves fabricated from these materials is reviewed. The success of carbon valves is considered within the context of the pathology associated with other previously and currently available prostheses.

INTRODUCTION

Exploration of the potential of carbon as a surgical implant biomaterial resulted during the 1960's from a convergence of medical studies of the resistance of materials to contact-induced blood clotting (thromboresistance) with engineering development of gas-impermeable and radiation-resistant coatings for nuclear reactor fuel particles. Serendipitously, electrically conductive graphite paint-coated specimens were found to be thromboresistant, even in experiments where an electrical charge was not applied. A collaboration then developed between the medical investigators under the direction of Dr. Vincent Gott, then at the University of Wisconsin, and the carbon group at General Atomic in San Diego, to study the interactions of pyrolytic carbon with blood and to relate thromboresistance to carbon structure and physical and chemical properties. The evolution of carbon development for medical application has been reviewed (Bokros et al., 1973; Bokros, 1977; Haubold et al., 1981) [1,2,3].

The primary clinical use of carbons has been in prosthetic heart valves. Nevertheless, carbons have been investigated for, and may someday find an important role in, a variety of cardiovascular, orthopedic, dental and soft tissue applications. It is estimated that, since clinical introduction in 1969, over 300,000 carbon heart valve components have been supplied for human implantation (Haubold et al., 1981) [3]. Carbons have been successful in this application due to their ability to allow fulfillment of the basic design principles for cardiac valve prostheses, as summarized in Table 1.

Table 1. Design Principles for Prosthetic Heart Valves

1. Little obstruction to forward blood flow when open (minimally stenotic) and close promptly and completely (minimally regurgitant).
2. Materials of construction must be easily fabricated, durable, non-thrombogenic, non-hemolytic and compatible with soft tissue.
3. Technically feasible to permit secure fixation in a physiologic location without deleterious local or systemic interactions.
4. Minimal discomfort to the patient including lack of noise.

The intent of this paper is to review the clinical status of carbon. Practically speaking, this is a review of LTI (low temperature isotropic) pyrolytic carbon in prosthetic heart valves. However, the utilization of carbon in any biomedical application is based on a unique combination of the ability to manipulate structure to give appropriate physical and chemical properties and tissue compatibility. Therefore, a discussion of the basic physical and biological properties of carbon is included to provide the foundation on which specific device development (heart valve prostheses and other) is based. The valve-related pathology of cardiac valve replacement is also discussed so that the success of carbon valves may be placed in the context of that of other previously and currently used prostheses. After the clinical results of specific configurations employing carbon are discussed, the possibilities of carbon application in other types of surgical implants are examined.

MATERIALS SCIENCE OF CARBONS

The properties of carbons are extremely structure-sensitive and the structure of carbonaceous materials may be closely controlled by meticulous attention to processing variables. In this section,the interrelationships among fabrication, structure and physical properties are summarized.

In nature, carbon occurs as organic molecules in living systems and as relatively amorphous coal, and as the two crystalline forms, diamond and graphite, in which the crystal lattice repeats over large distances. Carbon, however, may also exist in a spectrum of less crystalline structures. Poorly crystalline carbons may be prepared by 3 major processes: 1) by pyrolizing a gaseous hydrocarbon in a specialized furnace (the fluidized bed) leading to the low-temperature isotropic (LTI) pyrolytic carbons, 2) by pyrolizing a preformed polymeric body (vitreous or glassy carbon), or 3) by vacuum vapor deposition. LTI pyrolytic carbons have achieved widespread clinical use in large part because the structure and properties of these carbons may be carefully tailored and also because these carbons have the most favorable mechanical properties of any bulk configuration of carbon.

Fabrication and Structure of LTI Pyrolytic Carbons

A fluidized bed deposition system, shown schematically in Figure 1, allows the high-temperature decomposition of a hydrocarbon gas causing the deposition of carbon on the particles composing the bed. The particles are levitated by the incoming gas stream. Any other material which is placed in the bed and able to withstand the rigors of this process will also be coated. Hence, pyrolytic carbon is generally applied as a coating to heat-resistant substrates, such as graphite or refractory metals, preformed to the desired configuration. Figure 2 illustrates a cross-sectional photograph through a carbon heart valve ball. This illustration emphasizes that all pyrolytic carbon components of medical devices are composites of the substrate material and carbon. The coatings are usually approximately 1 mm thick. Control of the conditions of deposition (temperature, bed geometry, and the fluidizing gas composition and flow rate) leads to predictable and controllable structure (anistropy, density and crystal morphology) of the deposited carbon (Bokros, 1965; Kaae, 1971) [4,5]. The high flow rates required for fluidization of the bed are achieved by diluting the hydrocarbon gas with an inert carrier gas. The fluidized bed process also allows the introduction of other elements into the fluidizing gas and their co-deposition with carbon. For example, alloying with silicon is achieved by passage of the gas through methyltrichlorosilane (CH_3SiCl_3) (Kaae and Gulden, 1971) [6].

Although the as-coated surface of pyrolytic carbon is rough due to a mechanism of deposition which involves precipitation of carbon droplets from the gas phase, cardiovascular application generally requires a smooth surface; thus, most carbon device components are subjected to subsequent polishing procedures (Figure 3).

The bulk structure of pyrolytic carbon is best understood by comparing and contrasting it with that of graphite crystals (Figure 4). In graphite, the carbon atoms are linked together by strong covalent bonds to form large, planar, nearly-perfect hexagonal arrays. The layers are oriented specifically relative to each other so that there is a 3-dimensional order. Bonding between layers is predominantly of the van der Waals (weak) type and the well-known lubricating qualities of graphite depend on the ability of these layers to slide one upon the other. Because of the differential chemical bonding among the carbon atoms,the properties of the individual graphite crystallites are highly anisotropic; when these crystallites are large the overall structure has highly directional properties. In contrast, in the pyrolytic carbons,the layered planes are imperfect and contain vacant lattice-sites. As a result, there are cross-links

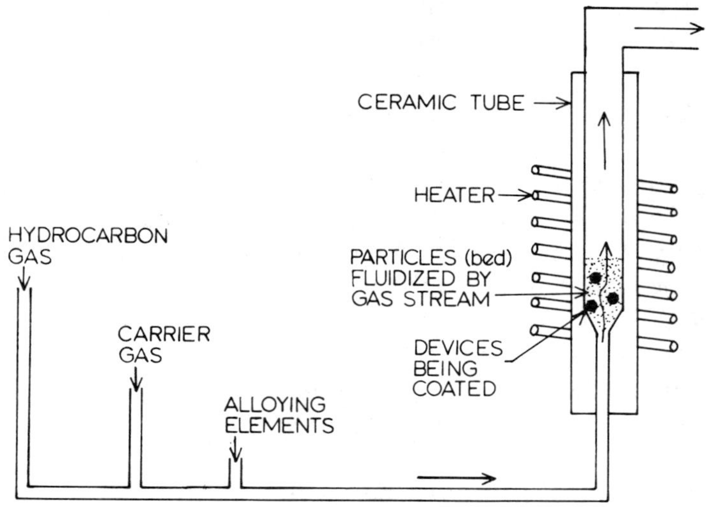

Figure 1. Schematic diagram describing fluidized bed coating process used to fabricate LTI pyrolytic carbon biomedical devices.

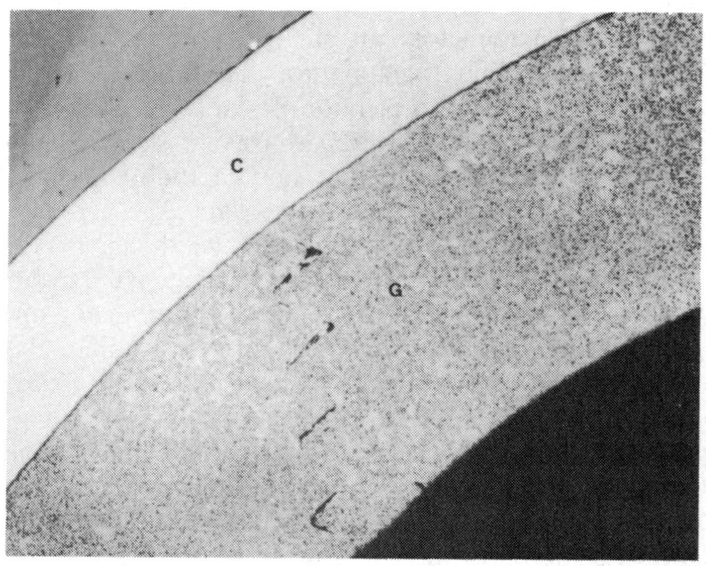

Figure 2. Cross-section of LTI carbon coating (C) on graphite substrate (G) in ball heart valve occluder configuration. The ball is hollow. (Courtesy of Carbomedics, Inc.).

among layers and the adjacent layers are not ordered with respect to one another. In general, the crystallites of pyrolytic carbon are very small (less than 50 Å) and randomly oriented in the bulk structure so that the aggregate is almost completely isotropic. The structure of pyrolytic carbons is often termed *turbostratic*. The properties of a particular carbon body depend on a) density, b) microstructure, c) crystallite size, d) degree of crystallite orientation, and e) presence of alloying elements (Bokros et al., 1973) [1].

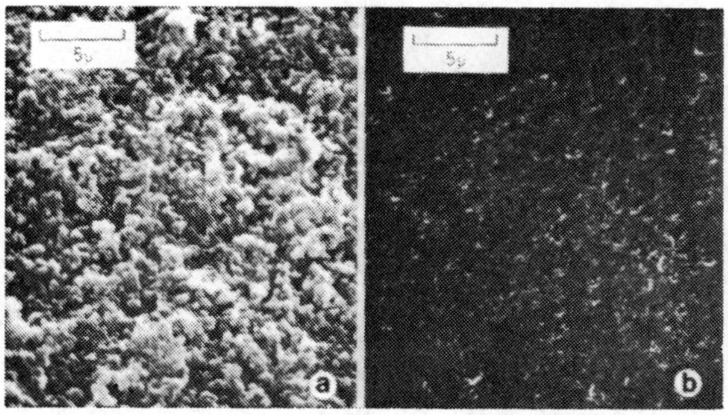

Figure 3. Scanning electron microscope photomicrographs of representative LTI carbon surfaces: A) As deposited (rough), B) Polished (smooth). (Courtesy of Carbomedics, Inc.).

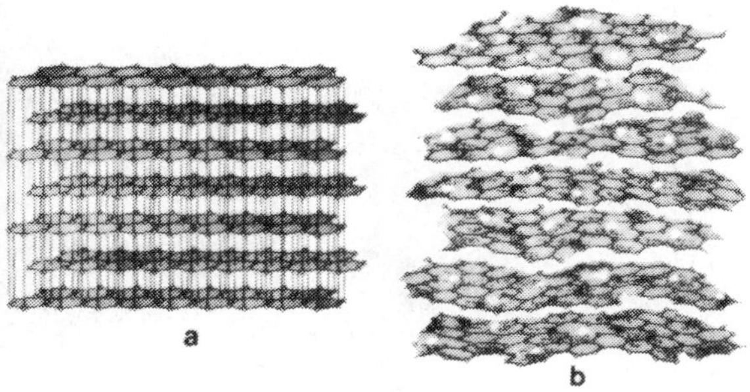

Figure 4. Structural comparison of graphite and LTI pyrolytic carbon. Note the three-dimensional order of the graphite crystal lattice (a) in comparison to the less crystalline (turbostratic) structure of pyrolytic carbon (b). [Reprinted from Ref. (1), Bokros et al., 1973, p. 106, courtesy of Marcel Dekker, Inc.].

Physical Properties of LTI Pyrolytic Carbon

The physical properties of importance for application in prosthetic heart valves and other surgical implant applications are fracture stress, toughness (energy to fracture), fatigue resistance and wear (abrasion) resistance.

Carbons have the unusual combination of high fracture strength with relatively low modulus of elasticity, as determined by Kaae (1971) [5]. The general configuration of the stress-strain curve for carbon as compared with those of other major materials classes is shown in Figure 5. The density-dependence of fracture strength is shown in Figure 6; the high fracture strength of LTI pyrolytic carbons is further enhanced by silicon alloying (Kaae, 1971; Kaae and Gulden, 1971) [5,6]. Values of 80-89,000 psi fracture stress and moduli of 2-3 million psi are typical for carbons prepared for heart valve components (which have a silicon concentration of 5-12%). Comparison of typical mechanical properties of LTI pyrolytic carbon with those of vitreous carbon and other types of carbon as shown in Table 2 indicates that the high strength and relatively low elastic modulus of LTI carbon results in a higher strain energy to fracture (toughness) than that for vitreous carbons (Kaae, 1972) [7].

Since heart valve prostheses must cycle approximately 40 million times per year without significant fatigue or abrasion damage, laboratory measures of materials durability are important. Studies of the fatigue resistance of pyrolytic (and vitreous) carbons indicated that the fatigue endurance limit was identical to the single cycle fracture stress, i.e., carbons do not fail in fatigue and unlike metals, polymers and some ceramics, progressive deterioration does not occur on cyclic loading (Schoen, 1973; Shim, 1974) [8,9]. This important property derives from the microstructure in that, unlike most crystalline solids, carbon does not contain mobile crystal lattice defects whose movement contributes to cumulative damage. Resistance to wear is greatest for the hardest carbon surfaces (strongest carbons) obtained through a combination of small crystallite sizes, high densities and silicon alloying (Shim and Schoen, 1974) [10]. Wear resistance of carbon-bearing-on-carbon systems is superior to that obtained with carbon-metal systems.

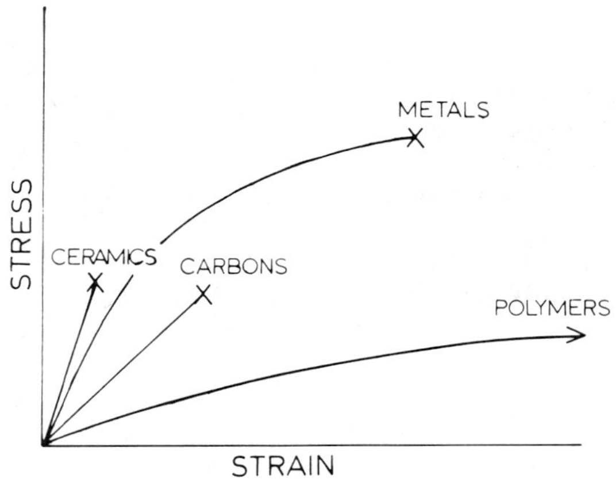

Figure 5. Comparison of stress-strain behavior of the major classes of materials. Carbons have a favorable combination of fracture stress and strain at fracture leading to a high toughness. (Reprinted from Schoen F. J.: Biomaterials. In Laskin, D. M.: Oral and Maxillofacial Surgery, Vol. 1. The biomedical and clinical basis for surgical practice, St. Louis, 1980, C. V. Mosby Co., p. 297, courtesy of C. V. Mosby Co.).

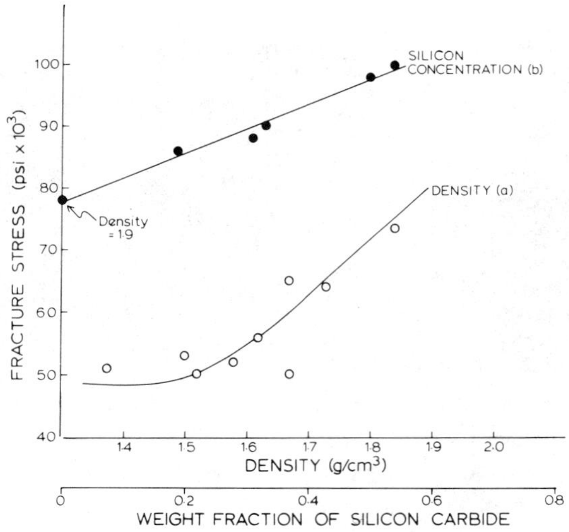

Figure 6. Fracture stress as a function of a) Density [data adapted from Ref. (5), Kaae: J. Nucl. Mat. 38:42, 1971] and b) Silicon concentration [data adapted from Ref. (6), Kaae and Gulden: J. Am. Ceram. Soc. 54:605, 1971].

Vitreous (Glassy) Carbons

Vitreous carbons are formed by the carbonization of thermosetting resins. A polymer precursor, preformed to the desired ultimate configuration, oversized according to a calculated degree of shrinkage, is pyrolized (baked) at a slow rate in a vacuum furnace, driving off volatile constituents and leaving a glassy-appearing carbonaceous residue. Such materials are characterized by a relatively low density (1.5 g/cm³) compared with that for the LTI pyrolytic carbons (usually 1.7-2.0 g/cm³). The purity obtainable is directly related to that of the precursor polymer, and structural defects may result from contaminants. While the fracture surface of LTI carbon is rough and reflects the nature of crack propagation around the droplets as the units of structure evident from Figure 3a, vitreous carbon has a smooth, concoidal fracture surface reflecting the ease of propagation of a crack through this material (Kaae, 1972) [7]. This leads to the relatively low strain energy to fracture (toughness) (Table 2).

Vacuum-Vapor Deposited Carbons

Fabrication or cost constraints may inhibit the use of LTI pyrolytic carbons under certain circumstances. For example, the relatively high temperatures required for fluidized bed deposition of LTI carbons prevents the use of this material as a coating for polymeric substrates for flexible prostheses (e.g., vascular grafts or catheters). Nevertheless, by using vacuum techniques, structurally analogous carbons may be deposited onto a substrate which is maintained at relatively low temperatures. The structures of such carbon coatings are highly variable and may be tailored to give structures which are amorphous or crystalline and granular or smooth.

Table 2. Representative Mechanical Properties of LTI, Glassy, and Vapor-Deposited Carbons*

Property	Glassy Carbon	Vapor-Deposited Carbon	LTI Carbon	LTI Carbon with Silicon (5-12%)
Density, g/cm^3	1.5	1.9	1.9	2.1
Crystallite size (L_c), Å	30	10	35	35
Flexural strength 1000 psi	20	80	70	85
Young's modulus, 10^6 psi	4.0	2.5	3.0	4.0
Strain to fracture, %	1.0	5.0	2.0	2.0
Fatigue limit/fracture strength	1.0	1.0	1.0	1.0
Strain energy to fracture, 100 psi	1	12	7	9

*Adapted from Bokros JC: Carbon biomedical devices. CARBON 15:355-371, 1977.

The coatings are generally very thin (0.5 to 1.0 microns) (Haubold et al., 1979) [11]. Nevertheless, some coatings may have properties equivalent to those of the LTI pyrolytic carbons (Table 2).

BIOCOMPATIBILITY OF CARBONS

The biocompatibility of carbons for cardiovascular application is considered below from 2 standpoints: blood/surface interaction and interfaces with solid tissue.

Blood/Surface Interaction

The delicate physiological balance between the fluidity of normally circulating blood and the initiation after vascular injury of powerful hemostatic mechanisms to avoid lethal hemorrhage is maintained by a complex interplay of factors which include intrinsic blood coagulability, flow dynamics and blood vessel endothelial surface reactivity. Alteration of any of these elements may shift the reaction toward either exuberant intravascular thrombosis on the one hand or uncontrollable hemorrhage on the other. Thrombosis in association with an implanted medical device is likewise a multifactorial problem involving blood biochemistry, flow and surface components. A heart valve substitute, for example, has a large, nonphysiological surface in contact with flowing blood. This in itself encourages thrombosis to some degree, since no artificial surface yet known approaches natural endothelium in its thromboresistance. With variable success, however, control of thrombosis complicating the use of blood-contacting prosthetic surfaces is effected by a combination of the use of relatively thromboresistant materials, manipulation of the reactivity of blood components by drugs, and the employment of valve designs which exploit the washing action of blood flow, and minimize turbulence, eddy currents and stagnation. Prevention of surface-induced thrombogenesis solely through manipulation of intrinsic plasma protein and platelet alterations with materials has not been satisfactorily achieved. Thus, the use of even relatively thromboresistant synthetic materials either in a poorly designed valve or in patients with normal coagulability may lead to disastrous thrombosis.

Although at present incompletely understood, the schema of interaction of blood and its components with nonphysiological surfaces may be described on a phenomenological basis (Baier, 1978) [12]. Experimental data indicate that under physiologically relevant hemodynamic conditions, the initial event (within a minute) occurring on exposure of foreign surfaces to rapidly flowing blood is the spontaneous adsorption of plasma proteins, especially fibrinogen. The formation of the adsorbed protein layer appears to be controlled primarily by the surface chemistry of the substrate and, to a lesser degree, by surface electrical charge and microscopic surface texture. By the time the protein film achieves a thickness of several hundred angstroms, *cellular thrombogenesis,* beginning with platelet adhesion to the first adsorbed plasma proteins, and subsequently *volumetric gelation* requiring the plasma coagulation factors, occur, potentially leading to the formation of a thrombus (a white thrombus, containing primarily fibrin and platelets such as generally forms in the arterial system). This is in contrast to *blood coagulation* which occurs in a slow- or non-flowing (or venous) system, involving almost completely volumetric gelation with large numbers of trapped erythrocytes (red thrombus).

Erythrocytes are probably late and relatively passive participants in the process of thrombus formation, although erythrocytes contain substances which, when released, enhance platelet adhesion and aggregation. There is recent evidence that blood leukocytes, formerly considered to be passive in surface-induced thrombogenesis, may play an active role in this process.

The blood compatibility of carbon has been investigated *in vitro,* and the early results were summarized by Bokros et al. (1973) [1]. More recently, Salzman et al. measured the adherence of platelets to carbon beads in a column on passage of platelet-rich plasma (Salzman et al., 1977) [13]. Adherence was high but release of platelet constituents was minimal. Treatment of the carbon with albumin led to both low retention and low release. This suggests a sort of conditioning or "passivation" of carbon to blood.

The classical canine superior vena cava ring implantation experiments of Gott demonstrated that smooth polished LTI pyrolytic carbons have excellent thromboresistance (Bokros et al., 1969) [14]. Implantation into the canine jugular vein produced similar favorable results. In general, the surfaces most compatible with blood *in vivo* are those of pure or silicon-alloyed LTI carbons that have been polished to remove the superficial roughness of the as-deposited state (Figure 3); the "rough" surfaces have impaired thromboresistance. Severe oxidation of the surface also reduced the thromboresistance in Gott's experiments, but pure or silicon-alloyed LTI carbons may be sterilized with ethylene oxide or steam without altering thromboresistance. Vacuum vapor-deposited carbons have also been shown to possess favorable thromboresistance in *ex vivo* flow models (Schultz et al., 1977) [15].

Why is carbon compatible with blood? Studies indicate that most surfaces compatible with blood have low surface energies (i.e., are hydrophobic). Carbon, despite its relatively high surface energy (50 dynes/cm, generally considered not thromboresistant) in the freshly prepared, clean, polished state, after exposure to blood for a short period of time, develops an altered surface that has a surface energy of 30 dynes/cm (considered to be in the thromboresistant range). Thus, contact with blood by some yet poorly understood mechanism alters the carbon surface toward compatibility, as measured by laboratory means. The view that blood compatible polymers must have low energy surfaces pre-implantation apparently does not apply in this case. Furthermore, chemical modifications of LTI carbon that markedly reduce thromboresistance (and soft tissue compatibility – to be discussed later) do not significantly alter the surface energy. This remains a puzzling issue.

Interactions with Solid Tissue

The initial result of placement of a biomaterial in solid tissue is *acute inflammation,* a physiologic response to injury. The histologic appearance of the acute inflammatory response is independent of the specific nature of the injurious agent (i.e., whether it is chemical, mechanical, circulatory, infectious). Nevertheless, the outcome of acute inflammation is in part dependent on the properties of the etiologic (causative) agent. The reaction may *resolve* if the noxious stimulus is removed and damaged tissue is regenerated (as in certain epithelia or bone); it may *repair* by scar formation if the damaged tissue cannot regenerate (as in muscle, nerve, or some types of connective tissue); or it may go on to *chronic inflammation* if the injurious agent persists. An intermediate level of reaction incorporating repair and chronic inflammation is *fibrous encapsulation.* This is the characteristic late reaction around a surgically implanted biomaterial (Coleman et al., 1974) [16]. In the most favorable case, the implant is surrounded by a thin, mostly avascular, layer of fibrous tissue (composed of collagen and fibroblasts, with a fine capillary network at its junction with normal tissue and minimal inflammatory cell infiltrate). The fibrous layer is in part caused by the surgery of implantation, and its thickness is in large part dependent on technique. The fibrous capsule serves to isolate the implant from the normal host tissues.

If tissue irritation and damage persist, a chronic inflammatory response ensues. In chronic inflammation, histologic examination reveals macrophages, lymphocytes, fibroblasts, collagen, and possibly necrotic tissue as well as other inflammatory cells. Chronic inflammation is characterized by the intensity of the reaction, type and number of inflammatory cells present, and the volume of tissue involved in the reaction.

The physical and chemical characteristics of the material are of primary importance in determining the relative degrees of repair and chronic inflammation. Composition, including the presence of contaminants or leachable toxic additives, and surface configuration must be ascertained. Fabrication history, especially that influencing degradation and corrosion behavior, may have a major effect on *in vivo* response. The physical form of the implant influences results; for example, sharp corners may induce substantially more response than flat surfaces (Wood, Kaminski, and Oglesby, 1970) [17]. The inflammatory capability of the recipient is also an important determinant of response.

Most of the published data on solid tissue response to carbon implants has been obtained during the investigation of carbon for orthopedic and dental prostheses. In general, the foreign body reaction is minimal.

We have investigated the soft tissue response to LTI pyrolytic and vacuum vapor deposited carbons in the rabbit paravertebral muscles (Schoen and Haubold, unpublished data). Implantation was by means of direct surgical incision of specimens 4 mm diameter × 40 mm length or the less traumatic percutaneous (through the skin) implantation of 1 mm diameter × 10 mm length specimens through 15 G needles (method of Autian, 1973) [18]. Tissue reaction was assessed at 10 days and 6 weeks in the latter experiments and at 6 weeks in the former. Some results are illustrated in Figure 7. The long term reactions using both models were qualitatively similar for implants of a specific carbon surface modification but the fibrous capsule was thicker after open surgical, than after percutaneous, implantation. Both smooth polished and as-deposited carbons were seen to be of equally low reactivity in this model (contrast to blood compatibility). Oxidized smooth polished carbons had a somewhat less favorable interaction with a substantially thicker and more cellular reaction despite the fact that the surface energies of these carbons were not substantially different from those of the pure polished LTI carbon (Schoen and Baier, unpublished observations). Vacuum vapor deposited carbons (coated on polyethylene substrates) were as nonreactive as polished LTI carbons.

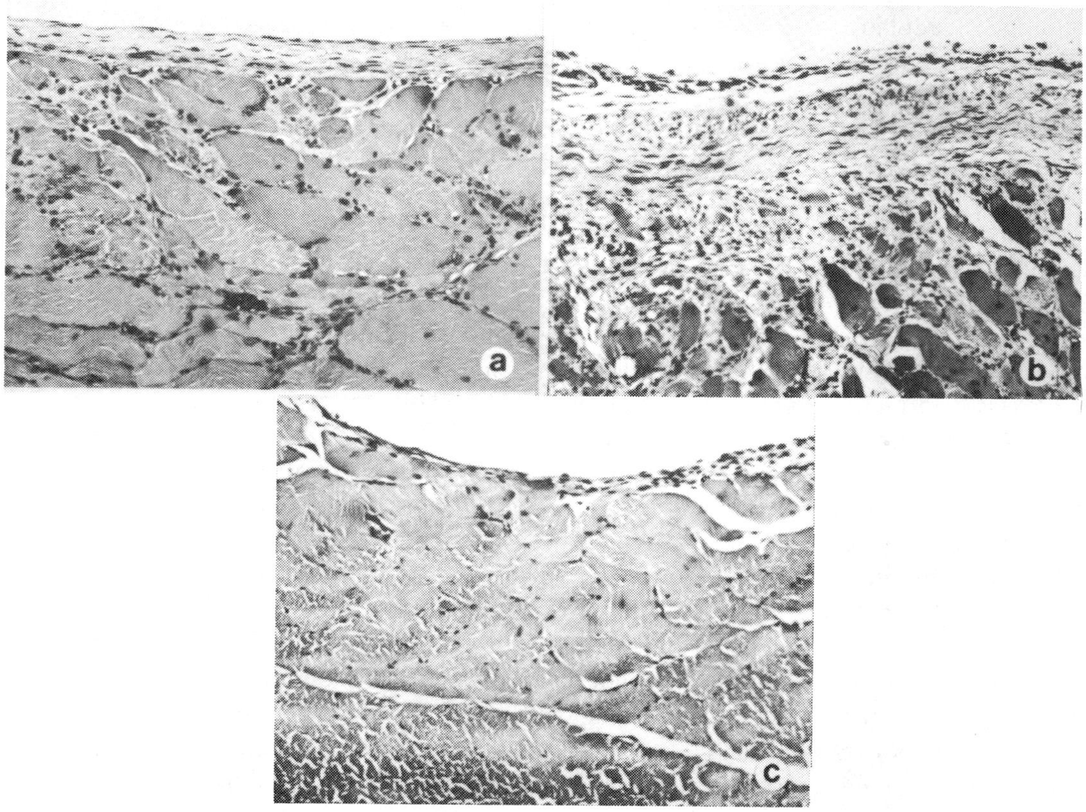

Figure 7. Photomicrographs of histologic appearance of experimental soft tissue reaction to carbons as assessed by implantation into rabbit paravertebral muscle. Six weeks duration. A) Smooth polished LTI carbon; open surgical implantation of cylinder, 40 mm in length × 4 mm diameter; B) Heavily oxidized LTI carbon; open surgical implantation of cylinder, 40 mm in length × 4 mm diameter; C) Smooth polished LTI carbon; percutaneous implantation through 15G needle of cylinder 10 mm in length × 1 mm diameter. Implant was at the top of each photo. Each section stained with hematoxylin and eosin; each magnification originally 168X.

CARBON HEART VALVE PROSTHESES

Pathology of Cardiac Valve Replacement

Cardiac valvular replacement has been widely available for almost 2 decades. It is estimated that over 700,000 individuals have received substitute heart valves and that approximately 40,000 such devices are currently implanted each year in the United States. Most patients so treated have benefited by enhanced functional capacity and prolonged survival. Surgical techniques and prosthetic design have undergone considerable evolution. Overall operative mortality is presently in the range of 5-10% at most institutions. Most early deaths are related to the poor condition of the heart with long-standing valvular disease or to surgical complications. In contrast, considerable late mortality (up to 50% of late deaths in some series) and morbidity are related to the prosthesis (Roberts et al., 1973; Schoen et al., 1981) [19,20].

Four major designs of cardiac valvular substitutes have been widely used. As shown in Figure 8, these are the caged-ball, caged-disk, tilting disk, and tissue valves (*bioprosthesis;* usually a tanned pig aortic valve mounted on a prosthetic stent).

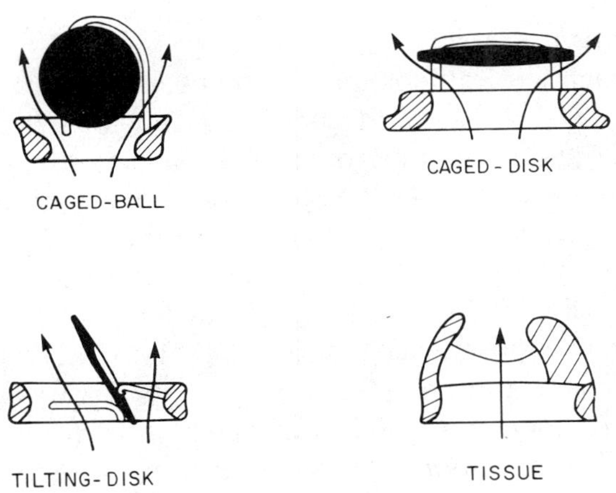

Figure 8. Schematic diagram of major available prosthetic cardiac valve configurations.

The most frequent clinically encountered complications of cardiac valve prostheses are listed in Table 3. The most frequent fatal valve-related complications in most clinical series are thromboembolic problems, with a representative incidence listed in Table 4. Thrombosis may lead to local occlusion of the prosthesis or to distant thromboemboli that may compromise blood flow to the heart, brain or kidneys. Valvular malfunction may result from a small thrombus or tissue fragment impairing movement of the occluder, or from materials degradation. Partial dehiscence (separation) of the suture line anchoring the valve occasionally occurs, leading to a paravalvular leak (regurgitation of blood around the prosthesis). Destruction of blood components on passage through the prosthesis, especially a degraded valve, or around the device when there is a paravalvular leak, leads to destruction of erythrocytes and may cause severe hemolytic anemia in some patients. Infective endocarditis (infection on the valve prosthesis) is a devastating and often fatal complication. The durability problems caused by materials degeneration which are encountered with some valve designs vary widely, as discussed below. In addition, all valves are to some extent intrinsically obstructive to forward flow. The significance of this feature in the extended outcome of patients with valve prostheses is not clear.

Each prosthesis configurational type is subject to the various complications listed above, but differences in materials of construction and in mechanisms of action of particular prostheses lead to marked differences in the frequency and nature of problems due to thrombogenesis, degradation, and hemodynamic abnormalities. Thromboemboli and durability considerations are both materials- and design-dependent, while valve hemodynamics and hemolysis are primarily design- rather than materials-dependent. The frequency and pathology of prosthetic valve endocarditis, on the other hand, are almost independent of

Table 3. Major Prosthesis-Related Complications

Obstruction
Dehiscence
Hemolysis
Thrombosis
Thromboemboli
Endocarditis
Degradation

Table 4. Thromboembolic Risk with Heart Valve Prostheses

	Starr Edwards (Non-Cloth-Covered Ball Valve)	Bjork-Shiley (Tilting Disk)	Porcine Heterograft (Tissue Prosthesis)
Mitral			
Local thrombosis	0.8*	2.4	0
Thromboembolism	5.8	4.8	5.2
Aortic			
Local thrombosis	0	0.7	0
Thromboembolism	5.0	2.2	2.0

Representative data adapted from Macmanus et al: J. Thorac. Cardiovasc. Surg. 76:788, 1978.
*Events per 100 pt. years.

specific valve materials and design considerations.

The history of durability problems, in particular, illustratrates the constraints involved. For example, the silicone ball occluder in early models of the Starr-Edwards and Smeloff-Cutter caged-ball prostheses was subject to lipid infiltration and subsequent ball variance, which often led to acute valvular malfunction and death. Of the 47 long-term survivors of aortic valve replacement at the University of Oregon between mid-1963 and mid-1964, ball variance was documented in 30 (64%) by 1970 (Hylen, 1971) [21]. At the National Institutes of Health, 11 of the 12 (92%) deaths in patients surviving more than 2 years after aortic valve replacement with early Starr-Edwards prostheses were caused by ball variance (Roberts and Morrow, 1968) [22]. Changes in polymer fabrication have eliminated this complication.

Cloth-covered caged-ball valves with metal poppets (designed to eliminate poppet wear and thromboembolism) suffer problems related to cloth wear by abrasion from the metal poppet and consequent hemolysis. In one series, 5 (2.5%) of 204 patients with cloth-covered metal ball Starr-Edwards prostheses were re-operated for consequences of cloth wear (Shah et al., 1978) [23]. Symptomatic embolism of the cloth covering the cage struts may be a secondary problem. A recently introduced modification of the cloth-covered ball valve prosthesis incorporates a metal track designed to eliminate direct contact of the metal ball with the cloth-covered cage (Macmanus et al., 1980) [24]; the long-term fate of this prosthesis is yet uncertain.

Wear of the caged disk valves has also been significant. Abrasion in this design is concentrated at critical points of the disk and struts. When extensive material loss occurs disk motion may become irregular. When 13 early Beall valves (Teflon disk and Teflon strut coating) implanted for periods greater than 29 months were recovered and analyzed at the University of Toronto, 12 (92%) had notching of the disk and focally complete denudation of the plastic coating on the struts (Silver and Wilson, 1977) [25]. Figure 9 illustrates wear on a Teflon Beall valve after 4 years implantation and also shows fragments of polymer in the heart muscle in such a patient with disk wear.

Tilting disk valves in general have had a good record with regard to durability (Roberts and Hammer, 1976) [26]. When tilting disk designs allow for disk rotation and minimal stress (e.g.,

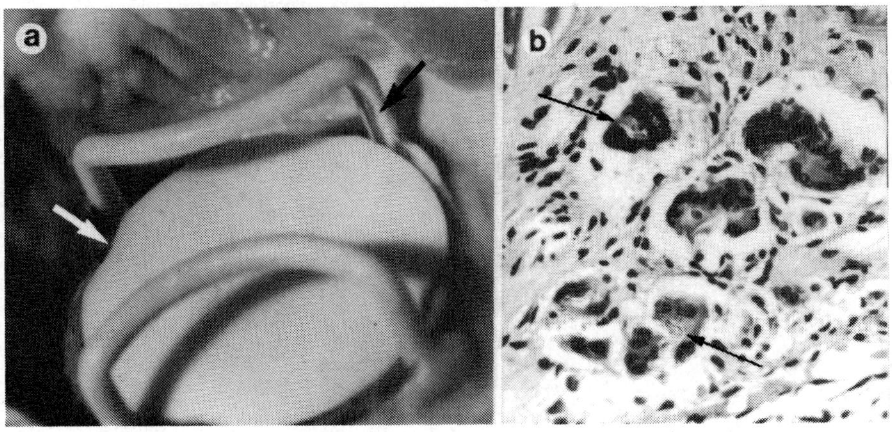

Figure 9. Disk variance: A) Gross photograph of Teflon Beall mitral valve prosthesis implanted for 4 years. Note notching of disk (white arrows) and focal denudation of polymer coating on cage strut (black arrow); B) Photomicrograph of heart section with embolized polymer fragments (arrows) eliciting foreign body giant cell reaction. Hematoxyln and eosin, originally 300×.

the Bjork-Shiley and Lillehei-Kaster valve prostheses) progressive mechanical failure is unlikely. However, designs which do not allow for disk rotation (e.g., the Wada-Cutter valve) may permit localized wear and its consequences, if sufficiently wear-resistant materials are not used.

The major valve prostheses used at the time of this writing are ball valve prostheses, especially the Starr-Edwards bare cage, silicone ball type, LTI pyrolytic carbon occluder tilting-disk prostheses, especially the Bjork-Shiley prosthesis, and the bioprostheses, especially the porcine glutaraldehyde-treated xenograft aortic valve.

For all mechanical valve prostheses lifetime anticoagulation is necessary to minimize the risk of thromboembolic complications. Violation of this principle may lead to complete thrombotic occlusion of a valve prosthesis, usually fatal, as shown in Figure 10. Nevertheless, anticoagulation therapy itself imposes a significant risk of hemorrhage that should not be underestimated. Bioprostheses have the important advantage that chronic anticoagulant therapy is not required except in patients with specific thromboembolic predisposition. However, degradation of bioprostheses after several years' implantation is now frequently encountered (Angell and Angell, 1980) [27]. Figure 11 illustrates the appearance of a bioprosthesis which has become calcified and developed a cuspal tear. Thus, although the potential for catastrophic failure of mechanical valves is well-documented, because of the uncertain durability of bioprostheses, the use of mechanical valves is indicated in many patients. Certainly, current interest in further development of mechanical valves is highly warranted.

Clinical Performance of Carbon-Containing Prostheses

This section summarizes the clinical results obtained with heart valve prostheses utilizing carbon components. Only those prostheses with reported data are included.

DeBakey Surgitool

The DeBakey Surgitool prosthesis is a caged-ball valve which has a silicon alloyed LTI

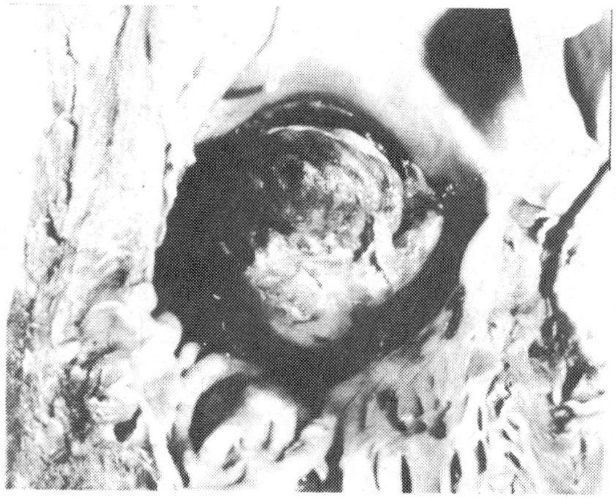

Figure 10. Gross photograph of outflow aspect of mitral valve prosthesis with sudden fatal complete thrombotic occlusion.

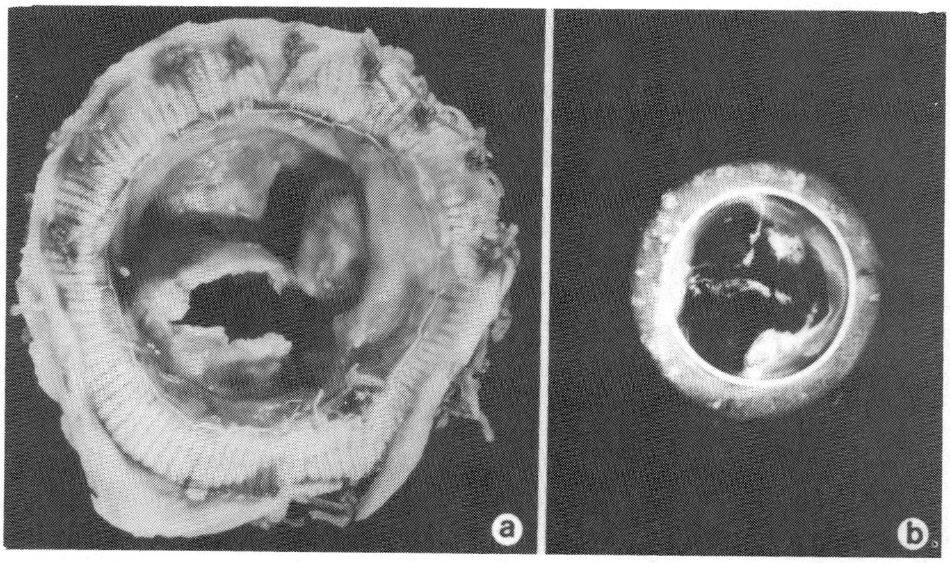

Figure 11. Failure of porcine heterograft bioprosthesis after 74 mos. A) Gross photograph showing cuspal tear; B) Radiograph of specimen in A) in identical orientation illustrating extensive calcification of cusps.

pyrolytic carbon poppet (Figure 12) with a bare titanium cage and a pyrolytic carbon orifice.

This valve prosthesis was never widely used. Two papers have reported series of 37 and 24 patients with DeBakey aortic prostheses (Scott et al., 1976; Paton and Pine, 1976) [28,29]. The thromboembolic rate was 3 and 6% per patient year, comparable to that of similar designs (see Table 4). There is no objective data on the DeBakey-Surgitool mitral (disk) prosthesis. These prostheses are no longer available (G. Carter, Medical Engineering, personal communication, 1981).

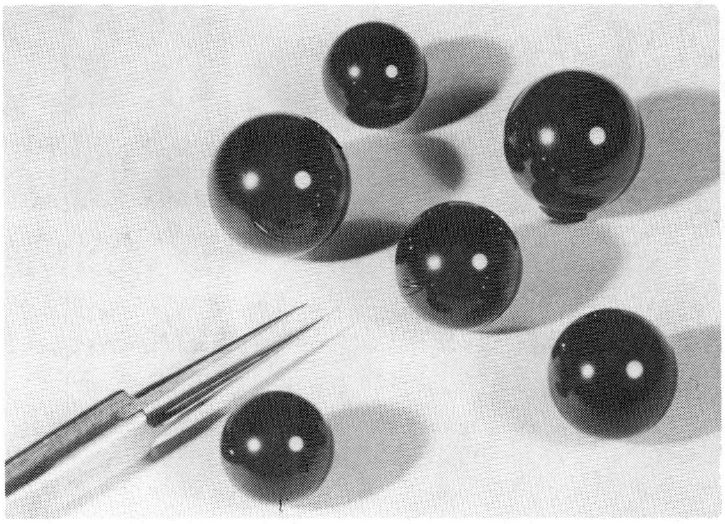

Figure 12. Carbon-coated ball occluders for DeBakey-Surgitool aortic valve prostheses. A cross-section of a representative ball is illustrated in Figure 2. (Courtesy of Carbomedics, Inc.).

Beall-Surgitool

The Model 105 Beall Surgitool mitral valve prosthesis with carbon disk and carbon-coated struts (Figure 13) was introduced in June, 1971 in an effort to eliminate the durability problems associated with the previous Teflon models (Models 103 and 104 – recall Figure 9). Strut fracture, both before and after implantation, was an early problem, but partial redesign (Model 106) and packaging alterations have eliminated this difficulty. Fernandez et al. (1976) [30] followed 100 patients receiving the Model 105 and 109 patients with the Model 104. Of 20 late deaths, 2 were due to thrombosis of the valve and 7 died of thromboemboli. However, it is not clear from that study which valve models were associated with the complications. Beall et al. (1973) [31] reported 4 thromboembolic complications in 175 patients receiving the Model 105 prosthesis.

The pyrolytic carbon Beall valve has not exhibited clinically significant progressive wear problems to date. We have had the opportunity to examine by scanning electron microscopy the bearing surfaces of the struts of 2 carbon Beall prostheses recovered after 4 and 7 years' clinical implantation (Schoen et al., 1981) [32]. The wear marking of a representative carbon strut from the valve implanted for 4 years is shown in Figure 14, compared with that of a Teflon Model 104 strut from a valve implanted for 34 days only. The wear of the plastic valve is far greater despite the fact that the duration of implantation is only a fraction of that of the carbon valve.

Cooley-Cutter

The early Cooley-Cutter caged-disk mitral valve prosthesis had a pyrolytic carbon disk and a set of titanium struts in each of the inflow and outflow areas (Wukasch et al., 1975) [33]. When the valve was open the occluder was restrained by the outflow cage; when it was

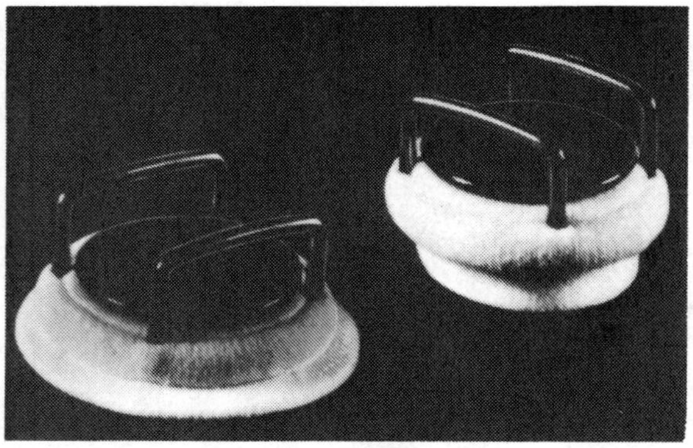

Figure 13. Beall-Surgitool mitral valve prostheses. Both regular (left) and "turtle-neck" sewing rings are shown. The "turtle-neck" configuration enhances fixation of the valve in the mitral annulus in some patients with distorted anatomy. (Courtesy of Medical Engineering Corp.).

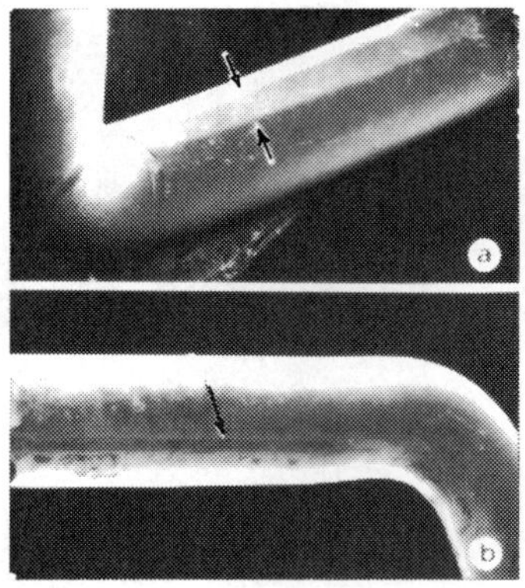

Figure 14. Comparison of wear on cage struts of Teflon and carbon Beall valves. A) Teflon model implanted for 34 days. Note the readily apparent wear track between the arrows; B) LTI carbon model implanted for 48 months. Note the superficial burnish (arrow). Magnification approximately 9X.

closed, the occluder rested against the cage in the inflow region,with its equator at the midpoint of the prosthetic annulus. With this design, the flow area in the open position equals the cross-sectional area of the occluder and the occluder used thus may be smaller than that of other disk valves with an equivalent orifice. Thus, resistance to forward flow is lessened. This full-flow orifice concept was originally adapted from the Smeloff-Cutter caged ball valve design. In 1975, a device incorporating a biconical carbon occluder in both aortic and mitral configurations was made generally available.

Although there have been no reported long-term studies of the Cooley-Cutter valves, preliminary results from Cooley's group (Wukasch et al., 1977) [34] indicated that the embolic rate was of the order of 7 to 8% per patient year (estimated) for both mitral and aortic prostheses. The valve is no longer available (Cutter Inc., personal communication, 1981).

Bjork-Shiley

The Bjork-Shiley valve consists of a stellite (cobalt-chromium alloy) cage with a disk which pivots around an eccentric axis in the plane of the valve orifice (Figure 15). The disk opening angle is 60° to the orifice plane. The disk, originally fabricated of Delrin, was later changed to pyrolytic carbon because of Delrin's propensity to absorb moisture and swell. The Bjork-Shiley prosthesis has been especially useful in those patients with a small aortic root but able to tolerate anticoagulation.

In general, the rate of peripheral emboli in the Bjork-Shiley mitral and aortic prostheses in anticoagulated patients is comparable to or lower than that of other contemporary aortic and mitral valve prostheses. Bjork and Henze (1979) [35] reported a rate of 4.2% per patient year with the pyrolytic carbon mitral prosthesis and 0.7% with the aortic. A recent analysis by Karp et al. (1981) [36] indicated an incidence of thromboembolism at least as favorable as that with other devices.

However, lightweight tilting-disk prostheses are particularly vulnerable to the conse-

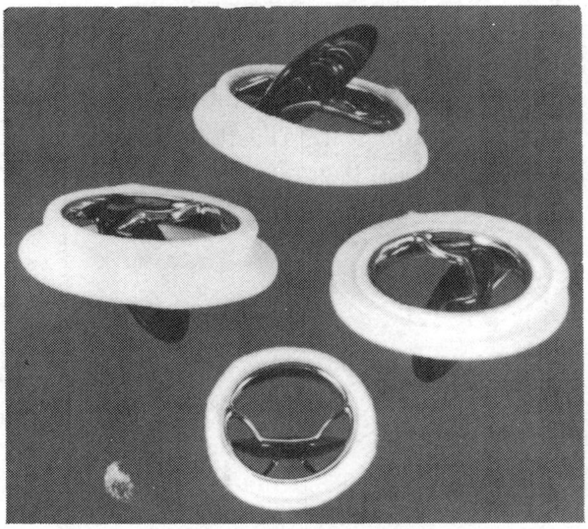

Figure 15. Bjork-Shiley prosthesis. Contemporary carbon design with modifications introduced to improve resistance to thrombotic occlusion. (Courtesy of Shiley Corp.).

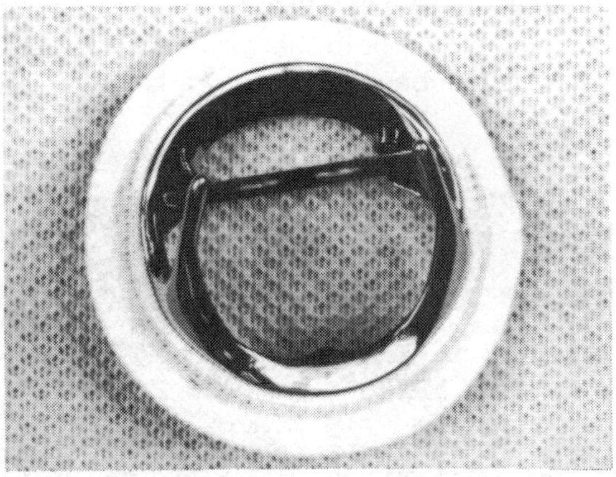

Figure 16. Lillehei-Kaster prosthesis.

quences of accumulation of minimal amounts of thrombotic material on the bare metal of the orifice and superstructure (Yoganathan et al., 1978; Karp et al., 1981) [37,36]. More than 100 cases of thrombosis have been reported with the early models; these cases comprise both mitral and aortic replacements in patients both with and without clinically adequate anticoagulation. This complication apparently relates to the design configuration of the prosthesis in which there exists an area of stasis at the outflow side of the disk edge at the minor orifice (Yoganathan et al., 1978) [37]. In an effort to circumvent this difficulty, the design has recently been revised (Bjork and Henze, 1979) [35] (Figure 15). No data has been reported as yet with the improved design.

Although strut fracture and subsequent disk embolization have occurred, such cases are rare and the overall durability characteristics have been excellent. Silver (1980) [38] examined 13 carbon Bjork-Shiley prostheses implanted for durations of up to 27 months. The minimal degree of wear observed would be unlikely to cause clinical dysfunction, even projected to very long times.

Lillehei-Kaster

The Lillehei-Kaster valve consists of a pivoting disk suspended in a titanium housing (Figure 16). The disk surfaces are completely flat. The outflow edge is guided in its pivoting arc by 2 metal projections extending from the valve ring. The disk is designed to open to an 80° angle relative to the plane of the valve orifice. However, angiographic studies have suggested that in the clinical situation the valve only opens to approximately 60° (Nitter-Hauge et al., 1971a) [39]. This valve originally underwent considerable *in vitro* and animal testing which indicated that wear rates, hemodynamics and level of hemolysis were favorable (Kaster et al., 1970) [40]. Lillehei (1977) [41] has summarized the early clinical results, including analysis of recovered clinical valves which have demonstrated a very low wear rate. As with the Bjork-

Shiley valve, acute catastrophic thrombotic occlusion may occur with the Lillehei-Kaster valve, despite anticoagulation.

A modified pivoting disk prosthesis has recently been developed, the Lillehei-Medical (Omniscience) valve in which the titanium components have been made smaller. In a further advanced design, both the valve occluder and body are fabricated from LTI carbon,and the sewing ring has been coated by a layer of vapor-deposited carbon (Figure 17). No data are yet available with either prosthesis.

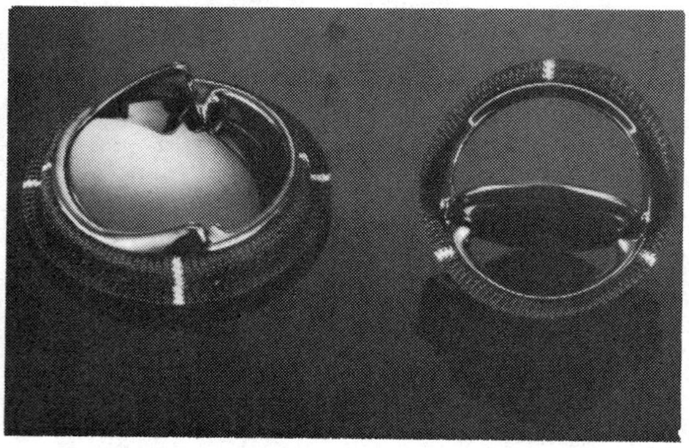

Figure 17. Omnicarbon prosthesis. In this tilting-disk prosthesis, all blood-contacting surfaces are carbon-coated. (Courtesy of Medical Incorporated.

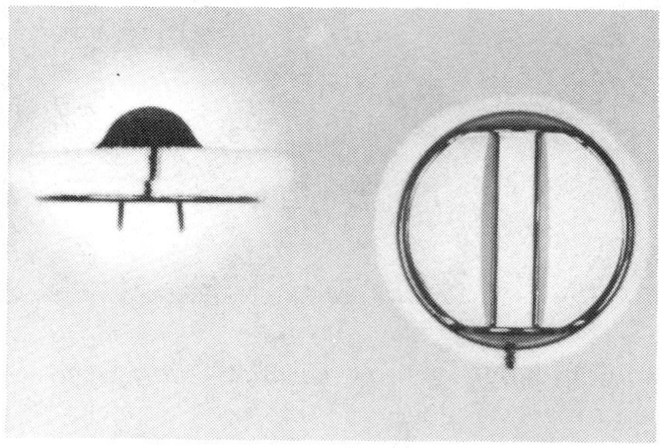

Figure 18. St. Jude Medical prosthesis. The hemi-disks and the housing are fabricated from carbon. (Courtesy of St. Jude Medical, Inc.).

St. Jude Medical

The St. Jude Medical cardiac valve prosthesis has an orifice ring, and 2 semi-circular discoid leaflets (Figure 18). The orifice ring and leaflets are composed of LTI pyrolytic carbon. The bileaflet design produces minimally impeded flow since the leaflets open to an angle of 85° to the plane of the orifice ring. The valve design is noteworthy for a relatively high flow orifice-to-tissue annulus diameter ratio; *in vitro* hemodynamics appear to be superior to those of other prostheses (Gabbay et al., 1980; Emery and Nicoloff, 1979; Hehrlein et al., 1979; Horstkotte et al., 1981; and Wortham et al., 1981) [42-46]. Extended clinical trials are in progress and the initial reports are encouraging.

The fact that this prosthesis has 2, rather than a single, moving occluders renders catastrophic failure unlikely, even when one disk becomes limited due to thrombotic buildup (Nunez et al., 1981) [47]. This potentially represents a very significant advantage of this prosthesis over other available tilting disk configurations. A major reservation, however, relates to the uncertain long-term durability (abrasion resistance) of the hemi-disk pivot-point contacts.

Hall-Kaster

The Hall-Kaster valve is a tilting disk valve with an S-shaped titanium disk guide strut with a disk stop (Figure 19). The disk is pyrolytic carbon-coated tungsten-impregnated graphite which has a central aperture and is fitted to the guide strut. The disk when in the open position divides the total valve orifice into 2 nearly equal parts. Initial clinical results indicate satisfactory function (Nitter-Hauge et al., 1979b) [48]. This prosthesis has recently been approved for general distribution (Medtronics, Inc., personal communication, 1981).

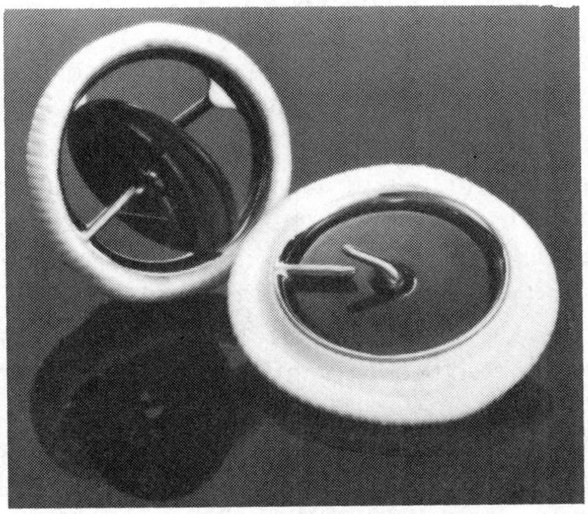

Figure 19. Hall-Kaster prosthesis. In this tilting disk design the disk has a central hole. (Courtesy of Medtronic Blood Systems, Inc.)

OTHER BIOMEDICAL APPLICATIONS OF CARBON

Some congenital and acquired left ventricular outflow tract obstructions may not be managed adequately with orthotopic prosthetic valve replacement. In an effort to aid such patients, the creation of a second low-impedance left ventricular outlet in the form of an apical left ventricle-to-aorta valved conduit has been developed. The left ventricular outlet connector must be rigid, compatible with myocardial tissue, thromboresistant and durable. LTI pyrolytic carbon was selected for this purpose. Norman et al., (1980) [49] reported 27 patients at the Texas Heart Institute with markedly decreased left ventricle-to-aorta pressure gradients and improved function after implantation of this device which carried approximately one-third of the cardiac output (Figure 20).

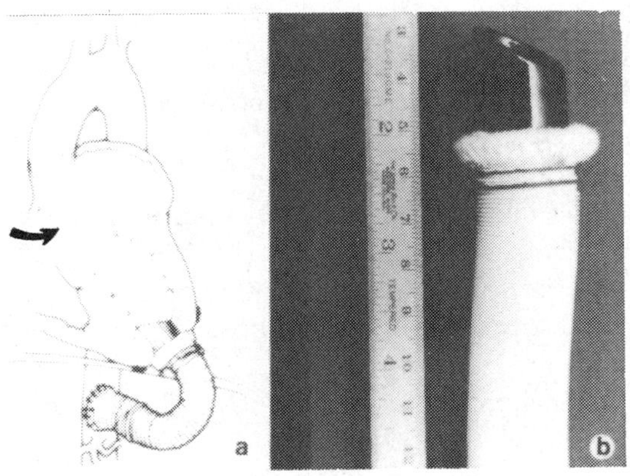

Figure 20. Apico-aortic conduit. Schematic diagram (A) illustrating surgically irreparable obstruction of the aortic outflow (arrow) and correction by prosthetic shunt (B) directing blood from left ventricular apex to abdominal aorta. There is generally a valve within the conduit allowing blood flow only away from the heart. (Courtesy of Carbomedics, Inc.)

Most circulatory assist devices in current use require flexible bladders. However, several centrifugal blood pumps utilizing all rigid blood-contacting components have been fabricated from LTI pyrolytic carbon and have been used in animals (Bernstein et al., 1974) [50]. The potential use of this device for temporary cardiac assist in humans is now being investigated.

Vacuum-vapor deposited carbon has been investigated as a coating material for 4 mm diameter vascular grafts (Sharp et al., 1978) [51] and for polymeric mesh tracheal prostheses

(Pizzoferrato et al., 1979) [53]. Clinical trials of the vascular grafts are in progress (Sharp and Teague, 1979) [52].

Through-the-skin leads for vascular access or electrical wires provide a particularly difficult situation since the tissue/material interface must be stable over long periods of time and resist both extrusion of the implant and invasion of infectious organisms. The optimum surface topography for long-term interfacial stability of percutaneous devices has not been determined; however, LTI and vitreous carbons have performed this function well for extended periods of time in certain configurations, as conduits for wires for neuromuscular (Mooney and Roth, 1976) [55], auditory, and visual prostheses (Eddington et al., 1978) [54] and as a device for maintenance of chronic vascular access (Golding et al., 1980) [56]. Conceivably, these same configurations could be utilized to transfer electrical or pneumatic power to an implanted cardiac assist device.

One particularly complex type of percutaneous device is the endosseous or subperiosteal dental implant. Both vitreous and LTI pyrolytic carbon dental implants have been used with some success over the last 10 years in the endosseous configuration (Bokros, 1977) [2]. Vacuum vapor-deposited carbons have been used extensively as a coating for metallic subperiosteal dental implants (Leake et al., 1979) [57].

ACKNOWLEDGMENT

The author is grateful to the following individuals for generously providing information and illustrative material: J. C. Bokros and A. D. Haubold, Carbomedics, Inc.; G. L. Carter, Medical Engineering Corp.; B. L. Dahlen, Cutter Laboratories, Inc.; M. C. Hufstutler, Jr., Medical, Inc.; D. Martin, Shiley, Inc.; C. J. Pakoy, St. Jude Medical, Inc., and J. Person, Medtronic Blood Systems, Inc. The author also acknowledges the technical assistance of R. G. Osol.

REFERENCES

1. Bokros, J. C., LaGrange, L. D. and Schoen, F. J.: Control of structure of carbon for use in bioengineering. IN *Chemistry and Physics of Carbon,* Vol. 9, Walker, P. L. and Thrower, P. (eds.), New York, Marcel Dekker, pp. 103-171, 1973.
2. Bokros, J. C.: Carbon biomedical devices. Carbon 15:355-371, 1977.
3. Haubold, A. D., Shim, H. S. and Bokros, J. C.: Carbon in medical devices. IN *Biocompatibility of Clinical Implant Materials,* Williams, D. F. (ed.), West Palm Beach, CRC Press, 1981 (In press).
4. Bokros, J. C.: The structure of pyrolytic carbon deposited in a fluidized bed. Carbon 3:17-29, 1965.
5. Kaae, J. L.: Structure and mechanical properties of isotropic pyrolytic carbons deposited below 1600°C. J. Nucl. Mater. 38:42-50, 1971.
6. Kaae, J. L. and Gulden, T. D.: Structure and mechanical properties of codeposited pyrolytic C-SiC alloys. J. Am. Ceram. Soc. 54:605-609, 1971.
7. Kaae, J. L.: The mechanical properties of glassy and isotropic pyrolytic carbons. J. Biomed.Mater. Res. 6:279-282, 1972.
8. Schoen, F. J.: On the fatigue behavior of pyrolytic carbon. Carbon 11:413-414, 1973.
9. Shim, H. S.: The behavior of isotropic pyrolytic carbons under cyclic loading. Biomat, Med. Dev. Art Org. 2:55-65, 1974.
10. Shim,H. S. and Schoen, F. J.: The wear resistance of pure and silicon-alloyed isotropic carbons. Biomat. Med. Dev. Art Org. 2:103-118, 1974.
11. Haubold, A. D., Shim, H. S. and Bokros, J. C.: Carbon cardiovascular devices. IN *Assisted Circulation,* Unger, F. (ed.), New York, Springer-Verlag, pp. 520-532, 1979.

12. Baier, R. E.: Key events in blood interactions at nonphysiologic interfaces – a personal primer. Artif. Org. 2:422-426, 1978.
13. Salzman, E. W., Lindon, J., Baier, D. and Merril, E. W.: Surface-induced platelet adhesion, aggregation, and release. Ann. NY Acad. Sci. 283:114-127, 1977.
14. Bokros, J. C., La Grange, L. D., Fadali, A. M., Vos, K. D. and Ramos, M. D.: Correlations between blood compatibility and heparin adsorptivity for an impermeable isotropic pyrolytic carbon. J. Biomed. Mater. Res. 3:497-528, 1969.
15. Schultz, J. S., Goddard, J. D., Ciankowski, A., Penner, J. A. and Lindenauer, S. M.: An ex-vivo method for the evaluation of biomaterials in contact with blood. Ann. NY Acad. Sci. 283:494-523, 1977.
16. Coleman, D. L., King, R. N. and Andrade, J. D. : The foreign body reaction: a chronic inflammatory response. J. Biomed. Mater. Res. 8:199-211, 1974.
17. Wood, N. K., Kaminski, E. J. and Oglesby, R. J.: The significance of implant shape in experimental testing of biological materials: disc vs. rod. J. Biomed. Mater. Res. 4:1-12, 1970.
18. Autian, J.: The new field of plastics toxicology – methods and results. CRC Crit. Rev. Toxicol. 1:1-40, 1973.
19. Roberts, W. C., Bulkley, B. H. and Morrow, A. G.: Pathologic anatomy of cardiac valve replacement: a study of 224 necropsy patients. Prog. Cardiovasc. Dis. 15:539-585, 1973.
20. Schoen, F. J., Titus, J. L. and Lawrie, G. M.: Autopsy-determined cause of death after cardiac valve replacement JAMA, 1982, in press.
21. Hylen, J. C.: Durability of prosthetic heart valves. Am. Heart J. 81:299-303, 1971.
22. Roberts, W. C. and Morrow, A. G.: Fatal degeneration of the silicone rubber ball of the Starr-Edwards prosthetic aortic valve. Am. J. Cardiol. 22:614-620, 1968.
23. Shah, A., Dolgin, M., Tice, D. A. and Trehan, N.: Complications due to cloth wear in cloth-covered Starr-Edwards aortic and mitral valve prostheses – and their management. Am. Heart J. 96:407-414, 1978.
24. Macmanus, Q., Grunkemeier, G., Housman, L., Maloney, C., Harlan, B., Lambert, L. and Starr, A.: Early results with composite strut caged ball prostheses. Am. J. Cardiol, 46:566-569, 1980.
25. Silver, M. D. and Wilson, G. J.: The pathology of wear in the Beall Model 104 heart valve prosthesis. Circulation 56:617-622, 1977.
26. Roberts, W. C. and Hammer, W. J.: Cardiac pathology after valve replacement with a tilting disc prosthesis (Bjork-Shiley type). A study of 46 necropsy patients and 49 Bjork-Shiley prostheses. Am. J. Cardiol, 37:1024-1033, 1976.
27. Angell, W. W. and Angell, J. D.: Porcine Valves. Prog. Cardiovasc. Dis. 23:141-166, 1980.
28. Scott, S. M., Sethi, G. K., Bridgman, A. H. and Takaro, T.: Experience with the DeBakey-Surgitool aortic prosthetic valve. J. Thorac. Cardiovasc. Surg. 21:483-486, 1976.
29. Paton, B. C. and Pine, M. B.: Aortic valve replacement with the DeBakey valve. J. Thorac. Cardiovasc. Surg. 72:652-656, 1976.
30. Fernandez, J., Morse, D., Spagna, P., Lemole, G., Gooch, A., Yang, S. S. and Maranhao, V.: Results of mitral valve replacement with the Beall prosthesis in 209 patients. J. Thorac. Cardiovasc. Surg. 71-218-225, 1976.
31. Beall, A. C., Jr., Morris, G. C., Jr., Noon, G. P. et al.: Clinical experience with an improved mitral valve prosthesis. Ann. Thorac. Surg. 15:601-606, 1973.
32. Schoen, F. J., Titus, J. L. and Lawrie, G. M.: Materials degeneration causing late failure of mechanical heart valve prostheses: problems and promise. IN *Implant Retrieval: Materials and Biological Analysis,* Weinstein, A., Gibbons, Dl., Brown, S. and Ruff, W. (eds.), Gaithersburg, Maryland, NBS Special Publication 601, National Bureau of Standards, pp. 269-282, 1981.
33. Wukasch, D. C., Sandiford, F. M., Reul, G. J., Jr., Hallman, G. L. and Cooley, D. A.: Complications of cloth-covered prosthetic valves: Results with a new mitral prosthesis. J. Thorac. Cardiovasc. Surg. 69:107-116, 1975.

34. Wukasch, D. C., Unger, F., Reul, G. J., Jr., et al.: Long-term results in cardiac valve replacement: Comparison of 6335 various type prostheses. IN *Second Henry Ford Hospital International Symposium on Cardiac Surgery,* Davila, J. C. (ed.), New York, Appleton-Century-Crofts, pp. 510-525, 1977.
35. Ten years' experience with the Bjork-Shiley tilting disc valve. J. Thorac. Cardiovasc. Surg. 78:331-342, 1979.
36. Karp, R. B., Cyrus, R. J., Blackstone, E. H., Kirklin, J. W., Kouchoukos, N. T. and Pacifico, A. D.: The Bjork-Shiley valve. Intermediate-term follow-up. J. Thorac. Cardiovasc. Surg. 81:602-614, 1981.
37. Yoganathan, A. P., Corcoran, W. H., Harrison, E. C. and Carl, J. R.: The Bjork-Shiley aortic prosthesis: flow characteristics, thrombus formation and tissue overgrowth. Circulation 58:70-76, 1978.
38. Silver, M. D.: Wear in Bjork-Shiley heart valve prostheses recovered at necropsy or operation. J. Thorac. Cardiovasc. Surg. 79:693-699, 1980.
39. Nitter-Hauge, S., Froysaker, T., Enge, I. and Hall, K. V.: Clinical and hemodynamic results after combined aortic and mitral valve replacement with the Lillehei-Kaster pivoting disc valve. Am. Heart J. 97:599-607, 1979. (a).
40. Kaster, R.L., Lillehei, W. and Starek, P. J. K.: The Lillehei-Kaster pivoting disc aortic prosthesis and a comparative study of its pulsatile flow characteristics with four other prostheses. Trans. Am. Soc. Artif. Int. Org. 16:233-243, 1970.
41. Lillehei, C. W.: Heart valve replacement with the pivoting disc prosthesis: Appraisal of results and description of a new all-carbon model. Med. Instrum. 11:85-94, 1977.
42. Gabbay, S., Yellin, E. L., Frishman, W. H. and Frater, R. W. M.: In vitro hydrodynamic comparison of St. Jude, Bjork-Shiley and Hall-Kaster valves. Trans. Am. Soc. Artif. Int. Org. 26:231-235, 1980.
43. Emery, R. W. and Nicoloff, D. M.: St. Jude Medical cardiac valve prosthesis. In vitro studies. J. Thorac. Cardiovasc. Surg. 78:269-276, 1979.
44. Hehrlein, F. W., Gottwik, M. G., Schlepper, M. and Fraedrick, G.: Heart valve replacement with the St. Jude Medical prosthesis – first clinical results –. Thorac. Cardiovasc. Surg. 27:187-189, 1979.
45. Horstkotte, D., Haerten, K., Herzer, J. A., Seipel, L., Bircks, W. and Loogen, F.: Preliminary results in mitral valve replacement with the St. Jude Medical prosthesis: comparison with the Bjork-Shiley valve. Circulation 64 (Suppl. II):II-203-II-209, 1981.
46. Wortham, D. C., Tri, T. B. and Bowen, T. E.: Hemodynamic evaluation of the St. Jude Medical valve prosthesis in the small aortic annulus. J. Thorac. Cardiovasc. Surg. 81:615-620, 1981.
47. Nunez, L., Iglesias, A. and Sotillo, J.: Entrapment of leaflet of St. Jude Medical cardiac valve prosthesis by miniscule thrombus: report of two cases. Ann. Thorac. Surg. 29:567-569, 1980.
48. Nitter-Hauge, S., Enge, I., Sembe, B. K. H. and Hall, K. V.: Primary clinical experience with the Hall-Kaster valve in the aortic position. Results at 3 months including hemodynamic studies. Circulation 60 (Suppl. I):I-55-I-62, 1979. (b).
49. Norman, J. C., Nihill, M. R. and Cooley, D. A.: Valved apico-aortic composite conduits for left ventricular outflow tract obstructions. A 4-year experience with 27 patients. Am. J. Cardiol. 45:1265-1271, 1980.
50. Bernstein, E. F., Cosentino, L. C., Reich, S., Stasz, P., Levine, I. D., Scott, D. R., Dorman, F. D. and Blackshear, P. L., Jr.: A compact, low hemolysis, non-thrombogenic system for non-thoracotomy prolonged left ventricular bypass. Trans. Am. Soc. Artif. Int. Org. 20:643-652, 1974.
51. Sharp, W. V., Teague, P. C. and Scott, D. L.: Thromboresistance of pyrolytic carbon grafts. Trans. Am. Soc. Artif. Int. Org. 24:223-227, 1978.
52. Sharp, W. V. and Teague, P. C.: ULTI carbon coated dacron grafts for small vessel replacement. IN *Proceedings of the 14th Bienniel Conference on Carbon,* Gatlinburg, Tennessee, June 1979, pp. 67-68.
53. Pizzoferrato, A., Leake, D., Michieli, S., Haubold, A. and Freeman, S.: Preliminary histologic evaluation of a biocompatible mesh for tracheal reconstruction. Biomat., Med. Dev., Art. Org. 7:321-331, 1979.

54. Eddington, D. K., Dobelle, W. H., Brackmann, D. E., Mladejovsky, M. G. and Parkin, J. L.: Auditory prostheses research with multiple channel intracochlear stimulation in man. Ann. Otol., Rhinol. and Laryngol. 87 (Suppl. 53):5-39, 1978.
55. Mooney, V. and Roth, A. M.: Advances in permanent percutaneous electrode systems. Biomat., Med. Dev., Art. Org. 4:171-180, 1976.
56. Golding, A. L., Nissenson, A. R., Higgins, R. and Raible, D.: Carbon transcutaneous access device (CTAD). Trans. Am. Soc. Artif. Int. Org. 26:105-109, 1980.
57. Leake, D., Reed, O. K., Armitage, J., Bokros, J. and Haubold A.: Carbon-coated subperiosteal dental implants for fixed and movable prostheses. J. Prosthet. Dent. 42:327-334, 1979.

Chapter 12

Development of Anionic Hemofiltration Membranes

Dr. R. L. S. Chang
Acurex Corporation
Energy & Environmental Div.
485 Clyde Ave.
Mountain View, CA 94042

ABSTRACT

The present study describes the development of anionic membranes that simulate the permselective properties of the glomerular capillaries for use as hemofiltration membranes. In particular, highly porous sulfonated polysulfone membranes (PSF) have been prepared. These PSF membranes have average fluxes of 35×10^{-5} ml/s cm^2 atm and have been shown to reject anionic dextrans to a greater extent, compared to neutral dextrans of the same hydrodynamic radius, over a range of sizes. In addition, urea has been shown to be freely permeable, while albumin is totally restricted. The high flux and increased permselectivity of these PSF membranes show promise as improved membranes for hemofiltration techniques.

BACKGROUND

The kidney plays an important role in the regulation of concentrations of various solutes in the physiological milieu as well as in the maintenance of extracellular volume. Through the process of filtration, excretion and reabsorption, the kidney retains useful ions and macro-molecules while metabolic wastes and toxic materials are eliminated. In the event of kidney failure, the fluid and electrolyte balance of the body is upset, concentrations of various toxic materials in the circulation build up, and this eventually leads to death. Every year, thousands of Americans suffering from kidney failure receive treatment from artificial kidneys and a great deal of effort is expended on the improvement of these devices.

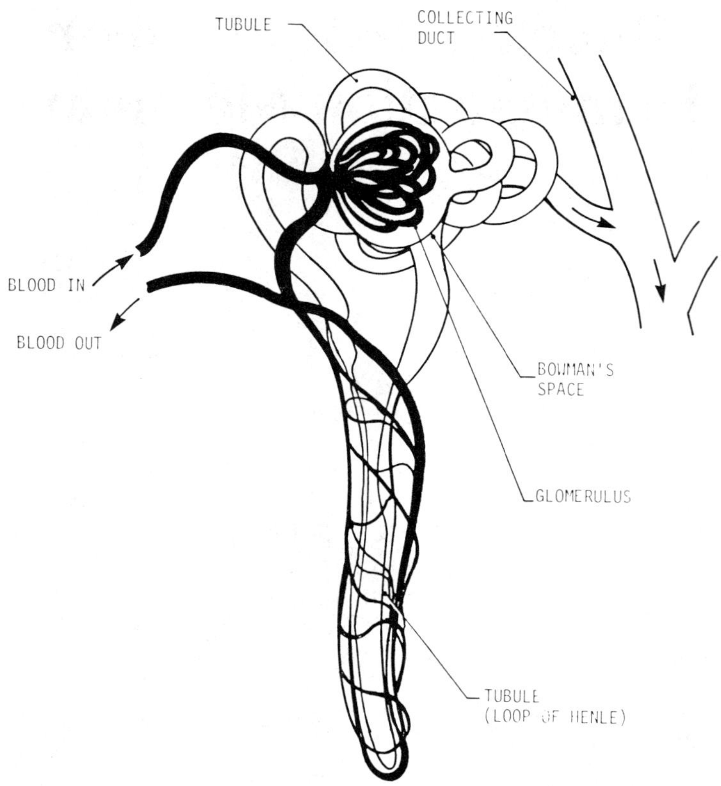

Figure 1. Schematic of the Nephron

While the kidney performs many complex functions not yet fully understood, it is generally agreed that the process of filtration, excretion and reabsorption takes place in numerous tubular units (one million or so in each human kidney) called nephrons. Detailed description of the many steps that take place from the beginning of the tubule where blood is first filtered to form filtrate to the end when urine is produced is given in many references [ref. 1, 2]. Essentially, the first step in the formation of urine takes place at the glomerular capillaries where blood entering the kidney is filtered under pressure into the proximal-most portion of the renal tubule called Bowman's capsule (Figure 1). One of the most remarkable features of the glomerular filtration process is the extent to which the glomerular capillary wall discriminates among different solutes, allowing some to pass freely, some partially, while completely restricting the passage of others. Earlier studies [ref. 3, 4, and 5] have found that the glomerular capillaries act like a porous membrane that allow small solutes to pass freely while restricting the passage of larger molecules according to their size. More recent investigations [ref. 6, 7 and 8] have found that the glomerular capillaries act as a "sieve" for solutes not only with respect to their size but with respect to their electrostatic charge as well. In fact, the glomerular capillary wall acts much like an anionic membrane, keeping the permeability of anionic solutes such as albumin much lower compared to a neutral molecule of similar size [ref. 7]. Figure 2 illustrates the permselectivity of the glomerular capillaries to dextran and anionic dextran sulfate. Note that a clearance of 1 indicates no restriction to solute transport while zero implies total restriction. Many types of kidney problems can be traced partially to the deterioration of the glomerular capillary wall and subsequent loss of its sieving ability. In some form of glomerulonephritis, for example, the resultant proteinuria observed can be attributed at least in part to the loss of anionic charge on the glomerular capillary wall which enables the passage of large amounts of albumin into the renal tubule [ref. 9]. To add to the complexity of the overall process, the filtrate that enters the renal tubule further undergoes a process of excretion and absorption of solutes and water before finally forming urine. The exact mechanisms involved are still not fully understood and a subject of much debate and research among different investigators. It becomes quite a challenge to mimick even one of the functions of the kidney in artificial devices, namely the maintenance of solute and water balance.

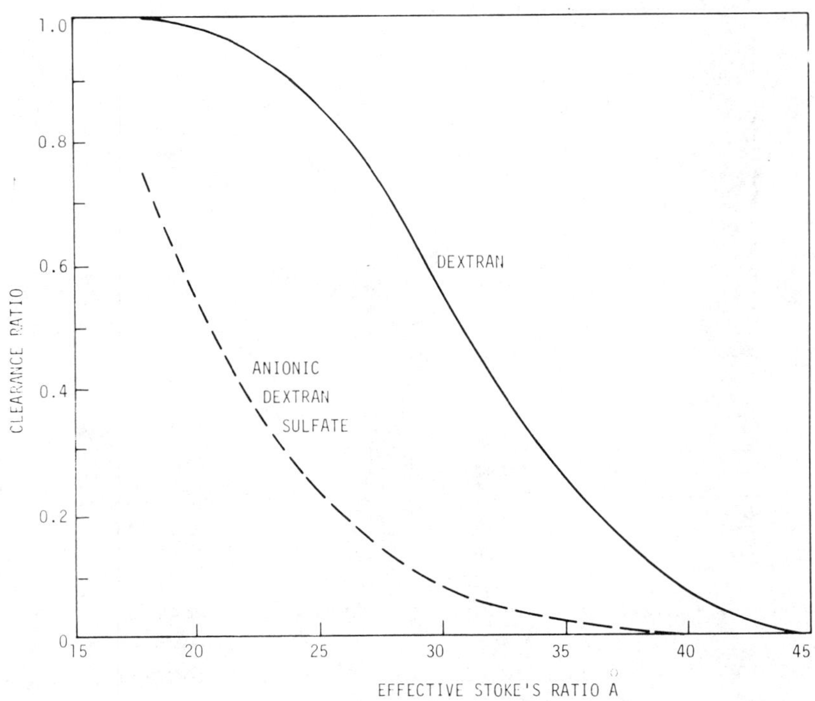

Figure 2. Comparison of Glomerular Capillary Permselectivity to Dextran and Anionic Dextran Sulfate

The most common treatment of kidney failure is hemodialysis [ref. 10, 11]. Blood is circulated through tubular or sheet membranes immersed in a dialysate bath. Solute removal from the blood side into the dialysate is controlled by adjusting the concentration of the solute in the dialysate. Solute removal takes place by diffusion across the membrane which is dependent on the concentration gradient of the solute. Excess water is removed by momentarily raising the hydrostatic pressure on the blood side. The membranes used have a molecular weight cut-off of about 5,000 so that while small ions as urea, uric acid and creatinine permeate relatively easily across the membrane, the transport of larger solutes decreases rapidly, reaching almost zero as the size of insulin (5,000 mol. wt.) is approached. Since the kidney removes solutes of much higher molecular weights as well, there has been much speculation whether some of these retained "middle-molecules" have any toxic properties associated with them [ref. 12 and 13].

An alternative approach under consideration recently removes solutes from the blood by a convective process called hemofiltration [ref. 14 and 15]. Solutes are removed primarily by bulk flow of plasma water from the blood side to the dialysate side induced by a hydrostatic pressure drop across the membrane, very much like what occurs across the glomerular capillary wall. Since no reabsorption of water occurs in the hemofiltration (compared to >99% reabsorption in the nephron) large amounts of fluid are added to the blood either before or after filtration. Useful ions are also added to the fluid since no reabsorption of ions takes place either in the artificial device. The hemofiltration membranes have a higher molecular weight cut-off compared to dialysis membranes but they encounter problems of protein loss across the membrane, many of which have unknown effects in the body.

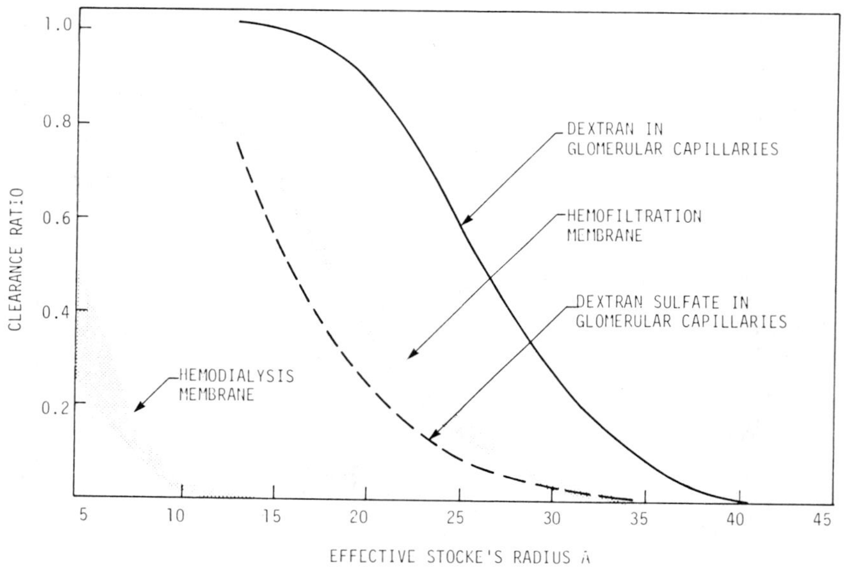

Figure 3. Comparison of the Permselectivity of Different Membranes

The problems encountered by hemodialysis and hemofiltration can readily be seen by comparing the membranes used with the properties of the glomerular capillaries (Figure 3). Membranes in artificial kidney devices are designed to selectively permeate molecules by size alone and does not have the permselectivity properties of the real kidney. Here again, clearance represents the relative permeability of solutes. A clearance of 1 indicates free permeation across the membrane and zero for complete restriction. It can be seen that the kidney is a more refined filter having high permeability while still being able to conserve useful materials by selectively permeating molecules with respect to both size and charge. Development of membranes with permselective properties which parallel those of the kidney could therefore significantly improve the usefulness and theraputic value of present artificial kidneys. On one hand, they could be highly permeable to small solutes, metabolic wastes and "middle" molecules and on the other, they can still conserve useful proteins such as albumin due to their electrostatic property. The higher permeability of these anionic membranes would also require less membrane surface area and thus more compact devices.

Another problem with existing membranes is they tend to clot blood over a period of time [ref. 18]. In addition to their more refined permselective properties, anionic membranes could have the additional important property of being less thrombogenic than conventional membranes. Studies [ref. 17] have shown that negatively charged polymeric surfaces are more thromboresistant than neutral or positively charged ones. Use of anionic membranes may therefore eliminate some of the problems associated with blood clotting in artificial kidney devices.

In summary then, anionic membranes with their refined permselectivity and thromboresistance could represent a significant advance in the improvement of present artificial kidney devices. Since acute and chronic kidney failures are important health problems today, better devices are constantly needed to improve the chances of survival for patients with renal diseases.

While little work is done to fabricate anionic membranes with properties adaptable for use in artificial kidneys, the properties and preparation of anionic membranes in general have been studied extensively. Most of the anionic membranes studied so far have been used for separating small ions. These are highly permselective membranes with complete restriction to large solutes. For example, anionic membranes were investigated for use in desalination processes for removing sodium chloride [ref. 18] and in ion exchange processes [ref. 19].

Membranes to be used for hemofiltration in artificial kidneys will have to be more "porous" to large solutes. Various methods for casting membranes and varying their "porosity" and permselective properties exists [ref. 20]. These methods, together with some newer techniques were studied to prepare suitable hemofiltration membranes.

METHODOLOGY

Membrane Formation Techniques

1) Membrane Casting – In general, most membranes were cast following the method of Loeb and Sourirajan [ref. 21]:

a) The polymer or mixture of polymers were first dissolved in suitable solvents.

b) The solution was poured onto a clean glass plate and a film was drawn on the plate with a casting knife (Gardner Lab, Inc., Bethesda, MD) set to a desired film thickness.

c) The film was dried for a fixed period of time under controlled conditions of temperature and humidity then quenched in a water bath where the membrane was floated off as a sheet.

In general, in order to increase the porosity (or permeability) of the membrane, fillers such as magnesium perchlorate, polyethylene glycol or a slow evaporating solvent such as dimethyl formamide was added. These tend to be leached out during the quenching process and make the membranes more permeable. The following factors were found to affect the final membrane properties during casting:

a) Type of solvent

b) Concentration of polymer solution

c) Type of filler added
d) Film thickness
e) Drying time
f) Humidity in room
g) Temperature in room
h) Temperature of quenching bath

For every new polymer or polymer combination used, the above conditions were adjusted by trial and error to obtain the optimum membrane.

2) Methods of Making Casting Solutions – Several methods for making anionic membranes were available. For example, a mixture of cationic and anionic polymers could be dissolved in a suitable solvent. The ratio of cations to anions being such as to make the overall membrane formed anionic. A mixture of neutral and anionic polymer could also be used. We found that these methods generally produce weak membranes or had undesirable filtration properties. The best membranes were formed by casting directly from anionic polymer solutions. Of the anionic polymers, the sulfonated polymers, polystyrenesulfonic acid, polyphenylene oxide sulfonate and sulfonated polysulfone were readily prepared and offered the most promise. Once prepared, they can be dissolved in a mixture of a highly volatile and a slow evaporating solvent and cast as membranes. In our experiments, sulfonated polysulfone produced anionic membranes with the best properties.

Sulfonated polysulfone was prepared by reaction of Polysulfone (PSF) (Union Carbide Corp., Bound Brook, NJ) with a sulfur trioxide triethyl phosphate complex, following the procedure below [ref. 22]:

A 2/1 sulfur trioxide (SO_3) triethyl phosphate (TEP) complex in 1-2 dichloroethane solution was prepared by adding 28.3 ml. SO_3 to a solution of 57.6 ml. TEP in 415 ml. 1-2 dichloroethane. The temperature of the solution was kept cool by adding the SO_3 slowly and using an ice bath. 100 ml. of this solution and 200 ml. of a solution of 15% polysulfone in 1-2 dichloroethane was added simultaneously via addition funnels to a stirred reaction kettle containing 220 ml. dichloroethane. The solutions were added to similar rates over a ten minute period. A heavy viscous precipitate resulted and stirring of the slurry was continued for 30 minutes. The slurry was then filtered, washed several times with 1-2 dichloroethane and dried in a vacuum oven at 60°C. The degree of sulfonation was determined by titration with 0.1 N tetramethyl ammonium hydroxide in methanol). For the procedure above, the degree of solfonation was found to be around 0.5.

Membrane Test Apparatus

The ultrafiltration experiments to measure membrane permeability were performed in a standard stirred ultrafiltration cell (Amicon Model 52) through which the test solutions were recirculated (Figure 4). A Masterflex peristaltic pump (Cole Parmer, Chicago, Ill.) was used to circulate the solutions. Pulsations in the flow were damped out with a surge tank. The cell has an effective area of 12.5 cm^2 and stirrer speeds were maintained at 1200 rpm to operate within turbulent fluid boundary conditions [ref. 23]. The filtration rate across the membrane was adjusted by the back pressure regulator and timed collections of the ultrafiltrate were made in a graduated cylinder. Samples from the reservoir and the ultrafiltrate were analyzed following techniques discussed previously.

Prior to testing the membranes for solute rejection characteristics each new batch of membranes were screened initially for their potential as effective filters by first studying their hydraulic permeabilities in nitrogen pressurized test cells with distilled water.

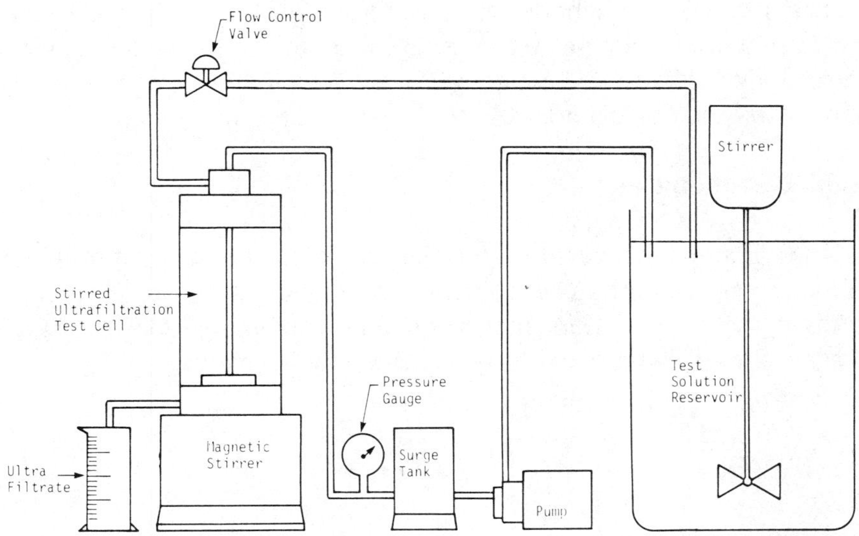

Figure 4. Ultrafiltration Test Apparatus.

Membranes with too high or too low hydraulic permeabilities or membranes that break easily are automatically rejected as potentially useful membranes. Test cells used in these experiments were simple dead end stirred cells obtained from Millipore (Millipore Model #XX4204710, 47 mm Stirred Cell, Bedford, Mass.).

Test Solutions

Test solutions were prepared in phosphate buffered saline containing 0.02 M phosphate buffer and 0.146 M sodium chloride. The following procedure is recommended for preparing the phosphate buffered saline:

19 ml 0.2 M $NaH_2PO_4 \cdot H_2O$
81 ml 0.2 M $Na_2HPO_4 \cdot 7H_2O$ dilute to 1000 ml
8.54 g NaCl

Solutes used include the following:

1) Urea – 0.1% solution, concentration read directly at 210 nm and by colorimetric determination with diacetyl monoxine read at 520 nm (Sigma Technical Bulletin #535, 1975).

2) Sucrose – 0.01% solution; concentration determined by colorimetric reaction with a sulfuric acid phenol reagent and read at 490 nm [ref. 6 and 24].

3) Inulin – 0.025% solution; concentration determined by the same method for sucrose.

4) Albumin – 0.1% solution; concentration read directly at 270 nm.

5) Dextran – Two narrow fractions of dextrans of $\bar{M}w$ 10,000 (T10) and 40,000 (T40) were used (Pharmacia Fine Chemicals, Inc., Piscataway, NJ). A heterogeneous mixture of dextran containing a relatively uniform distribution of dextran between $\bar{M}w$ = 10,000 and 40,000 was also prepared by mixing the T10 and T40 in the ration 1:1. The T10 and T40 solutions were 0.025% and the heterogeneous dextran 0.05%. All concentrations were determined by the same method for sucrose.

6) Dextran sulfate — A heterogeneous mixture of dextran sulfate was prepared by hydrolysis of a high molecular weight dextran sulfate ($\bar{M}w$ = 500,000) fraction from Pharmacia. Hydrolysis was carried out by adding 20 g dextran sulfate to 500 ml. water, adjusting pH to 1.5 with 37% hydrochloric acid and heating at 100°C for 10 minutes. The resultant solution was then diluted to 1 liter and the pH adjusted to 7 with sodium hydroxide.

Chromatographic Procedures

Sephadex G100 (Pharmacia) was used with an 0.05 N solution of ammonium acetate as buffer. The column was calibrated with standard techniques using blue dextran, dextran T10 and T20 fractions, cytochrome C, horseradish peroxidase and myoglobin [ref. 6]. Values of K_{AV} were plotted against log r_s (where r_s = Stokes-Einstein radius) where:

$$K_{AV} = \frac{(V_1 - V_o)}{(V_t - V_o)}$$

V_1 = elution volume of the solute
V_o = void volume of column determined by blue dextran
V_t = total volume of column
The Stokes-Einstein radius was assumed to be related to the diffusivity of the solute by:

$$D = \frac{RT}{6\pi\mu r_s}$$

D = diffusivity
μ = viscosity of solvent
R = gas constant
T = absolute temperature
The diffusivities of the standard molecules are well known and thus their effective radius can be obtained. The effective radius of unknown molecules are readily determined from their elution volumes.

In studies with the heterogeneous dextran and dextran sulfate solutions, samples were chromatographed on the gel columns and the concentrations of each fraction (each size) determined.

RESULTS

Anionic polymers such as sulfonated polysulfone are generally made into desalination and ion exchange membranes which are highly impermeable to all solute molecules and cannot be used for hemofiltration. The "porosity" of these membranes has to be increased by various techniques. Fillers such as magnesium perchlorate, polyethylene glycol and starch did not work. The problem is that solvents suitable for sulfonated polysulfone such as dimethyl formamide (DMF) and dimethyl sulfoxide (DSO) are both low in volatility. The membranes formed had to be dried in a heated oven and there is very little chance for porous pathways to form. More volatile solvents for sulfonated polysulfone are needed. Many solvents such as acetone, methanol, chloroform, cyclohexane, ethanol did not work. We found a mixture of 5 parts chloroform and 1 part methanol made an excellent solvent. However, membranes formed from solution of sulfonated polysulfone in this mixture by casting a film and quenching the partially dry membrane in water were impermeable. Adding a little dimethylformamide to the solution made the membrane permeable. The procedure we found to produce excellent anionic membranes with desired permeability properties is summarized below:

A 20% solution of sulfonated polysulfone in methanol/chloroform (1/5 by volume) was prepared and filtered. This solution and a methanol/chloroform solution (1/5 by volume) were mixed with dimethylformamide in the ratio 3:1.75:2.25 by volume. A membrane 5 mil thick was cast on glass plate, dried for 20 minutes and quenched in saturated salt solution.

It was found that the permeability of the membrane was highly sensitive to the ratio of the various solutions used and the degree of substitution of the polysulfone. Thus each factor must be taken into account and combined in proper quantities to produce the optimum membrane. Membranes we prepared are very stable and some have been tested for months without breakage. Hydraulic permeabilities of these membranes averaged around 35 × 10^{-5} ml/S cm^2 atm and are comparable to some of the high flux membranes in the market such as Rhone-Poulenc RP-AN69 (57 × 10^{-5} ml/S cm^2 atm). Values of solute rejection at different fluxes across the membranes are summarized in Tables 1 and 2 and average values plotted in Figure 5.

Table 1. Rejection Data at 25°C for Various Solutes Through Sulfonated Polysulfone

Urea (r_s = 1.8 Å)		Sucrose (r_s = 4.7 Å)		Inulin (r_s = 14 Å)	
*Jv x 10^4 (cm/s)	Apparent Rejection	Jv x 10^4 (cm/s)	Apparent Rejection	Jv x 10^4 (cm/s)	Apparent Rejection
0.22	0.0	0.27	0.06	0.25	0.34
0.54	0.0	0.54	0.06	0.71	0.32
0.88	0.0	0.89	0.07	1.00	0.35
2.08	0.0	1.95	0.07	1.38	0.35
2.78	0.01	2.83	0.08	2.30	0.35
3.53	0.04	3.30	0.21	3.8	0.36

Dextran T10 (r_s = 22 Å)		Dextran T40 (r_s = 45 Å)		Albumin (r_s = 34 Å)	
Jv x 10^4 (cm/s)	Apparent Rejection	Jv x 10^4 (cm/s)	Apparent Rejection	Jv x 10^4 (cm/s)	Apparent Rejection
0.3	0.46	0.25	0.97	0.26	0.97
0.6	0.47	0.62	0.96	0.64	0.98
0.95	0.48	0.89	0.96	1.10	0.99
2.00	0.45	1.37	0.97	2.17	0.99
2.75	0.49	2.35	0.97	3.2	0.98
3.9	0.45	2.66	0.97	3.8	0.99

*Transmembrane Volume Flux

For the solutes tested, it can be seen that the apparent rejections (R) are not strong functions of the transmembrane flux rate (Jv) in the range of Jv's tested. It has been shown that during ultrafiltration, solute R is a function of Jv, increasing with increasing Jv until a limiting constant value of R is reached above a certain Jv [ref. 23]. For the size of solutes we tested, this limiting value has already been reached within the range of fluxes used. The only exception to

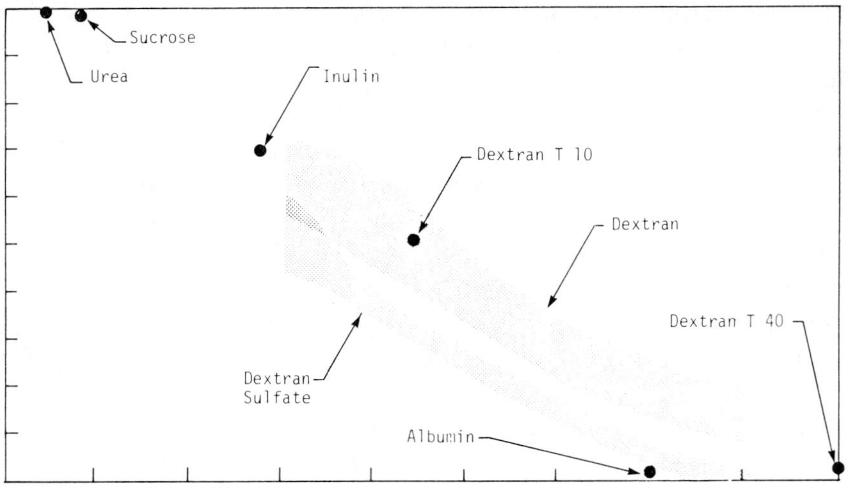

Figure 5. Permselectivity of Sulfonated Polysulfone Membranes.

Table 2. Rejection Data for Dextran and Dextran Sulfate Mixtures at 25°C Through Sulfonated Polysulfone.

Dextran

	Apparent Rejection		
Jv x 10^4 (cm/s)	1.50	1.70	2.00
Solute Radius (Å)			
15	0.28	0.43	0.32
20	0.31	0.54	0.45
25	0.56	0.66	0.53
30	0.66	0.75	0.63
35	0.76	0.83	0.71
40	0.81	0.87	0.75

Dextran Sulfate

	Apparent Rejection		
Jv x 10^4 (cm/s)	1.30	1.90	2.70
Solute Radius (Å)			
15	0.43	0.47	0.57
20	0.64	0.61	0.68
25	0.71	0.72	0.75
30	0.85	0.84	0.83
35	0.99	0.91	0.91
40	0.97	0.93	0.93

this are urea and sucrose. Urea, being a very small molecule, passes freely across the membrane without much restriction. Sucrose is slightly larger than urea and begins to show some dependence of rejection on transmembrane flux. The rise in rejection with flux, however, is slow. In general by referring to Figure 5 where average apparent rejections are used (plotted as 1-R versus solute radius r_s), a good comparison can be made of the relative permeabilities of various solutes across sulfonated polysulfone membranes. The clearance ratios obtained, while not exactly the same as for the glomerular capillary wall, are remarkably similar in terms of general permselective properties. Urea and sucrose are freely permeable while dextran T40 is almost totally restricted. Neutral molecules tend to have higher clearance ratios (less rejections) compared to anionic molecules of similar effective Stoke's radius. Albumin, for example, behaves more like dextran sulfate of the same size or a dextran of much larger size (dextran of 45 Å). Such a membrane will therefore demonstrate not only a solute size discrimination but a solute charge discrimination as well.

CONCLUSIONS AND RECOMMENDATIONS

Of the various techniques we experimented with in fabricating anionic hemofiltration membranes, the most promising is the casting of membranes directly from water insoluble anionic polymers. In order to use the membranes for application to hemofiltration suitable porosity must be imparted to the membrane by using a mixture of volatile and non-volatile solvents for making up the casting solution. The nonvolatile solvent can later be leached out during the quenching of the membrane in water. The finding of suitable combinations of solvents and polymer is really a trial and error process and the properties of the resultant membranes are strongly dependent on the polymer and the degree of substitution, the type of solvent and the combination of solvents used and the concentration of the casting solution. We found that other factors such as relative humidity, temperature, drying time and membrane thickness are not so critical for the sulfonated polysulfone membranes we prepared as long as we let the membrane dry long enough so that all the volatile solvents have essentially evaporated.

For use in actual applications, some support should be provided for the membranes to extend membrane life during operations. We have done some preliminary studies on casting the membrane directly on dacron mesh. The resultant membrane is extremely strong but we could not make the membrane very uniform. This possibility should definitely be explored under more controlled conditions. Since the membrane permselective properties are most probably a surface phenomena, an alternative is to make porous polysulfone membranes and then surface sulfonate the membrane. In this way, the polysulfone offers a strong support under the sulfonated surface layer.

The anionic membranes (sulfonated polysulfone) prepared up to now are very promising in that they did show dual preselective characteristics as we anticipated. They are capable of rejecting solutes with respect to both size and charge and thus add a new dimension to membrane perselectivity. Their range of perselectivity and their hydraulic permeabilities make them suitable candidates as hemofiltration membranes. At this point, the next steps should be to ensure strong membranes could be made either by use of supports or surface sulfonation and their fabricating a small hemofiltration device. The potential of improved hemofiltration therapy using these membranes exists and should be studied.

REFERENCES

1. Renkin, E.M. and J.P. Gilmore. Glomerular Filtration. In *Handbook of Physiology, Sec 8: Renal Physiology*. J. Orloff and R.W. Berliner, eds. Am. Physiol. Soc., Washington, DC, pp. 185-248, 1973.
2. Pitts, R.F. *Physiology of the Kidney and Body Fluids*. Chicago, Year Book Medical Publishers, Inc., 1970.
3. Pappenheimer, J.R. Passage of molecules through capillary walls. Physiol. Rev., vol. 33: 387-423, 1953.
4. Verniory, A., R. Dubois, P. Decoodt, J.P., Gassee, and P.P. Lambert. Measurement of the permeability of biological membranes. Application to the glomerular wall. J. Gen. Physiol., vol. 62: 489-507, 1973.

5. Arturson, G., T. Groth and G. Grotte. Human glomerular membrane porosity and filtration pressure: Dextran clearance data analyzed by theoretical models. Clin. Sci., vol. 40: 137-158, 1971.
6. Chang, R.L.S., I.F. Ueki, J.L. Troy, W.M. Deen, C.R. Robertson and B.M. Brenner. Permselectivity of the glomerular capillary wall to macromolecules II. Experimental studies in rats using neutral dextran, Biophys. J., vol. 15: 887-906, 1975.
7. Chang, R.L.S., W.M. Deen, C.R. Robertson, and B.M. Brenner. Permselectivity of the glomerular capillary wall III. Restricted transport of polyanions. Kidney Int., vol. 8: 212, 218, 1975.
8. Rennke, H.G., and M.A. Venkatachalam. Glomerular permeability: in vivo tracer studies with polyanionic and polycationic ferritins. Kidney, Int., vol. 11: 44-53, 1977.
9. Bennett, C.M., R.J. Glassock, R.L.S. Chang, W.M. Deen, C.R. Robertson and B.M. Brenner. Permeselectivity of the glomerular capillary wall, studies of experimental glomerulonephritis in the rat using dextran sulfate. J. Clin. Invest., vol. 57: 1287-1294, 1976.
10. Nose, Y. *The Artificial Kidney,* in *Advances in Biomedical Engineering and Medical Physics,* vol. 4, S.N. Levine, ed., N.Y., Wiley Interscience, 1971.
11. Babb, A.L., L. Grimsrud, R.L. Bell, and S.B. Layno. *Engineering Aspects of Artificial Kidney Systems,* in *Chemical Engineering in Medicine and Biology*. P. Hershey, ed., N.Y., Plenum, pp. 289-332, 1967.
12. Henderson, L.W., *Rationale and Evidence for the "Middle Molecule" in Uremic Man.* In Workshop on Dialysis and Transplantation. Am. Soc. Art. Internal Org., Washington, DC, pp. 69-75, 1972.
13. Scribner, B.H., P.C. Farrell, J. Milutinovic, and A.L. Babb. *Evolution of the Middle Molecule Hypothesis* in Proc. 5th International Congress of Nephrology, vol. 2, H. Villarreal, ed., Switzerland, S. Karger, pp. 190-199.
14. Colton, C.K., L.W. Henderson, C.A. Ford, and M.J. Lysaght. Kinetics of hemodiafiltration I. In vitro transport characteristics of a hollow fiber ultrafilter. J. Lab. Clin. Med., vol. 85: 355-371, 1975.
15. Henderson, L.W., C.K. Colton, and C.A. Ford. Kinetics of hemodiafiltration II. Clinical characterization of a new blood cleansing modality, J. Lab Clin. Med., vol. 85: 372-391, 1975.
16 Marshall, J.W., D.J. Shearn, R.J. Nothrun, J. Esterly, K.O. Nolph and J.F. Maker. "Adherence of blood components to dialyzer membranes." Morphological studies. Nephron, vol. 12: 157-165, 1974.
17. Murphy, P. Antithrombogenic properties of electrified polymers. Trans. Am. Soc. Artif. Internal Organs, vol. 13: 131-144, 1967.
18. Plummer, C.W., G. Kimura and A.B. La Conti. Development of sulfonated polyphemylene oxide membranes for reverse osmosis. U.S. Dept. of the Interior, Research and Development Progress Report No. 551, 1970.
19. Caplan, S.R., and K. Sollner. The influence of the characteristics of the activating polyelectrolyte in the preparation and on the properties of interpolymer ion exchange membranes. J. Colloid and Interface Sc., vol. 46: 46-66, 1974.
20. Lakshminarayanaih N. Transport Phenomena in Artificial Membranes. Chemical Reviews, vol. 65: 491-565, 1965.
21. Sourivajan, S. *Reverse Osmosis,* N.Y., Academic Press, 1970.
22. Noshay, A. and L. M. Robeson. Sulfonated Polysulfone, J. Appl. Polymer Sc., Vol. 20: 1885-1903, 1976.
23. Colton, C.K., S. Friedman, D.E. Wilson and R.S. Lees. Ultrafiltration of lipoproteins through a synthetic membrane. Implications for the filtration theory of atherogenesis. J. of Clin. Inves., vol. 51: 2472-2480, 1972.
24. Montgomery, R. Further Studies of the Phenol-Sulfuric acid reagent for carbohydrates. Biochem. Biophys. Acta, vol. 48: 591-593, 1961.

Chapter 13

Antithrombogenic Characteristics of Immobilized Urokinase on Synthetic Polymers

Takeshi Ohshiro, M.D.
Second Department of Surgery
Osaka University Medical School
1-1-50, Fukushima, Fukushima-ku
Osaka 553, Japan

ABSTRACT

Urokinase-treated sepharose revealed the fibrinolytic activity in both experiments of fibrinolysis method and hemoperfusion method. Then we tried to immobilize urokinase on the surface of polymeric materials, and to investigate the antithrombogenic characteristics in vitro and in vivo. The stronger fibrinolytic activity were obtained by immobilizing the grafted copolymer such as polyethylene imine and Gantrez in advance. HCl-etching was valid, too. Effective enzyme activity of immobilized urokinase was approximately 30% of same amount of soluble urokinase. The binding form of immobilized urokinase to nylon consist of stable ionic binding, peptide linking inactivated by some factors after repeated fibrinolysis test or long-term use and other sustained peptide linking. Immobilized urokinase was not almost affected by urokinase inhibitor, while soluble urokinase was inactivated. In disinfection, gamma ray irradiation done before immobilization of urokinase led to favorable result. On the antithrombogenic mechanism, I emphasized the three characterized points. Until today, we had the clinical applications of urokinase-treated polymeric materials in four medical fields such as intravenous catheterization, Handley's method in lymphedema, liquid drainage and vascular anastomosis. The findings were favorable.

Despite the dramatic advance of medical polymeric material, we can not get yet the clinically available material with high antithrombogenicity. This is one of the reasons why artificial organ is not put on the practical use. At present, a little attempt has been made to develop the new antithrombogenic material by the methods to immobilize anticoagulant substance, antiplatelet agent and fibrinolytic enzyme on the surface of polymeric materials. Among these methods, the last is interesting to us. One of the characteristics of the immobilized enzyme is that it is more stable than the free enzyme. On the base of it, the immobilized enzyme is able to stay in the human body for a long period of time and to display a good deal of enzyme activity by behaving like a catalyst. This characteristic was an incentive to commence the present study.

As already discussed, immobilized urokinase displayed fibrinolytic activity. In fact, this activity was demonstrated when it was immobilized on carriers such as CMC-hydrazide [1], agarose [2], graphite [3], sepharose [4,5], polymer Enzacryl [6]. However, a few problems must be solved before this technique is available clinically.

Described herein was the outcomes of the fundamental and clinical studies on urokinase-treated polymeric materials and discussed was the fibrinolytic mechanism of immobilized urokinase. The contents were divided into four items.

A. Fundamental experiment
B. Disinfection method
C. Animal experiment
D. Clinical application

A. FUNDAMENTAL EXPERIMENT

1. Experiment of Urokinase-Treated Sepharose

In order to study whether immobilized urokinase would reveal fibrinolytic activity or not, we carried out the preliminary experiments which used urokinase-treated sepharose.

1) Experiment by the Fibrinolysis Method (Figure 1)

A given amount of sepharose, to which urokinase was bound, was dropped on a fibrin plate, and fibrinolysis incubating at 37°C was observed serially with the lapse of time. In this experiment, streptokinase and plasmin, which were immobilized in the same way as urokinase, were used as reference enzymes.

Urokinase-treated sepharose had apparent fibrinolytic activity and the ring size increased linearly with time. Almost similar results were obtained in immobilized streptokinase and plasmin, but it must be supplemented that the fibrinolytic activity of plasmin was strongly inhibited when human plasma was added.

2) Experiment by the Hemoperfusion Method (Figure 2)

A closed circuit system was prepared for hemoperfusion, and the fibrinolytic ability of immobilized urokinase in blood was observed. Hemoperfusion was performed with preserved human ACD blood for 24 hours at room temperature. The volume of the circuit was 240 ml and the rate of hemoperfusion was 20 ml/min. The barrier filter of 40 μ mesh was filled with

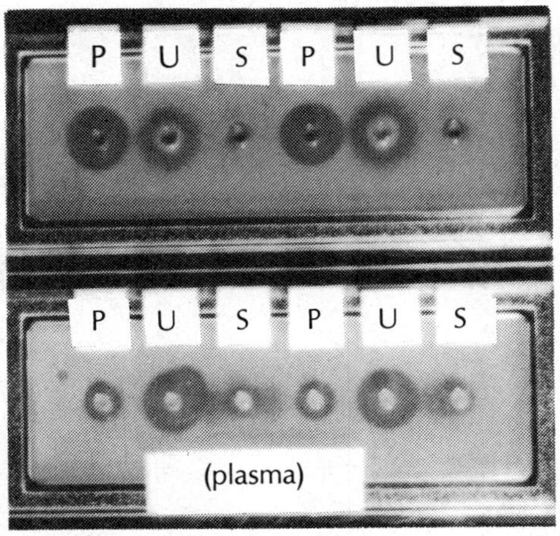

Figure 1. Experiment by fibrinolysis method. Among plasmin (P), streptokinase (S) and urokinase (U), which were bound to activated sepharose, urokinase-treated sepharose had the stronger fibrinolytic activity in fibrin plate to which human plasma was added.

sepharose to which urokinase was bound, in the amount of 25 ml in wet volume. Fibrin degradation product (FDP) and fibrinogen were measured by the hemoagglutination inhibition test and the weight method, respectively. Perfusion was also done, for comparative purposes, by use of soluble urokinase in an amount equivalent in enzyme activity to immobilized urokinase and by use of inactivated sepharose.

Time-course changes in the levels of FDP and fibrinogen in perfusate were followed up in the series of hemoperfusion using urokinase-treated sepharose (Sepharose-UK), soluble urokinase (Soluble UK) and inactivated sepharose (Sepharose), respectively. The FDP levels determined in each series 24 hours after the start of hemoperfusion were 320, more than 320 and 40 ug/ml, respectively. In other words, FDP increased in Sepharose-UK series and Soluble UK series and did not in Sepharose series. This outcome suggests that immobilized urokinase has almost the same fibrinolytic ability as soluble urokinase. On the other hand, the fibrinogen levels were reduced to 0, 80 and 0 mg/dl, respectively. Particularly in Sepharose-UK series and Sepharose series, fibrinogen completely disappeared during 24-hr hemoperfusion. It is supposed that fibrinogen was taken on sepharose, which consisted of a lot of minute particles, and degradated in Sepharose-UK series, and clotted in Sepharose series. By the way, time-course changes of erythrocytes, leucocytes, and platelets in blood under perfusion were also followed up. In the hemoperfusion using sepharose, leucocytes decreased rapidly after the start of hemoperfusion, while erythrocytes underwent practically no change. Platelets had already been decreased at the start.

This preliminary experiment concluded as follows:

(1) The fibrinolytic activity of urokinase is maintained after immobilization.
(2) Immobilized urokinase displays the fibrinolytic activity even in blood.
(3) Small particles like sepharose is an unsuitable carrier.

2. Experiment of Urokinase-Treated Polymeric Material

When we can make use of polymeric material as the carrier of immobilization, it is much convenient for clinical application.

1) Immobilization Method

Various types of polymeric materials such as nylon, polyester and polyvinyl chloride were employed as carriers.

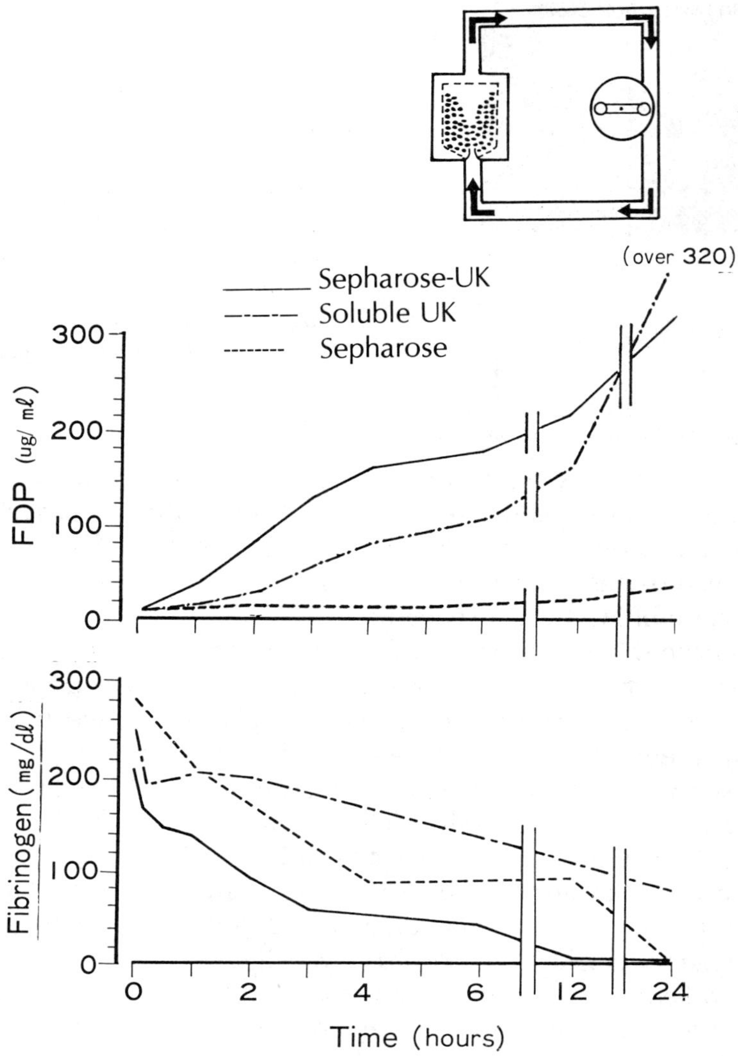

Figure 2. Experiment by hemoperfusion method. When human ACD blood was perfused through the filter filled with urokinase-treated sepharose (Sepharose-UK) or inactivated sepharose (Sepharose) in closed circuit, FDP in perfusate gradually increased in Sepharose-UK series but not in Sepharose series. Sepharose-UK series showed the almost same pattern as soluble UK series.

The immobilization process is as follows: material is

(1) etched 1-3 N HCl, NaOH or NaCl for one hour.
(2) dipped in 10 wt% polyethylene imine at 30°C for two hours under 5 wt% dicyclohexyl carbodiimide.
(3) dipped in 4 wt% Gantrez (maleic anhydride/methylvinyl ether copolymer) and 0.8 wt% 3-nitrophthalic anhydride at 30°C for five hours.
(4) dipped in 600 μ/ml urokinase solution at 30°C for one hour.

The binding map of each substance had been schematically shown in our past report [7]. The chemical reaction is shown in Figure 3.

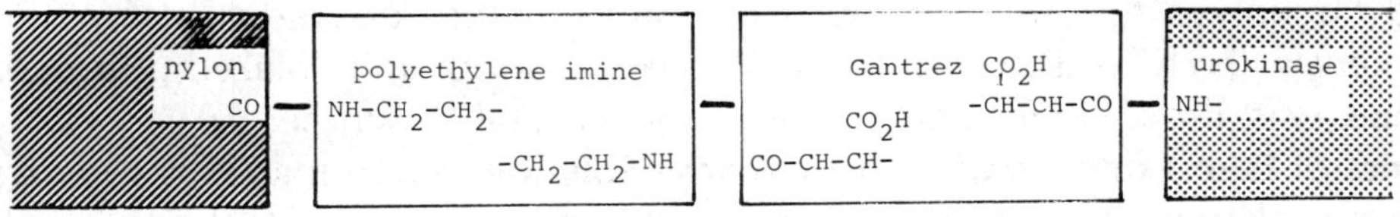

Figure 3. Chemical reaction of immobilization. It is supposed that immobilization is based on the binding of CO-NH, which is named peptide linking.

2) Immobilizable Amount of Urokinase

We performed experiments to study the following points with an eventual aim to ascertain a method of immobilizing more urokinase. In these experiments, nylon 6 was employed as a carrier among the various polymeric materials.

a) Effect of Grafted Copolymer. By means of modifying the immobilization process, five types of urokinase-treated nylon were prepared and a comparative study of their fibrinolytic abilities was made.

N-UK without HCl; after nylon is merely washed, urokinase is immobilized directly on the surface of nylon.

N-UK with HCl; after nylon is etched by HCl, urokinase is done in same.

N-PEI-UK; urokinase is immobilized to polyethylene imine which is linked with etched nylon.

N-PEI-G-UK; urokinase is immobilized to Gantrez which is further linked with polyethylene imine, done with etched nylon.

N-PEI-G-NP:UK; nitrophthalic acid are immobilized to Gantrez in parallel with urokinase.

This criterion, as a basis for comparison of fibrinolytic activity, was also used in other experiments unless otherwise specified.

Table 1. Comparison of Fibrinolytic Activity in Various Types of Urokinase-Treated Nylon

Type of Urokinase--treated Nylon	Fibrinolytic Activity (%)
N-UK without HCl	38 ±13
N-UK with HCl	49 ±11
N-PEI-UK	57 ± 23
N-PEI-G-UK	71 ± 18
N-PEI-G-NP:UK	100 ± 25

The result is shown in Table 1. The fibrinolytic activity of N-PEI-G-NP:UK is expressed as 100%. The stronger fibrinolytic activity was obtained by immobilizing polyethylene imine and Gantrez, which were adopted as grafted copolymers, and nitrophthalic anhydride together with them, which was an antiplasmin inhibitor. The main key is to form a grafted copolymer layer between urokinase and nylon for the purpose of considerably increasing the number of binding sites. Polyethylene imine and Gantrez were much better. Although the number of binding sites was theoretically expected to increase immensely, it was, in fact, no more than doubled experimentally. Nevertheless, it can be said that forming an intermediate layer is an effective means of facilitating immobilization.

b) Effect of HCl-Etching. Nylon materials were immersed in 3 N HCl for one hour before immobilization of urokinase. Nylon so pretreated with HCl showed a stronger fibrinolytic activity than that not pretreated. The fibrinolytic activity was augmented 20-40%. The results of repeated fibrinolysis test showed much the same pattern of gradual decrease (Figure 4). Pretreatment with HCl led to an increase in the amount of immobilized urokinase to nylon. HCl-etching was also valid for immobilizing a quantity of urokinase.

c) Effect of High Concentration of Urokinase Solution. Nylon materials were treated with ^{125}I-labeled urokinase in varying concentration. The amount of immobilized urokinase was determined with isotope counts. It did not practically change when a concentration below 2 mg% was used, but augmented almost linearly when a higher concentration was used (Figure 5). Thus, the higher the concentration was, the more urokinase was immobilized. The supplemented key is to get purified urokinase not mixed stable substance. This immobilized urokinase may be apt to release from carrier because of the loose binding form.

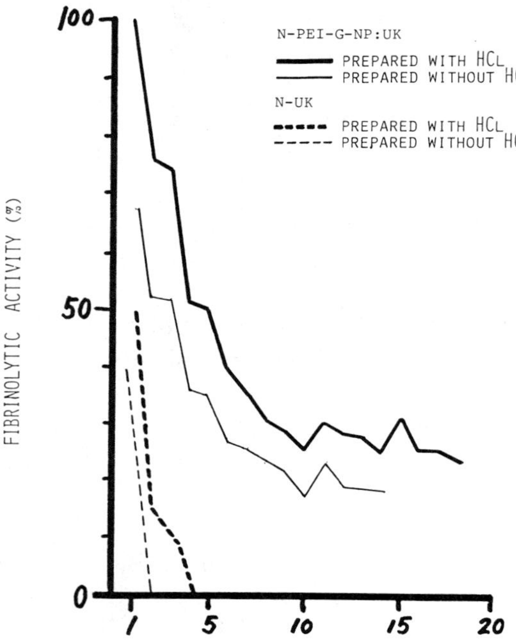

Figure 4. Effect of HCl-etching. Urokinase-treated nylon pretreated with HCl showed the stronger fibrinolytic activity than that not pretreated with HCl in repeated fibrinolysis test.

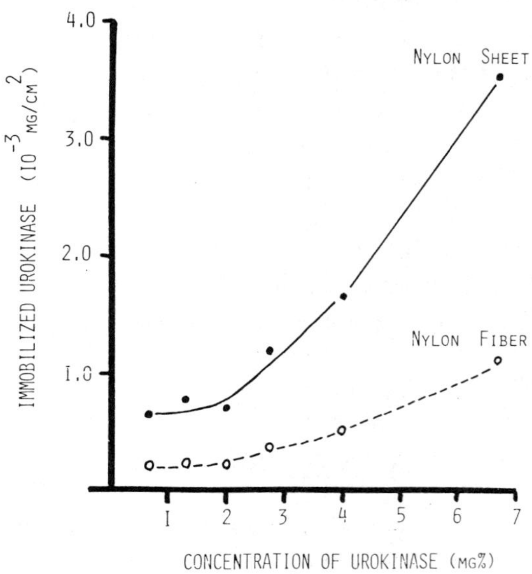

Figure 5. Effect of high concentration of urokinase solution. The higher concentration of urokinase solution was used for immobilization of urokinase, the more urokinase was immobilized on the surface of nylon carrier.

d) Effective Enzyme Activity of Immobilized Urokinase. In this study, the protein volume and the enzyme activity of immobilized urokinase had to be determined separately. Determination of the former was done by means of assaying the radioactivity of samples to which ^{125}I-labeled urokinase was immobilized and that of the latter by means of ascertaining the zymolytic activity according to the Glu-Gly-Arg-methylcoumarin 7-amide (MCA) method. The amount of immobilized urokinase, which was obtained from the radioactivity, was 1.5×10^{-3} mg/cm^2 which was equivalent to the fibrinolytic activity of 68 IU/cm^2. On the other hand, the fibrinolytic activity calculated from the zymolytic activity by the MCA method was 20 IU/cm^2. The ratio of the former to the latter was 7:2.

3) Repeated Fibrinolysis Test

This experiment, performed as one of the through processes which investigated the binding form of urokinase, gave the information on the maintenance of enzyme activity of immobilized urokinase. The sample of N-PEI-G-UK was selected as urokinase-treated nylon. Each sample was sufficiently washed with saline (pH 6.0), 1 M NaCl phosphate buffer (pH 8.0), 2% NH_4OH (pH 12.0) or 0.1 M K_2HPO_4 (pH 9.1). It is supposed that immobilized urokinase in physical adsorption and ionic binding is released from carrier by this washing process.

The fibrinolytic activities of these samples after repeated fibrinolysis test in standard human fibrin plate were examined (Figure 6). The findings revealed that these samples lost part of their fibrinolytic activities after being used several times. In fact, their fibrinolytic activities of fourth time test yielded by N-PEI-G-UK decreased to 20~30 mm^2 of fibrin lysis area, but maintained at same levels after further repetition. This maintained fibrinolytic activity seems to correspond to that of immobilized urokinase in peptide linking (= covalent binding).

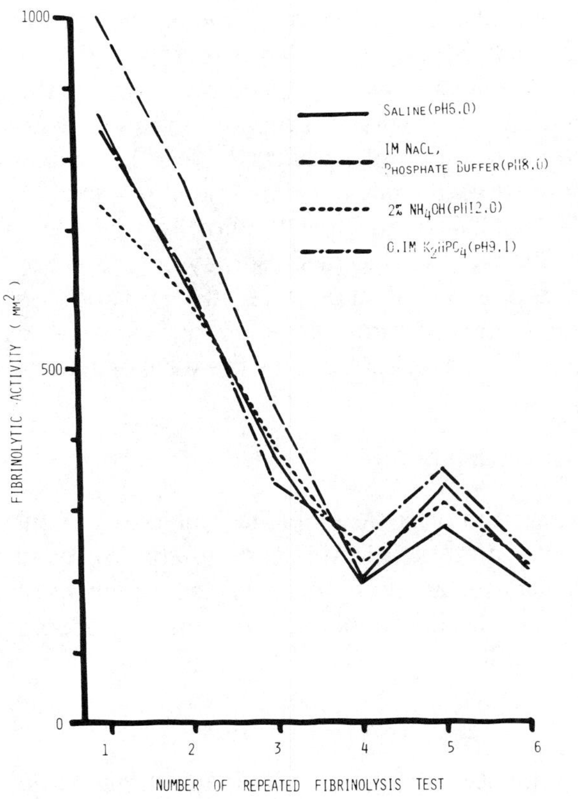

Figure 6. Repeated fibrinolysis test. Fibrinolytic activities of urokinase-treated nylons, washed with various kinds of solution to take off the urokinase which was immobilized in loose binding form, gradually decreased in repeated fibrinolysis test. Fibrinolytic activity was expressed as fibrin lysis area.

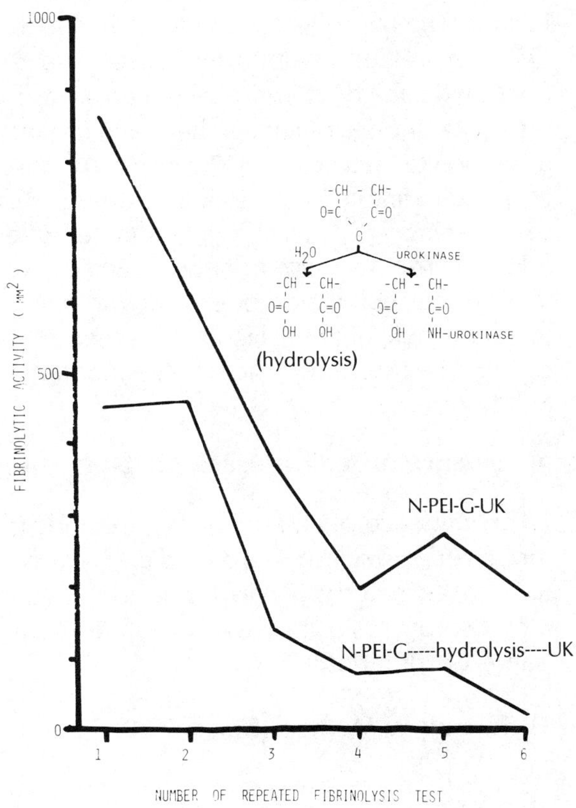

Figure 7. Comparison of fibrinolytic activities in two types of urokinase-treated nylon. Fibrinolytic activity of nylon on which urokinase were immobilized after hydrolysis reduced 120-220 mm^2 greater than that of regular urokinase-treated nylon.

3. The Binding Form of Urokinase to Polymeric Material

An interesting question concerning binding forms in immobilized urokinase to polymeric material remains. In order to study this question, two types of urokinase-treated nylon were employed in this experiment. The one was the complete preparation of urokinase-treated nylon. Another one was nylon having only those binding sites to which urokinase had not yet been immobilized, and being dipped in a physiological saline solution for three days prior to immobilization. This procedure intends to hydrolyze the physicochemical properties of the surface of nylon. It results in the sites for peptide linking (covalent binding) being blocked by hydrolytic reaction, as schematically shown in Figure 7. Following this process the nylon was immersed in urokinase solution and washed well with saline (pH 6.0), to release the unstable urokinase which is immobilized by the linkage of physical adsorption and ionic binding. Figure 7 compares the fibrinolytic activities of the above two samples. The former (N-PEI-G-UK) decreased after repeated fibrinolysis test and retained an activity of 200–300 mm^2. The latter (N-PEI-G . . . hydrolysis . . . UK) underwent a similar pattern to show an activity around 80 mm^2 in the fourth time test. The loss of activity in the latter was 120–220 mm^2 greater than in the former. The hydrolysis procedure yielded a reduction of 120 to 220 mm^2 in the fibrinolytic activity, expressed as fibrin lysis area. The reduced activity was considered to represent the fibrinolytic ability of immobilized urokinase in peptide linking, which was certainly one of the most vital modes of linkage between urokinase and nylon. The nylon preparation still showed a fibrinolytic activity of 800 mm^2 in the first of repeated fibrinolysis test. This can be mainly ascribed to stable ionic binding, although this linkage theoretically may have been released by the washing with 1 M NaCl phosphate buffer (pH 8.0), 2% NH_4OH (pH 12.0) or 0.1 M K_2HPO_4 (pH 9.1). The decrease of fibrinolytic activity after repeated fibrinolysis test may originate partially in the segregation or destruction of immobilized urokinase in peptide linking, in addition to stable ionic binding. Figure 8 is scheme of binding forms of immobilized urokinase on nylon carrier. We can expect the stronger fibrinolytic activity in early test but only the weaker activity in late test.

4. Influence of Anti-Urokinse Antibody and Urokinase Inhibitor

The influence of anti-urokinase antibody (antibody) and urokinase inhibitor (inhibitor) to immobilized urokinase were studied by the following methods. In this experiment, we used urokinase-treated polyvinyl chloride, soluble urokinase, anti-human urokinase antibody of rabbit serum (Green Cross Corporation in Japan) and urokinase inhibitor of human placenta (same Corporation).

1) Fibrinolysis Method (Figure 9,10)

In this method, measurement was performed by the fibrin lysis area in standard human fibrin plate.

When inhibitor was added to urokinase, soluble urokinase became unable to lyze fibrin, whereas immobilized urokinase retained nearly normal fibrinolytic activity. The performance of immobilized urokinase was similar in either of the following cases: In the first case, urokinase-treated polyvinyl chloride was immersed in inhibitor solution, and then it was placed on a fibrin plate. In the second case, the material was placed on a fibrin plate, and then inhibitor was dropped on it. By the way, antibody had no influence on the fibrinolytic activities of urokinase in two different forms under these conditions.

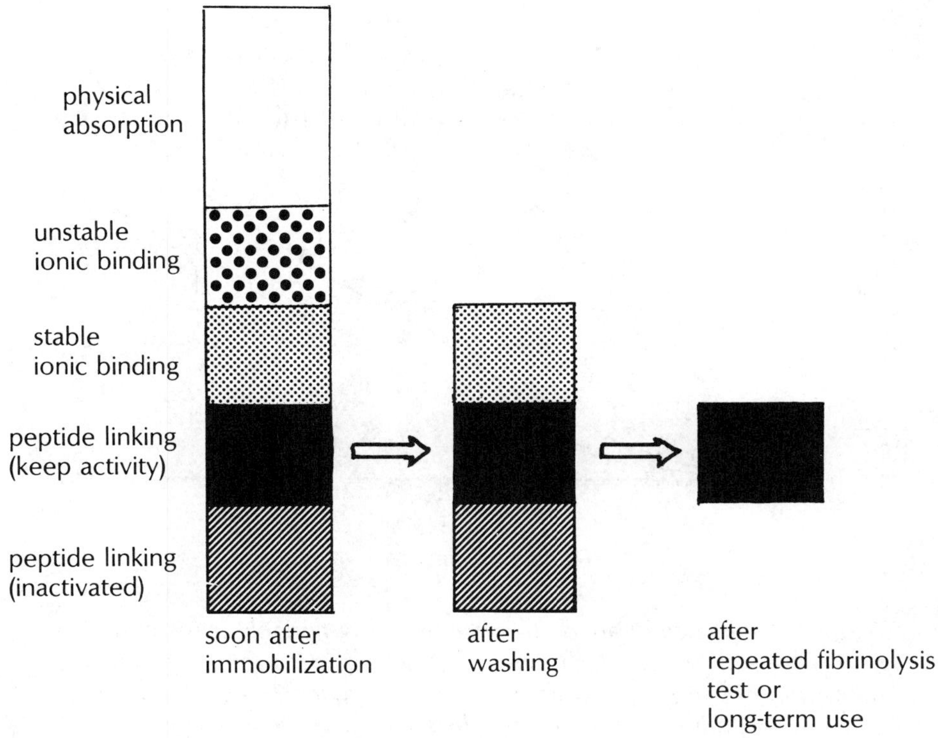

Figure 8. Scheme of binding forms of immobilized urokinase on the surface of nylon.

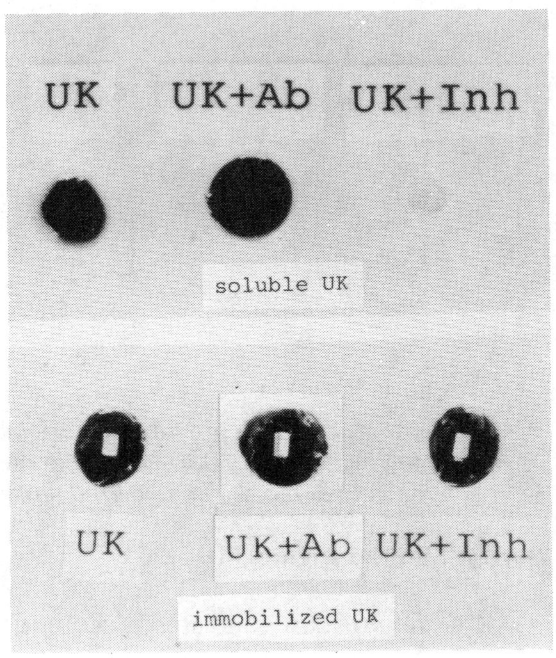

Figure 9. Influence of antibody and inhibitor in fibrinolysis method. When inhibitor (Inh) was added to soluble urokinase, its fibrinolytic activity disappeared, but enzyme activity of immobilized urokinase maintained in same treatment. Antibody (Ab)did not inhibit either of them.

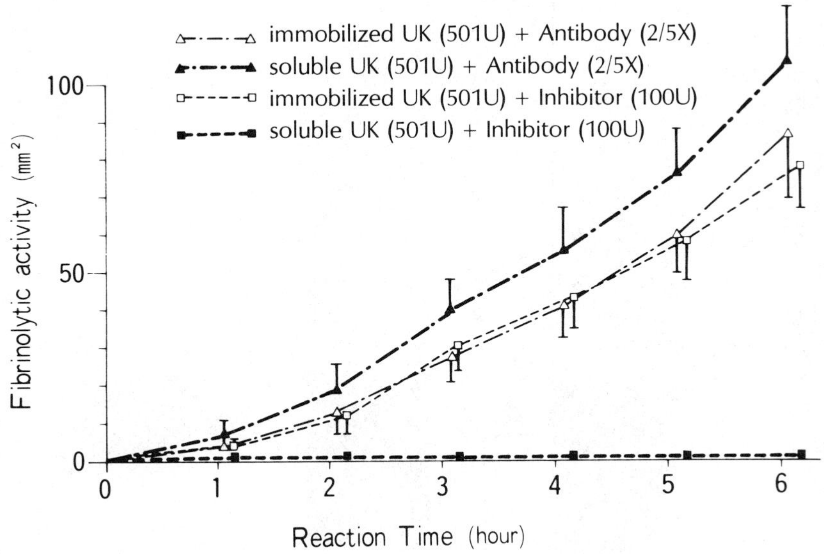

Figure 10. Influence of antibody and inhibitor in fibrinolysis method. This figure showed the serial changes of fibrin lysis area (mm²) in standard human fibrin plate which was performed in Figure 9. Soluble urokinase with inhibitor completely lost its fibrinolytic activity.

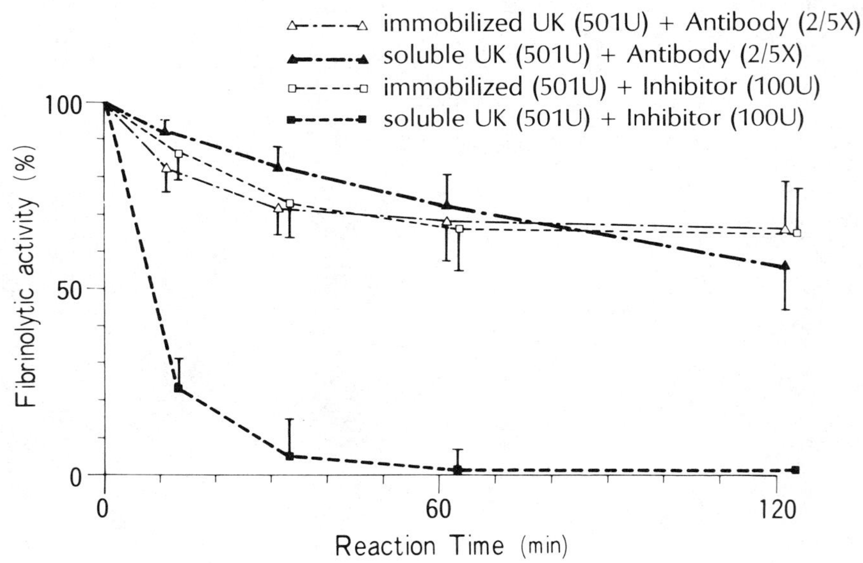

Figure 11. Influence of antibody and inhibitor in MCA method. 100 U of inhibitor completely neutralized 50 IU of soluble urokinase after 30 minutes incubation at room temperature, but not immobilized urokinase. Antibody did not inhibit either of them.

2) MCA Method (Figure 11)

MCA, a urokinase-mediated decomposition product of Glu-Gly-Arg-methylcoumarin-7 amide, was examined with a spectrofluorophotometer. Fifty IU of urokinase was used in two different forms, one was immobilized urokinase and the other was soluble urokinase. To this decomposition system, was added 2/5X of antibody, or 100 U of inhibitor.

After 50 IU of soluble urokinase was reacted with 100 U of inhibitor for 30 min at room temperature, the enzyme no longer exhibited fibrinolytic activity, while immobilized urokinase maintained its activity. It may be prudent, however, to add that when the amount of inhibitor was reduced, the extent of loss of the activity of soluble urokinase was lessened proportionally. By the way, antibody failed to inhibit the decompositive activities of urokinase in two different forms.

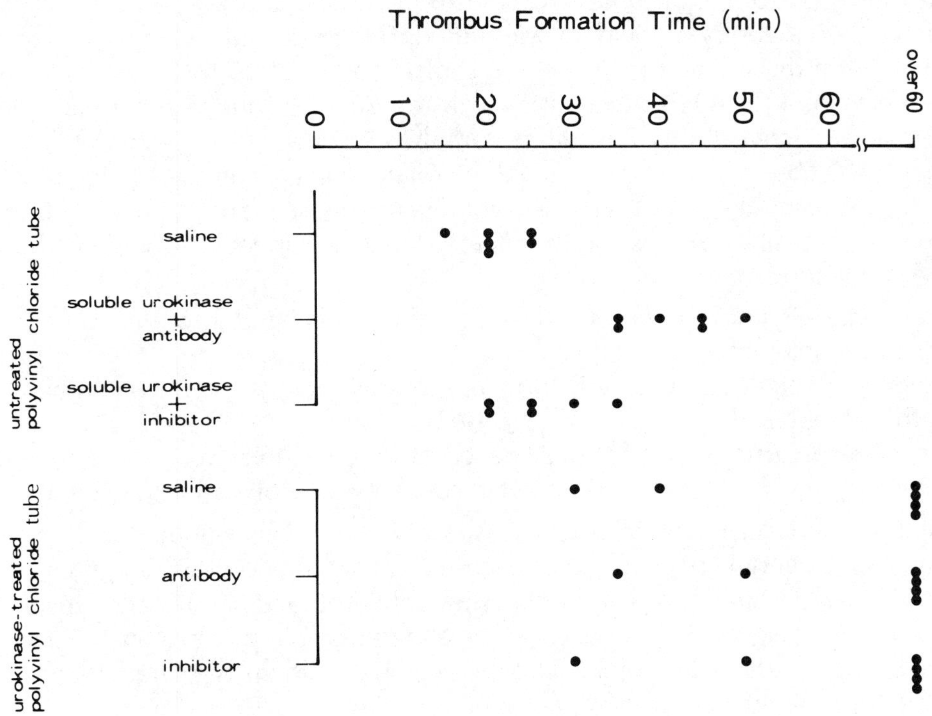

Figure 12. Influence of antibody and inhibitor in Chandler loop method. Thrombus formation time of untreated tube filled with blood containing soluble urokinase and inhibitor shortened about 20 to 35 minutes, but that of urokinase-treated tube filled with blood containing inhibitor exceeded 60 minutes.

3) Chandler Loop Method (Figure 12)

In this method, a tube coiled around an axle and filled with blood was rotated until blood lost its fluidity and formed its clot. And, the required time, that is, thrombus formation time was measured. The tube was 30 cm in length and 0.4 cm in diameter. We used two types of tubes, one was made of urokinase-treated polyvinyl chloride and the other of untreated polyvinyl chloride. One of the following was added to these tubes: equivoluminal physiological saline, 50 IU of soluble urokinase plus 2/5X of antibody, and 50 IU of soluble urokinase plus 100 U of inhibitor. The former tubes, meant by urokinase-treated tube, were not added soluble urokinase. After these treatments, each tube was filled with 0.2 ml of 3.8% citric acid, 1.8 ml of fresh whole blood and 0.2 ml of ¼ M $CaCl_2$. To sum up, we utilized three kinds of fillings for each of the two types of tubes.

In a series of experiments using untreated tubes filled with blood containing soluble urokinase and antibody, the thrombus formation time was a little longer than about 20 minutes in physiological saline series and about 25 minutes in soluble urokinase and inhibitor series. In experiments using urokinase-treated tubes filled with blood containing physiological saline, the thrombus formation time exceeded 60 minutes, and the same results were obtained when either antibody or inhibitor was added. FDP remained within normal level in two series in which the thrombus formation time shortened about 20 to 25 minutes, while it increased more than 50 μg/ml in other series with the delayed thrombus formation time. It is supposed that the increase of FDP resulted from the enzyme activity of immobilized or soluble urokinase. The fibrinolytic activity of soluble urokinase was depressed by inhibitor and that of immobilized urokinase was not. Whereas soluble urokinase is antagonized by urokinase inhibitor, immobilized urokinase is hardly affected. In this connection, one or more of the following explanations may be applicable:

(1) When urokinase is immoblized, its steric structure is changed into a form which hinders union with the inhibitor.
(2) The molecular weight of inhibitor is too large to draw near the surface of a carrier and to bind with immobilized urokinase.
(3) The surface of a carrier is not physically accessible to the inhibitor.
(4) The chance is small for the inhibitor to get in contact with urokinase when it is immobilized.

The failure of antibody to depress urokinase activity may be attributable to the facts that antibody titer is not enough to react to urokinase and that antibody binding sites are unidentical with or far away from enzyme activating sites. Inhibitor binding sites are considered identical with or closely neighboring to enzyme activating sites. Immobilized enzymes have many characteristics, compared with soluble urokinase. One of them is characterized by the insusceptibility to the influence of urokinase inhibitor.

B. DISINFECTION METHOD

The disinfection is an important problem in the clinical application of medical material. In the next experiments, we investigated the influence of antiseptic procedures to the fibrinolytic activity of immobilized urokinase, in order to establish the superior procedure.

1) Influence of Antiseptic Procedure

The experiment was performed in the sample of N-PEI-G-NP:UK, which was exposed to the five types of antiseptic procedures. The results were shown in Table 2. The activity was de-

Table 2. Influence of Disinfection to Fibrinolytic Activity of Urokinase-Treated Nylon

Antiseptic Procedure	Fibrinolytic Activity (%)
Control	100
Chlorhexidine alcohol (5-10 min)	90-95
Coction (100°C, 10-20 min)	10-30
Ethylene oxide gas (2 hrs)	40-70
Gamma ray (1.0-2.0 Mrad)	50-70
Electron beam (2.5 Mrad)	45-55

creased to 90-95% by submerging in 0.5% chlorhexidine alcohol for five to ten minutes, to 40-70% by treatment with 10% ethylene oxide gas for two hours, gamma rays (1.0-2.0 Mrad) or electron beams (2.5 Mrad), and to 10-30% by 100°C coction for 10 to 20 minutes. In consequence, 0.5% chlorhexidine alcohol showed a good performance, in that the fibrinolytic activity of the sample was almost unaffected. Its performance was followed by those of ethylene oxide gas, gamma rays and electron beams. In these procedures, the higher the temperature set is, the lower the fibrinolytic activity is. Out of the emergency measurement of disinfection, the submerging procedure in 0.5% chlorhexidine alcohol is better. The fibrinolytic activity of immobilized urokinase tolerated until 60 minutes (Figure 13), but that in the coction procedure did until 15 minutes (Figure 14).

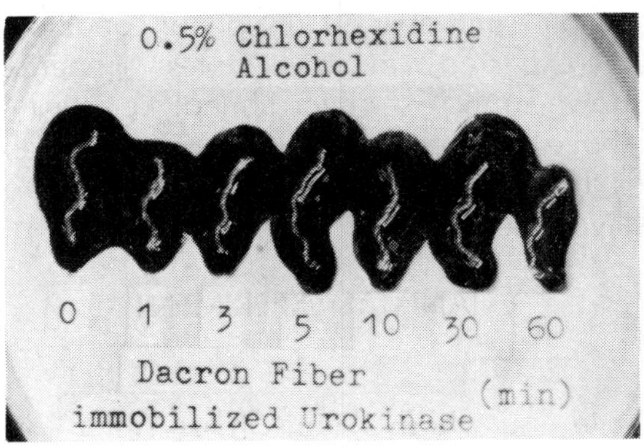

Figure 13. Influence of antiseptic procedure by alcohol. When urokinase-treated dacron was submerged in 0.5% chlorhexidine alcohol, its fibrinolytic activity tolerated until 60 minutes.

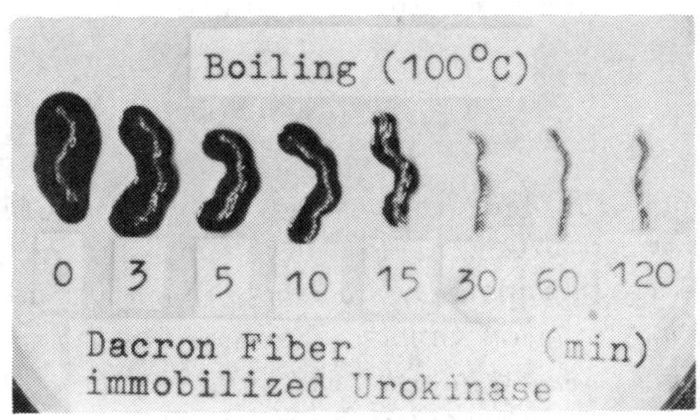

Figure 14. Influence of antiseptic procedure by coction. When urokinase-treated dacron was placed in boiling water, its fibrinolytic activity tolerated until 15 minutes.

2) Investigation of Gamma Ray Irradiation Method

In pursuit of a better result, it was attempted to disinfect nylon possessing binding sites where urokinase had not yet been immobilized. That is to say, the disinfection process

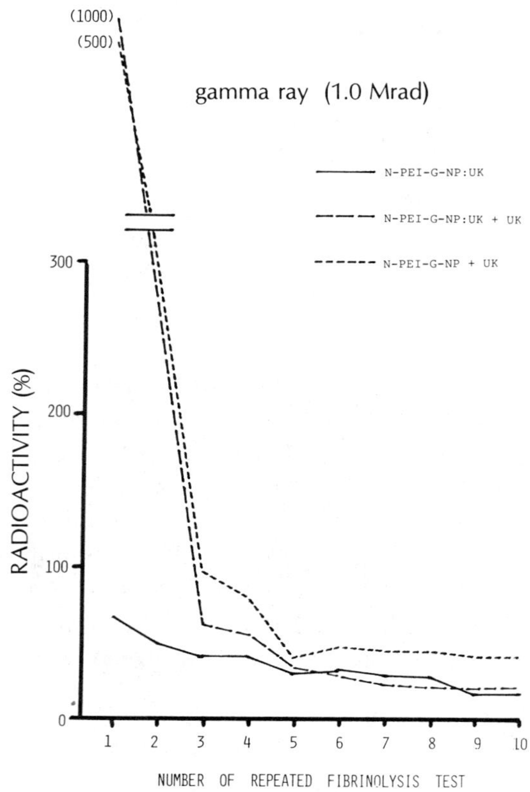

Figure 15. Fibrinolytic activities in three types of urokinase-treated nylon with the antiseptic procedure of gamma ray irradiation. Fibrinolytic activities of nylon samples, proceeded by irradiation, displayed in high level in the first time of repeated fibrinolysis test.

preceded the immobilization process. In this experiment, the gamma ray irradiation method was employed exclusively. This disinfection process was combined with the immobilization process in different ways and the following three types of nylon samples were prepared: 1) immobilization + irradiation (N-PEI-G-NP:UK), 2) immobilization + irradiation + immobilization (N-PEI-G-NP:UK + UK), and 3) irradiation + immobilization (N-PEI-G-NP + UK). Figure 15 shows the result of gamma ray irradiation method. The last two types, which were proceded by irradiation, exhibited high fibrinolytic activities ranging from, 1,000 to 500% when used for the first time of repeated fibrinolysis test. Their values fell to 60%~100% in the third time test, and subsequently maintained at around 20~40%. The gamma ray irradiation seems to play a part of increasing the binding sites of immobilization, which may be stable ionic binding. Compared with them, irradiation + immobilization (N-PEI-G-NP + UK) was better. In this type, urokinase was not exposed to the antiseptic procedure. Thus the enzyme could be immobilized in superior condition. As expected, nylon samples prepared showed much stronger fibrinolytic activity. Above all, gamma ray irradiation followed by the immobilization of urokinase led to favorable results.

C. ANIMAL EXPERIMENT

In our body, fibrinolysis system is controlled under the antagonistic function of antiplasmin. When antiplasmin becomes relatively active, fibrinolysis system does not work. Then, it is questionable whether urokinase-treated polymeric material artificially provided has the antithrombogenicity in vivo. The following animal experiments were performed to resolve this question.

1) Retention Test in Venous Vessel

A urokinase-treated nylon for vascular suture material with atraumatic needle was punctured and placed into the inferior caval vein of rat. After a five-minute retention, it was carefully extracted together with a fragment of the vein containing it, and the status of thrombus formation on the surface of nylon filament was examined.

Figure 16 is the photographs of urokinase-treated nylon and untreated nylon. The former is not apt to form thrombus, while the latter is easy to adhere fibrin membrane or buffy-coat clot. Table 3 shows the results of thrombus formation. Thrombus formation was unseen in 33.3% of the urokinase-treated nylon, while in only 8.3% of the untreated nylon. This means that the antithrombogenic effect of the former is approximately four times as great as that of the latter. It may be added, however, that thrombus formation of "membrane" grade was more frequent in both groups: the frequency was 59.2% in urokinase-treated nylon and 79.2% in untreated nylon. The thrombus formation on nylon filament may be rather related to the unskillful suture technique than the character of material, but immobilized urokinase on the surface of material can play one of the important roles not to adhere fibrin membrane or buffy-coat clot.

Same result was obtained in experiment in which venous wall of rat was continuously sewed by urokinase-treated nylon (Figure 17).

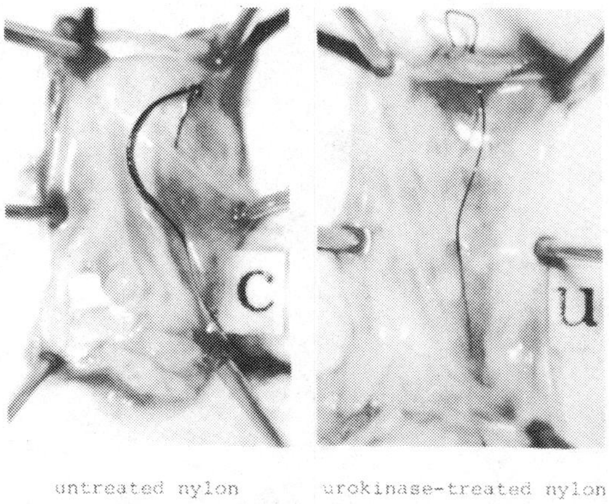

Figure 16. Photograph of nylon filament retained in inferior caval vein of rat. Untreated nylon was covered with fibrin membrane after five minutes, but urokinase-treated nylon was not.

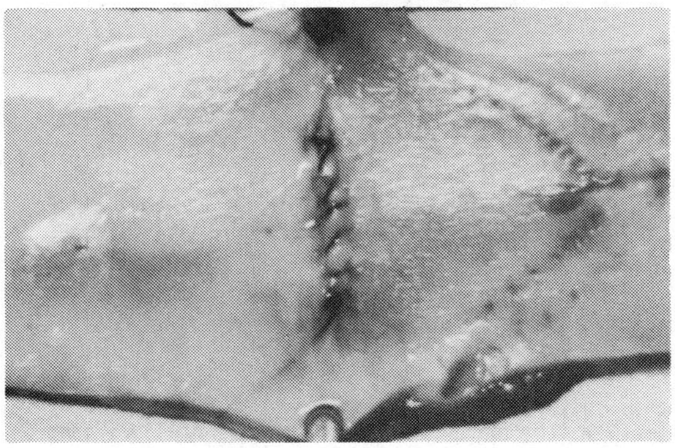

Figure 17. Photograph of nylon filament sewed venous wall of rat. Urokinase-treated nylon was almost intact without thrombus formation three days postoperatively.

We understand the significance of urokinase-treated polymeric material which has the antithrombogenicity in vivo, as follows. Blood coagulation incessantly occurs not only during the contact with foreign body but also with vascular vessel. But the reason why circulating blood can maintain its fluidity in vascular vessel is that it is on a dynamic equilibrium between coagulation and fibrinolysis systems. To be more precise, the endothelium of vascular vessel activates contact factor (Factor XII) for fibrin formation, but simultaneously acts as a trigger for the lysis of microfibrin so formed. The surface of urokinase-treated polymeric material is similar to the endothelium of vascular vessel with physiological antithrombogenicity, because the surface has the two characteristic functions to lead both coagulation and fibrinolysis phenomena. It is entirely physiological and rational to give the fibrinolytic activity to the surface of material.

2) Retention Test in Abdominal Cavity

Some pieces of ^{125}I-labeled urokinase-treated nylon were placed in the abdominal

Table 3. Thrombus Formation on Vascular Suture Material Made of Urokinase-Treated and Untreated Nylon

Vascular suture material	Thrombus (%)		
	none	membrane	clot
Urokinase-treated nylon	33.3	59.2	7.4
Untreated nylon	8.3	79.2	12.5

cavity of rat. The nylon sheets thus retained intraperitoneally were taken out one after another during 2 weeks for measurement of isotop counts. The radioactivity of each piece was shown in Figure 18. Given that the radioactivity before retention was 100%, it was 36 ± 16% on the first day and 21 ± 8% on the second day and subsequently, it maintained about 20%. This decreased pattern is similar to that in fibrinolytic activity of urokinase-treated nylon in repeated fibrinolysis test.

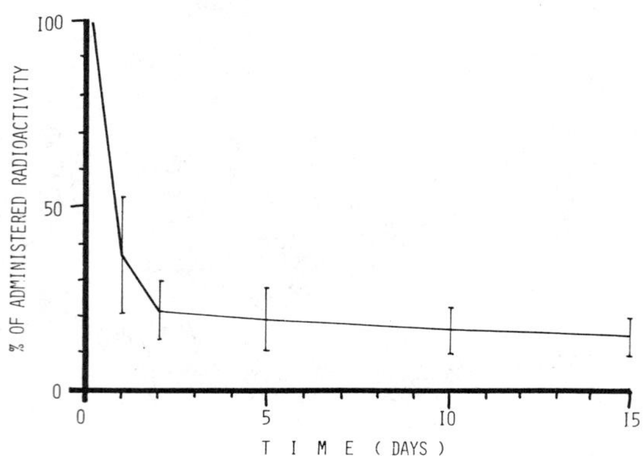

Figure 18. Radioactivity in ^{125}I-labeled urokinase-treated nylon retained in abdominal cavity of rat. Its radioactivity gradually decreased and maintained about 20% of administered radioactivity after two days.

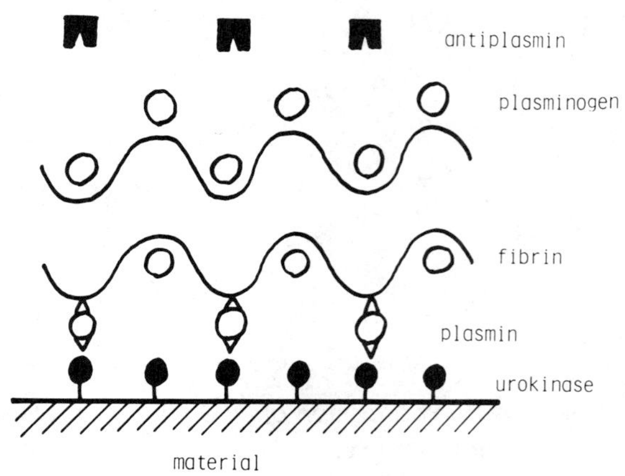

Figure 19. Scheme of antithrombogenic mechanism of urokinase-treated polymeric material.

3) Antithrombogenic Mechanism

The antithrombogenic mechanism (Figure 19) of urokinase-treated polymeric material may be interpreted, as follows: When blood gets in contact with the surface of material, Factor XII is activated and a lot of fibrin monomer are formed lastly. Then, plasminogen which has affinity for fibrin gathers around each fibrin monomer so formed. Consequently, urokinase converts plasminogen into plasmin to start fibrinolysis. This mechanism is characterized by the next points.

(1) Lysis of fibrin as seen on the surface of material occurs directly at the site of contact between the two, so that it is not affected by antiplasmin present in blood abundantly.

(2) The situation thus created on the surface of material has a close resemblance to the antithrombogenicity of endothelium in vascular vessel.
(3) Fibrinolysis uninterruptedly taking place on the surface of material is nothing but a localized phenomenon and it is never generalized.

D. CLINICAL APPLICATION

The possibility that urokinase-treated polymeric material had the antithrombogenicity in vivo was already foreseen by Kusserow [8]. This appeared to be supported by the present experiment. Then we started to have some clinical trials.

1. Utility of Urokinase-Treated Evatate Tube for Total Parenteral Nutrition in Fasting Patient

Because of the persistent strong desire of clinicians for the therapy of total parenteral nutrition, there is an increasing necessity for intravenously retained catheters, which are required to be at least durable, nontoxic, nonseptic and antithrombogenic. In an attempt to satisfy these requirements, catheters made of various different types of polymeric materials have been devised. The clinical usefulness of these devices has been recognized when used for a few days. However, their long-term use lasting for several weeks to several months does not necessarily lead to favorable results. This is because even polymeric materials have a defect in terms of the antithrombogenicity. Thrombogenesis is due to factors related to blood itself rather than polymeric material. Intrinsically, blood easily clots upon contact with foreign body. Catheters for intravenous retention are made of materials which are physicochemically stable, but they may still trigger blood coagulation system.

Here, we prepared urokinase-treated Evatate tube which was made of ethylene vinyl acetate copolymer. The catheter, 1.5 mm in diameter and 40-70 cm in length, has the fibrinolytic activity of 38.8 to 26.4 IU/10 cm of tube (ca 4 IU/cm^2) as shown in Figure 20. Its tip is blunted. A radiopaque line covering the whole length of it is drawn. The catheter is inserted in superior caval vein through right subclavian vein. In the presence of fibrin membrane attached to the surface of the catheter, it is judged that thrombus was formed. In some cases, it was examined by pullout venography, instead of macroscopic observation. The fibrinolytic activity was measured by MCA method. We tried them clinically in 55 patients.

Table 4 shows the clinical findings. Out of 55, 35 were in after operation, 12 in during serious illness and 8 in end stadium. Thrombi were formed during the use of six catheters (10.9%), while 49 (89.1%) were free from them (Figure 21). Bleeding from puncture eye, fever up from catheterization, and catheter occlusion from thrombus formation are generally known as complications associated with the use of conventional catheters. In our cases, a febrile condition was the only abnormality that might be ascribable to catheterization. It developed in no more than 5 cases and was present continuously after withdrawal of catheters. In view of these observations, we presumed that there was no correlation between thrombus formation and fever up. Although the fibrinolytic activity of Evatate tube decreased with the extension of retention period, it yet showed an activity of approximately 1.7 IU/10 cm of tube after one week and 0.3 IU/10 cm of tube after three weeks. Among the 55 catheters used, those to which clots were attached are shown with the mark * in Figure 22. As

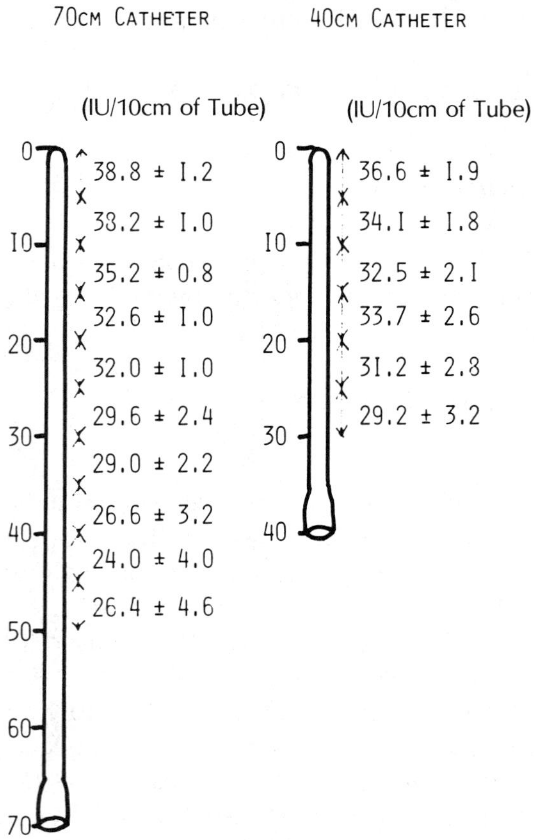

Figure 20. Fibrinolytic activity of urokinase-treated Evatate tube. Evatate tube had about 35 IU/10 cm of tube, which corresponded to about 4IU/cm². Enzyme activity was measured by MCA method.

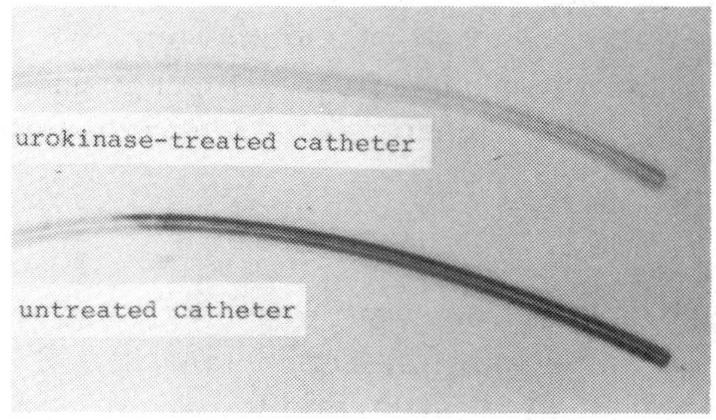

Figure 21. Photograph of Evatate tube used for intravenous catheterization. Urokinase-treated catheter had no thrombus, while untreated-catheter was covered with it.

seen therefrom, the thrombus formation correlated not with the retention period of catherization but with the fibrinolytic activity of Evatate tube. Of the six catheters that failed to prevent thrombus formation, five gave a value of less than 1 IU/10 cm of tube. There were a total of 24 catheters whose fibrinolytic activity lowered under 1 IU/10 cm of tube. The five catheters accounted for 20.8% of them. On the other hand, there were 27 catheters which gave a value above 1 IU/10 cm of tube and only one (3.7%) of them was associated with thrombus formation. The three catheters retained for 5, 32 and 64 days were subjected to tension tests and were found not to have been deteriorated in quality.

When thrombi are formed on an intravenously retained catheter, it becomes quite difficult to supply transfusions as planned and, to worsen the matter, the following complications may be induced: 1) thrombophlebitis, 2) venous occlusion (such as superior vena cava syndrome), 3) pulmonary embolism, and 4) pulmonary congestion. In the event a febrile condition has developed without any evident cause in patients with intravenous catheterization, such complications are suspected and catheters are removed and exchanged. For prophylactic purposes, we make it a rule to perform the catheter exchange periodically in patients under long-term therapy of total parenteral nutrition. It is unavoidable, however, that the catherization procedures impose much physical and mental burdens on those patients, their family members and surgeons. Naturally, it has been desired to lighten these burdens as far as possible. One of the promising methods is to immobilize antithrombogenic substances on the surface of catheter. Increasing attention has been paid to such devices for the following reasons:

1) Its preservation is easy and usage is simple.

Table 4. Utility of Urokinase-Treated Evatate Tube for Total Parenteral Nutrition in Fasting Patient

Clinical Cases	**55 (56.4 Years Old)**
Sex	
male	38 (69.1%)
female	17 (30.9%)
Used time	
after operation	35 (63.6%)
during serious illness	13 (21.8%)
in end stadium	8 (14.6%)
Purpose	total parenteral nutrition
Method	through subclavian vein
Retention period	16.1 ± 13.9 days (1-69 days)
Thrombus formation	
formed	6 (10.9%)
not formed	49 (89.1%)
Side effect	nothing

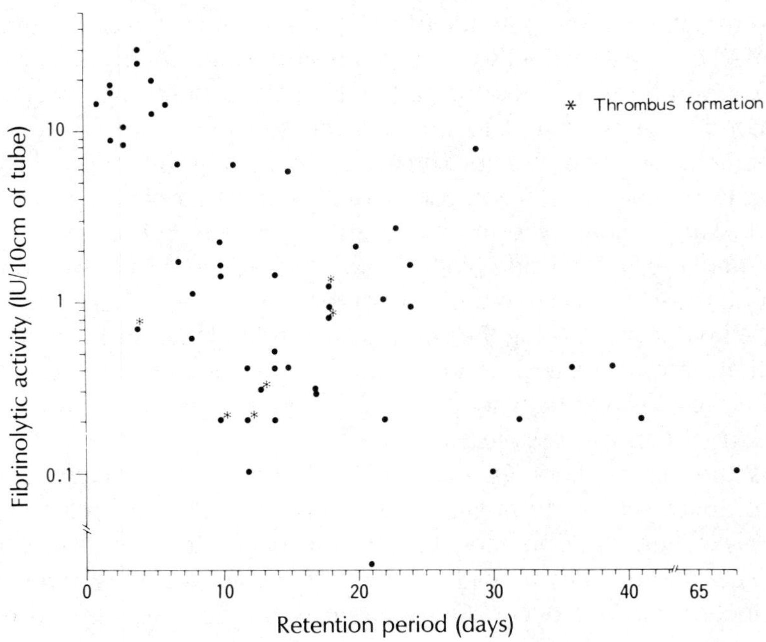

Figure 22. Fibrinolytic activity of urokinase-treated Evatate tube after catheterization. Its fibrinolytic activity gradually decreased in parallel with the retention period of catheterization.

2) It exerts a localized and sustained antithrombogenic ability.
3) It is rational and in addition economical.

Using urokinase-treated Evatate tube, we tested it at a clinical level. As touched upon earlier, the device was excellent in respect of not only antithrombogenicity but also security. These outcomes support the clinical usefulness of our catheter. In this work, the incidence of thrombus formation was as low as 6/55 (roughly 10%), which can be by far favorably compared with the incidence of conventional catheter (50-95%). The new catheter had the possibility of longer retention because it did not become fragile even during two months of retention. Examination of the six catheters disclosed that the thrombus formation occurred to only those whose fibrinolytic activity was much lowered. This fact well attests to the observations that thrombogenesis took place at a high incidence consequent upon the use of conventional catheter. Simultaneously, it strongly suggests the value of immobilizing antithrombogenic substances on the surface of catheter.

2. Utility of Urokinase-Treated Nylon Threads for Lymph Drainage in Lymphedema

Known as one of surgical operations to treat lymphedema is Handley's method which is to embed lymph drainage materials in edematous subcutaneous tissue. In this method, stagnant lymph is led to healthy subcutaneous tissue through the interspace provided within such materials and is absorbed there to return to the systemic circulation. Such materials are available in the form of threads, tubes or wicks made of silk, nylon or teflon. The passage of lymph through the interspace is smooth soon after embedding but is stopped by clotting of lymph and invasion of connective tissue after several weeks and, as a result, lymphedema develops again.

With a view to maintaining the patency of the interspace, we prepared urokinase-treated nylon threads twined of more than a thousand fibers and tested them clinically in 12 patients. In moderate cases, operations were performed by Handley's method only. First, small skin incisions were prepared at an interval of 15 cm in an affected limb. Threads were slided into the subcutis and embedded to creep by approximately 5 cm along the muscle layer, penetrating through the fascia. In severe cases, Thompson's method was employed in combination with Handley's method. Longitudinal incision covering the entire length of an affected limb was performed in the medial or lateral side. Pathological tissues were then excised together with part of the thickened muscle fascia in either side of the limb. After that a de-epitherialized dermal flap was formed without breaking the superficial lymph plexus and was enfolded into the muscle layer. At that time, threads were embedded in the subcutis, provided that they were passed through the muscle layer halfway (Figure 23). One of the threads was retained as near to the enfolded dermal flap as possible.

Table 5 shows the clinical findings. Out of 12, 4 were in primary type and 7 were in secondary type complicated by the radical operations of uterine or breast cancer. Eight patients obtained the excellent or good effect to reduce in circumference of affected limb (Figure 24). The sclerotic subcutaneous tissue with lymphedema was weakened even in 3 patients to whom such a reduction did not occur. One patient was made worse from the infection of embedded threads. Figure 25 displays the correlation of circumference and RI delayed rate of affected limb before and after operations. It is an intriguing question how long the fibrinolytic activity of urokinase-treated nylon threads is sustainable in vivo. In this study, the threads ten-

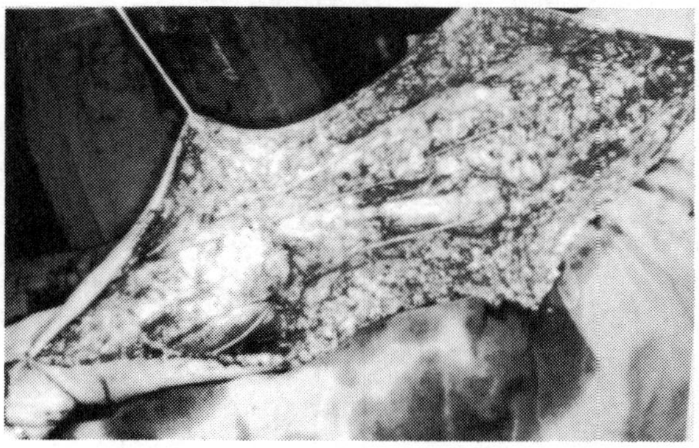

Figure 23. Photograph of Thompson's method combined with Handley's method for lymphedema. Three pieces of urokinase-treated nylon threads were embedded in subcutis.

Table 5. Utility of Urokinase-Treated Nylon Threads for Lymph Drainage in Lymphedema

Clinical cases	12 (41.5 years old)
Sex	
male	1 (8.3%)
female	11 (91.7%)
Classification	
primary	4 (33.3%)
secondary	7 (58.3%)
other	1 (8.3%)
unknown	0
Localization	
upper extremity	3 (25.0%)
lower extremity	9 (75.0%)
Clinical effect	
excellent	2 (16.7%)
good	6 (50.0%)
moderate	3 (25.0%)
poor	1 (8.3%)

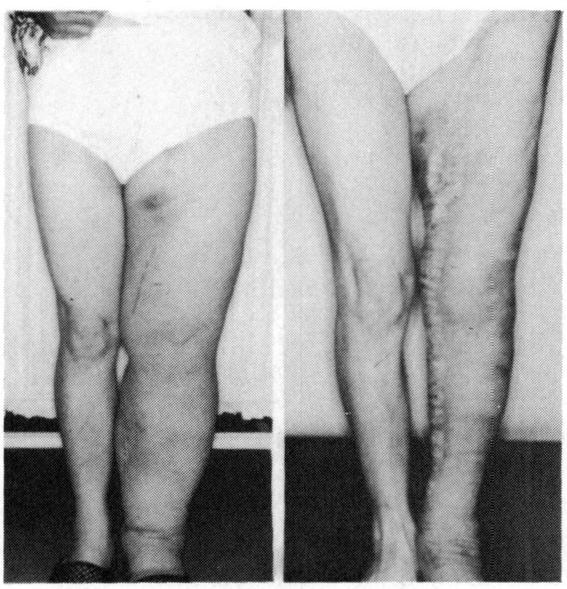

before operation after operation

Figure 24. Photograph of lymphedema before and after operation. This patient, 43 years old female, suffered from primary lymphedema and two years ago underwent Handley's method with silk fibers. But recurrence occurred. She underwent our operation, in combination method, shown in Figure 23. Left shows the recurrent finding and right does the improved finding one year postoperatively.

tively withdrawn 20 months postoperatively possessed about 5% of the original activity. This histological observations are briefed, as follows: Though connective tissues invaded into part of the interspace between fine fibers of nylon threads to occlude capillary lumens, the extent of invasion was mild. It was supposed that the threads had yet been functioning as lymphatic pathway at that stage (Figure 26).

The original Handley's method which embeds silk fibers has the two weak points that it has neither antithrombogenic ability nor valvular function. As possible resolutions to the problems involved, we made the following improvements:

1) Urokinase, one of fibrinolytic enzymes, was immobilized on the surface of nylon threads to have them acquire an antithrombogenic ability.
2) The partial portion of subcutaneously embedded threads was passed through the muscle layer. In this system, it is supposed that movement provides a valvular function.

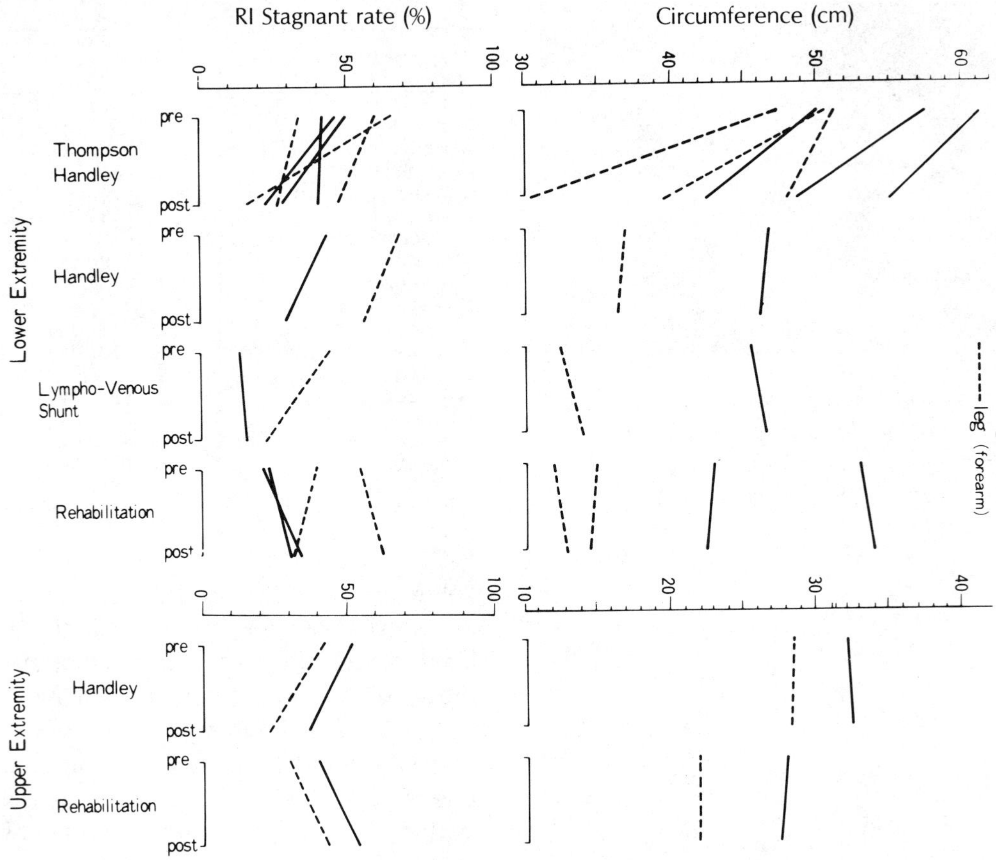

Figure 25. Correlation of circumference and RI stagnant rate in affected limb.

3. Utility of Urokinase-Treated Polyvinyl Chloride Tube for Liquid Drainage in Thoracic Surgery

Major surgery occasionally fails to draw off the liquid including hemorrhagic effusion through the drain inserted in advance, and we can often find the fibrin clots adhered to the hole of drain which stops to discharge. In thoracic surgery, these postoperative troubles cause the serious complications such as atelectasis, pneumonia, abscess, sepsis etc.

Now, we devised urokinase-treated polyvinyl chloride tube for liquid drainage and used them 29 times in 19 patients. Table 6 shows the clinical findings. The mean retention period of drainage was 5.9 days (3-15 days). Thrombi resemble to buffy-coat clot were observed in 4 tubes (13.8%), while not in 25 tubes (86.2%) (Figure 27). None of the patients suffered from any complications. The fibrinolytic activity of individual drain after retention was shown in Figure 28. The initial activity of 190 IU/10 cm of tube (ca 8 IU/cm^2) went down to 35 IU/10 cm of tube 6 days after retention. Four drains with buffy-coat clot remained in remarkably high activity.

It is generally known that thoracic and abdominal effusion possess the abundant amount of plasmin and keep the fluidity. It is difficult, however, to take off the clots which is once formed

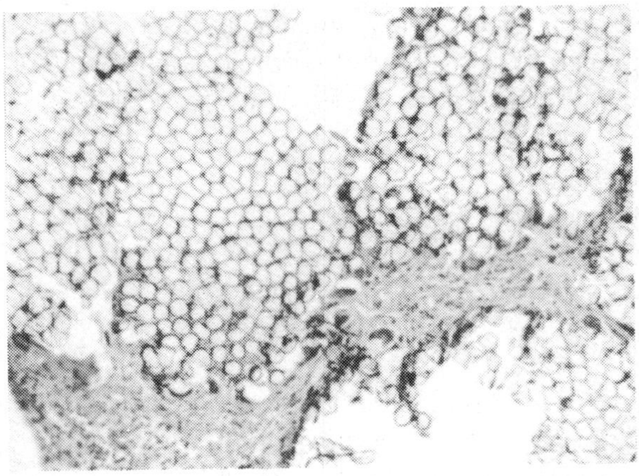

Figure 26. Histology of urokinase-treated nylon threads. A piece of nylon threads was tentatively withdrawn 20 months postoperatively. The invasion of connective tissue into interspace of nylon threads was mild.

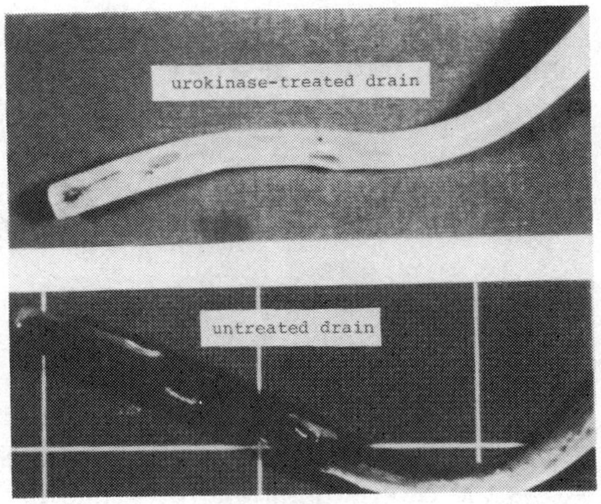

Figure 27. Photograph of drain used for liquid drainage. Urokinase-treated polyvinyl chloride drain had no thrombus, while untreated polyvinyl chloride drain was covered with it.

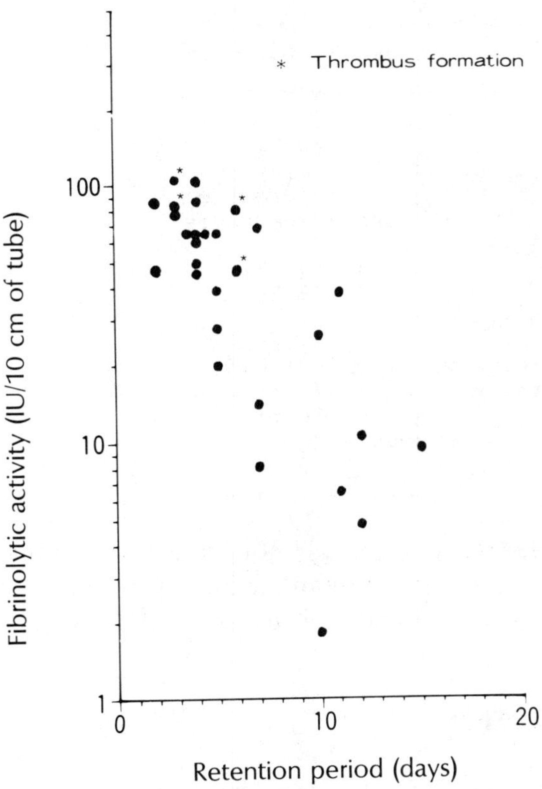

Figure 28. Fibrinolytic activity of urokinase-treated polyvinyl chloride drain after drainage. Its fibrinolytic activity gradually decreased in parallel with the retention period of drainage.

Table 6. Utility of Urokinase-Treated Polyvinyl Chloride Tube for Liquid Drainage in Thoracic Surgery

Clinical case	19 (60.8 y.o.)
Sex	
male	13 (68.4%)
female	6 (31.6%)
Purpose	drainage in thoracic surgery
Drainage period	5.9±2.8 days
Thrombus formation	
formed	4/29 (13.8%)
not formed	25/29 (86.2%)
Side effect	nothing

on the surface of drain. When the drainage from thoracic or abdominal cavity does not work within early postoperative days, surgeon is perplexed to reinsert another drain until the occurrence of complications. Urokinase-treated polyvinyl chloride tube seems to be beneficial.

4. Utility of Urokinase-Treated Nylon Filament for Arterial Anastomosis in Vascular Surgery

In microvascular surgery, minute thrombi formed on suture material become the cause of reocclusion. Then urokinase-treated nylon filament of 3-0 to 5-0 size were used for sewing the small vascular vessels.

This procedure was attempted 59 times in a total of 28 patients needing the reconstruction of iliac to femoral artery, sized with angiitis, arteriosclerosis, aneurysm or trauma. Table 7 shows the clinical findings. Three had bifurcated prosthetic grafts and 25 did straight ones, which were anastomosed by urokinase-treated nylon filament with atraumatic needle. During the mean follow up period of 2 years and 8 months, favorable blood flow was maintained in 20 cases (71.4%), while the prosthetic grafts were occlused in 8 cases (28.6%), consist of 3 in thromboangiitis obliterans and 5 in arteriosclerosis obliterans.

Table 7. Utility of Urokinase-Treated Nylon Filament for Arterial Anastomosis in Vascular Surgery

Clinical cases	28 (58.1 y.o.)
Sex	
male	24 (85.7%)
female	4 (14.3%)
Purpose	artery-prosthetic graft anastomosis
Prosthetic graft	
bifurcated graft	3 (10.7%)
straight graft	25 (89.3%)
Total number of anastomosis	
abdominal aorta	3/59 (5.1%)
common-external iliac artery	18/59 (30.5%)
superficial femoral artery	38/59 (64.4%)
Occlusion of graft	8 (28.6%)
Cause of occlusion	unknown

Although the real factor responsible for the reocclusion was not known, the urokinase-treated suture material was thought to have been useful for retarding thrombus formation on the suture line. Presumably, such a material will be beneficial, especially for suturing the venous wall.

CONCLUSIONS

The characteristic findings in our experiences on immobilized urokinase are briefly described, as follows:

1) Immobilized urokinase has a fibrinolytic activity.

2) The immobilizable amount of urokinase augments with increase in the number of binding sites of carrier.
3) This immobilized urokinase is partly released or inactivated after repeated fibrinolysis test.
4) The binding form between urokinase and carrier is due 20-30% to covalent binding and 70-80% to stable ionic binding.
5) The enzyme activity of immobilized urokinase is not almost injured by urokinase inhibitor.
6) Urokinase-treated polymeric materials show an antithrombogenic ability in vivo.

The necessity for antithrombogenic medical devices will further increase in future. Although it must be admitted that even our urokinase-treated polymeric material has both merits and demerits, we consider that the technique involved can be utilized in various related fields and hope that clinicians will find use for it as one of such devices.

REFERENCES

1. Ambrus, C. M., Roholt, O. A., Meyer, B. K. Enzymatic activity of insolubilized streptokinase (I-SK) and urokinase (I-UK). Fed. Proc. 31:267 Abs, 1972.
2. Deuth, D. G., Mertz, E. T. Activation of plasminogen with insoluble derivatives of urokinase. J. Med., 3:224, 1972.
3. Kusserow, B. K., Larrow, R. Use of surface bonded, covalently cross-linked urokinase as an approach to the creation of a Thromboresistant synthetic surface with fibrinolytic capability. Circulation, Suppl. 2:54, 1972.
4. Wiman, B., Wallen, P. Activation of human plasminogen by an insoluble derivative of urokinase. Structural changes of plasminogen with course of activation to plasmin and demonstration of a possible intermediate compound. Eur. J. Biochem, 36:25, 1973.
5. Ohshiro, T., Mukai, K., Koh, S., Sakamoto, S., Sugitachi, A., Murakami, F. Fibrinolytic therapy – The necessity and possibility of local fibrinolytic therapy. J. Med. Enzymol (Japan). 1:72, 1975.
6. Capet-Antonini, F. C., Grimard, M., Tamenasse, J. Properties of two types of solid-phase urokinase preparations. Thromb. Res, 2:479, 1973.
7. Ohshiro, T., Kosaki, G. Urokinase immobilized on medical polymeric materials: Fundamental and clinical studies. Artificial Organs, 4:58, 1980.
8. Kusserow, B. K., Larrow, R. W., Nichols, J. E. The surface bonded, covalently cross-linked urokinase synthetic surface. In vitro and chronic in vivo studies. Trans. Am. Soc. Artif. Intern. Organs, 19:8, 1973.

Chapter 14

Antithrombogenic Biomedical Materials Improved by Enzyme Immobilization Technique

Yoshiharu Miura
Department of Biochemical Engineering
Faculty of Pharmaceutical Sciences
Osaka University
Suita, Osaka, Japan

ABSTRACT

Thrombus formation is a serious unresolved problem in the clinical application of artificial organs. Thrombus is formed on the surfaces of biomaterials implanted in circulating blood; thrombus formation is triggered by both intrinsic and extrinsic coagulation factors, platelet aggregation and/or platelet adhesion onto the biomaterials surfaces.

Heparin has been found to be an effective systemic anticoagulant, since Heparin accelerates the neutralization rate of activated coagulation factors. Another systemic anticoagulant in current clinical use in Urokinase. Therefore, systemic administration of Heparin and Urokinase has been investigated to prevent thrombus formation on the surface of implanted biomaterials. Unfortunately, systemic administration of Heparin or Urokinase is rapidly eliminated from blood, and thus large concentrations of anticoagulant are required. Large amount administration of Heparin is known to cause bleeding, platelet aggregation and adhesion.

Antithrombogenic characteristics of biomaterials can be increased by enzyme immobilization techniques, since the pharmacological activity of immobilized enzyme is generally more stable than that of the native enzyme. This chapter reviews improvements of surface thrombogenicity by the enzyme immobilization technique through prevention of surface thrombus formation and platelet aggregation. Employing a cyanogen bromide activiation procedure, immobilization of anticoagulants was successfully applied to some biomaterials, such as PVA, poly HEMA and silicone-coated nylon.

I. INTRODUCTION

Thrombus formation is a serious problem at the surgical therapy and clinical application of artificial organs. Therefore, the need for the creation of high antithrombogenic biomaterials has been increasing. Thrombus formation is caused by blood coagulation, platelet aggregation and/or platelet adhesion onto foreign surfaces. Blood coagulation is now somewhat elucidated at the molecular level. The coagulation is triggered by both intrinsic and extrinsic causes and coagulation factors, i.e. clotting factors, are successively activated. Factor X, one of the coagulation factors, is at the intersection of the two pathways, intrinsic and extrinsic. Activated Factor X, Factor Xa, converts prothrombin to thrombin. At the last stage of blood coagulation, thrombin catalyzes the proteolysis of fibrinogen to fibrin and fibrin clot results. Antithrombin III (AT III) inactivates a number of the activated coagulation factors including Factor Xa and thrombin [1-4]. Urokinase has a fibrinolytic activity. Therefore, AT III and urokinase play the important roles for keeping the liquidity of blood.

The mechanisms of blood coagulation and platelet aggregation have been studied extensively in vitro, but there is little knowledge about the relationship of these mechanisms with thrombus formation. The clarification of mechanism of thrombus formation is very important for creating high antithrombogenetic biomaterials. Platelet adhesion onto foreign surfaces takes place as soon as the blood is in contact with the surfaces. The adhering platelets release some constituents such as ADP and serotonin, which apparently cause the subsequent platelet aggregation [5]. The aggregated platelets release phospholipids, which potentiate the activation of cascade reactions in blood coagulation pathway [6]. When platelets are altered in consequence of adhesion and aggregation, several blood coagulation factors may be released and adsorbed onto platelets and accelerate the coagulation [7].

Heparin has been found to be an effective anticoagulant, since heparin accelerate the neutralization rate of activated coagulation factors by AT III [8-11]. Therefore, the administrations of heparin as well as urokinase have been commonly done to prevent the thrombus formation. Those administered materials are, however, rapidly eliminated from blood and a large amount of them are required. The large amount administration of heparin causes bleeding, and platelet aggregation and adhesion [12,13].

The durability of antithrombogenetic activity of biomaterials can be increased by using the enzyme immobilization technique, since the activity of immobilized enzyme is generally more stable than that of native enzyme. In this review, the improvements of antithrombogenecity by the enzyme immobilization technique are discussed through preventions of blood coagulation and platelet aggregation.

2. CHARACTERISTICS OF IMMOBILIZED HEPARIN (I-HEP)

2.1 Introduction

The continuous administration of heparin is a common practice for preventing the blood coagulation. But the administration of heparin often brings about hemorrhage. Therefore, various anticoagulative biomaterials have been investigated in order to make heparin-administration unnecessary. Heparinized biomaterials have already been prepared by various techniques [14-23]. It is well known that heparinized biomaterials prepared by ionic binding exhibit good antithrombogenecity [20-22]. In materials so bound, however, heparin are eluted gradually into the blood stream, so the antithrombogenecity of these heparinized biomaterials disappear in a short time. In order to ensure durable antithrombogenetic effect, it is more desirable to obtain biomaterials that have tightly bound heparin and exhibit sufficient anticoagulative activity. Several biomaterials on which heparin was covalently bound have been prepared, but those had little antithrombogenetic activity. In this section, the anticoagulative characteristics of covalently immobilized heparin (I-Hep) is described, using the experimental results of author et al. [24].

2.2 Antithrombin Activity of Immobilized Heparin

The reactivity between I-Hep and thrombin was investigated by the following procedure. The remaining thrombin activities after the reaction with I-Hep were measured by means of the clotting time method using fibrinogen as a substrate, and also by a new method [25] in which a Tert-butoxycarbonyl-L-valyl-L-prolyl-L-arginine-4-methyl-coumarinyl-7-amide (peptide-MCA) was used as a low molecular-weight substrate. Bovine serum albumin was immobilized as a control preparation. No effect of control preparation on thrombin and Factor Xa was observed at all.

Thrombin binding to I-Hep was measured by the following procedure. Thrombin solution was incubated with I-Hep gel for 10 min at 37°C. After removal of I-Hep from the incubation mixture, the thrombin activity remaining in the solution was measured by the two assay methods. As shown in Table 1-A, only a small portion of thrombin activity remained in the

Table 1-A. Thrombin Activity Towards Peptide-MCA After Incubation with Immobilized Heparin.

	Remaining Thrombin Activity			
	Assay after I-Hep removal[a]		Assay without I-Hep removal[b]	
	Produced AMC (nmole/min)	%	Produced AMC (nmol/min)	%
Control	0.762	100	1.11	100
I-Hep	0.058	8	1.15	104

[a] I-Hep or control preparation, 10 mg dry weight of Sepharose 4B, suspended in 100 μl of 10 m*M* Tris-HCl buffer, pH 7.4 containing 0.145*M* NaCl, was allowed to react with thrombin of 44 μg in the buffer containing NaCl and 1% bovine serum albumin of 230 μl at 37°C for 10 min. The immobilized preparation was immediately removed from the reaction mixture after the reaction. The thrombin activity was calculated by the amount of AMC that had been produced in the reaction. The reaction solution of 100 μl was allowed to react with 0.1 m*M* peptide-MCA buffer solution of 1.0 ml at 37°C for 5 min.

[b] The immobilized preparation was allowed to react with thrombin of 65 μg at 37°C for 10 min, the removal of the preparation after the reaction was omitted. The remaining activity of the reaction mixture was measured.

solution, indicating that most of the enzyme was removed from the assay system together with I-Hep gel. When the removal of I-Hep from the incubation mixture was omitted, the total remaining activity of thrombin, both bound and soluble thrombin, could be measured. In the assay with a peptide-MCA, total activity of thrombin was not changed by the addition of I-Hep as shown in Table 1-A. This observation showed that the bound thrombin was as active as free one, because thrombin binding did occur to a large extent under the present conditions. In contrast, however, assay with fibrinogen as a substrates showed a significant decrease in thrombin activity as shown in Table 1-B. This decrease might be explained by poor substrate accessibility caused by gel structure around bound heparin molecules.

Table 1-B. Thrombin Activity Towards Fibrinogen After Incubation with Immobilized Heparin.

	Remaining Thrombin Activity			
	Assay after I-Hep removal[a]		Assay without I-Hep removal[b]	
	C.T. (sec)	Thrombin Activity (%)	C.T. (sec)	Thrombin Activity (%)
Control	14.6	100	13.4	100
I-Hep	66.9	10	46.4	16

[a] I-Hep or control preparation, 6 mg in the buffer of 300 μl, was allowed to react with thrombin of 1.5 units of 200 μl for 30 min, the immobilized preparation was immediately removed from the reaction mixture after the reaction. The remaining activity of the reaction solution was measured by the clotting time method using fibrinogen as a substrate.

[b] The removal of the immobilized preparation after the reaction was omitted, the activity of the reaction mixture was measured.

Table 1-C. Factor Xa Activity Towards Peptide-MCA After Incubation with Immobilized Heparin.

	Remaining Factor Xa Activity			
	Assay after I-Hep removal[a]		Assay without I-Hep removal[b]	
	Produced AMC (nmole/min)	%	Produced AMC (nmole/min)	%
Control	0.072	100	0.067	100
I-Hep	0.056	78	0.070	104

[a] The immobilized preparation, 10 mg in the buffer of 100 μl, was allowed to react with Factor Xa of 94 μg in 250 μl for 5 min. After the removal of the preparation from the reaction mixture, the remaining activity was measured using a peptide-MCA as a substrate.

[b] The immobilized preparation was allowed to react with Factor Xa of 87 μg for 5 min. After the reaction, the removal of the preparation was omitted and the activity of the reaction mixture was measured using a peptide-MCA.

2.3 Anti-Factor Xa Activity of Immobilized Heparin

Anti-Factor Xa activity of I-Hep was examined by the following method; Factor Xa was incubated with I-Hep, and the residual Factor Xa activity was measured by the two assay methods. One was the clotting time method, in which Factor VII and X deficient plasma was used as a substrate solution. The other method used tert-butoxycarbonyl-L-isoleucyl-L-glutamyl-glycyl-L-arginine-4-methyl-coumarinyl-7-amide (peptide MCA) as a substrate, and Factor Xa activity was measured by the amount of amino-4-methyl-coumarin (AMC) produced. Assays after removal of I-Hep from incubation mixture with Factor Xa show that Factor Xa, like thrombin, was bound to I-Hep as shown in Table 1-C. When the I-Hep gel incubated with Factor Xa was not removed from the incubation mixture, the activity of Factor Xa was not changed when assayed with a peptide MCA (Table 1-C), but was decreased in the clotting time assay method (Table 1-D). All the results with Factor Xa were quantitatively analogous to the results with thrombin. However, some differences were noted between Factor Xa and thrombin bindings. Thrombin was bound to I-Hep in much larger amounts than Factor Xa. I-Hep appeared to have a stronger affinity for thrombin than for Factor Xa.

2.4 Anticoagulative Activity of Immobilized Heparin in the Presence of Antithrombin III (AT III)

The inhibitions of the activated coagulation factors by I-Hep were investigated in the presence of AT III. Thrombin or Factor Xa was allowed to react with I-Hep in the presence or absence of AT III for various reaction times at 37°C. Similar experiments with soluble heparin or control immobilized preparation were also run. After the reaction, the removal of immobilized gel from the reaction mixture was omitted and the remaining activity of enzyme was measured by the clotting time method. The results are shown in Figure 1, which indicates that thrombin was progressively neutralized by AT III in the presence of control preparation and was instantaneously neutralized by AT III in the presence of soluble heparin. On the other hand, when thrombin was allowed to react with I-Hep in the presence of AT III, no synergetic effect on the thrombin neutralization was observed at all.

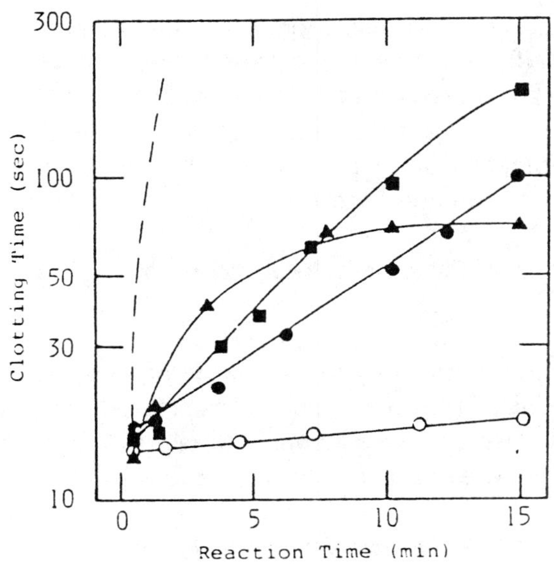

Figure 1. Neutralization of thrombin by AT III in the presence of immobilized heparin. The reaction of the following reaction mixture, in a final volume of 1000 μl: thrombin 5.0 units; the following materials; Tris-HCl buffer, pH 7.4, 10 mM; NaCl 0.145M and 0.8% bovine serum albumin, was carried out at 37°C for a defined reaction time. (–O–) Control preparation 7.58 mg; (–▲–) I-Hep 7.58 mg; heparin of 7.34 units was immobilized; (–●–) control preparation 7.58 mg + AT III solution 100 μl; (–■–) I-Hep 7.58 mg + AT III solution 100 μl. The remaining activity of an aliquot of the reaction mixture was immediately measured by the clotting time method. (—) Control preparation 7.58 mg + AT III solution 100 μl + soluble heparin of 7.34 units. After the reaction for 15 sec, the remaining activity was measured, the clot of the assay mixture was not formed at all and there was no detectable remaining activity of thrombin.

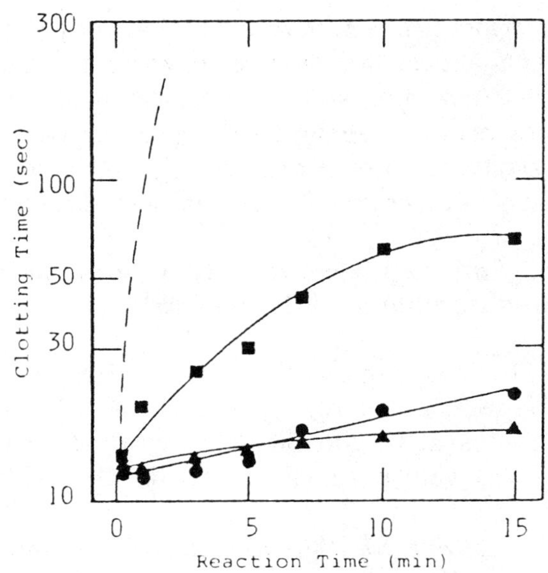

Figure 2. Neutralization of Factor Xa by AT III in the presence of immobilized heparin. The reaction of Factor Xa 175 μg and the following materials was carried out under the same conditions as Figure 1. except that Factor Xa was added instead of thrombin. (–▲–) I-Hep 7.58 mg; (–●–) control preparation 7.58 mg + AT III solution 100 μl; (–■–) I-Hep 7.58 mg + AT III solution 100 μl; (—) control preparation 7.58 mg + AT III solution 100 μl + soluble heparin of 7.34 units. After the reaction for 15 sec, the remaining activity was measured, the clot of the assay mixture was not formed at all and there was no detectable remaining activity of Factor Xa.

Table 1-D. Factor Xa Activity Towards Factor VIII and X Deficient Plasma after Incubation with Immobilized Heparin.

	Remaining Factor Xa Activity			
	Assay after I-Hep removal[a]		Assay without I-Hep removal[b]	
	C.T. (sec)	Factor Xa Activity (%)	C.T. (sec)	Factor Xa Activity (%)
Control	12.0	100	11.6	100
I-Hep	19.4	39	17.6	45

[a] The immobilized preparation of 5 mg in the buffer of 100 μl was allowed to react with Factor Xa of 500 μl for 5 min. After the removal of preparation from the reaction mixture, the remaining activity of the reaction solution was measured by the clotting time method using Factor VII and X deficient plasma as a substrate.

[b] The removal of the preparation after the reaction was omitted, the activity of reaction mixture was measured.

Figure 2 shows the results of the similar experiment for Xa neutralization. In the similar manner as above, the rate of Factor Xa neutralization by AT III was slow in the presence of the control preparation and was significantly increased in the presence of soluble heparin. In the presence of I-Hep, however, significant increase in the neutralization rate was not observed. From these observations, we anticipate that the cooperation of I-Hep and blood AT III will probably not increase the rates of neutralizations of thrombin and Factor Xa.

2.5 Anticoagulative Activity of Immobilized Heparin Previously Reacted with Antithrombin III, [I-Hep]-AT III

The anticoagulative activity of [I-Hep]-AT III was investigated by the following procedure. I-Hep was previously reacted with AT III. This particular I-Hep preparation was reacted with thrombin at 37 °C for 30 min. In the preincubation of I-Hep and AT III solution, the AT III bound to I-Hep with an affinity for heparin. The results of this experiment are shown in Table 1-E. The

Table 1-E. Thrombin Activity After Incubation with AT III Bound to Immobilized Heparin.

Materials	Remaining Thrombin Activity[b] C.T. (sec)	%
Control	13.9	100
I-Hep	29.8	31
[I-Hep]-AT III[a]	22.7	45

[a] [I-Hep]-AT III was prepared in the following manner: I-Hep, supended in 10 mM Tris-HCl buffer, pH 7.4 containing 0.145M NaCl, was allowed to react with a large amount of AT III solution at room temperature for one hour. The adsorbed AT III, except for the AT III bound to I-Hep by the affinity of I-Hep and AT III, was eluted and washed away on a glass filter with a large amount of the buffer containing 0.3M NaCl.

[b] Control preparation, I-Hep or [I-Hep]-AT III, 4.0 mg suspended in the buffer of 50 μl, respectively, was allowed to react with thrombin of 2.0 units in 200 μl at 37°C for 30 min. The remaining activity of 50 μl aliquot of the reaction mixture was measured by the clotting time method.

activity of the remaining thrombin was measured by the clotting time method after removal of immobilized preparation. After the reaction of thrombin with [I-Hep]-AT III, clotting time was 22.7 sec, which was longer than that with control preparation. This shows [I-Hep]-AT III could bind thrombin. However, thrombin activity was not neutralized instantaneously by [I-Hep]-AT III and there was no big difference in the clotting time between the cases of [I-Hep]-AT III and I-Hep. This suggests that [I-Hep]-AT III, unlike AT III and soluble heparin, had no synergetic effect on the neutralization of thrombin. We found that the synergetic effect could be prepared when AT III and heparin were preincubated prior to coimmobilization as shown in next section.

2.6 Effect of Immobilized Heparin on Plasma Recalcification Time (PRCT)

The effect of I-Hep on plasma recalcification time, PRCT, was also investigated. After the addition of the immobilized preparation to the citrated plasma, Ca^{2+} solution was added to the mixture and PRCT was measured. The prolongation of PRCT by I-Hep was observed as shown in Table 1-F.

Table 1-F. Prolongation of Plasma Recalcification Time by Heparin Immobilized on Sepharose 4B, PVA and Poly HEMA.

	Plasma Recalcification Time (sec)[a]			
	Sepharose 4B		PVA	Poly HEMA
	1.0 mg/20 μl	2.5 mg/50 μl	2.0 mg/50 μl	2.0 mg/50 μl
Control	140	150	110	120
I-Hep	180	360	110	170

[a] The immobilized preparation suspended in the buffer was added to the prewarmed citrate plasma of 200 μl and preincubated for 1 min at 37°C. 25m*M* Ca^{2+} solution of 200 μl was added to the mixture and PRCT was measured with a gentle agitation.

Using polyvinyl alcohol (PVA) and polyhydroxyethyl methacrylate (Poly HEMA) as immobilization carriers, the same experiments about the effect of I-Hep on PRCT were run in order to elucidate the influences of carrier properties.

Heparin was immobilized merely on the surface of PVA fibers, because PVA used had no pore structure. Heparin immobilized on PVA did not affect the plasma recalcification time as shown in Table 1-F. On the other hand, when Poly HEMA was used for immobilization carrier, the prolongation of PRCT was observed, but in a lower degree than when Sepharose 4B was used as a carrier.

2.7 Anticoagulative Characteristics of Immobilized Heparin

The role of heparin in promoting the reaction between AT III and several proteolytic enzymes has not been clearly understood. In the absence of AT III, the neutralizations of thrombin and Factor Xa by heparin are hard to observe. However, the rate of the reaction between thrombin and AT III is greatly increased in the presence of heparin [26,27]. Heparin is known to bind both AT III [28] and thrombin [29], and the following mechanisms have been proposed to explain the effect of heparin on the neutralization of thrombin. One model, which has been widely accepted, assumes that heparin forms a complex with AT III and transforms AT III into a more active AT III [30-32]. Another model suggests that heparin is bound first to thrombin and then the heparin-thrombin complex reacts with AT III [10,33,34]. In either case, the anticoagulative effect of heparin appeared to be mediated through AT III, the main inhibitor in blood.

Table 1-G. Effect of Heparin Immobilized on PVA, Poly HEMA and Sepharose 4B on Prevention of Blood Coagulation.

Carrier	Decrease of Thrombin Activity (Assay without I-Hep removal)		Prolongation of PRCT
	Peptide-MCA Substrate	Fibrinogen Substrate	
PVA (nonporous)	N.T.[a]	(±)[b]	(±)
Poly HEMA (porous)	N.T.[a]	(+)	(+)
Sepharose 4B (gel structure)	(−)	(++)	(++)

[a] Not tested.
[b] (++), (+), and (±) appearing in the Table represent the extent of decrease in thrombin activity, or of PRCT prolongation; the extent of effect of carrier is order here. (−) shows no decrease in thrombin activity.

The remaining activities of thrombin and Factor Xa measured by using peptide-MCA showed that I-Hep could bind to thrombin and Factor Xa but the activities of those enzymes were not decreased by the binding. However, when natural high molecular substrates were used in the assays of remaining enzyme activities, i.e., when the clotting time methods were employed, the decreases in enzyme activities were observed even in the reaction mixture of I-Hep and enzyme. This inconsistency might be caused by the following two phenomena: (1) the reaction between fibrinogen (or prothrombin) and thrombin (or Factor Xa) would be hindered sterically because the enzyme was bound to the immobilized heparin. (2) the influence of internal diffusion of high molecular-weight substrates might be more significant than that of artificial low molecular-weight substrates, peptide-MCA. In order to determine which is more probable, another set of experiments was run, using structurally different carriers, PVA and Poly HEMA. PVA used was fibrous, and heparin was immobilized only on the outer surface of PVA. Poly HEMA, made like sponge, had pore structure and the enzymes were immobilized also on inner surface. The extent of PRCT prolongation by immobilized heparin was dependent on carrier structure, as shown in Table 1-G. While the heparin immobilized on PVA scarcely prolonged PRCT, the heparin on Poly HEMA showed considerable prolongation. However, the degree of prolongation by heparin-Poly HEMA was much less than that of heparin-Sepharose 4B, which had a finer pore structure than Poly HEMA. The fact that the thrombin-heparin-PVA was active toward high molecular weight substrates suggests low possibility of steric hindrance. Thrombin inhibition and prolongation of PRCT by heparin-Sepharose 4B appear to be what one would expect from natural high molecular substrates that have low diffusivity within gel particle. It is well accepted that the participation of intraparticle diffusion of substrate in reactions decrease the apparent affinity of enzymes or that the apparent value of the Michaelis constant is increased by diffusional resistance. When thrombin was reacted with heparin-Sepharose 4B, most of the thrombin would be captured inside the gel particle because heparin retained its ability to bind thrombin. The bound thrombin was active, but most of it could not instantaneously react with a large substrate like fibrinogen. When a small substrate, like peptide-MCA was used for thrombin assay, this diffusion process was negligible and no inhibition of thrombin by heparin-Sepharose 4B was observed.

Heparin molecules, when immobilized onto CNBr-activated solid surface, retained their activity to bind thrombin and Factor Xa, but could not inhibit them, as described above. AT III which had previously been complexed with heparin molecules of I-Hep, unlike soluble heparin, failed to neutralize thrombin and Factor Xa at fair rate. These results apparently mean that the covalently heparinized biomaterials by CNBr-activation method are hardly able to inhibit the coagulation in the blood stream, ex vivo.

3. CHARACTERISTICS OF COIMMOBILIZED ANTITHROMBIN III AND HEPARIN (I-AT III·Hep)

3.1 Introduction

Heparin covalently immobilized on biomaterials has an ability to bind thrombin and Factor Xa, but these enzymes thus bound to I-Hep are still active as shown in the previous section. The instantaneous neutralization exhibited by AT III in the presence of soluble heparin was not observed when heparin was covalently immobilized. It was found, however, that heparin, when coimmobilized with AT III, exhibit much higher anticoagulative activity than immobilized heparin and/or immobilized AT III [35-37]. In this section, the anticoagulative characteristics of coimmobilized AT III and heparin (I-AT III·Hep) are discussed, comparing with I-AT III and I-Hep, according to our experimental results [35-37].

3.2 Comparison of Various Immobilized Preparations

Table 2. Various Preparations of Immobilized Heparin and Antithrombin III, and Their Anticoagulant Activity.

Preparation no.	Immobilization procedure	Abbreviation	Schematic expression	Anti coagulant activity
1	AT III and heparin were co-immobilized	I—AT III · Hep	—AT III —Hep	+ +
2	AT III and excess heparin were co-immobilized		—Hep —AT III —Hep	+ +
3	AT III was immobilized, heparin was bound to AT III		—AT III—(Hep)	+
4	Heparin was immobilized, AT III was bound to heparin		—Hep—(AT III)	+
5	AT III and heparin were immobilized separately	I—AT III + I-Hep	—AT III + —Hep	+
6	Bovine serum albumin was immobilized as a control gel	Control	—BSA	—

The anticoagulative activity was examined for various coimmobilized preparations and a mixed preparation of I-AT III and I-Hep, using the clotting time method. Results are shown in Table 2. Bovine serum albumin was immobilized as a control preparation, which showed no anticoagulative activity. As has been recognized, heparin has an affinity to complex with AT III, and in this state, heparin stimulate the anticoagulative activity of AT III up to 100-fold [30-32]. However, this cooperative phenomenon was not observed when heparin was covalently immobilized and incubated with free AT III, or when I-AT III was incubated with soluble heparin (Preparation 3 and 4). The same result was obtained with Preparation 5, which actually was a mixture of I-Hep and I-AT III. Only when AT III and heparin were preincubated and then coimmobilized in a complex form, was the stimulative effect preserved (Preparation 1 and 2).

3.3 The Effect of I-AT III·Hep on Plasma Recalcification Time (PRCT)

The effect of the coimmobilized preparation, I-AT III·Hep, on plasma recalcification time (PRCT) was compared with those of I-Hep and control preparation. The results are shown in Figure 3. Slight prolongation of PRCT was observed with both control and I-Hep, probably

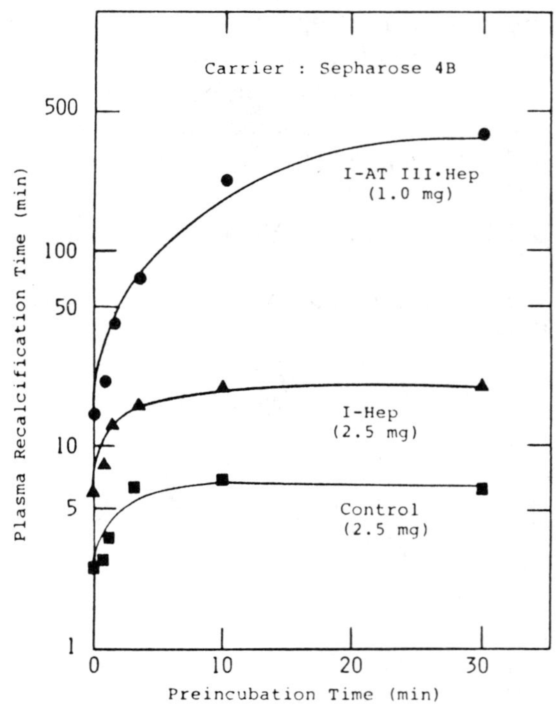

Figure 3. The prolongation of plasma recalcification time by co-immobilized antithrombin III and heparin. Control preparation or 2.5 mg of I-Hep suspended in 50 μl of 10 mM Tris-HCl buffer, pH 7.4 containing 0.145 M NaCl and 1 per cent serum albumin, or 1.0 mg of I-AT III·Hep in 20 μl buffer solution were mixed with 200 μl of freshly citrated bovine plasma. The mixture was incubated at 37°C for a definite time. After incubation 200μl to 25 mM Ca^{2+} solution were added to the mixture, and the plasma clotting time was measured.

because of adsorption phenomena of blood coagulation factors onto these preparations. I-AT III·Hep, upon incubation in citrated plasma, could significantly prolong PRCT, indicating that capture of the activated coagulation factors was much higher than in the cases of simple adsorption. Table 3 shows the effect of immobilization carriers. When PVA or Poly HEMA was used as a carrier for immobilization of heparin and AT III, the prolongation of PRCT was observed but to a somewhat lesser extent than when Sepharose 4B was a carrier. This should be due to the difference in carrier, especially in surface area per unit weight of carrier.

Table 3. Prolongation of Plasma Recalcification Time by Various Immobilized Preparations of Heparin and/or Antithrombin III.

Immobilized preparation	Carrier	Plasma recalcification time (min)			
		Sepharose 4B		PVA	Poly HEMA
		1.0 mg	2.5 mg	2.0 mg	2.0 mg
Control		3.0	2.0	5.7	4.3
I-Hep		3.4	6.1	6.0	5.8
I-AT III		3.8	9.2	7.3	5.0
I-AT III·Hep		20	No clot	8.0	7.8

Immobilized preparation (Sepharose 4B . 1.0 mg in 20 μl buffer solution or 2.5 mg in 50 μl buffer solution, PVA : 2.0 mg, and Poly HEMA : 2.0 mg in 20 μl buffer solution) was mixed with 200 μl plasma prewarmed at 37°C. After one min incubation, 200 μl of 25 mM Ca^{2+} solution were added to the mixture, and plasma recalcification time (PRCT) was measured. PRCT shown here was the mean of about 10 measurements.

While Sepharose 4B bound 6.0 mg of heparin per unit gram of carrier, PVA and Poly HEMA immobilized only 2.0 mg and 1.5 mg heparin per unit gram of carrier, respectively. Regardless of the binding capacity of carrier, coimmobilized preparations exhibited the best prolongation effect in all cases.

3.4 Antithrombin Activity of I-AT III·Hep

Thrombin plays an important role in fibrin clot formation, catalyzing the proteolysis of fibrinogen. Accordingly, antithrombin activity of heparin and/or AT III immobilized on Poly HEMA was measured: thrombin solution was incubated for 0 to 30 min with each immobilized preparation, which was then removed and the remaining thrombin activity was measured, using fibrinogen as a substrate. The neutralization of thrombin by I-AT III·Hep was almost instantaneous. In the incubation with I-AT III or I-Hep, the gradual decrease in thrombin activity was observed, but not with the control preparation as shown in Figure 4.

Table 4-A. Decrease of Thrombin Activity on Incubation with Immobilized Preparations of of Heparin and/or Antithrombin III.

Immobilized preparation	Remaining thrombin activity (per cent)	
	Assay after gel removal	Assay without gel removal
Control	100	100
I-Hep	56	100
I-AT III	67	73
I-AT III·Hep	56	63

Heparin and/or antithrombin III immobilized on Sepharose 4B gel was used. 10 mg of immobilized preparation were alolwed to react with thrombin (84 μg in 20 μl buffer solution) for 10 min at 37°C. The remaining activity of thrombin was assayed by using a peptide-MCA as substrate.

Table 4-B. Decrease of Factor Xa Activity on Incubation with Immobilized preparations of Heparin and/or Antithrombin III.

Immobilized preparation	Remaining factor Xa activity (per cent)	
	Assay after gel removal	Assay without gel removal
Control	100	100
I-Hep	76	87
I-AT III	67	89
I-AT III·Hep	34	36

Heparin and/or antithrombin III immobilized on Sepharose 4B gel was used. 10 mg of immobilized preparation were allowed to react with Factor Xa (114 μg in 20 μl buffer solution) for 5 min at 37°C. The remaining activity of Factor Xa was measured by the clotting time method, using Factor VII and X deficient plasma as substrate.

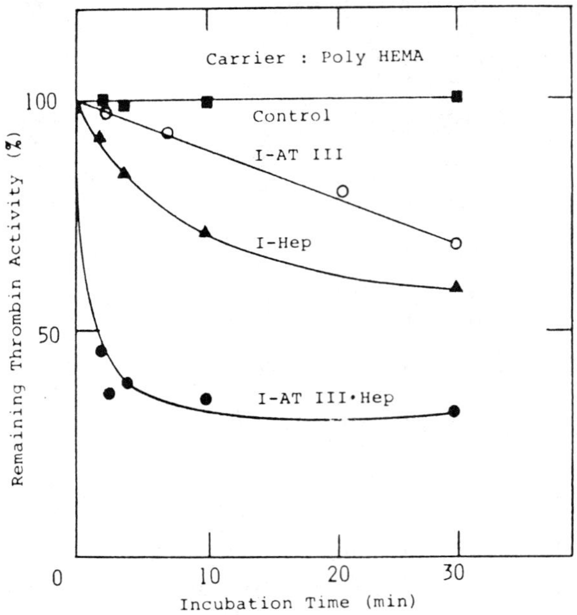

Figure 4. Decrease of thrombin activity on incubation with immobilized heparin and/or antithrombin III. 5 mg of immobilized preparation suspended in 200 μl buffer solution were mixed with 200 μl of thrombin solution (0.5 unit). After incubation for a definite time, the mixture was filtered and the thrombin remaining in the supernatant solution was assayed by the clotting time method.

Table 4-A shows the neutralization of thrombin on Sepharose 4B. In this experiment, remaining thrombin activity was measured in two different ways. In one series, after 10 min-incubation with each of the immobilized preparations, Sepharose 4B gel was immediately removed and thrombin was assayed in the supernatant solution. In the other series, thrombin activity was measured in the incubation mixture, thus both free and bound thrombin were subjected to assay. These experiments revealed interesting points; thrombin could bind to all types of immobilized inhibitors, I-Hep, I-AT III, and I-AT III·Hep; thrombin was inactivated when bound to I-AT III·Hep or I-AT III; no inactivation occurred on thrombin bound to I-Hep when a peptide-MCA was used as substrate as described in the previous section.

3.5 Anti-Factor Xa Activity of I-AT III·Hep

In order to evaluate the anti-Factor Xa activity of the immobilized preparations of heparin and/or AT III, Factor Xa solution was incubated with each immobilized preparation for 5 min at 37 °C, and the remaining activity was then assayed by a clotting time method using Factor VIII and X deficient plasma as testing solution (Table 4-B). Though both I-Hep and I-AT III decreased Factor Xa activity, the rate of neutralization by the coimmobilized preparation was much higher than that by I-AT III and I-Hep. Similar observations were obtained for thrombin neutralization. However, the rate of Factor Xa neutralization by I-AT III·Hep was somewhat higher than that of thrombin neutralization, as shown in Figure 5. The rate of Factor Xa neutralization by I-AT·III·Hep was approximately the same with the rates of Factor Xa and thrombin neutralizations by soluble AT III and heparin, as shown in Figure 5.

3.6 Anticoagulative Activity of I-AT III·Hep in the Presence of Both Factor Xa and Thrombin

I-AT III·Hep was found to be very effective, so far as the neutralization of a single enzyme, thrombin or Factor Xa, was concerned. In case of practical application of biomaterials to an

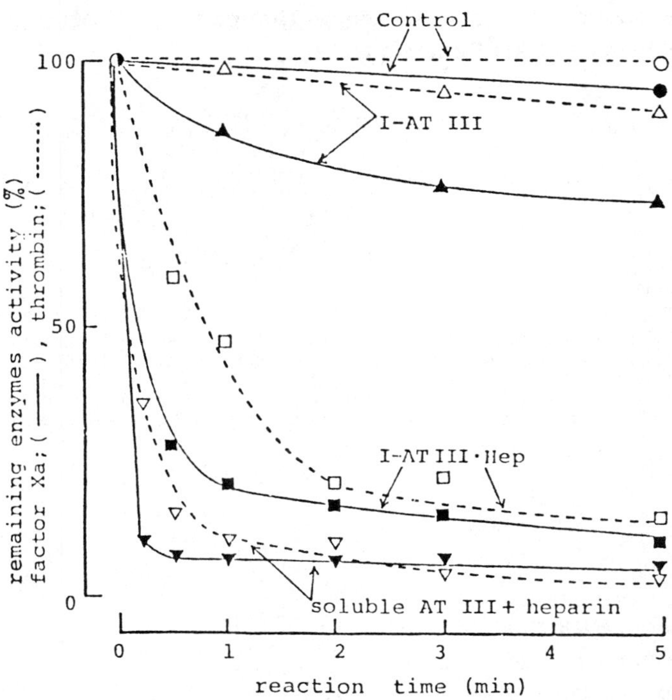

Figure 5. Neutralizations of thrombin and factor Xa by immobilized preparations, or soluble AT III and heparin. The immobilized preparation of 10 mg, or soluble AT III and heparin, equivalent to the amounts coimmobilized on 10 mg Sepharose 4B, was allowed to react with thrombin of 44 μg or factor Xa of 94 μg at 37°C for a definite time. The remaning enzyme activity in supernatant was measured using a peptide-MCA.

extracorporeal blood circulation system, the materials must be in contact with the blood in which coagulation factors would be activated, and the clotting be just ready to proceed. Thus, the evaluation of inhibitory activity of I-AT III·Hep in the presence of these activated factors is considered to be important. Among the activated factors in blood, thrombin and Factor Xa are the most important and consequently have been well studied. The activity of I-AT III·Hep was studied in the presence of these two enzymes. Figure 5 shows the result of such a study, where both Factor Xa and thrombin were allowed to react with a definite amount of I-AT III·Hep, the amount of neutralized Factor Xa was measured, and compared with the case of I-AT III·Hep and Factor Xa alone. The amount of neutralized Factor Xa was the same in both cases. Accordingly, it is concluded that there is no effect of thrombin on the neutralization of Factor Xa by I-AT III·Hep. The neutralization of thrombin by I-AT III·Hep was also examined in the presence and absence of Factor Xa. Contrary to the above case, the neutralization of thrombin was decreased by the presence of Factor Xa as shown in Figure 6. Table 5 shows the comparison in neutralized amounts of these two enzymes in three different ways of incubation with enzyme solution. When thrombin or Factor Xa was incubated with 5 mg of I-AT III·Hep, 9.0 μg or 15.3 μg of enzyme was neutralized, respectively. When a mixture of thrombin and Factor Xa was incubated with the same amount of I-AT III·Hep, 15.7 μg of Factor Xa were neutralized, but only a trace amount of thrombin was neutralized. The neutralized amount of Factor Xa by I-AT III·Hep when thrombin was absent was the same as when throm-

Table 5. Neutralization of Factor Xa and/or Thrombin Upon Incubation with Co-immobilized Heparin and Antithrombin III.

	Enzyme	Initial amount (μg)	Remaining activity after reaction (per cent)	Neutralized amount (μg)
1.	Factor Xa	41.5	62	15.7
	Thrombin	15.5	99	0.2
2.	Factor Xa	43.4	65	15.3
3.	Thrombin	18.7	52	9.0

Sepharose 4B was used as a crrier for immobilization. The specified amount of Factor Xa and/or throbin was allowede to react with 5 mg of I-AT III • Hep in 10 mM Tris-HCl buffer, pH 7.4 containing 0.145 M NaCl and 1 per cent bovine serum albumin. After reacting for 10 min, I-AT III • Hep was removed from the reaction mixture and the remaining enzyme activity was immediately measured using the peptide-MCA substrates.

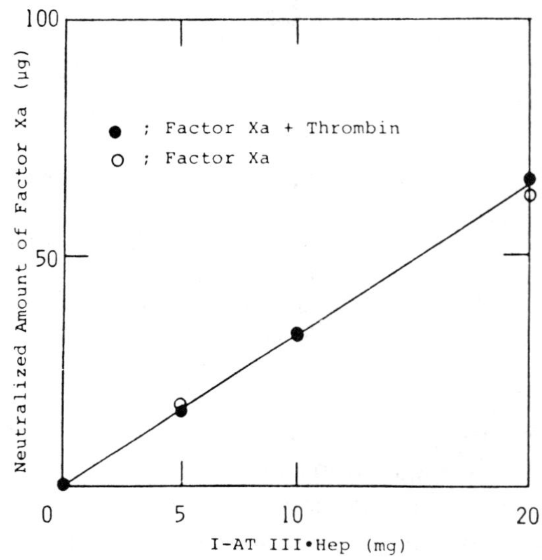

Figure 6. Neutralization of Factor Xa in the reaction of co-immobilized antithrombin III and heparin with Factor Xa and/or thrombin. The specified amount of I-AT III·Hep on Sepharose 4B was allowed to react with the enzyme mixture of Factor Xa 90 μg and thrombin 19 μg, or with 70 μg of Factor Xa alone at I-AT III·Hep 5 mg, Factor Xa 100 μg at I-AT III·Hep 10 and 20 mg, respectively. After reacting for 10 min, the I-AT III·Hep was removed from the reaction mixture and the remaining Factor Xa activity was immediately measured using the peptide-MCA as substrate.

bin was present. An additional experiment in which much larger amounts of thrombin were mixed with Factor Xa and the mixture was allowed to react with I-AT III·Hep, reinforced the above observation because no decrease in neutralized amount of Factor Xa was recognized even in the presence of excess thrombin. On the other hand, the neutralization of thrombin was not done by the presence of stoichiometrical amount of Factor Xa. It is, therefore, concluded that I-AT III·Hep can neutralize Factor Xa in preference to thrombin.

Through neutralizing 32 units of Factor Xa, 1 μg of AT III indirectly prevents the generation of 1600 NIH units of thrombin. To directly neutralize this amount of thrombin, 1000 μg of AT III are required. Much more AT III is necessary to inhibit the thrombin-fibrinogen reaction than is required to neutralize Factor Xa. Factor Xa is a more potent thrombogenic agent than thrombin itself. In this study, it was shown that a greater amount of Factor Xa than thrombin was preferentially and rapidly neutralized by I-AT III·Hep. The preferential and rapid neutralization

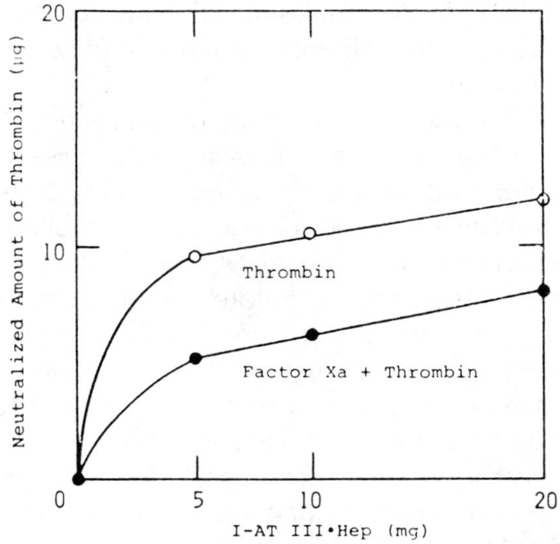

Figure 7. Neutralization of thrombin in the reaction of co-immobilized antithrombin III and heparin with Factor Xa and/or thrombin. The specified amount of I-AT III·Hep, Sepharose 4B, was allowed to react with the enzyme mixture of Factor Xa 10 μg and thrombin 20 μg, or thrombin alone 20 μg in the buffer solution. After reacting for 3 min, the I-AT III·Hep was removed from the reaction mixture and the remaining thrombin activity was immediately measured using the peptide-MCA as substrate.

of Factor Xa in presence of thrombin is very favorable for effective prevention of blood coagulation. Therefore, the coimmobilization of heparin and AT III would be a useful method to obtain antithrombogenic artificial biomedical materials.

4. CHARACTERISTICS OF IMMOBILIZED UROKINASE (I-UK)

4.1 Introduction

The administration of urokinase has been carried out to block the thrombus formation. However, the administrated urokinase is rapidly eliminated from blood and a large amount of urokinase is required to gain the therapeutic effect. Therefore, it is considered that the clinical utilization of the antithrombogenic biomaterials with immobilized proteins is available for prevention of thrombus formation. It is well known [38-51] that the urokinase immobilized onto surface of artificial polymers has a fibrinolytic activity and the biomaterials bearing urokinase are available for antithrombogenic biomaterials. In this section, the antithrombogenic characteristics of immobilized urokinase are described.

4.2 Immobilization of Urokinase

The fibrinolytic ability of immobilized uorkinase has been demonstrated using CMC-hydrazide [38], agarose [39], graphite [40,41], Sepharose [42,44,46], polymer Enzacryl [43] and polyanionic copolymer [43]. However, the quality of carrier materials, immobilization process and method and timing of disinfection must be investigated for the clinical application of immobilized urokinase. According to the research of Ohshiro and Kosaki [48], nylon, polyester (Dacron and Perplene) and polyurethane have quality desirable for clinical purposes.

The method for immobilizing urokinase on nylon was investigated by Ohshiro and Kosaki [48] and they obtained the following results. The amount of immobilized urokinase was increased efficiently by providing an intermediate layer of grafted copolymer. Polyethylene imine and Gantrez were adopted as grafted copolymers. Although the number of binding sites was theoretically expected to increase immensely, it was actually no more than doubled experimentally. The stronger fibrinolytic activity was obtained by immobilized nitrophthalic anhydride, an antiplasmin inhibitor, together with urokinase. Etching with HCl was also effective for immobilizing a quantity of urokinase. Fibrinolytic activity was augmented 20-40% by this method.

The method and timing of disinfection were also investigated by Ohshiro and Kosaki [48] and they had the following results. Disinfection was performed advantageously with 0.5% chlorhexidine alcohol without causing a great loss in the fibrinolytic activity of immobilized urokinase. Chlorhexidine alcohol was followed in performance by ethylene oxide gas, gamma rays and electron beams. A much better performance was displayed when gamma-ray irradiation was performed before immobilization of urokinase.

Watanabe et al showed [50,51] that collagen-synthetic polymer composite was adequately applicable as a support of immobilization of enzymes for the purpose of providing the material surface with some biological functions, and that urokinase-bearing composite had good fibrinolytic activity. Watanabe et al have been also investigating to replace various organs with that composite material experimentally and clinically. For example, the reconstructions of trachea, chest wall and esophagus were carried out by using that composite material. When such artificial organs are implanted into the body, bacterial infection may cause serious troubles. Watanabe et al [52] have, therefore, attempted to develop a new method of producing antibacterial biomaterials by immobilization of hen egg-white lysozyme and polypeptide antibiotic Polymyxin B onto that composite material.

4.3 Clinical Application of Immobilized Urokinase

It had already been reported by Kusserow [41] that urokinase-treated materials had an antithrombotic action in vivo. Ohshiro and Kosaki [48] found also that urokinase-treated nylon showed an antithrombotic action in vivo and urokinase-treated polymeric materials could be used for intravenous catheterization, vascular suture and lymph drainage. They showed [48] that urokinase-treated materials were retained in not only the abdominal cavity but also the inferior caval vein of rats. On the basis of those experimental results, these materials were clinically used, limiting to the three groups of patients described below.

The first group comprised 21 patients who underwent intraveous hyperalimentation. In this therapy, it is important to avoid plugging the catheter, which is retained in the vein, with thrombi. For intravenous catheterization, therefore, urokinase-treated nylon or Perplene tubes were used. Most of the patients were able to receive the therapy for the intended period of time. Almost no thrombi adhered to the tubes removed.

The second group consisted of ten patients with vascular disease of the small artery. In these patients, urokinase-treated nylon filaments were used for suturing the arterial wall. In two of the ten patients subjected to thromboendarterectomy, occlusion recurred. Although the real factor responsible for the reocclusion was not known, the urokinase-treated suture material was thought to have been useful for retarding thrombus formation in the sutural region. Presumably, such a material will be useful, especially for suturing the venous wall.

The third group was composed of seven patients with lymphedema. In these patients, urokinase-treated Dacron or nylon threads were used for lymph drainage. The drainage was conducted through capillary lumens formed in the interspace between individual fibers of the thread which was buried in subcutaneous tissue. The clinical effect of lymph drainage using these threads can not definitely be assessed without long-term follow-up. It may be mentioned, however, that it was remarkably effectively in the short-term study.

5. HIGH ANTITHROMBOGENICITY OF COIMMOBILIZED AT III·HEPARIN AND UROKINASE (I-AT III·HEP-UK) AND MIXED SYSTEM OF I-AT III·HEP AND I-UK, COMPARING WITH I-AT III·HEP AND I-UK

5.1 Introduction

It was described in the previous section that the artificial polymers bearing antithrombin III-heparin complex (I-AT III·Hep) have significant anticoagulative activity. Activated coagulation factors, such as Factor Xa and thrombin, were rapidly neutralized by I-AT III·Hep. The anticoagulative activity of I-AT III·Hep is due to binding of activated coagulation factors to I-AT III·Hep. Therefore, I-AT III·Hep does not catalytically inhibit the blood coagulation and the amount of neutralized coagulation factors is dependent on the amount of I-AT III·Hep. The antithrombogenic activities of the mixed system of I-AT III·Hep and I-UK and coimmobilized antithrombin III-heparin complex and urokinase (I-AT III·Hep-UK) were investigated by Miura et al [53], in order to create the biomaterials with high antithrombogenecity. In this section, the antithrombogenecity is compared between I-AT III·Hep, I-UK, a mixed system of I-AT III·Hep and I-UK, I-AT III·Hep-UK, using the research results of author et al [53].

5.2 Comparison of Antithrombogenetic Activity Between I-AT III·Hep, I-UK, and Mixed System of I-AT III·Hep and I-UK

Immobilized antithrombin III-heparin complex (I-AT III·Hep) showed a high antithrombogenetic activity; the blood thrombus formation of rabbit native of 0.8 ml was completely blocked by I-AT III·Hep of 10 mg, using Sepharose 4B as an immobilization carrier and Chandler's method [54] for measuring the thrombus formation time. When I-AT III·Hep less than 10 mg was used for the whole blood of 0.8 ml, the prolongation of thrombus formation time was observed but a complete block of thrombus formation was not accomplished as shown in Table 6-A.

Urokinase immobilized on Sepharose 4B (I-UK) exhibited the elongation of thrombus formation time. After the blood thrombus had been formed, reflowing of the coagulated blood sample was sometimes observed in the polymer tube containing I-UK. The antithrombogenic activity of I-UK, measured by prolongation of thrombus formation time, was less than that of I-AT III·Hep as shown in Tables 6-B and 7.

I-AT III·Hep of 5 mg and I-UK of 10 mg, respectively, prolonged slightly the thrombus formation time, but could not block the thrombus formation of native blood of 0.8 ml as shown in Table 6-B. On the other hand, thrombus formation was completely blocked by the mixture of I-AT III·Hep of 5 mg plus I-UK of 10 mg in all experimental runs. It was confirmed that the remarkable enhancement of antithrombotic function was brought about by the combined use of an anticoagulative function of I-AT III·Hep and a fibrinolytic function of I-UK.

5.3 High Antithrombogenetic Activity of the Coimmobilized Antithrombin III·Heparin Complex and Urokinase (I-AT III·Hep-UK)

Both antithrombin III·heparin complex and urokinase were coimmobilized on Sepharose 4B, and an antithrombotic function of I-AT III·Hep-UK was evaluated by Chandler's method [54]. I-AT III·Hep-UK whose anticoagulative activity was equal to half activity of I-AT III·Hep,

Table 6-A. Effect of Immobilized Antithrombin III-Heparin Complex on Thrombus Formation Time, Tested by Chandler's Method.

I-AT III·Hep (mg*)	Antithrombogenetic Activity: Number of Thrombus Formation Cases (TFT**: $\bar{x} \pm$ SD, sec)	Antithrombogenetic Activity: Number of Non-Formation Cases
None	4 (301 ± 30)	0
0.5	3 (273 ± 40)	1
1	3 (390 ± 60)	2
2.5	3 (416 ± 57)	1
5	7 (585 ± 186)	4
10	0	4

*; Dry weight of Sepharose 4B as an immobilization carrier.

**; Thrombus formation time of rabbit native blood of 0.8 ml was measured in the ring of polymer tube containing the specified amount of I-AT III·Hep suspended in Tris-HCl buffer (pH 7.4) containing 0.145 M NaCl (dry weight of Sepharose 4B 50 mg per ml of the buffer).

TFT: Thrombus formation time

Table 6-B. Antithrombogenetic Activity of Immobilized Urokinase and/or Immobilized Antithrombin III-Heparin Complex.

No.	Materials*		Thrombus Formation Time** (sec): in the presence of kaolin***	Thrombus Formation Time** (sec): in the absence of kaolin
1.	Control	10 mg	139	220
2.	I-U K	10 mg	170	370
3.	I-AT III·Hep	5 mg	390	550
4.	I-U K I-AT III·Hep	10 mg 5 mg	Non-Formation****	Non-Formation

*; Sepharose 4B was used as an immobilization carrier and the specified amount of immobilized preparation suspended in the buffer of 200 µl was previously poured into the polymer tube before the addition of rabbit native blood of 0.8 ml.

**; Thrombus formation time was measured by Chandler's method.

***; Thrombus formation time was measured in the ring of polymer tube containing 0.25 % kaolin suspension of 20 µl.

****; Thrombus was partially formed at 465 sec but the partial thrombus was disappeared subsequently.

Table 7. Antithrombogenetic Activity of Various Immobilized Preparations.

No.	Materials		Antithrombogenetic Activity: Number of Thrombus Foramtion Cases (TFT*: $\bar{x} \pm$ SD, sec)	Antithrombogenetic Activity: Number of Non-Formation Cases
1.	Saline	200 µl	12 (300 ± 83)	0
2.	Control	20 mg	14 (270 ± 116)	0
3.	I-U K	20 mg	14 (375 ± 261)**	1
4.	I-AT III·Hep	5 mg	7 (585 ± 186)	4
5.	(I-U K / I-AT III·Hep	20 mg / 5 mg	0	6
6.	I-AT III·Hep-UK	5 mg	0	5

*; Thrombus formation time of rabbit native blood of 0.8 ml was measured by Chandler's method using the polymer tube containing the specified amount of immobilized preparation suspended in the buffer of 200 µl

**; Reflowing of the once formed thrombus was observed in 4 cases.

was used in this study. The anticoagulative activity of immobilized preparations was measured by the neutralization of thrombin. And a fibrinolytic activity of I-AT III·Hep-UK was also equal to half activity of I-UK. I-AT III·Hep-UK also exhibited the high antithrombogenetic activity similar to the mixed system of I-AT III·Hep plus I-UK, as shown in Table 7. Thrombus formation was unseen in all runs of rabbit native blood containing I-AT III·Hep-UK of 5 mg, while I-AT III·Hep of 5 mg could prevent the thrombus formation only in 4 cases out of 11 experimental runs. I-AT III·Hep-UK having a half of antithrombin activity of I-AT-III·Hep per unit weight of Sepharose 4B and a half of fibrinolytic activity of I-UK, showed a higher antithrombogenetic activity compared with I-AT III·Hep and I-UK, respectively.

6. PREVENTION OF PLATELET AGGREGATION BY ENZYME IMMOBILIZATION TECHNIQUE

6.1 Introduction

It is well known that platelet adhesion and aggregation as well as blood coagulation are trigger steps for the thrombus formation. There are many factors causing the thrombus formation as described in section 1. In addition of these factors promoting thrombus formation, the shear stress to blood stream is the important factor for thrombus formation. Blood cells are sheared and often result in injury when blood is forced to flow through the artificial devices. It was reported [55,56] that the mechanical injury device, in vitro, produce very different functional and structural damage to platelets. The erythrocyte is subject to damage by shear stress. Hemolysis consequently occurred and hemoglobin- and many other constituents in erythrocyte are liberated into plasma [57,58]. It was observed in our work [59] that the platelet aggregation in sheared whole blood was produced by three in vitro devices; a peristaltic pump, a viscometer and a small cuvette with a shearing bar. But in sheared platelet rich plasma, no aggregation was produced and the adhesion of platelet on the surface was rarely produced by those devices. These phenomena suggest that the formation of platelet aggregation in circulating blood was not always caused by ADP released from platelet adhesion onto foreign surfaces. The mechanism of formation of platelet aggregates in sheared blood is discussed in this section.

The following two methods are available for preventing the thrombus formation originated from platelet function; (1) the use of agents preventing platelet adhesion and/or aggregation, like as aspirin, dipyridamol and prostagladins [60-62], (2) the removal of aggregation-inducing substance, which is liberated from injured erythrocyte and released from adherent platelet. The administration of those agents is clinically carried out. But the durability of antithrombogenic effect of those agents is low, since those agents are eliminated from blood in a short period. The durability of anti-aggregative activity can be increased by using the immobilization technique of enzyme which can catalyze the conversion of the aggregation-inducing substances. In this section, the prevention of platelet aggregation by immobilized enzyme is described through the experimental results of author et al [63].

6.2 Formation of Platelet Aggregates and Hemolysis in Sheared Blood

When the citrated whole blood was sheared by stirring bar at 500, 1000 and 1500 rpm, the formation of platelet aggregates was observed through a microscope. Neither erythrocyte was found in the aggregated platelet clumps, and nor fibrin clot was formed. When sheared stress was applied to the citrated platelet rich plasma (PRP), there was no platelet aggregates. The free platelet count (FPC) in sheared blood sample was measured in order to represent quantitatively the formation of platelet aggregates. The significant decreases in FPC were observed in the sheared whole blood but only a slight decrease in the sheared PRP, as shown in Figure 8. The addition of Heparin (3 units per ml) to the sheared citrated whole blood could

Figure 8. Reduction in free platelet count of sheared whole blood and sheared platelet rich plasma (PRP). Shear stress was applied to the citrated whole blood 0.75 ml by a stirring bar system at a rotation speed of 500 rpm (▲), 1000 rpm (●), 1500 (■), or 0 rpm (▼) as a control. Similarly shear stress was applied to the citrated platelet rich plasma at a rotation speed of 1000 rpm (O). After a definite time, free platelet count in the sheared blood samples was measured.

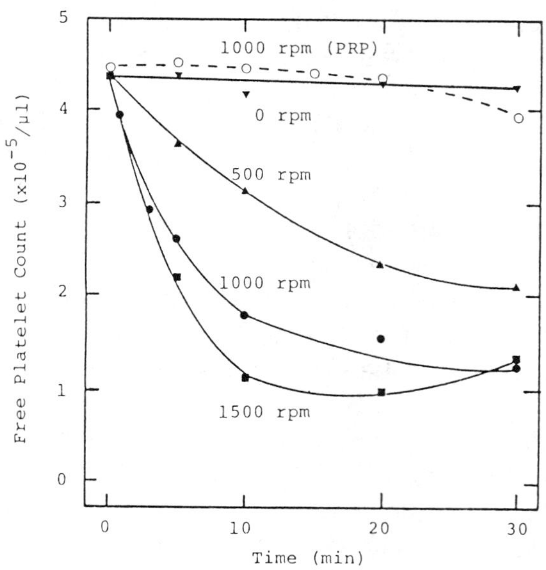

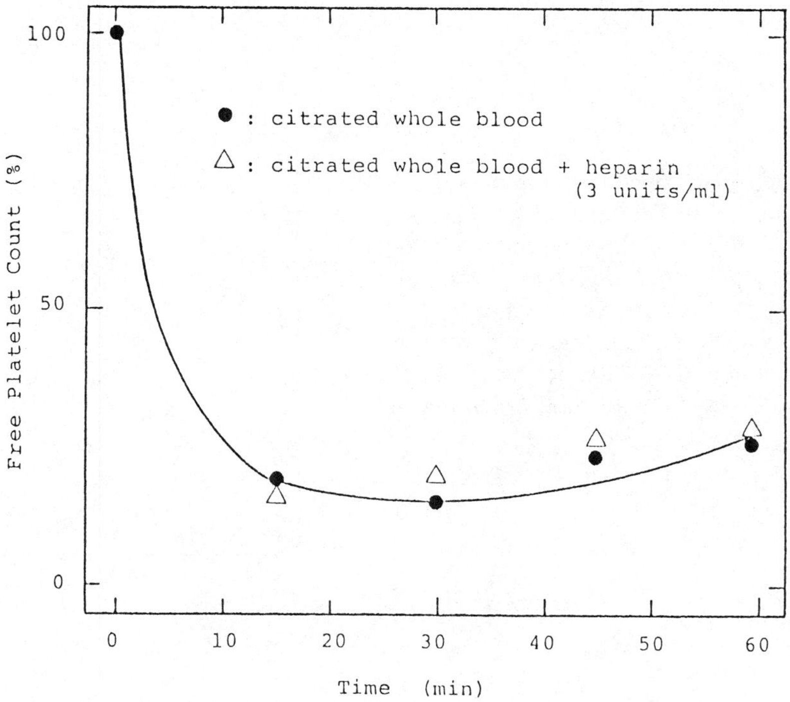

Figure 9. Effect of heparin on reduction in free platelet count of sheared citrate whole blood.

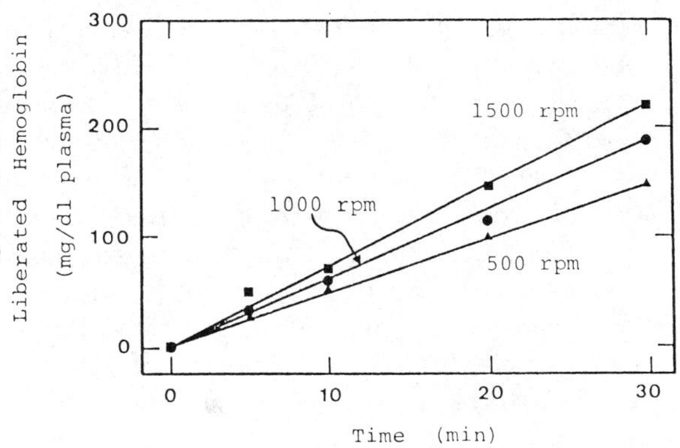

Figure 10. Hemolysis of sheared whole blood. Shear stress was applied to 0.75 ml of the citrated whole blood by a stirring bar system at a rotation speed of 500 rpm (▲), 1000 rpm (●), or 1500 rpm (■) for a definite time. Then the sheared blood was centrifuged at 2300 × g for 15 min and hemoglobin in plasma was measured.

not prevent the platelet aggregation as shown in Figure 9. This observation shows that thrombin is not involved in the platelet aggregation in sheared field of this experimental condition.

Hemolysis also occurred in the shear field. The amount of hemoglobin liberated into plasma under shear increased with increasing the rotation speed of stirring bar and shearing time as shown in Figure 10. Hemolysis of 0.15% occurred when shearing was carried out by stirring at 1000 rpm for 30 min.

6.3 Induction of Platelet Aggregation in Sheared Blood

Concentrations of ADP and ATP in sheared blood samples were assayed, since ADP-induced platelet aggregation had been suggested in the sheared whole blood. The results are

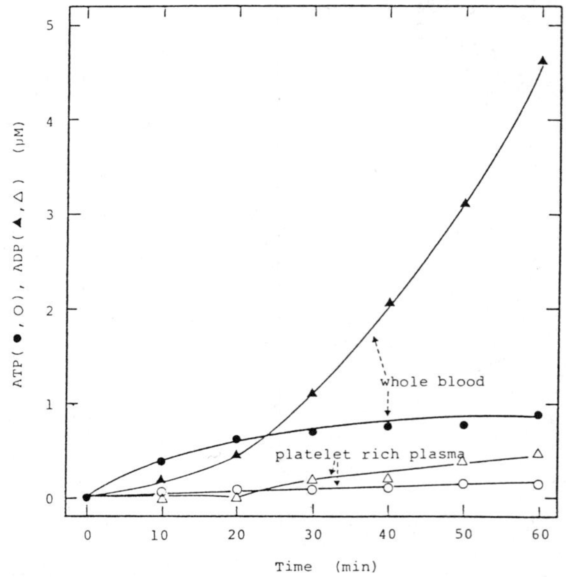

Figure 11. Extracellular concentrations of ATP and ADP in sheared whole blood and sheared platelet rich plasma. Shear stress was applied to the citrated whole blood or to the citrated platelet rich plasma by a stirring bar system at a rotation speed of 1000 rpm. After the specified time, the sheared blood sample was centrifuged at 2300 × g for 15 min. ADP (▲, △) or ATP (●, ○) concentration in plasma was assayed.

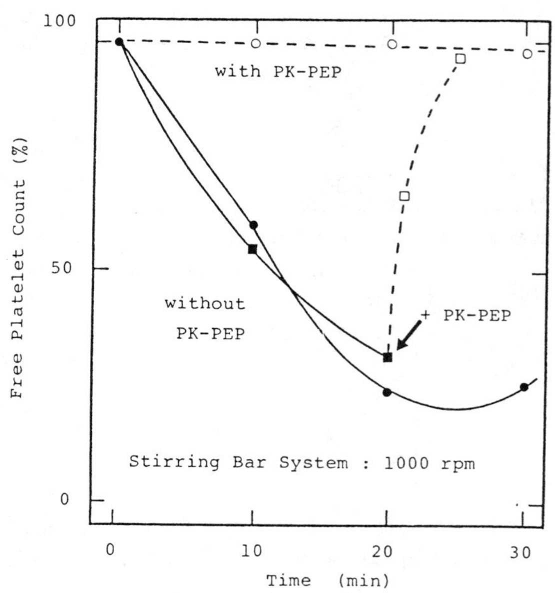

Figure 12. Effect of enzymatic conversion of ADP to ATP on reduction in free platelet count of sheared whole blood. Shear stress was applied to the following blood samples by a stirring bar system at a rotation speed of 1000 rpm and free platelet count was measured. The citrated whole blood with pyruvate kinase of 50 units per ml and phosphoenolpyruvate of 50 μM (○), and two whole blood samples without pyruvate kinase and phospohoenolpyruvate (●,■) were used. After 20 min of exposure time, 20 μl of pyruvate kinase (1925 units per ml) plus phosphoenolpyruvate (1.9 mM) solution was added only to one of the sheared blood sample. Initial free platelet count was 4.3 × 10^5 per μl in all blood samples.

shown in Figure 11. When citrated whole blood was sheared by stirring bar at a rotation speed of 1000 rpm, ADP concentration increased with shearing time and reached to about 5 μM after 60 min. ADP of these concentrations is enough to induce the primary platelet aggregation. On the other hand, the increase of ADP concentration was slight in the sheared PRP. Additionally, ATP concentration in plasma increased by giving shear stress to the whole blood, but the increase of ATP concentration was slight in PRP as shown in Figure 11. These results suggest that adenine nucleotides were liberated mainly from erythrocyte injured in the shear field.

Pyruvate kinase (PK) catalyzes the following reaction:

ADP + phosphoenolpyruvate (PEP) = ATP + Pyruvate where equilibrium constant ([ADP] [PEP]/[ATP] [Pyruvate]) is 1.55×10^{-4} at 30°C and pH 7.4. Figure 12 compares the time courses of FPC reduction in the stirring bar system (1000 rpm), in the presence and in the absence of pyruvate kinase plus phosphoenolpyruvate (PK-PEP), that is an enzymatic ADP-removal system. When the shear stress was applied to the citrated whole blood in which PK-PEP solution was previously added, no reduction in FPC was observed at all. When PK-PEP solution was added to the sheared blood in which FPC was reduced to 30% of initial count, platelet count was rapidly increased and was approximately restored to initial level. These observations indicate that the platelet aggregation in the shear field is caused by ADP, and so, the system which can eliminate ADP in plasma will be available to block the platelet aggregation and the thrombus formation.

6.4 Block of Platelet Aggregation in Sheared Blood by Immobilized Apyrase

It is considered from the previous described results that the artificial biomaterials with immobilized ADPase is available for prevention of platelet aggregation induced in the sheared field. Therefore, the immobilization of apyrase was carried out and the characteristics of the immobilized apyrase were investigated [63].

Blood cells were broken by means of homogenizer treatment or sonic treatment, and the blood cells extract (BCE) was obtained by centrifugation of broken cell. BCE induced the platelet aggregation in an aggregometer. The pattern of aggregation induced by BCE was similar to that of ADP-induced platelet aggregation. Heparin failed to inhibit the aggregation induced by BCE. When BCE of 28 μl obtained by the sonic treatment, containing hemoglobin of 1200 mg/dl, was added to citrated PRP of 250 μl in an aggregometer, platelet aggregation of 75% was observed as shown in Figure 13. The aggregation induced by BCE was lowered by soluble apyrase. Aggregated platelets were dissociated by the addition of soluble apyrase as shown in Figure 13.

The apyrase immobilized on Sepharose 4B and nylon fiber showed an activity of conversion of ADP to AMP. An activity yield was 75% at the immobilization of apyrase on Sepharose 4B. The aggregation-induced activity of BCE was reduced by apyrase immobilized on Sepharose 4B as shown in Figure 14. Apyrase immobilized on nylon also had an anti-aggregative activity similar with apyrase immobilized on Sepharose 4B for the platelet aggregation.

The immobilized apyrase was stable in the buffer and in the dry condition, respectively. The activity reduction of immobilized apyrase was scarcely observed when stored in 10 mM Tris-HCl buffer (pH 7.4) containing 0.145 M NaCl at 4°C, as shown in Figure 15. The apyrase immobilized on nylon was washed with distilled water, dried and stored in a desicator at room temperature for 8 days. The dried preparation retained 79% of the initial activity before drying and storage. The binding of apyrase on these carriers was very stable. There was no liberation of the immobilized apyrase from the carrier during the storage for several weeks at 4°C in the buffer.

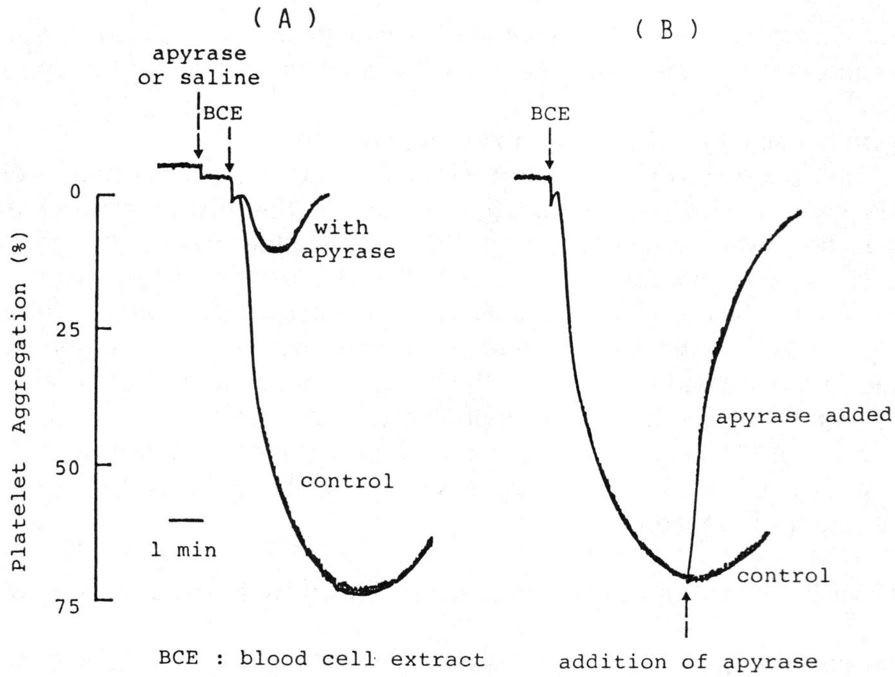

Figure 13. Depression of blood cells extract-induced platelet aggregation and disaggregation by apyrase. (A); 20 μl of saline or apyrase solution (7.7 units per ml) was added to 250 μl of citrated platelet rich plasma in a cuvette of an aggregometer. After 1.0 min, 30 μl of the blood cells extract was added and platelet aggregation (%) was measured. (B); Platelet aggregation was induced by the addition of 28 μl of the blood cells extract to platelet rich plasma. Then, when maximum platelet aggregation was observed, 20 μl of saline or apyrase solution was added.

Figure 14. Decomposition of platelet aggregation by immobilized apyrase. Blood cells extract of 10 ml was incubated with the immobilized materials (total dry weight of immobilized Sepharose 4B; 10 mg, suspended in saline of 0.1 ml) for a definite incubation period at 37°C. After the incubation, the reaction mixture was centrifuged at 1000 × g for 30 sec to remove the immobilized materials. 28 μl of the supernatant was added to 250 μl of platelet rich plasma in an aggregometer and platelet aggregation (%) was measured.

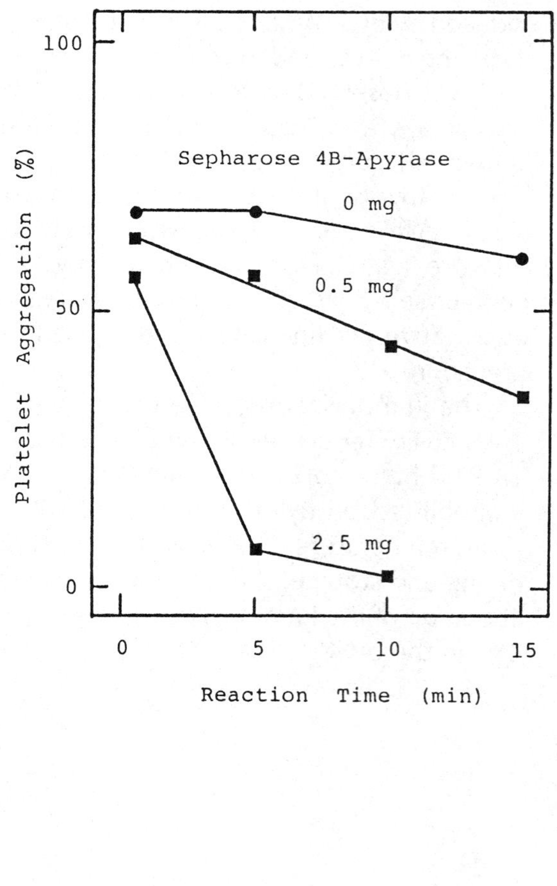

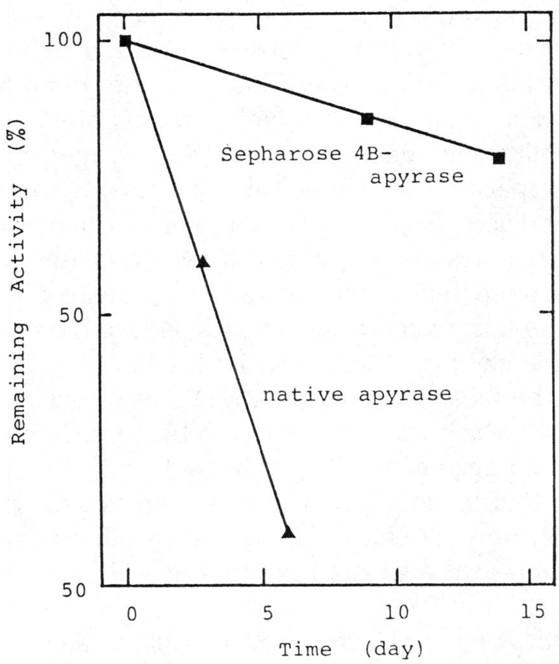

Figure 15. Stability of native and immobilized apyrase.

7. CONCLUDING REMARKS

It has been commonly considered that the AT III necessary for cooperation with heparin can be naturally supplied from blood, since AT III is present in blood. Thus, the immobilization of heparin has been proposed for obtaining antithrombogenic biomaterials [14-22]. It was found [24] that heparin covalently immobilized on biomaterials had an ability to bind thrombin and Factor Xa but these enzymes thus bound to the immobilized heparin were still active. This cooperative effect on the neutralization of Factor Xa and thrombin, i.e. the instantaneous neutralization exhibited by AT III in the presence of soluble heparin, was not observed when heparin was covalently immobilized. It was found [35-37], however, that heparin, when coimmobilized with AT III, exhibited much higher anticoagulative activity than immobilized heparin and/or immobilized AT III. Employing the activation procedure by cyanogen bromide, the coimmobilization was successfully applied to some biomaterials such as PVA, poly HEMA and silicone-coated nylon.

When two enzymes, Factor Xa and thrombin, are present, the coimmobilized AT III·Hep neutralize Factor Xa in preference to thrombin [37]. The neutralization of thrombin was inhibited by the presence of Factor Xa, but the neutralization of Factor Xa was independent of the presence of thrombin. The amount of Factor Xa neutralized was higher than that of thrombin. The rapid neutralization of Factor Xa in preference to thrombin is very favorable for the effective prevention of blood coagulation, since 1 unit of Factor Xa can catalyze the generation of 50 units of thrombin.

The immobilized urokinase (I-UK) had a fibrinolytic function and also showed the antithrombogenetic activity. However, the antithrombogenetic activity of I-UK was less than that of I-AT III·Hep. The coimmobilized AT III·Hep and urokinase (I-AT III·Hep-UK) showed much higher antithrombogenecity than I-UK and I-AT III·Hep, respectively [53]. The mixed system of

I-AT III·Hep and I-UK also showed a high antithrombogenetic activity. It was found that the cooperative utilizations of two different functions, anticoagulative and fibrinolytic functions, could increase the antithrombogenetic activity. Therefore, the coimmobilization of antithrombin III-heparin complex and urokinase and the combined use of I-AT III·Hep plus I-UK are very effective for giving high antithrombogenecity to artificial polymers, even when the polymers have low protein-binding capacity. The biomedical polymers of smooth surface cannot bind a large amount of protein, and accordingly it is difficult to obtain high activity of immobilized enzyme per unit of surface area. It is very important to overcome this defect in order to obtain the high antithrombogenic biomaterials. The immobilized proteins of high antithrombogenecity are needed to overcome this defect of the smooth surface biomaterials.

It was found that the platelet aggregation was induced principally by ADP liberated from the injured erythrocyte in the shear field and thereby FPC was significantly decreased. The enzymatic elimination of ADP, which was liberated from blood cells into plasma, was effective for the prevention of platelet aggregation in the sheared whole blood. Immobilized apyrase could effectively undergo the decomposition of ADP, and thereby prevent the platelet aggregation. The artificial polymers on which apyrase is immobilized, have an ability of preventing the platelet aggregation in the sheared blood and will be available as an antithrombogenic biomaterials.

One of the characteristics of immobilized enzyme is high stability. The administrations of anticoagulants and inhibitors of platelet function to human body don't have so long effect. This defect can be overcome by application of the enzyme immobilization technique. However, there are still many unsolved problems for creating the clinical applicable high antithrombogenetic biomaterials. Especially, the immunity and sterilization are very important problems which must be solved before the clinical application.

REFERENCES

1. Abligaard, U., "Binding of thrombin to antithrombin III", Scand. J. Clin. Lab. Inves., (24), 23, 1969.
2. Binder, B., "On the complex formation of Antithrombin III with thrombin", Thrombos. Diathes. haemorrh., (30), 280, 1973.
3. Jesty, J., "The inhibition of activated bovine coagulation factors X and VII by antithrombin III", Arch. Biochem. Biophys., (185), 165, 1978.
4. Jesty, J., "The kinetics of formation and dissociation of the bovine thrombin·antithrombin III complex", J. Biol. Chem., (254), 10044, 1979.
5. Thomas, O.P., Niewiarowski, S., and Ream, V.J., "Release of adenine nucleotides and platelet factor 4 from platelets of man and from other species", J. Lab. Clin. Med., (75), 607, 1970.
6. Joist, J. H. "Platelet factor 3 availability and the platelet release reaction", J. Lab. Clin. Med., (84), 474, 1974.
7. Miletech, J.P., Jackson, C.M., and Majerus, P.W., "Properties of the binding site on human platelets", J. Biol. Chem., (253), 6908, 1978.
8. Damus, P.S., Hicks, M. and Rosenberg, R.D., "Anticoagulant action of heparin", Nature, (246), 355, 1973.
9. Bjork, I. and Nordenman, B., "Acceleration of the reaction between thrombin and antithrombin III by non-stoichiometric heparin", Eur. J. Biochem., (68), 507, 1976.
10. Li, E.H.H., Fenton II, J.W. and Feinman, R.D., "The role of heparin in the thrombin-antithrombin III reaction," Arch. Biochem. Biophys., (175), 153, 1976.
11. Holmer, E., Soderstrom, G. and Anderson, L.-O., "Studies of the mechanism of the rate-enhancing effect of heparin on the thrombin-antithrombin III reaction", Eur. J. Biochem., (93), 1, 1979.

12. Mustard, J.F., "Factors influencing platelet function: adhesion, release, and aggregation", Pharmacol. Rev., (22), 97, 1970.
13. Joist, J.H. and Mustard, J.F., "Heparin, lysolecithin, and platelet function", <<Heparin; Structure, Function, and Clinical Implications>>, Bradshaw, R.A. and Wessler, S. ed., New York and London, Plenum Press, 255, 1975.
14. Schmer, G., "The biological activity of covalently immobilized heparin", Trans. Am. Soc. Artif. Int. Organs, (18), 321, 1972.
15. Hoffman, A.S., Schmer, G., Harris, C. and Kraft, W.G., "Covalent binding of biomolecules to radiation-grafted hydrogels on inert polymer surfaces", Trans. Am. Soc. Artif. Int. Organs, (18), 10, 1972.
16. Lagergren, H.R., and Ericksson, J.C., "Plastics with a stable surface monolayer of crosslinked heparin: Preparation and evaluation", Trans. Am. Soc. Artif. Int. Organs, (17), 10, 1971.
17. Yen, S.P.S. and Rembaum, A., "Complexes of heparin with elastomeric positive polyelectrolytes", J. Biomed. Mater. Res. Symp., (1), 83, 1971.
18. Goosen, M.F.A. and Sefton, M.V., "Heparinized styrene-butadiene-styrene", J. Biomed. Mater. Res., (13), 347, 1979.
19. Schmer, G., Teng, L.N.L., Cole, J.J., Vizzo, J.E., Francisco, M.M. and Scribner, B.H., "Successful use of a totally heparin grafted hemodialysis sytem in sheep", Trans. Am. Soc. Artif. Int. Organs, (22), 654, 1976.
20. Rembaum, A., "Heparin insolubilized with crosslinked agent", NASA Tech. Brief., 69-10299, 1969.
21. Merker, R.L., Elyash, L.J., Mayhew, S.H. and Wang, J.Y.C., "The heparinization of silicon rubber using aminoorganosilane coupling agents", Proc. Artificial Heart Program Conf. (AHP), 29, 1969.
22. Gott, V.L., Whiffen, J.D. and Dutton, R.C., "Heparin binding on colloidal graphite surfaces", Science, (142), 1297, 1963.
23. Iverius, P.H., "Coupling of glycosaminoglycants to agarose beads", Biochem. J., (124), 677, 1971.
24. Miura, Y., Aoyagi, S., Kusada, Y. and Miyamoto, K., "The characteristics of anticoagulation by covalently immobilized heparin", J. Biomed. Mater. Res., (14), 619, 1980.
25. Morita, T., Kato, H., Iwanaga, S., Takada, K., Kimura, T. and Sakakibara, S., "New fluorogenic substrates for thrombin, Factor Xa kallikreins and urokinase", J. Biochem., (82), 1495, 1977.
26. Bjork, I. and Nordenman, B., "Acceleration of the reaction between thrombin and antithrombin III by non-stoichiometric amounts of heparin", Eur. J. Biochem., (68), 507, 1976.
27. Holmer, E., Soderstrom, G. and Anderson, L.-O., "Studies on the Mechanisms of the rate-enhancing effect of heparin on the thrombin-antithrombin III reaction", Eur. J. Biochem., (93), 1, 1979.
28. Piepkorn, M.W., Lagunoff, D. and Schmer, G., "Heparin binding to antithrombin III: Variation in binding sites and affinity", Biochem. Biophys. Res. Commun., (85), 851, 1978.
29. Li, E.H.H., Orton, C. and Fienman, R.D., "The interaction of thrombin and heparin, proflavine dye binding studies", Biochem., (13), 5012, 1974.
30. Einarrson, R. and Anderson, L.-O., "Binding of heparin to human antithrombin III as studied by measurements of tryptophane fluorescence", Biochem. Biophys. Acta., (490), 104, 1977.
31. Anderson, L.-O., Engman, L. and Henninsson, E., "Crossed Immunoelectrophoresis as applied to studies on complex formation. The binding of heparin to antithrombin III and the antithrombin III-thrombin complex", J. Immunol. Methods, (14), 271, 1977.
32. Hooh, M., Bjork, I., Hoopwood, J. and Lindahl, U., "Anti-coagulant activity of heparin: Separation of high-activity and low-activity heparin species by affinity chromatography on immobilized antithrombin", FEBS Lett., (66), 90, 1976.
33. Machovich, R., "Mechanism of action of heparin through thrombin on blood coagulation", Biochem. Biophys. Acta, (412), 13, 1975.
34. Hatton, M.W.,C., Kaur, H. and Regoeczi, E., "The effect of heparin adsorbed on Sepharose-lysine on the inactivation of thrombin by anti-thrombin III", Biochem. Soc. Trans., (5), 1443, 1977.

35. Miura, Y., Miyamoto, K., Aoyagi, S. and Kusada, Y., "Anticoagulative activity of artificial biomedical materials with coimmobilized antithrombin III and heparin", Artif. Organs (Japan), (7), 193, 1978.
36. Y. Miura, Aoyagi, S. and Miyamoto, K., "The development of the anticoagulative artificial biomedical materials by coimmobilizing antithrombin III and heparin", Artif. Organs (Japan), (8), 288, 1979.
37. Miura, Y., Aoyagi, S., Ikeda, F. and Miyamoto, K., "Anticoagulant activity of artificial biomedical materials with coimmobilized antithrombin III and heparin", Biochimie, (62), 595, 1980.
38. Ambrus, C.M., Roholt, O.A. and Meyer, B.K., "Enzymatic activity of insolubilized streptokinase (I-SK) and urokinase (I-UK)", Fed. Proc., (31), 267, 1972.
39. Deuth, D.G. and Mertz, E.T., "Activation of plasminogen with insoluble derivatives of urokinase", J. Med., (3), 224, 1972.
40. Kusserow, B.K. and Larrow, R., "Use of surface bonded, covalently cross-linked urokinase as an approach to the creation of a thromboresistant synthetic surface with fibrinolytic capability", Circulation, Suppl., (2), 54, 1972.
41. Kusserow, B.K., Larrow, R.W. and Nichols, J.E., "The Surface bonded, covalently cross-linked urokinase synthetic surface. In vitro and chronic in vivo studies", Trans. Am. Soc. Artif. Intern. Organs, (19), 8, 1973.
42. Wiman, B. and Wallen, P., "Activation of human plasminogen by an insoluble derivative of urokinase. Structural changes of plasminogen with course of activation to plasmin and demonstration of a possible intermediate compound", Eur. J. Biochem., (36), 25, 1973.
43. Capet-Antonini, F.C., Grimard, M. and Tamenasse, J., "Properties of two types of solid-phase urokinase preparations", Thromb. Res., (2), 479, 1973.
44. Ohshiro, T., Mukai, K., Koh, S., Sakamoto, S., Sugitachi, A. and Murakami, F., "Fibrinolytic therapy – The necessity and possibility of local fibrinolytic therapy", J. Med. Enzymol. (Japan), (1), 72, 1975.
45. Ohshiro, T., Monden, M., Kosaki, G. and Takagi, K., "The study of nylon structure material immobilized urokinase", Artif. Organs (Japan), (6), 237, 1977.
46. Ohshiro, T., Sugitachi, A., Hong, S., Murai, K., Murakami, F., Kosaki, G. and Motoi, S., "Immobilization of fibrinolytic enzyme-fibrinolytic activity of immobilized urokinase linked to Sepharose 6B", Blood and Vessel (Japan), (9), 72, 1978.
47. Ohshiro, T., Takahashi, A., Mukai, K., Hong, D.S., Kosaki, G. and Takagi, K., "The study on available immobilization method of urokinase to nylon", Artif. Organs (Japan), (7), 210, 1978.
48. Ohshiro, T. and Kosaki, G., "Urokinase immobilized on medical polymeric materials: Fundamental and clinical studies", Artif. Organs, (4), 58, 1980.
49. Sugitachi, A., Kawahara, T., Takagi, K. Yabushita, Y., "Studies on antithrombogenecity of immobilized urokinase", Artif. Organs (Japan), (7), 214, 1978.
50. Watanabe, S., Shimizu, Y., Yamamoto, H., Teramatsu, T., Endo, J., Murachi, T. and Hino, T., "Immobilization of enzyme onto collagen-coated synthetic polymer support", Artif. Organs (Japan), (7), 206, 1978.
51. Watanabe, S., Shimizu, Y., Teramatsu, T., Endo, J., Murachi, T. and Hino, T., "Studies on collagen-coated synthetic polymer composite carrying immobilized urokinase", Artif. Organs (Japan), (8), 218, 1979.
52. Watanabe, S., Kato, H., Shimizu, Y., Teramatsu, T., Murachi, T. and Hino T., "Immobilization of hen egg-white lysozyme and poly-peptide antibiotic polymyxin B for producing antibacterial biomaterials", Artif. Organs (Japan), (9), 267, 1980.
53. Miura, Y., Aoyagi, S. and Miyamoto, K., "Antithrombogenetic activity of coimmobilized antithrombin III·heparin complex and urokinase", J. Biomed. Mater. Res., submitted.
54. Chandler, A.B., "In viro thrombotic coagulation of the blood", Lab. Invest., (7), 110, 1958.
55. Brown, C.H. III, Lemuth, R.F., Hellums, J.D., Leverett, L.B. and Alfrey, C.P. Jr., "Response of human platelets to shear stress", Trans. Am. Soc. Artif. Intern. Organs, (21), 35, 1975.

56. Hung, T.C., Hochmuth, R.M., Joist, J.H. and Sutera, S.P., "Shear-induced aggregation and lysis of platelet", Trans. Am. Soc. Artif. Intern. Organs, (22), 285, 1976.
57. Sutera, S.P., Croce, P.A. and Mehrjardi, M., "Hemolysis and subhemolytic alterations of human RBC induced by turbulent shear flow", Trans. Am. Soc. Artif. Organs, (18), 335, 1972.
58. Sakai, K., Saitoh, T., Ikeda, H., Suzuki, M., Azuma, N., Aoki, R., Inoue, N. and Iisaka, O., "Hemolysis by some mechanical effects", Artif. Organs (Japan), (6), 288, 1977.
59. Miura, Y., Aoyagi, S., Ikeda, F. and Miyamoto, K., "Release of adenine nucleotides and platelet aggregation response to extracellular ATP and ADP in sheared blood", Artif. Organs (Japan), (9), 314, 1980.
60. Kinlongh-Rathbone, R.L., Packham, M.A. and Mustard, J.F., "The effect of prostaglandin E_1 on platelet function in vitro and in vivo", British J. Haematology, (19), 559, 1970.
61. Moncada, S. and Korbut, R., "Dipyridamole and other phosphodiesterase inhibitors act as antithrombotic agents by potentiating endogenous prostacyclin", Lancet, (1), 1286, 1978.
62. Paccioretti, M.J. and Block, L.H., "Effects of aspirin on Platelet aggregation as a function of dosage and time", Clin. Pharmacol. Ther., (27), 803, 1980.
63. Miura, Y., Hirota, K., Fujino, T., Kitahori, F., Aoyagi, S. and Miyamoto, K., "Prevention of shear-induced platelet aggregation by immobilized apyrase," Artif. Organs (Japan), (10), 997, 1981.

Chapter 15

Hydrogels Grafted to Implant Surfaces with Atomic Hydrogen

Paul L. Kronick
The Franklin Institute
20th Street at Parkway
Philadelphia, Pa. 19103

ABSTRACT

Of several types of synthetic surfaces which have been explored for nonthrombogenic vascular implants, the water-swollen hydrogels were designed to mimic the naturally hydrophilic surface with its protein and glycosaminoglycan layers overlying the vascular endothelium. Preparing such linings which adhere to the subsurfaces of which the devices are made has proven to be very difficult. We have demonstrated that inert materials can be coated with polyacrylamide by the atomic-hydrogen method. Some blood proteins, such as fibrinogen and Factor XII, are absorbed to the hydrogel without loss of antigenic sites; in-vivo patency is prolonged in the vena-cava ring test, although not consistently in every sample; no acute or sub-acute toxic effects could be demonstrated. On the other hand, leucocyte adhesion and some hemolysis was observed in flowing blood in in-vitro stagnation-point flow and shear tests, respectively. It would appear that the benign interactions between polyacrylamide and blood, as a material property of the hydrogel, do not entirely compensate for effects of surface texture, which perturb laminar blood flow, and so increase the tendency of cell adhesion. On the basis of these observations, we have modified the coating process so that smoother films can be produced.

Supported in NHLBI-NIH contract No. NO1-HV-1-2017.

INTRODUCTION

It was generally realized, since the beginning of the program undertaken by the U.S. National Heart, Lung, and Blood Institute in 1964 to develop a totally implanted artificial heart, that the tendency of blood to clot on foreign surfaces would be a major obstacle to the clinical use of such devices. It has been assumed for some time that, even after materials have been found that satisfy the mechanical and chemical requirements of artificial organs, it may be necessary to coat them with something to make them compatible with blood. We have suggested (Kronick 1980) 10 requirements for such coatings which, together, are very difficult to satisfy:

1. They must be nonthrombogenic.
2. Their chemical and physical properties must be stable in physiological solutions, including lipids, and must be unaltered by physical forces such as shearing and stretching.
3. They must be applicable in thin layers.
4. They must not be toxic.
5. No introduction of solvents or swelling agents into substrata is permitted.
6. No excessive heating of substrata is permitted.
7. Reagents must be very fluid so that irregular surfaces (foams, fibers, and powders) can be coated.
8. Coatings must be uniform without holes, points, whiskers, or streamers.
9. The method of application must be adaptable to a variety of inert substrata and coating materials.
10. The coating process should be economically and technologically feasible for application to large surfaces, including dialysis and oxygenator membranes, blood-storage bags, and other mass-produced items.

The first requirement is best satisfied if the components of the blood, both solutes and formed elements, are indifferent to the presence of the foreign surface. Several thermodynamic criteria for such inert surfaces have been proposed. One possibility is that the free energy of adsorption of components of blood onto the surface should be zero or positive. Another is that the free energy for forming the interface between blood and the implant should be zero (otherwise the blood elements would tend to deposit on the surface to lower the area of the interface) (Andrade 1973). It would appear that either condition would be satisfied if the surface is chemically and physically similar to the aqueous solution. Therefore, water swollen polymers, hyhdrogels (Wichterle and Lim 1960), are candidates for vascular-implant interfaces.

Polymers of many different types have been widely used for coatings in intravascular devices. Application of hydrogels as nonthrombogenic coatings, however, introduces problems which are peculiar to this type of material, related to their incompatibility with likely structural polymers for the devices. Hydrogels are typically prepared from aqueous or very polar solvents, from which they must be spread in thin films upon nonpolar substrata such as polypropylene, silicone, or polyetherurethane. Because the two phases, hydrophilic and hydrophobic, have little mutual affinity, the interface is unstable and adhesion is poor. For this reason special methods have been developed, which in some cases are rather elaborate, to effect a physical or chemical bond between the hydrogel coating and the substratum.

Another problem arises in characterizing hydrogel coated materials. After a hydrophobic surface has been coated with hydrogel, a composite structure results in which the two components swell differentially when equilibrated with water. The result is a potential mechanical instability which may affect the performance of flexible parts such as pump diaphragms. Again, during the coating process, some components of thermoplastic substrata may migrate into the hydrogel layer, altering the nature of the hydrophilic product from that obtained in the absence of organic substrata. It is therefore necessary to analyze the chemical composition and the physical behavior of the coating *in situ*, even if it is only a few microns thick.

The potential of hydrogels as nonthrombogenic surfaces is based on their low interfacial tension with water as pointed out above. This parameter is minimized at a high water content of the gel. Therefore the surface coatings must be characterized by measurements of wetting angles as well as protein adsorption and blood-cell adhesion. To understand the structure and function of the coatings, it is also necessary to have data on water adsorption, interpenetration with substrata, chemical composition, crosslinking, and gel fraction.

The methods (Kronick, 1980) which have been used to prepare hydrogel coatings on organic polymer substrata include: simple casting and adhesion; formation of interpenetrating networks; chemical grafting initiated by ceric ion from solutions of hydrogel monomer onto the substratum; ultraviolet irradiation; ionizing radiation; and activation of monomer vapor with atomic hydrogen or ozone. Devices for vascular applications are fabricated with extraordinary care from medical-grade polymers, which should be of the highest purity. Immersion of such items in liquids for the purpose of coating them exposes them to the risk of imbibing dissolved impurities, which might be difficult to remove later. Vapor-coating methods meet this drawback, since impurities are all volatile and present in a very dilute form. Another advantage of vapor coating is that complex shapes can be treated with rapid penetration of reagents into crevices without local stirring. The slight volatility of HEMA permits it to be deposited onto plastic surfaces from its vapor at reduced pressure. Yamauchi (1975) described such a method, in which polyvinyl chloride was first activated with a mixture of 1.4% ozone in oxygen. HEMA was then deposited on the surface from the vapor and polymerized by heating at 98°C at 5 torr. A concomitant increase in thromboresistance was reported.

Oxygen and ozone probably activate polymeric surfaces by forming reactive oxides or peroxides. Such reactions lead to degradation and oily products. Atomic hydrogen, on the other hand, results largely in hydrogen abstraction, leading to metastable free radicals and internal crosslinks. Although degradation proceeds as well as crosslinking, in all polymer substrates examined so far (polymeric hydrocarbons, silicones, polyetherurethanes, polyesters, polystyrene, and others) the net change was an increase in network formation (Hansen and Schonhorn 1966). The lifetimes of the free radicals are distributed over a range from seconds to days, and so can be used to initiate grafted polymer chains if a monomer is introduced to them shortly after they are formed.

The vapor of atomic hydrogen is extremely reactive, forming free radicals in solid polymers to a depth of approximately 10^{-5} cm. Ingalls and Ward (1961), treating finely divided polystyrene with atomic hydrogen, formed an average radical concentration of 10^{-3}M with lifetimes of about 2 hr at room temperature. Results from radiation grafting show that this is fully adequate to initiate grafting polymerization reactions with large yields. The active vapors are stable enough to be conducted several feet along internal surfaces to be treated, which are located remote from the vapor-activating apparatus. Thus the choice of this apparatus can be arbitrary: a microwave discharge, an electric arc, or simply a heated filament. In the equipment which we use, (Kronick 1975, 1979) a 1:1 mixture of hydrogen and helium at 3 torr flows through an intense electrical discharge in a 100-W microwave cavity, where some of the hydrogen is dissociated into its atoms. It flows into a chamber where the sample to be treated is located, at which point it is 3% dissociated, giving a vapor with 10^{-8}M atomic hydrogen.

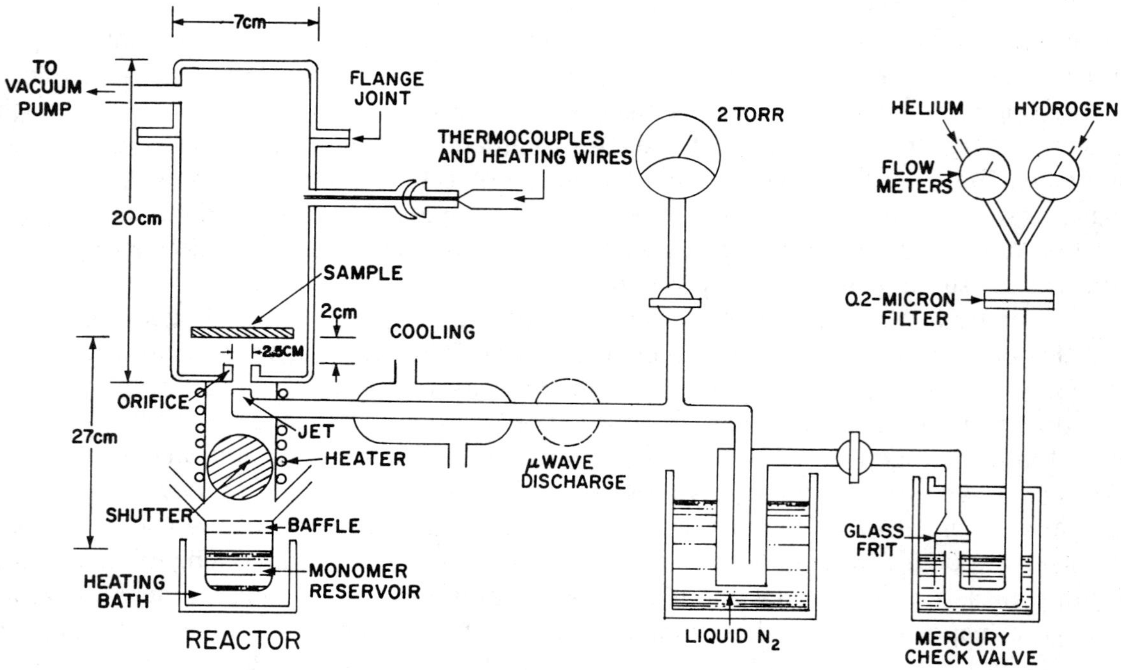

Figure 1. Active-Vapor Grafting Apparatus. Separately metered vapors of hydrogen and helium are mixed, filtered, and introduced into the vacuum system through the mercury check-valve, which is a fritted filter funnel inverted in a pool of mercury. In the discharge region the helium is ionized, exciting the hydrogen also. The high temperature and energetic collisions cause the hydrogen to dissociate into atoms. This activated vapor is introduced into the sample-treatment reactor. At the bottom of the reaction assembly, monomer is distilled through the baffle, shutter, and reactor port onto the sample. In the treatment, a sample is mounted in the reactor, the system is filled with hydrogen-helium at atmospheric pressure, and the system is pumped down and backfilled with hydrogen-helium 3 times. It is extremely important that no oxygen remain in the system, and that the system not leak, because of the danger of explosion of the mixture if its composition reaches an explosion limit when the discharge is on. The monomers are brought to temperature with the shutter closed. The program of monomer-atomic hydrogen can be chosen at will, with the port opening simultaneously with the ignition of the discharge, or alternating with it.

2. METHODS AND MATERIALS

2.1 VAM Active-Vapor Coating Technique

The reactor and vapor handling train is shown in Figure 1. Helium and hydrogen flow from their respective tanks into the system at atmospheric pressure and at rates of 300 and 271 cm^3/min, respectively. After passing a 0.4-micron filter the gas mixture is introduced into the vacuum system through the mercury check valve. Mercury vapor from the check valve is removed by the liquid-nitrogen trap packed with molecular sieve. An electrical discharge is excited at 100 W with 2450 MHz microwaves, using a tuned cavity described by Broida and Chapman (1958). The gap in the microwave cavity accommodates a 1-cm glass tube. A blast of air from a fan on the outside of the heated portion of the tube prevents it from melting. The linear velocity of the gas in the tube is 2×10^5 cm/sec. The hydrogen partially dissociates in the dicharge and travels a distance of 12 cm along a section of tubing which is water-cooled and coated on the inside with phosphoric acid to suppress recombination of the atoms, arriving at the sample position near the orifice of the reactor in about 40 microsec and passing completely through the reactor in 3 msec. Since the lifetime of atomic hydrogen under our conditions is typically about 1 sec (Thrush, 1968), decay of the reactive species is negligible.

The reactor in Figure 1 consists of a heated monomer source, intermittent shutter, microwave discharge, active-vapor jet, and sample locations. The shutter operates on a 6-sec open-closed cycle, with adjustable "open" and "closed" phases of the 6-sec cycle. Atomic hydrogen enters the sample compartment throughout the cycle, the shutter regulating the accessibility of monomer.

The uniformity of the atomic hydrogen concentration in the reactor was observed by the darkening of a glass rod coated with solid molybdic anhydride, placed along a long diagonal of the reaction chamber in Figure 1. Under the generation conditions described above, the rod turned uniformly green-black along its length, confirming that the distribution of hydrogen atoms was uniform in the reactor volume.

Attempts to use a platinum thermocouple to routinely monitor the atomic hydrogen when the apparatus was in use failed as soon as monomer vapors were introduced into the system, which poisoned and eventually coated the platinum with a black film. The temperature of the thermocouple, which was raised by the hydrogen recombination reaction catalyzed on its surface, gradually fell from 98°C to ambient.

Although the active hydrogen was uniformly distributed, the deposition of polymer decreased rapidly with distance above the orifice. We found that the best distance for coating 5-cm squares uniformly was 2 cm from the orifice, because the non-volatile monomers condensed on the wall of the apparatus beyond this distance and were therefore lost from the vapor. At shorter distances the hydrogel deposited preferentially in the center of the square.

2.2 Concentration of Active Hydrogen in the Vapor

Atomic hydrogen concentration was measured separately by substitution of a trap containing a 10^{-3}M solution of potassium ferricyanide in glycerol (Figure 2) for the reactor (Figure 1). Active vapor was bubbled through this trap after it emerged from the electrical discharge. The concentration of ferricyanide was measured at 420 nm before and after the active hydrogen was bubbled through, the amount reduced by the $H^{\cdot}$ being determined by difference, using the absorption coefficient of 1000 $M^{-1}cm^{-1}$ (Czapski and Stein 1960). The concentration of atomic hydrogen in the vapor was found to be 2.6×10^{-8}M. Except for the substitution of glycerol for water, made necessary because of the reduced pressure, the procedure follows that of Navon and Stein (1966).

2.3 Composition of Monomer Vapor

The composition of monomer vapor is indirectly controlled by that of the reservoir and its

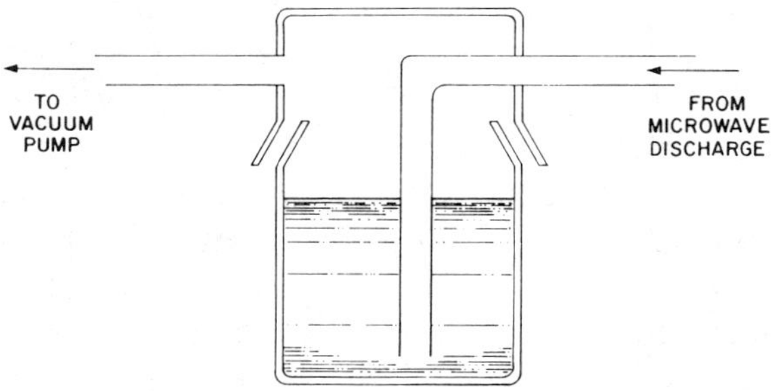

Figure 2. Small active-vapor reactor. This reactor can replace the larger one shown in Figure 1 for special applications, such as introducing the active vapor under the surface of a liquid.

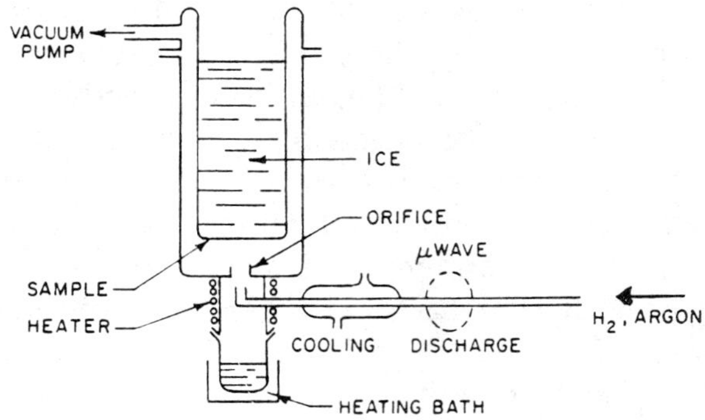

Figure 3. Active-vapor reactor for cooling the substratum. The specimen to be coated with hydrogel is attached to the lower surface of the cold finger while it is subjected to the monomer and active vapors.

temperature. A distillation curve was constructed with either hydroxyethyl methacrylate-ethylene glycol or acrylamide-ethylene glycol mixtures. In the distillation assembly various mixtures were distilled up to a cold finger and condensed into a collection vial. The compositions were determined from the refractive index at 30.0°C determined with an Abbe' refractometer.

2.4 Temperature of the Reaction Zone

A thermometer was suspended inside the reactor, observable from the outside. The reservoir contained 30% acrylamide in ethylene glycol. Without water running through the cooling section, the temperature reached 40°C; with water, 30°C. The temperature could be controlled exactly by the introduction of a cold finger into the reactor (Figure 3).

2.5 VIP Active-Vapor Initiated Polymerization

A large number of experiments were done with a simpler method (called VIP) than the grafting with vapors of atoms and monomers (VAM) described above. When the monomer was HEMA, it was found that hydrophobic surfaces could be wetted with organic solutions of the monomer and crosslinker (ethylene glycol dimethacrylate). Items covered with such liquid films of the monomer solution could be placed in the apparatus shown in Figure 1 and were treated with the active hydrogen with no additional cross flow of monomer from the reservoir. An advantage of this method was that it was not limited by the availability of monomer at the surface to be coated, while the active hydrogen, as shown above, persisted at considerable distance from its point of generation. Therefore it was possible to coat larger objects uniformly without modifying the apparatus, except for making it larger or longer.

2.6 Photopolymerization Post-Treatment

Samples can be given a final coat of pAAm applied by the photochemical method described by Oster (1960). The surface of the sample was first coated with VAM-pHEMA or VAM-pAAm by the method described in Section 2.1, which we denote the VAM (vapor of atoms and monomer) method. The sample was then either soaked in 2.5 g/l ferric chloride at ph=2 or was exposed to benzophenone vapor for 17 hr. at room temperature in a sealed container. It was then immersed in a solution of 50% AAm, 0.2% MBA and exposed to 100-W quartz medium-pressure mercury arc filtered through borosilicate glass and 1 cm of aqueous (25 g/l) copper sulfate, which removed heat and far-ultraviolet radiation. In some cases the sample was rotated in the solution at 1 Hz during the illumination for better coating uniformity while supported at the focus of an elliptical reflector. The exposure was for 5 min. In these treatments the hydrated ferric ions or benzophenone molecules were excited by the violet light and subsequently abstracted hydrogen atoms from the surface of the underlying VAM film; the radicals formed thereby in the VAM film reacted to initiate the polymerization of the AAm in the vicinity of the surface, continuing the coating with pAAm in a conventional photopolymerization reaction.

2.7 Materials

Polyetherurethanes (PEU) were obtained as cast films, tubes, or coated implant rings all from Stanford Research Institute (SRI). Polypropylene (PP) vena-cava rings were obtained from the Medical Product Division of Gulf General Atomic Corp. This source also supplied the blank rings which were later coated with PEU, and implant rings for the Kusserow renal-embolism test. Polypropylene film was Hercules N400, 250 microns thick. Teflon film (25 micron thick) was obtained from AIN Plastic, New York. These substrata were rinsed with alcohol and distilled water before further use. The PEU contained a fluorescent impurity, not apparently leachable into water, which was not identified.

Acrylamide (AAm) and N,N'-methylene bisacrylamide (MBA) were supplied from the Research Laboratories of Polysciences, Inc., triply recrystallized; ethylene glycol dimethacrylate (EGDMA), from Monomer-Polymer Laboratories, Inc., and hydroxyethyl methacrylate (HEMA), from Rohm and Haas, Inc.; The HEMA was redistilled at 2 torr and 72-75°C.

2.8 Purity of Monomer

The purified HEMA must be analyzed extensively for impurities by spectroscopy and gas-liquid chromatography (glc). HEMA (Rohm and Haas) as supplied has a yellow tinge with an absorption shoulder at 290 nm (abs. coef. = 1.3 cm^{-1}) due to a non-volatile impurity absent from all distilled products (Figure 4). The first distilled fraction, boiling at 63° at 2 torr, does not have the 290-nm-absorbing impurity, but does have a volatile impurity absorbing weakly at 330 nm (Abs. coef. = 0.05 cm^{-1}). This is absent from later fractions.

EGDMA, which codistills with HEMA, causes some gelation in the purified monomer. When this monomer was dissolved in CCl_4, in which polyHEMA gel is insoluble, a precipitate formed which could be measured as turbidity, causing an increase in slope of the absorbance-wavelength curve in the near-UV (Figure 4).

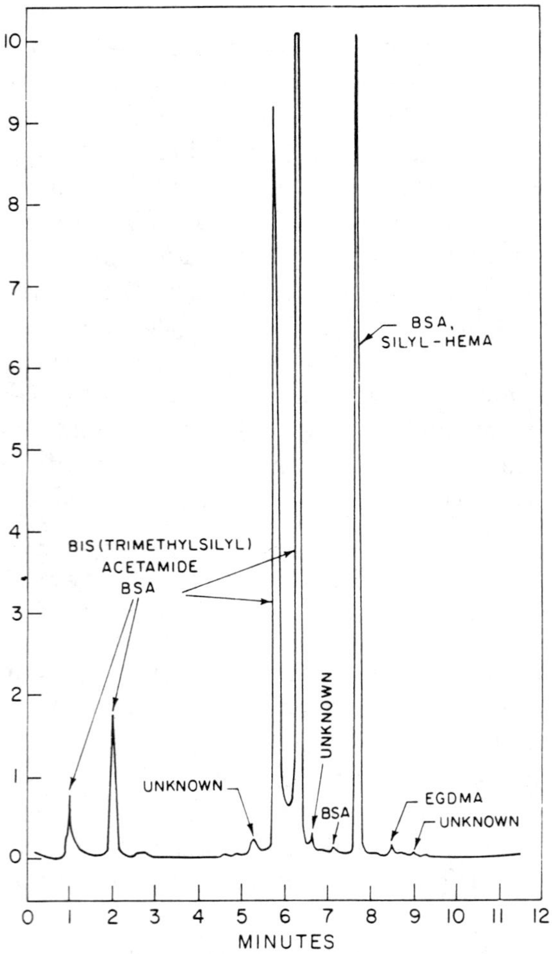

Figure 5. Gas-liquid chromatograph of distilled HEMA after reaction with BSA. Details are given in the text.

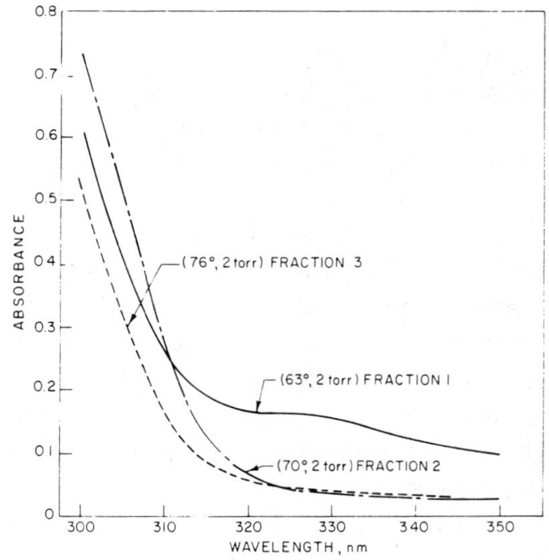

Figure 4. Turbidity of precipitated-gel suspensions in (2:3) (HEMA/CCl_4) mixtures.

A third fraction (72°C, 2 torr) from a vacuum distillation of Rohm and Haas HEMA was reacted with 5X excess bis-trimethylsilyl acetamide (BSA). A clear, colorless mixture resulted which became slightly yellow when allowed to stand for several hours. This was injected into the Hewlett-Packard model 5700 glc under the following conditions: column, 4 ft. dual glass, 10% Silica Gum Rubber USC98; injector temp, 100°C; flame-ionization detector temp, 300°C; column temp 80°C; hold at 80°, 4 min; heating rate, 32°C/min; hold at 270°C, 4 min; carrier gas, N_2.

There is no HEMA peak (Figure 5), but a peak due to EGDMA, an impurity even in freshly distilled HEMA, appears. From the structure it is seen that there is no active hydrogen available for silylation by BSA reagent, nor is there in diethylene glycol dimethacrylate. Three unknown peaks were recorded, but no assignment can yet be made. Six peaks common to the BSA reagent appear; one of these is coincident with the HEMA-ether peak. No other large peaks were found that could be assigned to the silyl-HEMA product.

The effect of HEMA monomer is to inhibit both the aggregation of platelets and the release of granules, even when stimulated with thrombin (Kronick and Rembaum 1977).

3. RESULTS AND DISCUSSION

3.1 Water Content of Hydrogels Prepared by the VAM Process

3.1.1 pHEMA

VAN-pHEMA films were prepared on glass, and their weights were monitored continuously on a Cahn electrobalance while water or other solvents were being absorbed from the vapor. Glass cover slips (1 in × 2 in) were washed in dichromate, tap water, distilled water, and ethyl alcohol, and dried at 110°C to constant weight. They were then supported in the treatment chamber (Figure 1) exposed to flowing vapors of HEMA, hydrogen atoms, hydrogen and helium for 1 hr, and weighed again to obtain the weights of the films. For these samples, the shutter remained open the entire time. There was no crosslinker in these mixtures. To determine solvent uptake, the films were then suspended from an arm of the microbalance in a chamber filled with 90% solvent-saturated air, counter-balanced by a clean glass coverslip in the same chamber (swollen film weight).

There was no observable weight gain when the solvent in the vapor phase was water. The swelling of four different samples in DMF vapor, with higher affinity than water, is shown in Table 1.

Table 1. Swelling of VAM PolyHEMA Films by DMF

Wt of Swollen Film	Thickness (wt x 1g/cm^3)	Wt. Solvent	Swelling (Wt. Solvent/ Wt. Swollen film)
4.10 mg	3.14	3.89 mg	95%
4.10	3.14	3.30	81%
3.85	2.95	2.10	55%
5.10	3.91	3.35	66%

The same procedure was used for preparing each of the four films. The variation of swelling among them shows that there is some aspect of the process which is not now subject to our control. Also, the swelling in DMF, a powerful swelling agent, is small, even allowing for possible biaxial constrant due to the adhesion to the glass. (VIP polyHEMA actually is lifted from the glass by DMF swelling as by water, as seen in Figure 6). This indicates a very high degree of cross linking. The lack of swelling in water is especially significant, for it shows that the VAM-pHEMA films, although chemically they are polyHEMA, did not form hydrogels.

Although they are not hydrogels, the VAM-polyHEMA films nonetheless have very hydrophilic surfaces. Contact angles for such coatings on a series of polypropylene Kusserow renal-artery rings were 13.8°, 7.7°, 3.2°, and 4.8°. That blood clotting on the samples was not inhibited by the VAM-polyHEMA serves to indicate that mere hydrophilicity of the

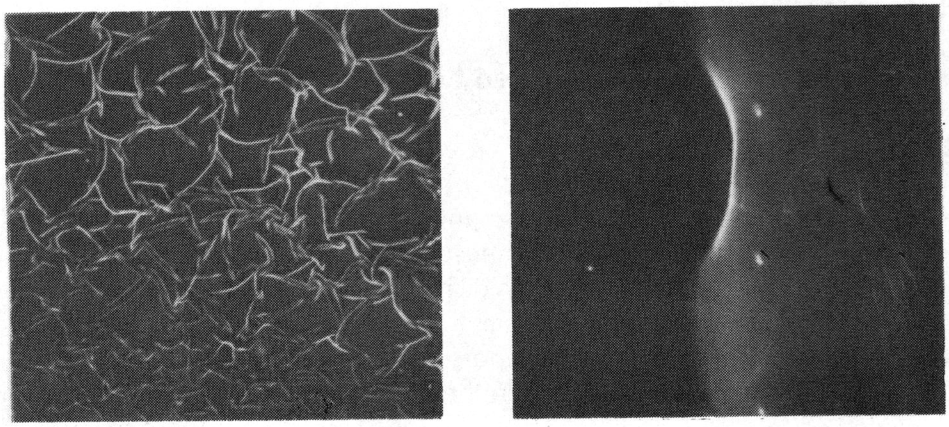

Figure 6. Scanning electron micrographs of surfaces of VIP-pHEMA films prepared on glass plates. 0.2 ml of a solution of 1:3/HEMA:CCl_4 was placed on a glass microscope slide and placed in the sample position in the active-vapor treatment apparatus and treated with atomic hydrogen for 10 min. (The CCl_4 was included because it had been used as a penetrating solvent to coat PEU.) After the film was allowed to swell to equilibrium in dimethylformamide vapor, it was dried in vacu, gold plated, and examined in the SEM.

surface is not a significant property of polyHEMA for determining its behavior in vascular implants.

3.1.2 Water Content of VAM-pAAm Hydrogels Prepared with Varying Amounts of Atomic Hydrogen in the Vapor

An experiment similar to 3.1.1 was done using acrylamide. The reservoir contained AAm monomer only. The treatment chamber was heated to about 50°C to prevent crystals from forming. The resulting polymer was completely soluble in water; no network formed.

A series of pAAm films was prepared by introducing a mixture of AAm, EGDMA and non-volatile solvent into the flowing active hydrogen and allowing the mixture to polymerize on cooled polyethylene substrata on the end of the cold finger of the apparatus in Figure 3. In the reservoir were 3 g AAm, 0.15 ml EDGMA, 2 ml ethylene glycol, and 0.5 g CuCl to inhibit polymerization in the reactor, heated to 75°C. The collected products for each hydrogen concentration were extracted with water and alcohol, dried at 110°C, and weighed. The amounts of water which the samples absorbed were then determined by equilibrating them with saturated water vapor in the evacuated Cahn electrobalance chamber. The degrees of swelling in the samples are shown in Table 2; no trend is perceptible.

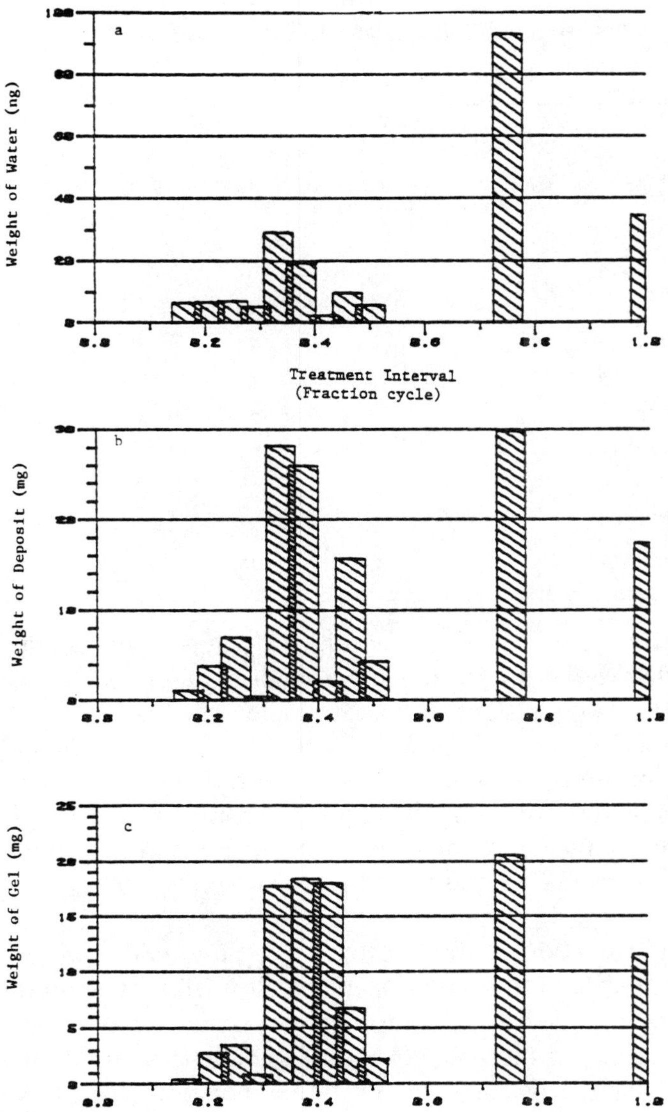

Figure 7. Properties of VAM-pAAm on polypropylene as function of program of opening of the shutter in Figure 1. Polypropylene films were placed in the substratum position in the reactor and treated with intermittent opening and closing of the shutter. The usual 6-sec cycle was maintained, but the portion of each cycle during which the shutter was open was varied from 1 to 6 sec. For each sample, the total time during which the shutter was open remained the same, so the total treatment time varied from 20 to 120 minutes. After the treatment the samples were removed from the reactor and analyzed for a) absorbed water, b) total deposit, and c) insoluble portion of the deposit by the method described in detail in Section 3.1.3. In d), gel fraction = (weight of final dry gel)/(weight of original deposit), in which the original deposit includes low molecular weight polymer, unconverted monomer, and glycerol, whereas the dry gel comprises the insoluble network only. Each treatment condition was run in duplicate. The water fraction = (weight of water absorbed after 17 hr)/(weight of dry gel + weight of water absorbed after 17 hr).

3.1.3 Water Content of VAM-pAAm Hydrogels Prepared with Intermittent Monomer-Hydrogen Cycles

The reactor shown in Figure 1 was used. The substrata were films of polypropylene (Hercules N400, 0.25 mm thick), cleaned with alcohol.

The Karl-Fischer titration was used to determine the water content following ASTM specification E203-64. A standard 10.33-cm^2 area was cut from each film after deposition of the gel. After the films had been soaked for 18 hrs. in water, they were blotted with filter paper under a uniformly applied pressure of 8.85 g/cm^2 for 10 sec. Each sample was then placed in a closed electrolytic-conduction cell fitted with two platinum electrodes containing methanol made anhydrous with Karl-Fischer reagent and was then titrated with the Karl-Fischer reagent: an anhydrous solution of SO_2 and iodine in pyridine. The reaction is

$$SO_2 + I_2 + 3C_5H_5N + CH_3OH + H_2O = C_5H_5NHSO_4OH + 2C_5H_5NHI$$

Table 2. Swelling of Active-Hydrogen Polymerized Polyacrylamide Crosslinked with EGDMA

Concentration of Active Hydrogen in vapor	Dry Weight of pAAm	% Water in Swollen Gel
1×10^{-9}M	4.8 mg	28
2	3.75	31
3	2.55	40
4	2.4	33
5	12.75	41
6	26.20	34
7	42.55	37
8	2.75	35
9	9.90	36
10	2.20	36

The end point for the titration is marked by a rapid increase in conductivity due to the formation of the salts. The titration was standardized with 10 ml of methanol containing 6.8 mg water (Harleco Standard Solution), which was equivalent to 14.8 ml Karl-Fischer reagent.

After the titration, which is non-destructive, the sample was washed for 17 hrs. in water and dried to constant weight at 100%C. These data gave the weights of the initial deposits, the insoluble gels, and the water contents of the hydrogels. The large variations in yield (Figure 7b) were found to be due to droplets of monomer from the reservoir being transported up to the substratum. This was eliminated later by inserting a baffle just below the shutter to trap unvaporized material.

In Figure 7d the gel fractions and water fraction of the hydrogels prepared with various cycles are compared. The variances in water fraction seemed to be smaller with the shutter open for less than 4 sec. (2/3 cycle). There was, however, no apparent dependence of either gel or water content on the treatment cycle. We therefore chose to operate the apparatus with the 2/3-cycle shutter-open interval, which gives convenient total running times. Many of our preparations, however, were performed before this information was obtained, and, in fact, before the shutter was introduced. These were of course carried out with the 100% open cycle.

Since there was no dependence of water content on treatment cycle, we combined all the data and determined the frequency distribution of water contents among the samples. This distribution is plotted in Figure 8. It has a maximum at 70% water, which was shown by experience with polyacrylamide hydrogels (Ratner and Hoffman 1974) to be satisfactory for biocompatibility.

3.1.4 Water Content of VIP-pHEMA

A thin film VIP polyHEMA was prepared on glass. A cover slip was hung in the reactor while HEMA was distilled onto it forming a liquid film. The reservoir was cut off, and the atomic hydrogen was turned on for 5 minutes, polymerizing the film. After having been ex-

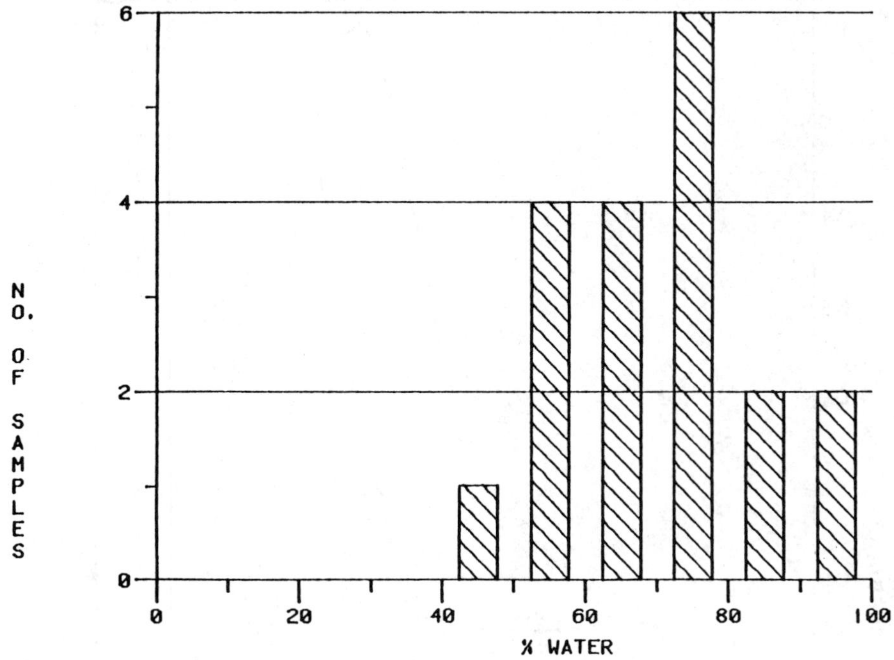

Figure 8. Frequency distribution of water contents of a series of VAM-pAAm hydrogels on polypropylene. The samples are the same as in Figure 10, treated as a random sample, since there appeared no correlation between treatment conditions and water content. As can be seen from the distribution, the most probable water content from the treatment is 70% water, based on total weight of hydrogel.

tracted with water and dried, the VIP film weighed 0.108 mg/cm² corresponding to a (dry) thickness of about 1 micron. The coated slide was then hung from the arm of a Cahn recording microbalance and equilibrated with water on the Cahn balance, gaining 9.48% in weight. When, however, the sample was actually immersed in water, blotted, and air-dried briefly, it gained 29%.

The experiment was repeated on a larger sample of uncrosslinked polyHEMA weighing 20 g which, not being supported on a glass plate, was free to change its dimensions. The result was the same: 15% swelling when equilibrated with water vapor, and 30%, with liquid water. We observe from these results that much of the swelling of polyHEMA in liquid water may be non-thermodynamic, perhaps an effect of capillarity in pores, and that the VIP films are equivalent in affinity for water to bulk-polymerized polyHEMA.

3.2. Spectroscopic Probes of Water Structure in pHEMA Coatings

3.2.1 Solvatochromic Dye Probe Merocyanine 540

The interior polarity of pHEMA films on PEU was observed in the changes in the absorption spectra of the dye and of water taken into them. Merocyanine 540 (Eastman No. 14014) shifts its maximum to the blue, with attenuation, in polar solvents (Figure 9). The solvatochromic properties of dyes of this type have been described previously (Brooker et al., 1965). A thick

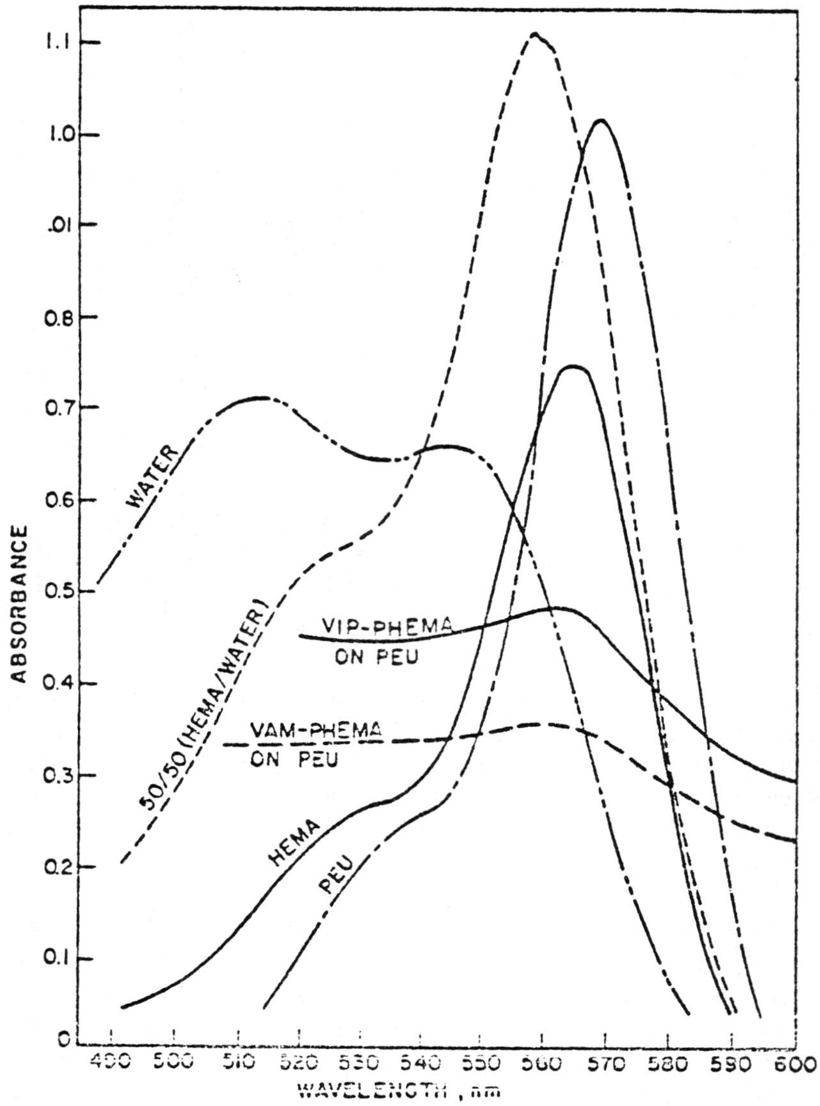

Figure 9. Visible absorption spectra of merocyanine 540 in various media for comparison with spectra in hydrogels. Sheets of PEU 3-(1000/425)/(70/30)-1-X, 0.12 mm thick, were treated with VAM-pHEMA for 15 min to make the surface hydrophilic. They were then dipped in 1:1 HEMA:water, which spread evenly over the surface. After the sheets were drained, they were replaced in the reactor with the reservoir empty and treated with active hydrogen for 30 min, to polymerize the VIP-pHEMA coating. The amounts of pHEMA, determined gravimetrically, were 14 mg for the VAM-pHEMA and 23 mg for the VIP coating, over an area of 19.4 cm². These weights were determined on the samples as they were taken from the reactor. Since the gel fractions of VIP-pHEMA on PEU were not found to exceed 40% (4 samples), these values may be at least double the true weights of hydrogel. The treated films were supported on 200-mesh stainless-steel screens and were soaked in dimethylformamide to dissolve the PEU and dyed in saturated ethanolic merocyanine 540 for 30 min. The samples were then washed 5 min in water, blotted, and placed in the sample compartment of a Cary 14R spectrophotometer to obtain the spectra.

sheet of PEU 3-(1000/425) (70/30)-1-X was grafted with polyHEMA by the VAM and VIP processes. The sheets were supported between two 200-mesh stainless steel screens and extracted for 5 days with frequent changes of dimethylformamide. An untreated sheet was completely dissolved in this way. After dissolution of the PEU substrate the samples were dyed in aqueous Mercyanine 540. The spectra in Figure 11 have their maxima at 558 nm as does 50-50 HEMA-water. The pure polyurethane maximum is at 570 nm.

Although we have shown by silver penetration, (q.v. Section 3.4.1) that mixing between HEMA and PEU occurs during the surface coating, the present observations show that the two networks – pHEMA and PEU – are not covalently attached, and that most of the PEU is still soluble in DMF and not crosslinked. When the PEU is dissolved away, the remaining pHEMA has the polarity, when swollen with water, of a HEMA-water solution.

3.2.2 Near-Infrared Spectrum of Water

Since the state of water may be the determinant of the biocompatibility of hydrogels (Bruck, 1972), we also measured its near-IR spectrum in these films. The theory of this determination is based on a recent reinterpretation of the spectrum (Bonner and Choi 1974). The exact position of the (V_2 + V_3)-combination band of water at about 2 micron depends on whether hydrogen bonds form through one or both hydrogens. The first case gives rise to 2 bands, below 1900 nm and above 1940 nm respectively; the symmetrical case gives a single band at 1905-1945 nm. In a mixture, the bands are resolvable by fitting three superposed Gaussian curves to the observed spectrum.

We cast slabs of polyHEMA 0.54 mm thick between 0.2 mm microscope coverslips, which themselves gave negligible absorbance in this spectral region. Various polymerization mixtures were used incorporating different amounts of water up to 40%. The spectra appear in Figure 10. The resolved spectral components varied little in wavelength from one composition to another, including pure water. The relative intensities of the components, however, did vary, showing more of the symmetrical bonding in the drier samples. This data is being analyzed more fully and will be published later. We see here, however, no indication that differences in thrombogenicity among hydrogels with different amount of water are due to variations in the structure of the water.

3.3. Primary Molecular Weight (Uncrosslinked Homopolymer)

Polyacrylamide without crosslinker was prepared on a cold finger at the sample position of the reactor in Figure 5. The reservoir was charged with 3 g acrylamide, 2 ml ethylene glycol (diluent) and 0.5 gm cuprous chloride (added as a nonvolatile inhibitor), and was maintained at 75°-80° for 1.5 hr., during which time active hydrogen flowed through the polymerization system at a pressure of 2-3 torr. The partial pressure of the hydrogen was varied over a tenfold range by adjusting the flow in several experiments, to obtain polymer prepared with different amounts of active-hydrogen initiator. The performance of this system had been previously analyzed with a platinum thermocouple, the temperature of which varied linearly with the partial pressure of the hydrogen. The polymer product, which was soluble since no cross linker was present, was collected as a solution in ethylene glycol on the end of the glass cold finger.

These solutions were then diluted ten-fold with methanol to precipitate the polymer,

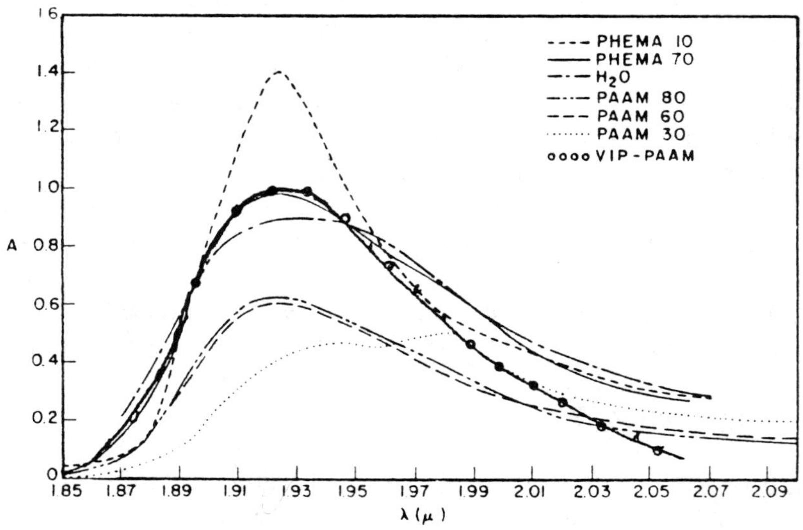

Figure 10. Adsorption spectra of water in hydrogels in the overtone-vibration (near infrared) region. Mixtures of HEMA and water containing 0.2% (w/v) ammonium persulfate were polymerized in the same configuration from aqueous mixtures of AAm containing 0.4% ammonium persulfate and 0.2% tetramethylethylenediamine at room temperature. The VIP-pAAm sample was prepared by coating a 4-cm² sheet of PEU 3-(1000/425) (70/30)-1-X, spread on a microscope coverslip, with VAM-pHEMA to make it hydrophilic, and then spreading on it 20 ul of a solution 1:1:1;0.01 acrylamide:glycerol:water:MBA and treating with atomic hydrogen in the apparatus in Figure 1 (reservoir empty) for 1 hr. The PEU had a coating of 10 u, based on final weight gain, before swelling in water. Before placing the specimen in the spectrophotometer, it was washed with water, blotted, and covered with a second coverslip. Spectra were obtained in a Cary 14R spectrophotometer.

which was filtered on a tared funnel and weighed. The polymer was redissolved in distilled water and added to an Ubbelohde dilution viscometer for viscosity measurements on serial dilutions.

The molecular weights of soluble polyacrylamide were calculated from the inherent viscosity determined at 25°, using the Mark-Houwink equation (Ishige & Hamiliec 1973):

$$[\eta] = 6.80 \times 10^{-4} M^{n\ -0.66}. \qquad (1)$$

The molecular weights of polyacrylamide samples polymerized with different concentrations of atomic hydrogen in the vapor are listed in Table 3.

In a free-radical system which is polymerizing without chain transfer, every molecule continues to grow until it is terminated by combining with another growing molecule. According to Flory's theory of free-radical polymerization, the degree of polymerization is then given by:

$$\text{Constant} \times H^{o-1/2}$$

Table 3. Viscometric Determination of Molecular Weight of Active-Hydrogen Polymerized Polyacrylamide

Relative Active Hydrogen Concentration	Inherent Viscosity	M_n
1	1.3	95,000
3	1.04	66,000
4	0.43	18,000
5	0.54	25,000
6	0.78	43,000
7	0.39	14,000

in which H° is the atomic-hydrogen concentration in the condensed phase. The molecular weight therefore decreases with increasing concentrations of active hydrogen. This is in agreement with the data in Table 3, although the data is not precise enough to estimate the constant in (2). We have determined that the concentration of the atomic hydrogen is about $2.8 \times 10^{-8}M$ in the vapor. It is not known how this correlates with the concentration in the condensed phase, which, from the low molecular weight of the product, appears to be higher than usual for the conventional polymerization system, which yields typical values of molecular weight of over 10^6 Dalton.

3.4. Interpenetration of Hydrogel and Substratum

In all the hydrogel grafting reactions, a hydrogel monomer fluid is introduced to a polymeric substratum. Depending upon the intermiscibility of the two components, the fluid monomer can penetrate the substratum and form a graft copolymer in the bulk as well as at the interface. The product can vary from substratum macromolecules with dependent polar sidechains to interpenetrating hydrogel-substratum polymer networks. This effect has been reported for polyacrylamide-coated silicone rubber which has been grafted by ionizing radiation while immersed in a concentrated aqueous solution of the monomer (Gelding 1978). These treated surfaces were shown to contain both silicone and acrylamide, rather than the pure acrylamide.

3.4.1 Method

The interpenetration profiles can be examined by electron-probe analysis of cross-sections of treated samples. To carry out this analysis, a series of conventional pAAm samples were polymerized with different amounts of cross-linker to vary the degree of water uptake in the series. The samples were equilibrated with aqueous solutions of a low molecular-weight solute which contained a heavy atom. For example, solutions 0.1M in KCl, KBr, or $AgNO_3$ were used. The samples were lyophilized, fractured and examined with a scanning electron microscope in its energy-dispersed X-ray (EDX) mode. THe X-ray fluorescence characteristic of the heavy atom was counted and was calibrated against the amount of water imbibed by the sample at equilibrium, measured gravimetrically (Figure 11). Water contents were varied over the range 50 to 90 percent. To study an unknown sample, it was soaked in one of the above solutions, lyophilized, and fractured. The fracture surface was examined by scanning electron

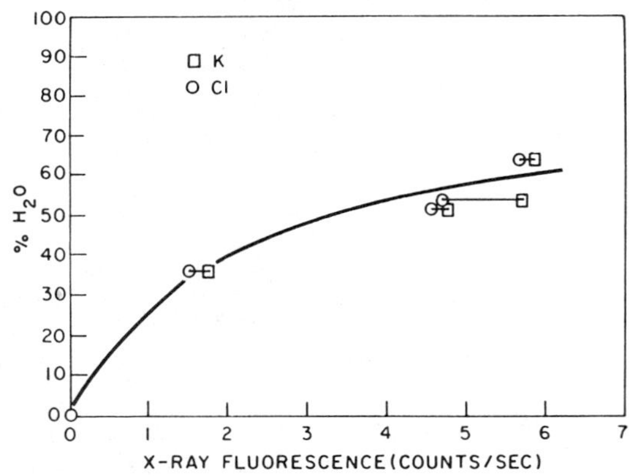

Figure 11. Polyacrylamide was prepared in sealed tubes by warming 20% aqueous acrylamide with 0.4% ammonium persulfate and various amounts of MBA from 0.6% to 2% (w/w) at 70°C for 2 hr. The rods were cut into slices, which were soaked in 0.1 M KCl. After five days the slices were further cut into small slivers which were vacuum dried, lightly gold plated, and probed with the electron beam of the SEM in its EDX mode. The X-ray fluorescence was counted with a Si(Li) detector set to discriminate characteristic K or Cl X-rays. The water contents in the slices were determined by thermogravimetric analysis weighing while heating in a Model 200 Dupont thermal analyzer between room temperature and 150°C. The weight-loss curve reached its plateau between 110°C and 150°C.

microscopy and also in the energy-dispersed X-ray mode, as above. The X-ray emission was compared to the calibration curve obtained with the conventional samples to determine the amount of aqueous and gel phases and the collapse of the gel during drying, which would increase the local concentration of fluorescent solute. The method is the more sensitive the heavier the atom, silver emitting more X-rays than potassium.

3.4.2 Results

Three samples prepared in different ways are shown in Figure 12, sectioned and stained by the silver-penetration method, showing a progression of water penetration. Sample 12A, consisting of VAM-pAAm on polypropylene, has a discrete layer of hydrogel, sharply demarcated from the substratum. The intense white field in the EDX map shows a high water content. Polyetherurethane block copolymer (Stanford Research Institute 3-(1000/435) (70/30)-1-X) treated with VIP-pAAm shows deep penetration,with lower water absorption 10 to 20% even near the surface (Figure 12B). This surface is hydrophilic, however, and dyes deeply with aqueous crystal violet.

The deepest penetration is observed with PEU coated with VAM-pAAm (Figure 12C). In Figure 12C is shown a silver-penetration scan of a sample prepared on a film of PEU only 0.1mm thick, cast on a microscope cover slip. In Figure 12D the coated PEU is compared with untreated PEU. The height of the scan above the horizontal axis is proportional to the amount of silver. Increasing distances measured to the left of the vertical bar indicate distances into the treated sample; increasing distances measured to the right of the vertical bar in Figure 12D and E represent distance into an untreated sample. The silver-ion concentration rises at the surface to a peak and then levels off in the treated sample; in the untreated PEU there is only a slight rise due to background. In Figure 12E the treated sample is compared with a piece of solution polymerized pAAm (from 57% AAm, 3% EGDMA, 40% water, with persulfate-amine initiator). The scan on the right is for the pAAm-PEU graft copolymer; that on the left, for the solution-polymerized sample. It is seen that the graft copolymer swells in water more than does the conventional pAAm containing 40% water. The penetration occurs all the way into the depth

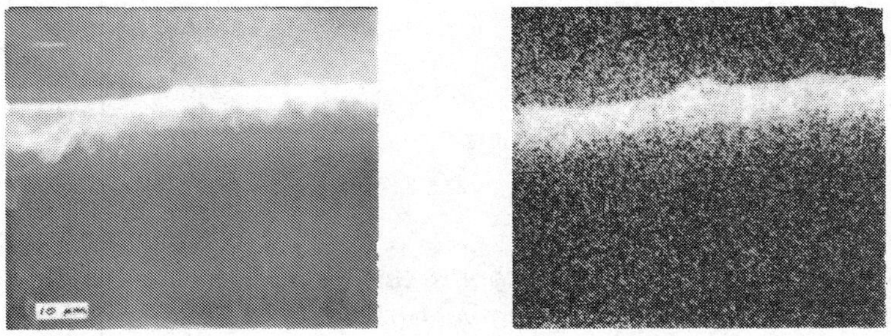

Figure 12A Polypropylene film coated with VAM-pAAm was soaked to equilibrium in 0.1 M $AgNO_3$, rinsed quickly, and fractured while frozen in liquid nitrogen. The fracture face, cross section through the film, is shown in SEM and in the EDX electron-probe analysis after drying in the vacuum of the metal-deposition apparatus.

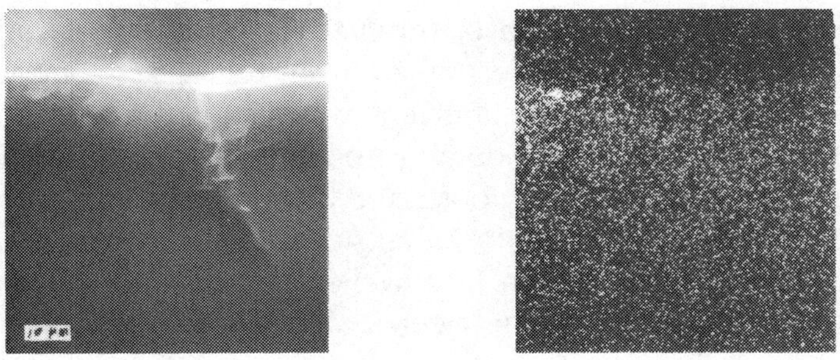

Figure 12B. VIP-pAAm on PEU 3-(1000/425)/(70/30)-1-X. The PEU film (200 um) was soaked in a mixture of 1.2 g AAm, 50 mg bis, 8 ml ethylene glycol, and 32 ml methoxyethanol. After the volatile methoxyethanol was evaporated, the sample was treated with atomic hydrogen for 2 hr in the reactor of Figure 1. The density of silver counts (white dots) is similar to that in a piece of pAAm containing between 10 and 20% water and mounted on the same stub.

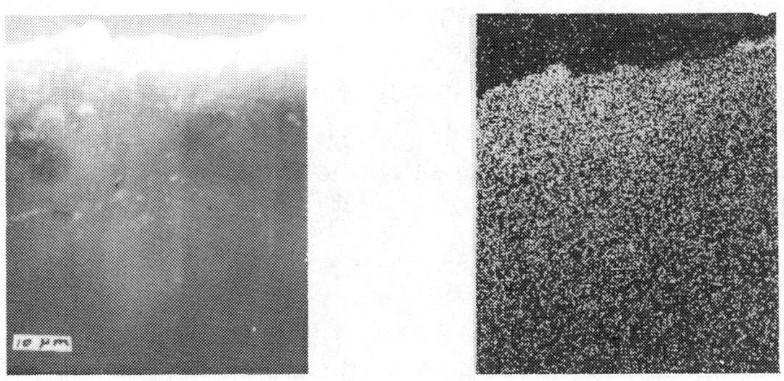

Figure 12C. VAM-pAAm on same PEU as in (B), examined as in (A). Conditions were: reservoir, 3g AAm, 0.1 g EGDMA, 3 g ethylene glycol, 0.5 g CuCl at 80°C; sample cooled with ice (Figure 5); treatment with mixed vapors from reservoir and atomic hydrogen for 15 min. The amount of material added on this reaction was 44.5 mg onto a sample area of 4.9 cm^2, corresponding to an apparent coating 90 u thick.

Figure 12 continued.

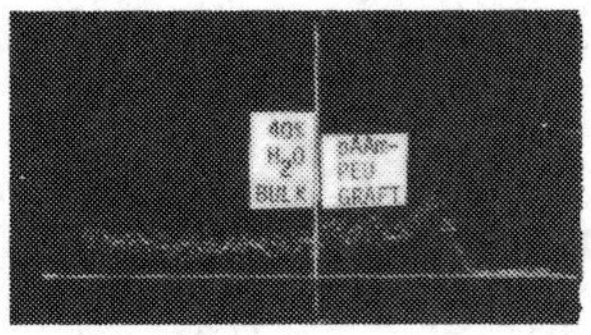

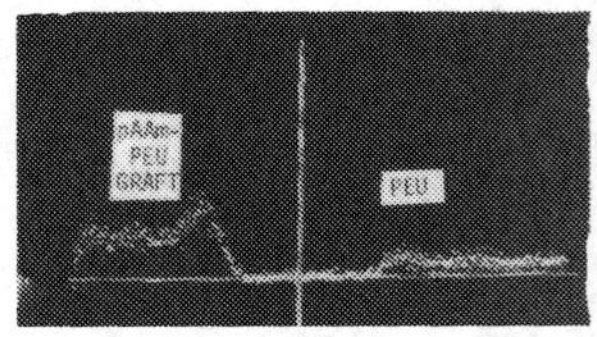

Figure 12D, Same sample as in (C), compared with uncoated PEU which was also soaked in 1 M $AgNO_3$. In (D) the amount of Ag is plotted vs distance into the film, as explained in Section 3.4.1.

Figure 12. Water penetration into vapor-grafted pAAm hydrogel coatings. Parts A–D show conditions with increasing penetration of the coatings into the substratum.

of the substratum. With this thin film backed by the glass coverplate we evidently obtain a system in equilibrium with the vapor phase. The high degree of modification was evident in the swelling of the films, which would delaminate from their glass supports.

Although we did not measure it quantitatively, we observed that the permeability of the grafted films to water is also raised considerably above that of PEU, as would be expected if the absorption is increased. This was demonstrated by a rapid lowering of the water wetting angle of one side of the film when only the other side was exposed to a humid atmosphere. The PEU-pAAm graft copolymer of Figure 12D swelled homogeneously when wet. Measured directly the volume swelling was 100% between water and the 50% relative humidity of the room air.

Therefore, although it was not anticipated, the hydrogel structure depends, not only on the method of preparation, but also on the substratum. PEU is a particularly troublesome substratum because of interpenetration with the hydrophilic polymer. The VAM process, especially, causes deep penetration, but also the VIP process does, when penetrating solvents are used.

The FMIR spectrum of a VIP-pHEMA film on PEU is shown in Figure 13. The PEU was SRI 3-(1000/425) (70/30)-1-X. We estimate the thickness of the film to be 5 u, thick enough to mask the infrared bands of the underlying substratum. The aromatic "fingerprint"region, however, shows through in the coated sample with undiminished intensity from that in the uncoated one. New bands appear, at 2.75-3.3 um (—OH, H_2O) and 5.7-6.0 um (=CO), showing the presence of the pHEMA. This result confirms that the surface of the material was a copolymer rather than pure pHEMA.

3.5. Surface Texture and Microtopography

Microtopographies of VIP coatings prepared from a series of mixtures of HEMA and water, on a series of PEU's of varying "hardness," or penetrability, varying from the soft 3-2000-1-E to the hard 3-1000-2-X, are shown in Figure 14. For any PEU formulation, as the water content of the monomer in which the substratum is soaked is increased from 30% to 70%, the texture becomes rougher, more granular, and with ridges lying deeper and closer together. This

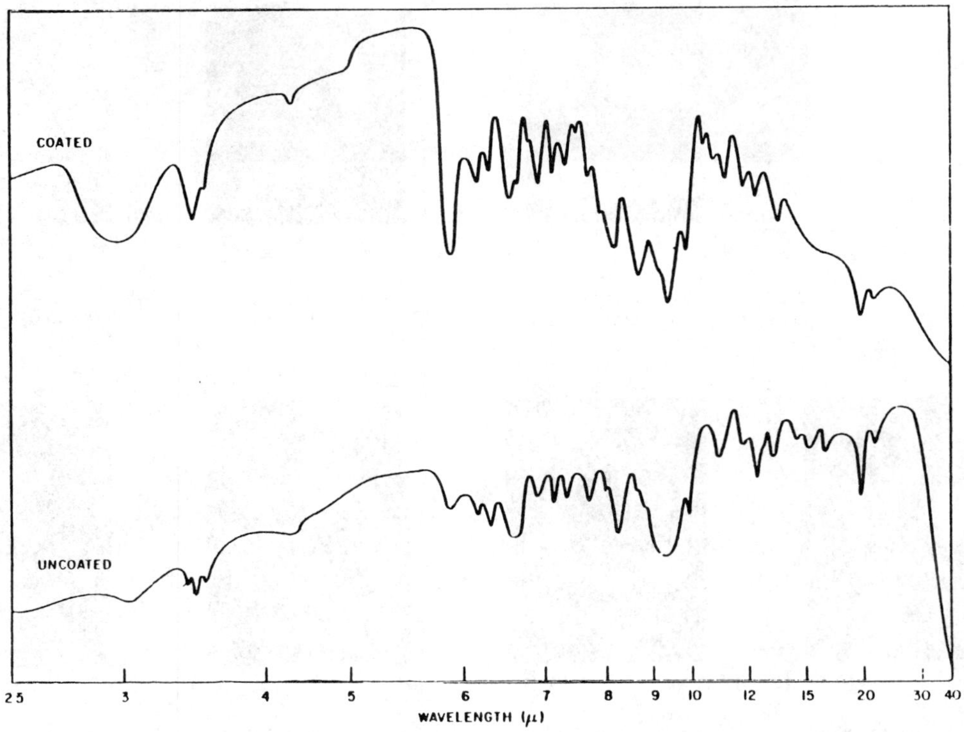

Figure 13. Infrared spectrum of VIP-pHEMA on PEU. The PEU was soaked for 5 min in a solution containing 500 ml HEMA, 10 ml EGDMA and 340 ml CCl_4, drained without blotting, and treated with atomic hydrogn for 1 hr. The weight gain was 2×10^{-4} g/cm^2, corresponding to a coating thickness of 5 u. The non-hydrated film was clamped to a KRS-5 (thallium bromide) frustrated multiple internal reflectance plate in a Wilks mounting and scanned with a Perkin-Elmer Model 521 infrared spectrometer. The spectrum of untreated PEU is also shown.

variation is also seen as the hardness of the polymer increases. Both of these variables depend in the same way on the penetration of the monomer mixture into the substratum: the deeper the penetration, apparently, the smoother the surface. Here we show that the surface texture of a penetrating hydrogel depends on the properties of the substratum.

The microtopography of VIP coatings on an impenetrable substrate, while not dependent on the underlayer, show features which, perhaps like those on penetrable substrata, seem to arise from differential dimensional changes between the surface and the underlayer. When we ran the polymerization reaction, without grafting, on microscope cover-slips in the reactor (Figure 3) we obtained VIP-pHEMA on glass, which looks at first glance like VIP-pHEMA grafted onto polyetherurethane surfaces. It is smooth when viewed at 3000 × (Figure 6).

All VIP samples are hazy in appearance, which we believe is due to the surface features seen in the SEM. This haziness on PEU appears in seconds after the atomic hydrogen is turned on; on glass, only after the slide is wet.

The texture of VAM films depends upon the monomer and upon process variables, but not on the substratum. VAM-pHEMA is very smooth, shown after a swelling-drying cycle with the solvent dimethylformamide in Figure 15. Although it was shown earlier that the water uptake of VAM-pHEMA is small (cf. Section 3.1.1), it is hydrophilic and absorbs the dye crystal violet

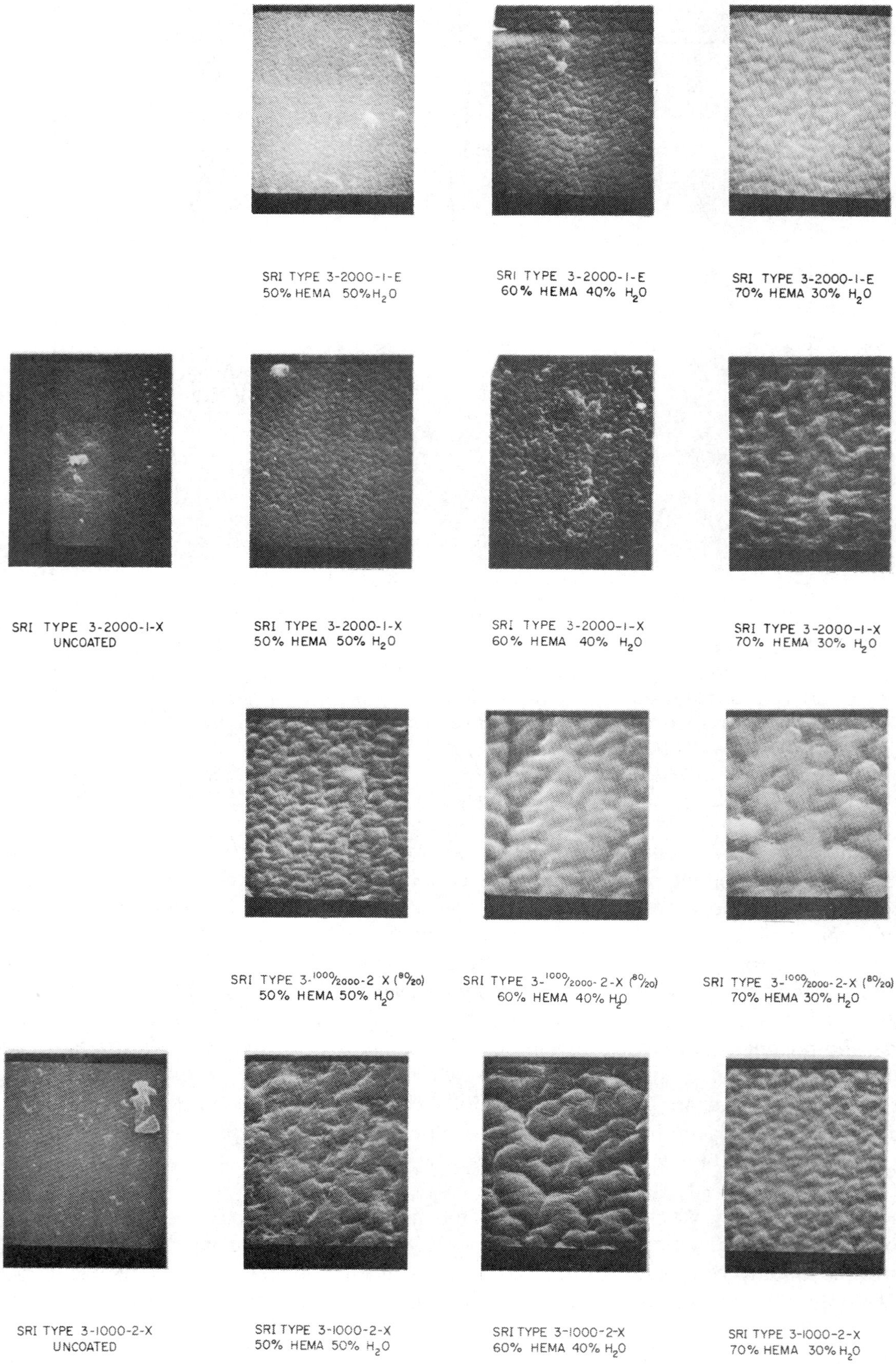

Figure 14A. pHEMA.

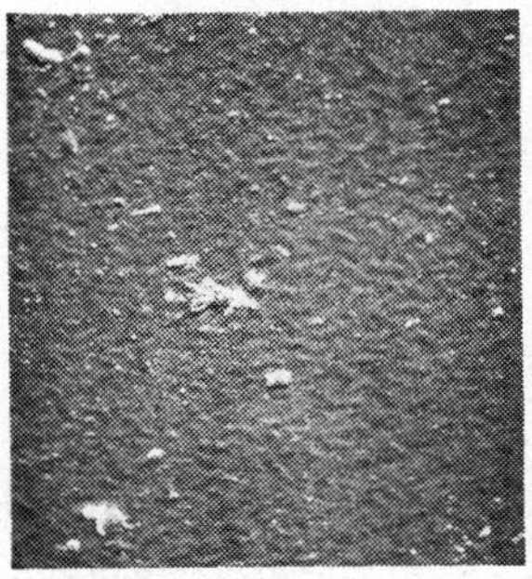

SRI TYPE 3-2000-I-E
ACRYLAMIDE COATED

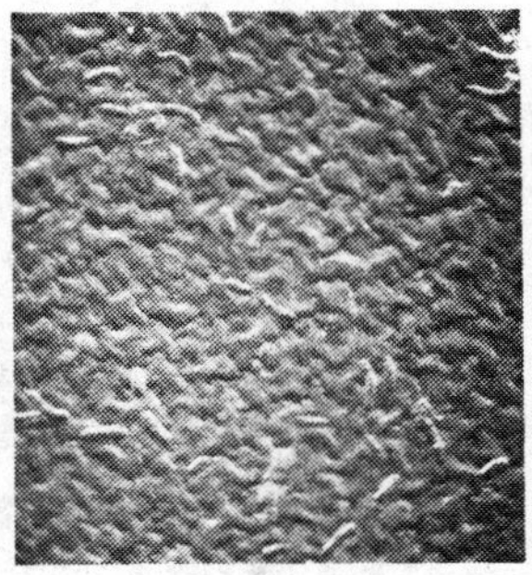

SRI TYPE 3-2000-I-X
ACRYLAMIDE COATED

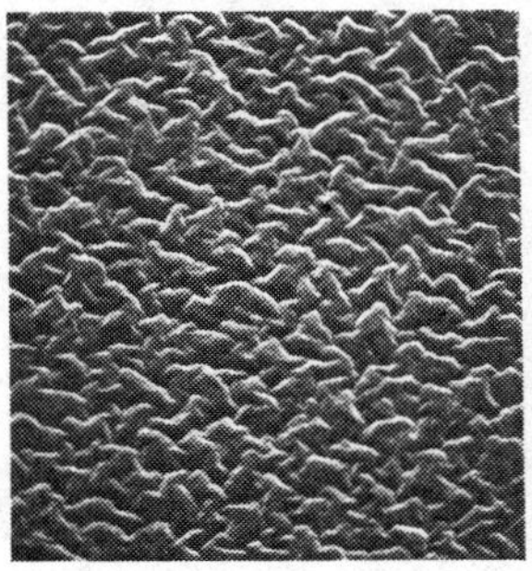

SRI TYPE 3- 1000/2000 2-X (80/20)
ACRYLAMIDE COATED

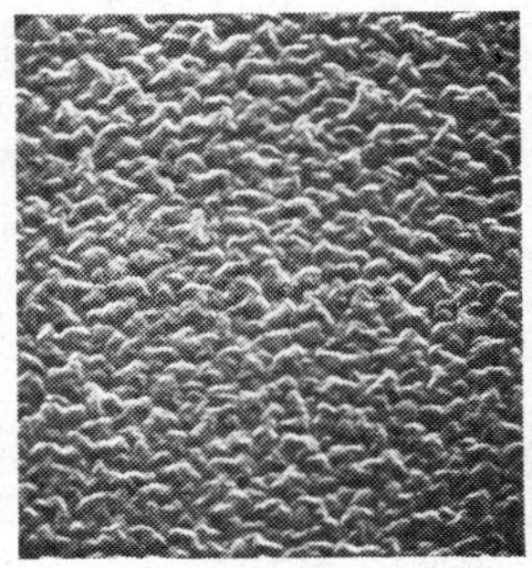

SRI TYPE 3-1000-2-X
ACRYLAMIDE COATED

Figure 14B. Polyacrylamide.

Figure 14. Scanning electron micrographs of surfaces of VIP coatings on PEU. The pHEMA coatings were prepared by soaking PEU films in various aqueous solutions of HEMA, as indicated, and then treating with atomic hydrogen for 2 hr, washing thoroughly with water, drying in a vacuum metallizing apparatus, and depositing a 200-A film of gold. The pAAm coatings were applied by dipping in a solution of AAm:ethylene glycol:2-methoxyethanol/3:10:40, drying in vacuo for 30 min, and treating with atomic hydrogen for 2 hr.

from aqueous solution to give large, evenly dyed areas (Figure 16). The smoothness of the surface and the ability of the vapor to penetrate geometrically complex objects is exemplified in Figure 17. Here we have coated VAM-pHEMA onto samples of Parylene-coated polypropylene microfibers obtained from the Union Carbide Corp. The thickness of the microfibers and the space between them are the order of a few microns. These hydrogel coatings must be thin enough so that they do not block the spaces between the microfibers,

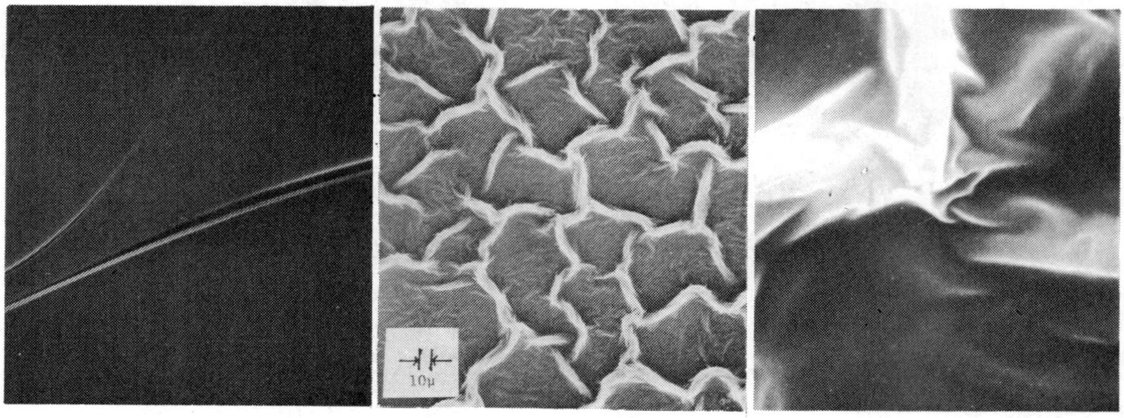

Figure 15. A glass microscope cover slip was cleaned in dichromic acid, water and alcohol, flamed, and dried at 110°C. The apparatus in Figure 1 was used to coat with VAM-pHEMA for 1 hr with the shutter open during the entire time. It was then hung on a Cahn balance in 90% saturated dimethylformamide vapor until the equilibrium weight was reached. The film weighed about 4 mg, corresponding to 3 μ thickness. (A) Film with a scratch revealing its thickness. (B) Film after having been soaked in dimethylformamide and dried.

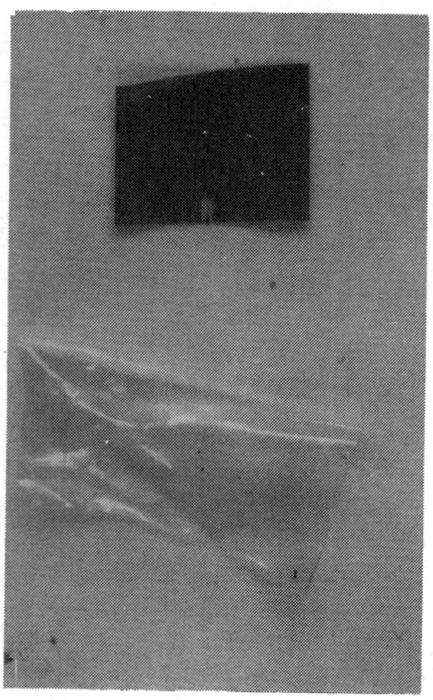

Figure 16. "Springy polypropylene" film untreated and treated with VAM-pHEMA. After being treated with the 100% shutter-open cycle for 1 hr, the sample was washed in water, dyed for 15 min with saturated aqueous crystal violet, washed, and dried. The untreated film was dyed similarly.

and thus the entry of endothelial or other cells to be grown on them. This demonstration of grafting vaporized HEMA represented breakthroughs in several respects: it offers a means of (1) producing very thin hydrogel coatings, (2) even on very inert substrates such as unoxidized Parylene, and (3) using more economical and readily available inhibited HEMA monomer, of which only the vapor is used for grafting.

The glassy quality of the VAM-pHEMA films was probably due to the introduction of the many free radicals into the monomer and forming polymer by the very reactive H-atoms. Attempts were made to control the cross linking by increasing the amount of HEMA in the vapor. To this end the reservoir temperature was set at 58°C and the reservoir was moved up to a position 75 mm below the substratum. The reservoir in these cases was a 30-ml beaker of monomer mixture placed up in the reactor chamber in Figure 1 and provided with its own heating coil and thermocouple. The substrata were polypropylene vena-cava rings. After the VAM-treatment, the sample was held in the active hydrogen with HEMA vapor for 30 minutes. A coating which received aqueous crystal violet well resulted. The HEMA was distilled rapidly in this preparation to give a thick coating, seen in cross section at 1000X in Figure 18A. Here the light area is the coating, sloping

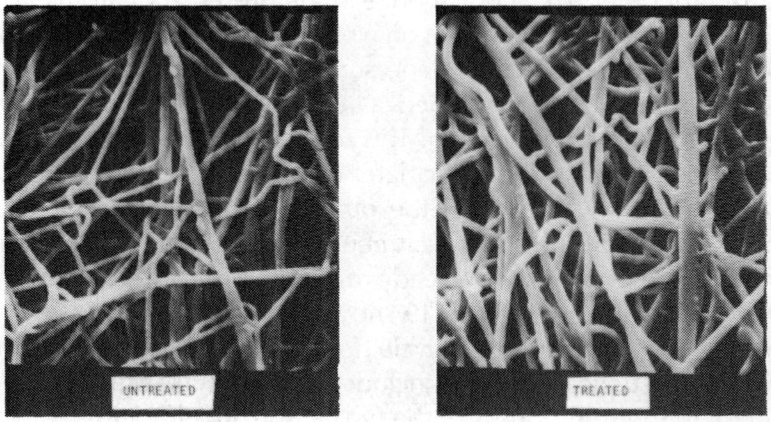

Figure 17. Microfibers coated with VAM-pHEMA. The microfibers, 1-5 μ thick, were polypropylene coated with Parylene (polyxylylene), prepared by the Union Carbide Co. laboratories. These were placed in an early form of the apparatus in Figure 1, consisting of the reactor provided with an alembic which held the HEMA surrounding the sample position. Because of the proximity of the monomer to the substratum, external warming was not required. The product accepted the dye crystal violet; the untreated fibers did not.

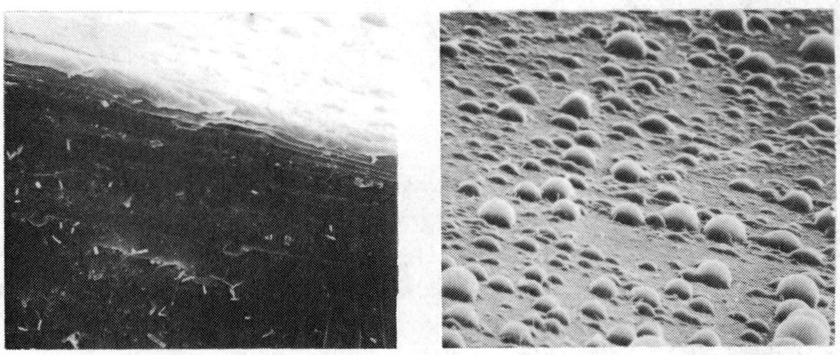

Figure 18. Scanning electron micrograph of a thick coating of VAM-pHEMA on polypropylene. A 50-ml beaker was wrapped with nichrome heating wire and supported in the reactor of Figure 1 above the inlet port. Current for the heater and a thermocouple were supplied via the feedthrough at the side of the reactor. The sample, a polypropylene vena-cava ring, was suspended 75 mm above the beaker. The treatment with flowing atomic hydrogen was carried out for 30 min with the HEMA at 58°C. After the reservoir was removed from the reactor, the sample was post-treated with atomic hydrogen for 30 min to continue the polymerization.

away from the viewer, at right angles to the cut edge of the sectioned ring. The surface is not smooth, but is covered with tiny droplets after the sample is soaked in water (Figure 18B); these can be seen also in Figure 18A. Obviously nucleated condensation must be occurring, forming droplets of monomer which polymerize in the presence of atomic hydrogen. We do not at present know the nature of the nuclei on which the droplets form, but they must correspond to nonuniformities in the polypropylene surface.

The treatment described above included a reaction with atomic hydrogen after initial deposition to complete the polymerization. This reaction was effective only at the surface of the film. In many cases the resulting product later disintegrated into flakes and streamers as it was loosely attached in a few spots. On the other hand, it was easier to control discrete hydrogen-monomer phases of the short treatment cycles than to change the balance of the amounts of monomer and hydrogen in a steady reaction. It was for this reason that the shutter shown in Figure 1 was introduced. Figure 19 shows SEM of Teflon sheets coated with VAM-pAAm by means of a 16.7% shutter-open cycle, following the procedure given in METHODS. Although the textures are typical, we have included rare defects in the field to show that they exist and to accentuate the smoothness of the typical surrounding surfaces. The basal coating thickness is 4 microns, with a 0.1 micron modulation. This texture resembles that of presently used polyvinyl chloride catheters.

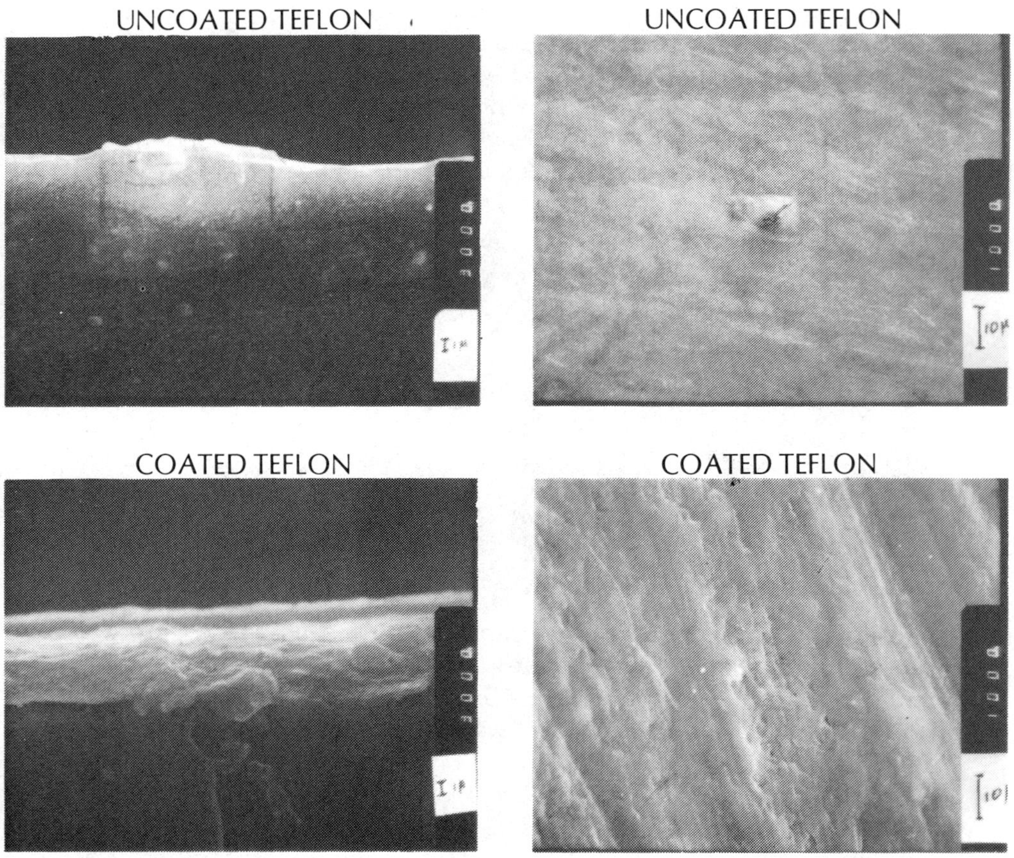

Figure 19. VAM-pAAm on Teflon. A sheet of Teflon was treated with AAm with 1:1/AAm:glycerol in the reservoir, which was at 78°C, the shutter being open during the whole cycle. Imperfections such as that shown in the untreated film were infrequent, being singular for the 0.5 cm ^{2} sample examined, but of course it could cause a wedge thrombus in the stagnation-point flow experiment. The texture of the coated surface was typical.

3.6 Biocompatability

The main purpose of our project was to prepare specimens for evaluation in various biocompatibility tests performed by co-contractors in the Biomaterials Program. Several hundred samples were prepared covering most of the tests pioneered by this Program: the vena-cava ring implant test, blood element deposition on spinning disks, in a stagnation-point flow chamber or in a helical-flow chamber, static adsorption of plasma proteins, flow erosion, shear-induced hemolysis, renal embolism, critical surface tension, tensile tests and cell and tissue toxicity. The tests for which we actually obtained results, for some of the samples submitted, were the vena-cava and renal-artery ring implantations, the stagnation-point flow and spinning-disk adsorption experiments, static adsorption of plasma proteins, and toxicity.

3.6.1 In-Vivo Tests

The vena-cava ring results are summarized for the various types of coatings in Table 4.

Table 4. Results of Vena-Cava Ring Tests on Hydrogel Coatings

Sample Batch	Sample Type*	2-hr Clot	2wk Death	2wk Clot	2wk Small Clot	2wk Clear
129-41	VIP-HEMA-PEU	0	0	2	3	1
129-50	" " "	3	0	0	0	0
129-56	" " "	0	0	4	1	3
132-42	VIP-pAAm-PEU	0	1	0	0	1
132-45	VIP-pAAm-PEU	0	4	0	0	0
132-55	VIP-pHEMA-PEU	0	1	0	0	0
132-657-5	VIP-PHEMA-PEU	0	0	0	2	0
1321-61	VAM pAAm-OpAAm-PP	2	10	2	1	2
13.9-42	VIP-pAAm	2	0	0	1	1
31-13	pAAm-PEU-Thick	2	0	2	0	0
31-55	VAM-pAAm-OpAAm-PP	2	7	2	1	1
PLS 37-57	VAM pAAm on PP	1	4	4	2	0
PLS 37-61	VAM pAAm on PP	0	3	3	5	1
SRI	PEU Blank	0	2	0	0	5
SRI	PEU Blank	1	2	1	2	2
SRI	PEU Blank	0	1	0	2	0

* PP = Linear polypropylene; OpAAm = photopolymerized AAm after treatment as described in Section 2.6

It has been observed that this test is poorly reproducible (Mason 1979), and the results for SRI PEU 3-(1000/425) (30/70)-1-X is consistent with this observation. This material serves as a blank, although a better control would be a well-characterized surface, which was not available for testing. It appears that every possible result was observed for this material. The same comment can apply after it was coated with the hydrogels. The earliest three batches of samples submitted, to the Gott group at Johns Hopkins University, had an appreciable fraction which lasted more than two weeks (129-41, 50,56). This coating was VIP-pHEMA on the above PEU. In batches 129, the HEMA was applied to the rings by dipping; batch 132-67-5 was prepared by dipping in a mixture of HEMA:CCl_4/5:1, a penetrating solvent. At the time the experiments were done, we thought the results were promising, but the sample was statistically not valid, in view of the results for the (presumably) more uniform PEU blanks. The results for VIP-pAAm on PEU (batches 132-42, 45 and 55) should be interpreted in the same light.

Larger numbers of samples were tested for the VAM-pAAm preparations. The results are again distributed, with most of the materials causing clots or death in less than two weeks. The surfaces of these samples, which were prepared without the baffle in place in the apparatus in Figure 1, were not smooth (Figure 19), and so the results could depend on hydrodynamic influences more than those of the PEU blanks.

3.6.2 Extracororeal Tests

A number of samples were treated, after the active-vapor grafting, with a photopolymerization step described in the Section 2.6, including sample batches 31-55 and 1321-61 in Table 4. These coatings were tested on sample sheets of PEU mounted on a spinning disk in an extracorporeal chamber connected to a dog (Kochwa et al. 1977). Four-minute tests for platelet adhesion in this apparatus gave, for two samples, 4.0 and 0.4 cell per 900 u^2, compared to 17.0 cells/900 u^2 for untreated PEU.

Determinations were also made on adsorption of proteins from single-protein solutions. In these experiments, carried out in the laboratories of Dr. Leo Vroman et al. (1977), the disks were immersed in normal human plasma, and the adsorbed proteins were measured either immunologically or by their ability to correct the clotting behavior of human blood deficient in one or another clotting factor. Tests were run for fibrinogen adsorption, fibrinogen "conversion," and adsorption of Factors IX and XII and 7S-gamma-globulin. Some Factor XII was adsorbed, correcting deficient plasma by 7.8%; adsorbed Factor XI corrected by 37.9%. A single sample showed no adsorption of any of these proteins; this sample had the thickest polyacrylamide coating.

Although fibrinogen and gamma globulins deposit onto many surfaces within 1 sec. the pAAm-grafted material showed no immunochemical evidence of the protein after 5 sec., but it did appear after 10 min. in a platelet-adhesive ("unconverted") form.

Stagnation-Point Flow Test (Petschek et al. 1968)

VAM-pAAm samples on PEU were prepared with the substratum either at room temperature or cooled with ice. An additional set of samples were post-treated with photopolymerized pAAm, as described in Section 2.6. No qualitative differences were seen among these preparations, and the data were treated together by Avco-Everett Laboratories. At low-shear conditions, white blood cells were observed over the whole test area, as were scattered platelet aggregates. At high shear (beta between 31 and 175 mm^{-1} sec^{-1}) shear limited white-cell circle appeared, implying that it would require high arterial blood flow to prevent white cell deposition on the surface of the material. Platelet wedge thrombi were prevalent over the whole surface, which are always due to bumps on the surface. These were easily observed under a microscope, and were due to swelling of the hydrogel. They were absent on dry samples.

VAM-pAAm on polypropylene, again post-treated by the photopolyermization of AAm, also gave a bumpy surface, with resulting wedge thrombi at all shear conditions. When one of the thrombi was removed, PMN's were observed firmly attached to the underlying surface. Subsequently, the post-treatment was improved to yield a smoother surface. In these samples, the white-blood-cell circle appeared at intermediate values of shear in 5-10 min., indicating that these cells display moderate adhesion to the surface, not enough to permit affixation under arterial conditions. Although these surfaces were not actually prepared by vapor grafting, the product hydrogel should have been identical to bulk-polymerized 50% pAAm, to which cells should not attach at all according to the hypothesis in Section 1; the present stagnation-point flow test results cast doubt on this hypothesis.

3.6.3 Toxicity

VAM-pAAm polypropylene film was coated on both sides for implantation into tissue, tissue-culture-agar overlay tests, hemolysis, and growth inhibition of cells. The results are summarized as showing the samples to be noncytotoxic, nonhemolytic, and noninhibiting. The Material Science Toxicity Laboratory at the University of Tennessee, who carried out the tests reports: "No significant acute or subacute tissue response to the implanted material (Y-5884) was observed. A response of *1* for the Histopathologic Rating (observed in one implant site at 1 week) is not considered a significant toxic response since that rating is obtained in 5-10% of negative control implants."

The results of the implantation are summarized in Table 6.

When these samples were examined by our electron-probe analysis, penetration of the aqueous salt (in this case KBr) was observed to 20 micron. The surface texture was the same as described earlier for polyacrylamide on polypropyene. Thus the films evaluated in those toxicity tests were thicker than those usually tested with blood.

REFERENCES

1. Andrade, J. D., Medical Instrumentation 7:110 (1973).
2. Bonner, O. D. and Choi, Y. S., J. Phys. Chem. 78:1723 (1974).
3. Broida, H. P. and Chapman, M. W., Anal. Chem. 30:2049 (1958).
4. Brooker, L. G. S., Craig, A. C. Heseltine, D. W., Jenkins, P. W. and Lincoln, L. L., J. Am. Chem. Soc. 87:2443 (1965).
5. Bruck, S. D., J. Biomed, Mater. Res. 6:173 (1972).
6. Bruck, S. D., Biomaterials, Medical Devices, and Artificial Organs 1:79 (1972).
7. Currie, C. L. and Thrush, B. A., Trans. Farad. Soc. 64:390 (1968).
8. Czapski, G. and Stein, G., J. Phys. Chem. 64:291 (1960).
9. Detwiler, T. C. and Feinman, R. D., Biochem 11:2462 (1973).
10. Gelding, D. K., Green, G. F., Annis, D. and Wilson, J. G., Trans. Soc. Art. Int. Organs 24:411 (1978).
11. Halpern, B. D., Solomon, O. and Chowhan, D. G., Polymer Studies Related to Prosthetic Cardiac Materials which are Non-Clotting at a Blood Interface. Contract No. NO1-HV-6-1124. National Heart and Lung Institute, National Institute of Health, Bethesda, MD. Annual Report June 1976. PB 255 913/AS.
12. Hansen, R. H., and Schonhorn, H., Polymer Lett. 4:203-209 (1966).
13. Ingalls, R. B. and Wall, L. A., J. Chem. Phys. 35:370-1 (1961).
14. Ishige, T. and Hamielec, A. E., J. Appl. Polymer Sci. 17:1479 (1973).

15. Kochwa, S., Litwak, R. S., Rosenfield, R. E. and Leonard, E. F., Ann. N.Y. Acad. Sci., 283:457-472 (1977).
16. Kronick, P. L. "Fabrication and Characterization of Grafted Hydrogel Coatings as Blood Contacting Surfaces," M. Szycher and W. J. Robinson, Eds., *Synthetic Biomedical Polymers,* Technomic (1980).
17. Kronick, P. L. and Jimenez, S. A., Thrombosis Res. 9:553 (1976).
18. Kronick, P. L. and Rembaum, A., J. Biomed. Mater. Res. Symp. 8:39 (1977).
19. Kronick, P. L., Polymer Preprints 16(2):441-445 (1975).
20. Mason, R. G., Working Group on Blood-Material Interactions, Final Report to Devices and Technology Branch, NHLBI-NIH, May, 1979.
21. Navon, G. and Stein, G., J. Phys. Chem. 70:3630 (1966).
22. Oster, G., Brit. Patent 856, 884, Dec. 21, 1960.
23. Petschek, H. E., Adamis, D. and Kantrowitz, A. R., Trans. Amer. Soc. Artif. Int. Organs 14:256 (1968).
24. Raab, M., Pelzbauer, Z., Hanacek, J. and Stol, M., J. Poly Sci. C. 38:221 (1972).
25. Ratner, B. D. and Hoffman, A. S., J. Appl. Polymer Sci. 18:3183 (1974).
26. Vroman, L., Adams, A. L., Klings, M., Fischer, G. C., Munoz, P. C. and Solensky, R. P., Ann. N.Y. Acad. Sci. 283:65-76 (1977).
27. Wichterle, O. and Lim, D., Nature 185:117 (1960).
28. Yamauchi, J., Japan. Kokai Patent No. 75-38790 4/10/75.

III

Current Topics in Biomaterials

Chapter 16

Pathology Assessments in Human Polymeric Implants

James M. Anderson, Robert L. Druet, Yezid Gutierrez and Rimma Slobodkin
Department of Pathology
Case Western Reserve University
Cleveland, Ohio 44106

ABSTRACT

The retrieval and evaluation of polymeric implants and devices and tissues removed from humans can provide the opportunity to determine various aspects of the tissue/implant interaction of a given implant. Obviously, human implantation is the ultimate goal of the science and technology of biocompatible polymers and, as such, it can provide information on factors related to the polymeric implant and tissues at the implant site which may compromise the biocompatibility of the implant. In addition, information derived from the retrieval and evaluation of polymeric implants from humans can provide correlative information relating to in vitro and in vivo studies in other species. The cases presented here are uncommon to rare in their occurrence but address the need for the development of a better understanding of the implant/tissue interaction. These cases include fibrous capsule formation, the interface in total joint prostheses, wear and degradation of cardiovascular and orthopedic prostheses and implant associated infections.

This work was partially supported by a National Institutes of Health Research Career Development Award, HL-00779 (J.M.A.).

The ultimate test for biocompatibility of a polymer, device or prosthesis is human implantation. While biomedical polymers and medical devices are tested under various *in vitro* and *in vivo* conditions, the correlation between such examinations as they relate to their respective performance in the human body is often poor. Thus, while basic and clinical scientists have used a wide and varied number of sophisticated techniques to appreciate or determine the suitability of a given polymer for a given implant application, the question of the correlation of these studies to the actual performance in the human body still remains.

The retrieval and evaluation of polymeric implants and tissues removed from humans offers an opportunity to appreciate the various aspects of the biocompatibility of a given implant. The biocompatibility, or tissue/implant interaction, may be different due to subtle and not so subtle differences between the experimental animal used for the biocompatibility studies and the human regarding physiology, hematology, healing response, etc. The retrieval and evaluation of implants from humans can thus provide a unique perspective and information relating to the ultimate end use. While it is not the purpose of this paper to present or identify the varius modes or mechanisms by which polymeric implants may fail when implanted in humans, the evaluation of polymeric implants from humans can provide information on selective factors related to the polymeric implant which may lead to a compromise in the biocompatibility of the implant and an inappropriate implant/host interaction. This information is important in the design and development of so-called second generation materials or devices.

Since the onset of the use of devices and materials in reconstructive surgery in humans, clinical and basic science investigators have been interested in the evaluation of these devices and materials. An excellent example of one of the early monographs which still remains a classic in its area is the monograph by S. A. Wesolowski published in 1962 [1]. Numerous monographs and reviews are now available which deal with biocompatibility of specific types of prostheses [2-9]. In addition, sufficient interest and effort in the retrieval and evaluation of human implants led to a national conference dedicated to advances in this field [10].

An Implant Retrieval and Evaluation Program has been developed in the Department of Pathology at Case Western Reserve University. The objective of this Program is to analyze, whenever possible, the tissue response and document any material changes of implants recovered by the Department's Autopsy and Surgical Pathology services. In addition to individuals in the Department of Pathology, members of the Department of Macromolecular Science and the Department of Biomedical Engineering also assist in the evaluation of these implants.

Over the past nine years, 4,182 autopsies performed in the Department of Pathology, University Hospitals, Case Western Reserve University, have yielded 761 implants. These 761 implants were removed from 627 patients showing that some patients had more than one implant. The overall percentage for this nine year period is 18%. Table 1 shows the statistics for each individual year and it can be seen that from eight to 31% of the autopsies yield implants. In addition, we have also retrieved and examined implants through the Surgical Pathology service. In 1981, the Surgical Pathology service has provided 135 implants, in 1980 the Surgical Pathology Service provided 161 implants and in 1979, 116 implants. The vast majority of these cases also provided tissue which has permitted us to examine the tissue/implant interaction and obtain more meaningful information about the biocompatibility of the device or implant.

The common types of implants found at autopsy are presented in Table 2. Various types of catheters have also been included as implants as they have a predilection toward infection,

Table 1. Autopsy Implant Retrieval and Evaluation

Year	Autopsies	Autopsies with Implants Number	Autopsies with Implants Percentage	Implants Number	Implants Percentage
1972	560	47	8	64	11
1973	517	46	9	49	9
1974	497	60	12	73	15
1975	450	67	15	72	16
1976	432	39	9	40	9
1977	424	75	18	96	23
1978	477	75	16	101	21
1979	400	86	22	107	27
1980	425	132	31	159	37
TOTAL	4182	627	15%	761	18%

Table 2. Types of Implants Retrieved at Autopsy

Total Hips	Intubation Tubes
Total Knees	Tracheotomy Tubes
Total Ankles	
Finger Joints	Umbilical Artery Catheters
Orthopedic Nails	Umbilical Vein Catheters
Orthopedic Pins	Hyperalimentation Catheters
	Venous Catheters
Cardiac Valves	
Pacemakers	CSF Shunts
Vascular Grafts	Soft Tissue Implants
Septal Defect Patches	Breast Augmentation Implants
Arterial-Venous Shunts	IUDs
	Artificial Testicles

that is, their ability to serve as a nidus or pathway for bacteremia or septicemia. The implants retrieved at autopsy come from both children and adults and rarely has an implant been associated with patient morbidity or mortality. The implants retrieved from the Surgical Pathology service, however, are usually associated with patient morbidity.

It is not the purpose of this paper to elucidate the numerous factors that may lead to an inappropriate implant-host interaction, requiring the removal of an implant. Such an undertaking far exceeds the space available and with this constraint in mind, several selected cases from our implant retrieval and evaluation program will be presented, illustrating various types of implant pathology and more importantly, the problems associated with various aspects of implant biocompatibility. Specifically, we will deal with certain aspects of the all important interface between the implant and the adjacent tissue.

FIBROUS CAPSULE FORMATION

The extent and duration of tissue reactions to polymeric implant materials is important in assessing biocompatibility. In general, the ideal foreign body reaction in soft tissue to a polymeric implant is one in which the acute inflammatory response (polymorphonuclear leukocytes, exudation and hyperemia) is minimal and fibrosis and eventual encapsulation of the implant by fibrous tissue occurs rapidly [11-14]. Interaction of the tissue with the polymeric implant may result in a continuation of the chronic inflammatory phase or lead to increased fibrosis. This increased fibrosis or over-development of the fibrous capsule may involve adjacent organs or tissues and lead to adverse reactions [15,16].

Fibrous capsule formation with subsequent contraction of the fibrous capsule around the implant is a frequent complication of mammary augmentation [17]. The etiology of this phenomenon remains unknown although investigators have sought to show the dependency of fibrous capsule contraction on migration of silicone from the implant and the presence of myofibroblasts in the capsule [18-20]. It has recently been shown that capsule thickness or vascularity, collagen alignment, presence of foreign bodies or the presence of an inner cell layer of macrophages did not correlate with the clinical finding of firmness in mammary augmentations [21].

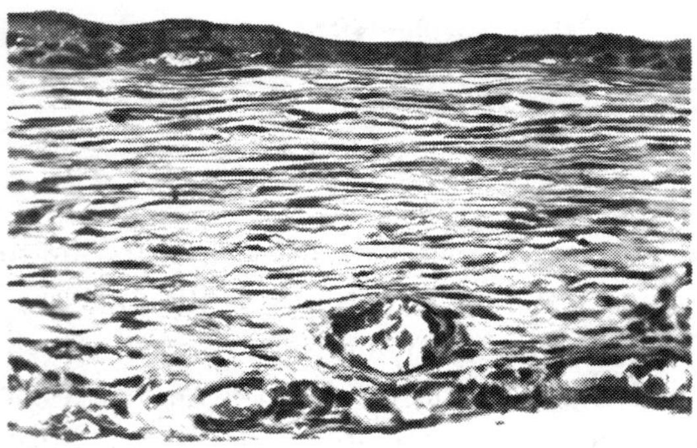

Figure 1. Fibrous Capsule Surrounding Silicone Rubber Implant. The implant/tissue interface is at the top of the photograph. Note the relative lack of vascularization of the implant/tissue interface and in the fibrous capsule. (X320, original magnification).

The role of movement of the breast prosthesis on fibrous capsule development is unclear, although it is generally accepted that implant movement leads to a thicker fibrous capsule. Figure 1 shows the general type of fibrous capsule which forms around silicone implants. Three distinct zones can be identified. The thickness and composition of the implant-tissue interface zone may vary depending on the motion of the implant. This zone usually contains mononuclear leukocytes, macrophages and fibroblasts. The second zone, the fibrous capsule, is composed of longitudinally oriented fibroblasts and collagen fibers. The third zone is at the outer edge of the fibrous capsule and contains numerous capillaries. The location of these capillaries is distinctive and the avascularity of the implant-tissue interface zone and the fibrous capsule is noteworthy. In our experience, the thickness of the fibrous capsule surrounding breast implants is thicker in the caudal areas as opposed to the cephalad areas, indicating the possible role of motion and/or stress in the development of the fibrous capsule.

We have seen several cases in which normal fibrous capsule development around commonly used implants led to complications. In two of these cases, the fibrous capsule surrounding an aorto-femoral vascular graft and polymethylmethacrylate bone cement from the acetabular component of the total hip prosthesis, respectively, have also encapsulated a ureter leading to obstruction of the urine flow from the kidney to the bladder by extrinsic compression of the ureter. In each of these cases, the fibrous capsule formation is normal, that is, it is no different histologically from fibrous capsules which form around biocompatible polymeric prostheses. It should be noted that these complications resulted from surgical error, *i.e.* the lack of consideration of the healing response to these devices.

THE INTERFACE IN TOTAL JOINT PROSTHESES

The various types of orthopedic implants and devices recovered through the autopsy service are listed in Table 2. However, the greatest number of orthopedic cases comes through the surgical pathology service where the largest number of problems involve total joint revision. Total joints retrieved include hips, knees, ankles, metacarpal-phalangeal and elbows. As these cases are usually retrieved with associated tissue, an appreciation of the tissue-implant interaction can be readily obtained.

In describing the components of total joint prostheses and their interaction with adjacent tissues, many authors identify the articulating interface (metal/polymer), the metallic prosthesis – polymethylmethacrylate bone cement interface and the bone cement-bone interface. Unfortunately, the bone cement-bone interface may be transient with a fibrous capsule eventually interposing itself between the bone cement and the bone to create the bone cement-fibrous capsule-bone interface [22,23]. In the case of total joint prostheses where *in situ* polymerizing methlymethacrylate is used as bone cement, this fibrous capsule formation may be accelerated by the heat of polymerization or the toxicity of the monomer, both of which may lead to localized tissue destruction and cell death [24,25]. These changes in the bone and tissue can lead to an inflammatory response with the result being fibrous capsule formation and eventual loosening of the prosthesis. Figure 2 shows a retrieved femoral component of a total hip prosthesis and a hemisected portion of the femur in which the prosthesis had been implanted. Several features are noteworthy. First, the implant bed is lined by fibrous tissue which is interposed between the bone cement and the trabecular bone. Secondly, large areas of the surface of the bone cement are relatively smooth indicating poor fixation. In considering the most optimum of situations where only the normal tissue response is present, this normal response may lead to fibrous capsule formation and eventual loosening of the prosthesis. Aseptic loosening is the most frequent postoperative complication of total joint replacement in the weight-bearing extremities. In general, the peak incidence occurs early, zero to two years postoperatively, or late, beyond four years postoperatively.

Our efforts have been directed at examining these retrieved implants with the specific aim of delineating the biologic mechanism of failure. In particular, we have sought to differentiate the microscopic findings at the cement-bone interface in early loosening, usually less than one year, and late loosening, greater than four years. Twenty-three loose total joint prostheses (10 hips, 12 knees and 1 ankle) were evaluated. The time postoperatively prior to symptoms was greater than four years in 12 patients, and less than one year in seven patients. The radiographic findings included a radiolucent line around the cement-bone interface and in several cases fracture of the cement and/or metallic component. Microscopically, five criteria were utilized for evaluation of the cement-bone interface. These criteria are thickening of the fibrous capsule, osteoid formation on the trabecular bone at the interface, cement particulate in the fibrous capsule, and reorientation and hypertrophy of the trabecular bone at the interface [26].

Early loosening was predominantly characterized by osteoid formation, thickened fibrous capsule at the interface and the trabeculae were randomly oriented to the cement interface. Early loosening can result from excessive loading of the cement-bone interface with possible trabecular fractures combined with undesired features in the preparation and insertion of the cement. Micromotion leads to a thickened fibrous capsule. During the early postoperative course, the randomly oriented trabecular bone may act as a sufficient energy absorbing medium between the cement and cortical bone unless unduly stressed. With time, the trabeculae respond to stress by reorientation and hypertrophy.

Aseptic loosening which occurs after four years implanation may be related to the reorientation and hypertrophy of the trabeculae at the cement-bone interface. During remodelling,

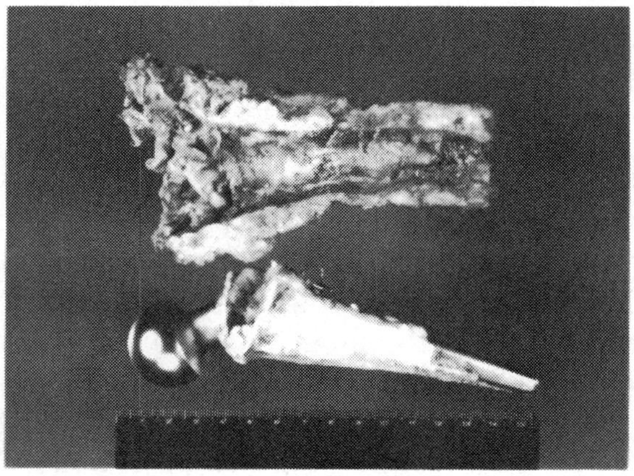

Figure 2. Femoral Prosthesis with proximal portion of femur (implant bed). Note fibrous tissue which lines the implant bed and the relatively smooth areas on the bone cement.

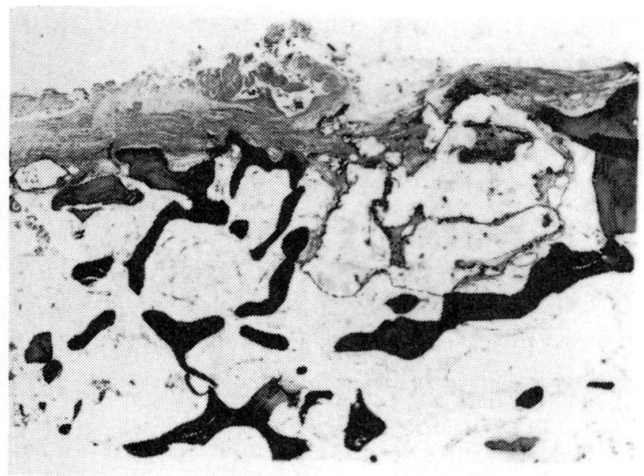

Figure 3. The bone cement/fibrous capsule/bone interface in late loosening. The bone cement is not present. (X20, original magnification).

unequal trabecular resorption or new bone formation may result in stress concentrations creating fractures of the trabeculae and/or cement. Late loosening was characterized by reorientation of the trabeculae to being parallel to the cement interface with marked trabecular hypertrophy. Frequently, the diameters of the trabeculae adjacent to the interface were two to six times that of more distant trabeculae. There was also an increased incidence of cement particulate in the fibrous capsule. The cement particulate at the interface ranged from 300 to 600 microns in thickness. Figure 3 shows several large irregular zones, indicative of polymethylmethacrylate bone cement particulate, immediately beneath the fibrous capsule and interfacing with the trabecular bone. The trabecular bone exhibits some hypertrophy and reorientation. This implant was removed after 4.5 years for loosening. Examination of the interface of the non-loose component in late loosening revealed the same trabecular hypertrophy and reorientation, but minimal cement particulate and a thin fibrous capsule. The microscopic findings in early and late loosening are summarized in Table 3.

Table 3. Microscopic Findings at the Bone Cement/Fibrous Capsule/Bone Interface in Early and Late Loosening of Total Joint Prostheses

Criteria	Early	Late
Fibrous capsule thickening	++++	+
Osteoid	++	+
Cement Particulate	0	+++
Trabecular Reorientation	0	++++
Trabecular Hypertrophy	0	++++

WEAR AND DEGRADATION

Numerous cardiovascular implants are used routinely in surgery today, but problems associated with these implants still remain [27]. The first problem confronting the pathologist is the correct identification of the prosthesis. Fortunately, publications are available which provide the pathologist with a means for the correct identification of heart valves, pacemakers and vascular grafts [28-30]. From a materials point-of-view, the ability of polymeric materials in functioning implants such as heart valves and total joint prostheses to withstand wear is inadequate at best. Since prosthetic heart valves were first introduced, wear of the component parts has ranked with nonthrombogenic behavior as major criteria for the acceptability of candidate materials for prosthetic heart valves. Third body wear of the articular surfaces in total joint prostheses is also a major problem. Wear or variance of prosthetic heart valve occluder balls or discs have presented problems since prosthetic heart valves were first introduced [31]. In recent years, there have been several reports describing the erosion and subsequent emobilization of ball occluders from cage-ball cardiac valve prostheses [32,33]. Figure 4 shows a Braunwald-Cutter aortic prosthesis which exhibits marked occluder variance and loss of fabric from the struts of the cage. The constant impact of the ball occluder on the fabric covering the sewing ring and struts leads to fabric loss. The continued loss of fabric increases the distance between the struts allowing for possible ball emoblization. The silicone rubber occluder wears from repeated contact with the bare metal struts. The wear particles from the silicone rubber occluder and the Dacron strut and sewing ring fabric can embolize. We have observed this phenomenon in several cases from our Implant Retrieval and Evaluation Program.

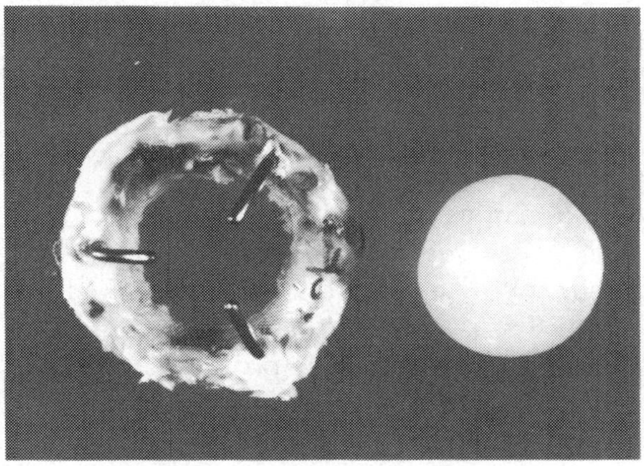

Figure 4. Braunwald-Cutter Prosthetic Aortic Heart Valve with marked occluder wear and loss of fabric from the struts of the cage.

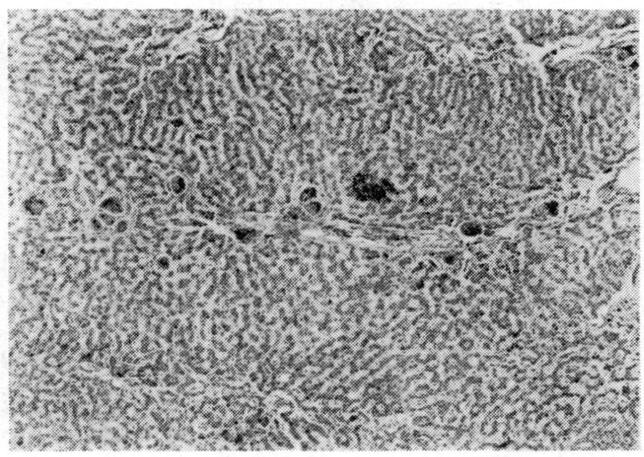

Figure 5. Periportal foreign body giant cells containing silica (filler) and/or polydimethylsiloxane in the liver. (X55, original magnification).

Associated with this finding has been the presence of characteristic perivascular foreign body giant cells containing refractile, irregular, nonbirefringent material in the liver (Figure 5), spleen and kidneys. The material in the foreign body giant cells could not be stained with hematoxylin and eosin, PAS or trichrome stains. Secondary X-ray dispersion analysis with scanning electron microscopy showed the presence of the K α and K β peaks for silicon. While it is unclear whether the silicon is from polydimethylsiloxane or silicon dioxide, the identification of silicon within these perivascular foreign body giant cells coupled with the marked variance of the silicon occluder balls is strong evidence for the emobilization of wear particles from the occluder ball. Wear products of the Dacron sewing rings have also been identified in distant organs such as the brain and liver.

The long-term chronic degradation of a prosthetic material may also take place, leading to a chronic inflammatory response with fibrosis [34]. This phenomenon has been seen in a case where an Ivalon® (cross-linked polyvinyl alcohol) patch has been used to close a ventricular septal defect. Seven years following implantation, the Ivalon® patch showed focal degradation with calcification and fibrosis, foci of lymphocytes were present suggestive of a chronic in-

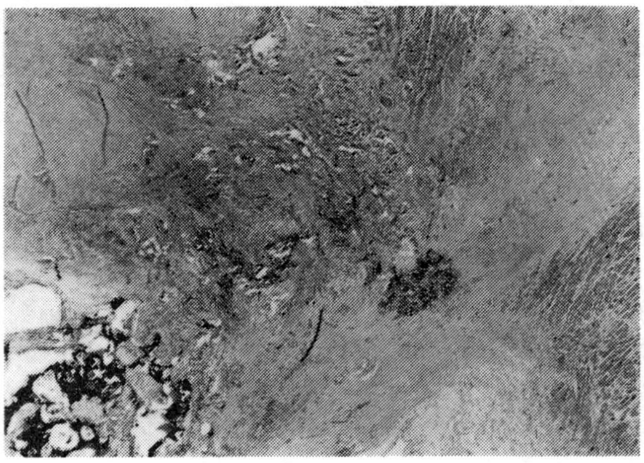

Figure 6. Focal degradation and calcification of Ivalon® . Foci of chronic inflammation are present in the fibrous tissue at the implant/tissue interface (center of the photograph) and cardiac muscle is at the top and right of the photograph. (X20, original magnification).

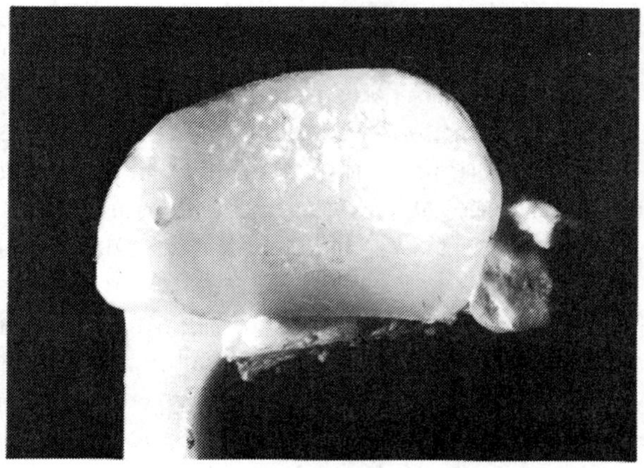

Figure 7. Marked wear of the articular surface of the high density polyethylene tibial component of a total knee prosthesis. Polymethylmethacrylate bone cement particulate is present in the surface.

flammatory response to the material and/or its degradation products (Figure 6). The poor biocompatibility of Ivalon® is well documented in human and animal studies [34-36].

A common finding from failed hip and knee prostheses is wear particles from the polymeric and metallic components that have migrated into the synovium of the joint capsule [37,38]. Third body wear can be a major problem in the function of total joint prostheses. Figure 7 shows the articular surface of the tibial component of a total knee prosthesis. Marked wear is obvious and polymethylmethacrylate bone cement particulate is embedded in the surface of the high density polyethylene tibial component. The pseudocapsule surrounding the joints and joint spaces in cases exhibiting marked wear contain polyethylene and polymethylmethacrylate bone cement particulate. This is shown in Figure 8 where large macrophage or foreign body giant cell lined vacuoles and numerous foreign body giant cells are present. With standard tissue processing for histology, the bone cement particulate is dissolved out of the tissue leaving only the spaces. Polyethylene particulate usually remains in the tissue during this processing and several particles can be seen in the vacuoles in Figure 8. Wear of the metallic components can also occur with subsequent migration of the metallic particulate into the pseudocapsule. Figure 9 shows the synovium of a pseudocapsule with chronic synovitis and metallic particulate in macrophages in the synovium and subsynovium.

IMPLANT ASSOCIATED INFECTIONS

The infectious susceptibility of implants remains as a major unsolved problem in the area of implants [39,40]. Implants may serve as a route for the entry of an infectious agent or may serve as a preferential site for the deposition of the agent with subsequent growth, embolization, if in the cardiovascular system, or infiltration into adjacent tissue. In many of these cases, removal of the prosthesis is necessary to achieve a cure.

Nearly every type of prosthesis used in humans has been associated with serious infections. These include orthopedic prostheses (joint space or bone infections), prosthetic heart

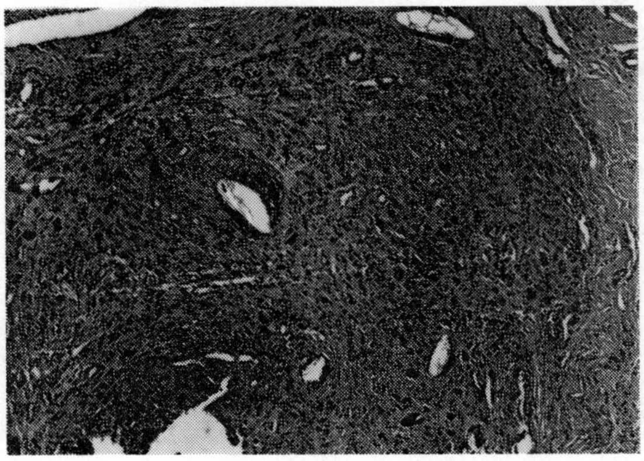

Figure 8. Polyethylene and polymethylmethacrylate bone cement particulate in the pseudocapsule of a total knee prosthesis (X50, original magnification).

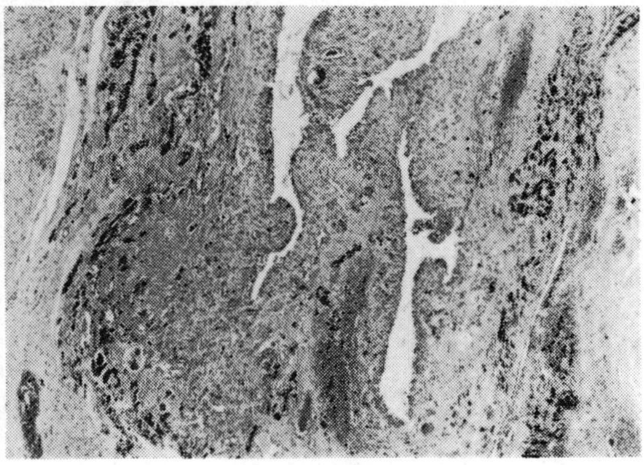

Figure 9. Metallic particulate in the pseudocapsule of a total hip prosthesis with marked third body wear of the articular surfaces of the femoral and acetabular components. (X37, original magnification).

valves (endocarditis), vascular prostheses (graft infections and bacteremia), intraocular lens prostheses (endophthalmitis), hemodialysis (hepatitis, bacteremia and shunt site infections), cerebrospinal fluid shunts (ventriculitis), and all types of catheters [41-43]. In many cases, fulminant infectious processes may be present in patients who present clinically with minimal signs and symptoms. Compromised and immunosuppressed patients requiring life-support systems and other invasive implants, especially catheters, are susceptible to infections.

A major consideration in the etiology and therapy of infections associated with prostheses is the capability of the prosthesis to function as a nidus for the dissemination of the infectious agents. These devices may also provide microorganisms with a protected site that is relatively inaccessible to the cellular and humoral elements of the inflammatory response as well as bacteriocidal or other pharmacologic agents. Each type of implant presents a different combination of variables related to the etiology and development of an infectious process. Little is known about the etiologic, bacteriologic, pathologic, clinical and pharmacokinetic variables which influence the development, extent and duration of prosthesis-related infections.

Moore and coworkers have demonstrated the importance of neointima development on reducing the infectious susceptibility of cardiovascular implants [44,45]. Figure 10 shows a cross-sectional portion of an expanded polytetrafluoroethylene vascular graft which has been used as an arterio-venous shunt for dialysis. A bacterial stain was used on the tissue section which was used to obtain this photograph. The irregular dark black clumps of material present within the vascular graft and immediately beneath the luminal surface (bottom of photograph) are aggregates of Staphylococci. This was confirmed by culture. The ability of organisms to penetrate prostheses is insidious and poorly understood. It is obvious from Figure 10 that surgical resection and removal may represent the only definitive procedure to obtain a cure.

CONCLUSIONS

The cases presented here are uncommon to rare in their occurrence but they represent factors which must be addressed in determining the biocompatibility of polymeric implants in

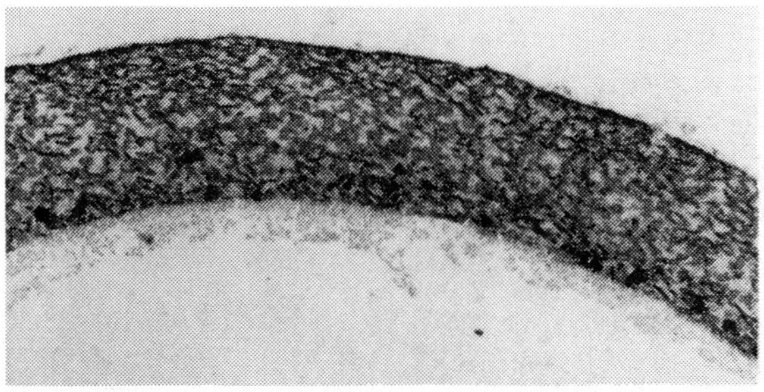

Figure 10. Staphyloccal aggregates in expanded polytetrafluoroethylene vascular graft. Lumen of the graft is at the bottom. (×38, original magnification).

humans. From another viewpoint, the altered implant/tissue interactions presented in these cases offer an opportunity to the polymer scientist who wishes to examine these complex problems. Included in these problems is an elucidation of those tissue and material variables which lead to variations in fibrous capsule formation. Little research has been done in this area and yet, since almost all human implants are partially or totally encapsulated, this area would appear to be of importance in determining the biocompatibility of human implants. The other major area which appears to be common to the majority of implants is the infectious susceptibility of implants. As better materials and more sophisticated devices are implanted in humans, new problems in the biocompatibility of these materials and devices will appear as a result of the improved functional longevity of the materials and devices. These so-called second generation problems will be recognized and solved by a better understanding of the tissue/implant interaction.

REFERENCES

1. Wesolowski, S. A., "Evaluation of Tissue and Prosthetic Vascular Grafts," Charles C. Thomas, Springfield, Illinois, 1962.
2. Sawyer, P. N. and Kaplitt, M. J., editors, "Vascular Grafts," Appleton-Century-Crofts, New York, 1978.
3. Dardik, H., editor, "Graft Materials in Vascular Surgery," Year Book Medical Publishers, Chicago, Illinois, 1978.
3. Syrett, B. C., and Acharya, A., editors, "Corrosion and Degradation of Implant Materials," American Society for Testing and Materials, Philadelphia, Pa., 1979.
5. Chapchal, G., editor, "Arthoplasty of the Hip," G. Thieme, Stuttgart, West Germany, 1973.
6. Total Joint Arthoplasty Symposium in Mayo Clinic Proceedings, *54*, 557-601, 1979.
7. Lefrak, E. A. and Starr, A., "Cardiac Valve Prostheses," Appleton-Century-Crofts, New York, 1979.
8. Williams, D. F., editor, "Fundamental Aspects of Biocompatibility," Volumes I and II, CRC Press, Inc., Boca Raton, Florida, 1981.
9. Gebelein, C. G. and Koblitz, F. F., editors, "Biomedical and Dental Applications of Polymers," Plenum Press, New York, 1981.
10. Weinstein, A., Gibbons, D., Brown, S. and Ruff, W., editors, "Implant Retrieval: Material and Biological Analysis," National Bureau of Standards Special Publication 601, U.S. Government Printing Office, Washington, D.C., 1981.
11. Coleman, D. L., King, R. N., and Andrade, J. D., The foreign body reaction: a chronic inflammatory response, J. Biomed. Mater. Res., *8*, 199-211, 1974.

12. Ocumpaugh, D. E. and Lee, H. L. Foreign body reactions to plastic implants, J. Macromol. Sci. Chem., *4A*, 595-613, 1970.
13. Rigdon, R. H. Tissue reaction to foreign materials, Crit. Rev. Food Sci. Nutr., *7*, 435, 1975.
14. Frisch, E., Functional considerations in implant design, Medical Device and Diagnostic Industry, *3(7)*, 23-26 (1981).
15. Hirsch, S., Robertson, H. and Gornowsky, M., Arterial occlusion secondary to methylmethacrylate use, Arch. Surg. (Chicago), *3*, 204, 1976.
16. Casagrande, P. and Darahy, P., Delayed sciatic nerve entrapment following the use of self-curing acrylic, J. Bone J. Surg., *53A*, 167-169, 1971.
17. Vinnick, C. A., Spherical contracture of fibrous capsules around breast implants, Plast. Reconstruc. Surg., *58*, 555-560, 1976.
18. Baarker, D. E., Retsky, M. I., and Schultz, S., "Bleeding" of silicone from bag-gel breast implants, and its clinical relation to fibrous capsule reaction, Plast. Reconstruc. Surg., *61* 836-841, 1978.
19. Rudolph, R. et al., Myofibroblasts and free silicon around breast implants, Plast. Reconstruc. Surg., *62*, 185-196, 1978.
20. Wagner, H., Beller, F. K. and Pfautsch, M., Electron and light microscopy examination of capsules around breast implants, Plast. Reconstruc. Surg., *60*, 49-55, 1977.
21. Gayou, R. M., A histological comparison of contracted and non-contracted capsules around silicone breast implants, Plast. Reconstruc. Surg., *63*, 700-707, 1979.
22. Willert, H.-G., Ludwig, J. and Semlitsch, M., Reaction of bone to methacrylate after hip arthoplasty, J. Bone and Joint Surg., *56-A*, 1368-1382, 1974.
23. Reckling, F. W., Asher, M. A., and Dillon, W. L., A longitudinal study of the radiolucent line at the bone-cement interface following total joint-replacements procedures, J. Bone and Joint Surg., *59-A*, 355-358, 1977.
24. Reckling, F. W. and Dillon, W. L., The bone-cement interface temperature during total joint replacement, J. Bone and Joint Surg., *59-A*, 80-82, 1977.
25. Jefferiss, C. D., Lee, A. J. C. and Ling, R. S. M., Thermal aspects of self-curing polymethylmethacrylate, J. Bone and Joint Surg., *57-B* 511-518, 1975.
26. Anderson, J. M., Goldberg, V., and Green, D., unpublished results.
27. Silver, M. D. Cardiac pathology — a look at the last five years. II. The pathology of cardiovascular prosthesis, Hum. Pathol., *5*, 127-138, 1974.
28. Silver, M. D., Datta, B. N. and Bowes, V. F, A key to identify heart valve prosthesis, Arch. Pathol., *99*, 132-138, 1975.
29. Chun, P. K. C. and Nelson, W. P., Common cardiac prosthetic valves, radiologic identification and associated complications, JAMA, *238*, 401-403, 1977.
30. Morse, D. and Steiner, R. M., "The Pacemaker and Valve Identification Guide," Medical Examination Publishing, Garden City, N.Y., 1978.
31. Byrne, J. P., Behrendt, D. M., Kirsch, M. M. and Orringere, M. B., Replacement of heart valves by prosthetic devices, in *Pathobiology Annual,* Vol. 7, H. L. Ioachim, ed., Appleton-Century-Crofts, N.Y., 1977, p. 83.
32. Hameed, K., Ashjaq, S. and Waugh, D. O. W., Ball fracture and extrusion in Starr-Edwards aortic valve prosthesis with dissemination of ball material, Arch. Pathol., *86*, 520-524, 1968.
33. Ridolfi, R. L. and Hutchins, G. M., Detection of ball variance in prosthetic heart valves by liver biopsy, Johns Hopkins Med. J., *134,* 131-140, 1974.
34. Hawe, A., Late deterioration of intracardiac Ivalon sponge patches, J. Thorac. Cardiovasc. Surg., *58*, 87-91, 1969.
35. Chen, R. W., Musser, A. W. and Postlethwait, R., Alterations of and tissue reaction to polyvinyl alcohol sponge implants, Surgery, *66*, 899-906, 1969.
36. Harrison, J. H., Swanson, D. S. and Lincoln, A. F. A comparison of the tissue reactions to plastic materials, Dacron Ivalon sponge, Nylon, Orlon and Teflon, Arch. Surg. (Chicago), *74*, 139-144, 1957.

37. Willert, H. G., and Semlitsch, M., Reactions of the articular capsule to wear products of artificial joint prostheses, J. Biomed. Mater. Res., *11,* 157-164, 1977.
38. Crugnola, A., Lowell, A. S. and Radin, E., Polymeric debris in synovium after total joint replacement: histological identification, J. Bone and Joint Surg., *59-A,* 860-862, 1977.
39. Stamm, W. E., Infections related to medical devices, Ann. Intern. Med., *89,* 764-769, 1978.
40. Duma, R. J., editor, "Infections of Prosthetic Heart Valves and Vascular Grafts," University Park Press, Baltimore, 1977.
41. Reinarz, J A., Nosocomial infections, Clinical Symposia (CIBA Pharmaceutical Co., Summit, N.J.) *30(6),* 2-32, 1978.
42. Maki, D. G., Goldmann, D. A., and Rhame, F. S., Infection control in intravenous therapy, Ann. Intern. Med., *79,* 867-887, 1974.
43. Maki, D. G., Rhame, F. S., Mackel, D. C. and Bennet, J. V., Nationwide epidemic of septicemia caused by contaminated intravenous products: epidemiologic and clinical features, Amer. J. Med., *60(4),* 471-485, 1976.
44. Goldstone, J. and Moore, W. S., Infection in vascular prostheses, clinical manifestations and surgical management, Amer. J. Surg., *128,* 225-233, 1974.
45. Roon, A. J., Malone, J. M., Moore, W. S., Bean, B. and Campagna, G., Bacteremic infectability: a function of vascular graft material and design, J. Surg. Res., *22,* 489-498, 1977.

Chapter 17

Immune Responses to Glutaraldehyde-Treated Xenografts

P. K. Bajpai, Ph.D.* and M. L. Salgaller
University of Dayton
Dayton, Ohio 45469

ABSTRACT

Glutaraldehyde-treated tissue valve xenografts have been claimed as an excellent choice for replacing malfunctioning human heart valves. These tanned tissue valves exhibit excellent hemodynamic function in the absence of anticoagulant therapy. However, the immunologic potential of these tanned tissue prostheses has not been clearly resolved. Reports on the ability of glutaraldehyde to mask some and unmask other antigens coupled with lack of studies using tanned modified antigens in the testing system were instrumental in designing studies on the immunogenicity of glutaraldehyde-modified tissues.

Porcine heart valve and bovine pericardial tissues were treated with 0.5% glutaraldehyde (pH 7.4) for two weeks. Immunogenicity of untanned and tanned porcine heart valve and bovine pericardial tissue homogenates and xenografts were studied in rabbits using morphological as well as the following immunological procedures; capillary tube agglutination, gel diffusion, micro-complement fixation, indirect hemagglutination, macrophage migration inhibition, leucocyte migration inhibition and skin reaction tests.

Review of the literature and the results of immunogenicity studies indicate that: A) glutaraldehyde stabilization delays the eventual degradation of the tissue xenografts; B) glutaraldehyde treatment alters some antigens and enhances the immunogenic properties of other tissue determinants; C) tanned tissue xenografts are capable of evoking humoral, cellular and autoimmune respones; D) indirect hemagglutination, micro-complement fixation and leucocyte migration inhibition procedures can be used to monitor immune responses to tanned tissues in humans.

*Also Physiology Program, Wright State University, Dayton, Ohio 45435.

1. INTRODUCTION

Glutaraldehyde, or 1,5 pentanedial is a dialdehyde (Figure 1) and in solution consists of a mixture of monomers and a high percentage of low molecular weight polymers. At room temperature the components of glutaraldehyde include acryclic monohydrates, dihydrates and free aldehydes. The alpha and beta-unsaturated aldehydes result from loss of water after hemi-acetal condensations. Free aldehyde side groups of glutaraldehyde make it an ideal agent for cross-linking proteins. According to Peracchia and Mittler polymeric rather than monomeric forms of glutaraldehyde cross-link biological material [1]. Glutaraldehyde reacts with N-terminal amino groups of some peptides, alpha amino groups of amino acids, phenolic and imidazole groups of tyrosine and histidine derivatives, epsilon amino groups of lysine and hydroxyl, sulfhydrl and guanidine groups [2,3].

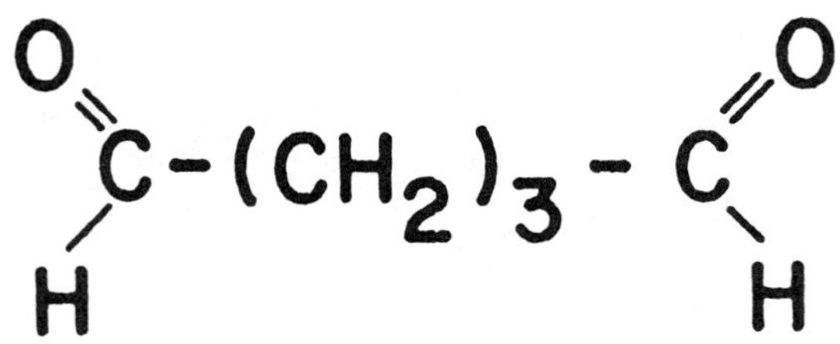

Figure 1. Structure of glutaraldehyde.

Two major mechanisms have been postulated by which glutaraldehyde reacts with tissues. According to one concept, glutaraldehyde reacts with tissues by forming protein pyridinium salt cross-links. On the other hand, Woodroof is of the opinion that glutaraldehyde stabilizes tissues by forming Schiff base intermediates and secondary amines at physiological pH and temperature [2,3].

Since interactions with glutaraldehyde cause a wide variety of intra-molecular cross-linkages and configurational alterations, it has been used to insolubilize and stabilize various kinds of biologic materials [4,5]. Glutaraldehyde was originally used to tan leather [2]. Perhaps the greatest use of glutaraldehyde at present is as a fixative for preparing biologic materials for histochemistry and electron microscopy [4]. During the mid-seventies glutaraldehyde was used as a potent bactericidal agent [5]. The precise mechanism by which glutaraldehyde acts as a sterilizing agent has yet to be clearly elucidated. Thomas is of the opinion that glutaraldehyde kills bacteria by interacting with the proteins and mucopeptides of the bacterial cell wall and/or spore coat and forming a lattice highly impermeable to water and nutrients [5]. Glutaraldehyde is cytotoxic in concentrations of 10-15 μg/ml. The bactericidal properties of glutaraldehyde increase with increase in pH, reaction time and concentration of the dialdehyde [6]. Glutaraldehyde has also been used to sterilize food [2].

Use of glutaraldehyde as a cross-linking agent for tissue implants started in the sixties [2]. Since stabilization by means of glutaraldehyde was postulated to protect biologic materials from degradation by enzymes, macrophages and microorganisms, it was assumed that glutaraldehyde treatment would also render biological material inert, non-viable, non-antigenic and non-immunogenic [2,7]. However, glutaraldehyde has been used to prepare immobilized but active enzymes and/or antigens, vaccines and polymeric immunogenic allergens [1,4,6]. A brief review of these uses of glutaraldehyde will provide the reader the rationale for investigating the immunogenic role of glutaraldehyde stabilized tissues.

2. GLUTARALDEHYDE STABILIZED ANTIGENS, ANTIBODIES AND ENZYMES

Glutaraldehyde treatment has been used to obtain stabilized protein derivatives for performing procedures which could not be conducted efficiently with soluble monomeric forms. Various concentrations of glutaraldehyde have been used to stabilize bovine serum albumin, human serum proteins and immunoglobulin type IgG [2,6]. Glutaraldehyde treatment did not alter the antigenicity of these proteins and the stabilized derivatives were used as immunoadsorbants for isolation of specific antibodies or antigens [2]. Thus, use of glutaraldehyde was advocated for polymerization of cellular membrane antigens and isolation of membrane antibodies [2,6].

Glutaraldehyde stabilization also decreases the leakage of IgG from sepharose-immunoadsorbants to trace levels without significantly hindering the antigen binding and enzyme activity [8]. Glutaraldehyde-treated cells have been used for immunocytochemical analysis and visualization of porcine brain microtubules in electron micrographs [4]. Tubules treated with 0.5% (w/vol) glutaraldehyde were injected into rabbits to produce antigen-specific antibodies [4]. Antibodies obtained against the treated antigen reacted less severely with untreated brain tubulin [4]. Antibody to glutaraldehyde-treated porcine brain tubulin (GTPT), purified by affinity column chromatograph, bound specifically to microtubules in glutaraldehyde-stabilized tissue culture cells (Figure 2). The anti-GTPT antibody-cytoplasm interactions produced brilliant, uniform fluorescent filaments [4].

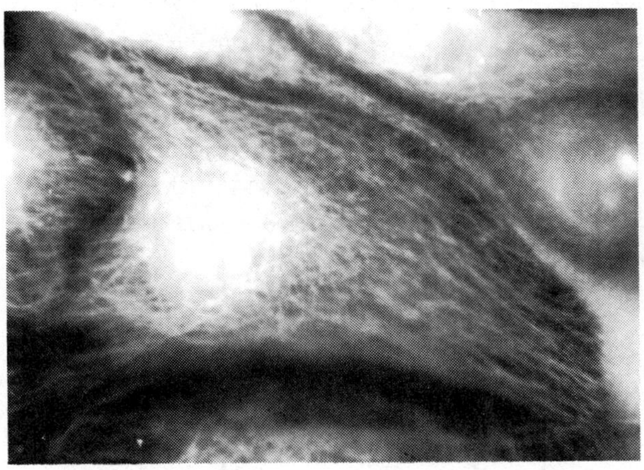

Figure 2. Indirect immunofluorescence of PTK_1, cells after treatment with antibody specific for glutaraldehyde-treated porcine brain tubulin showing fine lattice of microtubules visible around the nucleus in a glutaraldehyde fixed cell: Original magnification 1950x (Courtesy of Dr. B. S. Eckert).

Horseradish peroxidase conjugated antibodies prepared by glutaraldehyde coupling procedure retain 70% of their native enzyme activity and have been used effectively in immunoassays and histochemical procedures [9]. Use of other cross-linking agents has resulted in the loss of enzyme activity and inability to produce specific antibodies [5,10]. Glucomylase, cross-linked to chiton by means of glutaraldehyde, is two times more active than glucomylase absorbed on chiton [2].

Glutaraldehyde stabilization renders glucocerebrosidase loaded erythrocytes less susceptible to lysis without inactivating the entrapped enzymes. Glutaraldehyde treatment also allows the cells to be removed quickly from the circulation for macrophage processing. Since Gaucher's disease is characterized by an inherited deficiency of the enzyme glucocerebrosidase, use of glutaraldehyde stabilized enzyme loaded erythrocytes results in the quick delivery of the enzymes to the spleen and liver [10]. According to Deloach, the macrophages process the glutaraldehyde stabilized and unstabilized enzyme loaded cells in the same proportion [11].

3. GLUTARALDEHYDE STABILIZED CELLS

Glutaraldehyde treatment of erythrocytes does not interfere with the ability of the cell to absorb specific antibodies. However, it does reduce the ability of the erythrocyte to agglutinate in the presence of ABO specific antisera [12]. Glutaraldehyde treated sheep erythrocytes preferentially induce the cellular immune response, a normal secondary immune response and a low to undetectable primary immune response [2,13].

Leshem and Naor showed that while the mice injected with glutaraldehyde treated sheep erythrocytes were unable to induce primary immune response they elicited a specific secondary immune response [13]. The immunological memory in these mice was directed specifically to the erythrocyte membrane determinants and not to the new antigenic sites which may have been induced by glutaraldehyde treatment. They concluded that since glutaraldehyde stabilized erythrocytes were not processed in a normal manner by the macrophages, they were not available for the macrophage-dependent primary immune response. Macrophages of mice challenged simultaneously with untreated and glutaraldehyde treated erythrocytes phagocytose and digest the two types of cells independently of each other [14]. While most of the untreated erythrocytes are digested by 48 hours the same macrophage takes 100 hours to digest the glutaraldehyde treated erythrocyte. According to Ramos and coworkers, alteration in digestion time of glutaraldehyde stabilized cells is probably responsible for the suppression of primary immune response. Mice, primed with glutaraldehyde stabilized sheep erythrocytes, develop an early helper function mediated by the thymocyte dependent (T) cells. Since transfer of immunity to irradiated recipients from mice treated with glutaraldehyde stabilized cells can only be induced by the transfer of T-cells, it is apparent that the fixed nature of the antigenic determinants on the stabilized cell selectively stimulates the activity of T helper cells [14].

Glutaraldehyde stabilized tumor cells or cell membrane rich fragments have been used to protect experimental animals against viable tumors [2,16]. Frost and coworkers injected mice with untreated and glutaraldehyde treated methylcholanthrene-induced sarcoma cells or membrane rich tumor cell fragments. After 14 days they challenged the injected mice with viable tumor cells and screened for development of tumors. Immunizations with glutaraldehyde stabilized tumor cells or fragments protected the animals from developing tumors on injection of viable tumor cells [16]. Immunizations with glutaraldehyde stabilized hamster polyoma cells also induce cellular immunity in Syrian hamsters [17]. According to Tomecki, sensitized lymphoid spleen cells obtained from animals injected with glutaraldehyde treated tumor cells destroyed tissue culture target cells after 48 hours of incubation when the ratio of attacking to target cells was at least 50:1 [17]. Failure to detect antibodies in the serum of animals immunized with glutaraldehyde treated cells or cell fragments has prompted some investigators to propose that glutaraldehyde modifies the cellular antigens to preferentially engage the cellular immune system [15,16,17].

Some investigators have not been able to induce immunity with injections of glutaraldehyde treated cells. Price and his associates failed to induce an immune response in rats with injections of glutaraldehyde treated rat hepatoma cells [2,18]. However, glutaraldehyde stabilized rat hepatoma cells did display the presence of tumor specific antigen by various serologic tests. Subsequent studies using mice showed that immunizations with tanned X-irradiated meth A cells did not impair the immunogenicity of glutaraldehyde treated cells [18]. Since rats are capable of inducing immune responses against other glutaraldehyde stabilized antigens, differences in species cannot explain the discrepancies observed by Price and coworkers [2,19,20]. Furthermore, similar discrepancies have also been noted in mice with the use of different antigens. Mice primed with 0.013 to 0.13% glutaraldehyde tanned allogeneic lymph node cells do not induce a primary lymphocytotoxic antibody response, whereas mice primed with similar tanned preparations of P815 allogeneic tumor cells retain their immunogenic capabilities [21]. Thus, differences in antigens and/or pathways of inducing immunity probably account for the above discrepancies [2].

Glutaraldehyde in final concentrations of 0.013M has also been used to prepare vaccines since it inactivates bacteria and toxins without impairing their immunogenicity [22]. Injections of glutaraldehyde treated bacteria induce high titers of antibodies [22]. Cross-linking of p-amino-phenol (PAP) with N-acetylmuramyl-L alanyl-D-isoglutamine (MDP) by means of glutaraldehyde restores several biologic activities including antibody production and non-specific resistance against *Kleibsella* infection [23].

4. GLUTARALDEHYDE STABILIZED ALLERGENS

For many years investigators have tried to depress allergen sensitivity and increase allergen-specific antibody response by chemical treatment of the allergens. Glutaraldehyde treatment of allergens such as ragweed pollen reduces the ability of the allergen to react with cell-bound reagins and increases the synthesis of allergen-specific IgG-immunoglobulins [2,24]. Glutaraldehyde stabilized pollen extracts also retain their capacity to induce the formation of allergen-specific antibody (IgG) in rats [25]. Differences in antibody (IgG) titers were not observed when rabbits were immunized with untreated and glutaraldehyde treated timothy pollen extracts [25].

However, pollen specific antibodies (IgG) induced by glutaraldehyde stabilized pollen immunizations block skin reaction in pollen sensitive humans [25]. Immunizations with grass and pollen allergen decrease the severity of allergic rhinitis [26]. Administration of glutaraldehyde treated allergens also reduce the symptoms of allergic reactions such as sneezing, dyspnea, and nasal discharge and blockage. A glutaraldehyde stabilized timothy grass pollen extract has also been prepared for intranasal immunizations. Anti-allergen IgE levels increased in the patients receiving placebo treatment, while anti-timothy grass pollen IgE, IgM, and IgG antibody levels increased in patients treated with glutaraldehyde modified pollen extract [26].

Antigen AgE is the major but not the only allergen in ragweed extract and complex fractionation procedures make it difficult to obtain large quantities of purified AgE [27]. Hence, Patterson and his associates polymerized a more complex fraction of ragweed extract by means of glutaraldehyde [24]. They reported that glutaraldehyde modification lowered the allergenicity but maintained the immunogenicity of the allergen (Figure 3). The reduction in allergenicity was attributed to the reduced number of antigenic determinants displayed on glutaraldehyde modified ragweed antigen, the decreased ability of large polymers to diffuse and bridge IgG antibody on skin mast cells, and the lower molar concentration of glutaraldehyde treated allergen per unit weight [24].

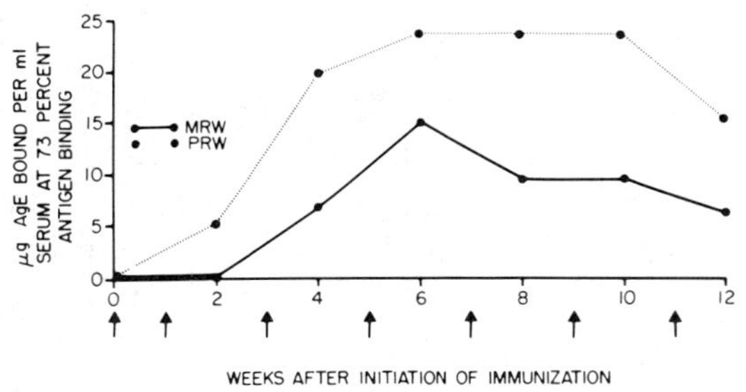

Figure 3. Seventy-two hour passive cutaneous transfer titers (means) with the use of sera from rabbits immunized with untreated monomeric ragweed antigens (MRW) and glutaraldehyde-treated polymeric ragweed antigens (PRW). Arrows indicate immunizations (Courtesy of Dr. R. Patterson).

5. GLUTARALDEHYDE STABILIZED MAMMALIAN TISSUES

Although the major components of vascular tissues are collagen, elastin, glycoproteins, mucoproteins and soluble proteins, collagen forms the bulk of the tissues. Whereas cartilage contains collagen type II, skin and parenchyma of several organs contain collagen type I and type III. Immune response against collagen has been demonstrated by several of the following procedures; complement fixation, passive hemagglutination, immunofluorescence, incorporation of tritiated thymidine into lymphocytes, macrophage migration inhibition, radioimmunoassay and skin reaction [2]. Homologous, heterologous and denatured type I mammalian skin collagens show extensive cross-reactions and are capable of inducing both cellular and humoral immune responses [28]. The ability of denatured collagen to cross-react and induce cellular sensitivity suggests that it's helical determinants are not involved in eliciting immune responses [28]. On implantation, collagen induces a chronic inflammatory response and eventually is degraded by the host [2].

Before using stablized vascular heterografts, a large number of investigations were conducted with homografts [2,29,30]. Usually the procedure used to investigate the immunogenicity of venous homografts dictated the conclusion whether the venous homograft was mildly antigenic or antigenic. However, there seems to be general agreement that venous homografts are antigenic.

Animal studies conducted in the early sixties indicated a very high rate of aneurysms in bovine arterial heterografts [30]. Thus, use of tanned bovine arterial arterio-grafts was advocated in the late sixties. Defalco conducted extensive immunological studies with a clear supernatant antigen (0.64 mg/ml protein) prepared by centrifuging the cross-linked and insolubilized bovine carotid artery homogenate at 12,000 rpm. In contrast, untreated clear antigen (3.64 mg/ml of protein) was prepared by centrifugation of the homogenate at 3,000 rpm. Since the clear supernatant from tanned bovine arteries did not induce an immune response and react in serological reactions, it was concluded that tanned bovine arteriografts were not immunogenic [31]. However, high rate of infection, early incidence of thrombosis, aneurysmal degeneration, lack of length, inadequate diameter and high cost discouraged the use of tanned bovine arterio-grafts [2].

Since then, other investigators have also used supernatants or soluble extracts of tanned as well as untanned tissues to test the immunogenicity of cross-linked insolubilized tissues [32,33]. Esato and associates used human umbilical cord vein as canine arterial bypass grafts and reported that the immunogenicity of the grafts was effectively suppressed by stabilizing the veins with 0.5 to 1% glutaraldehyde [34]. Infiltration of glutaraldehyde-treated porcine heart valve xenografts with mononuclear cells, lymphocytes and macrophages (Figure 4)

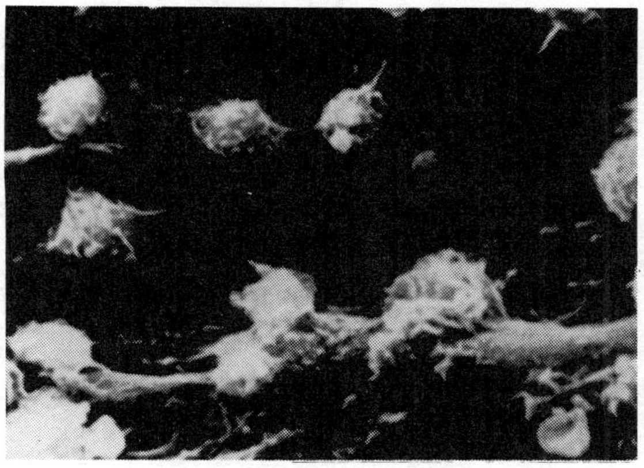

Figure 4. Scanning electron micrograph of a porcine heart valve xenograft showing macrophages on the outflow surface of a valve implanted for 3 months in a patient. Original magnification X 1200. (Courtesy of Dr. V. J. Ferrans).

along with degeneration of the tanned bioprostheses suggest that the immune system does not spare the tanned xenografts [35,37].

Antigenic challenge of sensitized lymphocytes can induce the production of biologic mediators. These mediators can modulate connective tissue metabolism by releasing lymphokine-fibroblast activating factor (FAF) which helps in the synthesis of collagen and lymphokine-macrophage activating factor (MAF) which helps in the destruction of collagen [36]. Since cross-linking of the tissue delays degeneration of collagen, it is possible that the formation of new connective tissue, due to an immune involvement overcomes the destructive process. We have observed induction of immune responses as well as encapsulation and degradation of glutaraldehyde-stabilized porcine aortic valve and bovine pericardial tissue heterografts in rabbits [27,37,38].

Glutaraldehyde cross-links and insolubilizes biologic materials [3]. Hence, absence of or trace amounts of insolubilized or tanned antigen is expected to be found in the supernatants of soluble extracts of tanned tissues. Tests, including skin reactions, conducted with such extracts reveal very little information about the immunogenicity of an insolubilized tissue. Using fine particulate antigen preparations of tanned porcine aortic valve and bovine pericardial tissues for immunization and serological testing, we have shown induction of humoral as well as cellular immune responses against tanned tissues in rabbits [27,37,38].

Makkes and his associates treated isologous and homologous muscle fragments with 2% glutaraldehyde for seven days at 37°C. They then dried the tanned tissue and packed it in 15mm long and 3.6mm inside diameter polyethylene tubes having four 0.6mm diameter holes in the sides. The ends of the tubes were sealed with wax. Control empty tubes and tubes containing untreated tissues or tanning agents as well as tubes containing tanned tissues were implanted subcutaneously in the forelegs of three month old rats [19,20]. Leakage of the tanned tissues induced a chronic inflammatory response (Figures 5 and 6) accompanied by the presence of granulocytes, giant cells, lymphocytes and eosinophils (Figures 5, 6, 7 and 8). Eosinophils play a major role in chronic reactions to antigens [19,20,39]. It is apparent that although the bulk of the tanned tissue was inside the polyethylene tubes, leakage of small amounts of tanned tissue into the surrounding tissue was sufficient to invoke an active immunological response [37].

6. GLUTARALDEHYDE STABILIZED TISSUE VALVES

Major manufacturers of tanned tissue heart valves use glutaraldehyde concentrations ranging from 0.2 to 0.625% for stabilizing tissue valve xenografts [37]. Glutaraldehyde stabilized tissue heart valves are dead, hence on insertion they shrink, degenerate and calcify with time [40,41]. Followups of patients who have received glutaraldehyde-treated porcine heart valve

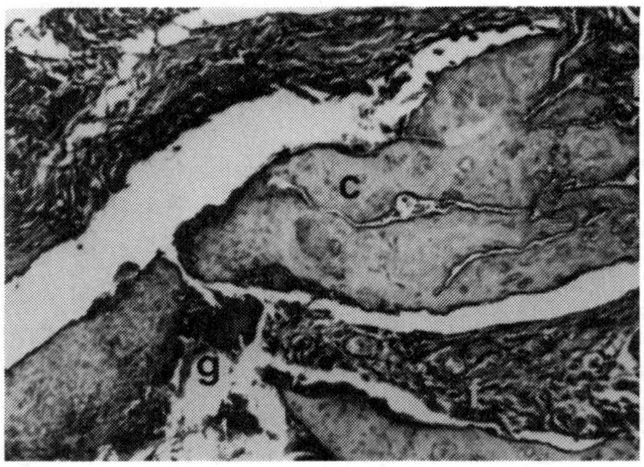

Figure 5. Microphotograph of a section of tissues surrounding a tube filled with glutaraldehyde-fixed isologous muscle tissue after 35 days of implantation showing conglomeration of granulocytes (C), multinucleated giant cell (g) and ingrowth of fibrous tissue (f). Original magnification X63, Hematoxylin-Phloxin stain. (Courtesy of Dr. P. Ch. Makkes).

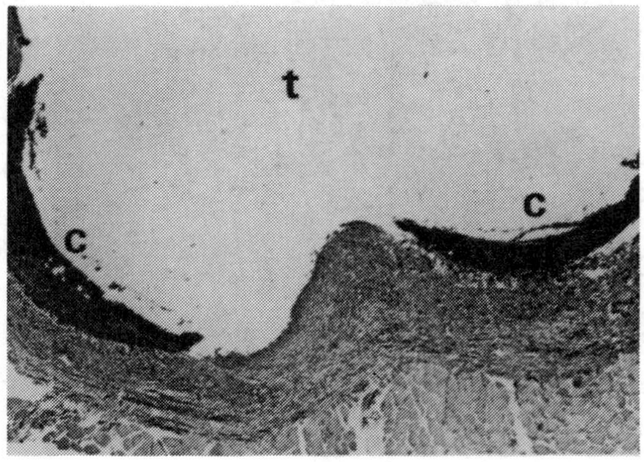

Figure 6. Microphotograph of a section of tissues surrounding a tube filled with glutaraldehyde-fixed homologous muscle tissue after 14 days of implantation showing original location of tube (t) and conglomeration of granulocytes (c). Original magnification X10, Hematoxylin-Phloxin stain (Courtesy of Dr. P. Ch. Makkes).

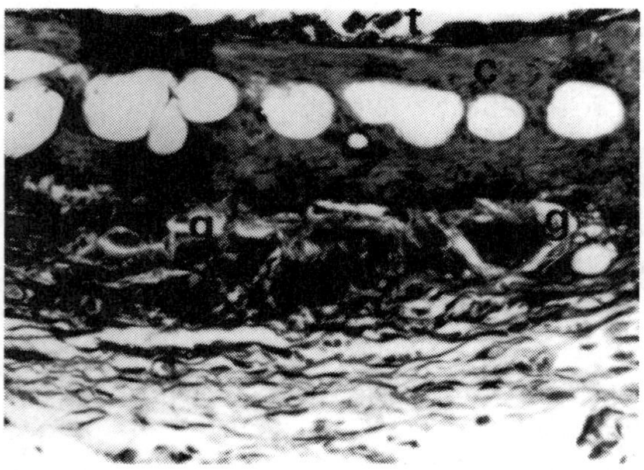

Figure 7. Microphotograph of a section of tissues surrounding a tube filled with glutaraldehyde-fixed isologous muscle tissue after 21 days of implantation showing original location of tube (t), conglomeration of granulocytes (C), and multinucleated giant cells (g). Original magnification X160, Hematoxylin-Phloxin Stain. (Courtesy of Dr. P. Ch. Makkes).

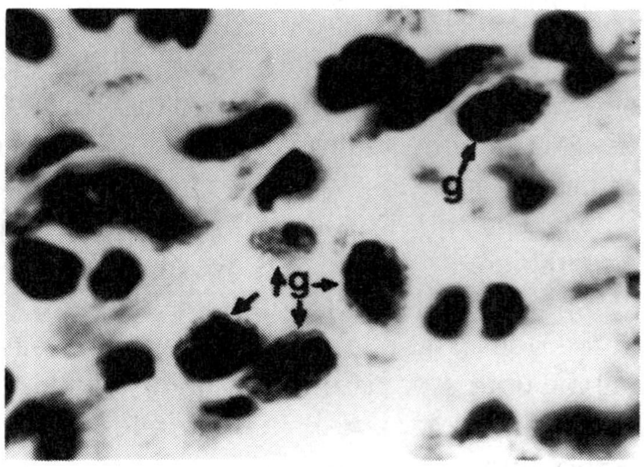

Figure 8. Microphotograph of a section of tissue (higher magnification of Figure 6) surrounding a tube containing glutaraldehyde-fixed homologous muscle tissue after 14 days of implantation showing eosinophilic granulocytes (g). Original magnification X630, Giemsa Stain. (Courtesy of Dr. P. Ch. Makkes).

(GTPHV) xenografts show incidence of collagen degeneration, paravalvular necrosis, calcification, infiltration of mononuclear cells, lymphocytes and macrophages (Figure 4), cardiac myopathy and diseases unrelated to the prostheses [35,42,43].

Some of the factors which favor the induction of an immune response are protein, carbohydrate, lipoprotein, or glycoprotein conformation, disgestibility, accessibility to determinants, large size and surface area, higher stability and polymeric conformation [37]. Glutaraldehyde stabilizes and crosslinks proteins, polymerizes biologic material, delays but does not prevent the digestion process and masks some and unmasks other determinants. Hence, it is logical to expect that glutaraldehyde treated tissue valves should evoke an immune response. However, only a few investigators have studied the immunogenicity of tanned valve xenografts [7,27,32,33,37,44].

Carpentier and his colleagues were the first to replace human heart valves with tissue heart valve xenografts. They preserved the xenografts in organic mercurial salt solution or 4% formalin [7,37]. On implantation in patients, these xenografts showed thinning of the tissue, denaturation of collagen and elastin, and inflammatory and immunologic type of cellular reactions [7,37]. However, presence of antibodies either to the muscle or valve tissue in the sera of these patients was not detected by tanned cell and immunofluorescent procedures [7,37]. This promoted Carpentier's group to study the antigenic nature of porcine heart valves. They used routine immunological techniques and observed that the cell, mucopolysaccharide, protein and structural glycoprotein components of the porcine valve had the highest degree of antigenicity while elastin and collagen were the least antigenic [7,37]. Subsequently, Carpentier's group developed a procedure including washing or electrodialysis, oxidation and glutaraldehyde treatment to eliminate cells and soluble proteins, denature glycoproteins and stabilize collagens [7,37]. However, high incidence of late post-operative failure associated with rips, perforations and calcifications of the oxidized glutaraldehyde tanned porcine heart valve xenografts prompted them to drop the oxidation step from the tanning procedure [37].

Frolova and his coworkers reported high titers of antibodies against extracts of untreated valves and low titers of antisera against water soluble extracts of GTPHV xenografts. Ouchterlony gel-diffusion tests conducted with anti-UTPHV sera showed four distinct bands against UTPHV extracts and two reaction bands against soluble extracts of GTPHV tissues. These data enabled Frolova and associates to conclude that glutaraldehyde blocked some antigenic detrminants and did not induce the formation of new determinants [32]. Since the immunogenic response in the host implanted with a tanned tissue xenograft will be against the tanned insoluble tissue rather than fresh untreated tissue, antigens used to test the immunogenicity of tanned tissues must be comprised of a mixture of particulate and water soluble extracts of tanned tissue. Similar extracts of untreated tissues should also be used to detect cross-reactivity and common antigenic determinants between the untreated and treated tissues.

6.1. Glutaraldehyde Treatment and Preparation of Antigen

Porcine heart aortic valves and bovine pericardial tissue were obtained fresh from the slaughter house in cold normal saline. Untreated porcine heart valves were trimmed to remove undesirable tissue. The pericardial tissues were cleaned of excess fat and fiber, then placed in Travenol Tis-u-sol for five hours. The porcine aortic valves and the pericardial tissues were rinsed in saline then quick frozen until use. The trimmed bovine pericardial tissues and porcine heart aortic valves were tanned by placing them in 0.5% glutaraldehyde (pH 7.4) for two weeks. The tanned tissues were rinsed once with normal saline before quick freezing [37].

Untanned porcine heart aortic valves (UTPHV), glutaraldehyde-treated porcine heart aortic valves (GTPHV), untanned bovine pericardial tissue (UTBPT) and glutaraldehyde-treated bovine pericardial tissue (GTBPT) were diced in chilled phosphate buffered saline (PBS) pH 7.4. The diced tissues were centrifuged in cold for 10 minutes and resuspended in PBS. Washed, diced tissue was then homogenized in cold by means of a Polytron Homogenizer (Brinkman Instruments, Inc., N.Y.). Subsequent homogenizations were accomplished with a Virtis Homogenizer (Precise Instrument Co., Wisconsin), a sonifier (Heat Systems Co., N.Y.), and Tri-R Stir. R. Homogenizer (Tri-R Instruments, N.Y.). Final homogenate was filtered through cheesecloth and the filtrate was used for immunizations. Cheesecloth filtrate was subsequently filtered through a Whatman No. 1 filter paper. The resulting filtrate contained a fine particulate antigen suspension and this was used for serological procedures [37,38].

6.2 Immunogenicity Studies

In the initial investigation, rabbits were immunized with either untanned porcine heart valve and bovine pericardial tissue homogenates in Freund's Adjuvant. Antibodies to untreated and glutaraldehyde-treated antigens developed after seven weeks of immunization. Presence of anti-porcine heart valve and anti-bovine pericardial tissue antibodies were detected by means of capillary tube agglutination test. Titers of anti-untanned tissue and anti-tanned tissue antibodies were in the same range in the four experimental groups. Intravenous antigenic challenge with corresponding antigens ten weeks after the initial immunization resulted in the induction of anaphylactic response in immunized rabbits. Non-immunized rabbits did not exhibit an anaphylactic response on intravenous challenge with tanned or untanned antigens (Figures 9 and 10). Anaphylactic reactions were manifested by changes in respiratory depth and frequency and P and R voltage amplitudes as well as occurrences of nodal beats, atrial fibrillation, and premature ventricular contractions or a combination thereof (Figure 11). These initial studies suggested that tanned antigens were capable of inducing immune responses and that the anaphylactic response in the immunized animals could result in both respiratory and cardiac failure [37]. Both cardiac and pulmonary dysfunctions have been reported as contributing factors in the mortality of patients implanted with tanned tissue xenografts [42].

Villa and coworkers studied the immunogenicity of glutaraldehyde-treated porcine heart valves by injecting mice intraperitoneally twice with valvular homogenates (prepared by means of a Potter apparatus) in aluminum phosphate gel at 10 day intervals and testing the sera by means of cytotoxicity tests using porcine lymphocytes as target cells [44]. They reported low to no immunogenic response in mice injected with tanned valvular tissue homogenates. Several factors can contribute to the type of response observed by Villa and coworkers [44]. In our investigation we observed a positive response after 50 days of repeated immunizations at weekly intervals. Villa and associates collected the sera for testing from mice six days after the second immunization (20 days). According to several investigators, tanned tissues are processed in a different manner and at a slower pace than untanned tissues [13,14]. Their test was primarily designed to detect immune responses generated against histocompatibility (HC) antigens of the procine heart valve. Besides HC antigens the porcine heart valve contains many other antigenic determinants [7,37]. According to several investigators, glutaraldehyde either modifies or alters the antigenic determinants [14,15,16,17,24]. Hence,

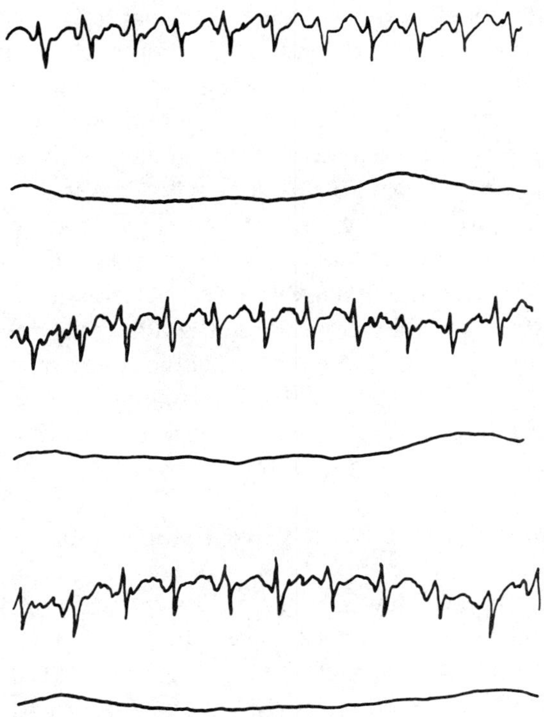

Figure 9. Electrocardiograms (ECG) and respiration of a non-immunized rabbit challenged intravenously at week 10 with a 1 mg untreated porcine heart valve extract (UTPHV). A. Normal reading, B. Five minutes after phosphate buffered saline injection (I/V), C. Five minutes after 1 mg UTPHV extract injection (I/V) showing no change in the ECG or respiration patterns. (From Bajpai, P.K., Immunogenicity of tanned tissue valve xenografts in Biomaterials and Reconstructive Surgery. C. V. Mosby & Co., St. Louis, MO. Chapter 47. 1982)

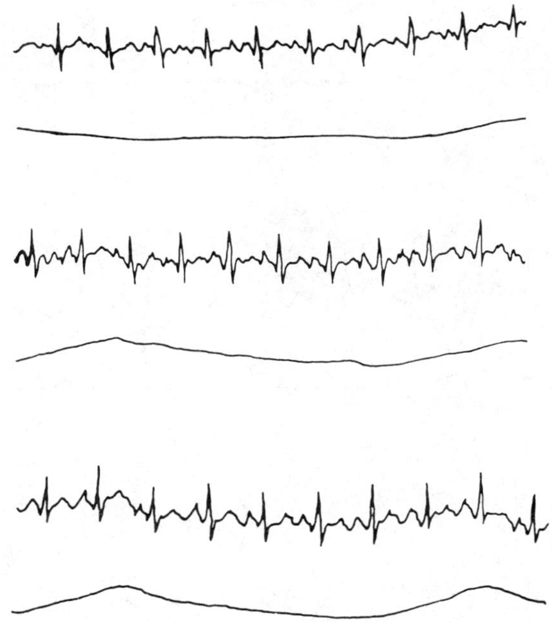

Figure 10. Electrocardiograms (ECG) and respiration of non-immunized rabbit challenged at week 10 with 1 mg glutaraldehyde-treated bovine pericardial tissue (GTBPT) extract (I/V). A. Normal reading, B. Five minutes after phosphate buffered saline injection (I/V), C. Five minutes after 1 mg GTBPT extract injection (I/V) showing no change in the ECG patterns. (From Bajpai, P.K., Immunogenicity of tanned tissue valve xenografts in Biomaterials and Reconstructive Surgery. C. V. Mosby & Co., St. Louis, MO. Chapter 47. 1982)

testing of the sera obtained from animals immunized or grafted with tanned tissues should yield antibodies specific to tanned tissues and these, depending on the nature of the antigen, may or may not cross-react with antigens of untreated tissues. After seven weeks of immunization we tested the sera of rabbits immunized with tanned and untanned porcine heart valve extracts by means of complement fixation test. Sera obtained from UTPHV injected rabbits showed titers of 100 to 375 units against UTPHV antigens and 0 to 25 units against GTPHV antigens. Sera obtained from GTPHV injected rabbits showed titers of 5 to 200 units against GTPHV antigens and 0 to 100 units against UTPHV antigens. In each case higher titers were obtained with corresponding antigens than with non-corresponding antigen. Three separate cross-reacting GTPHV and UTPHV antigenic determinants were identified by double diffusion gel precipitation test [38]. Anti-UTPHV and GTPHV sera did not react with porcine kidney or liver extracts. Heart valves contain type I collagen. These collagens, whether they are

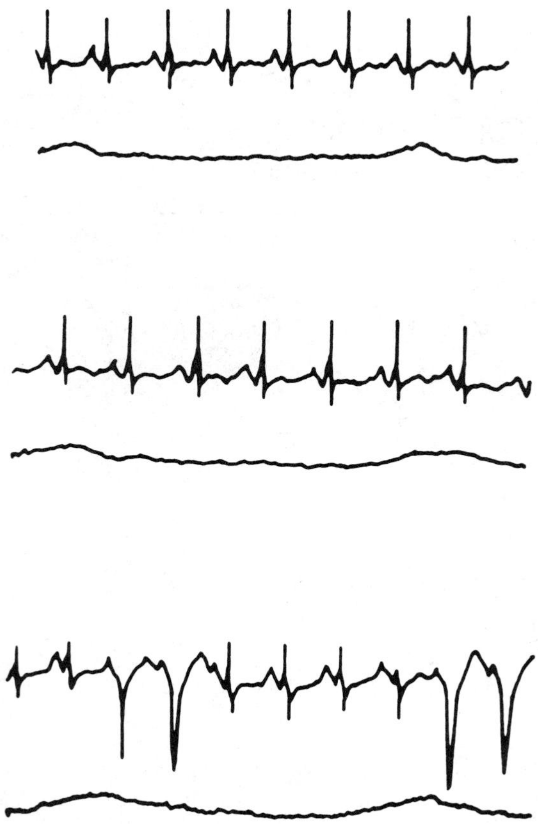

Figure 11. Electrocardiograms (ECG) and respiration of a rabbit immunized with glutaraldehyde-treated porcine heart valve (GTPHV) extract and challenged intravenously at week 10 with 1 mg GTPHV extract. A. Normal reading, B. Five minutes after phosphate buffered saline injection (I/V), C. 135 seconds after 1 mg of GTPHV injection (I/V) showing coupled premature ventricular contractions. (Reproduced from Slanczka, D. J. and Bajpai, P. K., IRCS Med., Sci. 6, 421, 1978).

allogeneic, xenogeneic or denatured are capable of inducing both humoral and cellular responses [37]. Since the preliminary investigation conducted on tanned tissues in our laboratory indicated that glutaraldehyde treatment does not render the tissue immunologically inert and because glutaraldehyde delays enzymatic digestion, subsequent investigations were designed to study whether tanned tissue grafts were immunogenic or non-immunogenic. The grafts were implanted in the abdominal area in order to avoid cardiac surgery and formation of cardiac autoantibodies.

6.2.1. Porcine Heart Valve Tissue Grafts

Mature New Zealand White rabbits were grafted subcutaneously in the abdominal region with three 1 × 2 cm strips of UTPHV or GTPHV xenografts. Grafts were removed from each tissue-implanted rabbit at monthly intervals for histopathological examination.

6.2.1.1 Pathology. All implanted porcine tissues were encapsulated by the recipient tissue. Maximal encapsulation was observed 3 months after the initial implantation. Morphological examination of all excised grafts showed persistent inflammation with focal necrotic loci and phagocytosis of both untreated and glutaraldehyde-treated graft particulates by foreign body cells (Figures 12 and 13). It was evident that glutaraldehyde fixation delayed the degeneration process but was unable to prevent the processing of tanned tissue by the recipient's defense system. Both encapsulation and degradation can be promoted by sensitized lymphocytges [36]. Villa and associates grafted fresh and untanned porcine heart valvular tissues in cutaneous pouches on the backs of inbred C57B1 and DBA mice for 50 days [44]. They observed that the implants of fresh, untreated porcine heart valvular leaflet underwent progressive resorption over the 50 day duration of their investigation [44]. In our study, untanned dead tissue also underwent progressive resorption and was almost resorbed by the end of 3 months [37]. Villa and coworkers reported that the tanned tissue did not resorb and that there was no infiltration of the tanned leaflet by inflammatory cells. However, the leaflet was surrounded by granulocytes and lymphocytes [44]. We also did not observe thinning of the tanned graft but did observe erosion of the borders of

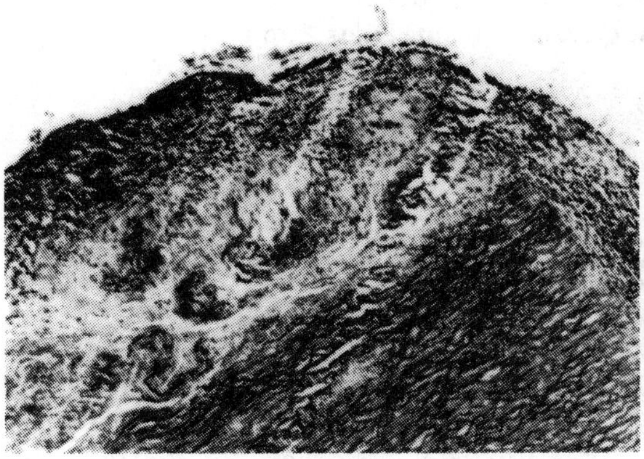

Figure 12. Photomicrograph of a section of untreated porcine heart valve xenograft (UTPHV) implanted in a rabbit showing chronic inflammation with focal areas of necrosis and foreign body cells. Original magnification X70. (Reproduced from Bajpai, P. K., Stull, P. A., Anderson, J. M., IRCS Med. Sci., 8, 519, 1980).

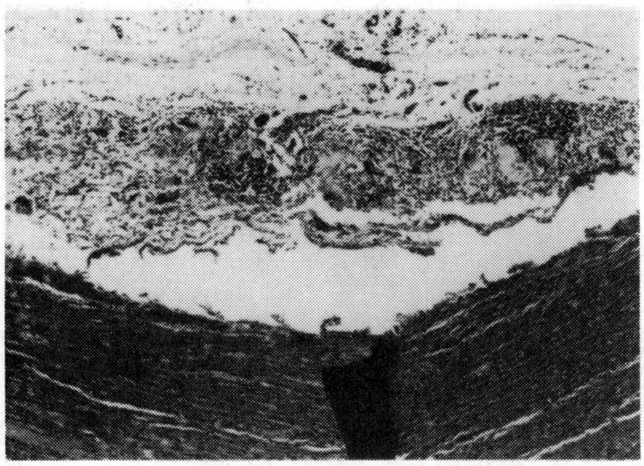

Figure 13. Photomicrograph of a section of glutaraldehyde-treated porcine heart valve xenograft (GTPHV) implanted in a rabbit showing chronic inflammation with focal areas of necrosis and foreign body cells. Original magnification X55. (Reproduced from Bajpai, P. K., Stull, P. A., and Anderson, J. M., IRCS Med. Sci., 8, 519, 1980).

the graft by inflammatory cells [37,38]. Makkes and coworkers [19,20] observed a similar phenomenon around implants of polyethylene tubes containing tanned muscle tissue in rats and attributed the presence of granulocytes, lymphocytes and eosinophils to a chronic inflammatory immunogenic response (Figures 5, 6, 7 and 8). Meritt and coworkers observed an increase in the number of eosinophils around metal implants in animals and individuals sensitive to the implanted metal [39]. Meritt and associates postulated that the increase in eosinphils was due to an eosinophilic chemotactic factor produced by T cells and confirmed the presence of cell mediated immune response against the metal by a leucocyte migration inhibition test [39]. Majority of the rabbits implanted with tanned and untanned tissues in our investigations have also shown positive humoral and cell mediated immune responses [37,38].

Spray and Roberts conducted a follow-up on 51 patients implanted with GTPHV xenografts. They observed that GTPHV xenografts implanted for less than two months showed infiltration of plasma proteins, penetration of erythrocytes in surface crevices, deposition of fibrin, and presence of macrophages, giant cells, and platelets. Two month biopsies of implanted GTPHV xenografts revealed progressive disruption of the valve collagen, erosion of the valve surface, platelet aggregation, lipid accumulation, calcium deposition and bacterial contamination [37,43]. They also reported that the greatest reaction occurred in a 14 day GTPHV implanted patient whose earlier GTPHV xenograft had failed 56 months after implantation [37,43]. Thus, Spray and Roberts concluded that GTPHV xenografts were probably antigenic [37,43]. They were also of the opinion that the incidence of rejection suggested that the host may have been sensitized to the bioprosthetic antigen [37,43].

6.2.1.2. Humoral Response. Circulating antibodies were detected by means of microcomplement fixation test in the sera of grafted rabbits eight weeks after implantation of the xenografts (Table 1). Rabbits grafted with GTPHV xenografts developed anti-GTPHV antibodies, likewise rabbits implanted with UTPHV xenografts developed anti-UTPHV antibodies

Table 1. Antibody Titers of Sera Obtained from Sham-Operated Controls and Rabbits Grafted with Either UTPHV or GTPHV Implants Using Complement Fixation Procedure (CF)

Weeks of Implantation	Antigen Used in C.F.	Sera from Control Rabbits and Rabbits Implanted with Porcine Heart Valve Xenografts		
		Controls (7)	UTPHV (5)	GTPHV (5)
0	UTPHV	0	0	0
	GTPHV	0	0	0
8	UTPHV	0	20-160	20-40
	GTPHV	0	0-10	10-20
12	UTPHV	0	20-80	40-80
	GTPHV	0	0-10	20-40

( ) Number of surviving rabbits in each group.

[Modified from Bajpai, P.K., Stull, P.A., and Anderson, J.M., IRCS. Med. Sci., 8, 519, 1980].

(Table 1). Sera obtained from two rabbits implanted with UTPHV xenografts cross-reacted with GTPHV antigens whereas antisera obtained from each rabbit grafted with GTPHV xenografts reacted with UTPHV antigens. Sham-operated rabbits did not develop antibodies against either UTPHV or GTPHV antigens. Villa and associates [44] observed for antibodies in sera of mice grafted with fresh porcine heart valves or tanned valve leaflets after 20 days of implantation by means of a lymphocytoxicity test [44]. They reported that fresh porcine heart-valve leaflet grafts induced the synthesis of antibodies which were cytotoxic to porcine lymphocytes whereas the grafts of tanned porcine heart valve leaflets did not induce the formation of antibodies cytotoxic to porcine lymphocytes [44]. Since glutaraldehyde masks some and unmasks other determinants, it is likely that glutaraldehyde suppresses the immune response to histocompatibility (HC) antigens. Glutaraldehyde has been used to decrease the virulence of bacteria and allergenicity of allergens, and augment the synthesis of antibodies [22,24,25,26]. Hence, testing for antibodies to histocompatibility antigens alone does not rule out the nonimmunogenicity of other antigens in the tanned porcine heart valvular tissue. It is unlikely that a dead tissue will be rejected. However, implantation of dead tissue can induce hypersensitivity as well as production of antibodies against implanted dead tissue antigenic determinants [19,20,37].

Sheikh and his associates reported that of 35 patients implanted with tanned porcine heart valve xenografts, 58% showed antibodies to soluble extracts of untreated porcine heart valve tissue and 32% showed cell-mediated immune response [33]. However, they also observed that of 20 patients who had bypass heart surgery 35% showed antibodies to untreated porcine heart valve tissue [33]. Hence, they suggested that cardiac autoantibodies resulting from cardiac surgery cross-reacted with porcine heart valve tissue extracts [33]. Since porcine tissue have substance 'A' probably a majority of the 35% bypass heart surgery patients had natural anti-A antibodies in their plasma [37]. Glutaraldehyde treatment enhances (4x) the inherent ability of porcine heart valve antigens to bind human anti-A antibodies [45]. Since both mechanical and biological degradation of GTPHV xenografts occur in patients, GTPHV antigens released in the circulation can augment the synthesis of anti-porcine heart tissue valve antibodies and/or cardiac autoantibodies [37]. Generation of anti-GTPHV antibodies in 'A' blood group patients can also lead to thrombus formation [37]. Release of minute amounts of glutaraldehyde stabilized 'A' type substance from the implanted GTPHV xenografts probably increases the titers of anti-A antibodies in patients implanted with tanned porcine tissue valves. These in turn can either cause further degradation of the implanted tanned porcine heart valve or provide protection by forming a coating of immunoglobulin on the valve. Intravenous injection of minute amounts of purified A and B substances isolated from animal sources have been reported to increase the titers of anti-A and anti-B isoantibodies respectively [46]. Cross-reacting polymerized GTPHV antigens in circulation can also form immune complexes with circulating natural anti-A antibodies, cardiac autoantibodies or anti-GTPHV antibodies and cause pathogenesis in heart and other organs of the body [37].

Many patients implanted with heart valve prosthesis die of myocardial failure unrelated to their prosthesis [41]. Some of these patients had coronary artery disease, other focal areas of myocardial fibrosis [41]. Silver questioned whether death due to cardiomyopathy of patients with heart valve prosthesis was iatrogenic [41]. Literature reviewed so far seems to suggest that death due to cardiomyopathy in patients implanted with tanned tissue valves could be iatrogenic in origin.

6.2.1.3. Cell-mediated Immune Response. According to several investigators fixation and/or alteration of antigens by glutaraldehyde may preferentially engage the cellular elements of the immune system [15,16,17]. Since both macrophage migration inhibiting factor and skin reaction tests use the antigen in question as a component of the testing system, these two tests were selected for monitoring the cellular immune responses induced by UTPHV and GTPHV xenografts. Macrophage migration inhibition factor is released by sensitized lymphocytes in the presence of sensitizing antigens.

In the presence of GTPHV antigens, lymphocytes obtained from either UTPHV or GTPHV grafted rabbits significantly ($P<.01$) inhibited the migration of macrophages from the agar droplet (Table 2). Lymphocytes obtained from the control rabbits did not inhibit the migration of macrophages (Table 2).

Skin induration of 5mm or more, 48 hours after the intradermal injection of antigen in rabbits was recorded as a positive reaction [37,38]. One month after the removal of all xenografts, rabbits implanted with UTPHV xenografts gave positive reactions on intradermal challenge with UTPHV antigens (10 ± 2mm). Rabbits grafted with GTPHV xenografts also gave positive skin reactions on intradermal challenge with GTPHV antigens (8 ± 1mm). Two months after the retrieval of xenografts, rabbits grafted with either GTPHV or UTPHV xenografts gave positive skin reactions with non-corresponding UTPHV and GTPHV antigens respectively [37]. Induction of cell-mediated immune response has also been reported in patients implanted with Hancock GTPHV xenografts [33]. Sheikh and coworkers reported that of 35 patients implanted with Hancock GTPHV xenografts, 32% showed cell-mediated immune response by means of leucocyte adherence inhibition test [33]. Sheikh's group used soluble extracts of UTPHV tissues in the leucocyte adherence inhibition test instead of GTPHV particulate extracts [37]. Literature reviewed so far seems to suggest that tanned tissues, though dead, are immunogenic and not biologically inert.

6.3.1. Bovine Pericardial Tissue Heart Valves

A five year study of 160 patients implanted with glutaraldehyde-treated bovine pericardial tissue (GTBPT) valve showed that the functional integrity of the valve was retained up to 56

Table 2. Migration Distance (Blocks) and Percent Migration Inhibition of Macrophages when Cultured with Lymphocytes Obtained from Rabbits Implanted with UTPHV and GTPHV Grafts in the Presence and Absence of GTPHV Antigens

	Lymphocytes From					
Rabbit[2] #	UTPHV Grafted Rabbits			GTPHV Grafted Rabbits		
	Migration Distance[1] in		Percent Inhibition	Migration Distance in		Percent Inhibition
	Control Media	GTPHV Media	of Migration	Control Media	GTPHV Media	of Migration
1.	20.0 ± 0.6	16.0 ± 0.6	20.0[x]	17.4 ± 0.4	14.0 ± 0.5	19.5[x]
2.	16.0 ± 0.3	15.1 ± 0.9	5.6	23.0 ± 0.5	20.7 ± 0.5	10.0[x]
3.	18.6 ± 0.5	16.5 ± 0.3	11.3[x]	22.7 ± 0.9	18.9 ± 0.3	16.7[x]
4.	19.9 ± 0.4	17.0 ± 0.4	14.6[x]	22.0 ± 0.5	18.0 ± 0.4	18.2[x]
5.	21.3 ± 0.3	21.1 ± 0.6	0.9	14.0 ± 0.5	12.9 ± 0.9	8.0
Mean of Means.	19.1	17.1	10.5[x]	19.8	16.9	14.5[x]

[x] Inhibition of macrophage migration significant at P<.01.

[1] Average migration distance has been expressed as Mean ± Standard Error of Mean of 4 replicates.

[2] Two rabbits in each of the grafted groups died during the investigation due to miscellaneous causes including surgery, anesthesia, etc.

[Reproduced from Bajpai, P.K., and Stull, P.A., IRCS. Med. Sci. 8, 642, 1980].

months [47]. According to Tandon and coworkers, GTBPT valves exhibit excellent hemodynamic function in the absence of anticoagulant therapy and their transvalvular gradient is superior to tanned porcine tissue heart valves [47].

Heynan's group constructed heart valves from autologous dog pericardial tissues and treated them with 87% glycerol for five minutes at 37°C [48]. On implantation in dogs, the valves were covered with a thin layer of fibrin including platelets, erythroblasts, erythrocytes, plasma cells and/or immunoblast-like cells [48]. According to Heynan and coworkers, the appearance of precocious but durable immunocompetent cells suggested that the glycerol treatment was responsible for the local immune reaction [48]. Glycerol is known to contain glutaraldehyde as a contaminant and probably was responsible for modifying the tissue [37]. Immunofluorescent reactions of plasma cells and valvular tissue with anti-dog immunoglobulin also suggested that the glycerol treatment of the autologous graft was responsible for inducing a local and temporary autoimmune disease [37,48].

According to Kasp-Grochowska, anti-bovine heart valve sera reacts with several components of the human heart [49]. Anti-bovine heart valve sera reacted with the endocardium, plate of the valve, connective tissue of the arterial walls and reticulin around the muscle fibers of mitral valve and myocardium [37,49]. Anti-bovine heart valve sera obtained after prolonged immunization also reacts with fibroblasts, endothelial cells and myocardium of the heart [37,49].

Since GTBPT valves, like their porcine counterparts, cannot be repaired and are apt to degrade with the passage of time, we considered it necessary to determine whether glutaraldehyde-treated bovine pericardial tissue xenografts were immunogenic or non-immunogenic.

Earlier we had investigated the immunogenicity of tanned bovine pericardial tissue homogenates by means of capillary tube agglutination test [37]. Before conducting investigations with pericardial tissue xenografts, the immunogenicity of untanned and tanned bovine pericardial tissue homogenates was confirmed by immunizing rabbits and determining the presence of anti-UTBPT and GTBPT antibodies in rabbit sera by means of an indirect hemagglutination test using antigen coated tannic acid 'O' human cells [27].

Mature New Zealand White rabbits were grafted subcutaneously on the abdominal musculature with three 1 × 2cm strips of untreated (UTBPT) or tanned bovine pericardial tissue xenografts (GTBPT). Control rabbits were grafted with 1 × 2cm strips of dialysis tubing. Dialysis tubing and grafts were retrieved after 90 days of implantation for morphological examination.

6.3.1. Post-Operative Morphology

Implantation of untanned and tanned bovine pericardial tissue xenografts did not impair the health of the rabbits over the 100 days of the investigation. Gross examination of the retrieved xenografts did not reveal thinning of the GTBPT implants. All GTBPT xenografts had adhered to the adjacent muscle and connective tissue and were encapsulated by the host tissue. All untreated (UTBPT) xenografts were resorbed by the host [27]. These results are in accordance with observations reported earlier on the fate of UTPHV and GTPHV xenografts [37,44]. Data reported by us and others suggests that glutaraldehyde treatment delays the degradation process of the implanted tissue xenografts [37,44].

6.3.2. Humoral Response

Humoral responses to dialysis tubing, UTBPT and GTBPT xenografts were monitored by means of indirect hemagglutination procedure [37,45]. Anti-UTBPT antibodies were observed in the sera of five rabbits implanted with UTBPT xenografts 30 days after implantation (Table 3). Rabbits implanted with sterile dialysis tubing did not develop antibodies against either UTBPT or GTBPT antigens. Sera obtained from six GTBPT implanted rabbits showed the presence of anti-GTBPT antibodies 30 days after implantation of the xenografts (Table 3). Maximum titer of anti-GTBPT antibodies was observed 60 days after the implantation of GTBPT xenografts. Highest titers of anti-UTBPT antibodies were recorded 90 days after the implantation of UTBPT xenografts (Table 3). Sera obtained from seven rabbits implanted with GTBPT xenografts cross-reacted with UTBPT antigens 60 days after the implantation of xenografts whereas sera obtained from three rabbits implanted with UTBPT xenografts cross-reacted with GTBPT antigens 90 days after the implantation of the xenografts (Table 3). These data once again confirm our earlier findings that tanned tissue xenografts are immunogenic [37,48]. In this investigation, glutaraldehyde treatment of bovine pericardial tissue seemed to enhance the induction of humoral immune response [27]. Implantation of rabbits with GTBPT xenografts produced antibodies largely specific for GTBPT antigens (Table 3) implying that glutaraldehyde treatment may have conferred new antigenic determinants on the tanned tissue. According to Onica and coworkers, glutaraldehyde modified compounds remain antigenic due to development of new antigenic determinants [50]. The data obtained on the immunogenicity of tanned tissues in our laboratories supports the view of Onica and coworkers [27,37,50]. Anti-GTBPT antibodies cross-reacted very poorly with UTBPT antigens (1:4) and vice versa suggesting that

Table 3. Antibody Titers of Sera Obtained from Sham-Operated Controls and Rabbits Implanted with Either UTBPT or GTBPT Xenografts Using Indirect Hemagglutination Test (HIT)

SERUM OBTAINED FROM ANIMALS IMPLANTED WITH: # of Rabbits	RANGE OF ANTIBODY TITERS 0*		30		60		90	
	UTBPT[a]	GTBPT[a]	UTBPT	GTBPT	UTBPT	GTBPT	UTBPT	GTBPT
DIALYSIS TUBING (8)	0	0	0	0	0	0	0	0
UTBPT XENOGRAFT (8)	0	0	0-4	0	0-4	0	4-256	0-4
GTBPT XENOGRAFT (8)	0	0	0	0-16	0-4	16-256	4- 64	16-256

* Days after implantation of dialysis tubing and xenografts.

a Antigen used in HIT.

[Modified from Salgaller, M.L., and Bajpai, P.K., IRCS. Med. Sci., 9, 672, 1981].

only a few antigens retain their original antigenic specificity in tanned bovine pericardial tissues (Table 3).

6.3.3. Cell-Mediated Immune Response

Cellular immune responses against untanned and tanned bovine pericardial tissues were monitored by skin reaction and leucocyte migration inhibition (LIF) tests [27]. Macrophage migration inhibition test (MIF) was replaced by LIF test since it can be conducted with the cells obtained from the buffy coat of peripheral blood of animals as well as humans [27]. Meritt and coworkers have used both LIF and skin reaction tests for detecting immune reactivity to metal implants in rabbits and humans [39]. Leucocyte migration inhibiting factor (LIF) released by sensitized lymphocytes in the presence of sensitizing antigens specifically inhibits the migration of polymorphonuclear leucocytes [27].

After sixty days of xenograft implantation, migration of leucocytes obtained from GTBPT grafted rabbits was significantly inhibited by GTBPT antigens (Table 4). Both GTBPT and UTBPT antigens significantly inhibited the migration of leucocytes obtained from GTBPT grafted rabbits 90 days after the implantation of xenografts (Table 4). Migration of leucocytes obtained from rabbits implanted with sterile dialysis tubing (controls) was not inhibited by either UTBPT or GTBPT antigens (Table 4). Leucocytes obtained from rabbits implanted with UTBPT xenografts did not show inhibition of migration by either UTBPT or GTBPT antigens after 60 days of xenograft implantation (Table 4). However, after 90 days of xenograft implantation both UTBPT and GTBPT antigens significantly inhibited the migration of leucocytes obtained from UTBPT grafted rabbits (Table 4).

Skin induration of 5mm or more 48 hours after antigen challenge indicates the presence of cellular immune responses mediated by T cells. Ninety days after xenograft implantation, seven of eight UTBPT grafted rabbits (5.77 ± 0.40mm) and five of eight GTBPT grafted rabbits (5.82 ± 0.65mm) gave a positive skin reaction 48 hours after the administration of corresponding UTBPT and GTBPT antigens (Table 5).

These observations suggest that although glutaraldehyde treatment confers some new

Table 4. Percent Migration Inhibition of Leukocytes when Cultured with White Blood Cells Obtained from Rabbits Implanted with UTBPT and GTBPT Grafts in the Presence of UTBPT and GTPBT Antigens

WHITE BLOOD CELLS FROM ANIMALS IMPLANTED WITH:	DAYS OF IMPLANTATION	NUMBER OF RABBITS	% MIGRATION INHIBITION ± SEM IN THE PRESENCE OF:	
			UTBPT ANTIGEN	GTBPT ANTIGEN
DIALYSIS TUBING	0	8	0.0 ± 0.0	0.0 ± 0.0
	30	8	0.0 ± 0.0	0.0 ± 0.0
	60	8	3.4 ± 4.2	0.0 ± 0.0
	90	8	1.1 ± 3.9	2.0 ± 3.6
UTBPT XENOGRAFT	0	8	0.0 ± 0.0	0.0 ± 0.0
	30	8	0.0 ± 0.0	0.0 ± 0.0
	60	8	15.1 ± 7.8	0.0 ± 0.0
	90	8	40.4 ± 4.5*	26.6 ± 4.1*
GTBPT XENOGRAFT	0	8	0.0 ± 0.0	0.0 ± 0.0
	30	8	1.0 ± 6.1	0.0 ± 0.0
	60	8	7.0 ± 6.8	34.6 ± 6.8*
	90	8	42.5 ± 3.2*	53.8 ± 5.3*

* Significant at P < 0.05

[Reproduced from Salgaller, M.L., and Bajpai, P.K., IRCS. Med. Sci., 9, 868, 1981].

Table 5. Skin Reactions of Rabbits Implanted with UTBPT and GTBPT Grafts 48 Hours After Injection of UTBPT and GTBPT Tissue Homogenates

RABBITS IMPLANTED WITH:	DAYS OF GRAFT IMPLANTATION	NUMBER OF POSITIVE REACTORS	INDURATION DIAMETER OF POSITIVE REACTORS IN MILLIMETERS ± SEM
DIALYSIS TUBING	0	0/8	-
	30	0/8	-
	90	0/8	-
UTBPT XENOGRAFT	0	0/8	-
	30	0/8	-
	90	7/8	5.77 ± 0.40
GTBPT XENOGRAFT	0	0/8	-
	30	0/8	-
	90	5/8	5.82 ± 0.65

[Reproduced from Salgaller, M.L., and Bajpai, P.K., IRCS. Med. Sci. 9, 868, 1981].

specificity to the treated tissue, it fails to modify all the antigenic determinants of the bovine pericardial tissue [27]. The differences in the degrees of specificity between the humoral and cellular immune responses are probably due to higher specificity of immunoglobulins and lower specificity of T cells [27].

7. CONCLUSION

Review of the literature and the results of immunogenicity studies conducted in our laboratory indicate that tanned tissues are immunogenic. Perhaps our greatest contribution has been in terms of developing *in vitro* procedures which can be performed with untanned and tanned antigens using components of peripheral blood from humans. Since glutaraldehyde treatment delays biologic processing of the xenografts and the immune response usually declines in older patients, it would help substantially to know what age group of patients has the highest degree of immune reactivity, what is the percentage of reactors in older and younger patients, whether there is any correlation with blood group antigens and/or antibodies and how long after implantation of the xenograft the patients test positive for humoral and/or cell-mediated immune responses [37].

ACKNOWLEDGEMENTS

Acknowledgements are due to: The Dept. of Biology and Research Council of the University of Dayton, Dayton, Ohio 45469. To Dr. J. M. Anderson for interpreting photomicrographs of tissue sections, D. J. Slanczka for technical assistance, Robin Bajpai for editing the manuscript and Ann Feldmann for typing this manuscript.

REFERENCES

1. Peracchia, C. and Mittler, B.; New glutaraldehyde fixation procedures; J. Ultrastructure Res.; 39; 57-64, 1972.
2. Bajpai, P. K.; Antigenicity of glutaraldehyde stabilized biological materials; In: Biomaterials in Reconstructive Surgery; Editor, Rubin, L. R.; St. Louis, Mo.; C. V Mosby & Co.; 243-251, 1983.
3. Woodroof, E. A.; Use of glutaraldehyde and formaldehyde to process tissue heart valves; J. Bioeng.; 2; 1-9, 1978.
4. Eckert, B. S. and Snyder, J. A.; Combined immunfluoresence and high voltage electron microscopy of cultured mammalian cells, using an antibody that binds to glutaraldehyde-treated tubulin; Proc. Natl. Acad. Sci.; 75; 334-338, 1978.
5. Thomas, S.; Effect of high concentration of glutaraldehyde upon bacterial spores; Microbios. Letters; 4; 199-204, 1978.
6. Avrameas, S., Ternynck, T. and Guesdon, J. L.; Coupling of enzymes to antibodies and antigens; Scand. J. Immunol.; 8 (Supple. 7); 7-20, 1978.
7. Carpentier, A.; From valvular xenograft to valvular bioprosthesis (1965-1977); Med. Instr.; 11; 98-101, 1977.
8. Kowal, R. and Parsons, R. G.; Solubilization of protein immobilized on sepharose from leakage by glutaraldehyde cross-linking; Anal. Biochem.; 102; 72-76, 1980.
9. Nygren, H., Hansson, H. and Lange, S.; Studies on the conjugation of horseradish peroxidase to immunoglobin G via glutaraldehyde; Medical Biology; 57; 187-191, 1979.
10. Boorsma, D., Steerfkerk, I., and Kors, N.; A Quantitative comparison of two peroxidase conjugates prepared with glutaraldehyde or periodate and a fluorescein conjugate; J. Histochem. Cytochem.; 24; 1017-1025, 1976.

11. Deloach, J., Peters, S.,Pinkard, O., Glew, R. and Ihler, G.; Effect of glutaraldehyde treatment of enzyme-loaded erythrocytes; Biochemical et Biophysica Acts; 496; 507-515, 1977.
12. Herz, F. and Kaplan, E.; Effect of glutaraldehyde fixation on erythrocyte agglutinability; Proc. Soc. Exp. Biol. Med.; 114; 1017-1019, 1973.
13. Leshem, B. and Naor, D.; Studies on the immune responses to fixed antigens. IV. Recall of immunologic memory with fixed antigens; Israel, J. Med. Sci.; 16; 25-32, 1980.
14. Ramos, A., Zavala, F. and Hoecker, G., Immune response to glutaraldehyde-treated cells. I. Dissociation of immunological memory and antibody production. Immunology; 36; 775-780, 1979.
15. Kahan, M., Berman-Goldman, R., Saltoun, R. and Naor, D.; Studies on the immune response to fixed antigens; J. Immunol.; 117; 16-22, 1976.
16. Frost, P., Edwards, A. and Sanderson, C.; Discussion paper: The use of glutaraldehyde-fixation for the study of the immune response to syngeneic tumor antigen; Ann. N.Y. Acad. Sci.; 276; 91-96, 1976.
17. Tomecki, J.; The influence of immunization of syrian hamsters with tumor cells treated with glutaraldehyde on transplantation immunity and the cytotoxic effect of lymphocytes on polyoma tumor cells. Archivum. Immunologiae et Therapiae Experimentalis; 27; 209-216, 1979.
18. Price, M. R., Dennick, R. G. and Law, L. W.; Effect of heat and glutaraldehyde upon the immunogenicity of Meth-A sarcoma cells; Br. J. Cancer; 40; 663-665, 1979.
19. Makkes, P. Ch., Thoden van Velzen, S. K. and Vandenhoof, A., Response of the living organism to dead and fixed enclosed tissue; Oral Surg.; 46; 131-144, 1978.
20. Makkes, P. Ch., Thoden Van Velzen, S. K. and Vandenhooff, A.; The response of the living organism to dead and fixed dead enclosed homologous tissue; Oral Surg.; 46; 296-306, 1978.
21. Milton, J. D.; The effect of glutaraldehyde fixation on the immunogenicity of allogeneic lymphoid and tumor cells; Immunology; 41; 715-721, 1980.
22. Relyveld, E. H., Girard, D. and Desormeau-Bedot, J. P., Procede de fabrication de vaccins a l'aide du glutaraldehyde; Ann. Immunologie, Hungaricae; 17; 21-31, 1973.
23. Parant, M., Damais, C., Adibert, F., Parant, F., Chedid, L., Sache, E., Lefrancier, P., Choay, J. and Lederer, E., In vivo and in vitro stimulation of non-specific immunity by the B-D-P Aminophenyl glycoside of N-acetylmuramyl-L-Alanyl-D-Isogutamine and an oligomer prepared by cross-linking with glutaraldehyde; J. Infectious Diseases; 138; 378-386, 1978.
24. Patterson, R., Suszko, I. M., Leiss, C. R., Pruzansky, J. J. and Bacal, E.; Comparison of immune reactivity to polyvalent monomeric and polymeric ragweed antigens; J. Allergy Clin. Immunol.; 61, 28-35, 1978.
25. Moran, D. M., and Wheeler, A. W.; Chemical modification of the crude Timothy grass pollen extract; Int. Arch. Allergy. Appl. Immunol.; 50; 693-708, 1976.
26. Johansson, S. G. O., Deuschl, H. and Zetterstrom, O.; Use of glutaraldehyde-modified timothy grass pollen extract in nasal hyposensitization treatment of hay fever; Int. Arch. Allergy, Appl. Immunol.; 60; 447-460, 1979.
27. Salgaller, M. L.; Immunogenicity of glutaraldehyde-treated bovine pericardial tissue xenografts; M. Sc. Thesis; University of Dayton, Dayton, Ohio, USA, 1981.
28. Trentham, D. E., Townes, A. S., King, A. H., and David, J. R.; Humoral and cellular sensitivity to collagen in type-II collagen induced arthritis in rats, J. Clin. Invest.; 61; 89-96, 1978.
29. Hiratzka, L. F. and Wright, C. B.; Experimental and clinical results of grafts in the venous system. A current review; J. Surg. Res.; 25; 542-561, 1978.
30. Rosenburg, N.; The bovine arterial graft and its several applications; Surg. Gynecol. Obstet.; 142; 104-108, 1976.
31. Defalco, R. J.; Immunologic studies of untreated and chemically modified bovine carotid arteries; J. Surg. Res.; 10; 95-100, 1970.

32. Frolova, M., Barbarash, L., Gudkova, R. and Karpinskaya, J.; Effect of method of conservation on immunogenicity and antigenic composition of xenograft heart valve tissues; Bulletin Eksperimental noi Biologii i Meditsiny; 73; 306-309, 1973.
33. Sheikh, K. M., Tascon, M. A., and Nimni, M. E.; Autoimmunity in patients with Hancock valve implant and bypass heart surgery; Fed. Proc. Amer. Soc. Exp. Biol.; 39; 472, 1980.
34. Esato, K., Shintani, K., and Yasutake, S.; Modification and morphology of human umbilical cord vein as canine arterial bypass grafts; Ann. Surg.; 191; 443-451, 1980.
35. Ferrans, V. J., Spray, T. L., Billingham, M. E. and Roberts, W. C.; Structural changes in glutaraldehyde-treated porcine heterografts used as substitute cardiac valves. Am. J. Cardiol.; 40; 1159-1184, 1978.
36. Wahl, S. M. and Wahl, L. M.; Lymphokine modulation of connective tissue metabolism. Annals. N.Y. Acad. Sci.; 332; 411-422, 1979.
37. Bajpai, P.K.; Immunogenicity of tanned tissue valve xenografts; In: Biomaterials in Reconstructive Surgery; Editor, Rubin, L.R.; St. Louis, MO., C. V. Mosby & Co.; 734-752, 1983.
38. Bajpai, P. K., Russo, D. A., Slanczka, D. J. and Weiskettel, L. E.; Immunogenicity of glutaraldehyde-treated tissues used in heart valve replacement; In: Advances in Biomaterials, 3; Editors, Winter, G. D., Gibbons, D. F. and Plenk, H.; United Kingdom; John Wiley & Sons, Inc.; 603-612, 1982.
39. Meritt, K., Mayor, M. B., and Brown, S. A.; Evaluation of sensitivity to metallic implants; In: Evaluation of Biomaterials; Editors, Winter, G. D., Leray, J. L. and Degroot, K.; London, John Wiley & Sons, Ltd.; 315-324, 1980.
40. Broom, N. D.; Fatigue-induced damage in glutaraldehyde preserved heart valve tissue; J. Thorac. and Cardiovas. Surg.; 76; 202-211, 1978.
41. Silver, M. D.; Late complications of prosthetic heart valves; Arch. Pathol. Lab. Med.; 102; 281-284, 1978.
42. Fishbein, M., Gissen, S., Collins, J., Barsamian, E. and Cohn, L.; Pathologic finding after cardiac valve replacement with glutaraldehyde-fixed porcine valves; Am. J. Cardiol.; 40; 331-337, 1977.
43. Spray, T. L., and Roberts, W. C.; Structural changes in Hancock porcine xenograft-cardiac valve bioprosthesis; Adv. Cardiol; 22; 241-251, 1978.
44. Villa, M. L., DeBiasi, S. and Pilotto, F., Residual heteroantigenicity of glutaraldehyde-treated porcine cardiac valves; Tissue Antigens; 16; 62-69, 1980.
45. Russo, D. R.; Studies on the antigenicity of porcine intima. M.Sc., Thesis; University of Dayton, Dayton, Ohio, USA 1979.
46. Witebsky, E., Klendshoj, N. and McNeil, C.; Potent typing sera produced by treatment of donors with isolated blood group specific substances. Proc. Soc. Exp. Biol.; 55; 167-170, 1944.
47. Tandon, A. P., Smith, D. R., Mary, D. A. S. and Ionescu, M. I.; Sequential hemodynamic studies in patients having aortic valve replacement with the Ionescu-Shiley pericardial xenograft; Ann. Thor. Surg.; 24; 149-155, 1977.
48. Heynan, Y. G., Dureau, G. and Eloy, R.; Immediate consequences and long term biological consequences of the glycerol-pretreatment of the autologous pericardial valves. Proceedings. First World Biomaterials Congress Vienna (Baden), Austria; April 8-12; 2.9, 1980.
49. Kasp-Grochowska, E., Kingston, D. and Glynn, L. E.; Immunology of bovine heart valves II. Reaction with connective tissue components; Ann. Rheum. Dis.; 31; 290-297, 1972.
50. Onica, D., Margineanu, I. and Dobre, M.; Antigenic specificity of glutaraldehyde-treated rabbit albumin; Molecular. Immunol.; 17; 783-789, 1979.

Chapter 18

The Pathogenesis of Porcine Xenograft Valve Calcification

Robert J. Levy, M.D.
The Department of Cardiology
The Children's Hospital Medical Center, Boston
and the Department of Pediatrics
Harvard Medical School, Boston

ABSTRACT

Porcine xeongraft valve calcification has emerged as a major clinical problem affecting the use of these bioprostheses. Valvular calcification occurs more frequently in children than adults, and very often results in prosthesis failure. Although renal or parathyroid disorders may predispose to xenograft calcification, in most cases, no predisposing conditions exist. Furthermore, host immune response to the xenograft valve has not been shown to be the basis of valvular calcifications. Pathologically, the xenograft valve calcifications are predominantly localized in the spongiosa region of the valves, occurring there along the collagen fibrils. Thrombus related calcifications also occur to a lesser extent, and cellular events appear to be unrelated to the calcific deposits. Biochemical research has demonstrated the occurrence of vitamin K-dependent calcium binding proteins containing gammacarboxyglutamic acid (Gla) in both clinical and experimental specimens of xenograft valve calcification. However, experimental studies have not as yet demonstrated prevention of valvular mineralization with vitamin K antagonism.

Grant Support: NIH Grant HL 24463 and American Heart Association Grant-in-Aid 81760.

THE PATHOGENESIS OF PORCINE XENOGRAFT CALCIFICATION

The glutaraldehyde preserved porcine aortic valve xenograft has come into wide use as a cardiac valve prosthesis [1-3]. This bioprosthesis offers the chief advantage of freedom from anticoagulant usage, plus central orifice flow and good mechanical durability. However, calcific degeneration [4-9] has emerged as a major complication affecting long term usage of the xenograft valves, and is of concern both with respect to guidelines for future use of these valves, as well as the care of past recipients. Currently, the determinants of xenograft calcification are incompletely understood. The present paper will explore a number of aspects of research into this area including: the biochemical basis for valve preparation; the clinical scope of the calcification problem; immunologic considerations; pathological observations; biochemical research into clinically retrieved specimens; and experimental approaches.

Bioprosthesis Development

Serious interest in developing tissue valvular prostheses began with the work of Carpentier and his colleagues [10, 11]. Initial attempts to preserve xenografts with formalin were unsuccessful because of inadequate mechanical durability [10]. The tanning agent glutaraldehyde ($CHO(CH_2)_3CHO$) was ultimately chosen as the preservative of choice [11] because of its ability to form intrafibrillar collagen crosslinks, interconnecting lysyl and hydroxylysyl side chains [12-15]. The nature of the crosslinking reaction is incompletely understood; Schiff base formation as well as aldol condensation are thought to be important mechanisms in crosslink formation. Periodate treatment to oxidize glycosaminoglycans was tried as an additional improvement of the glutaraldehyde procedure, and has been abandoned [11]. Variations in the concentration of glutaraldehyde followed by mechanical fatigue testing, plus bacteriacidal considerations have resulted in the current preservations conditions, which consist of initial preservation in .2-6% glutaraldehyde buffered at physiologic pH (7.4) in phosphate buffers, followed by storage in buffered 0.1-0.25% glutaraldehyde.

No steps in the preservation procedure are known either experimentally or theoretically to potentiate calcification. Of the valvular collagen lysinyl residues, approximately 75% are thought to be available for cross linkages [15]. Of these about one quarter are only involved in unipoint bonds [15], and could theoretically attract cations such as Ca^{++}. However, since the epsilon amino groups of lysine are thought to be important sites for phosphate linkages [16] it could be argued that glutaraldehyde crosslinking would eliminate, in large part, this group of hydroxyapatite nucleation sites, and thereby protect against calcification. Finally a possible underlying problem relevant to calcification could be the fact that glutaraldehyde can irreversibly, crosslink other proteins to valvar collagen [12-15]. Therefore minute amounts of plasma proteins could be cross-linked to the valvular collagen, and then function as calcium binding sites, and/or hydroxyapatite nucleation sites.

Bioprosthesis Calcification: Clinical Determinants

In recent years, porcine xenograft valve calcification (Figure 1) has been the subject of numerous case reports and clinical series [4-9]. Documented porcine xenograft calcification has occurred as early as two weeks after valve replacement [8], and has been noted by Sanders et al to be present in over 50% of valve retrievals, two years post-

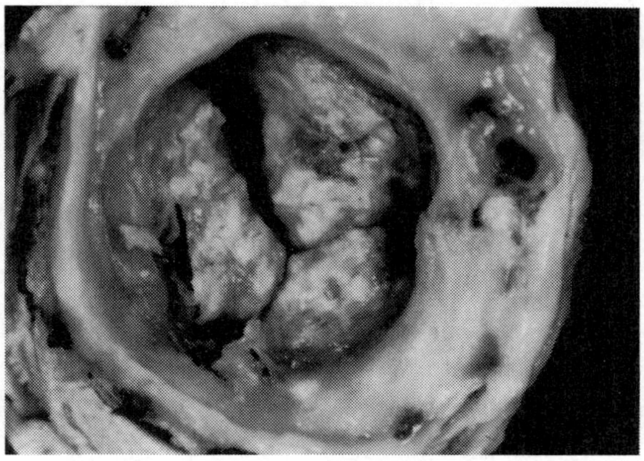

Figure 1. A calcified porcine xenograft valve retrieved from the mitral position after 34 months in place in a 13 year old patient.

operation [4]. Valvular calcification has occurred in some patients with seemingly predisposing conditions such as renal, and parathyroid disorders [6] but in most cases, no obvious underlying metabolic problems exist.

A number of reports have documented that porcine xenograft calcification occurs more frequently in children [4,5,7]. This is of interest, since calcific atherosclerotic disease [17] and calcific aortic stenosis [18] are both pathologic phenomena of late adulthood. This implies that relevant pathogenic hypotheses should consider endocrinologic, developmental considerations. For example, growing children have serum phosphate levels, alkaline phosphatase, and parathyroid hormone levels that are higher in younger children up to the onset of puberty, and then drop to much lower adult values [19,20]. Furthermore, urinary excretion of gammacarboxyglutamic acid (Gla) a calcium binding amino acid, found in the vitamin K dependent calcium binding proteins (see below) reflects the metabolism of Gla containing proteins [21,22] and is greatly increased in younger children compared to adults with a precipitous drop occurring by early adolescence [21,22]. Perhaps these phenomenon are in some way related to the necessary conditions for bioprosthesis calcification.

Xenograft Calcification: Valvular Pathology

Two types of calcium deposits are typically noted on the affected valves. The first, so called extrinsic, or thrombosis related calcification (Figure 2), is noted on the surface of the leaflets and is probably an early phenomenon not related to prosthesis failure [5]. In this setting of extrinsic calcification, hydroxyapatite deposits have been seen to originate in the mitochondria of platelets and leukocytes. Intrinsic calcification occurs deep in the leaflets with the heaviest deposits noted in the central spongiosa region of the valves. The spongiosa of nonpreserved aortic valves is typically rich in glycosaminoglycans (GAG) which in bone development are thought to function as inhibitors of mineralization [23]. The glutaraldehyde preservation procedures extract the GAG's as noted histologically [5], and this observation has led to the speculation that the diminution of GAG content may in fact predispose to mineral deposition via inhibitor removal.

Intrinsic calcification (Figure 3) is seen to occur along the collagen fibrils of the valve stroma [5] in much the same way that collagen calcification occurs in bone mineralization [16] and in experimental calciphylaxis [24]. Associated cellular elements appear to have little relation to

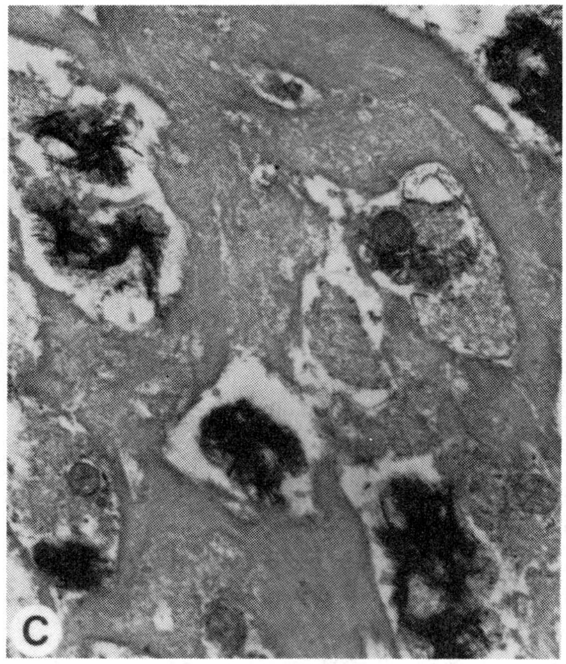

Figure 2. Transmission electron micrography (×37000) of extrinsic xenograft valvular calcification with remnants of platelets trapped in fibrin mesh (F). Reprinted with permission from Ferrans et al Am. J. Cardiol 46:721-734, 1980.

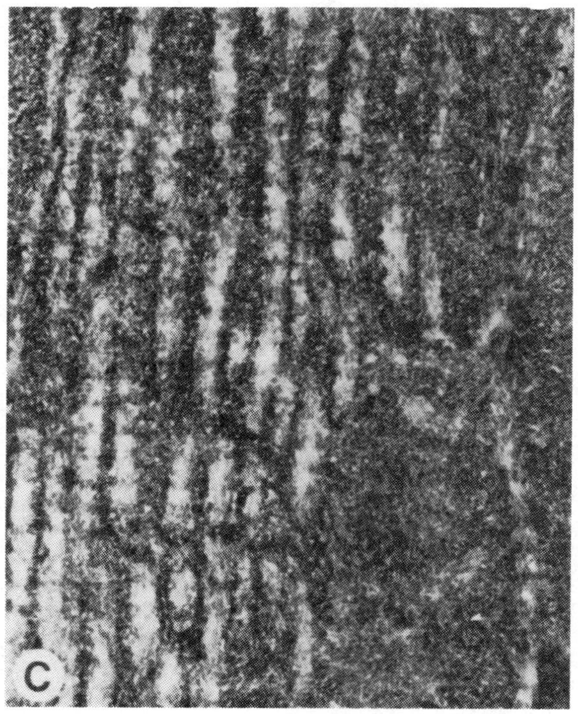

Figure 3. Transmission electron micrography (×60000) of intrinsic xenograft valvular calcification with calcific deposits occurring between collagen fibrils. Reprinted with permission from Ferrans et al Am. J. Cardiol 46:721-734, 1980.

the calcium deposits [25,26]; in fact, the histiocytes, leukocytes, fibroblasts, and giant cells are noted almost at random in explanted leaflets, and have lead a number of investigators to speculate that these elements may in fact represent an immune response to the porcine antigens, perhaps responsible in part for the collagenous degeneration noted histologically, apart from calcification.

Etiologic Considerations: Immune Aspects

Clinical usage of the xenograft valves has been, with rare exceptions, free from a clinically significant immune response. Several pathologic series demonstrate cellular-immune activity suggestive of rejection like phenomenon but no documented cases of xenograft valve rejection have been reported. Sheikh and coworkers noted both a cellular and humoral response specific to porcine heart valve tissue in 58% of 35 postoperative patients undergoing valve replacement with a glutaraldehyde preserved valve [27]. They further observed that 7 of 20 patients postoperative cardiopulmonary bypass for other types of heart surgery also developed circulating antibodies to porcine aortic valve tissue, suggesting cross reactivity with cardiac autoantibodies [27]. Rocchini et al [26] reported abnormal immune parameters associated with porcine xenograft failure, including hypergammaglobulinemia, bone marrow plasmacytosis, and several instances of immunofluorescence detectable antibody deposition in the valvular tissue. They also noted that the cellular response seen histologically reflects, in most cases, a foreign body immune response with numerous histocytes, plasma cells, giant cells, and some instances of granuloma formation. They hypothesized that accelerated tissue damage as a result of the immune response could lead to calcification, although no evidence for this exists.

Bajpai has studied the immunogenicity of glutaraldehyde preserved porcine aortic leaflet valves via a number of immunoassay techniques [28,29]. His work demonstrates that the preserved porcine valvular tissue experimentally elicits both humoral and cellular immune responses [27,28]. Of further interest is the recent demonstration of human blood group A antigen on the porcine valve surface [30]; this would suggest an aspect of immune tolerance in some cases, as well as explain the presence of immunoprecipitants. A more detailed consideration of immune aspects can be found in Dr. P.K. Bajpai's chapter in this work.

Clinical Porcine Xenograft Valve Calcification: Biochemical Studies

Recent work in this laboratory has demonstrated the presence of a unique class of vitamin K dependent calcium binding proteins in xenograft valvular calcifications. Background in this area began with the discovery by Stenflo of gammacarboxyglutamic acid (Gla) a calcium binding amino acid, occurring at the calcium binding sites of the amino terminal region of the prothrombin molecule [31]. Subsequent work [32] has shown that the biosynthesis of Gla in prothrombin is a vitamin K-dependent, enzymatic, post-translational carboxylation of specific glutamic acid residues, and that vitamin K antagonism results in inhibition of Gla synthesis, decreased calcium binding and the formation of the anticoagulated state (Figure 4). These

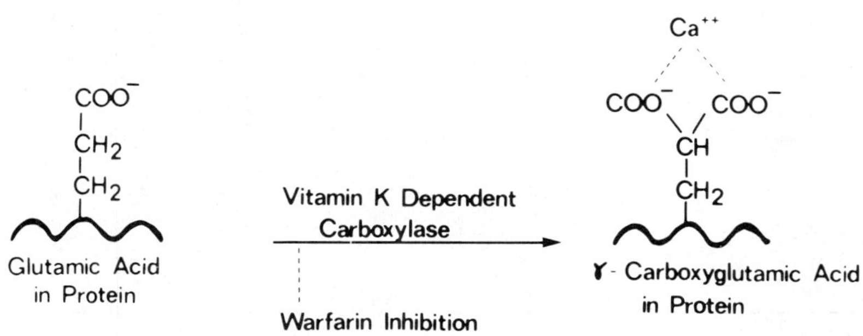

Figure 4. A representation of the post-translational, vitamin K-dependent enzymatic carboxylation of specific glutamic acid residues to form gammacarboxyglutamic acid (Gla).

discoveries prompted Hauschka, Lian, and Gallop [33] to their discovery of the vitamin K-dependent calcium binding protein, osteocalcin. Osteocalcin is the most abundant non-collagenous protein of bone [33,34]. Its biosynthesis is also vitamin K-dependent in a directly analogous manner to prothrombin [34]. Currently the biologic function of osteocalcin is unknown, but it is thought to regulate normal mineral deposition.

Table 1. Gla Containing Proteins According to Tissue [44].

Normal Tissues	Gla Containing Proteins
Liver	Prothrombin; Coagulation factors: VII, IX, X
Bone	Osteocalcin
Kidney	Partially characterized
Spleen	Uncharacterized
Pathologic Tissues	
Atherosclerotic Plaque	Osteocalcin, Atherocalcin
Cardiac Valvular Calcification	Osteocalcin, and other partially characterized
Renal Calculi	Partially characterized
Subcutaneous calcification	Uncharacterized

Gla containing proteins were also demonstrated to occur in a wide variety of other normal tissues, and pathologic calcifications (see Table 1) including calcified atherosclerotic plaque [35,36] and calcified cardiac valves [37], including porcine xenograft valve calcifications [37,38]. In the valvular calcifications [37,38] Gla content correlated with tissue calcium concentrations, both in calcific aortic stenosis as well as bioprosthesis calcification (Table 2 and

Table 2. Aortic Valvular Gla, and Calcium Analyses-Clinical Results.

Diagnosis	No. Valves	Patient Age (years)	Gla (nm/mg protein)	Ca^{++} (nm/mg protein)
Normal Human	2	15,77	0.0	36.0,164.2
Noncalcified Congenital Aortic Stenosis	3	12-18	0.0	68.2-335.0
Calcific Aortic Stenosis	4	52-77	2.0-10.6	2080-16197
Calcified Aortic Valve Homograft	1	7	8.3	9.80
Unimplanted Porcine Xenograft Leaflet	2	--	0.0	108,146
Noncalcified xenograft Explants	2	18,21	0.0	282-306
Calcified Xenograft Explants	6	10-14	4.3-18.3	7527-30441

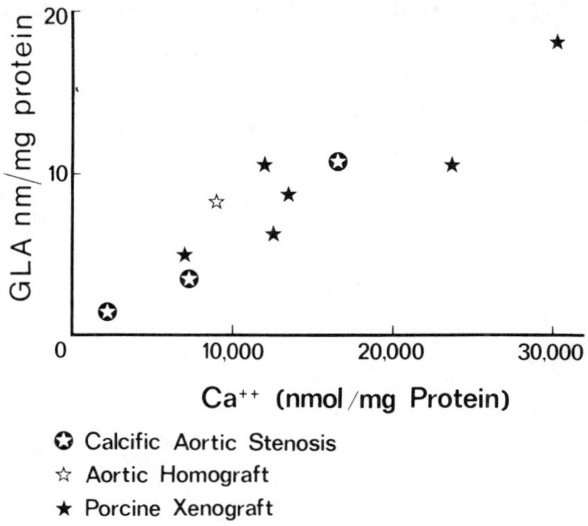

Figure 5. Gla versus calcium content in calcified aortic valves. Gla and calcium are expressed as nanomoles per mg protein.

Figure 5). Gla content in clinically calcified valves compares well with the levels found in mineralized bone. Complete identification of the Gla containing proteins occurring in xenograft valve calcifications remains to be determined. However, work to date in this laboratory [39] has demonstrated the presence of osteocalcin in porcine xenograft valve calcifications of levels of 2.7 to 22.3 ng/mg accounting for .02 to .05% of the total Gla; no osteocalcin is detectable in control tissue. Furthermore, no immunoreactive prothrombin is detectable in the pathologic material. Work in our laboratory has led to the identification of a high molecular weight Gla containing protein in calcific atherosclerosis, known as atherocalcin [36] for which an immunoassay is currently under development. This should permit the identification, if present, of atherocalcin in calcified xenograft valves.

Experimental Porcine Xenograft Calcifications

Very recent work has demonstrated the occurrence of porcine xenograft valve calcifications in a variety of experimental settings in both the circulation [40] and in extracirculatory sites [41]. These calcifications occur progressively and work in this laboratory (Figure 6) demonstrates the same relationship with increasing Gla containing protein levels associated with increasing calcium content noted in clinical retrievals (Figure 7 and Table 3). Of interest is the

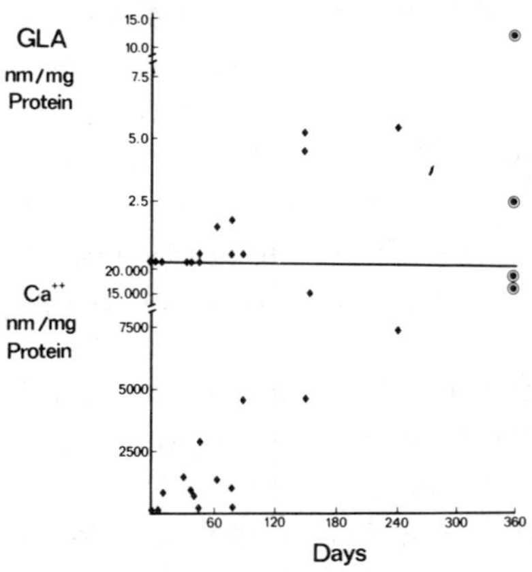

Figure 6. Chronologic accumulation of calcium and Gla in porcine xenograft valve explants from calves. ◆ indicates warfarin therapy (prothrombin time = 2× control); ● indicates no anticoagulation therapy.

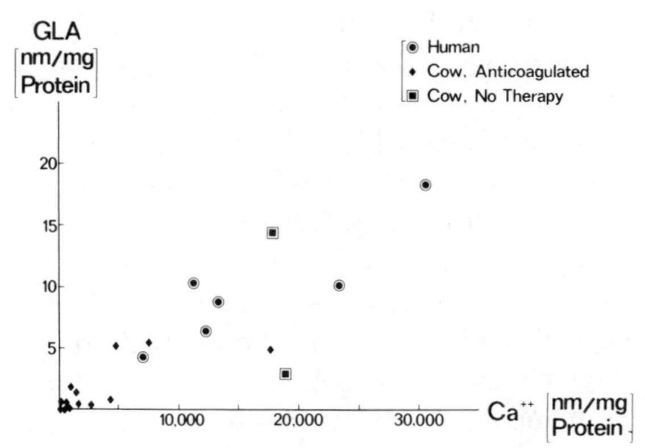

Figure 7. Comparative Gla and calcium levels in bovine and human porcine xenograft valve explants.

Table 3. Biochemical Analyses of Porcine Bioprostheses – Bovine Retrievals.

Porcine Xenograft Valves	No.	Duration	Ca^{++} (nm/mg protein)	Gla
Unimplanted Controls	2	--	108-146	0.0
Bovine, Calcified*	8	44d-12 mos	1000-7300	0.0-5.3
Bovine Noncalcified*	5	8d-78d	116-880	0.0-.28
Bovine, No Warfarin	2	1 year	17377-18037	2.5-14.5

* On Warfarin anticoagulant therapy, prothrombin time = 2 x control.

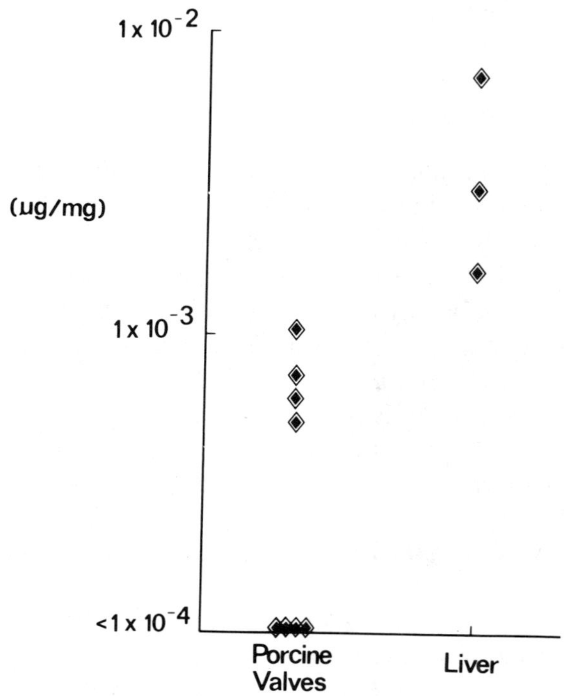

Figure 8. Tissue warfarin levels comparing drug content of calf xenograft valve explants with liver.

work by Levy and Bernhard therapy [40] in which a series of bovine explants were studied from calves on warfarin anticoagulant. These studies showed that warfarin anticoagulant therapy failed to abolish calcification, although possibly less calcium was present by comparison to explants from clinical material and control calves. This phenomenon may be due in part to insufficient warfarin tissue levels as documented by high pressure liquid chromatography [42] which demonstrated drug levels of warfarin in the valves an order of magnitude below those found in liver (Figure 8). Systemic vitamin K antagonism is, therefore, probably not the way to probe this aspect since the anticoagulant effects of this approach would always limit sufficient dosages.

Subcutaneous valve implants in rabbits lead to valvular calcification which resembles the clinical phenomenon in the circulation very closely, including the development of calcium deposits along the collagen fibrils, and maximal deposition in the valve spongiosa [41]. Gla containing proteins were also present in the explanted valves at levels comparable to clinical retrievals. Work done in collaboration with Dr. Julie Glowacki of Children's Hospital has further documented that in the rat, porcine xenograft valve leaflets not only calcify subcutaneously (over a two week period), but stimulate osteogenesis in bone defect implants [43]. The rat implants, regardless of site, also develop the accumulation of Gla containing proteins with mineralization. This work emphasizes that glutaraldehyde preserved porcine leaflets are potent stimuli of mineral deposition, and can stimulate the process in a variety of settings. Finally, recent work in our laboratory has also demonstrated the occurrence of osteocalcin in rat subcutaneous valve calcifications as noted above in clinical material.

SUMMARY AND CONCLUSIONS

Porcine xenograft valve calcifications represents a major complication associated with the use of these bioprostheses. However, research, both clinical and experimental has shed light on a number of important aspects, which should govern the direction of further productive work in this field. Clinically, valvular calcification occurs much more frequently in children than adults and pathologically involves calcium deposition in a manner analogous to bone mineralization and experimental calciphylaxis. This strongly suggests an endocrinologic basis at least, in part, determining the events of this process. Furthermore, the presence of vitamin K dependent Gla-containing proteins, and in particular the bone protein osteocalcin, in the valvular mineralization, suggests a link between this type of pathologic calcification and bone mineralization. Experimental warfarin anticoagulant therapy has little impact on this process and other means of regulating Gla containing protein synthesis will have to be sought to study the control of this process. Finally, new model systems, producing porcine xenograft calcifications subcutaneously should facilitate progress toward the solution of this problem.

REFERENCES

1. Carpentier A., DeLoche A., Relland J. Six year followup of glutaraldehyde preserved heterografts with particular reference to the treatment of congenital valve malformation. J. Thorac. Cardiovasc. Surg. 68:771-782, 1974.
2. Cohn L.H., Koster J.K., Mee R., Collins J.J. Long-term follow up of the Hancock bioprosthetic heart valve; a six year review. Circulation 60:I:87-92, 1978.
3. Albert A.M., Brant L.R., Schechter F.G. Seven year experience with mounted porcine valves. Ann. Surg. 185: 7170721, 1977.
4. Sanders S.P., Levy R.J., Freed M.D., Norwood W.I., Castaneda A.R. Use of Hancock porcine xenografts in children and adolescents. Am. J. Cardiol. 46:429-438, 1980.
5. Ferrans V.J., Bryce S.W., Billingham M.E., Jones M., Ishihara T., Roberts W.C. Calcific deposits in porcine bioprostheses: structure and pathogenesis. Am. J. Cardiol. 46: 721-734, 1980.
6. Fishbein M.C., Gissen S.A., Collins J.J., Barsamian E.M., Cohn L.H. Pathologic findings after cardiac valve replacement with glutaraldehyde fixed porcine valves. Am. J. Cardiol. 40:331-337, 1977.
7. Kutsch L.M., Oyer P., Shumway N., Baum D. An important complication of Hancock mitral valve replacement in children. Circulation 60:I:87-92, 1978.
8. Lamberti J.J., Wainer B.H., Fisher K.A., Karunaratni H.B., Al-Sadir J. Calcific stenosis of the porcine heterograft. Ann. Thorac. Surg. 28:28-32, 1979.
9. Forfar J.C., Colter L., Merrit G.N. Severe and early stenosis of porcine heterograft mitral valve. Br. Heart J. 40:1184-1187, 1978.
10. Binet J.P., Carpentier A., Langois A., Duran C., Colvase P. Implantation de valves heterogenes dans le traitement des cardiopathies aortiques. CR. Acad. Sci. 261:4733-5734.
11. Carpentier A., Lemaigre G., Robert L., Carpentier S., DuBost C., Biological factors effecting long term results of valvular heterografts. J. Thorac. Cardiovasc. Surg 58:467-483, 1969.
12. Korn A.H., Feairheller S.H., Filachione E.M. Glutaraldehyde: nature of the reagent. J. Mol. Biol. 45:525-529, 1972.

13. Richard F., Knowles J. Glutaraldehyde as a protein cross linking reagent J. Mol. Biol. 37:231-233, 1968.
14. Robertson E.A., Schultz R.L. The impurities in commercial glutaraldehyde and their effect on the fixation of brain. J. Ultrastruct. Res. 30:275-287, 1970.
15. Bowes J.H., Carter C.W. The interaction of aldehydes with collagen. Biochem. Biophys. Acta. 168:341-352, 1968.
16. Glimcher M.J., Composition, structure and organization of bone and other mineralized tissues and the mechanism of calcification in Gleep RO, Astwood EB, Aurbach GP, Geiger SR eds. Handbook of Physiology. Endocrinology. Washington D.C., American Physiological Society, 7:25-116, 1976.
17. Langou R.A., Huang E.K., Kelley M.J., Cohen L.S. Predictive accuracy of coronary artery calcification and abnormal exercise test for coronary disease in asymptomatic men. Circulation 62:1196-1203, 1980.
18. Campbell M. Calcific aortic stenosis and bicuspid aortic valves. Brit. Heart J. 30:606-616, 1968.
19. Tanner J.M., Whitehouse R.W. Clinical longitudinal standards for height, weight height velocity, weight velocity, and stages of puberty. Arch. Dis. Child 51:170-179, 1976.
20. Round J.M. Plasma calcium, magnesium, phosphorous and alkaline phosphatase in normal British school children. Brit. Med. J. 3:137-140, 1973.
21. Levy R.J., Lian J.B. γ-carboxyglutamate excretion and warfarin therpy. Clin. Pharm. and Therap. 25: 562-570, 1979.
22. Gundberg C.M., Lian J.B., Gallop P.M. A new method for the detection of γ-carboxyglutamate acid at the nanomole level in *Vitamin K-Metabolism and Vitamin K-dependent Proteins* ed. J.W. Suttie. University Park Press; Baltimore 153-156, 1980.
23. Termine J.D., Mineral chemistry and skeletal biology. Clin. Orthop. 85:207-241, 1972.
24. Bovin G., Tochon-danguy, H.J. Etude chez le rat due calcinose cutanee induite par calciphylaxis locale. Ann. Biol. Animal Bioch. Biophys. 16:869-878, 1976.
25. Spray T.L., Roberts W.C. Structural changes in porcine xenograft used as substitute cardiac valves. Gross and histologic observations in 51 glutaraldehyde preserved Hancock valves in 41 patients. Am. J. Cardiol. 40:319-330, 1977.
26. Rocchini A.P., Weesner K.M., Heidelberger K., Leren D., Behrendt D., Rosenthal A. Porcine xenograft valve failure in children: an immunologic response. Circulation 64:II:162-171, 1981.
27. Skeikh K., Tascon M., Nimni M. Autoimmunity in patients with Hancock valve implant and bypass heart surgery. Fed. Proc. 39:472, 1980.
28. Bajpai P.K., Stull P.A., Anderson J.A. Immunogenicity of glutaraldehyde cross linked porcine heart valve xenografts. IRCS Medical Science 8:519-520, 1980.
29. Bajpai P.K., Stull P.A. Glutaraldehyde cross linked porcine heart valve xenografts and cell mediated immune response. IRCS Medical Science 8:642-643, 1980.
30. Russo D.R. Studies on the antigenecity of porcine intima. M.S. Thesis University of Dayton 1979.
31. Stenflo J., Fernlund P., Egan W, and Roepstorff P. Vitamin K-dependent modification of glutamic acid residues in prothrombin. Proc. Natl. Acad. Sci. USA 71:2730-2733, 1976.
32. Suttie J.W., Jackson C.M. Prothrombin: structure, activation, and biosynthesis. Physiol. Rev. 57:1-70, 1977.
33. Hauschka P.V., Lian J.B., Gallop P.M. Direct identification of the calcium binding amino acid, γ-carboxyglutamate in mineralized tissue. Proc. Natl. Acad. Sci. USA 72:3925-3929, 1975.
34. Lian J.B., Friedman P.A. The vitamin K-dependent synthesis of carboxyglutamic acid by bone microsomes. J. Biol. Chem. 253:6622-6626, 1978.
35. Lian J.B., Skinner M., Glimcher J.M., Gallop P.M. The presence of carboxyglutamic acid in the proteins associate with ectopic calcification. Biochem. Biophys. Res. Commun., 71:349-355, 1976.
36. Levy R.J., Lian J.B., Gallop P.M. Atherocalcin a carboxyglutamic acid containing protein from atherosclerotic plaque. Biochem. Biophys. Res. Commun. 91:41-49.
37. Levy R.J., Zenker J.A., Lian J.B. Vitamin K-dependent calcium binding proteins in aortic valve calcification. J. Clin. Invest. 65:563-566, 1980.

38. Levy R.J., Sanders S.P., Lian J.B. Retrieval analysis of calcific degeneration of tissue valves in *Implant Retrieval: Material and Biologic Analysis* Eds. A. Weinstein, D. Gibbons, S. Brown, W. Ruff. U.S. Government Printing Office: Washington, D.C. 339-348, 1981.
39. Levy R.J., Gundberg C.M. The presence of the bone specific protein, osteocalcin in calcified atherosclerotic plaque, and mineralized heart valves. Circulation: abstracts, in press, 1981.
40. Levy R.J., Bernhard W.F. Porcine xenograft calcification and vitamin K-dependent processes. Circulation 62:II:237, 1980.
41. Fishbein M., Levy R.J., Nashef A., Ferrans, V.J., Dearden L.C. Goodman A.P., Carpentier A. Calcification of cardiac valve bioprostheses: histologic ultrastructural and biochemical studies in a subcutaneous implantation model system J. Thorac. Cardiovasc. Surg. in press 1981.
42. Fasco M.J., Piper L.J., Kominsky, L.S. Biochemical applications of a quantitative high pressure liquid chromatographic assay of warfarin and its metabolites. J. Chromatog. 131:365-373, 1977.
43. Glowacki J., Levy R.J. Unpublished observations.
44. Gallop P.M., Lian J.B., and Hauschka P.V. Carboxylated calcium binding proteins and vitamin K. N. Eng. J. Med. 302:1460-1466, 1980.

Chapter 19

Wear Analysis of Retrieved Prostheses

Dr. Judith M. Dowling
Department of Medicine
Bioengineering Group for the Study of Human Joints
University of Leeds
England

ABSTRACT

The articulating surfaces of acetabular sockets from 23 Charnley total hip replacements (THR) have been examined to identify the in vivo wear mechanisms for ultra high molecular weight polyethylene (UHMWPE) sliding against stainless steel and to determine why the plastic wears faster in vivo than in vitro. Optically, it is observed that wear of the socket is confined to one area: transmission electron microscopy reveals that initially the plastic wears by a mechanism of adhesion but later (after about 7 years of use) by one of surface fatigue. Laboratory wear tests have shown that similar mechanisms operate in vitro and therefore cannot account for the higher clinical wear rate of the UHMWPE. These higher clinical wear rates are discussed with regard to variation and magnitude, patient activity and certain deformation processes which may operate in vivo but not in vitro. It is proposed that compressive creep deformation accounts for much of the so called clinical wear rate, at least initially, and this hypothesis is supported by results from preliminary creep tests on UHMWPE acetabular cups.

1. INTRODUCTION

Professor Sir John Charnley (National Hip Centre, Wrightington Hospital, Wigan) has been inserting a particular type of total hip replacement (THR) for about 20 years. Although the design details have been modified over the years, the Charnley THR consists essentially of a 316L stainless steel femoral prosthesis and an ultra high molecular weight polyethylene (UHMWPE) acetabular cup, Figure 1. Replacement of arthritic hips with artificial ones, especially the metal-plastic type of THR, is very successful according to the judgements of both surgeons and patients [1,2,3]. Typically the success rate for hip replacement is better than 90%, a cautious estimate but quoted values are dependent upon such things as the method of assessment, definition of success and length of follow-up [4,5,6]. A clinical failure may be difficult to define but the main causes of mechanical failure are loosening of a component, fracture of the femoral component and body reaction to wear debris, with loosening considered the most serious problem [5,7,8,9].

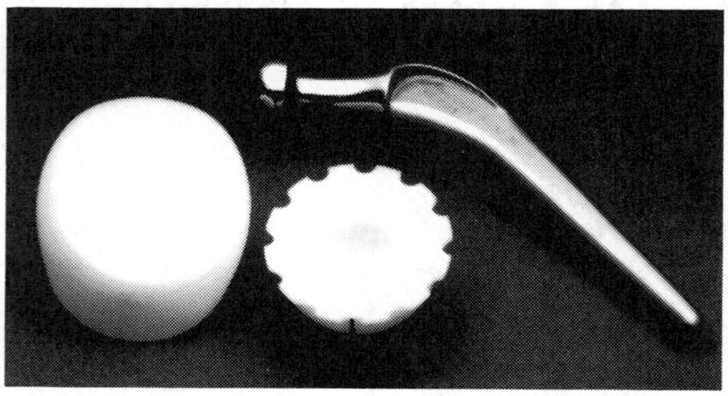

Figure 1. Charnley Total Hip Replacement. The acetabular cup on the left is the current design, the "brim" being trimmed to size during surgery.

On its own, wear of the plastic acetabular cup is not expected to result in wearing out of the socket and hence, early replacement [5,9]. However, since the majority of patients undergoing THR surgery are over the age of 60 years and on the whole are not very active, it would be surprising if wear of UHMWPE was a problem. If similar THR are inserted into younger and more active patients, the UHMWPE cup may have a higher wear rate and have to be replaced within the lifetime of the patient [5,10]. At the moment, little is known about the long term wear and deformation behavior of UHMWPE in the elderly patient and even less concerning its behavior in the younger patient. Certainly there is evidence to suggest that UHMWPE has a higher wear rate in young, active, male patients who have normal function post operatively but such information is limited [11].

Thus it is important to investigate the wear and deformation of UHMWPE with a view to understanding its long term behavior not only in the young but also in the elderly whose life expectancy is increasing. In the last few years many papers have been published on laboratory wear tests of UHMWPE and Clarke has discussed the results from a number of these and their relevance to the clinical use of the plastic [12]. Laboratory tests on their own are not sufficient to predict the long term wear for a number of reasons: the test conditions are usually very simple and do not simulate the conditions in the body, they are accelerated and of a short duration, some methods give misleading or erroneous estimates of wear [12,13]. To ascertain the in vivo response, it is better to examine UHMWPE prosthetic components after use in the body and preferably from patients whose artificial joints have provided trouble-free service, i.e. no mechanical or clinical problems, and are therefore representative of the majority of used THR.

For the past six years such a survey has been conducted by the author. Over the years, Professor Sir John Charnley has collected removed Charnley THR which have been donated by his patients on their death and this collection has been made available for examination. The aims of the survey were to identify the in vivo wear and deformation mechanisms for the plastic socket and how these change with time, to investigate the discrepancy between reported clinical and laboratory wear rates and to examine the effect of patient variables on socket wear.

2. EXPERIMENTAL DETAIL

2.1 Specimen Data

Acetabular sockets from 23 removed THR were examined, the service age of a hip ranging between 1 and 14 years. All the THR are of the Charnley type illustrated in Figure 1. The cup is machined from block UHMWPE and has a 22 mm diameter socket with a wall approximately 10 mm thick. The femoral stem is machined from forged 316L stainless steel and has a highly polished head which is hemispherical with a diameter of 22 mm. Acrylic cement is used to anchor both components to the bone.

All the prostheses had been inserted at Wrightington Hospital and, with one exception, had been removed at post mortem. The exception was an acetabular cup which had been removed at the same time as the loose femoral component even though the cup was not loose. This cup was the only one not stored in formaldehyde as were the rest because they had been removed with bone and joint capsule intact.

The 23 prostheses came from 18 patients of which half had only one hip replaced and half had both hips replaced but not necessarily both with Charnley THR. Of the bilateral patients, eight had 2 Charnley THR and one had one Charnley THR and one Mckee THR. The Mckee prosthesis was not examined and nor was one hip from each of three bilateral patients. In the latter group, the hip prostheses were not available for examination in two cases whilst the third was inserted just one month prior to the patient's death. Table 1 gives a break down of the patients and their hip replacements: in the middle column, each patient in a particular grouping is identified by a label of the type 1HB, 2HB and so on; the end column gives the total number of sockets examined in each group.

Table 1. Specimen Data

Grouping	Patients in Group	Number of THR Examined in Group
1 Hip replaced: Charnley THR	1HB, 4HB, 5HB, 7HB, 11HB, 13HB, 15HB, 16HB, 17HB	9
2 Hips replaced: Both Charnley THR	2HB, 3HB, 8HB, 10HB, 21HB	10
2 Hips replaced: Only 1 Charnley THR	12HB	1
Others: 2 Charnley, only 1 examined	6HB	1
Others: 2 Charnley, only 1 available for examination	9HB, 14HB	2

Table 2. Details of Weight, Age, Activity and Socket Age for Each Patient

i) Category C patients

Patient Socket	Hip	Sex	Patient age at operation (y)	Patient weight (kg)	Patient activity	Other remarks	Socket age (y)	(m)
6HB	L	F	70	92.3	Walking limited	Obese; limp	1	2
10HB	R	F	71	44.6	Just able to walk	Rheumatoid joints, artificial knee; two sticks.	2	5
9HB	L	F	75	60.9	Walking limited	Limp; stooped; housework 1 stick.	5	0
1HB	R	M	64	65.5	Walking limited	Gross limp; rheumatoid joints; retired.	5	2
10HB	L	F	67	44.6	Just able to walk	Rheumatoid joints; artificial knee, two sticks.	6	3
2HB	R	F	65	61.4	Walk normal	Light housework; 1 stick	7	1
2HB	L	F	65	61.4	Walk normal	Light housework; 1 stick	7	5
4HB	R	F	73	67.5	Senile; stroke	Retired; 1 stick; stroke at 2 yrs; senile at 5 yrs.	8	0
21HB	L	M	66	57.3	Walk normal	Left knee stiff; bad chest; ex-whaler; shore work.	8	10
8HB	L	F	60	50.2	Walking limited	Housework; 1 stick.	8	11
8HB	R	F	60	50.2	Walking limited	Housework; 1 stick.	9	1
11HB	R	F	76	66.8	Senile; obese; doddery.	Little housework.	10	1
21HB	R	M	62	57.3	Walk normal	Left knee stiff; bad chest; ex-whaler; shore work.	12	9

ii) Category B patients

Patient Socket	Hip	Sex	Patient age at operation (y)	Patient weight (kg)	Patient activity	Other remarks	Socket age (y)	(m)
12HB	L	M	74	65.5	Walk normal	Slight limp, retired; 1 stick.	9	8
14HB	L	F	74	50.1	Walk normal	Light housework; 1 stick.	9	8
3HB	L	F	75	46.4	2-3 mile/day	Light housework; 1 stick	9	9
3HB	R	F	75	46.4	2-3 mile/day	Light housework; 1 stick	9	11

iii) Category A patients

Patient socket	Hip	Sex	Patient age at operation (y)	Patient weight (kg)	Patient activity	Other remarks	Socket age (y)	(m)
5HB	L	M	70	73.2	Golf every day	General practitioner; 7 mile walk; very active.	3	8
13HB	L	M	61	81.8	Retired	Excellent range of movement	7	8
17HB	R	M	67	-	Did everything	Company director; played golf	8	5
16HB	L	M	59	-	Active farmer	Still engaged in heavy manual work.	8	6
7HB	L	F	77	59.1	Very active for age	Lived alone; all housework; 1 stick.	11	5
15HB	R	F	71	75.6	Not very energetic	Housework; excellent result	13	3

2.2 Patient Data

For the 18 patients in the survey, medical records were available with reference to their hip. These records contained detailed reports of each patient's progress pre and post-operatively, the post-operative follow ups continuing for many years, often up to death. Details of each patient's age, weight and activity (post operatively) are given in Table 2. The patients have been divided into three groups (A, B or C) according to a grading system used at Wrightington Hospital [1,14]. A, indicates that the patient has a unilateral hip condition and that all other systems related to walking are normal. B, indicates that the patient has a bilateral hip condition and all other systems related to walking are normal for the patient's age. C, indicates that there exist factors other than hip, or hips, which affect the function of walking. Examples of other factors in C patients are rheumatoid arthritis of the knee, heart disease, gross obesity, senility: all these could reduce the function of walking below normal even though the hip joints were perfect. When using this grading system, the letter B or C must not be taken to mean that a patient has two artificial hips: a B patient may have a bilateral condition where one hip is arthritic whilst the other has had an arthroplasty [14].

In addition to the medical records, Professor Sir John Charnley provided data on wear rates for the sockets. The depth of wear had been determined by profilometer measurements of castings for the majority of the sockets; 5 wear rates were calculated from post operative radiographs.

2.3 Socket Examination

As the removed acetabular cups are used by Charnley for his own histological research, non-destructive techniques had to be used and this limited the survey to a surface examination of the worn sockets. The macroscopic features of wear were studied with the naked eye and a hand lens. To reveal the microscopic features, transmission electron microscopy, using a two stage replication technique, was necessary. Two stage replication is a method which enables a surface to be examined without damaging it or having to section the bulk sample. Another advantage of this method is that surface topography of very smooth surfaces may be examined at a higher resolution than is often obtainable in a scanning electron microscope [15].

The replication procedure for the socket surfaces was as follows:

i) A square (about 1 mm × 1 mm) of thin Bex film is softened in acetone and pressed onto the surface.
ii) When dry, the Bex replica is removed, turned upside down and "shadowed" by evaporating a heavy metal, at an angle of 30° onto the surface. This increases contrast by accentuating surface topography.
iii) Next a thin layer of carbon is evaporated onto the replica surface in a planar fashion.
iv) Finally, the Bex film is dissolved away in acetone as it is not stable in the electron beam. The resulting carbon square or replica is ready for examination in a conventional transmission electron microscope (CTEM).

The optical examination and preparation of Bex film replicas were conducted at Wrightington Hospital, the metal and carbon evaporation being carried out at Leeds University. The carbon replicas were also examined at Leeds University using either a Philips EM300 or a JEOL 100CX, both operated at 100 kv.

2a : OPTICAL RECORD

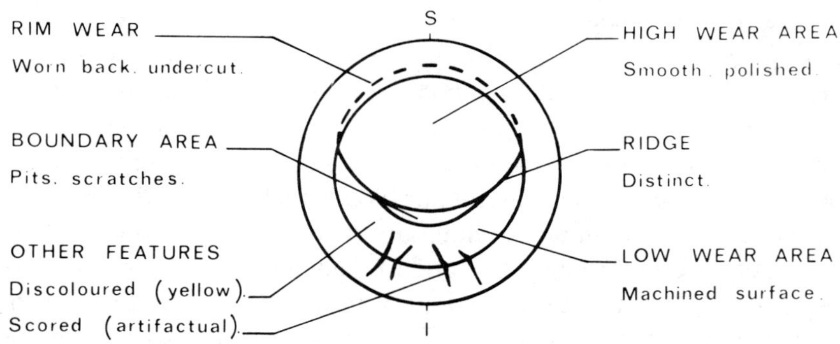

2b : REPLICA RECORD

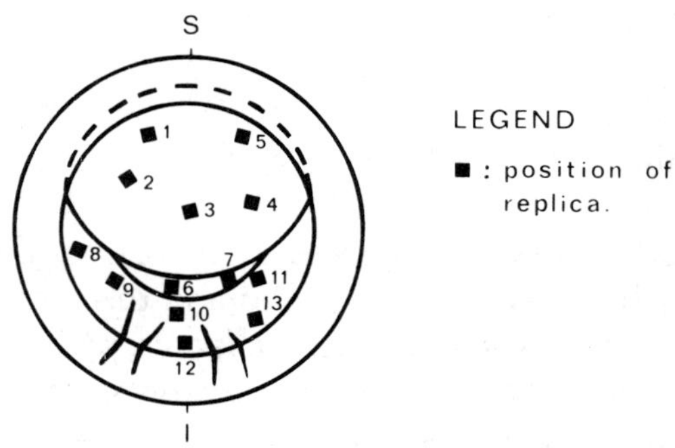

2c : PATIENT DATA

PATIENT	:	16 HB MALE
HIPS REPLACED	:	LEFT ONLY
AGE AT OPERATION	:	59 years
AGE OF UHMWPE CUP	:	8 years 6 months
OCCUPATION	:	ACTIVE FARMER
ACTIVITY	:	HEAVY MANUAL LABOUR

Figure 2. Record sheet for a used acetabular cup. 2a, schematic plan of features visible to naked eye; 2b, record of approximate position of each replica on socket; 2c, patient and socket data. (Abbreviations: S, superior; I, inferior).

To record the optical features and positions of the numerous replicas on each acetabular cup, a schematic mapping system was devised. The optical features were sketched on a plan of the socket, an example of which is seen in Figure 2a. The approximate positions of the replicas were recorded on a separate plan on which had been drawn the optical features, Figure 2b. Using this method, it was possible to correlate the wear and deformation features seen in the CTEM with those observed optically.

3. OPTICAL APPEARANCE OF WORN SOCKETS

The appearance of the articulating surface of a worn acetabular cup is well illustrated by the socket from patient 16HB in Figure 2. This male patient was 59 years old when his left hip was replaced with a Charnley THR, Figure 2c. Post-operatively, he continued to run his farm and was capable of heavy manual labor such as lifting sacks of grain. Eight and a half years later, the artificial hip was replaced with another Charnley THR when the original femoral stem became loose. Patient 16HB is still alive and, at the time his original left socket was examined, was actively involved in farming.

All the sockets examined had two features in common: an area of high wear and an area of low wear, Figure 2a. The high wear area is a smooth, well polished region on the superior part of the socket: here the original turned surface is no longer visible. On the inferior part of the socket, the grooves of the original machined surface are visible in the low wear area.

These observations imply that contact between femoral head and cup, and hence wear, is confined to one area of the socket. This is not unexpected considering the loading geometry of the hip joint. The acetabular cup is inserted at an angle of 45° to the body vertical, Figure 3a. When standing or walking, a joint force may be considered to act downwards at 10°-15° to the vertical and is the resultant of the body weight and the force exerted by the abductor muscles. Thus, when weight is put onto the hip during walking, there will be contact between femoral head and acetabular cup in the superior region of the articulating socket surface i.e. the region above the plane XY which passes through a diametral plane of the head and is perpendicular to the joint force. Since the main contact area lies above XY then the main wear scar should also lie above XY and will be approximately hemispherical in shape. Consequently, a region of high wear is observed on the superior part of a removed socket whilst the inferior part is little worn because there is little or no contact there.

In socket 16HB, the superior part was quite deeply worn, the depth of wear being 2.33 mm as measured from a casting of the socket at removal. Between the high and low wear area was a distinct step or ridge, Figure 2a. This ridge is a direct consequence of wear being confined to one part of the socket and hence the loading geometry of the hip. During the THR's years of service, the machining marks are gradually worn away on the high wear area of the socket by the continual rubbing of the femoral head as it bores its way into the socket wall. The direction of wear will tend to be parallel to the line of action of the joint force and so the femoral head effectively bores a new socket for itself along this direction. The observed ridge on a deeply worn socket is then merely the lower edge or rim of this new socket, Figure 3b.

In the boundary region at the ridge, areas of pitting and scratching are frequently seen: socket 16HB has just such an area on the low wear side of the ridge, Figure 2a. These boundary areas are associated with sockets which have been in use for several years, particularly in patients who have been very active, and may arise from the impacts of femoral

3a

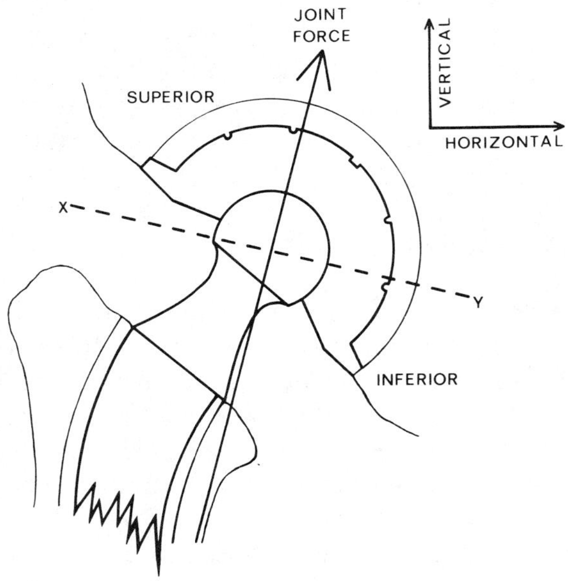

3b

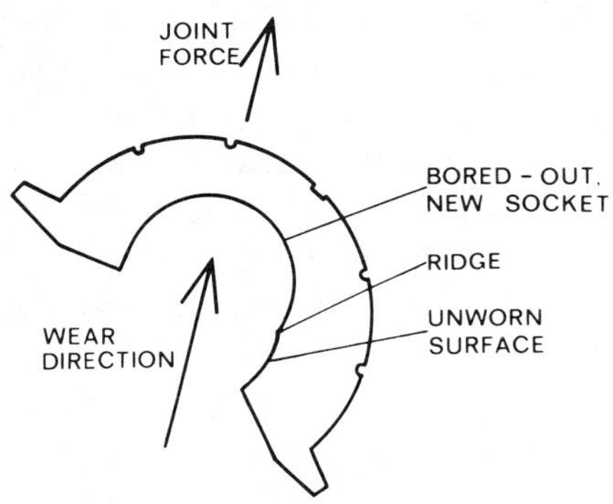

Figure 3. Loading geometry for artificial hip in vivo. 3a, vertical section through right hip, body center line is to right of diagram; 3b, formation of ridge and "new" socket as result of loading geometry (acetabular cup has the same orientation as in 3a).

head against the ridge as the head slides in its new socket. Likewise, rim wear is associated with very active patients and impingement of the femoral head against the socket flange: rim wear is usually confined to the high wear area, Figure 2a.

Socket 16HB shows two features which were not observed on the other 22 sockets: discoloration (yellowing) of the plastic in the low wear area and deep scoring. The former is indicative of degradation of the polymer whilst the latter is the inevitable damage done to the socket during its removal at revision surgery. Removal damage, which possibly includes some of the scratching observed on the socket surface, is absent from the other sockets because the method of their removal at post-mortem was such that they were not extracted from the bone.

Socket 16HB is typical of sockets which were used in vivo for 7 years or more and also sockets which originated from active patients. When sockets worn for less than 7 years, or removed from sedentary patients, are examined, the wear scars on the superior part are shallower and the ridge is indistinct or not detectable by sight or touch. Pitting and scratching near the ridge tend to be absent especially in sockets from sedentary patients; the same is true for rim wear.

Finally, regardless of the period of use, the surface of the femoral head was always highly polished and resembled that of an unused femoral prosthesis. On the whole, the used heads appeared to be almost scratch-free and no interference effects were observed which might be indicative of a transfer layer of UHMWPE adhering to the metal surface.

4. TRANSMISSION ELECTRON MICROSCOPY (TEM)

For the description of the microscopic features of in vivo wear, the TEM results will be presented in two sections. One section will deal with those sockets which have been used for less than 7 years, the other the remainder. In both sections, the observations will be described in general terms and electron micrographs from a variety of sockets will be shown and not just from socket 16HB.

4.1 Sockets Used for Less than 7 Years

In the polished high wear area, TEM shows that the surface is microscopically smooth but covered with smears and thread-like pulls, Figures 4 and 5. Both smears and pulls are thought to be indicative of wear by adhesion [16]. As the metal head slides in the socket, parts of the UHMWPE surface adhere to the metal: the polymer is stretched out locally into a thin thread which eventually breaks, leaving a permanently deformed pull or smear on the surface of the plastic. The smears and pulls in Figures 4 and 5 are not lined up in a particular direction. Such random orientation is to be expected in view of the complicated sliding motion of the femoral head in its socket [13].

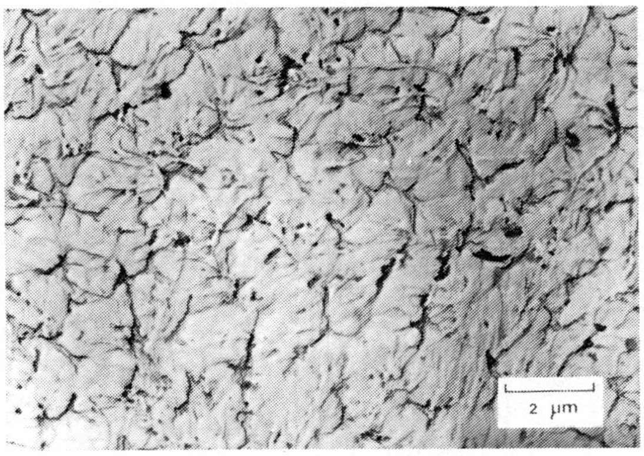

Figure 4. Adhesive smearing on high wear area. Left socket (age: 5 2/12y) from patient 1HB. TEM; 2 stage replica.

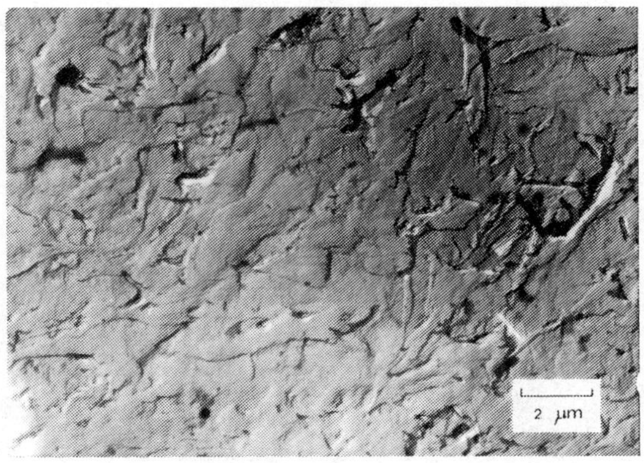

Figure 5. Adhesive pulls on high wear area. Left socket (age: 1 2/12y) from patient 6HB. TEM; 2 stage replica.

In the low wear area, the microscopic grooves on the turning marks are visible, Figure 6. Some smearing and flattening of the grooves is apparent and this implies that some wear or contact has occurred here, at least initially.

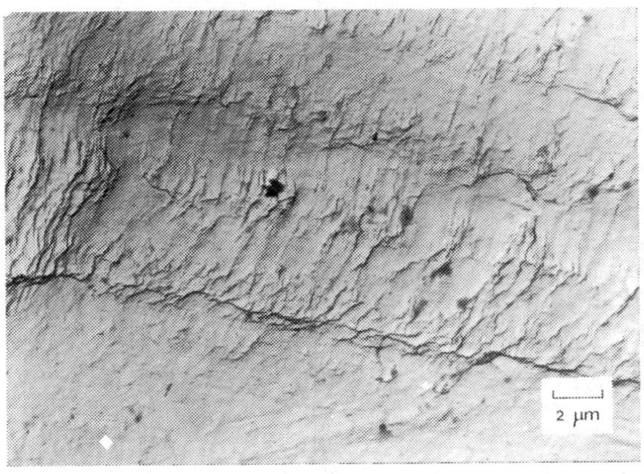

Figure 6. Micro-grooves on machined surface of low wear area. Left socket (age: 1 2/12y) from from patient 6HB. TEM; 2 stage replica.

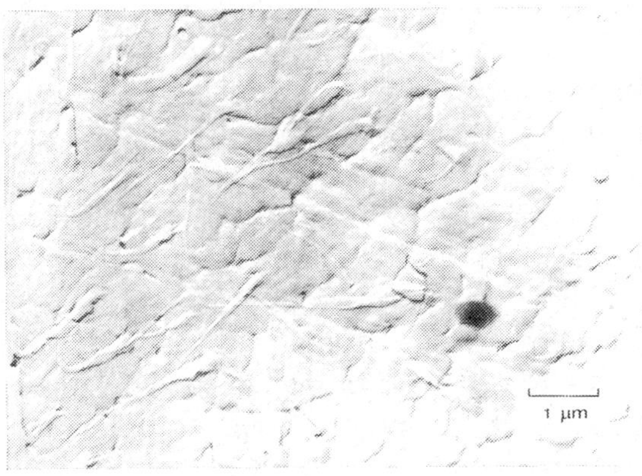

Figure 7. Scratches made in vivo. Left socket (age: 8 6/12y) from patient 16HB. TEM; 2 stage replica.

Scratches are sometimes seen in the high and low wear areas, a proportion of the scratches having been introduced during handling of the sockets after removal at post-mortem. Figure 7 shows a scratch in the high wear area: the scratch is shallow with a width much less than a micrometer and lying across the scratch are several pulls. The positions of these adhesive features suggest that the scratch has been made in vivo: subsequent sliding of the femoral head has partially obliterated the scratch [13].

4.2. Sockets Used for More than 7 Years

After 7 or 8 years of use, additional microscopic features are seen in the high wear area. These take the form of fine short cracks, no more than a few micrometers long, Figure 8. Because the contrast at the edges of adhesive pulls and smears resembles that of the cracks, these fine cracks are not easily identified.

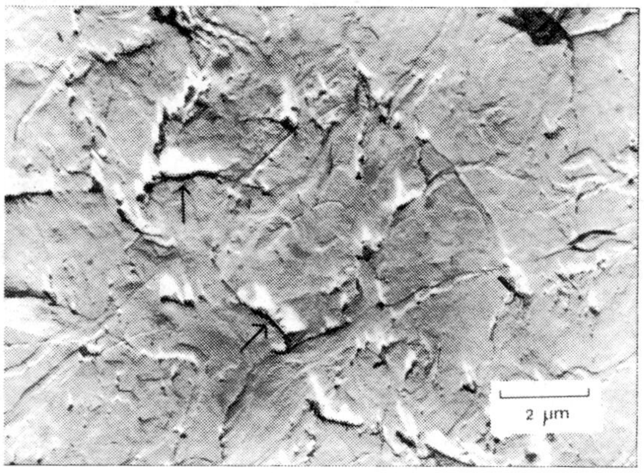

Figure 8. Fatigue cracks (arrowed) in high wear area. Left socket (age: 9 8/12y) from patient 12HB. TEM; 2 stage replica.

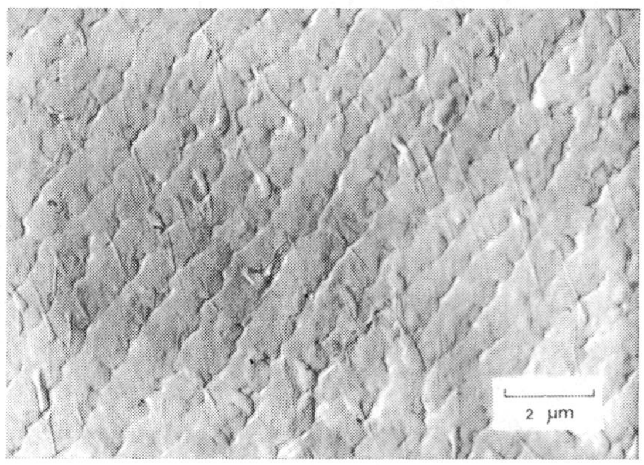

Figure 9. Parallel ripples in high wear area. Left socket (age: 8 6/12y) from patient 16HB. TEM; 2 stage replica.

In other sockets, parallel ripples are seen, Figure 9. In this particular socket (16HB), the ripples were nearly continuous over the entire area of each replica from the high wear area. Whether or not the ripples were parallel across the entire wear scar is not known because the orientation of one replica relative to another is lost during the specimen preparation. As well as the ripples, large bald patches are seen and these could range in size from 10 μm to 200 μm across, Figure 10. Although continuous ripple formation was observed in very old sockets such as 7HB, in younger sockets patches of ripples were observed in a background of pulls and smears and the bald patches were usually absent.

The parallel ripples are a curious phenomena and not expected considering the complicated sliding patterns of the hip. But the ripples, bald patches and fine cracks are all believed to be the result of a surface fatigue mechanism [13,16]. The parallel ripples may be connected with a type of fretting fatigue because similar features have been observed on fretted aluminum surfaces, however the authors could provide no explanation for ripple formation [17]. The bald patches are thought to be areas of the socket surface where the polymer has spalled or flaked off.

In the low wear area, again the remains of the original machined surface are seen but near

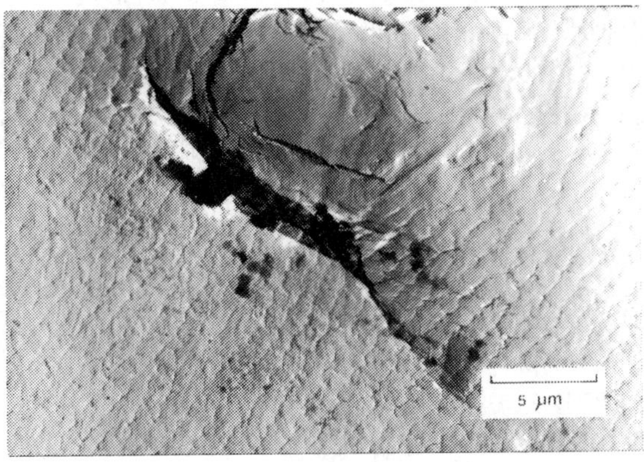

Figure 10. Part of spall in high wear area. Left socket (age: 8 6/12y) from patient 16HB. TEM; 2 stage replica.

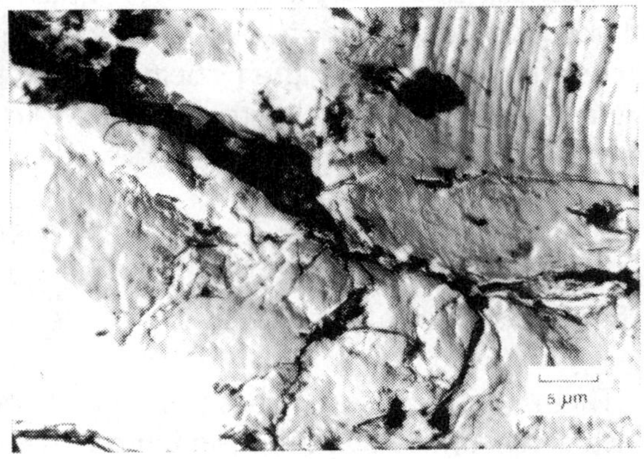

Figure 11. Wrinkling of surface near ridge. Right socket (age: 12 9/12y) from patient 21HB. TEM; 2 stage replica.

the ridge the surface often appears rumpled or wrinkled, Figure 11. It has been suggested that these wrinkles are the result of creep deformation of the socket [13]. If creep of the UHMWPE is occurring in the high wear area, flow of the plastic towards the low wear region is expected. To accommodate this extra material the surface buckles there because it is the only free surface, the rest being constrained by the cement anchoring the prosthesis. Alternatively, the wrinkling of the surface near the ridge may just be plastic deformation produced by impacts of the femoral head against the ridge.

In those sockets which have pitted areas near the boundary, TEM shows that these regions are rough and pitting and scratches are seen, Figure 12. Such roughened areas are also typical of very heavy rim wear where flaking and pitting is observed optically.

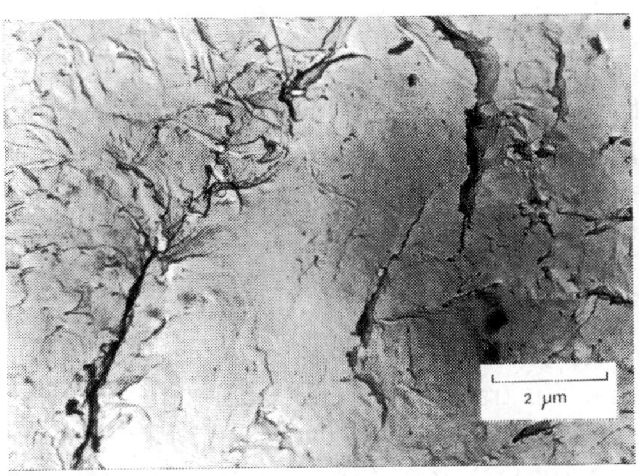

Figure 12. Pitting at border area. Left socket (age: 5 2/12y) from patient 1HB. TEM; 2 stage replica.

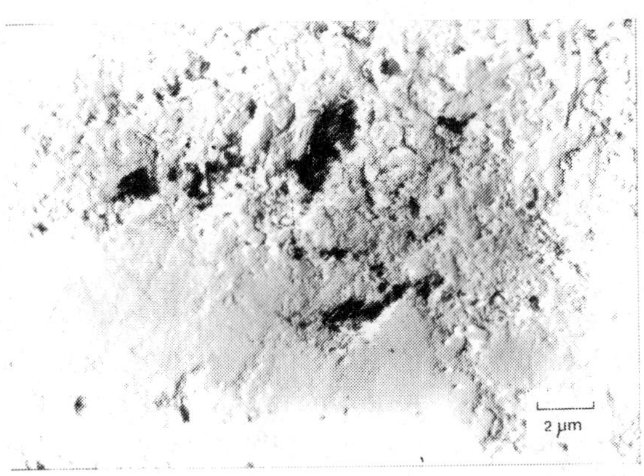

Figure 13. Pitting in discolored area of 16HB. TEM; 2 stage replica.

Socket 16HB differed from the other 22 sockets in that the low wear area was yellow instead of the more usual off-white. Electron micrographs from the yellow area show that the surface has a "corroded" appearance, Figure 13. The appearance of the cracks suggests that the normally chemically inert UHMWPE has been chemically attacked. Yellowing of UHMWPE is linked with degradation and hence weakening of the plastic, thus if some degradation has occurred in this socket then chemical attack should be expected. However, the extent of degradation is probably limited to just a thin surface layer in this socket, because the deeply worn high wear was not discolored.

5. DISCUSSION

5.1 In Vivo Wear Mechanisms

The microscopy survey has shown that socket wear is confined to the superior part of the articulating surface and here the femoral head effectively bores out a new socket for itself. In the description of the optical features, the direction of wear, and hence bore, was taken to be parallel to the line of action of the joint force and at the angle of 10°-15° to the vertical towards the body center line, Figure 3b. In practice, this is often not the case [10]. A study of wear direction in 59 sockets has shown that the most common direction was upwards and outwards (64.4%) whilst in 32.2% of the sockets the wear direction was vertical but that only 3.4% (2 sockets) was in the expected 10° direction. However, the amount of wear in the sockets was often less than 2 mm and this made accuracy of the true wear direction to be no better than ±10°.

The micro-topography suggests that initially the UHMWPE socket wears by a process of adhesion but, after about 7 or 8 years of use, a surface fatigue mechanism operates. Similar observations, regarding wear mechanisms, have been made by Brown [16]. During accelerated laboratory wear tests of UHMWPE sliding on polished stainless steel (dry) using loads and sliding speeds akin to those in the hip, the plastic wore by adhesion at first. After long sliding times, the wear rate increased and fine surface fatigue cracks were seen on the worn plastic surface. Initially the wear rate was 2.2×10^{-7} mm^3 N^{-1}m^{-1} but it increased to 3.6×10^{-7} mm^3 N^{-1} m^{-1} at the onset of surface fatigue. When these results are interpreted in terms of a 22 mm THR, the average wear rate is roughly 0.02 mm per annum and the onset of fatigue is predicted to occur after 5 to 10 years of in vivo use [13,16].

A major difference between in vivo and in vitro worn surfaces is the appearance of the metallic counterface. The removed femoral components had heads which were bright and shiny with no evidence that polymer was adhering to the surface. Transferred layers of polymer are often seen on metal counterfaces sliding against plastics, these layers being characteristic of adhesive wear and indeed the counterfaces in the dry wear tests were covered with a transferred layer of UHMWPE [18]. However, it should be remembered that in vivo the THR is not a dry bearing and that lubricants can hinder the formation of transfer layers [19]. Certainly there is some laboratory evidence that this transfer is inhibited in plastic/metal hips. McKellop, investigating the effects of lubricants on the friction and wear of UHMWPE on 316L, found that when the tests were run in baths of serum the metal surfaces were bright and shiny and resembled those of removed prostheses [20]. Initially, on addition of fresh serum, the friction and temperature increased and this was accompanied by the formation of a heavy transfer layer on the metal counterface. After several hours, the friction and temperature dropped to normal levels and the transfer layer was slowly rubbed away to leave a clean, metal surface. In saline and water, transfer layers were formed and were stable more or less throughout the tests.

With regard to the long term wear phenomena of surface fatigue cracks and spalls these have not been commonly observed in other surveys of removed prostheses [21,22,23,24]. Probably, this merely reflects the ages and conditions of the available prostheses and the method of examination. In many surveys, the prostheses are examined in scanning electron microscopes and these may not have sufficient resolution to reveal the fine scale detail on the smooth surfaces of worn sockets [15]. In others, the available prostheses have been used for only a few months and thus surface fatigue would not be observed. In yet others, cups have been removed because of loosening and infection [21,22,23]. Where prostheses have been removed because of loosening, there is much evidence that the articulating surfaces have been abraded by acrylic cement debris and thus these prostheses are probably not representative of the many prostheses which provide trouble free service.

5.2. Patient Variables and Wear

In the description of the worn sockets, the effect of a patient's activity on the wear features was alluded to. In general, the features of long term usage such as a deep wear scar, fatigue cracks, ripples and spalls are present after 7 years of use. If the patients were arranged in chronological order of socket age, exceptions to this generalization would be noticed. However, regrouping the patients according to their category of A, B or C does demonstrate that this statement is generally true, Table 3. In Table 3, each group of patients has been arranged in order of socket age; where a patient has 2 THR, each socket is entered separately. For each socket, there is a brief description of the owner's potential or achieved mobility which is taken from the detailed information in Table 2. The remainder of the table contains data on absence or presence of the long term or heavy wear features (ridge and fatigue topography) and clinical wear or penetration rates. The latter were obtained by measuring castings of the post-mortem sockets except in the cases of 9HB and 8HB in category C, 14HB in category B and 7HB in category A. These 5 penetration rates were estimated from the patients' radiographs taken some years before their death: the time of measurement is indicated by X - R, followed by the number of years, in the column for penetration depth.

Looking first at the grade B and C patients, indistinct and slight ridges are observed after 7 years but equally ridges are absent in some of the oldest sockets, 11HB, 12HB and 14HB. Admittedly, the observation of a ridge depends on the author's ability to detect one by sight or touch but the measured penetration depths tend to agree with the qualitative assessment. When there has been more than 1mm depth of wear, the ridge has been detected: thus no ridge was discerned in patient 12HB because the penetration depth was less than 0.55mm. When the B and C sockets are studied for the appearance of fatigue features, there is better agreement: all sockets over 8 years old shows some sign of surface fatigue wear.

Turning to the category A patients, it is seen that even in the cup used for 3 8/12 years there is an indistinct ridge. Unfortunately, the next socket in this group was used for nearly 8 years so no firm predictions may be made about the onset of fatigue. However, apart from the first socket, the A sockets showed definite ridges and indicators of fatigue wear and thus it seems reasonable to suggest that fatigue may occur early in these active patients than in the more sedentary B and C patients.

When the penetration rates are studied it is seen that these are higher in the A sockets than in the C sockets, whilst the B sockets show 2 high rates and 2 low rates. The reason for this more rapid wear in the A patients is the high level of their activity [25,26]. On the whole, these

Table 3. Summary of Wear Features, Penetration Depth and Rate in Relation to Socket Age

Socket	Patient Activity	Socket age (y)	(m)	Penetration depth (mm)	Penetration rate ($mm \cdot y^{-1}$)	Ridge present?	Fatigue features?
i) Category C patients							
6HB(L)	Walking limited	1	2	Measurements not valid		no	none
10HB(R)	Just able to walk	2	5	0	0	no	none
9HB(L)	Walking limited	5	0	X-R : 4y 0	0	no	some ripples
1HB(R)	Walking limited	5	2	1.13	0.22	indistinct	none
10HB(L)	Just able to walk	6	3	0.55	0.09	no	some ripples
2HB(R)	Walk normal	7	1	0.75	0.11	only low wear section available	
2HB(L)	Walk normal	7	5	1.20	0.16	yes	none
4HB(R)	Senile; stroke	8	0	0.9	0.11	indistinct	ripples, spalls
21HB(L)	Walk normal	8	10	0.8	0.09	inferior section missing	ripples
8HB(L)	Walking limited	8	11	X-R : 5y 0	0	slight	some ripples
8HB(R)	Walking limited	9	1	X-R : 5y 0	0	no	ripples
11HB(R)	Senile; obese; doddery.	10	1	0.85	0.08	no	some ripples
21HB(R)	Walk normal	12	9	1.12	0.09	yes	ripples
ii) Category B patients							
12HB(L)	Walk normal	9	8	0.5	0.05	no	cracks
14HB(L)	Walk normal	9	8	X-R : 4.5y 0	0	no	some spalls and cracks
3HB(L)	2-3 mile/day	9	9	2.58	0.26	yes	cracks
3HB(R)	2-3 mile/day	9	11	3.38	0.36	yes	cracks
iii) Category A patients							
5HB(L)	Golf every day	3	8	0.53	0.14	indistinct	none
13HB(L)	Retired	7	8	measurements not valid		yes	ripples
17HB(R)	Did everything	8	5	0.5	0.07	yes	ripples some cracks
16HB(L)	Active farmer	8	6	2.33	0.27	yes	ripples cracks + spalls
7HB(L)	Very active for age	11	5	X-R : 10y 1.0	0.10	yes	ripples + spalls
15HB(R)	Not very energetic	13	3	2.88	0.22	yes	ripples + cracks

patients have led lives which are no different from people unaffected by joint disease: two of the A patients played golf, one was a farmer, another an elderly but independent spinster, Table 2. Amongst the category C patients, the level of activity is limited by rheumatoid arthritis, senility, obesity: many of them walked with the aid of a stick, some had limps, and for many, light housework was the extent of their capabilities, Table 2. Some of the patients had limiting factors which were more debilitating than others and this must be remembered because it may account for some unexpected observations. For example, in the category B sockets 12HB and 14HB show little sign of wear (0.5mm and 0mm) but the 3HB sockets were deeply worn (2.58mm and 3.38mm) and all four had been in use for 10 years. Referring to Table 2, patients 12HB and 14HB appear to have been relatively sedentary whereas patient 3HB claimed she could walk 2 to 3 miles a day. Therefore in general terms, we may say that a normal healthy individual with one THR will wear out her acetabular socket faster than a patient with one or two THR *plus* some debilitating factor [26].

5.3 In Vivo Penetration Rates

Although variation in socket penetration may be explained qualitatively in terms of the patient's activity and mobility, these arguments do not provide a satisfactory explanation for the discrepancy in magnitude between clinical and laboratory wear rates. As discussed in section 5.1, the wear mechanisms appear to be identical for in vivo and dry, in vitro conditions: wear by adhesion first and surface fatigue wear later. However, the dry in vitro tests predict an average wear rate of 0.02mm per annum whereas the penetration rates in Table 3 range from 0 to 0.4mm per annum. A more comprehensive study has estimated that the average clinical penetration rate is 0.07mm per annum over the first 9 years of use [11]. Of the 491 sockets in the survey, 63.5% had less than 0.06mm per annum of wear and 4% had more than 0.18mm per annum. With regard to the age of the patients, 52 were under 50 years of age, 339 were aged 50 to 69 and 100 were over 70. When wear rates from wet in vitro tests are considered, the discrepancy in wear rates appears even greater. McKellop has calculated that, in serum, UHMWPE will wear at a rate of about 0.002mm per annum [20]. This value was considered to provide an indication of the minimum wear rate which might be expected in vivo.

The high wear rates observed clinically have been attributed to many causes such as wear by three body abrasion, stress cracking and degradation, microstructural imperfection and creep [21,22,23,27,28,29]. Three body abrasion occurs when hard particles are trapped between rubbing surfaces: the hard particles severely abrade or scratch the surfaces and produce a wear rate higher than that of ordinary abrasion. In artificial hips, it is generally accepted that three body abrasion occurs when acrylic cement particles or bone debris is trapped in the joint cavity. Such debris may be the result of surgical technique but is more commonly observed in artificial joints removed because of loosening [22,23]. Whether the loosening has produced the cement debris or debris, introduced at time of implantation, has led to loosening through increased friction is not easily answered. Be that as it may, the net result is a heavily scratched articulating surface on both metal and plastic and debris embedded in the surfaces, Figures 14 and 15, a topography not observed in this survey.

Degradation and stress cracking may well be closely linked: degradation reducing the chemical resistance of UHMWPE to stress cracking, the conjoint action of stress and a non corrosive fluid. Indicators of these were not detected in the survey except in one instance: the socket of 16 HB showed discoloration in the low wear area. Another example of a socket which may have been degraded or undergone stress cracking is shown in

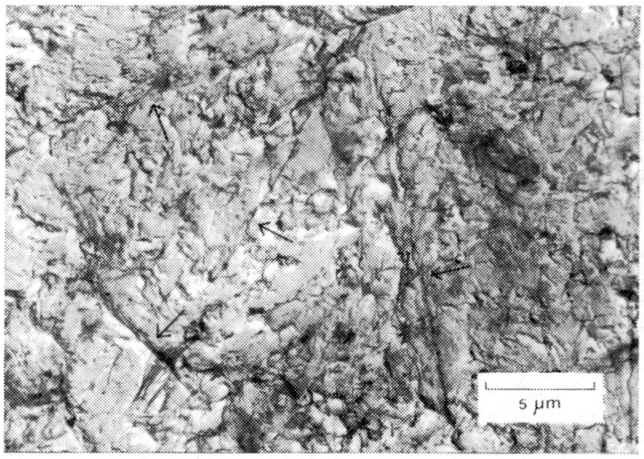

Figure 14. Scratches (arrowed) on abraded UHMWPE socket. Socket removed for loosening; acrylic cement and bone debris in joint cavity (joint not from Charnley Collection). TEM; 2 stage replica.

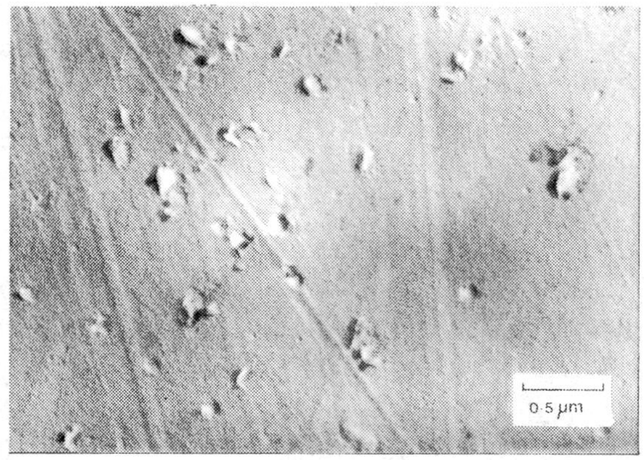

Figure 15. Scratches and embedded particles on abraded femoral head. Femoral component of socket in Figure 14. TEM; 2 stage replica.

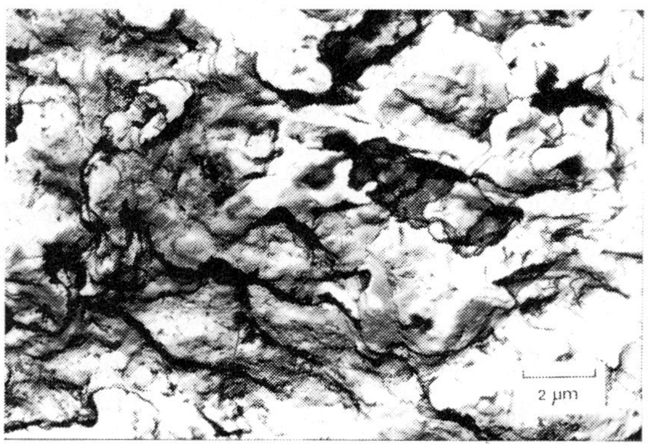

Figure 16. UHLMWPE socket degraded in-vivo. Socket removed because of broken femoral stem and infection. Socket colored orange on removal. (Joint not from Charnley Collectin). TEM: 2 stage replica.

Figure 16. This is a rare example where the socket was grossly discolored, the discoloration extending into the socket walls: infra-red spectroscopy has indicated that the plastic was degraded in vivo [30].

The presence of microstructural imperfections, such as voids and unduly high amounts of low molecular weight polymer, have been detected in UHMWPE prostheses [21,23,27]. The voids and low molecular weight fraction are formed during manufacture of the plastic: the low molecular weight fraction during polymerization, the voids arising from incomplete compaction of the powder into bulk form. Examination of used prostheses in section has revealed that the voids provide an easy path for cracks and fissures and are associated with severe wear as is the presence of large amounts of the low molecular weight polymer [21,23]. The size and distribution of the voids appears to vary from prosthesis to prosthesis and thus from batch to batch of UHMWPE [21]. Similarly, the amount of the low molecular weight fraction varies from prosthesis to prosthesis. High wear rates for prostheses have been attributed to these imperfections [23].

Recently, the author has investigated the creep deformation of UHMWPE at 37°, using Charnley acetabular cups and compressive loads [28]. Cyclic and static tests have shown that the plastic does creep under loads experienced in vivo and the resulting permanent deformation may account for the discrepancy between clinical and laboratory wear rates. Preliminary results indicate that permanent thinning of the cup wall, arising from compressive creep, proceeds at a rate of 0.04mm per annum over the first 10 years. Now the previously quoted in vitro rates of 0.002 to 0.02mm per annum were determined by weight loss of the test specimens so these values will not include a creep component. Addition of the in vitro wear rate to the in vitro "creep" rate gives an overall penetration rate of about 0.06mm per annum, and this is close to the reported clinical value of 0.07mm per annum. Thus it has been proposed that creep plays a major role in the penetration of an UHMWPE cup by a metal femoral head, at least in the first few years [28].

Of the proposed mechanisms leading to high wear rates in vivo, only creep and microstructural defects seem to be applicable to this survey of sockets which have operated in normal sliding conditions. Assuming microstructural defects are present in most prostheses and they exacerbate wear processes then a similar exacerbation of creep must be expected. Presumably, the magnitude of these effects will be a function of the size and distribution of the defects both creep and wear rates increasing with defect density. If this is so, then the high clinical penetration rates of 0.4mm per annum might arise because some prostheses have a higher than average defect density. Likewise, the surfaces of these sockets may show a greater degree of polymer spalling, assuming that spalls are formed by the spread of sub-surface cracks.

8. CONCLUSIONS

Examination of 23 Charnley acetabular cups has shown that in vivo wear is confined to the superior part of the socket and this is a direct consequence of the loading geometry of the hip joint. After about 7 or 8 years of use, a deep wear scar may be seen with the naked eye. In the heavily worn area, the surface is smooth and well polished. Initially, the UHMWPE wears by adhesion but after 7 years or so, a surface fatigue mechanism operates. This observed wear behavior is typical of UHMWPE sockets removed from hips with *normal sliding* conditions. In the presence of bone or cement debris, three body abrasive wear will occur and this is associated with abnormal conditions such as loosening.

The observed clinical penetration rates for the sockets vary from 0 to 0.4mm per annum and are much higher than predicted by laboratory wear tests. The variation can be explained qualitatively by the differing activities of the patients: the highest wear rates were observed amongst those patients who lead very active lives post operatively, whilst the lowest ones were associated with sedentary individuals.

Laboratory studies have indicated that creep deformation may account for much of the observed high clinical penetration rates. Other mechanisms, such as three body abrasion and degradation, were discounted as these were not observed in the surveyed sockets from normal sliding conditions. However, the presence of microstructural imperfections is considered to be important in determining the rate of wear of UHMWPE. It seems likely also that these defects will influence the creep behavior of the plastic.

REFERENCES

1. Griffith, M. J., Seidenstein, M. K., Williams, D., and Charnley, J., Eight Year Results of Charnley Ar-

throplasties of the Hip with Special Reference to the Behaviour of the Cement, Clin. Orthop., 137, 24-36, 1978.

2. Symposium: Statistics on Total Hip Replacement, Clin. Orthop., 95, 2-262, 1973.
3. Weaver, J. K., Activity Expectations and Limitations Following Total Hip Replacement, Clin. Orthop., 137, 55-61, 1978.
4. Burton, K. E., Wright, V. and Richards, J., Is the Claim for a High Success Rate for Total Hip Replacement Justified, Res. Psychol. Med., 2, 311-312, 1979.
5. Swanson, S. A. V., The State of the Art in Joint Replacement, Part 3: Results, Problems and Trends, J. Medical Engng. and Techn., 16-20, January 1978.
6. Dobbs, H., Survivorship of Total Hip Replacements, J. Bone Jt. Surg., 62-B, 168-173, 1980.
7. Hirsch, C., Clinical Problems in Total Hip Replacements, J. Biomed. Mater. Res. Symp., 5 (2), 227-244, 1974.
8. Willert, H. -G., and Semlitsch, M., Reactions of the Articular Capsule to Wear Products of Artificial Joint Prostheses, J. Biomed. Mater. Res. 11, 157-164, 1977.
9. Dumbleton, J. H., Elements of Hip Joint Prosthesis Liability, J. Med. Engng. and Techn., 341-346, November 1977.
10. Charnley, J., Rate of Wear in Total Hip Replacement, Clin. Orthop., 112, 170-179, 1975.
11. Griffith, M. J., Seidenstein, M. K., Williams, D. and Charnley, J., Socket Wear in Charnley Low Friction Arthroplasty of the Hip, Clin. Orthop., 137, 37-47, 1978.
12. Clarke, I. C., Wear of Artificial Joint Materials 1, Friction and Wear Studies: Validity of Wear Screening Protocols, Engng. in Med., 10, 115-122, 1981.
13. Dowling, J. M., Atkinson, J. R., Dowson, D. and Charnley, J., The Characteristics of Acetabular Cups Worn in the Human Body, J. Bone Jt. Surg., 60-B, 375-382, 1978.
14. Charnley, J., The Numerical Grading of Hips, Centre for Hip Surgery, Wrightington Hospital, International Publication No. 20, December 1968.
15. Keown, S. R., Chapter 8: Specimen Preparation for Transmission Electron Microscopy, Modern Physical Techniques in Materials Technology, Editors: Mulvey, T. and Webster, R. K., London, Oxford University Press, 94-115, 1974.
16. Brown, K. J. and Atkinson, J. R., The Wear of UHMWPE and a Preliminary Study of Its Relation to the In Vivo Behaviour of Replacement Hip Joints, Wear, 40, 255-264, 1976.
17. Alic, J. A. and Hawley, A. L., On the Early Growth of Fretting Fatigue Cracks, Wear, 56, 377-389, 1979.
18. Atkinson, J. R., Mechanical Properties and Wear Behavior of Plastics in Relation to Their Use in Prostheses, Br. Polym. J., 7, 93-107, 1975.
19. Teer, D. G. and Arnell, R. D., Chapter 5: Principles of Tribology, Editor: Halling, J., London and Basingstoke, The Macmillan Press Ltd., 94-127, 1978.
20. McKellop, H., Clarke, I. C., Markolf, K. L. and Amstutz, H. C., Wear Characteristics of UHMWPE: A Method for Accurately Measuring Extremely Low Wear Rates, J. Biomed. Mater. Res., 12, 895-927, 1978.
21. Gibbons, D. F., Anderson, J. M., Martin, R. L. and Nelson, T., Wear and Degradation of Retrieved UHMWPE and Other Polymeric Implants, ASTM STP 684, 20-39, 1979.
22. Hastings, G. W., In Vivo Wear Properties of UHMWPE Used in a Total Knee Prosthesis, Wear, 55, 1-9, 1979.
23. Rose, R. M., Crugnola, A., Ries, M., Cimino, W. R., Paul, I. and Radin, E. L., On the Origins of High In Vivo Wear Rates in Polyethylene Components of Total Joint Prostheses, Clin. Orthop., 145, 277-286, 1979.
24. Rostoker, W., Chao, E. Y. S. and Galante, J. O., The Appearance of Wear on Polyethylene – A Comparison of In Vivo and In Vitro Wear Surfaces, J. Biomed. Mater. Res., 12, 317-335, 1978.
25. Dowling, J. M., Atkinson, J. R., Dowson, D. and Charnley, J., The Influence of Patient's Weight and Level of Activity on Service Lives of Charnley Prostheses, 3rd Int. Conf. on Plastics and Medicine in Surgery, Enschede, The Netherlands, The Plastics and Rubber Institute, London, England, 1979.

26. Dowling, J. M., Atkinson, J. R., Dowson, D. and Charnley, J., Chapter 3: Characterisation of Worn Polyethylene Acetabular Cups in Relation to Service Time in the Human Body, Mechanical Properties of Biomaterials, Editors: Hastings, G. W. and Williams, D. F., Chichester, John Wiley and Sons Ltd., 39-52, 1980.
27. Rose, R. M., Nusbaum, H. J., Schneider, H., Ries, M., Paul, I., Crugnola, A., Simon, S. R. and Radin. E. L., On the True Wear Rate of UHMWPE in the Total Hip Prosthesis, J. Bone Jt. Surg., 62-A, 537-549, 1980.
28. Atkinson, J. R., Dowling, J. M. and Cicek, R. Z., Materials for Internal Prostheses: the Present Position and Possible Future Developments, Biomaterials, 1, 89-96, 1980.
29. Traveniuo, S. Z. M., Irregularities in the Wear of Plastics Materials in the Hip Joint, Plastics and Rubber, 1, 194-196, 1976.
30. Furber, P. K., Chp. 14: Discussion of Results – Wear of Oxidatively Degraded UHMWPE Against EN58J, Ph.D. Thesis: The Wear of Semi-Crystalline Polymers, The University of Leeds, England, 112-120, 1978.

Chapter 20

Prosthesis Materials and Devices – A Review

John H. Dumbleton, Ph.D.
Director of New Product Technology (Europe)
Howmedica International Inc.
Raheen, Limerick, Ireland

ABSTRACT

The tribological implications of using joint prostheses are discussed with the emphasis placed on wear. An indication of the manner in which joint prostheses were developed is given and the performance and failures of the early materials combinations is reviewed. The different ways in which failure can occur are given.

A description of the levels of wear testing is made with attention to the factors to be considered in test machine design. Techniques of wear measurement are given for in vitro and in vivo evaluation.

The performance of combinations in use such as ultra high molecular weight polyethylene against various metallic alloys and against alumina is detailed as well as the performance of polyoxymethylene against cobalt-chromium-molybdenum alloy. Attention is given to results obtained on laboratory wear test machines, joint simulators and clinically and the degree of agreement among the various findings is made.

Unresolved questions in the wear performance of joint materials are given and the future progress of the field described.

1. INTRODUCTION

1.1 Tribology and Implants

Tribology is the science which involves friction, lubrication and wear which are processes manifested by the interaction of surfaces in relative motion. Although the main impact of tribological studies has been in engineering, there are many examples of interaction between moving surfaces in the body. Perhaps the most obvious example concerns the joints which must articulate under high loads for many millions of cycles during a life-time; the operating conditions are especially rigorous for joints at the knee and at the hip. Other situations involving motion are the movement of the lungs in the pleural cavity and the motion of tendons during muscle pull.

With the increasing use of implants to replace or augment body components or organs, the subject of the tribological performance of these devices has had to be addressed. Thus there has been great interest in the friction performance of artificial hip joints, in the wear of heart valve replacements, in the wear of artificial teeth and in the wear of joint replacements in general. Usually there has not been the same degree of interest in lubrication due to the fact that lubrication mechanisms for devices are likely to be very different from those occurring naturally in the body. However, wear situations with devices can occur which do not naturally occur in the body. Multicomponent devices are employed for fracture fixation and relative motion between device components can lead to wear. Fretting between screw heads and bone plates is an example of this phenomenon.

Although there are many areas of interest regarding the tribology of implants, the focus here will be on implants in the orthopaedics area. Furthermore the discussion will be on the performance of joint replacement prostheses rather than on the tribological problems of trauma devices such as bone plates. The interest in joint replacements as regards performance has been primarily in the area of wear and secondarily in the area of friction; there has been little interest in joint lubrication. This emphasis will be followed here.

1.2 Joint Prostheses

The performance of the natural joints is superb. Lubrication of the cartilage by synovial fluid results in a joint which can perform under a wide variety of conditions. Typically loads of four times body weight are applied across the weight-bearing joints of the lower extremity during walking and significant loads occur across the joints of the hand and arm in activities such as lifting, grasping and turning. The excellence of lubrication is seen in the low friction coefficient which typically is in the range 0.003-0.015. Wear is often low and cartilaginous surfaces last a lifetime of over 70 years. However, the performance of a joint may be compromised by disease, accident or abnormal useage. Should the damage be severe then surgical intervention may be indicated and one of the more successful treatments is the excision of the diseased or damaged joint and its replacement with a prosthetic joint.

The history of joint replacements goes back to the nineteenth century and indications of the develoment of joint prostheses have been given by Scales [1] and Walker [2]. However success in joint replacement was not reproducibly achieved until 1960 when Charnley employed acrylic cement for fixation of total hip components. Since that time joint replacement procedures have become widespread with prostheses replacing the joints of the hip, knee, ankle, elbow, shoulder, wrist, fingers and thumb. In many cases the performance of these devices has been equivocal but outstanding success has been achieved for hip joint replacement. Table 1 gives the estimated number of total joint replacements in the United States alone for the years 1972-1976 [3] and it will be seen that the emphasis in joint replacement is at the hip followed by the knee with a smaller but growing number of replacements at the other joints. This reflects not only the greater success in hip replacements but also the greater degree of incapacitation resulting from disease or injury at the hip. As higher performance is achieved with prostheses for the other joints the number of implantations should grow considerably.

Table 1. Estimated Number of Total Joint Replacements in the United States in the Years 1972-1976 [3]

JOINT	1976	1975	1974	1973	1972
Hip	80,000	80,000	77,500	75,000	55,000
Knee	40,000	32,500	20,000	10,000	4,000
Other	10,000	8,500	6,500	3,800	2,500

2. THE DEVELOPMENT OF JOINT PROSTHESES

The history of the development of joint prostheses has been one of materials development although changes in design have occurred. It has also been recognized that there is a materials/design interaction and that materials which perform well with one design may show less satisfactory behavior in a different configuration or joint location. Since most of the experience with joint prosthesis development was for the hip, with this experience applied later to the development of other joints, the discussion will center around changes in hip prosthesis materials and design.

Changes in material for total hip prostheses are shown in Table 2. Prior to the materials presented wood, ivory and other materials had been employed in hip surgery [1]. A distinction should be made between total joint replacement in which the femoral head and the acetabulum are replaced and a hemiprosthesis which replaces only the femoral side of the joint and so bears against the cartilage of the acetabulum. In the case of a hemiprosthesis wear of the articular cartilage can occur but this aspect will not be discussed further since it is related to biomechanical aspects of joint function rather than the performance of the material used for the prosthesis. Recent design changes have employed bicentric prostheses which attempt to confine the motion within the device while minimizing the motion between device and articular cartilage.

Many of the changes in materials listed in Table 2 were due to wear considerations. By 1960 it was found that gross wearing-out of a component could occur as with polytetrafluoroethylene (PTFE) acetabular cups. Attempts to increase the wear resistance by using silica-filled PTFE did not improve the wear performance of the joint. At that stage ultra

Table 2. Materials Combinations Employed for Total Hip Prostheses and Hemiprostheses

FEMORAL COMPONENT	ACETABULAR COMPONENT	RESULT
Stainless steel (EN58J)	Polytetrafluoroethylene (PTFE, Teflon)	Failure due to creep, wearing out and tissue reaction (teflonoma)
Stainless steel (EN58J)	Silica-filled Teflon	Failure with high wear of the cup and wear of the metallic component
Cobalt-chromium-molybdenum (Co-Cr-Mo) alloy in cast form	Cast Co-Cr-Mo alloy	Still used but phased out due to loosening (high friction or tissue reaction to wear debris)
PTFE or Ultra high molecular weight polyethylene (UHMWPE) [1]	Cartilage	Failure due to high wear of the polymer
Co-Cr-Mo alloy	Cartilage	Still used. Long term wear of the cartilage
Polyethylene Terephthalate [1] (PET, Polyester)	Co-Cr-Mo alloy	Failure due to wear, tissue reaction
Co-Cr-Mo alloy	PET	Better than above but dropped due to better performance of UHMWPE
UHMWPE [1]	Cast Co-Cr-Mo alloy	High wear of head
Cast Co-Cr-Mo alloy [2]	Polyoxymethylene (polyacetal, Delrin)	Used with success in one design
Stainless Steel (EN58J, 316LVM) Co-Cr-Mo alloy [3] MP-35N [4]	UHMWPE [5]	Most widely used combination
Ti-6Al-4V alloy	UHMWPE	Used to some extent. Question over wear rate
Alumina [1]	UHMWPE	Used on a restricted basis
Alumina [1]	Alumina	Used on a restricted basis
Stainless steel (23Cr-9Ni-5Mn)	UHMWPE	No reports. Appears satisfactory

1 Femoral head material, stem metallic

2 Metal head and stem with Delrin trunnion

3 Cast, forged and powder metallurgical processes now used

4 Co-Cr-Mo alloy head on MP-35N stem

5 Machined and directly moulded UHMWPE now used

high molecular weight polyethylene (UHMWPE) was employed and since that time total hip prostheses have used UHMWPE as the material of choice.

Although UHMWPE was employed with great success other polymers were also tried as prosthesis components. Polyethylene terephthalate (PET) and later surface modified PET were used in some designs. These polymers showed high rates of wear that, while not giving wearing-out of the prosthesis, allowed sufficient production of wear debris to be liberated so that tissue reaction necessitated device removal.

At an early stage in the development of total hip prostheses all-metal devices were used consisting of a cobalt chromium molybdenum alloy. Although such devices were successful in the short and medium term it has been recognized that a high degree of loosening and systemic responses have been associated with all-metal prostheses. The majority of prostheses today are of the metal/plastic variety and all-metal devices are little used for joint replacement.

Experience over some 20 years total hip replacement has given other information on the role of materials selection and design on the wear behavior. For example it has been found that polymers which perform satisfactorily as components with concave bearing surfaces perform less well when the bearing surface is convex. Polymers show high wear rates when bearing against articular cartilage.

The materials combinations employed most widely for total hip prostheses have stainless steel (316LVM), cobalt chromium molybdenum alloy (cast, forged or produced by powder metallurgical techniques) or MP-35N, a multiphase cobalt-nickel alloy, for the femoral component with UHMWPE as the acetabular cup. For some 10 years polyoxymethylene (POM) has been used in total hip replacement but the use has largely been restricted to one particular design. A titanium alloy, Ti-6Al-4V, has been used on a restricted basis for the femoral component and high purity alumina components have been used either as alumina-alumina or alumina-UHMWPE combinations. Carbon fiber filled UHMWPE has been used on a limited basis for acetabular cups. Recent changes in materials have been made to increase the strength of the femoral component and have not been carried out because of wear considerations. A recent introduction has been the use of a modified stainless steel for the femoral component.

Table 3 gives examples of total hip prosthesis designs and configurations typically used at the present time. These examples are representative of the large variety of designs available. There is far greater restriction in the number of materials combinations employed.

By and large the discussion of materials can be carried over to the knee and to other joints except that there is even more uniformity in the materials combinations employed. The majority of devices use cast cobalt chromium molybdenum alloy in combination with UHMWPE although 316LVM stainless steel has been used on a limited basis. In a similar manner to at the hip the useage of all-metal prostheses, often in a hinge configuration, has been superceded by metal/plastic devices. Carbon fiber filled UHMWPE has been employed on a restricted basis. In general the materials experience is much more limited than for the hip. Knee prostheses were only widely used after 1970 and successful replacement at joints other than the hip and knee is a later development still. Problems such as loosening have demanded most attention for joints other than the hip from the onset. Prostheses have often not remained in place long enough to determine whether or not wear was a problem. However, at the knee some experience has been gained and it may be stated that the wear of UHMWPE is not as satisfactory as when used at the hip because of the higher bearing pressure and due to the ready ingress of acrylic cement.

For joint replacement materials, combinations and designs have evolved since the time of first widespread joint replacement. Most experience has been gained for total hip replacement and a restricted number of materials combinations have been employed. Additions to this number in the alloy area have been due to reasons other than wear. However the use of alumina ceramics was specifically to provide even lower rates of wear than for metal/polymer combinations. There is some experience at the knee but attention is focused at design rather than at materials combinations due to problems with loosening. At the other joints there is very limited experience. Again the prevention of loosening occupies most attention and efforts are chiefly directed in the design area. At the present time materials combinations developed for the hip have been carried over to the knee and to the other joints but it may be necessary to develop combinations specifically for these other joint applications. Further details of materials development are given elsewhere [4,5]. Figure 1 shows the configuration of prostheses used to replace some of the joints of the body.

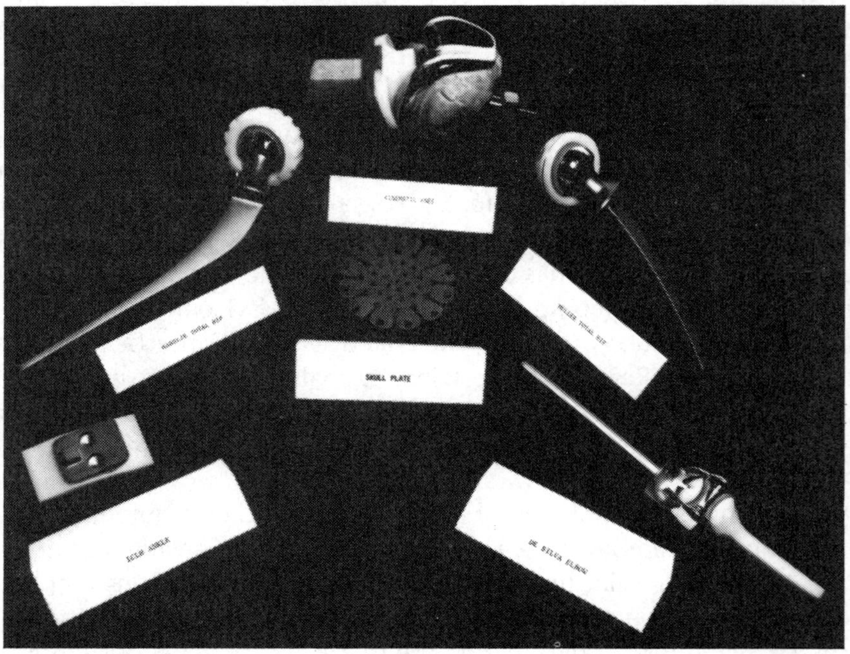

Figure 1. Some examples of total joint prostheses.

3. WEAR AND FRICTION

3.1 Joint Prosthesis Failures

Early in the development of joint prostheses failures due to wear were encountered. However changes in materials have greatly increased the wear resistance and failures due to other causes have become evident. Most experience has been accumulated with total hip replacement. For such prostheses there are many causes of failure [4] but the main causes are infection, loosening or fracture. Wear is no longer a cause of failure in the short-term but may contribute to prosthesis removal in the long-term [5].

In the hip prosthesis wear failures fit into several categories. Gross wearing out of acetabular cup materials leads to the femoral head bearing against bone giving pain. Substantial wear but of a lower magnitude can give rise to the restriction of motion, impingement of the femoral neck of the prosthesis against the acetabular cup and subsequent cup loosening. Generation of wear debris in sufficient quantities can give gross rejection as in the case of teflonomas or can lead to tissue necrosis and subsequent prosthesis loosening [6]. With metal-on-metal devices the wear debris gives rise to sensitivity effects and has been associated with device loosening. Longer-term reactions to wear debris may be found [5]. It will be noted that the effects of wear have shifted from mechanical failure to the prospect of longer-term biological failure as improved materials have been employed.

As has been mentioned the experience with joints other than the hip has been shorter. Infection and loosening are the main difficulties but presumably the effects of wear debris would be encountered if prostheses were in place for a sufficient period of time. At the knee, even in the short term, substantial damage of UHMWPE tibial components has been noted from the entrapment of acrylic bone cement between the joint surfaces. Such a phenomenon had been noted at the hip but due to the different geometry of the device caused much less of a problem. Thus it is possible that wear problems other than those met at the hip will be found at the knee and other joints. This follows from the differing joint prosthesis geometry and the different joint conditions.

Failures due to friction are not widespread but the possibility of such failures led to the development of different designs of prosthesis. Thus the Charnley total hip prosthesis employs a femoral head of only 22mm diameter to give a small frictional moment whilst the Christiansen prosthesis employs a trunnion bearing so that motion between the head and the cup is reduced. The possibility of loosening due to high frictional moments has also been mentioned in connection with all-metal total hip prostheses since it has been known for some time that the coefficient of friction for the metal-on-metal combination was about ten times higher than for metal-polymer combinations. Again this was a reason for the phasing out of metal-on-metal devices. For joints other than the hip loosening is a major problem usually met in the short-term but this appears to be due to the inadequate fixation of the joint components because of poor bone stock and anatomical constraints rather than because of high frictional torques. Nonetheless most prostheses for the knee and other joints are of the metal/plastic variety.

3.2. Reasons for Friction and Wear Measurement

The frictional forces between joint prosthesis components no longer are a concern from the point of view of joint performance. Thus the measurement of friction coefficient is not a major objective of any materials evaluation. However, the evaluation of the coefficient of friction and frictional moments is of interest especially in the evaluation of a new material for joint prosthesis use and in the evaluation of designs of prosthesis.

The measurement of wear is perhaps more significant. In the short-term at the hip joint wear is not a problem but there is interest in the long-term performance of joint prostheses and in the effects of accumulation of wear debris in the tissues. This concern could lead to the introduction of materials with even lower wear rates than the materials at present used; alternatively the search could be for materials of higher biocompatibility which would be tolerated in greater quantities in the tissue.

Apart from the evaluation of the long-term performance at the hip there is interest in the evaluation of the wear behavior of materials at the other joint locations. Thus at the knee the contact stresses are considerably higher than at the hip. Wear of the knee prosthesis is also complicated by the presence of acrylic bone cement. The performance of a material at the knee or at the other joints may not follow the extrapolation of experience with that material at the hip joint requiring testing of an established material under the specific conditions of the application.

Wear measurement may also be required for any new material combination introduced for joint prosthesis use. The more recent changes in materials have not been on the basis of reduced wear but for other reasons such as increases in fatigue strength. In the case of one material, MP-35N, introduced as a femoral stem component to give increased fatigue strength, this problem was avoided by having the bearing surface of an already accepted material but this course of action leads to other problems. Besides performance advantages changes in materials may follow from market pressures or manufacturing advantages.

Thus although high rates of wear are no longer a problem in joint prostheses there are ample reasons for the measurement of wear. Friction measurements are often made as an adjunct to wear measurements. Apart from scientific interest in wear measurement and in the interest in performance measurement, in certain countries wear measurement as a qualification procedure may be mandated by the appropriate government ministry. Product liability laws also play a role in deciding on the level of pre-market testing and evaluation. All of these factors ensure that the wear evaluation of new and existing materials combinations and designs will be carried out.

4. LEVELS OF WEAR MEASUREMENT

4.1 Material versus Device

The evaluation of a material combination for use in joint replacements must be distinguished from the evaluation of a device. Study of a material usually takes place in the laboratory and the wear behavior is evaluated over a variety of conditions. All that can be gathered from a study of this nature is that a material combination is or is not promising for joint prosthesis use. Accelerated tests are often used so that many test conditions can be covered in a manageable time frame. However acceleration of the tests may lead to invalid results unless the relationship between the accelerating variable and the wear lifetime is understood. An advantage of materials testing is that the degradation of the material may be investigated but such tests should not be combined with wear tests due to complex interactive effects. Materials tests may be carried out on simple test machines but the penalty for this is that there may be difficulty in extrapolating the results to the end-use.

Testing of a device is more costly than the testing of a material since evaluation must be done on a joint simulator. The use of a specific device places constraints on the generality of the test which may not be extrapolated to other devices of different design even at the same joint location. However device testing is the only way to fully evaluate a material in the end-use configuration. As has been pointed out a material may work well at one location but fail or perform less well at another (see Table 2 for UHMWPE). Testing of a device on a joint simulator does not guarantee that the prosthesis will perform well in the body and this can only be ascertained by *in vivo* studies in which the prosthesis is implanted and followed under carefully controlled conditions.

Table 3. Some Configurations of Total Hip Prostheses

CONFIGURATION	EXAMPLE
Metallic femoral stem and UHMWPE acetabular cup	Charnley, Muller
Trunnion bearing prosthesis, metallic stem and Delrin acetabular cup	Christiansen
Metallic femoral stem with cone taper fixation of alumina head with UHMWPE acetabular cup or alumina cup	Muller, Lindenhof
Surface replacement with metallic femoral shell and UHMWPE acetabular cup	Wagner

4.2 Parameters Measured

In the evaluation of the performance of a material or a device the performance is monitored by measuring the friction and wear. For a material the friction coefficient is evaluated whereas for a device the frictional force, torque or moment is measured.

The rate of wear is evaulated in the steady state and also a measure of the degree of wear during the wearing-in should be noted although the latter parameter may simply reflect the nature of the test and test conditions. Observation of the sliding surfaces is useful for establishing the mechanisms of wear which may allow prediction of the wear behavior at longer sliding times. Collection and characterization of wear debris is important since the size and shape of the wear particle can influence the biological interaction; the wear rate will indicate the quantity of material liberated into the tissues.

4.3 Levels of Testing

There are a progression of tests which can be used to evaluate a material and a device. The advantage in moving to a higher level of testing is that the test more closely resembles the human situation. The disadvantage is the greater complexity, time and cost of the test procedure. The levels of testing are as follows:

(i) laboratory wear testing machine – this approach is employed to screen materials although attempts have been made to predict the wear rates of devices *in vivo* from such simple *in vitro* tests.

(ii) laboratory joint simulator – although an *in vitro* test the evaluation is on a joint prosthesis. The problem of the measurement of wear on a device has not been solved in a routine fashion. Tests are complex compared to wear testing on materials and machine costs are high.

(iii) animal studies – testing on materials or devices may be undertaken. Materials tests are for biocompatibility. Studies on tissue response to particulate matter, simulated wear debris, may be carried out. Device testing may be done in animals but the connection between this and device performance in a human is problematic. Animal testing is costly. Devices may be removed after use to examine wear and to see if degradation occurred.

(vi) clinical trials – this involves the use of the device in patients under carefully controlled conditions and is usually the last step before wide-spread introduction of the prosthesis. Even after the general introduction of the device much valuable information on device performance can be obtained including the examination of removed implants.

The advantages and disadvantages of each level of testing are given in Tables 4-8. A general comment is that the divisions between the levels of testing have been emphasized for clarity and some overlap could occur. The more closely the *in vivo* conditions are reproduced the more difficult it is to measure the wear. Not all of the testing levels need be employed in the introduction of a new material or device and this depends on the novelty of the introduction.

Table 4. Laboratory Wear Testing

ADVANTAGES		DISADVANTAGES
Simple, low cost		Simplicity means that only some aspects of the in vivo situation are reproduced. Cost increases rapidly if more faithful reproduction of conditions required.
Geometry can be varied to reproduce different contact pressure distributions.		
Constant load	simplify interpretation of results	
Oscillation or rotation at different speeds but only simple motion in more cases.		Cannot reproduce physiologic loads or load profiles. Velocity profile not matched. Full motion degrees of freedom not produced.
Joint fluid may be used or other physiologic fluids.		Difficulties of changing fluid characteristics with time or preservatives must be used.
Many different conditions may be used to investigate material.		Extrapolation of the results on a material to a design or in-vivo performance is not direct due to differences in condition and the lubrication regime from in vivo situation.
Acceleration of the test may be done to obtain results for long sliding distances in a short time.		
Wear mechanisms may be identified and wear debris examined.		Wear mechanisms may be typical of wear test configuration only. Amount of wear debris usually very small.
May be used to examine degradation on samples from laboratory, animals or humans.		Extrapolation not direct to in vivo situation.
Special machines may be built to produce large volumes of debris for testing		Size and nature of debris is determined by the machine and may not be typical of the debris produced by a prosthesis

Table 5. Laboratory Simulation Machines

ADVANTAGES	DISADVANTAGES
Load profile and magnitude can be simulated. Joint fluid or other physiological fluid may be used.	High cost. Only one type of joint may be used, i.e. simulators are usually for hips, knees and so on. If a universal simulator is constructed the cost is prohibitive.
Tests may be done on designs in the end-use configuration. Wear debris may be collected. Wear mechanisms may be determined. Some acceleration of testing can be done.	Although some acceleration is possible, tests usually are undertaken in real time. Thus a considerable time is required to get results. The situation is even worse on a universal simulator since many different types of prostheses may be waiting for testing.
Effect of degradation on performance may be investigated. Simulator may be used for other tasks than wear measurement, e.g. creep, motion versus position of prosthesis, fixation, torque measurements.	In vivo situation not strictly simulated but the simulation aspects may lead to false security since it may be assumed that the in vivo situation is fully reproduced.
	In general wear cannot be accurately measured. Amount of wear debris small and difficult to collect.

Table 6. Animal Studies

ADVANTAGES	DISADVANTAGES
May be used for degradation tests on material.	No acceleration possible.
May be used for testing effect of wear debris - either debris produced specially and introduced into tissue or joint cavity or wear debris produced by the prosthesis (examination of surrounding tissue).	Debris usually obtained from powder fraction or from specially constructed machine and may not be typical of wear debris.
May be used for testing biocompatibility.	
May be used for wear testing and overall performance evaluation of prostheses.	Loading not controlled and not known. Prosthesis must be miniaturised and design may need modification to anatomy.
Overall advantage is that tests are done in vivo.	Overall disadvantage is cost since animals are expensive. However, tests such as biocompatibility may be done on small animals. Good facilities needed for surgery and animal care. Supply may be a problem.

Table 7. Clinical Trials

ADVANTAGES	DISADVANTAGES
Studies carried out on actual device under in vivo end-use conditions. Performance can be measured. Ex-vivo devices may be examined.	Complicated to set up a full trial. Protocol and documentation needed. In some countries, government health ministry permission required.
Results may be used to introduce prosthesis to other countries or areas.	Centres may not fill in or return documentation.
Possibility of continuing follow-up and evaluation to long implantation times after clinical trial has ended, i.e. extension into general use phase.	Cost may be high.

Table 8. General Use Evaluation

ADVANTAGE	DISADVANTAGE
Prosthesis evaluated under widely differing condition.	More centres involved. Greater difficulties of data collection than with clinical trial.
Possibility of obtaining greater supply of ex-vivo devices for examination.	Hidden costs of evaluation may be high in terms of personnel commitment.

5. WEAR TESTING AND EVALUATION

5.1 Conditions and Characterization

In order to adequately evaluate a material or a device for use as a joint replacement, the conditions of the test must resemble the conditions of use. For a joint prosthesis the following information is useful in setting up a test: loads, load variation with joint movement, number of motions with the range of motion about each axis, angular velocity of joint motion about each motion axis, nature of any lubricant present. Not all of this information is readily available but a summary of information has been made along with indications of how to calculate joint forces [7].

It should be noted that full characterization of materials and devices must be made. Test conditions and the nature of the experiment should be described. In the past results have been published with incompletely characterized on even uncharacterized materials and with incomplete descriptions of the test procedure. This has led to confusion and an inability to compare the results from different groups. A check-list of factors to be considered has been given [8].

Table 9. Wear Testing Machines Employed for the Evaluation of Joint Materials

Machine	Geometry (No. samples)	Materials	Motion	Load	Speed	Liquid	Temper-ature	Wear measurement
(9)	Ring on conforming block (1)	Metal/plastic stationary plastic block	89 cycles/min oscillation through 86.5 degrees	6.42 MN/m^2	10.5 cm/s	Mineral oil	32°C	Height change. Weight loss
(10)	Pin-on-disc (pin end flat) (1)	Metal/plastic stationary plastic pin	Rotation and translations not synchronised Rotation 1 cycle/min longitudinal motion 130 stroke/min (3.75 cm stroke) Transverse motion 7.5 cm/min	9 kg. to give 3.17 MN/m^2	as under motion	water 0.5% gelatine Synovial fluid	28°C	Depth of a witness groove
(11)	Disc-on-plate	Metals, plastics and ceramics combinations	Rotation	0-270 kg up to 10 MN/m^2	500-20,000 cm/min	water	37°C	Wear scar
(12)	Ball-on-flat	Metal/Metal	Reciprocating	6kg(on 22 mm dia. ball)	0.1 cm/s	Dry, Synovial Fluid, Water, Ringers solution, Hip fluid. Hyaluronic acid.		Wear scar
(13)	Ball-on-flat	Metal/Plastic	Oscillation of metal ball	2.3kg (on 22 mm dia. ball)	0.2 cm/s	water	RT	wear scar
(14)	Disc on conforming body (1)	Metal/plastic ceramics	Rotation	0.3 MN/m^2	40 cm/s	Dry, water	-	weight loss
(15)	Annulus-on-flat	metal/plastic	Stationary plastic Oscillation through 110 degrees	To give 3.45 MN/m^2	7.6 cm/s	Water, blood, plasma	RT	Height change
(16)	Pin-on-disc (spherical end 2 cm dia.) Also journal-on-bush machine (1)	metal/plastic metal pin	Rotation	-	-	Bovine serum	-	wear track
(17)	Disc-on-flat (disc edge with radius 0.2 cm). (1)	metal/carbon carbon/carbon	Rotation of disc at 60 rev/min	2.2g	2.5cm/min	water	RT	wear scar
(18)	Pin-on-flat (pin with flat end) (12)	metal/plastic ceramic/plastic	Reciprocating 100 c/min	3.45-6.90 MN/m^2	500 cm/min	Bovine serum	RT	weight loss
(19)	Pin-on-disc (pin dia. 2cm) (1)	Various materials	Rotation	100 N	5 cm/sec	Bovine serum	RT	wear scar
(20)	Tri-pin-on-disc (flat end pin) (3)	metal/plastic plastic pin	Rotation	155 N to give 17 MN/m^2	24 cm/sec	Dry water	RT	Weight loss. Height Change
(21)	Cylinder in a conforming trough, also non-conforming (1)	Metal/plastic with metal cylinder	Oscillation through 45 degrees	445 N for half-cycle Zero other half.	0.5 cycle/s	water	37°C	Volumetric wear
(22)	Annulus-on-flat (1)	Ceramic/ceramic	Oscillation ± 25 degrees	To give 20 MN/m^2	1 cycle/s (≈ 1.7 cm/s)	-	-	wear scar
(23)	Pin-on-flat (flat end pin) (6)	Metal/plastic Metal flat moves	Reciprocating, stroke 2.5 cm	To give 0-10 MN/m^2 on/off	5 cm/s	water serum	RT 37°C	Height change. Weight loss.

5.2 Wear Testing Machines

Many different types of wear testing machines have been used to evaluate materials for joint prosthesis use. A list of machines is given in Table 9. There is no agreement on a standard machine for wear evaluation but in the United Kingdom draft standards have been made for a pin-on-disc geometry with a metal spherically-ended pin bearing against a flat polymer disc. In the United States a draft standard has been presented for a reciprocating pin-on-flat geometry in which a flat-ended polymer pin bears against a metal or ceramic flat. The pin-on-disc machine has a rotational motion while the pin-on-flat machine has a linear motion. These machines are not totally satisfactory for testing ceramic against ceramic combinations and here an annular contact machine has been suggested.

Different methods have been used to measure wear. These methods include height change, dimensions of wear scar, volumetric wear and weight loss. Dimensional measurements suffer from the problem of creep for polymeric materials while weight loss measurements have the difficulty of allowing for liquid uptake by the polymer.

In the weight loss technique the sample is weighed before and after the wear test. The weight change ΔW is given by:

$$\Delta W = -(\Delta W)_{\omega} + (\Delta W)_{1} \qquad (1)$$

where $-(\Delta W)_{\omega}$ is the weight loss due to wear and $(\Delta W)_{1}$ the weight increase due to liquid adsorption: $(\Delta W(_{1})$ is obtained from "soak-control" specimens [18].

For linear dimensional change $\Delta 1$ there are several components that must be separated to give the change due to wear $(\Delta 1)_{\omega}$:

$$\Delta 1 = -(\Delta 1)_{\omega} - (\Delta 1)_{c}\, (\Delta 1)_{1} \pm (\Delta 1)_{t} \qquad (2)$$

where $-(\Delta 1)_{c}$ is the dimensional change due to creep, $(\Delta 1)_{1}$ is the change due to liquid adsorption and $\pm\, (\Delta 1)_{t}$ the length change due to thermal expansion or contraction.

Apart from disagreement over the geometry of the test machine there has been some variation in the test conditions adopted. It is widely accepted that a fluid should be present but there is no agreement on the type of fluid; recent tests have tended to emply synovial fluid, however. The length of test has been the subject of some discussion. The length of test has been increased in recent studies to simulate several years of use. It has been estimated that approximately 2.5×10^{4} m of sliding represent one year of use at the hip.

A summary of test conditions and geometry is given in Table 10.

5.3 Joint Simulators

The general conditions for joint simulators are given in Table 11. The type of simulator depends on the nature of the prosthesis to be evaluated. Simulators have been built to test total hip prostheses, knee prostheses and prostheses for the other joints. Most work has been carried out on hip prostheses, less work on knee devices and little work on prostheses for other joints [6].

Some of the simulators available to test total hip prostheses are listed in Table 12. In

Table 10. Conditions for Wear Testing Machines

Geometry of Contact	:	Annulus-on-flat) Flat-on-flat) Ball-on-flat) Cylinder-in-through) choice of material for moving components
Load	:	Constand load chosen to give a nominal contact pressure of 3.45 MN/m^2 or 6.90 MN/m^2 (500 psi or 1000 psi).
Type of motion	:	Reciprocating (linear) Oscillating Unidirectional (rotational)
Velocity or Frequency	:	0.01 - 0.05 m/s 1 c/s
Length of stroke	:	0.01 - 0.05 m
Liquid	:	Absent Distilled water Saline Ringers or Hanks solution Serum (human or animal) Plasma Synovial fluid (animal)
Temperature	:	20°C 37°C

Table 11. Conditions for Joint Simulators

Geometry of contact	:	Determined by prosthesis
Load	:	Variable following published load curves. One component, two components or three components applied
Type of Motion	:	Flexion-extension) Abduction-adduction) magnitudes as published Internal-external rotation)
Velocity or frequency	:	Velocity profiles as published Frequency 1 c/s
Liquid	:	Distilled water Saline Ringers Hanks solution Serum (human or animal) Plasma Tynovial fluid (animal)
Temperature	:	37°C 20°C

Table 12. A Listing of Simulators for the Hip Joint

CHARACTERISTIC	M.I.T. SIMULATOR (24)	CINCINNATI SIMULATOR (25)	MUNICH SIMULATOR (26)	IMPERIAL COLLEGE SIMULATOR (27)	HOSPITAL FOR SPECIAL SURGERY SIMULATOR (28)
No. of test positions	One	One	One	One	One
Load	Mech. System	Servo-hydraulic	Hydraulic	Mechanical	Pneumatic
(a)No. of axes	One vertical axis	One vertical axis (offset)	One vertical axis	One vertical axis	One vertical axis
(b)Profile	As published (21)	as published (23)	Double peak	Cyclically varying	Double peak
(c)Amplitude/baseline/profile changes	Load approx. 250kg. Ability to change not stated	Up to approx 350kg Amplitude change easy. Profile change with difficulty.	Can be varied	Up to approx 450kg Can be varied in amplitude.	Not stated
Motion :	Mech. system	Mech. system	Hydraulic actuators	Mechanical	Mechanical
(a)No. of motions	One (flexion-extension)	One (flexion-extension)	All three motions	One (flexion-extension) but other motions available	One (flexion-extension)
(b)form of motion	As published (22)	Sinusoidal	Not stated	Probably sinusoidal	Probably sinusoidal
(c)ability to change motion	not stated	Amplitude change only	Can be varied	Adjustable amplitude	± 30 degrees.
Speed	30 c/min	Up to 60 c/min	Stepless variation	Up to 90 c/min	Not stated
Temperature	R.T.	R.T.	37°C	Variable as desired	37°D
Liquid	Any liquid	Any liquid	Any liquid	Any liquid	Any liquid
Wear	Dimensional change/debris collection	Single location change (cup thickness)	Dimensional	Wear debris collection	Wear debris collection
Friction measurement	Yes	No	On all axes	Yes	Yes

general hip joint simulators have been complicated and costly but there have been attempts to reduce the complexity of the machine while retaining adequate simulation of the device function. Clarke [29] has reviewed some of the experience with hip joint simulators at different centers and has described a ten-channel simulator which has the virtue of simplicity while preserving most of the desirable features of a hip joint simulator. In this machine hip joints are tested in bovine serum with two degrees of motion under a varying load to simulate the load experienced by a hip joint during ambulation.

There have been rather fewer knee simulators constructed. Table 13 lists some of the knee simulators along with operating characteristics. Knee prostheses must be tested on specially constructed machines since the motion at the knee is more complicated than that at the hip.

Table 13. A Listing of Simulators for the Hip Joint

CHARACTERISTIC	M.I.T. KNEE SIMULATOR (30)	TWENTE KNEE SIMULATOR (31)	SYRACUSE KNEE SIMULATOR (32)	RICHARDS KNEE SIMULATOR (33)	LEEDS KNEE SIMULATOR (34)
No. of test positions	One	One	One	One	One
Load: (a)No. of axes	Hydraulic one, along tibia	Pneumatic one, along tibia	Mechanical Dead weight plus quadricens force	Hydraulic one, along tibia	- Two, axial and anterior-posterior
(b)Profile	as published(35)	as published	Simulates stance & swing phase	as published(36)	as published (23)
(c)Amplitude/base-line/profile change	256kg used. Can be changed	Up to 10 x body weight. Can be changed	Not given	Typically 7 x B.W. Can be changed	-
Motion	Hydraulic actua-tors, four-bar	Mechanical, four-bar linkage	Hydraulic	Hydraulic	Mechanical
(a)No. of motions	All three mot-ions	Flexion-extension passive rotation	Flexion-extension	Flexion-extension internal-external rotation	Flexion-extension fixed axis
(b)Form of motion	as published(35)	as published	Simulates physio-logic	as published(37)	as published
(c)Ability to change motion	Not stated but probable	Not stated but probable	Adjustable but load also changes	Adjustable	can be changed
Speed	40 steps/min variable	0-3.1 c/s	About 1 c/s	1 c/s	1 c/s
Temperature	Not stated	not controlled	Room temperature	$37^{o}C$	-
Liquid	any liquid	any liquid	Dry	calf serum	-
Wear measurement	not stated	not stated	Visual	weight loss	-
Friction meas-urement	about three axes	not stated	none	none	-
Special features	only flexion-extension &joint force need be controlled	can test natural knees	- -	Computer contro-lled force and	Computer con-trolled force

Machines constructed to evaluate prostheses for joints other than the hip or knee are much simpler in construction. In some cases other types of simulator may be adapted. One difficulty in testing these other joints is the comparative lack of information on the joint operating conditions [38].

As has been mentioned above, the difficulty in the measurement of wear increases the closer the test becomes to the actual in-use conditions. Many different methods of measuring wear have been employed with joint simulators, some of these methods are still in the development stage. No method is completely satisfactory. The list of methods is as follows [38]:

(i) weight loss measurements – this is the classical method of measuring wear and is the most straightforward to interpret if certain problems can be overcome. The first difficulty was discussed earlier and concerns the absorption of liquids by the polymer. The second problem is to mount the component so that there is ready removal for measurement while giving stability under the high loading during the test. The mounting arrangement must be such that material is not lost during the removal of the component and, in addition, it is necessary to locate the component accurately each time it is remounted. Due to these difficulties it is only recently that workable methods have been developed.

Treharne et al. [39] described the measurement of wear on an UHMWPE tibial component tested as part of a prosthesis on a knee simulator. The method was a development of that of McKellop et al. [40] employed in the wear testing of materials. Special mounting fixtures ensured that the tibial component could be removed and remounted after weighing. A control sample was employed to obtain the amount of fluid uptake which was used to correct the weight change on the wear sample to give the weight loss due to wear. The procedure was found to be accurate to within ±0.01 mg.

Clarke [29] has described a system for use on a multi-channel hip joint simulator in which specially designed fixtures allow the acetabular cup to be removed for weighing. Soak-control specimens in identical fixtures are used to correct for fluid absorption.

(ii) Dimensional measurement of wear – the difficulties with this method are as for the dimensional measurement of wear on wear testing machines with the added complication of the geometry of the device. Attempts have been made to employ a control sample to account for the deformation due to creep. However, in most studies employing this method of measurement it has been accepted that the measurements give a combined picture of creep and wear.

The earliest measurements were of the single-point type in which the thickness of the component was measured at the location of greatest wear [25]. However, measurement of the thickness change of UHMWPE acetabular cups over the entire surface has been carried out using an electro-mechanical depth gauge [24]. This technique has recently been extended by coupling the measuring head to a computer to automatically produce a contour map of the cup.

An alternative technique has been employed at the Royal National Orthopaedic Hospital, Stanmore in which measurements are made on a replica of the cup using a profilometer. Originally plaster of paris was used but more recently silicone rubber has been employed.

(iii) measurement by the collection of wear debris – several techniques have been utilized for the collection of wear debris as a means of evaluating the wear of prosthesis components. Simple filtering of the test fluid was used in several evaluations of joint prostheses but the technique did not gain wide acceptance [38].

More recently there has been a resurgence of interest in the use of wear debris collection as a wear measuring technique. Rose et al. [41] developed a technique by which wear debris could be separated from serum or other body fluid. The method involved denaturing the fluid with potassium hydroxide followed by filtration to obtain the particulate matter which would include blood debris as well as wear particles. A density gradient column was used to separate the wear particles from the debris. In this way wear amounts down to a fraction of a milligram could be measured. Although this method does allow wear to be measured it is time-consuming and difficult and has not been adopted elsewhere.

Ferrography is a technique developed for the analysis of metallic particles in lubrication oil. Separation of the particles by size is carried out by passing the liquid between the poles of a magnet having a very high field gradient. A change in the technique has allowed it to be extended to non-magnetic particles by utilizing a prior treatment in a magnetic ion solution. The method has been used to study wear particles from around prostheses in patients but has not yet been used with joint simulators [42].

(iv) optical methods – holographic interferometry has been used on a trial basis to measure the dimensional changes in acetabular cups and tibial components [43,38]. Several different techniques have been employed. Dual index holographic contouring shows the greatest promise but while qualitative demonstration of the wear and deformation is straightforward the quantification is more difficult. The optical techniques work best for surfaces which are planar or nearly so and are best applied to components such as tibial plateaux. There is greater difficulty in using the techniques on a component such as an acetabular cup.

There is no one technique which has been standardized for the measurement of wear of prostheses tested on simulators. Methods involving debris collection are involved and are not likely to be widely used. Holographic methods are still in the development stage and although success is likely with tibial components the outcome is less certain with components having a high degree of curvature. Optical methods measure dimensional changes and so include the deformation contribution. Direct dimensional measurements may be made. Computer controlled profile measurements are still being developed. Such measurements again include a deformational component. Recent improvements in weight loss measurements hold promise for this technique. Overall evaluation of a device, however, will require not only the measurement of wear but also the study of the degree and location of deformation. Thus there will be a need for both weight loss and dimensional measurements to be made.

5.5 In Vivo Evaluation

The advantage of *in vivo* evaluation of a joint replacement is that the device is tested under the end-use conditions but this is offset by the difficulty in the measurement of wear while the prosthesis is in place. Devices can be removed for examination but this cannot be done as a routine measure; devices are removed due to compromise of the mechanical function or because of a biological reaction often manifested as pain. The evaluation of a device in an animal is mainly to show safety and so most of the *in vivo* and *ex vivo* studies of wear have been done with patients. It may be noted that in contrast to laboratory wear testers and joint simulators, where friction may be measured as part of the evaluation procedure, friction is not measured *in vivo*.

In vivo wear has been evaluated by roentogenographic methods. In principle wear could be measured by the collection of debris but this would require aspiration of the patient, a procedure only carried out if there is a problem requiring removal of fluid for bacterial culture or other purposes. The ferrographic technique is not likely to become widespread. A study of removed implants also allows the estimation of wear but as has been mentioned this is not a routine procedure. It must be emphasized that examination of a removed implant and roengenographic measurement *in situ* are dimensional techniques which give deformation as well as wear. There is no satisfactory way of separating the two components of dimensional change. In the past it has been assumed that changes in dimension measured after long times of implantation reflect wear since creep may be assumed to level off but this has by no means been proven.

Roengenographic measurements have been employed with total hip prostheses with polymeric acetabular cups. For the Charnley prosthesis a metal marker wire is fixed to the acetabular cup in the coronal plane (polar wire position). In the Muller prosthesis the acetabular cup employs an equatorial marker wire. The distance between the femoral head and the marker wire is used to give the reduction in thickness of the acetabular component after correction for magnification and other factors. Thus the technique gives one measurement only, the reduction in thickness of the cup in the direction of greatest wear. Further details of the technique and measurements are given elsewhere [44]. X-ray techniques have not been employed with prostheses other than the hip due to geometrical considerations.

Ex vivo examination of all types of devices has been carried out. An advantage of such an examination is that the overall pattern of wear and deformation may be obtained.

5.6. Techniques Employed

Information on the wear of joint prosthesis components and on materials has been obtained by a wide variety of techniques. Many materials have been evaluated on laboratory wear testing machines. Fewer materials, as part of devices, have been examined on joint simulators. Very few materials combinations have been studied *in vivo*. The majority of data have been gathered with respect to total hip implantation. In the following discussion the results mentioned will pertain to total hip replacement with only cursory mention of knee prostheses and replacements at the other joints.

In examining the data there are several questions to be borne in mind:

(i) 316LVM stainless steel or cast Co-Cr-Mo alloy bearing against UHMWPE have been the most widely used combinations. What is the wear rate of UHMWPE and can predictions on the performance in the body be made from measurements made on laboratory testing machines or on joint simulators?

(ii) variations in the standard materials have been made. For example Co-Cr-Mo alloy components have been produced by forging and by powder metallurgy techniques. UHMWPE components have been produced directly from powder rather than by machining from block material. Carbon fiber filled UHMWPE components have been produced with the object of reduction of creep. What are the effects of these changes on the wear rate?

(iii) with the standard materials different designs and sizes have been used. What are the effects of design change on the wear rate? If acrylic bone cement particles are trapped between the joint surfaces, what is the effect on the rate of wear?

(iv) POM has been used for a restricted number of designs. Is the wear rate of POM higher or lower than that of UHMWPE and should this polymer be employed as a joint prosthesis material?

(v) other materials have recently been introduced for total hip replacement. Femoral components of Ti-6Al-4V alloy have been employed. Laboratory studies have indicated that high rates of wear of UHMWPE may be encountered against this alloy. Are these reports correct and under what conditions is the high wear encountered? Is the same effect to be found with prostheses in patients? It has further been reported that the wear is exacerbated by the ingress of acrylic debris and there is interest in seeing whether this effect is found *in vivo*.

Alumina ceramics have been used in alumina/alumina and in alumina/UHMWPE combinations and the basis for this was the reduction in wear expected. A review of the performance of these combinations is of importance to see whether the expectations are borne out in practice.

The above represent just some of the areas which require examination. Rather than to consider the wear of materials in the context of techniques, the approach will be to consider the information available from a variety of measurements on each combination in turn. Where possible performance at joints other than the hip will be considered.

6. WEAR RESULTS FOR MATERIALS AND DEVICES

6.1 Established Alloys/UHMWPE

6.1.1 Wear Test Results

Cast Co-Cr-Mo alloy and 316LVM stainless steel sliding against UHMWPE have been extensively evaluated over the past 10 years due to the widespread use of these combinations in joint prostheses. There have been wide variations in the results reported due to different starting material e.g. irradiated or non-irradiated UHMWPE, test geometry, test conditions or method of wear measurement. These results have been examined for validity and summarized [45,46,47].

There appears to be little difference in the wear of UHMWPE whether cast Co-Cr-Mo alloy or 316LVM stainless steel counterfaces are used. For example McKellop et al. [40] at a pressure of 6.90 MPa found the wear of UHMWPE to be 0.20 $mm^3/10^6$ cycles (equivalent to 0.65 μm/year) against stainless steel and 0.17 $mm^3/10^6$ cycles (0.55 μm/year) against Co-Cr-Mo alloy. These results are in line with the findings of other studies but considerably higher wear rates have been published for UHMWPE, some 50 times higher, for studies on other types of wear testing machines. It may be noted that even these higher results are indicative of very low wear rates in an absolute sense. McKellop has remarked "... we concluded that the very low polyethylene wear in our laboratory wear study corresponds to the minimum potential wear rate *in vivo* ..." [46]. However, it may be argued that a wear test machine is satisfactory if it allows combinations to be ranked even if it is not possible to calculate the wear rate to be expected for that combination in service. This is, in fact, what Clark [47] and McKellop [46] now argue. Since by far the largest series of combinations have been examined by McKellop the results obtained in this series will be presented. This allows the performance of combinations of materials to be evaluted.

As mentioned the wear of UHMWPE in irradiated form is little different whether stainless steel or cast Co-Cr-Mo alloy is used as a counterface. There are, however, variations on the processing of the cobalt base alloys since, to improve fatigue strength, forging and powder metallurgy techniques have been employed. At 3.45 MPa wear rates of 0.17 $mm^3/10^6$ cycles were obtained for UHMWPE/forged Co-Cr-Mo alloy and 0.14 $mm^3/10^6$ cycles for UHMWPE/Co-Cr-Mo alloy produced by powder metallurgy techniques [40]. These wear values are not statistically different. Thus the changes in processing do not affect the wear rate of UHMWPE; the wear rate against the cast material is 0.17 $mm^3/10^6$ cycles at 6.90 MPa.

UHMWPE components may be modified in various ways. Irradiation is used for sterilization and this causes cross-linking which could alter the wear rate. Irradiation also introduces carbonyl groups which cause the polymer to absorb a higher level of fluid than in the unirradiated state. Early results either showed no change in wear rate or an increase by about a factor of two. Recent results support the contention that irradiation causes an increase in the wear rate of UHMWPE [40].

Molding of UHMWPE components from powder is an alternative processing technique to machining the components from block. It has been shown that the wear of molded and machined specimens is virtually identical [40].

Carbon fiber reinforced UHMWPE has been used in those components where creep was a problem due to high contact stresses. Early results gave very high wear rates after initial low rates of wear due to abrasion caused by break-down of the composite in which fibers were released. Later results did not show this behavior and wear rates either the same as for the unreinforced material or even lower were found [45]. Recent results have shown that the surface of the composite can become gray and roughened due to the release of carbon fibers at and near the surface. Somewhat higher wear rates than for the unreinforced polymer were found and it was estimated that the carbon fiber reinforced material would give a wear rate some 4 times that of the unreinforced UHMWPE. The situation regarding the performance of the carbon fiber reinforced material is as yet not resolved.

6.1.2 Simulator Results

There have been few results published for hip prostheses and of those published the wear data have been published in comparative terms. However, Rose et al. [41] tested standard Charnley and Muller prostheses of cast Co-Cr-Mo alloy against UHMWPE over simulated implantation periods of 1 and 10 years. Six prostheses were tested for the one year simulation. In four cases it was possible to collect UHMWPE wear debris and the wear varied from 0.3 mg to 10.2 mg. Assuming a contact area of 5 cm^2 the measurements gave a wear depth of 0.0006-0.02 mm but a total recession of 0.035-0.1 mm was found showing that most of the dimensional change was due to deformation. In the 10 year simulation wear debris were collected for the last year of simulation. One prosthesis gave 1.1 mg and the other 0.76 mg corresponding to wear depths of 0.003 and 0.002 mm.

Hip simulator results have been reviewed elsewhere [29,38]. It is interesting to note that results have been given for carbon fiber reinforced UHMWPE indicating that the wear rate is at least a factor of 4 lower than that of unreinforced UHMWPE [48].

Recent results have been published for knee simulation studies on five types of knee prosthesis with a cast Co-Cr-Mo alloy/UHMWPE combination of materials. An RMC design showed the lowest wear rate of 1.48 mg/10^6 cycles (equivalent to one year of use in the body) while the highest wear was from a UCI-type design which gave a wear rate of 30.3 mg/10^6 cycles [39].

Limited results have also been given on the performance of UHMWPE and carbon fiber reinforced UHMWPE at the knee, hip and ankle. In all cases the wear of the reinforced material was lower by at least a factor of two. The wear rate was highest at the hip and about the same at the knee and ankle for UHMWPE. Results on the hip joint simulator were also given for UHMWPE and the carbon fiber reinforced material bearing against different metal components [48]. Tables 14, 15, and 16 show the data. The wear data for carbon reinforced UHMWPE have yet to be confirmed by other studies.

Table 14. The Wear of UHMWPE and Carbon Fiber Filled UHMWPE on a Hip Joint Simulator

Acetabular Cup Material	No. of test cycles	wear rate (g/cycle)
UHMWPE	3.1×10^6	3.80×10^{-8}
UHMWPE	1.8	4.78
UHMWPE	2.2	2.00
C-PE 10 percent	3.5	3.80×10^{-9}
C-PE 10 percent	2.7	4.40
C-PE 10 percent	1.8	4.40
C-PE 15 percent	3.5	5.20
C-PE 20 percent	3.5	4.80

Table 15. The Wear of UHMWPE and Carbon Fiber Filled UHMWPE at the Hip, Knee and Ankle in Simulation

Test Machine	Wear Rate ($mm^3/10^6$ cycles)	
	UHMWPE	C-PE
Hip Simulator	25.1	6.55
Ankle Simulator	6.10	3.18
Knee Motion Simulator	6.54	1.50

Table 16. The Effect of Counterface Material on the Wear of UHMWPE and Carbon Fiber Filled UHMWPE on a Hip Joint Simulator

Femoral Component	Diameter	Wear Rate ($mm^3/10^6$ cycles)	
		UHMWPE	C-PE
316L SS	28mm	25.3	6.07
H.I.P. Co-Cr-Mo	28	16.0	5.73
Ti-6Al-4V	28	26.0	-
MP 35N	28	41.9	12.5
Alumina	32	6.74	5.01

In comparing the simulator results for UHMWPE it may be seen that the wear rates differ considerably from a low of 0.3 mg to a high of 25 mg at the hip. However, even the highest wear rate is still a low wear rate in absolute terms. The results for prostheses at the knee and ankle show wear rates in the same range.

6.1.3 In Vivo Results

The measurements of wear *in vivo* has only been done for the UHMWPE acetabular components of total hip prostheses. The measurements only give the total of wear and deformation and are subject to great error unless much care is taken. A review is given elsewhere [44]. For the Charnley total hip prosthesis the most recent data are for a follow up period of 7-9 years. The average "wear" was 0.59 mm giving an average of 0.07 mm/year (70μm). Of the 491 hips surveyed, 312 sockets showed less than 0.06 mm/year dimensional change but 20 had worn at 0.24 mm/year. Data have also been presented for patients with Muller prostheses, which differ from the Charnley prosthesis is having a 32 mm diameter femoral head as against a 22 mm diameter head. The Muller device employs a cast Co-Cr-Mo alloy femoral head while 316L stainless steel is used for the Charnley prosthesis. For 57 patients treated with the Muller prosthesis with follow-up of 2-4 years a "wear" rate of 0.05-0.4 mm/year was found.

6.1.4 Ex Vivo Results

There have been many studies carried out on removed components. Total hip prostheses, total knee devices and prostheses from other joint have been examined. Reference is made to the most recent examinations [44,49,50].

Rose et al. [49] examined 15 total hip prostheses and 35 total knee prostheses which had been in place for up to 8 years. A wide range of designs was included in the removed knee group but only two designs of total hip prosthesis were examined. Attention was directed at the wear of the UHMWPE components. It was found in many cases that acrylic bone cement particles were embedded in the UHMWPE components and in a few cases bone particles were embedded. The trapped debris appeared to be responsible for the formation of craters in the polymer however the nature of the fabrication process of UHMWPE components is essentially a sintering process in which the polymer particles bond together and incompletely sintered material can easily be removed from the surface to form a crater irrespective of the presence of acrylic cement. Fatigue wear of UHMWPE was associated with the presence of low molecular weight polymer at the surface.

Clarke [50] examined a group of some 30 retrieved UHMWPE sockets with 6 months to 8 years follow-up. There were no examples of gross wear and the cups varied in appearance from highly polished minimal wear to moderate surface disruption due to the ingress of acrylic bone cement. Also given in this publication is a review of other findings. Thus the appearance of the cups was stated to be similar to those examined by Dowling and co-workers. Reports were given of cases of fracture of the acetabular component. In one series of 34 hips, 6 showed severe wear and 1 had broken into five fragments. There have been several other reports of fracture and also cases of severe acetabular cup wear [see 50].

Severe deformation and damage on UHMWPE tibial components has been reported [50]. Contributing factors include the presence of bone cement, the presence of bone chips, malpositioning of the device and impact of the prosthesis against bone. Scaring, cracking and pitting have been reported and in some cases fracture of the tibial component occurred.

For a removed ankle prosthesis component in UHMWPE there was extensive wear, wrinkles, cracks and pits. The contralateral joint had a similar prosthesis but with carbon fiber reinforced UHMWPE and this component showed much less wear [see 50].

There have been many more studies of removed components than those mentioned here. One problem with such reports is the anecdotal nature of the material. However, the removal of prostheses does afford an opportunity to examine the device. As a generalization it may be stated that with UHMWPE against stainless steel or Co-Cr-Mo alloy the removal is almost invariably for loosening and is not a direct consequence of wear. There is a great variety of appearances on removed components ranging from an unused appearance to a highly damaged appearance. The appearance of UHMWPE components from the knee invariably shows higher damage than components from the hip. The *ex vivo* studies have highlighted the damage caused by acrylic bone cement and other third bodies and have indicated the existence of fracture as a failure mechanism. Fracture had not been considered up to that time because of the ductility of UHMWPE and its existence points to the possibility of a degradation effect. Examination of removed components has also directed attention to the fabrication of UHMWPE components and the manner in which surface damage is a consequence of polymer morphology. Study of removed components has not allowed the rate of wear of UHMWPE to be established.

Examination of the metallic component has been carried out at the same time that the UHMWPE components have been studied. The wear of the metallic component is very low compared to that of the polymer component and the appearance usually indicates only burnishing or slight scratching.

6.1.5 Laboratory Evaluation and Clinical Results

It is only for the combinations stainless steel/UHMWPE or cast Co-Cr-Mo/UHMWPE that there is possibility of reaching a conclusion on the appropriateness of laboratory evaluations for predicting clinical results for it is only for these combinations that sufficient work has been done at each level of evaluation.

One approach is to calculate the rate of wear expected for a total hip prosthesis from the wear rate measured on a laboratory wear testing machine. In carrying out this calcualation there are several assumptions:

(i) it is assumed that for half the walking cycle the contact pressure at the hip is 3.45 MPa and for the other half of the cycle the pressure is zero.
(ii) the sliding distance under load per walking cycle is given by $d\theta/2$ where θ is the flexion-extension angle and d is the diameter of the femoral head. For a Charnley prosthesis this angle is 60 degrees and the head diameter is 22 mm.
(iii) it is assumed that the femoral head wears out a path equal to the diameter of the femoral head diameter.
(iv) that the wear rate in the laboratory reflects the wear rate *in vivo* where the load and speed vary throughout the walking cycle.

With the above assumptions the volume of wear per year is given by:

Volume = (penetration rate) (sliding distance) (area of femoral head)

or

$$V = \frac{\pi}{8} w\theta n d^3 \qquad (3)$$

where n is the number of walking cycles per year which may be taken as 1×10^6. For a Charnley prosthesis the volume of UHMWPE produced per year is 0.12 mm^3 or 0.11 mg if the wear rate is taken from the work of McKellop et al. as 0.15 μm per one million cycles (equivalent to a sliding distance of 5×10^7 mm).

The results from the extrapolation of wear test data are in fair agreement with the results obtained by Rose et al. [41] on simulation. To make this comparison n may be taken as 1.8×10^6 and for a Muller prosthesis d equals 32 mm. The weight loss calculated is found to be 0.65 mg.

The results from radiographic methods of evaluation indicate much higher rates of wear. Taking some of the more recent results for the Charnley device the average penetration of the head into the cup was 0.07 mm/year but some cups showed lower wear and a few cups much higher wear. Assuming that the wear volume equals the area of the femoral head times the depth of penetration gives a wear volume of approximately 25 mm^3 (density of UHMWPE may be taken as 0.94 giving a weight loss of about 23.5 mg).

Thus the *in vivo* wear rates appear to be larger than the wear rates measured on laboratory testing machines by a factor of about 200 (cf. 0.12 mm^3 versus 25 mm^3). A similar discrepancy is found for the lowest of the simulator wear rates but for the highest wear rate the factor is only two.

McKellop [46] has argued that there are several reasons for this discrepancy:

(i) the total penetration measured on radiographs includes an unknown amount of deformation. Tests under laboratory conditions have shown high rates of creep especially in the first few years of use [51].

(ii) the reported range of penetration rates represents the average of all the penetration rates observed. For many of the devices examined no penetration could be measured and for 28 percent of the devices the penetration was 50 μm per year or less.
(iii) the highest penetration rates may have been due to poorly-formed polyethylene, acrylic cement particles or excessive creep.

It is true that variability in the UHMWPE may be responsible for the highest "wear" rates seen possibly via a degradation effect due to interaction with body fluids which could also lead to fracture in extreme cases, a phenomenon occasionally seen in the body.

The effect of acrylic cement in increasing the rate of wear is not known. Although this possibility has been mentioned many times there have been no definitive experiments. Rovell et al. [52] have reproduced the surface patterns seen *ex vivo* by placing cement between articulating surfaces of a prosthesis under test but were not able to provoke an increase in the wear rate. There is no evidence to suggest that the wear rate of UHMWPE does increase due to the presence of bone cement despite the high degree of surface damage caused by acrylic particles.

It is likely that a large part of the penetration seen on X-ray is due to deformation. The results of Rose et al. [41] gave a value for penetration due to deformation about 10 times greater than the penetration due to wear.

Apart from the factors discussed there are several areas where there can be error in extrapolating from the laboratory wear rates to *in vivo* wear rates.

These errors include:

(i) the fact that the test is conducted under constant load while in the hip joint the load varies during the walking cycle.
(ii) the fact that the test is conducted with unidirectional motion while the motion is complex at the hip joint. Velocities and accelerations of the sliding surfaces are encountered at the hip joint which are not reproduced on the wear test machine.
(iii) the test being carried out on well-chosen polymer samples. Presumably defects of the type found in some acetabular components are avoided. In addition tests are carried out under clean conditions with no third body abrasion.
(iv) the assumption of parameters such as the number of walking cycles per year and the distance of sliding for each walking cycle.

Thus, the wear rate from radiographic measurements could be taken as a fraction of the lowest "wear" rate of 50 μm per year on the assumption that acrylic cement and other factors could cause the higher "wear" rates seen while the lowest "wear" rates represent the most favorable conditions as in a laboratory wear situation. Deformation could be as much as 80 percent of the penetration so that the wear would be some 10 μm per year. Now turning to the laboratory wear test situation the prediction is wear of 0.12 mm^3 per year which represents a penetration of approximately 0.35 μm per year. This figure can be increased by a factor of two since the contact stress might be 6.90 MPa rather than the 3.45 MPa assumed in the calculation. In addition a further factor of two could easily be introduced by doubling the sliding distance for one year of use. The wear rate of 0.15 μm/million cycles is at the low end of the values found by McKellop et al. and a further factor of two could be assumed. With these corrections the wear rate from the laboratory tests would be about 3 μm per year. It can be seen that the wear predictions from the laboratory tests can be forced to fit the modified predictions from *in vivo* measurements but the question is whether or not such a procedure is at all worthwhile. It may be noted that simulator results fit quite well with the radiographic measurements if it is assumed that the latter measurements include a high percentage of deformation.

The *ex vivo* examination of total hip prostheses indicates that in many cases the wear is very low. This adds weight to the approach of taking the lowest penetration rates as the basis for comparison with the laboratory wear studies.

6.2 The Wear of UHMWPE Against Ti-6Al-4V

6.2.1 Introduction

The alloy Ti-6Al-4V has been investigated for use as a femoral component material because it is readily worked to give high mechanical strength and high fatigue strength. It has been argued that the modulus of elasticity of this alloy, which is only half that of 316LVM stainless steel or Co-Cr-Mo alloy, allows greater transfer of stress from the prosthesis to the bone which is beneficial for osteogenesis. Higher stresses in bone cement may be generated, however, metal sensitivity has not been demonstrated for patients with this alloy. Whatever the merits of these arguments the above reasons provided a driving force for the introduction of this alloy and so it was necessary to examine the wear behavior of the combination Ti-6Al-4V/UHMWPE.

6.2.2 Laboratory Studies

The wear behavior has been examined on wear test machines and on simulators and the results have been reviewed by Dumbleton [38,44], Clarke et al. [53] and Rostoker and Galante [54].

Two types of behavior have been shown on laboratory wear test machines. In the first type the wear of UHMWPE is unremarkable and is about the same as for combination with other metallic alloys in common use. Even though there are differences in the absolute wear rate of UHMWPE between different studies, the wear of UHMWPE against Ti-6Al-4V and against stainless steel or Co-Cr-Mo alloy could be compared and were found to be close in value [38]. For example McKellop et al. [46] found that the wear of UHMWPE for one million cycles was 0.20, 0.08 and 0.14 mm^3 against 316 stainless, Ti-6Al-4V and hot pressed Co-Cr-Mo alloy respectively. Nitrided Ti-6Al-4V alloy gave slightly higher wear rate of 0.27 mm^3/million cycles for UHMWPE.

The second type of behavior involves the catastrophic wear of the UHMWPE polymer along with surface damage to the titanium alloy counterface and the production of large quantities of black debris. This type of behavior has been well described in the various studies of Rostoker and Galante [54]. It was proposed, based on these results, that the high wear rates were due to breakdown of the oxide surface layer on the titanium alloy. Thus treatment by growth of the layer by passivation or the use of nitriding treatments could lead to more stable surface layers.

Further complication of the picture ensued from the investigation of the wear of UHMWPE against Ti-6Al-4V alloy in the presence of acrylic bone cement. Before the placement of the cement particles between the surfaces the wear was normal but rapidly rose to a high value with the addition of the bone cement. There was high damage to the polymer and to the titanium alloy and a black deposit formed. This behavior was found for UHMWPE against unmodified Ti-6Al-4V surfaces but did not occur with nitrided Ti-6Al-4V alloy or for other alloys such as cast Co-Cr-Mo alloy or stainless [46]. It may be noted that the author was unable to reproduce the high wear situation for UHMWPE against titanium alloy even in the presence of acrylic bone cement; catastrophic wear could only be initiated if a very hard third body such as alumina powder was introduced between the sliding surfaces.

In a recent review Clarke et al. [53] point to three investigations on wear testing machines which found high wear of UHMWPE and three which did not. In the case of experiments with acrylic bone cement two studies showed high wear and one did not. The picture from wear testing is, therefore, confused.

An equally confusing situation exists from hip simulator studies. According to Clarke et al. [53] several of the studies are not relevant either because of inappropriate test conditions or because the objective was not to measure wear; for example the objective of one study was to generate wear debris for biological evaluation of compatibility. In the one study judged as being relevant scarring and black discoloration was observed and this was judged to be a negative comment on the wear behavior.

In the case of acrylic bone cement contamination three studies were described [53]. In one study breakdown was observed but in the other two studies only normal behavior was seen. In the first case the simulator was really a wear testing machine since a constant load and uniaxial motion were employed. The author has introduced acrylic cement particles between the joint surfaces on a multi-stage hip joint simulator without observing high wear of the UHMWPE acetabular cup when rubbing against a Ti-6Al-4V alloy femoral component.

That the castastropic wear of UHMWPE against Ti-6Al-4V is caused by breakdown of the surface layer of the alloy has been demonstrated by Rostoker and Galante [54], who examined the wear against titanium alloy, in water and in bovine serum and compared the results to those obtained with 316LVM stainlees steel. Simply polished titanium alloy gave high rates of wear of UHMWPE but the wear rate could be brought down to the levels seen with other alloys by growth of the surface layer either through oxidation in air or by immersion in an oxidizing acid (passivation). Presumably the growth and stabilization of the surface layer on titanium alloy would play a role in resisting the abrasive effect of acrylic bone cement.

6.2.3 In Vivo Results

The use of Ti-6Al-4V alloy in joint prostheses is not widespread and has largely been confined to femoral components of total hip prostheses. Mixed cast Co-Cr-Mo alloy/titanium alloy devices have been used and are found in some custom-made devices. There have not been any reports of abnormal wear rates of UHMWPE acetabular cups when employed with Ti-6Al-4V femoral components. Clark et al. [53] have commented on a series of some 300 total hip implantations in which the UHMWPE/Ti-6Al-4V alloy combination were used. In eight instances the devices were either removed for other causes or inspected after being in place for times of 11 to 57 months. There was no evidence of metallic sludge, black staining or other abnormal wear phenomenon. The *in vivo* performance was excellent.

6.2.4 Comparison of In Vitro and In Vivo Results

The study of the wear rate of UHMWPE against Ti-6Al-4V alloy has not received as much attention as the wear of UHMWPE against other alloys. Attention has mainly been focused on the abnormally high rates of wear found under some circumstances. From the studies in which the abnormal wear was not found it would appear that the wear rate of UHMWPE against titanium alloy is about the same as against other alloys in common use.

The discrepancy among the different studies lies in the manner in which the titanium alloy surface was treated prior to testing breakdown of the layer can lead to abrasive third body wear. If a stable layer exists the wear behavior is unremarkable. The existence of a stable layer should also avoid breakdown due to the ingress of bone cement.

There have not been any cases of catastrophic wear reported in clinical use and this is probably due to the fact that devices receive a passivation treatment prior to packaging; this would give a stable surface layer. The behavior demonstrated in the laboratory in those cases of abnormally high wear is thus an artefact since it is a consequence of inappropriate preparation of the titanium alloy specimens but it does demonstrate what could happen should the surface layer on the prosthesis be damaged.

6.3 The Wear of Polyoxymethylene

6.3.1 Introduction

Polyoxymethylene (POM) and in some cases copolymers have been used for a considerable time in joint replacements on a restricted basis but in substantial quantities. POM is much harder than UHMWPE and so is less subject to large creep deformations. In addition, components of POM may be made by injection molding whereas UHMWPE is either formed by compression molding or by machining; thus there are advantages to using POM especially for components of complex shape. The use of this class of materials has been reviewed [4,55] and the early background will not be covered here. At the present time POM is employed for a trunnion bearing and an acetabular cup in the Christiansen total hip prosthesis, for an acetabular cup on a selected number of Stanmore total hip prostheses and in copolymer form for the isoelastic hip prosthesis.

6.3.2 Laboratory Wear Results

The question whether POM has a higher wear rate than UHMWPE when sliding against a metal counterface has involved some attention over a period of some 15 years without a definitive answer being given. McKellop [46] listed five studies of the wear of Delrin®, a homopolymer, against different counterfaces. In four of the studies the wear was worse than that of UHMWPE and in one case better. However, of these four studies one did not quantitatively evaluate the wear and in another the wear was only slightly higher than that of UHMWPE. Dumbleton [44] has pointed out that the wear of Delrin is high unless a protein containing fluid such as plasma is employed. Dumbleton, [44,55] found that the wear of Delrin was approximately 80 percent that of UHMWPE but McKellop [46] cited his own earlier work in which the wear of Delrin was as much as 200 times greater than the wear of UHMWPE. It has recently been pointed out that the wear rate of Delrin 150 obtained by Dumbleton was about 25 μm/million cycles at 3.45 MPa against 60 μm/million cycles for McKellop [55]. The discrepancy lay in the measurement of the wear of UHMWPE since the value given by Dumbleton was about 50 μm/million cycles while that given by McKellop was 1 μm/million

® Du Pont de Nemours

cycles. Furthermore the highest rate of wear was found by McKellop at a surface pressure of 6.90 MPa and was 600 μm/million cycles as against 3 μm/million cycles for UHMWPE. The question is whether the wear results of McKellop are valid and whether such wear rates would cause a problem *in vivo*.

The situation has been reviewed by McKellop [46] who now states that the earlier very high wear rates were partly caused by periods of high friction on the wear test machine during which the temperature also increased at the sliding surfaces. The data collected at 6.90 MPa were invalid. However it was felt that the wear rates at 3.45 MPa were valid. As noted above the wear rate for Delrin 150 at 3.45 MPa is close to that found by Dumbleton.

The wear of acetal copolymers has been evaluated in several studies. It is generally agreed that the wear of the copolymer is far higher than that of the homopolymer.

Few simulation studies of the wear of total hip devices with Delrin components have been carried out [55]. Early work gave a wear rate lower for a Delrin acetabular cup than for an UHMWPE cup. Simulation studies with the Christiansen prosthesis did not show any abnormal wear and thickness measurements made an UHMWPE and on Delrin acetabular cups gave similar results [55].

6.3.3 In Vivo Results

Since 1970 the Christiansen total hip prosthesis has been used in some 10,000 cases. There have been no reports of high rates of wear. Removed devices have been examined and the tissues from around the device studied. High levels of wear debris have not been seen. Further details on the experience are given elsewhere [55,44].

The results with the Christiansen prosthesis are in marked contrast to those obtained with the Stanmore prosthesis. This is a conventional total hip prosthesis with a cast Co-Cr-Mo alloy femoral component and a plastic acetabular cup for which UHMWPE is normally employed. For some 70 prostheses scales [56] has stated that Delrin 150 was used. At a recent follow-up 55 patients were examined. Six cups were removed. All cups were loose. In two cases the femoral components were loose. Some removals were due to pain which typically began 8-12 months post-operatively. X-rays showed gross wear of the cup and histology revealed birefringent particles and an active cellular response with giant cells and necrosis around the particles. Patients other than the six have clinical symptoms and more removals are expected. On removal penetration rates of between 0.71 and 1.76 mm/year were found corresponding to volumetric wear rates of 468 to 866 mm^3/year.

Morscher et al. [57] report on the clinical results with the isoelastic prosthesis. However, this is not a prosthesis involving the wear of the copolymer since a metallic femoral head is used. Interesting laboratory results are reported in which the lowest wear rates were obtained for acetal/polyethylene sliding pains.

6.3.4 In Vitro and In Vivo Results

There is reasonable agreement regarding the wear rate of POM in the form of Delrin 150 as determined on laboratory wear testing machines. Taking the results of McKellop [46] who gives the wear rate of Delrin 150 as 34 times that of UHMWPE and employing similar calculations as previously a wear volume of 4 mm^3/year is predicted. This is an exceedingly small volume of wear; even increasing some of the factors in the calculation would give a wear rate of no more than 20 mm^3/year.

Results from simulator studies are not of any use since quantitative measurements were not made or the test conditions were not optimum.

Clinical results are confusing. The wear rate is low for Delrin 150 in the Christiansen prosthesis and this is what would be predicted from the laboratory tests. For the Stanmore prosthesis the wear rates are 100 times higher than predicted in the laboratory. It must be remembered that the volumetric measurements include a deformation component but the creep of Delrin is low compared to that of UHMWPE and a reduction of the "wear" rate by 20 percent would be the maximum expected. There are several possible explanations. The Stanmore device has a femoral head size of 25 or 29 mm whereas the Christiansen has a head size of 37 mm. Thus the surface pressures will be higher for the Stanmore prosthesis. However, calculations show that the stress is very high for the trunnion on the Christiansen prosthesis and high wear of this component is not seen. An alternative explanation is that Delrin was not employed in the Stanmore prosthesis but that the copolymer was used; this would explain the high wear rates seen.

6.4 The Wear of Alumina

6.4.1 Introduction

In recent years high purity alumina has been employed in total hip prostheses. Two combinations have been used: alumina/alumina and alumina/UHMWPE. Problems have been found with all-alumina sliding combinations due to fractures and high wear in some cases. Only the wear of alumina/UHMWPE devices will be considered.

6.4.2 Laboratory Wear Results

There have been various reports on the wear of UHMWPE against high purity alumina [45]. These reports indicate that the wear of UHMWPE against alumina may be as little as one-tenth that of UHMWPE sliding against metallic alloys. McKellop et al. [40] reported on other studies which showed that UHMWPE against alumina gave less than one-half the wear rate of the polymer against the commonly used alloys. McKellop et al. [40] in their own studies found that the wear rate of UHMWPE against alumina was as low as, but not lower than, the wear rate against metallic counterfaces.

Simulator studies reviewed in [40] give wear rates from UHMWPE against alumina down to one-twentieth the wear rate against metallic alloys. Clarke [29] reported on other simulator studies which indicated that the wear of UHMWPE against alumina was about one half the wear rate of UHMWPE/metallic combinations.

6.4.3 In Vivo Results

There have been few reports on the performance of UHMWPE/alumina total hip prostheses. Early radiographic measurements on five Muller prostheses with alumina heads and UHMWPE cups gave an average penetration rate of 0.1 mm/year for followup times of 12 to 38 months. Results on UHMWPE cups with cast Co-Cr-Mo alloys heads gave a penetration rate of 0.2 mm/year for the first three years and 0.1 mm/year for the following three years [44]. The implication is that the wear with alumina is lower but the number of patients is too small and the followup time too short to be sure.

6.4.4 In Vitro and In Vivo Results

Laboratory wear tests and simulator tests indicate that the wear of UHMWPE against alumina is no higher than and is probably lower than the wear against metallic alloys in use. This conclusion seems to be borne out by clinical useage but the results available are too limited for firm conclusions.

7. LABORATORY PREDICTION AND CLINICAL PERFORMANCE

There have been many investigations of the friction and wear of different materials combinations; combinations either used and discarded, combinations in use or combinations contemplated for use in joint prostheses. Testing and evaluation have been studied at different levels including the wear testing of materials, simulator testing of materials/device combinations, animal studies and clinical study. Animal studies are of more relevance for testing biocompatibilty rather than evaluating the performance of a device.

It must be stated that many of the materials and designs placed in service in the early days of joint replacement were either not tested prior to implantation or were tested in a cursory fashion. The following were identified as unsuited for clinical use and were subsequently withdrawn from clinical use: PTFE as an acetabular cup, PET as a femoral head, POM as a femoral head, UHMWPE as a femoral head and bearing against articular cartilage; all-metal prostheses have all but disappeared from the market.

There has been a recent resurgence in the testing of some of these materials since it was felt that one way of judging the correctness of a test was in its ability to differentiate between materials which were withdrawn from service due to high wear rates and those materials giving satisfactory performance. Among others this type of approach has been employed by McKellop [46] for wear testing of PTFE, PET, POM and UHMWPE, which under the same conditions gave wear rates of 322, 160, 9.4 and 0.2 mm^3/one million cycles at 6.90 MPa. This rating of materials is in line with clinical performance. Clarke [29,58] has examined PTFE and UHMWPE acetabular components on a hip joint stimulator. In the initial study the PTFE cup wore at a rate of 2100 mm^3/year or a depth of penetration of 3.4 mm per year. This penetration value agrees well with the typical rate of penetration of 2 mm/year found clinically. The wear of the UHMWPE cup was judged to be too slight for measurement. However, the later study gave wear rates of 80 mm^3 per million cycles for UHMWPE against Co-Cr-Mo alloy equivalent to 0.1 mm per year penetration.

In discussing the relevance of laboratory tests the combinations UHMWPE/Co-Cr-Mo alloy, UHMWPE/316LVM stainless steel, UHMWPE/Ti-6Al-4V, UHMWPE/alumina and POM/Co-Cr-Mo alloy were discussed. The performance of these combinations will be reviewed.

For UHMWPE against Co-Cr-Mo alloy (cast, forged or produced by powder metallurgy techniques) the wear is low and cannot be differentiated from the wear against 316LVM stainless steel. It matters little whether machined or directly formed UHMWPE components are used. Many different values have been obtained for the wear rate of UHMWPE on wear testing machines but the most recent studies indicate exceedingly low wear rates which predict *in vivo* wear rates perhaps 100 times lower than those observed. On the other hand there are considerable errors in the *in vivo* wear rates and in the extrapolation of wear test results so that the two sets of data can be forcefitted together at a penetration rate of 10 μm/year. The picture is further confused by the simulator results. The data of Rose et al. [41] cover a wide range but fit into the gap between the *in vivo* measurements and the wear test predictions. However, the latest results [58] indicate a penetration of about 0.1 mm/year, a value in excellent agreement with the *uncorrected* radiographic measurements which supposedly contain a large deformation component. If these latest results are correct the implication is that the radiographic measurements provide a good basis for the evaluation of the wear rate. In addition it must be supposed that wear rates based on the collection of wear debris are subject to error by incomplete collection and the results from the wear test machine are not only much lower than the *in vivo* results but also are much lower than the simulator results.

The wear of carbon fiber filled UHMWPE has been shown to be of the same order as the wear of the unfilled polymer. Clinical results are awaited.

The wear of UHMWPE against Ti-6Al-4V alloy is low and is about the same as for UHMWPE against the commonly used alloys. High rates of wear are seen if breakdown of the surface layer occurs; this has happened in laboratory wear situations with samples for which the surface layer was not stabilized. Clinical and laboratory tests show normal wear when there is appropriate surface preparation. Recent simulator results give the wear of UHMWPE against Ti-6Al-4V alloy as 102 mm^3 per year compared to 80 mm^3 per year against Co-Cr-Mo alloy [58].

The wear of UHMWPE against alumina appears to be about the same as for UHMWPE against metallic alloys with the tendency for the wear against alumina to be slightly less. Clinical results also suggest this but there is little information available.

The wear of POM against metallic alloys is somewhat higher than the wear of UHMWPE but the wear rate is low. Clinically there is one extensive series in which wear is not a problem but definitive measurements have not been made. In a smaller series wear has been a severe problem which would not have been predicted from laboratory wear rates. The reason for this high wear rate is not known.

There is a need for wear testing on simple machines and a joint simulator but the extrapolation of the results to the *in vivo* situation is neither simple nor straightforward. Many of these points are covered elsewhere [4]. Clarke [47] has examined the validity of wear screening protocols and has recommended multiple long-term tests of each material combination at different sets of conditions. McKellop [46] considers his machine to be capable of indicating those materials with wear resistance clearly adequate for clinical use, those obviously inadequate and possibly those which fall in between these two classes and which require further testing. Clarke [29] has stated that there is "a practical and exciting role ahead for hip joint simulators" and it has been indicated that the hip joint simulator developed provides a reliable method for determining the effect of materials and design on the wear of prostheses [58]. These are all positive statements but considerable standardization and testing are required before the results of wear testing and simulation can be accepted as giving a quantitative indication of performance rather than merely a qualitative ranking.

Besides the matters covered it is clear that there is as yet no answer on the effect of acrylic bone cement on the wear of UHMWPE. The existence of high wear rates of UHMWPE *in vivo* which are found in some cases has not been explained, neither has the fracture of some components. There are factors which have not been adequately explored and hence have not yet been included or considered in *in vitro* tests.

It may never be possible to give a wear rate which will allow a material to be definitely recommended for use in a prosthesis. The biological factors have not been discussed here but failures due to high levels of wear debris have been reported for different materials [5]. What is defined as high depends on the nature of the material, the debris size and the quantity of material liberated per unit time. Thus biological testing must be done to decide on the level of debris that can be tolerated by the tissues for each material. In practice the engineering approach has been to strive for a wear rate as low as possible. More sophisticated techniques are desirable if a prosthesis lifetime of some 30 years is required.

Most of the discussion of joints has been in terms of total hip prostheses. There has been little simulation work carried out on prostheses for the knee and for the other joints. As the implanted lifetime of these devices becomes longer there will be a need to develop simulation techniques for these joints and to develop techniques of wear measurement for *in vivo* evaluation.

8. CONCLUSION

The study of wear of materials for joint replacement has been under way for some 20 years but there is still a wide variety of machines and simulators employed. The results show that the wear rate of UHMWPE at the hip is very low provided the correct configuration of component is used. There is a discrepancy between the wear rates produced in the laboratory for UHMWPE and the wear rates obtained *in vivo*. Simulator results are confused with the latest data tending to reinforce the radiographic findings.

For UHMWPE it matters little whether alumina, 316LVM stainless steel, Co-Cr-Mo alloy or Ti-6Al-4V is used as a counterface material.

The wear of POM is low but not as low as the wear of UHMWPE. There is, as yet, no explanation for high wear rates found in one clinical series.

There is a tendency to standardize laboratory wear testing and hip joint simulation. Little testing for joints other than the hip has been carried out but is to be expected in the future.

For prediction of the performance at long times of implantation it is essential to carry out biological evaluation in conjunction with wear evaluation.

REFERENCES

1. Scales, J. T., "Arthroplasty of the Hip Using Foreign Materials: A History," *in "Lubrication and Wear in Living and Artificial Human Joints," Proc. Instn. Mech. Engrs., 181* pt. 3J, 63-89, 1966-1967.
2. Walker, P. S., "Human Joints and Their Artificial Replacements," Charles C. Thomas, Springfield, Illinois, 1978.
3. Hori, R. Y., Lewis, J. L., Zimmerman, J. R. and Compere, C. L., "The Number of Total Joint Replacements in the United States," Clinical Orthopaedics and Related Research, *132,* 46-52, (1978).
4. Dumbleton, J. H., "Tribology of Natural and Artificial Joints," Elsevier, Amsterdam (1981).
5. Dumbleton, J. H. and Black, J., "Some Long Term Complications of Total Hip Replacements," *in* "Complications of Total Hip Replacement," Ling, R. (ed), Churchill Livingston, Edinburgh, to be published.
6. Swanson, S. A. V. and Freeman, M. A. R. (eds), "The Scientific Basis of Joint Replacement," Pitman Medical, Tunbridge Wells, Kent (1977).
7. Dumbleton, J. H., "Tribology of Natural and Artificial Joints," Elsevier, Amsterdam (1981), Chapter 4.
8. Dumbleton, J. H., "Tribology of Natural and Artificial Joints," Elsevier, Amsterdam (1981), pp. 140-147.
9. Amstutz, H. C., "Polymers as Bearing Materials for Total Hip Replacement: A Friction and Wear Analysis," J. Biomed. Mater. Res., 3, (1968), 547-568.
10. Charnley, J., "The Wear of Plastics Materials in the Hip Joint," Plastics and Rubber, 1, (1976), 59-63.
11. Galante, J. O. and Rostoker, W., "Wear in Total Hip Prostheses," Acta, Orthop. Scand., Suppl., 145 (1973).

12. Walker, P. S. and Erkman, M. J., "Metal-on-Metal Lubrication in Artificial Human Joints," Wear, 21 (1972), 377-392.
13. Walker, P. S. and Erkman, M. J., "Variables Affecting Polymer Wear in Artificial Human Joints," Lieng-Huang Lee (ed), in Advances in Polymer Friction and Wear, Vol. 58, Plenum Press, New York, 1974, 553-565.
14. Beutler, H., Lehmann, M. and Staehli, G., "Wear Behaviour of Medical Engineering Materials," Wear, 33 (1975), 337-350.
15. Dumbleton, J. H., Shen, C. and Miller, E. H., "A Study of the Wear of Some Materials in Connection with Total Hip Replacement," Wear, 29, (1974), 163-171.
16. Scales, J. T. and Lowe, S. A., "Choosing Materials for Bone and Joint Replacements," M. Jayson (ed) in Total Hip Replacement, London, Sector Publishing, 1971.
17. Shim, H. S. and Schon, F. J., "The Wear Resistance of Pure and Silicon-Alloyed Isotropic Carbons," Report of the General Atomic Company, San Diego, October 1973.
18. McKellop, H., Clarke, I. C. and Markolf, K., "Friction and Wear Evaluation of Prosthesis Materials using a 12-Channel Screening Device," Proc. 21st SAMOE Meeting, Los Angeles, 1976, 508-521.
19. Ungethum, M., "Requirements of Operational Tests and Test Results in Total Hip and Knee Arthroplasty," M. Schaldach and D. Hohmann (eds), in Artificial Hip and Knee Joint Technology, Springer-Verlag, Berlin, 1976, 493-518.
20. Dowson, D., Atkinson, J. R. and Brown, D., "The Wear of UHMWPE with Particular Reference to its use in Artificial Human Joints," Lieng-Huang Lee (ed) in Advances in Polymer Friction and Wear, Vol. 58, Plenum Press, New York, 1974.
21. Trent, P. S. and Walker, P. S., "Wear and Conformity in Total Knee Replacement," Wear 36, (1976), 176-187.
22. Ungethum, M., Report on activities in the Munich Biomechanics Laboratory.
23. Dumbleton, J. H., unpublished work.
24. Weightman, B. O., Paul, I. L., Rose, R. M., Simon, S. R. and Radin, E. L., "A Comparative Study of Total Hip Replacement Prostheses," J. Biomechanics, 6, (1973), 299-311.
25. Dumbleton, J. H., Miller, D. A. and Miller, E. H., "A Simulator for Load Bearing Joints," Wear, 20, (1972), 165-174.
26. Ungethum, M., "Requirements of Operational Tests and Test Results in Total Hip and Knee Arthroplasty," in Artificial Hip and Knee Joint Technology, M. Schaldach and D. Hohmann (eds), Springer-Verlag, Berlin, 1976.
27. Swanson, S. A. V., Freeman, M. A. R. and Heath, J. C., "Laboratory Tests on Total Joint Replacement Prostheses," J.B.J.S., 55B, (1973), 759-773.
28. Walker, P. S. and Salvati, E., "The Measurement and Effects of Friction and Wear in Artificial Hip Joints," J. Biomed. Mater. Res., 4, (1973), 327-342.
29. Clarke, I. C., "Wear of Artificial Joint Materials, *IV* Hip Joint Simulator Studies," Engineering in Medicine, in press.
30. Paul, I., Rose, R., Simon, S. and Radin, E., "The MIT Knee Joint Simulator," presented at a one-day Meeting on Simulation, Leeds, January, 1976.
31. Private communications, R. Bosma, University of Twente, Holland.
32. Shaw, J. A. and Murray, D. G., "Knee Joint Simulator," Clinical Orthopaedics and Related Research, 94, (1973), 15-23.
33. Young, R. W., Young, S. R. and Treharne, R. W., "Simulation of the Knee Joint using a Computer Controlled System," Trans. 25th ORS, 3, 1979.
34. Dowson, D. and Wright, V., "Bioengineering at Leeds," Instn. Mech. Engrs., 7, (1978), 63-65.
35. Kettlekamp, D. B. and Masca, R., "Biomechanics and Knee Replacement Arthroplasty," Clinical Orthopaedics and Related Research, 94, (1973), 8-14.
36. Seirig, A. and Arvikar, R. J., "The Prediction of Muscular Load Sharing and Joint Forces in the Lower Extremities During Walking," J. Biomechanics, 8, (1975), 89-102.

37. Streitman, A. J. and Pugh, J. W., "The Design and Implementation of a Simple Effective System for Gait Analysis," Bull. Hosp. Jt. Dis., 38, (1977), 31-34.
38. Dumbleton, J. H., "The Tribology of Natural and Artificial Joints," Elsevier, Amsterdam, (1981), Chapter 8.
39. Treharne, R. W., Young, R. W. and Young, S. R., "Wear of Artificial Joint Materials. III Simulation of the Knee Joint Using a Computer-Controlled System," Engineering in Medicine, *10,* 137-142, (1981).
40. McKellop, H., Clarke, I., Markolf, K. and Austutz, H., "Friction and Wear Properties of Polymer, Metal and Ceramic Prosthetic Joint Materials Evaluated on a Multichannel Screening Device," J. Biomed. Mater. Res., *15,* 619-653, (1981).
41. Rose, R. M., Schneider, H., Ries, M., Paul, I., Crugnola, A., Simon, S. R. and Radin, E. L., "A Method for the Quantitative Recovery of Polyethylene Wear Debris from the Simulated Service of Total Joint Prostheses, "Massachusetts Institute of Technology Report, August 1978.
42. Mears, D. C., Hanley, E. N., Jr., Rutkowski, R. and Westcott, V. C., "Ferrography: Its Application to the Study of Human Joint Wear," Wear, *50,* 115-125 (1978).
43. Atkinson, J. T. and Lalor, M. J., "Holographic Interferometry Applied to Minimal Wear Measurement," presented at the First European Congress on Optics Aplied to Metrology, Strasbourg, September 1977.
44. Dumbleton, J. H., "Tribology of Natural and Artificial Joints," Elsevier, Amsterdam, (1981), Chapter 9.
45. Dumbleton, J. H., "The Tribology of Natural and Artificial Joints," Elsevier, Amsterdam, (1981), Chapter 7.
46. McKellop, H., "Wear of Artificial Joint Materials 11 Twelve-Channel Wear-Screening Device: Correlation of Experimental and Clinical Results," Eng. in Medicine, *10,* 123-136, (1981).
47. Clarke, I. C., "Wear of Artificial Joint Materials In Friction and Wear Studies: Validity of Wear Screening Protocols," Eng. in Medicine, *10,* 115-122 (1981).
48. Greer, K. W., "Four Years of Wear Testing Experience on Three Joint Simulators," presented at Eleventh International Biomaterials Symposium, Clemson, April-May, (1979).
49. Rose, R. M., Crugnola, A. N., Cimino, W. R. and Ries, M. D., "The In Vivo Performance of Polyethylene Components of Total Joint Replacements," *in* "Implant Retrieval: Material and Biological Analysis," National Bureau of Standards, Special Publication, 601, (1981).
50. Clarke, I. C., "Wear of Polymeric Implants – Clinical Reality, Retrieved Implants and Laboratory Predictions," *in* "Implant Retrieval: Material and Biological Analysis," National Bureau of Standards, Special Publication 601, (1981).
51. Atkinson, J., Dowling, J. and Cicek, R., "Materials for Internal Prostheses: The Present Position and Future Developments," Biomaterials, *1,* 89-96, (1980).
52. Revell, P. A., Weightman, B., Freeman, M. A. R. and Vernan Roberts, B., "The Production and Biology of Polyethylene Wear Debris," Arch. Ortho. Traum. Surg., *91,* 167-181, (1978).
53. Clarke, I. C., McKellop, H. A., McGuire, P., Okuda, R. and Sarmiento, A., "Wear of Ti-6Al-4V Alloy," Biomechanics, in press.
54. Rostoker, W. and Galante, J. O., "The Influence of Titanium Surface Treatments on the Wear of Medical Grade Polyethylene," Biomaterials, *2,* 221-224, (1981).
55. Dumbleton, J. H., "The Behaviour of Acetals as Implant Materials," *in* "Biomaterials in Reconstructive Surgery," Rubin, L. (ed), The C. V. Mosby Company, St. Louis, Mo., in press.
56. Scales, J., Private Communication.
57. Morscher, Bombelli, R., Schenk, R. and Mathys, R., "The Treatment of Femoral Neck Fractures with an Isoelastic Endoprosthesis Implanted Without Bone Cement," Arch. Orthop. Traumat. Surg., *98,* 93-100, (1981).
58. McKellop, H., Redfern, F., Okuda, R. and Clarke, L., "Correlation of Hip Joint Simulator Wear Tests with Clinical Experience," to be presented at the 8th Annual Meeting of the Society for Biomaterials, April 24-27, (1982).

Chapter 21

Accelerated Fatigue Testing of Elastomers in Blood and Related Environments

Dr. Carl R. McMillin
Contract Manager
Monsanto Research Corporation
1515 Nicholas Road
Dayton, Ohio 45418

ABSTRACT

There are presently no short-term in vitro *fatigue tests available that can predict long-term* in vivo *performance of elastomers in physiological environments such as circulatory assist devices. Thus, the introduction of new and better elastomers for cardiovascular applications is hampered in the development stage by lack of data on which materials to commercialize. After development, new materials are also slow to be used because of lack of data comparing them to elastomers presently being used. To remedy this lack of information, the National Institutes of Health have sponsored several contracts aimed at developing accelerated fatigue tests for elastomers. At Monsanto Research Corporation, a wide variety of fatigue tests have been investigated, primarily using a constant strain fatigue test machine constructed in our laboratory. In most of these fatigue tests, the strain is increased daily until failure occurs.*

Although blood is generally considered to be a very corrosive environment, our tests indicate that it actually extends the fatigue life of elastomers compared to air or water environments. A combination of fatigue tests using both cut-initiated and uncut test specimens appears to provide the most predictive information. Longer term fatigue tests are being started to validate the short-term fatigue test results.

This work has been funded with Federal funds from the Department of Health, Education, and Welfare under contract numbers NO1-HV-7-2918 and NO1-HV-02909. The contents of this publication do not necessarily reflect the views or policies of the Department of Health, Education, and Welfare, nor does mention of trade names or commercial products imply endorsement by the U.S. Government.

BACKGROUND

The development of cardiac assist devices and other instrumentation and components which come in contact with the cardiovascular system requires materials which will perform in a physiological environment. One particularly difficult application is the diaphragm for blood pumps, which requires an elastomer to undergo cyclic deformation and/or flexing while in contact with blood.

Currently, few data are available on the fatigue properties of elastomers cycled at body temperature and in contact with blood. Artificial heart device applications are particularly demanding of elastomers since even a three-year implantation of a heart will involve in excess of 10^8 cycles.

Evaluation of the fatigue properties of elastomers suitable for cardiovascular application is currently a long, and therefore, costly proposition. This is especially true if the fatigue tests are to be conducted in contact with blood.

The objectives of this program are to develop short term *in vitro* fatigue test methodologies that will predict long-term *in vivo* performance of elastomers used in cardiac assist devices and to evaluate the fatigue life of candidate materials for potential use in these applications.

To meet these objectives, the National Institutes of Health initially funded three 3-year projects, each with the same objectives but using different experimental approaches. These projects were conducted at the National Bureau of Standards (Dr. Penn), Washington University (Dr. Kardos), and Monsanto Research Corporation (Dr. McMillin). Additional three-year research efforts are now progressing at Washington University and Monsanto Research Corporation. The results of the research conducted at Monsanto Research Corporation (MRC) are presented in this paper.

MATERIALS AND MATERIALS CHARACTERIZATION

Many studies, particularly in the life sciences area, are not reproducible because small quantities of unique materials were used in the research. A commitment was made when the present program began to fully characterize the elastomers utilized in the development of accelerated fatigue tests. At the start of the program, the Principal Investigators of the fatigue test development projects selected a limited number of candidate materials to be produced in quantity, characterized, and used for testing in each of the laboratories. Procurement, quality control, and initial characterization responsibilities were divided among the laboratories.

The materials selected to evaluate alternate approaches for accelerating fatigue tests included elastomers at that time in use in circulatory assist devices – Hexsyn® , Biomer® , and Avcothane-51® as well as more readily obtainable elastomers – butyl rubber and Pellethane® 2363-80A. A detailed description of these materials follows:

Hexsyn® is a sulfur-vulcanized hydrocarbon rubber, essentially a polyhexene, made by Goodyear Tire and Rubber Company, Akron, Ohio. Hexsyn (covered by U.S. patent numbers 3,993,769 and 3,991,262) is polymerized from a mixture of 95% hexene-1, 3% 4-methyl-1, 4-hexadiene and 2% 5-methyl-1,4-hexadiene using a Ziegler-Natta heterogeneous polymerization with Et_3Al, $TiCl_4$, and VCl_4. This gum rubber is then compounded and vulcanized using a traditional accelerated, high crosslink efficiency mixture as follows:

	Parts-per-hundred resin
Polymer	100
IASF carbon black	50
Zinc oxide	2
Steric acid	2
Sulfur	2
Tetramethyl thiuram disulfide	1
2-Mercaptobenzothiazole	0.5

The vulcanized rubber is extracted with an acetone/toluene mixture and dried prior to any testing.

Biomer® is the trade name for a polyether urethane of the Ethicon Corporation, Sommerville, New Jersey. Biomer is generally prepared as a 30% by weight solution in dimethyl acetamide (DMA). The solution is suitable for dip casting and is usually vacuum oven dried prior to use. For this project, it is fabricated into sheet form by Thoratec Labs Corporation, Emeryville, California.

Avcothane-51® – The trade name for a block copolymer of 90% polyether urethane and 10% poly (dimethylsiloxane) of the Avco Everett Company, Everett, Massachusetts. Avcothane is film, cast from a 11-15% by weight solution of a 2:1 mixture of tetrahydrofuran (THF) and dioxane (DXE). The solution is suitable for dip casting. For this project, it is fabricated into sheet form by Avco Everett.

Butyl Rubber – A carbon black filled compound of isobutylene-isoprene (butyl) rubber designated as National Bureau of Standards standard reference material 388j. NBS synthesized, compounded, and vulcanized the material and supplied it in sheet form to MRC through Dr. R. W. Penn of the National Bureau of Standards.

Pellethane® CPR 2363-80A – The trade name and product number for an extruded thermoplastic, polyether urethane elastomer, of the Upjohn Company, Torrance, California. This material was generously supplied by the CPR Division of the Upjohn Company in North Haven, Connecticut.

The quantity of these materials needed for all of the intended fatigue testing research was estimated to be 10 m^2 each. Since this is about two orders of magnitude greater than the amount of these specialized materials generally manufactured at any one time, a substantial manufacturing effort was required prior to any fatigue testing.

These materials have been extensively characterized. A summary of some of their properties determined at Monsanto Research Corporation is shown in Table 1.

The number of materials being treated has been expanded in order to ascertain if fatigue test relationships developed for the five materials cited above will hold for a wide variety of materials. The additional elastomers currently being tested are listed below.

Silicone – A commercial sheet silicone rubber of the Graindyk Manufacturing Company.

EPDM – Goodyear Versigard® rubber; a commercial sheet EPDM rubber.

Polyurethane – B. F. Goodrich CU-85 Novitane® commercial sheet polyurethane rubber.

Natural Rubber – Goodyear Pureten® Rubber Style 40TG; a commercial sheet natural rubber.

Neoprene – Goodyear Wingprene® ASTM grade commercial sheet neoprene rubber.

SBR – B. F. Goodrich SBR-75 commercial sheet styrene-butadiene rubber.

Nitrile – Goodyear Chemigum® ; a commercial sheet butadiene-acrylonitrile rubber.

Table 1. Properties of Candidate Materials

Property	Hexsyn	Biomer	Avcothane	Pellethane	Butyl
Tensile strength (psi)					
37°C	1,740			7,830	
23°C	2,060			7,050	
Elongation (%)					
37°C	284			380	
23°C	321			353	
Elastic modulus (psi)					
100% @ 37°C	456	357	354	730	277
100% @ 23°C	490				
300% @ 37°C	607	583	631	935	354
300% @ 23°C	646				
Hardness (Shore A)					
at 23°C	67				59
Density (g/cc)					
at 37°C	1.047	1.041		1.114	1.109
at 25°C	1.074	1.049		1.116	1.117
Tear strength (lb/in.)					
Graves @ 37°C	-			258	
Graves @ 23°C	105			333	
Tear strength (lb/in.)					
Trouser @ 37 °C	15	55	210	53	110
Tear energy at 37°C (in.-lb/in./in.)	32	319	2,350	147	839
Glass transition temperature					
Differential scanning calorimetry (DSC) (maximum endotherm - °C)	-52	-72	-57	-57	-70
Crystalline melt [DSC and thermal mechanical analysis (TMA)]	48°C	0°C (DSC only)			
Decomposition temperature					
in air (°C)	342	200		250	195
in helium (°C)	402	130		250	177
Linear coefficient of expansion by TMA (in./in./°C)	8.4×10^{-4}				
Storage modulus (10^8 dynes/cm^2					
@ 37°C at 11 Hz	2.27				
@ 23°C	1.72				
Loss modulus (10^7 dynes/cm^2)					
@ 37°C at 11 Hz	2.47				
@ 23°C	3.93				
Damping (tan Δ)					
@ 37°C at 11 Hz	0.109				
@ 23°C	0.144				
Residual solvents					
(acetone, ppm)	<3				
(toluene, ppm)	80 to 1,540				
Single cycle tension set (%)					
100% strain @ 37°C	5.7			13.3	
100% strain @ 23°C	6.1			6.7	
20% strain @ 37°C	3.6			3.2	
20% strain @ 23°C	3.6			1.2	
Stress relaxation (psi)					
100% strain @ 37°C	21.6			24	
100% strain @ 23°C	23.0			24	
20% strain @ 37°C	22.7			9.4	
20% strain @ 23°C	24.3			8.2	

Continued

Table 1. Properties of Candidate Materials (Continued)

Property	Hexsyn	Biomer	Avcothane	Pellethane	Butyl
Swelling ratio (size increase)					
Hexane (23°C)	1.9				
Cyclohexane (23°-37°C)	2.8-3.1				3.25-3.24
Toluene (23°-37°C)	2.5-2.5				
Blood (23°-37°C)	1.04-1.05				1.003-1.01
Phenotole (23°-37°C)	1.46-1.55				
Reduction in 100% modulus after 5 cycles to 250% strain (% of original)	18.5			48.3	
Molecular weight uncrosslinked gum (gel permeation chromatorgaphy/light scattering)					
Mw	781,000				
Mn	468,000				
Mz	970,000				
Intrinsic viscosity (uncrosslinked gum) in dl/g	5.25				
Permeability to water mg·mm/sec·m²	24.6	1022	588	375	14.0
Critical surface tension at 37°C (dynes/cm)					
Dan series	42				
Ethanol/water series	27				
Mixed glycols	25				
ASTM series	27				
Cytotoxicity to human D98S cells					
As received	Positive	Negative	Negative	Negative	Positive
After extraction	Negative	Negative	Negative	Negative	Negative
Mutagenicity (Ames test)					
Direct contact	Negative	Negative	Negative	Negative	Negative
Extract	Negative	Negative	Negative	Negative	Negative
100 psi oxygen exposure for 112 days (% increase in 100% modulus)	12.9		12.0	7.8	7.0
Fatigue test permanent set (%)					
100% extension @ 37°C	22	8	27	17	18
150% extension @ 37°C	43	14	54	45	38

(Concluded)

Santoprene – Monsanto Company Santoprene® ; a commercial sheet thermoplastic rubber based on polypropylene.

All materials are stored in a refrigerator maintained at 4°C prior to use. This refrigeration slows some aging processes and shields the materials from ultraviolet light.

FATIGUE TESTS

In the literature, it is easy to observe that different types of fatigue tests rank materials in different orders. Thus, to predict a material's behavior for specific long-term end-use applications, it is important to select the correct fatigue test.

Most early artificial hearts and left ventricular assist devices consisted of a hemispherical diaphragm alternately inflated and deflated by compressed air. The controls generally regulated the amount of pressure and vacuum applied to the device. In this case, the elastomeric diaphragm was exposed to an alternating stress or force. That is, in each cycle a stress of 2 kg, for example, would be applied to the diaphragm. This type of device would best be modeled by a constant stress fatigue test. Creep tests would tend to rank the candidate materials in the same order as constant stress fatigue tests.

More recently, the National Institutes of Health have been emphasizing hearts and assist devices capable of mechanical or electrical operation. Most of these devices have a pusher plate that moves back and forth to displace the diaphragm a fixed (but adjustable) distance, generally independent of the pressure of each stroke. The fatigue test which most closely mimics this condition will deform the test specimens to a fixed deformation or strain. This is the type of fatigue test machine that Monsanto Research Corporation has constructed for this program.

The difference in results from stress versus strain fatigue tests can be very significant. A material that has a low modulus of elasticity (stretches easily) will generally survive long-term fatigue to a fixed strain, but under conditions that apply a stress, they elongate, reducing their cross-sectional area, and fail much more rapidly. Conversely, a high modulus (stiff) elastomer will be able to withstand a higher repetitive stress, but if forced to deform, it will have a shorter fatigue life. An extreme example of this comparison would be a toothpick that can survive constant stress fatigue (and creep) but instantly fails in constant strain tests, versus a soap bubble that can easily withstand constant strain tests but instantly fails in constant stress (or creep) tests.

Fatigue Machine Design

In order to conduct accelerated fatigue tests in a number of environments including blood, a fatigue testing machine had to be designed and constructed to provide the following parameters:

- Large number of test positions
- Constant strain fatigue test
- Variable and controlled temperature ($<0°C$ to $>100°C$)
- Ability to withstand corrosive environments such as blood
- Ability to use only a small volume of medium for tests (human blood is expensive)
- Variable rate of testing (60 to 240 cycles/minute)
- Variable strain (zero to 260% elongation)
- Ability to use standard 5-inch "dog bone" tensile strength test specimens

The design of the wobble plate fatigue tester which meets the above criteria is shown in Figures 1 to 3. It requires approximately 30 units of blood (about 15 liters) to conduct fatigue

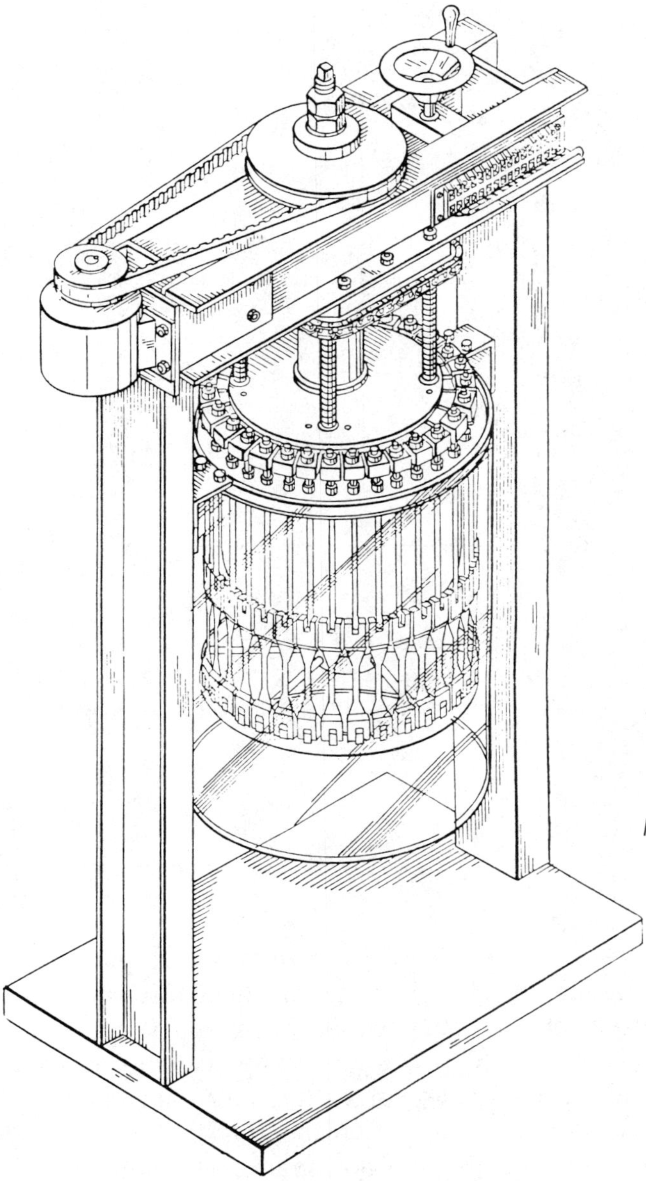

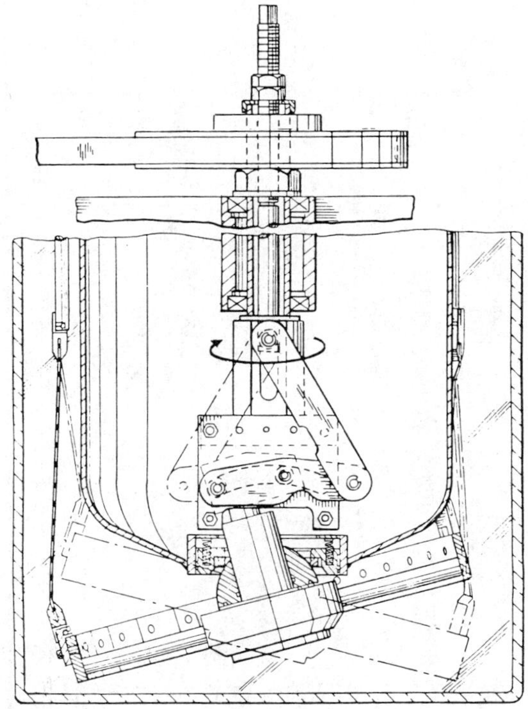

Figure 2. Operation of the Monsanto wobble plate fatigue tester.

Figure 1. Monsanto wobble plate fatigue tester.

tests in this environment. All exposed parts are made of 316 stainless steel to avoid corrosion problems.

Uniaxial Fatigue Test Methods

Conventional fatigue tests apply a specified strain (or stress) to the test specimens in a cyclic manner and record the cycles required until failure. These values are then generally plotted on a log type of paper (or Weibull distribution paper) at different strain (or stress) levels versus cycles to failure. The primary problem with this type of test is the long time required to generate the data at lower strain levels.

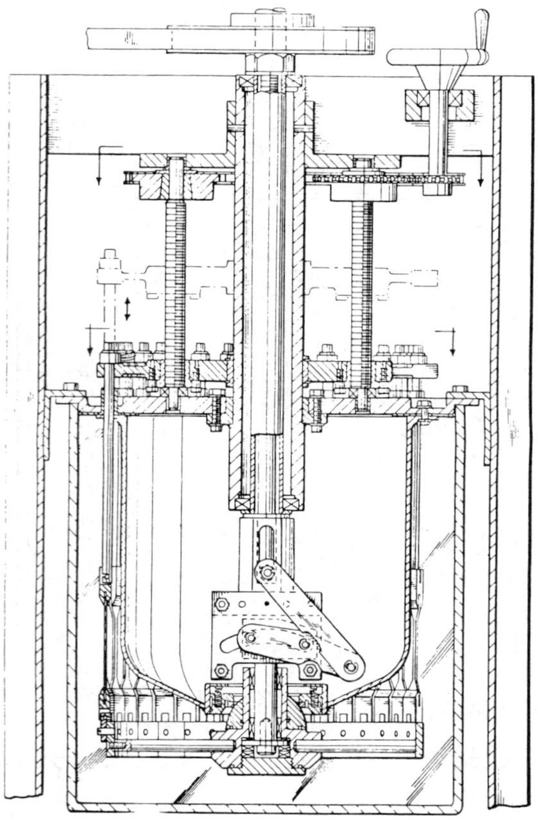

Figure 3. Internal design of the Monsanto wobble plate fatigue tester.

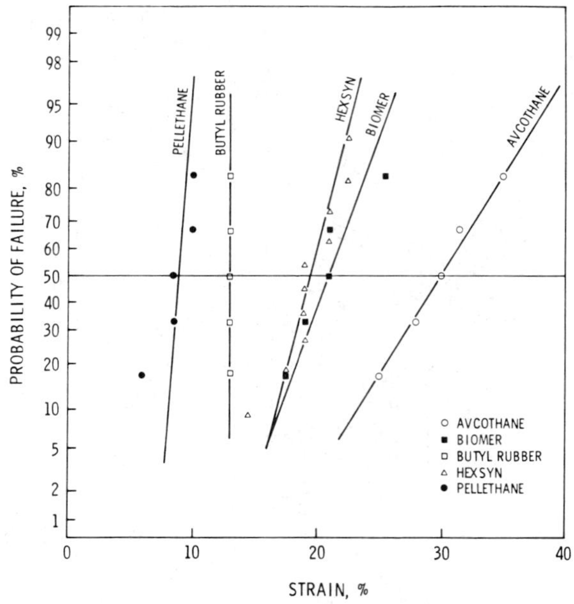

Figure 4. Cumulative distribution function for a step increasing strain fatigue test cycled at 120 cpm in distilled water at 37°C using cut-initiated specimens.

One possible method of accelerating the fatigue test involves increasing the strain (or stress) in either discrete steps of in a progressive manner [1,2]. This type of fatigue test has now been used for testing steel, polystyrene, polymethyl methacrylate, nylon, and reinforced plastic [3]. Although some deviations have been noted [2,4], this type of test has the advantages of speed, elimination of long-term run-outs, and reduction of scatter of the data near the endurance limit. One potential problem with all methods that use a higher than end-use strain or stress is the possibility that the failure mechanism changes at higher strains, which may lead to erroneous predictions. However, all accelerated fatigue tests suffer from this potential difficulty; conditions for all of them vary from real life.

An increasing strain was used to accelerate the test for all of the uniaxial fatigue data generated at MRC to date. This can easily be seen in Table 2 where the maximum cyclic strain is increasing from 1.7% on day 1 to 35% on day 20. These data are then plotted as cumulative probability to failure versus percent strain at failure, as shown in Figure 4. Regression lines are then fit to the data. The strain at 50% probability of failure is then used for all comparisons of data.

Design of Stress Concentration (Cut-Growth) Fatigue Tests

In order to conduct cut-growth fatigue tests similar to the uncut tests shown above, standard

Table 2. Chronological Fatigue Life for Avcothane-51, MRC Lots 141265 and 1412690 Cut-Initiated Specimens, Cycled at 120 CPM in Distilled Water at 37°C

Testing day	Percent cyclic strain	Specimens failed	Accumulated cycles
1	0-1.7		
2	0-3.5		
3	0-5.2		
4	0-7.0		
5	0-8.5		
6	0-10.0		
7	0-11.5		
8	0-13.0		
9	0-15.0		
10	0-17.0		
11	0-19.0		
12	0-21.0		
13	0-22.8		
14	0-24.6	*(0302511)	2,332,800
15	0-26.3		
16	0-28.0	*(060515)	2,678,400
17	0-29.8	*(060762)	2,851,200
18	0-31.5	*(Rej. "J")	3,024,000
19	0-33.3		3,196,800
20	0-35.0	*(060762)	3,369,600

ASTM D-412C tensile specimens were cut with a razor blade using the fixture shown in Figure 5. This fixture allows a precise 1-mm cut in the gage center of each specimen. Cut specimens are then cycled at 120 cycles/minute while the strain level is periodically increased.

Uniaxial Fatigue Test Results

Increasing temperature decreases the modulus of elasticity of rubber materials at the same time that accelerated chemical effects occur. In our constant strain fatigue test, it has been found that the effect on the modulus is significantly more important than chemical degradation effects, as shown in Figure 6. Thus, failure occurred much more rapidly at 4°C than at 37°C or 60°C. This may be one manner in which fatigue tests can be accelerated. Extreme care must be taken, however, to assure that the tests remain valid, even at 4°C, since the glass transition temperatures (Tg) of the candidate materials are different. Extrapolating data taken close to the Tg of one material to end-use conditions may not be the equivalent of reduced temperature testing of other materials with much lower glass transition temperatures.

Another set of fatigue tests showed that there was no effect of oxygen on the fatigue life of the uncut test specimens, as shown in Figure 7. On the other hand, fatigue tests using test specimens with 1-mm cut in the side showed a substantial decrease in fatigue life in the presence of oxygen, as shown in Figure 8. The dependence on oxygen for the cut-initiated tests is believed by MRC to be significant. Fatigue literature indicates that low stress or strain fatigue results are generally oxygen dependent, while high stress or strain (shorter duration) tests are not oxygen

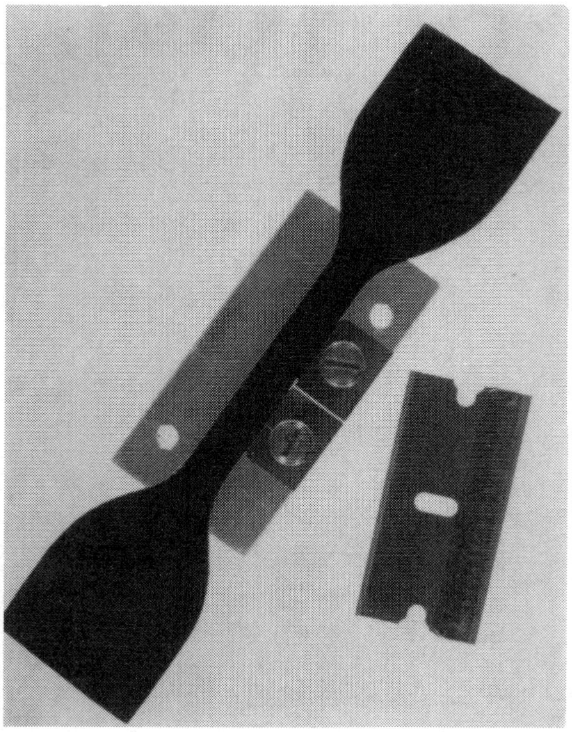

Figure 5. Specimen cutting fixture.

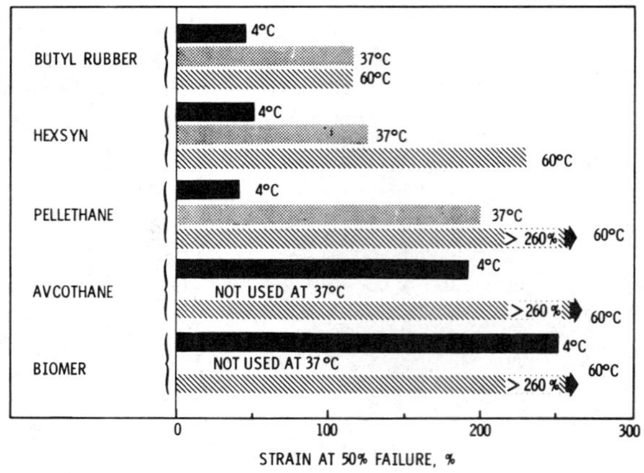

Figure 6. Strain at 50% failure for uncut specimens tested in saline solution.

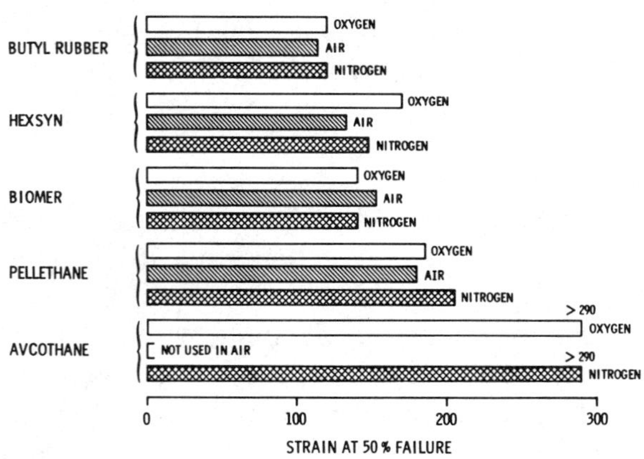

Figure 7. Oxygen influence upon uncut specimens from step increasing strain fatigue tests cycled at 120 cpm and at 37°C.

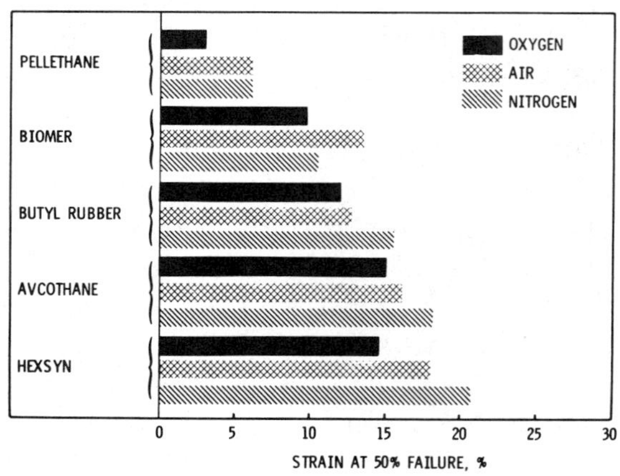

Figure 8. Oxygen influence upon cut-initiated specimens from step increasing strain fatigue tests cycled at 120 cpm and at 37°C.

dependent [5]. The period of testing was approximately three to six weeks in both tests. One hypothesis we are investigating is that unless accelerated fatigue tests demonstrate an oxygen dependence, they are probably representative of the wrong portion of the fatigue life curve and will probably not properly predict long-term results. Further research on the significance of oxygen dependence on the validity of predictive accelerated fatigue tests will be conducted by MRC.

Environmental effects also need to be considered when developing fatigue testing methodology. The human body presents an unbelievably corrosive environment for foreign materials. The best stainless steels, cobalt alloys, and even platinum undergo pitting, cracking, and failure when used *in vivo*. It is little wonder that the physical properties of polymers are generally degraded after *in vivo* implantation [6-8].

MRC has evaluated the effect of fatigue testing of candidate cardiovascular materials in human blood versus fatigue testing in air and saline – all at 37°C (Figures 9 and 10). Whole human blood was chosen as one of the mediums for testing at 37°C, in spite of the difficulties associated with this testing.

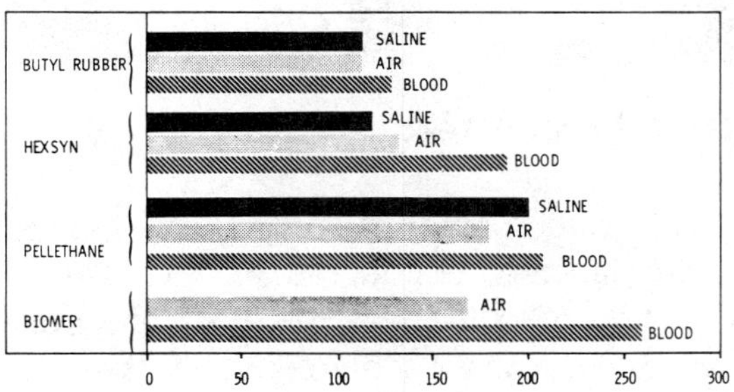

Figure 9. Strain at 50% failure in fatigue tests conducted at 37°C on uncut specimens.

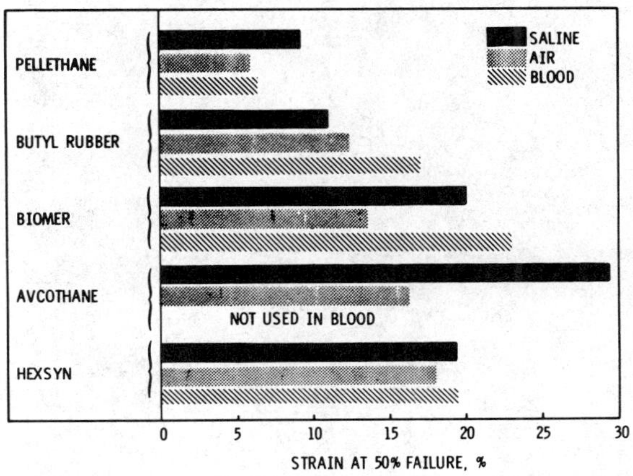

Figure 10. Strain at 50% failure in fatigue tests conducted at 37°C on cut-initiated specimens.

We used outdated human CPD (citrate-phosphate-dextrose) blood from the Dayton Community Blood Center. At 21 days, CPD blood still retains 78% survival of the red blood cells and would fairly well simulate *in vivo* physiological conditions. During these tests, many enzymes and proteins may denature and/or precipitate. Even after suffering that trauma, the resulting fluid is more suitable for material testing than other pseudo-physiological fluids since it still contains most of the salt, lipids, hormones, oligomers, nucleotides, saccharides, etc., found in whole blood *in vivo*.

We have found that blood used in our fatigue tester needs to be changed about once a week. We routinely add penicillin, streptomycin, and mycostatin to the blood to prevent bacterial and mold growth. Also, heparin and/or ethylene diamine tetracetate (EDTA) (a calcium chelator) are added to prevent blood clotting. In spite of these precautions, the viscosity of the blood begins to increase and microbiological growth begins to occur after about one week. The instrument is therefore drained, cleaned with a mild soapy solution, and refilled on a weekly basis.

Results from our fatigue tests have shown that, in the one- to two-month accelerated fatigue tests, blood is a *less severe* environment than saline or air. This may be due to adsorption of the blood components into the microcracks, resulting in reduced stress concentrations. More work is anticipated to study the effect of blood on the fatigue life of elastomers.

All of the above results were generated by tests in which the cyclic strain was started low and gradually increased until all of the specimens broke. Longer term fatigue tests at different, discrete, strain levels are planned for the future.

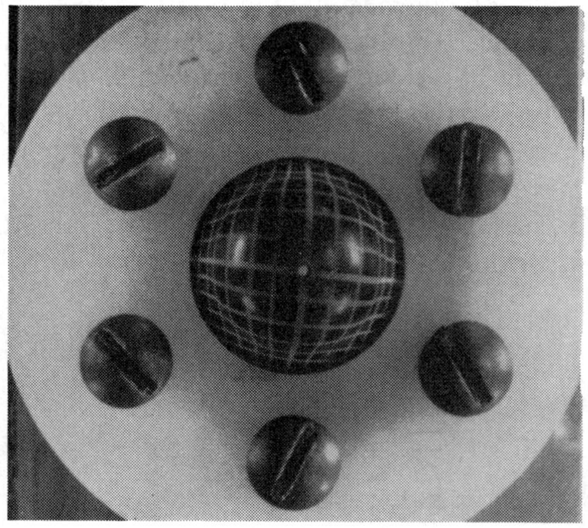

Figure 12. Hexsyn specimen with a hot pinhole stress concentrator mounted in the biaxial fatigue testing machine.

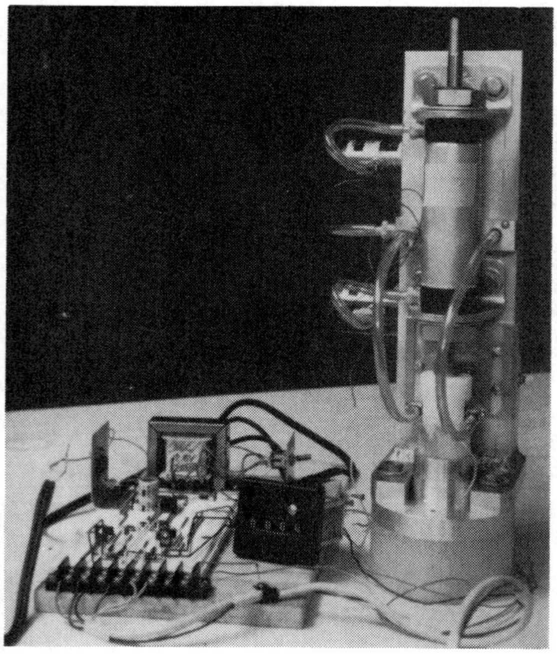

Figure 11. Biaxial fatigue testing machine in the manufacturing stage.

Biaxial Fatigue Testing

A limited amount of biaxial fatigue testing has been conducted at MRC. A biaxial testing machine was designed and built (Figure 11) using a Teflon plunger as the driving mechanism. Figure 12 shows two views of a specimen being fatigued. When controlled defects were introduced into the biaxial test specimens, it was found that a smooth hole (made with a hot pin) did not appear to affect the results substantially, while a rough hole (made with a cold pin) caused early failure of the specimens. The rough holes were not reproducible. The most reproducible type of defect resulted from a controlled razor blade cut or cross made while the specimen was slightly deformed. The overall results obtained with this testing machine ranked the elastomers in the same order as the unaxial fatigue testing machine.

Ranking of the Candidate Cardiovascular Materials

Results from our accelerated fatigue tests and static mechanical/physiological tests have confirmed our assumption that a durability ranking of the selected materials with respect to their usefulness in cardiovascular devices is decidedly influenced by the type of testing methodology selected. Table 3 is a comparison of five candidate materials' relative rankings using five test methodologies. The asterisk denotes the material with the longest durability or highest resistance to the particular test method indicated. All of the five materials tested were found to be superior in one of the five tests cited in Table 3. Thus, all five materials being tested could be argued to be the superior elastomer currently being tested. This illustrates the difficulty of ranking candidate materials.

Table 3. Relative Ranking Is Influenced by the Test Selected

Elastomer	Cut-growth air @ 37°C	Uncut blood @ 37°C strain at 50% failure	Uncut N_2 @ 37°C	Uncut air @ 37°C	Cut-growth fixed strain cycle 1 hr. failure strain
Hexsyn	18*	190	150	125	30
Biomer	12	260*	140	150	25
Avcothane	16	---	>290*	---	--
Pellethane	6	210	205	175*	12
Butyl	12	140	110	115	>45*

*The material with the longest durability or highest resistance to the particular test method indicated.

Care must be taken to assure that the correct types of tests are used to rank materials for specific applications. For example, most recently designed circulatory assist devices utilize a pusher plate mechanism in which the pusher plate is displaced a predetermined distance. This type of device would best be modeled by a constant strain fatigue test. Materials which creep and have high permanent sets tend to fail more rapidly on a constant stress fatigue test but last a longer time in constant strain fatigue tests. The bending and compression of finger joint prostheses or the rolling of the side material in pusher plate circulatory assist devices may not be well modeled by either of the above tests.

CONCLUSIONS

After extensively characterizing and fatigue testing the five candidate materials, I have some opinions on their usefulness in cardiovascular applications:

Biomer — This material performs well under a variety of experimental conditions and should be considered for use in most cardiovascular applications. Particular advantages are the low permanent set, high resistance to creep, and generally good fatigue resistance. Disadvantages include a relatively high permeability to fluids, a necessity to be film cast in multiple layers as the only method of fabrication, and an uncertainty as to the effect of thickness on performance (better fatigue results were obtained with the thinner films).

Hexsyn — Performance varies from adequate to very good in a variety of fatigue tests, and Hexsyn should be considered for use in most cardiovascular applications. Particular advantages include low permeability to fluids, the ability to be compression molded (good for high volume applications), low cost of the raw materials, and ready availability from more than one supplier in medical grade material. Disadvantages include an intermediate amount of permanent set, lower resistance to creep, lower modulus of elasticity (which may be an advantage in some applications), and low tear strength (although Hexsyn has a high resistance to cut growth in fatigue).

Avcothane — This material performs exceptionally well in most constant strain fatigue tests and should be considered for use in most cardiovascular applications. A particular advantage is its fatigue test performance under a variety of conditions. Disadvantages include a very high permeability to fluids, a very high permanent set, a very low resistance to creep, a high cost of materials, and a necessity to be film cast in multiple layers under rigid controls available only at the material suppliers' facilities.

Pellethane – This material performed satisfactorily in some of the fatigue tests and should be considered for some cardiovascular applications, particularly in noncritical locations. Advantages of this inexpensive, commercially available thermoplastic include its ability to be formed into parts by a wide variety of methods such as extrusion, blow molding, injection molding, or film casting. In fatigue situations without stress concentrators, Pellethane's performance was similar to that of Biomer. From our tests, if a thick part were required, Pellethane should be considered. Disadvantages include a rapid decrease in fatigue resistance in the presence of cuts or other stress concentrators. Its permeability to fluids is similar to Biomer's, but it has a slightly higher permanent set and lower resistance to creep. Although Pellethane is probably the most inexpensive material tested, it is not available in a specific, closely controlled, medical grade.

Butyl rubber – This material generally had the least endurance in fatigue tests, but it may be adequate for some cardiovascular applications. Advantages include less sensitivity to stress concentrators than Pellethane, a very low permeability to fluids, a moderate creep resistance and widespread availability at low cost. Disadvantages include a relatively low fatigue resistance compared to the elastomers specifically designed for these applications. The rubber tested was not designed for medical applications and had standard rubber additives and modifiers that were cytotoxic unless the material had been extracted after manufacture.

EXTENSION OF TESTING TO OTHER ELASTOMERS

In order to expand the number of test materials in the program, eight commercial rubber materials of different generic types were obtained in sheet form as cited earlier. Physical properties have now been measured on these materials. Shore "A" hardness values of these materials ranged from 42 for natural rubber to 85 for a polyurethane and are tabulated in Figure 13. Silicone rubber had the highest permeability to water (ASTM D-814-55) and nitrile and natural rubbers the lowest. The polyurethanes (both Pellethane and the Goodrich) had the highest tensile properties (ASTM D-412-68) whereas, as expected, the silicone rubber had the lowest. The tensile properties of the candidate materials are tabulated in Figure 14.

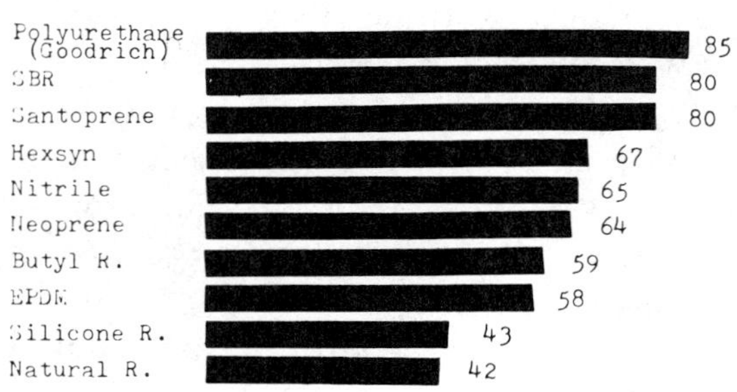
Polyurethane (Goodrich)
85
SBR
80
Santoprene
80
Hexsyn
67
Nitrile
65
Neoprene
64
Butyl R.
59
EPDM
58
Silicone R.
43
Natural R.
42

Figure 13. Hardness of materials to be tested (Shore "A").

Uncut fatigue failure with increasing strain at 37°C in air was measured using the wobble plate fatigue tester. Excellent agreement with previously obtained 50% failure strain data was seen for the control samples (Pellethane and butyl). The strain at 50% failure was the highest for Santoprene and the lowest for SBR and nitrile (Figure 15).

Research is continuing with accelerated fatigue tests being conducted on the new materials under a variety of conditions. Also, longer term fatigue tests are planned at a number of strain levels to help validate the accelerated fatigue test methodology developed in this program.

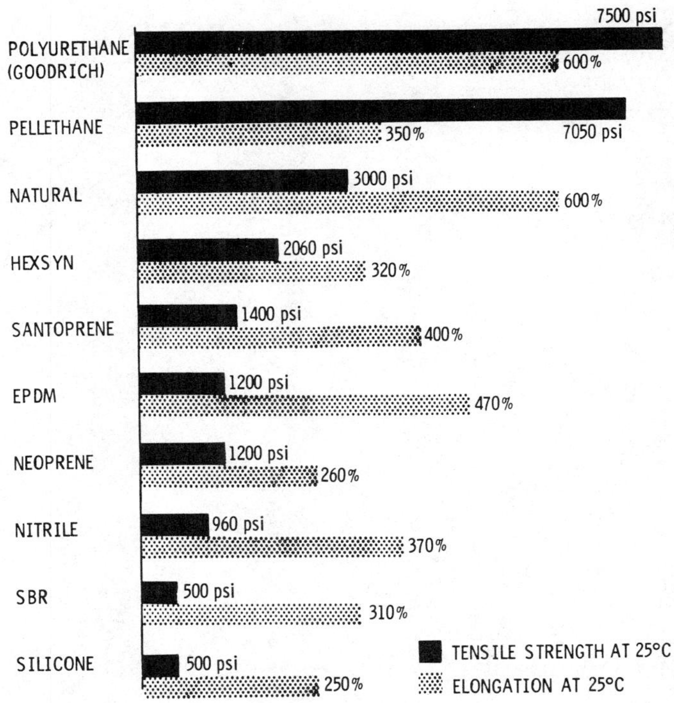

Figure 14. Tensile and elongation properties for new materials.

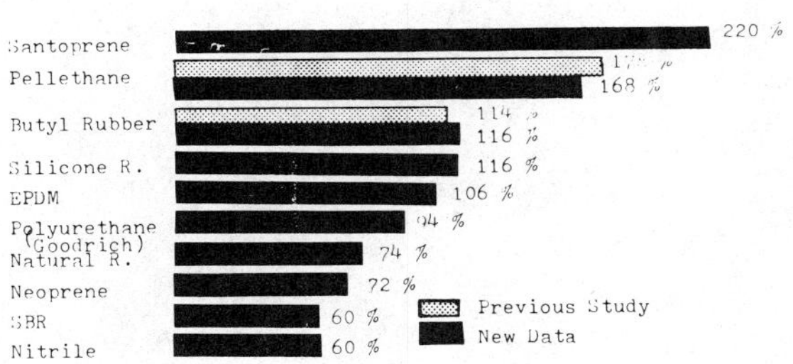

Figure 15. Uncut fatigue failure – increasing strain at 37°C in air (strain at 50% failure).

REFERENCES

1. Lazar, L. S. Accelerated Fatigue of Plastics. ASTM Bulletin, 67-72, February 1957.
2. Weibull, W. Fatigue Testing and Analysis of Results. Pergamon Press, New York, 1961.
3. Thorkildsen, R. L. In: Engineering Design for Plastics, E. Baer, ed. Reinhold Publishing Corp., New York, 1964.
4. Prevorsek, D. C. and Brooks, M. L. Fatigue Under Complicated Load Histories. Law of Cumulative Damage. J. Appl. Poly. Sci. 11:925-927, 1967.
5. Lake, G. J. Corrosive Aspects of Fatigue. Rubber Age 104: 39-49, 1972.
6. Noishiki, Y. Biochemical Response to Dacron Vascular Prosthesis. J. Biomed. Mater. Res. 10:759-767, 1976.
7. Mayhan, K. G., et al. Analysis of a Silicone Elastomer Heart Ball Valve. J. Biomed. Mater. Res. 7:405-418, 1973.
8. Sawyer, R. N., et al. Implantation Characteristics of Metal-Backed Polymercoated Heart Valves: Biophysical Scanning and Transmission Electron Microscopic Studies. Trans. Am. Soc. Artif. Intern. Organs 20:692-702, 1974.

Chapter 22

Survey of Clinically Important Wound Closure Biomaterials

C. C. Chu, Ph.D Assistant Professor
Department of Design & Environmental Analysis
Martha Van Rensselaer Hall
Cornell University, Ithaca, NY 14853

ABSTRACT

Virtually every operation requires the use of materials to close the wound for subsequent successful healing. The material must retain adequate strength during the critical period of healing; it should also induce minimal tissue reaction that might interfere with the healing process. The complexity involved in wound healing calls for different types of wound closure materials. In general, they are divided into three major categories: suture materials, tissue adhesives and surgical staples. The chemical, physical, mechanical, and biological properties of the first two categories are reviewed. The purpose is to present the most recent research work in this area for not only assisting medical professionals in the reliable selection of these wound closure materials but also providing polymer scientists and engineers with a coherent view of this interdisciplinary field. The ultimate solution of choosing wound closure materials will likely be a compromise of chemical, physical, mechanical and biological properties for optimum performance. Continuous research in this area is highly desirable, particularly in the development of absorbable suture materials, better understanding of the biodegradation mechanism, anti-infection would closure biomaterials, and more biocompatible tissue adhesives.

A. INTRODUCTION

Wound closure biomaterials concern every surgeon. Virtually every operation requires the use of materials to close the wound for subsequent successful healing. The proper closing of the wound can influence the success of the operation. Many complications such as infection, wound dehiscence, and sinus formation occur in the wound closure line. The wound closure materials required depend to some extent on the type of wound to be closed. However, the material must retain adequate tensile strength during the critical period of healing; it should also induce minimal tissue reaction that might interfere with the healing process.

The complexity involved in wound healing, such as the involvement of more than one type of tissue in the wound, the various degrees of wound strength during the process of healing, the exposure of the materials to body fluids, or the variety of surgical wounds each with its own healing problems, call for different types of wound closure materials. The choice of these materials is based largely on the type of wound and the surgeon's preference.

In general, wound closure biomaterials are divided into three major categories: suture materials, tissue adhesives and staplers. The former have received the most attention and are widely used in wound closure, while the use of tissue adhesives is still being debated. The stapler system facilitates anastomosis with minimal trauma necrosis or interruption of tissue function.

A suture, by definition, is a strand of material, either natural or synthetic, used to ligate blood vessels and to approximate tissue together. According to records, the ancient Egyptians used linen as a suture material as far back as 2000 B.C. Since then, numerous materials have been used as ligatures and sutures: iron wire, gold, silver, dried gut, horse hair, strips of hide, bark fibers, silk, linen, and tendon. Among them, catgut and silk dominated the suture market until 1930. The introduction of steel wire and synthetic fibers like nylon and polyester during and after World War II greatly expanded the chemical composition of suture materials. Today the surgeon can choose between a large number of suture materials with various chemical, physical, mechanical, and biological properties. During the early 1970's, the successful introduction of two synthetic absorbable suture materials, Dexon® and Vicryl® , opened a new chapter for suture materials. Owing to their precisely controlled manufacturing processes and uniform and reproducible properties, these materials have received a great deal of attention from both surgeons and researchers. Recently a new experimental synthetic absorbable suture material, Polydioxanone, has been reported [1], and will soon be available, commercially.

Coover discovered tissue adhesives in the mid-1950's. Although they are not as popular as suture materials, particularly in the United States, they have a unique role in wound closure biomaterials. Unlike sutures, which hold the wound together mechanically, tissue adhesives chemically bond to the wounded tissues. Some surgeons prefer tissue adhesives over suture materials in certain types of surgery, such as joining blood vessels and closing lacerated solid organs. The special environment of tissues, their regenerative capacity, biodegradability, and tissue reactions to biodegradable products, however, make tissue adhesives more difficult to develop. The most representative tissue adhesives come from the homologs of alkyl-α-cyanoacrylate. They are used most frequently in the anastomosis of blood vessels and the small and large intestine. Other applications, like the treatment of fragile tissues in liver, spleen, and kidney wounds, and in repairing ophthalmological, genitourinary, and cardiovascular systems have also been reported [2,3].

Even though tissue adhesives have certain advantages over suture materials, such as hemostatic capability and the lesser degree of tissue deformation which is important in plastic surgery, sutureless closure of operation wounds with these adhesives is still quite unsatisfactory. The use of a stapler system in wound closure is relatively new. It allows accurate apposition with minimal tension and time and can be removed easily. It also has good cosmetic results. Much more research needs to be done before a final conclusion can be drawn about tissue adhesives and staplers.

As a result of recent progress in this field, medical professionals are faced with an increasing challenge in selecting the proper wound closure biomaterials from a vast number of available biomaterials. The traditional way of choosing wound closure materials, particularly with suture materials (largely based on habit and the surgeon's training background), is becoming gradually inappropriate. The purpose of the present chapter is to survey the properties (e.g., chemical, physical, mechanical, and biological) of wound closure biomaterials. This will not only assist medical professionals in the reliable selection of these materials, but will also provide polymer chemists and engineers with a coherent view of this field and useful information for the future design of even better wound closure materials.

B. SUTURE

An ideal suture should have the following properties:

- Handle comfortably and naturally
- Minimum tissue reaction
- Adequate tensile strength and knot security
- Be unfavorable for bacterial growth and easily sterilized
- Nonelectrolytic, noncapillary, nonallergenic, and noncarcinogenic

These properties should be achieved jointly by the two components of a suture – the needle and the thread.

B.1 Surgical Needle

The needle must be able to carry suture materials through tissue with minimum trauma. It should be sharp enough to penetrate tissue easily and be corrosion-resistant. A properly balanced needle is important for smooth handling as well as to prevent it from breaking under various degrees of stress. Needles are normally made of stainless steel. Although numerous types are available, they basically have three components: the point, the body, and the eye. The basic shapes of the point are cutting, tapered, spatula, or blunt. A taper point has no cutting edge. It is used for less resistant tissues such as intestine and dura mater. A spatula point has a cutting edge in the horizontal plane. It is a multi-purpose needle and is used both in soft and tough tissues. A cutting point has three cutting edges, two in the horizontal plane, one in the vertical plane. There are normal and reverse cutting points. Both are used in tough tissue like skin, tendon, and ligament. The blunt point has a rounded end. It is used where either cutting or piercing could damage the function of the tissue, for examples with parenchymatous and friable tissues (e.g. liver & kidney). Figure 1 illustrates the various types of points. The surgeon should select the type of needle point that is appropriate for his specific use.

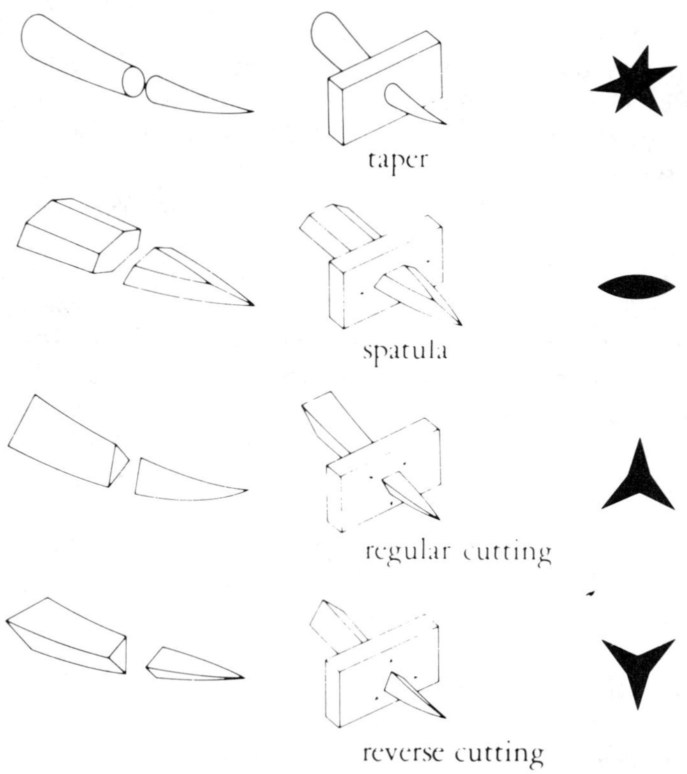

Figure 1. The type of needle point. (Courtesy of Dr. Holmlund et al., Ref. 31).

Regardless of size, the body has the following configurations: oval, round, triangular, or flat. The needle may be straight or curved, depending on the accessibility of the tissue to be closed. In the curved needle, the curvature can be 1/4, 3/8, 1/2, or 5/8" wide.

There are three types of eye: closed, swaged, and split (French). The closed eye (ordinary, round, and square) is similar to a household sewing needle. French-eye needles have a slit from inside the eye to the end of the needle. The swaged eye (sometimes called eyeless) causes less tissue disruption and damage than the closed-eye needle when it passes through the tissue, due to the direct attachment of the needle to the suture material. This type is increasingly popular, but is more expensive.

The thread component of a suture is probably more important than the needle in terms of the functional of a wound closure material because the thread remains in the wound to carry out its function – i.e. to maintain the opposition of the tissue. Therefore, the rest of the chapter deals largely with the thread, which people are usually referring to when they talk about suture materials.

B.2 Classification of Suture Materials

In terms of their performance, suture materials are generally classified into two broad categories: absorbable and non-absorbable. Absorbable suture materials lose their entire tensile strength within two to three months; those which retain their strength longer than two to three months are non-absorbable. The absorbable suture materials are catgut (collagen sutures derived from sheep intestinal submucosa), reconstituted collagen, polyglycolic acid (PGA), and its lactide copolymers. The non-absorbable sutures are divided into the natural fibers (i.e., silk, cotton), and man-made fibers (i.e., polyethylene, polypropylene, polyamide, polyester, and stainless steel.

Suture materials are also classified according to their size. Currently, two standards are used to describe the size of suture materials: USP (United States Pharmacopoeia) and EP (European Pharmocopoeia). The former is more commonly used. In USP standard, the size is represented by a series combination of two arabic numbers: a zero and any number other than zero, like 2/0-5/0. The higher the first number, the smaller the suture material is. Sizes greater than 0 are denoted by 1, 2, 3, and so on. This standard size also varies with the type of suture material, as shown in Table 1.

Table 1. Suture Size Classification

USP size codes		EP size codes (mm.)	Suture diameter in mm.
Nonsynthetic absorbable materials	Non-absorbable and synthetic absorbable materials	Absorbable and Non-absorbable materials	Min. - Max.
	11/0	0.1	0.01 - 0.019
	10/0	0.2	0.02 - 0.029
	9/0	0.3	0.03 - 0.039
	8/0	0.4	0.04 - 0.049
8/0	7/0	0.5	0.05 - 0.069
7/0	6/0	0.7	0.07 - 0.099
6/0	5/0	1	0.10 - 0.14
5/0	4/0	1.5	0.15 - 0.19
4/0	3/0	2	0.20 - 0.24
3/0	2/0	2.5	0.25 - 0.29
2/0	0	3	0.30 - 0.39
0	1	4	0.40 - 0.49
1	2	5	0.50 - 0.59
2	3	6	0.60 - 0.69
3	4	7	0.70 - 0.79
4	5	8	0.80 - 0.89
5	6	9	0.90 - 0.99
6	7	10	1.00 - 1.09

In EP standard, the code number ranges from 0.1 to 10. The corresponding minimum diameter (mm) can be easily calculated by taking the code number and dividing by 10. EP standard does not separate natural from synthetic absorbable sutures as USP does. Table 1 summarizes both EP and USP standards.

In terms of the physical configuration of the suture materials, they can be classified into monofilament, multifilament, twisted, and braided. Suture materials made of nylon, polyester and stainless steel are available in both multifilament and monofilament forms. Catgut, reconstituted collagen, and cotton are available in twisted multifilament form, while polyglycolic acid, poly(glycolide-lactide), and silk are available in braided multifilament configuration. Polypropylene suture material exists in monofilament form. Stainless steel metallic

Table 2. A List of Commercially Available Suture Materials

Generic Name	Trade Name	Physical Configuration	Surface Treatment	Manufacturer
Catgut	catgut or surgical gut	twisted multifilament	plain & chromic	A.E. D/G, SSC
Reconstituted Collagen	collagen	twisted multifilament	plain & chromic	E.
Polyglycolic acid	Dexon	braided multifilament	-	D/G
Poly(glycolide-lactide) (Polyglactin 910)	Vicryl	braided multifilament	with & without an absorbable coating	E.
Silk	Surgical Silk	braided multifilament	tru-permanizing	E.
Silk	Dermal	twisted multifilament	tanned gelatin (or other proteins)	E.
Silk	Virgin Silk	twisted multifilament	-	E.
Silk	Silk	braided multifilament	silicone	E & D/G
Silk	Silk	braided multifilament	paraffin wax	SSC
Cotton	Surgical Cotton	twisted multifilament	-	E.
Cotton	Cotton	twisted multifilament	-	D/G
Linen	Linen	twisted multifilament	wax	SSC & E.
Polyester	Ethibond	braided multifilament	polybutilate	E.
Polyester	Mersilene	braided multifilament	-	E.
Polyester	Ethiflex	braided multifilament	teflon	E.
Polyester	Dacron	braided multifilament	No	D/G
Polyester	Ti-cron	braided multifilament	silicone	D/G
Polyester	Silky Polydek	braided multifilament	teflonized	SSC
Polyester	Sterilene	braided multifilament	teflonized	SSC
Polyester	Tevedek	braided multifilament	teflonized	SSC
Polyester	Astralen	braided multifilament	teflonized	A
Polyester	Mirafil	monofilament	-	BM
Polyamide (Nylon 6, & 66)	Ethilon	monofilament	-	E.
Polyamide (Nylon 6, & 66)	Nurolon	braided multifilament	yes	E.
Polyamide (Nylon 66)	Surgilon	braided multifilament	silicone	D/G
Polyamide (Nylon 66)	Dermalon	monofilament	no	D/G
Polyamide	Sutron	monofilament	-	SSC
Polyamide (Nylon 6)	Supramid	core-sheath	-	A
Polyamide (Nylon 6)	Perlon	core-sheath	-	PTA
Polypropylene	Prolene	monofilament	-	E.
Polypropylene	Surgilene	monofilament	no	D/G
Polyethylene	-	monofilament	no	D/G
Stainless Steel	Surgical stainless steel	mono & twisted multifilament	-	E.
Stainless Steel	Flexon	twisted multifilament	-	D/G
Stainless Steel	-	mono & twisted multifilament	-	D/G
Stainless Steel	Stainless steel	mono & twisted multifilament	-	A. SSC

A: Astra
D/G: Davis & Geck
E: Ethicon
SSC: Societe Steril Catgut
BM: Braun Melsungen

suture materials can be obtained in either monofilament or twisted multifilament configurations. Another unique physical configuration of suture materials is made of polyamide (nylon 6) and has the tradename Supramid® . It has a twisted core covered by a jacket of the same material. Table 2 summarizes all suture materials that are available in the United States and Europe, their generic and trade names, physical configurations, and manufacturers.

B.3 Chemical Structure and Manufacturing Processes

B.3.1 Absorbable Suture Materials

B.3.1.1 Catgut. Plain catgut was described as early as 175 A.D. The basic constituent is collagen. It is derived from the submucosa of sheep intestines or serosa of bovine intestine. The jejunum and ileum portions of the intestine of sheep or beef are split into two or more longitudinal ribbons, and then the mucosa muscularis and other unwanted layers are removed by chemical and mechanical treatments. The remaining portion is treated in diluted formaldehyde to block the $-OH$ and $-NH_2$ groups on collagen in order to increase the strength and the resistance to enzyme attack. Several ribbons are then twisted into strands, dried, machine ground, and polished by a centerless grinder to a correct and smooth size. This grinding and polishing process can produce unpredictable amounts of weak points and local tearing of fibrils. Thus, fibrils could fray during use. Reproducible strength is also difficult to achieve.

The resulting untreated catgut suture is called plain catgut. If the plain catgut is further tanned in a bath of chromium trioxide, it is called chromic catgut, a variant first developed by Lister in 1840. There are two types of chromicizing processes: Tru and Surface Chromicizings. The former is done to each ribbon before it is spun into strands while the latter is conducted on the finished strand. This treatment would alter the color of plain catgut from a yellowish-tan shade to a darker shade of brown. Depending on the concentration of chromic bath and duration of chromicizing, mild and extra chromic catgut are available. Of course, the degrees of absorption and tissue response are also affected by the severity of tanning process. Chromic catgut suture is generally more resistant to absorption and causes less tissue reaction than plain catgut suture.

B.3.1.2 Reconstituted Collagen. Reconstituted collagen sutures are prepared from the long flexor tendons or beef. The tendon is cleaned, frozen, sliced, treated with ficin, and then swollen in dilute cyanoacetic acid. The resulting viscous gel is extruded through a spinerette into an acetone bath for coagulation. The coagulated fibril is stretched, twisted, and dried or treated with chromic salts before twisting and drying. These sutures are similar in appearance to catgut. They are made only in fine sizes, and thus are almost exclusively used in microsurgery.

B.3.1.3 Polyglycolic Acid and Poly(glycolide-lactide). Polyglycolic acid (PGA) was the first synthetic absorbable suture. It was developed by Davis and Geck. This suture is polymerized from the cyclic dimer of α-hydroxyacetic acid, more commonly called glycolic acid. Glycolic acid exists in sugar beets, unripe grapes, and wheat and barley leaves. Most higher plants utilize glycolic acid in photo-respiration. On heating, glycolic acids form cyclic dimers, called glycolides, more readily than other hydroxy acids due to the formation of stable, ring-strain free six-member ring anhydrides. Glycolide exists in two polymorphic forms, α and β, depending on the crystallization temperature (Tc) during purification. The α form obtained at

$42°C < Tc < 82.5°C$ is thermodynamically stable and less sensitive to moisture than the β isomer, which is stable below 42°C [4]. Thus, the α isomer is preferred for the preparation of high molecular weight PGA.

PGA can be polymerized either directly or indirectly from glycolic acid. The direct polycondensation produces a polymer of $\overline{M}n$ less than 10,000 because of the requirement of a very high degree of dehydration (99.28% up) and the absence of monofunctional impurities [5,6]. For PGA of molecular weight higher than 10,000 it is necessary to proceed through the ring-opening polymerization of the cyclic dimers of glycolic acid.

Numerous catalysts are available for this ring-opening polymerization. They include organometallic compounds and Lewis acids [6,7]. For biomedical applications, stannous chloride dihydrate or trialkyl aluminum are preferred. The mechanism of polymerization is believed to be cationic melt polymerization if stannous chloride dihydrate (in the presence of alcohol) is used, or nucleophilic attack of a carbanion on one of the glycolide carbonyls if the trialkyl aluminum is used, as shown in Figure 2 [4,8]. The activation energy and heat of polymerization are 20.7 and 6.3 Kcal/mole, respectively [7]. No polymer could be obtained by γ-irradiation in all conditions.

The resulting polymer having $\overline{M}w$ from 20,000 to 140,000 is suitable for fiber extrusion and suture manufacturing. The fiber is stretched above its glass transition temperature (36°C), heat-set for improving dimensional stability and inhibiting shrinkage, and subsequently braided into final suture forms of various sizes [9].

The lactide-glycolide copolymer suture material, sometimes called polyglactin 910, is also randomly copolymerized in the same fashion. For copolymers high in glycolic acid (such as polyglactin 910 absorbable suture which contains a 90/10 molar ratio of glycolic to lactic acid), Lewis acid catalysts are preferred [7].

Lactic acid, due to its one asymmetric carbon, has two optical isomers, L(+) and D(−). It is present as either an intermediate or an end product in carbohydrate metabolism. The six-membered cyclic dimers of lactic acid, called lactides, are also optically active. They exist in L(−), D(+), and meso forms. The polyglactin 910 absorable copolymer suture is polymerized from L(−) lactide rather than other optical or racemic isomers. Copolymer sutures from glycolide and D.L. racemic lactide can shrink up to 50%, while the copolymer sutures prepared from either D. or L. pure lactide isomer exhibit very low shrinkage [9,10].

Both PGA and polyglactin 910 are semi-crystalline polymers. The crystal structure of the former has been extensively studied by x-ray diffraction methods [11]. PGA was found to exhibit an orthorhombic unit cell with dimensions a = 5.22 Å, b = 6.19 Å, and c (fiber axis) = 7.02 Å. The planar zigzag-chain molecules form a sheet structure parallel to the ac plane, as shown in Figure 3, and do not have the polyethylene type arrangement. The molecules between two adjacent sheets orient in opposite directions. The tight molecular packing and the close approach of the ester groups might stabilize the crystal lattice and contribute to the high melting point of PGA (224-227°C). The specific gravities of PGA are 1.707 for a perfect crystal and 1.50 in a completely amorphous state [12]. The heat of fusion of 100% crystallized PGA is reported to be 12 KJ/mole or 45.7 cal/gram [7].

In the case of lactide-glycolide copolymer, the regularity of the chain stacking in the sheets is disturbed because of the existence of a lactide comonomer whose methyl group must affect the chain packing along the b axis [11]. The broadening of the reflections in the copolymer demonstrates this. Such disorder in the b direction (the direction in which sheets stack) of the copolymer might contribute to the difference in the biodegradation phenomena between the copolymer and the homopolymer sutures.

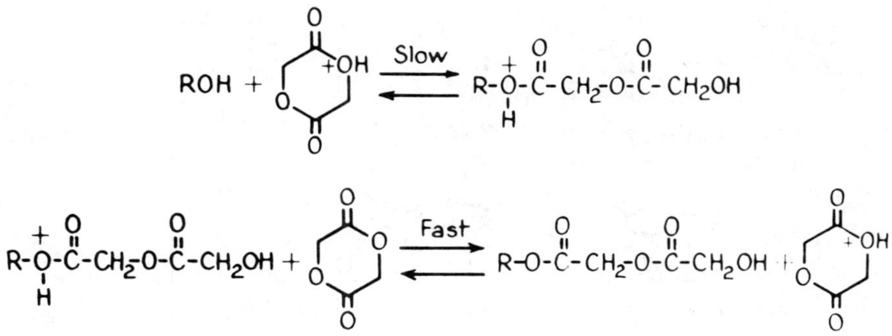

Figure 2a.

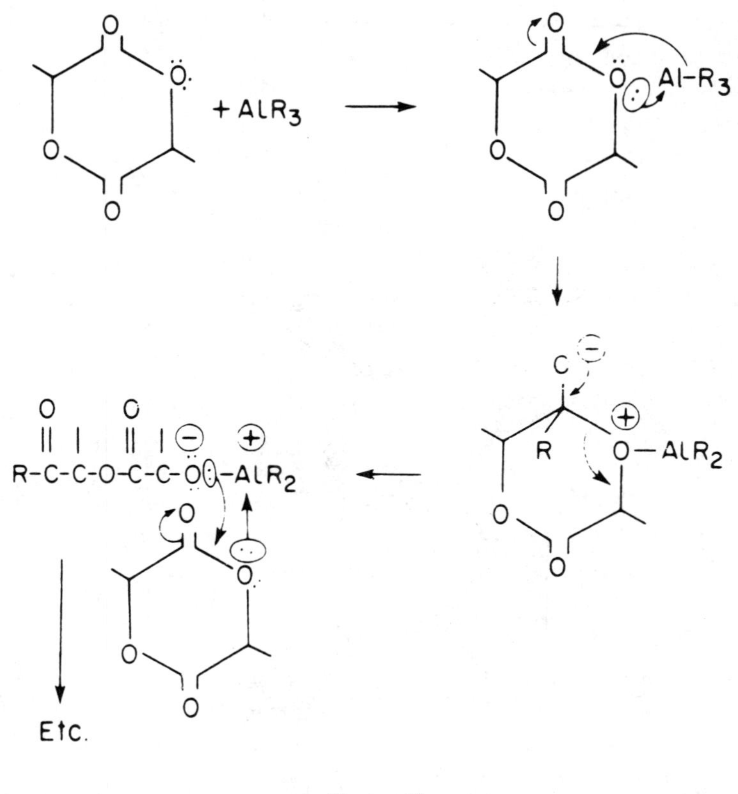

Figure 2b.

Figure 2. Polymerization mechanism of polyglycolic acid. (a) cationic, (b) nucleophilic. (Courtesy of Drs. Frazza & Wise et al., Ref. 4 & 6).

B.3.2 Non-absorbable Suture Materials

B.3.2.1 Silk. Silk is one of the three major fibrous proteins (the others are wool, and collagen). Silk is crystalline and oriented in an axial direction. The actual fiber protein is called fibroin, while the gummy substance that holds the fiber together is called sericin. As it is spun

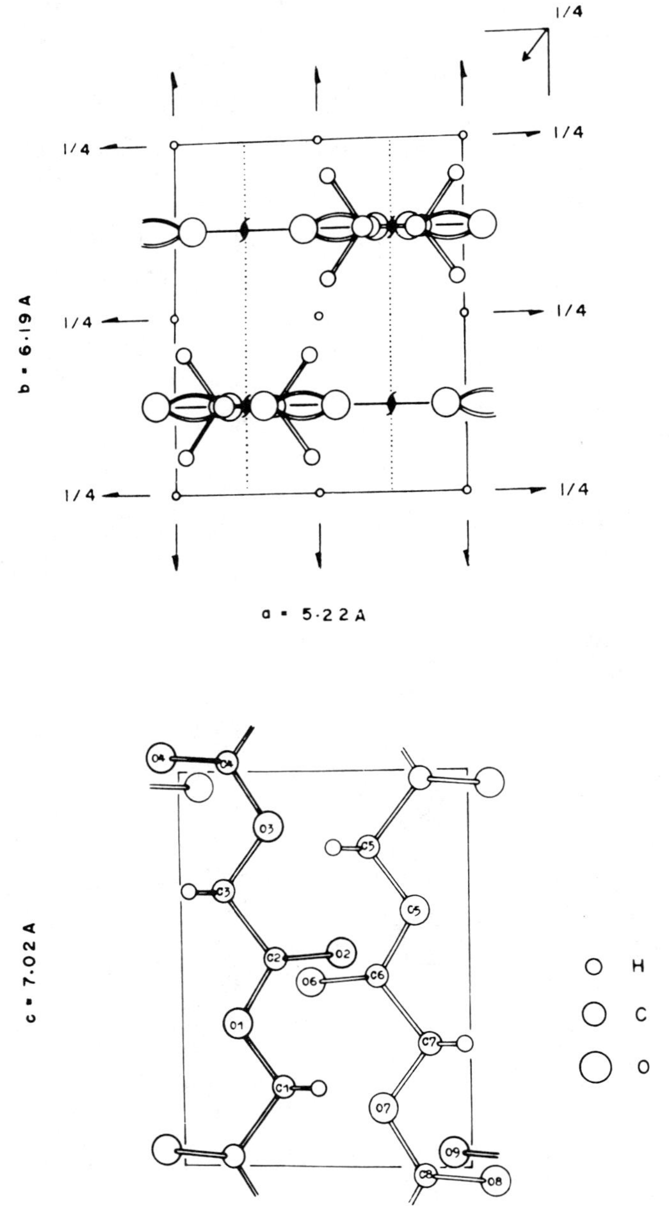

Figure 3. Crystal structure of polyglycolic acid. (Courtesy of Dr. Chatani et al. Ref. 11).

by the silkworm, silk fiber consists of two triangular filaments stuck together with sericin. In contrast to wool and the other α-keratins, silk does not contain sulfur-containing amino acid residues like cystine, and is composed mainly of Gly, Ala, and Ser residues with relatively small amounts of the more bulky side chains. The amino acids with bulky side chains cannot be accommodated within the three-dimensional, ordered structure. Thus, disordered amorphous regions co-exist with the crystalline ones. Cross-sectional views of silk fiber show somewhat irregular triangular shape.

The mechanical properties of silk closely correlate with the fraction of bulky side groups present and thus with the crystalline-amorphous ratio. The crystalline portion of the polypeptide chains in silk are in the extended zigzag β-conformation. Neighboring chains are antiparallel to one another, and a pleated sheet is formed. The Gly residues lie on one side of the sheet and the Ser and Ala on the other. There is an axial repeat of 7 Å, corresponding to two amino-acid residues. The fibroin molecules, which are about 1400 Å long, tend to be oriented parallel to the fiber axis, and the material is moderately crystalline. The molecules with simple and regularly packed side groups form the crystalline regions, while the chain segments with bulky side groups do not crystallize easily and thus form the major part of the amorphous regions. This arrangement bears an important relationship to properties such as moisture absorption and biodegradation which occur mainly in the amorphous regions of silk.

All silks are not, however, chemically identical. Different silkworm species produce fibrous proteins that contain different sequences and proportions of amino acids. These compositional differences in turn influence the mechanical properties of the fibers. The most common form of silk, produced by the silkworm Bombyx mori, has a predominant six residue sequence Gly-Ser-Gly-Ala-Gly-Ala, which repeats itself for long distances along the chain. This sequence accounts for a large proportion of the amino acid residues that are present. The identity of the silkworm species used for making silk suture materials is not publicly available, but is suspected to be the most common silkworm, Bombyx mori.

The process of making silk sutures has not been disclosed by the manufacturer. It is believed, however, that the raw silk fibers from the cocoon are cleaned first by removing the natural waxes and gums. The cleaned silk fibers are then either twisted or braided to form the suture strand. Silk has a relatively high standard moisture regain of 11%. Various types of surface treatments are used to render it non-capillary, serum proof, or incapable of the ingrowth of tissue cells, or all of these. Tissue ingrowth is prevented by encasing the twisted silk fibers in a nonabsorbing coating of tanned gelatin or other protein substances. The trade name of this treated silk suture is Dermal.

B.3.2.2 Cotton and Linen. Basically, there are three types of cotton, classified according to length: short staple (3/8–3/4 inch), intermediate-length staple (13/16–11/4 inch), and long staple fibers (1-1/2–2-1/2 inch). Cotton sutures are made from long staple fiber. The raw cotton fibers are first separated from their seeds (called ginning), cleaned, and blended to ensure a spun yarn of uniform quality. Then they go through carding and combing processes which continue to separate and align the fibers for evenness, smoothness, fineness, and strength. Slivers from the carder or the comber are finally processed through roving and spinning. The amount of twist and the size of the yarn are introduced and controlled during the spinning process. The purpose of twist is to maintain the integrity of the strand to keep it from fraying during use.

The cross-sectional shape of cotton fiber varies from a U-shape to a nearly circular form. The fiber has a natural twist called convolutions, and a long staple cotton has about 30 twists per inch. This twist facilitates the spinning of cotton fiber. Cotton is 10 to 20% stronger when wet than dry, and its strength can be increased by a process called mercerization. Cotton is a relatively high density fiber with a specific gravity of 1.54 (polyester-1.38, nylon-1.14). It absorbs moisture well and its moisture regain is 7 to 8%. Microorganisms such as fungi can grow on cotton fiber and eventually deteriorate it.

Linen is made from twisted long staple flax fibers. The first step in preparing flax fibers is called retting, which loosens the bark from the stem, followed by breaking and scutching. The resulting flax fibers go through a hackled process before they are ready for spinning.

The properties of flax fiber are about the same as those of cotton, except for the wicking ability. Wicking ability, commonly known as capillary effect, is important in suture design. Flax fiber has higher wicking ability than cotton, and hence moisture travels readily along the fiber.

The basic structural unit of cotton and flax is cellulose. The skeleton of the cellulose chain consists of successive β-linkages of glucose rings at their number one and number four carbon positions. The three OH-groups on each ring in the chain have an important influence on the properties of the cellulose molecule. They contribute to the high moisture absorbency and melting point. Due to the large number of H-bonds, the cellulose crystal is extremely stable. Since it decomposes before it melts, cellulose cannot be melt-spun, nor can it be dissolved in water or any ordinary solvents.

B.3.2.3 Polyester Suture Material. Almost all polyester sutures are made of polyethlyene terephthalate, HO–[OC–⌬–COO–CH_2–CH_2–O]$_n$–H, which in turn is polymerized from ethylene glycol, HO–CH_2CH_2–OH and terephthalic acid, HOOC–⌬–COOH, (or dimethyl terephthalate in the case of Terylene®). Polymerization is conducted in a vacuum at a high temperature. The first stage involves the formation of low molecular weight oligomers through ester interchange. The oligomers are then polycondensed further to build up high molecular weight polyester. The second stage is carried out at about 270°C and reduced pressure (0.5 torr).

The resulting polyester chips are melt-spun into round cross-sectional shaped filaments. The filament is then hot-stretched (above its Tg 80°C) to about five times its original length. Further crystallization occurs during the hot drawing. Depending on the degree of drawing, polyester yarns of either normal strength or high tenacity can be obtained. The molecular weight of PET that is capable of making fibers is on the order of 20,000. Unlike the simple zigzag structure of polyethylene and nylon, the poly(ethylene terephthalate) molecule has an extended rectilinear shape, the plane of the benzene rings being parallel to the (100) plane [13]. The –COO– group is out of the plane of the benzene rings by 12° and the ethylene glycol residue by 20°. In a stretched fiber the axes of the molecular chains are inclined in relation to the fiber axis in such a way that the (230) plane remains vertical and the inclination of the (001) plane to the fiber axis increases. For a fiber annealed at 210°C and relaxed, the angle between the fiber axis and the crystal axis is 5°.

The benzene ring, together with its two associated C–C bonds, forms a single rigid structure. Consequently, the chain is rigid and less flexible than nylon and polyethylene. This accounts for the slow rate of crystallization and high melting point (265°C). The melt-spun filaments are thus largely amorphous before drawing. The maximum rate of crystallization of amorphous PET occurs at 190°C. The stereochemical structure of the PET chain changes during crystallization. The ethylene glycol residues of crystalline and oriented amorphous PET chain acquire a transconfiguration while the same residues in amorphous PET possess mainly gauche conformation with a small portion of transconformation [14].

The physical structure of PET is also winding speed-dependent during the melt spinning process. PET yarns wound at a speed slower than 4,000 meters per minute exhibit an amorphous structure, while at a higher speed, the structure changes from amorphous to semicrystalline [15].

B.3.2.4 Polyamide Suture Materials. The most successful aliphatic polyamide that polymer scientists have synthesized is nylon, which was a product of the genius of Wallace H. Carothers. Nylon is basically polymerized either from polycondensation of a dicarboxylic acid and a diamine, or through a ring-opening polymerization of appropriate lactams. Although there are numerous types of nylon, such as nylon 3, 4, 5, 6, 7, 8, 9, 11, 12, 66, 610, only 66 and 6 are used to make suture materials. The former is more popular in the United States, while the latter is used in Europe. They are readily identified by a simple numeral system:

$$\underset{\text{diamine}}{H_2N(CH_2)_nNH_2} + \underset{\text{dibasic acid}}{HOOC(CH_2)_{m-2}COOH} \rightarrow \underset{\text{Nylon 66 if n and m = 6}}{\left[HN(CH_2)_nNHCO(CH_2)_{m-2}CO \right]}$$

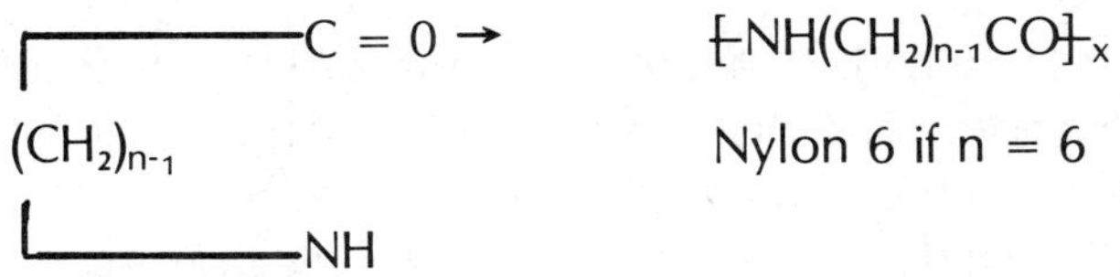

Nylon 66 is made from adipic acid, $HOOC(CH_2)_4COOH$, and hexamethylene diamine, $H_2N(CH_2)_6NH_2$. These two chemicals, dissolved separately in methanol, are mixed and nylon salt, $H_3H^+\ (CH_2)_6NH_3^+\ {}^-OOC(CH_2)_4COO^-$, is precipitated. Equal moles of adipic acid and diamine are important for achieving high molecular-weight nylon 66. Because of the increasing price of oil, alternative syntheses of raw materials for making nylon salt have been explored, including cereal products, notably bran and husks, and butadiene [16].

Nylon salt is melted under an inert gas atmosphere to prevent discoloration. Acetic acid is added as a stabilizer during polycondensation. No catalyst is needed for polymerization; suitable conditions are a temperature of 280°C and four hours. The molten polymer is extruded in ribbon form, which is quenched with cold water in order to reduce the crystal size, and then cut into chips. The extent of polymerization is determined by the residual moisture content. A vacuum should be applied if high molecular weight nylon is desirable [17]. Nylon 66 can also be made by interfacial polycondensation [17]. The reaction takes place at the interface between a diamine water solution and a dicarboxylic acid chloride in a water-insoluble solvent. The reaction is rapid and a precise amount of the reactants is unnecessary. This method obtains high molecular weight nylon 66. Nylon 66 of molecular weight 12,000 to 20,000 is suitable for melt-spinning into fibers.

Nylon 6 is made from caprolactam:

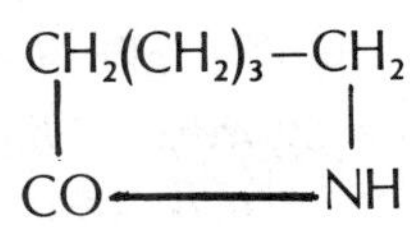

Two alternative methods are used [16]. The first method involves the liquifying and heating of caprolactam under high pressure. The resulting nylon 6 polymer chain consists of an average of 200 repeating units. The second method needs about 10% water and is carried out at a high temperature with a controlled release of steam. There are three reactions in the second method of polymerization: addition, condensation, and hydrolysis [17].

Addition:

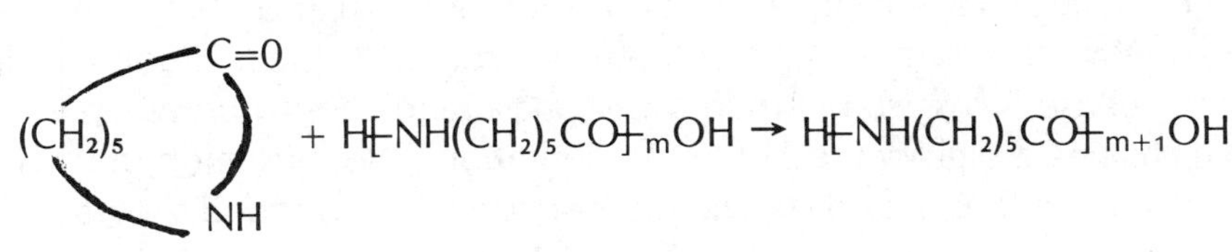

Condensation: $$H[NH(CH_2)_5CO]_mOH + H[NH(CH_2)_5CO]_nOH \rightarrow H[NH(CH_2)_5CO]_{m+n}OH + H_2O$$

Hydrolysis: 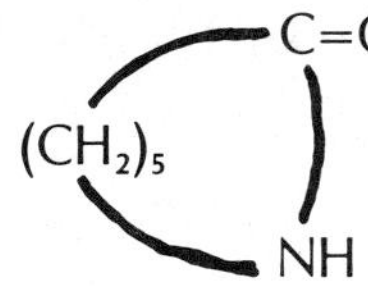 $+H_2O \rightarrow H_2N(CH_2)_5COOH$

The major growth mechanism of nylon 6 is the addition reaction, while nylon 66 is made by condensation reaction. Thus, the polymerization of nylon 6 is expedited in the presence of aminocaproic acid. The second method is easier to control, but it takes longer than the first one. Nylon 6 is also made anionically. The resulting polymer, however, has a very high molecular weight and is not as thermally stable as that made by the second method. Thus, it is not directly applicable to injection molding or extrusion [17]. Whichever polymerization method is used, nylon 6 contains about 10% extractable monomers and cyclic oligomers which act as plasticizers and are preferably removed for biomedical uses by water washing or vacuuming.

The resulting nylon 66 or 6 chips are then melt-spun into a cooling chamber in which nylon filaments form. In the case of nylon 66, the filaments are run through a steam chamber to wet them before they are wound. This treatment eliminates the undesirable extension of the yarns after they reach equilibrium by absorbing moisture from the air. The wound yarn is further cold-drawn by stretching about 400% in order to acquire better strength. During this cold-drawing process, vegetable oil is applied to the yarn as a lubricant and is washed off afterwards.

In the case of nylon 6, the same process of melt-spinning as for nylon 66 is used except that the steam chamber is not suitable. The relatively high residual concentration of monomers in nylon 6 would make the filaments sticky and adhere to one another if steamed. The filaments are normally drawn to 350-400%. Higher drawing can be achieved if a stronger fiber is needed. It is well recognized in fiber technology that by increasing the draw ratio (the ratio of the speed of output and input feed rollers), both tensile strength and elastic modulus increase, while the elongation at break decreases. If the molecular weight of nylon 6 is between 20,000 and 25,000, hot-drawing is used.

Unlike PET, both nylon fibers are fairly crystalline when they are spun. The crystal structures of nylon 66 and 6 fall into three categories: α, β, and γ phases. Almost all the commercially important nylons exist in either the α or β phase.

Even-even polyamides such as nylon 66 exist mainly in the α phase, which is more stable than β phase and is characterized by the progressive stacking of planar sheets (parallel to ac plane) of H-bonded molecules to meet the requirement of completely strain-free H-bonding [18]. The molecules in the crystalline region are in the fully extended zigzag conformation and the adjacent molecules have the same directionality (parallel) for strain-free H-bonding as shown in Figure 4. The structure is triclinic, with a = 4.9 Å, b = 5.4 Å, c (fiber axis) = 17.2 Å, and one chemical repeat per unit cell. The perpendicular distance between H-bonded sheets is 3.6 Å, while the normal distance between chains within a H-bonded planar sheet is 4.2 Å. The beta phase is less stable than the α phase and cannot be reliably determined except in samples having a high degree of axial orientation. The formation of the β phase is thought to be due to the up-and-down staggering of successive H-bonded sheets. Others postulate initial

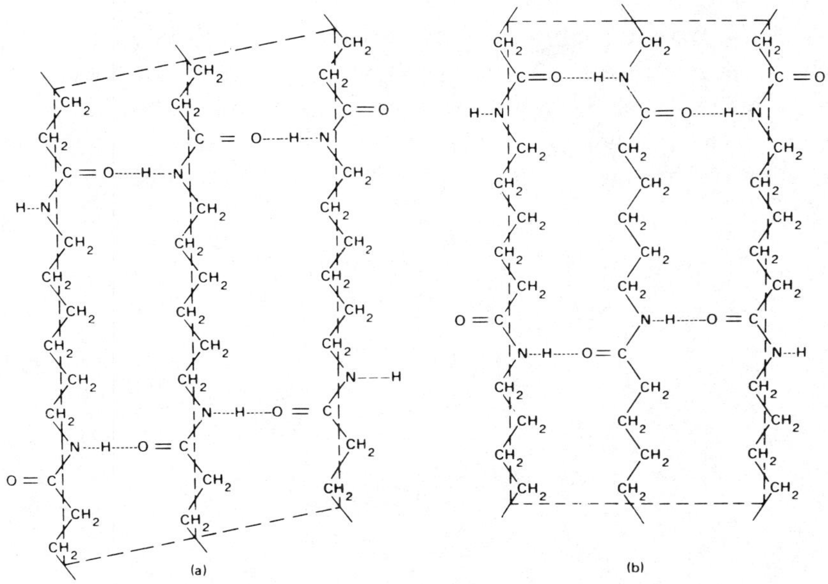

Figure 4. Ordered chain conformation for polyamides. (a) Nylon 66, (b) Nylon 6. (Courtesy of Dr. Bunn et al., Ref. 18).

stages of ordering and the presence of unrelated small crystallites.

Unlike nylon 66, H-bonded sheets of the α phase of nylon 6 involve adjacent molecules arranged in opposite directions (antiparallel) so that all the H-bonds are free of strain. Figure 4 illustrates these parallel and antiparallel chain conformations. Other even nylons from nylon 8 up, however, crystallize into the γ phase. H-bonds in the γ phase are between parallel molecules (like nylon 66). This forces the chains to twist slightly in order to realize strain-free H-bonds and hence, assume a puckered or pleated conformation. Consequently, the unit cell if γ phase is about 2% shorter. Nylon 6 assumes the γ phase after an iodine treatment, while most chemically untreated nylon 6 exists predominantly in α form [19].

The unstable β and γ phases can be converted into the α phase by improving crystallinity and orientation, namely drawing and annealing [19]. The relative amount of the α to γ phases is also found to depend on the winding speed in the spinning process [20]. Indications are that the γ phases are mainly generated from orientation-induced nuclei at speeds higher than 2500 meters per minute. Drawing at high ratios facilitates a γ to α transition. Due to the complex morphology of nylon 6, crystallinity values from density measurement (which are based on the additivity of the amorphous and crystalline phases) are thus inaccurate.

B3.2.5 Polypropylene. Polypropylene suture materials are made from isotactic polypropylene, which is polymerized from propylene with a Ziegler-Natta catalyst. The Z-N catalyst consists of a transition metal halide (e.g., $TiCl_3$) with a reducing agent (e.g., AlR_3). Ziegler-Natta catalyst systems are quite complex, and the exact structure of the catalysts cannot be determined precisely [21]. Many factors could influence the activity of the catalyst, such as the crystal structure, the molar ratio of the components, the aging of the complex, impurities, and the temperature of preparation [22]. The general polymerization kinetics are similar to other types of addition polymerization. The stereoregularity of the resulting polypropylene is controlled by the propagation step, which consists of repeated insertion of the propylene monomer into the carbon-transition metal bond through the polarization mechanism. This mechanism (Figure 5), normally called bimetallic mechanism, provides for an active site which can complex an incoming propylene monomer and maintain the end group of the growing polymer chain in a position suitable for propagation. Other mechanisms, like the monometallic one, involving an active site in which the transition metal assumes an octahedral configuration, are also proposed [23]. It is at present, difficult to distinguish the two mechanisms.

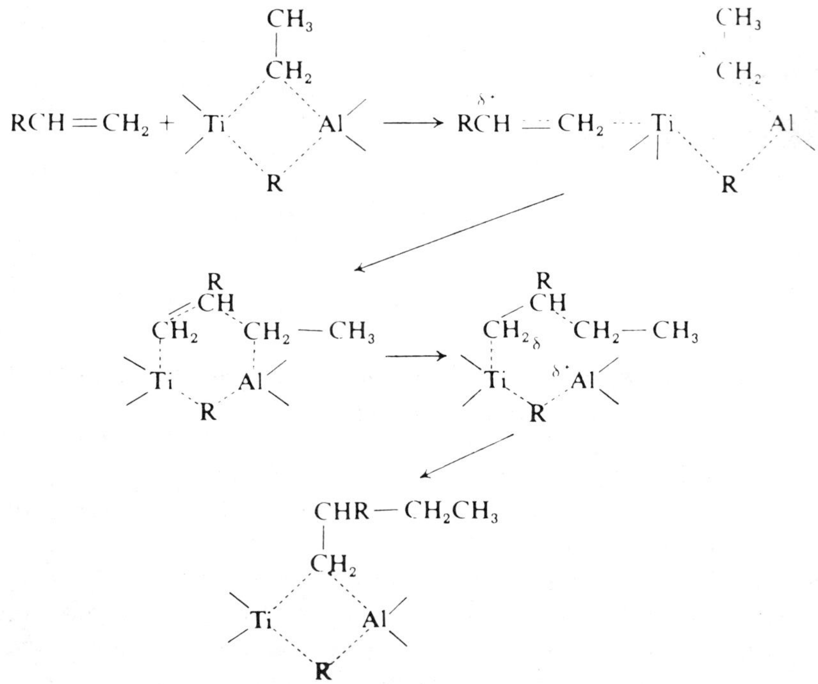

Figure 5. Bimetallic mechanism of polypropylene. (Courtesy of Dr. Kaufman et al., Ref. 22).

The resulting isotactic polypropylene has a molecular weight of about 80,000 and is melt-spun and drawn into fiber form like polyamides and polyesters do. The crystallinity is 50% before melt-spinning decreases to 33% after spinning and before drawing, and increases to 47% after drawing. Annealing increases the crystallinity further to 68% [16].

Due to the steric position of the CH_3 group in propylene, either a regular (isotactic and sydiotactic) or irregular (atactic) chain configuration can result. If atactic, it cannot crystallize and is a grease. In the isotactic form (CH_3 group on the same side of the backbone), the chain cannot assume a planar zigzag form as polyethylene and nylon 66 do, because of the bulky size of $-CH_3$. As shown in Figure 6, the chain thus twists into a helix form with three chemical repeat units per turn and packs into a monoclinic unit cell. The helix form permits the best inter- and intra-molecular packing of side groups. Within a limited temperature range and in the presence of certain foreign nuclei, isotactic polypropylene can be crystallized into a hexagonal unit cell.

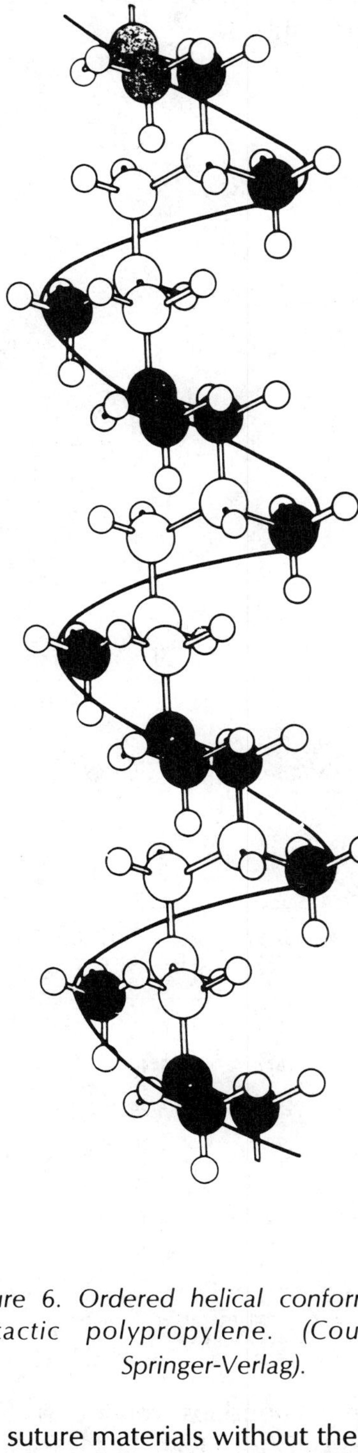

Figure 6. Ordered helical conformation of isotactic polypropylene. (Courtesy of Springer-Verlag).

B.4 Mechanical Properties of Suture Materials

Since the major function of suture materials is to hold the wound until it heals, these materials experience the same kinds of mechanical forces as the wound does. It is often literally true that the life of a patient hangs by a tiny thread. Suture strength is a complicated issue. An optimal utilization of suture materials is based on a proper balance/match between tissue strength and suture strength. Two factors must be considered in this connection.

First, consider the kind of tissue. It is well-recognized that the suture-holding strength of most soft tissues depends on the amount of fibrous tissue they have. Thus, the spinal cord and brain will scarcely support sutures due to their minimal amounts of fibrous connective tissue, while skin and fascia are the toughest of the soft tissues. The seromuscular coat of the intestinal wall is easily torn by sutures unless the tough, fibrous submucosa are sewn. Second, consider the health of the sewn tissue. Tissues become friable with acute inflammation. If the suture is too tight, particularly with a fine suture, it could cut through the inflammatory tissue.

The mechanical properties of fibrous polymers that are important for suture uses include: 1) tensile properties; 2) tensile strength retention; 3) stiffness and flexibility; and 4) knot strength and security. Each will be discussed in the following sections.

B.4.1 Tensile Properties

Although the properties of knotted sutures are a better representation of the in vivo condition, tensile properties of straight sutures give a better fundamental characterization of different suture materials without the complications arising from the knot. Detailed reports on the tensile properties of suture materials like stress-strain curves, elastic moduli, work of rupture and stress-relaxation are sparse [24,25]. A recent comprehensive study of the tensile properties of seven commonly used suture materials, employing a new grip device, is the beginning of an awareness of the importance of such a fundamental characterization of suture materials [24]. The results of that study are summarized in Figure 7 and Table 3.

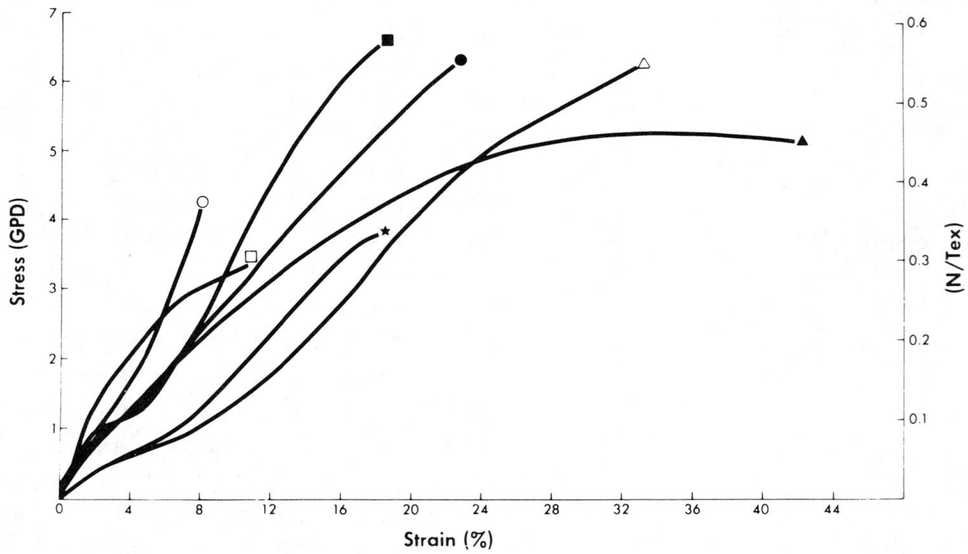

*Figure 7. Stress-strain curves of 2-0 suture materials. O - Mersilene; ● - Dexon; □ - Silk; ■ - Vicryl; Δ - Ethilon; ▲ Prolene; * - Nurolon.*

Table 3. Mechanical Properties of Suture Materials

Suture (2-0)	Yield Stress (GPD)	Breaking Stress (GPD)	Yield Strain (%)	Breaking Strain (%)	Modulus of Elasticity	Specific Work of Rupture (N/Tex) x 10^{-2}
Dexon	0.80 (0.77)	6.30 (6.2)	1.9 (1.9)	22.6 (26.3)	55 (53)	6.63
Vicryl	0.97 (0.98)	6.55 (6.28)	1.8 (1.9)	18.4 (20.8)	67.5 (64)	5.46
Mersilene	1.20 (1.25)	4.20 (4.08)	2.7 (2.9)	8 (8.2)	53 (47.5)	1.32
Silk	1.33 (1.22)	3.43 (3.35)	1.9 (1.90)	11.5 (13.1)	79.0 (78.5)	2.36
Nurolon	0.34 (0.325)	3.80 (3.75)	1.6 (1.8)	18.2 (21)	21.0 (19.5)	2.80
Ethilon	0.41 (0.38)	6.25 (5.88)	2.2 (2.4)	33 (37)	20.0 (19.0)	8.96
Prolene	0.52 (0.40)	5.14 (5.0)	1.2 (1.2)	42 (43.2)	58.5 (38.5)	14.69

* Data from yarn grip tests except those parentheses which are from conventional grip tests.

† For those who are interested in N/Tex is 1 GPD = 0.08825 N/Tex.

It is evident from Figure 7 that a wide range of stress-strain relationships were observed in the seven commonly used sutures. Tenacity ranged from 3.43 GPD for silk, 4.3 GPD for Mersilene, and 5.14 GPD for Prolene, to 6.55 GPD for Vicryl. The breaking strain ranged from 8.9% for Mersilene, 11.5% for silk, and 18.2% for Nurolon, to 42.0% for Prolene. A summary of important mechanical properties of these sutures tested on both yarn and conventional grips is listed in Table 3.

Yield stress and strain are the correspondent stress and strain at the yeild point on the stress-strain curve. Materials start to deform permanently after the yield point; they cannot recover their original dimensions after the removal of the external force. The modulus of elasticity is equal to the slope of the stress-strain curve at the origin, and is a measure of the resistance to elongation before the yield point. The reciprocal of this property is called compliance.

Suture materials can, thus, be grouped according to these mechanical properties. On the basis of yield stress, Nurolon, Ethilon,and Prolene have the lowest yield stress (0.34-0.52 GPD), Dexon and Vicryl are in the middle (0.80-0.97 GPD), while Mersilene and silk have the highest yield stress (1.20-1.33 GPD). When grouped on the basis of breaking stress, the order is different. Dexon, Vicryl, and Ethilon are then the strongest (6.30-6.25 GPD), Prolene is in the middle (5.14 GPD), while silk, Nurolon, and Mersilene are the weakest (3.43-4.30 GPD). In terms of breaking strain, Mersilene and silk exhibit the lowest values (8 and 11.5%, respectively), Vicryl and Nurolon higher and similar values (18.4 and 18.2%, respectively), and Ethilon and Prolene the highest values (33 and 42%, respectively). These seven commonly used sutures also have wide ranges of moduli of elasticity. The order of increasing modulus of elasticity is Ethilon, Nurolon, Mersilene, Dexon, Prolene, Vicryl, and silk; the values range from 20 GPD to 79 GPD. Dexon, Mersilene, and Prolene have close moduli of elasticity. The geometric form of sutures does not appear to have any significant effect on the modulus of elasticity as evidenced from the small difference in elastic modulus between braided nylon (Nurolon) and monofilament nylon (Ethilon).

Specific works of rupture of the seven suture materials are also given in Table 3. Specific work of rupture of fibrous materials is defined as: Specific work of rupture

$$W_s = \frac{\text{work of rupture}}{(\text{mass/unit length}) \times \text{initial length}}$$

Work of rupture is defined as the amount of energy needed to break a material (sometimes called toughness) and is represented by the area under the stress-strain curve. It measures the ability of a material to withstand sudden shocks of a given energy. The material will be broken if the amount of energy from a sudden shock exceeds the work of rupture of the material. In a clinical situation, the coughing and vomiting will impose this kind of sudden shock on the suture material. In order to compare different materials, work of rupture should be normalized to take account of the various masses of different materials. Hence, specific work of rupture, which is the amount of energy needed to break a material of unit mass, should be used. There is a wide difference in specific work of rupture among the seven sutures, and the values range from 1.32 N/Tex for Mersilene to 14.69 N/Tex for Prolene – an almost tenfold difference. Specific works of rupture are about four times as great for sutures of the same chemical nature, but different geometrical configuration, such as Nurolon and Ethilon.

The shape of the stress-strain curves, along with the related mechanical properties extracted from the curves, provide important data for characterizing suture materials better. These shapes reveal a literal and overall discrimination of suture materials that is difficult to obtain by breaking strength and size specification alone. They are particularly helpful for discriminating among suture materials that have similar strengths or elongations. Although Dexon, Vicryl, and Ethilon behave similarly from the standpoint of breaking strength, these sutures exhibit very different stress-strain relationships, particularly in yield stress, breaking strain, and modulus of elasticity. Likewise, Nurolon and Vicryl have very similar breaking strains but show almost totally different stress-strain curves. Silk and Nurolon have similar specific work of rupture, but different stress-strain characteristics. Mersilene, Dexon, and Prolene have similar moduli of elasticity, but their stress-strain curves behave differently. Even the same materials (such as sutures of Nylon, Ethilon, and Nurolon) behave quite differently from each other in stress-strain curves as a result of their different geometrical configurations. Suture materials can, thus, be classified into several broad categories: 1) relatively hard and brittle, such as Mersilene and silk, 2) relatively strong and ductile, such as Dexon, Vicryl, and Ethilon, 3) relatively weak but ductile and tough, like Prolene, and 4) relatively weak, ductile, and soft, like Nurolon.

These examples, and data cited above, strongly suggest that suture materials having a few similar or even identical mechanical properties (i.e., breaking stress), are actually very different from each other in terms of overall performance. Therefore, more useful and complete information, such as stress-strain curves, could provide a better ground for discriminating between different suture materials for specific uses, even though they have some nominal similarities. For example, judging from the mechanical properties alone, Nurolon and Ethilon, due to their low moduli and high strains, are considered to be less appropriate than others for suturing wounded tissues that are relatively inelastic and constrained, like bone and tendon. Prolene and Ethilon are believed to be suitable for closing tissues having large elongation capabilities, such as skin (78% ultimate elongation) and cardiac muscle (63.8%).

The difference in distensibility of different materials, however, can be compensated by employing various suture techniques. For example, elongation of a suture material will not result in a wide separation of the wound cleft if a very short loop is used. Yield stress and strain data along with modulus of elasticity extracted from the stress-strain curves might also be important for sutures in closing surgical wounds having severe edema. Due to the swelling of these wounds, sutures will be elongated; the degree of elongation depends on the level of swelling. If the suture is elongated beyond its yield point, the suture is permanently deformed. When the edema is recessed (corresponding to the removal of external force) the suture might not be able to closely approximate the wound edge, due to the inability of the suture to recover its original dimension fully. Since modulus of elasticity is a measure of the resistance of the material to deformation before yield point, a suture having high modulus of elasticity (hence, less compliance) is less likely to yield to the swelling pressure of the wound. Consequently, cutting through the sewn tissue may result.

The ultimate solution for choosing suture materials of the right mchanical properties for closing specific wounds might be to select a material whose stress-strain has the best match with the stress-strain curve of the tissue to be sewn. The availability of stress-strain curves of suture materials, like the one shown in Figure 7, is ideal for such a task. Of course, other properties such as tissue reactions, wound condition (i.e., infection), knot security, hand, and degree of absorption should also be considered, along with the suture's mechanical properties. The final selection will likely be a compromise of these properties for optimum performance.

Due to different testing conditions, size of suture materials, and unit of strength, it is almost impossible to list all suture materials completely, particularly those from different authors and labs, which are not given in Figure 7 and Table 3, and compare their mechanical properties. Thus, only a qualitative comparison of the above-mentioned seven suture materials with other suture materials will be given.

Among all suture materials stainless steel sutures show the highest tensile breaking strength (113-162 Kg/mm^2) and moduli of elasticity (8.4 × 10^3—1.17 × 10^4 Newton), but the smallest elongation at break (2%) [25,26]. Its poor handling characteristics have limited the use of stainless steel despite its strength. Linen sutures behave like steel and are more rigid than most other suture materials. They have a modulus of elasticity of 5.63 × 10^3 Newton, elongation at break of 3%, and a tensile breaking strength of 65 Kg/mm^2. Cotton suture is the weakest suture. It has only a 46 Kg/mm^2 tensile breaking strength when tested dry [26]. Of course, slightly higher values would be expected when it is tested wet. Among the absorbable sutures, Holmlund reported that both plain and chromic catgut sutures have almost the same stress-strain properties as PGA sutures. But their poor handling properties and intense inflammatory reaction (see the section on biological property) make them less desirable than PGA.

B.4.2 Retention of Tensile Strength

Because suture materials stay either temporarily or permanently inside the body, they are subjected to various types and degrees of biodegradation, particularly in view of the hostile environment of the body. Due to the breakdown of molecules, suture materials often lose their original tensile strength with time. The retention of their tensile strength and the rate of tensile strength loss are vital factors in their usefulness in wound healing. For non-critical surgical conditions such as small vessel ligature or the coaptation of uncomplicated wounds in rapidly healing tissues, the rate of loss of tensile strength is probably of little importance. For more critical surgical wounds, however, the difference among suture materials in the rate of loss of tensile strength may be highly significant, particularly in tissues slow to heal such as tendons and ligaments, and for those with neoplasia, hypoproteinemia, etc. In a few situations, suture materials must retain strength for the lifetime of the patient, e.g. a synthetic graft sutured to the aorta.

Since the loss of tensile strength of a suture material depends on the animal species, type of tissue, size of suture material, and the testing condition, the reported data vary considerably. Figures 8 and 9 show the percent retention of tensile breaking strength of both absorbable and nonabsorbable suture materials in rabbits and rats, respectively [27]. Polyglactin 910 sutures retain better tensile strength than chromic catgut and PGA during the initial 14 days in vivo; PGA is slightly inferior to chromic catgut sutures during this period, and remains so until 21 days. Chromic catgut retains the best tensile strength after 15 days. It is generally recognized that the results of catgut are erratic. In contrast, Katz and Turner found that PGA sutures were two to three times stronger than the values obtained with medium chromic catgut at 7 and 11 days in all sizes, and only size 4-0 & 1 PGA sutures were not statistically higher at 15 days in rabbits [28]. Thus, medium chromic catgut sutures lost strength at a much faster rate for the first 11 days than did PGA sutures. This discrepancy in the rate of tensile strength retention of PGA and catgut sutures may be due to either the different degree of chromicizing process of catgut sutures that different investigators used or an unexplained biologic difference among animals and patients.

Among nonabsorbable suture materials, braided polyester and monofilament polypropylene sutures have the best retention of tensile strength. There is virtually no loss of strength during the period of 390 days. Postlethwait observed the same result in his five years implantation study [39]. Braided silk sutures, however, lost almost all of their strength in the same period, and this loss is more severe during the first 56 days (65% of original tensile

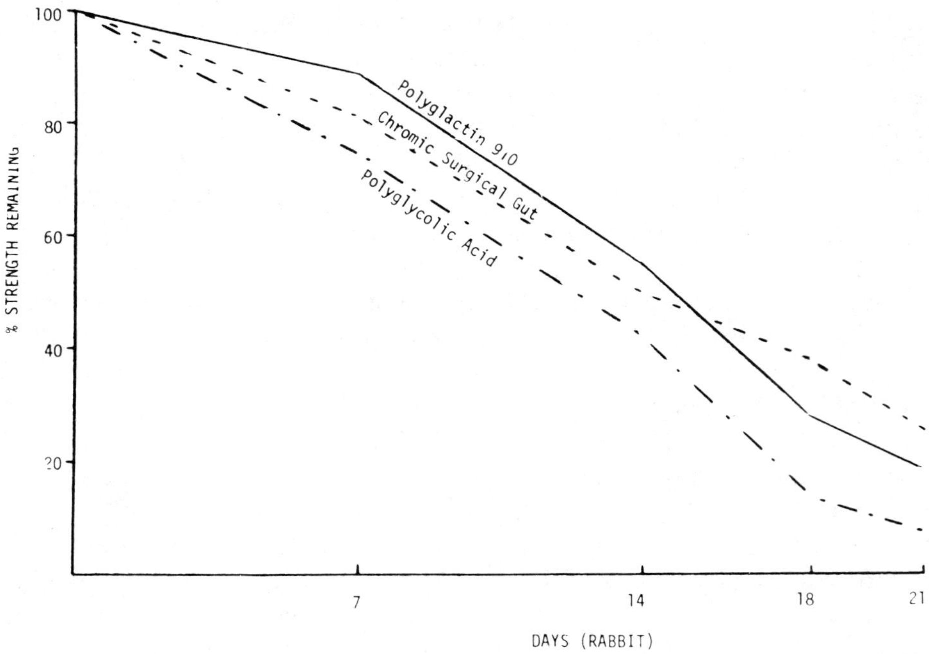

Figure 8a. Retention of tensile breaking strength of absorbable suture materials. (Courtesy of Dr. Salthouse et al., Ethicon, Inc.).

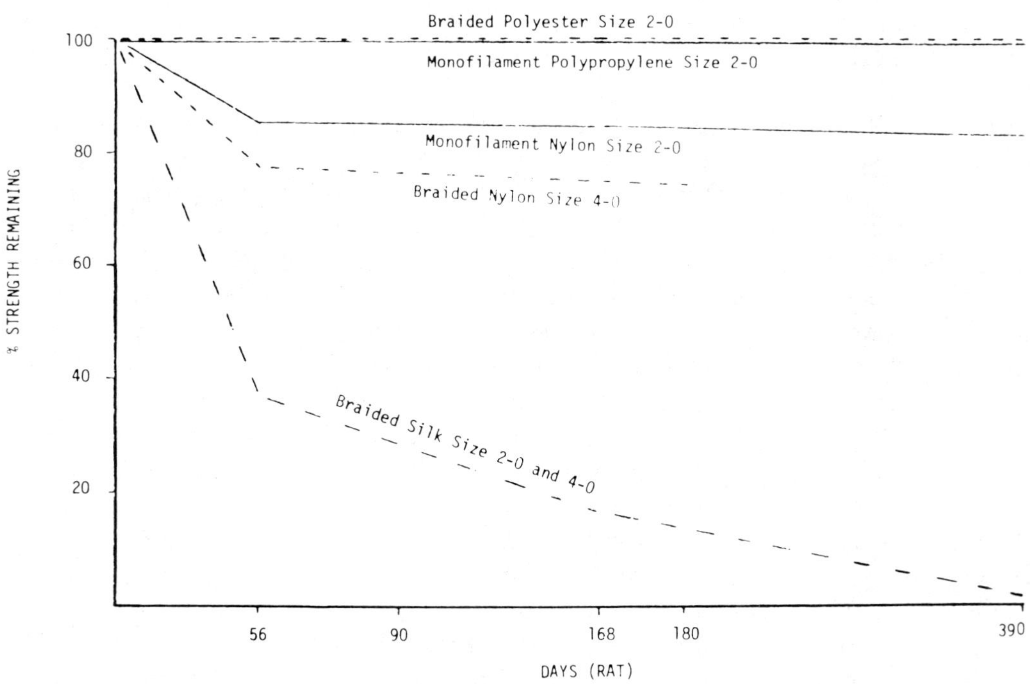

Figure 8b. Retention of tensile breaking strength of nonabsorbable suture materials. (Courtesy of Dr. Salthouse et al., Ethicon, Inc.).

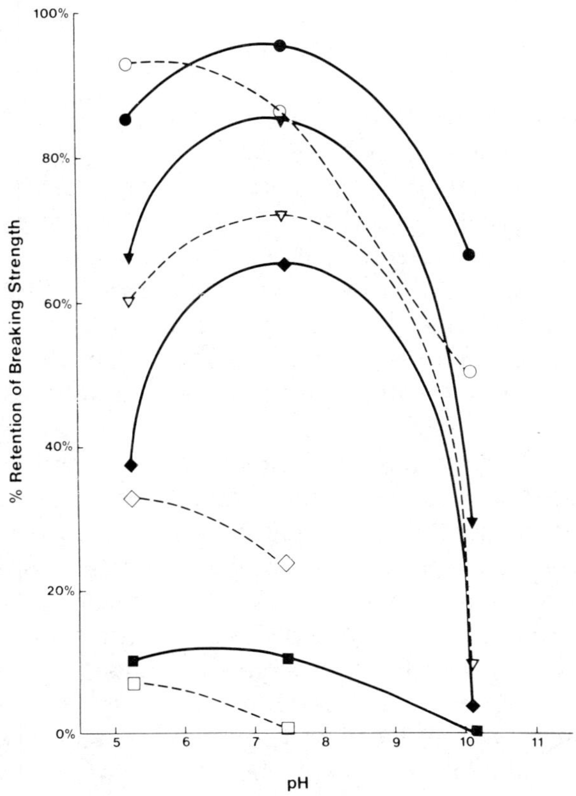

Figure 9. The effect of pH on the in vitro retention of tensile breaking strength of 2-0 PGA and polyglactin 910 sutures. Broken lines - PGA; Solid lines - Polyglactin 910; Circle - 7 days; Inverted triangle - 14 days; Diamond - 21 days; Square - 28 days.

strength lost). No strength could be measured after two years. Cotton sutures lose approximately half their tensile strength by the end of the first year, and this remains more or less constant during the second year. Nylon sutures fall between the above two categories. After an initial drop of strength, they remain relatively constant thereafter. Body enzymes like lysozymes may be responsible for the in vivo degradation of the amide linkages in the nylon molecules. Monofilament nylon sutures are slightly better than multifilament nylon. Furthermore, nylon 6 appears to retain strength slightly better than nylon 66 sutures. The difference, however, is clinically insignificant.

It is important to recognize that suture materials with the same chemical structure but from different manufacturers frequently have different mechanical properties due to the variety of manufacturing techniques. Different mechanical properties are observed even in suture materials with the same chemical structure and manufacturer. This is particularly true with new suture materials because manufacturers constantly improve the manufacturing process –

for economic reasons and/or better quality control – as more information becomes available. Thus, it is critically important to know the history and background of suture materials before comparing them. Such a task is often difficult due to the manufacturer's failure to release proprietary information.

B.4.3 pH Effect

So far, the study of the pH effect on the retention of tensile strength of suture materials is sparse and focuses on synthetic absorbable sutures. It is important to understand the pH dependent degradation of suture materials, particularly absorbable ones, because suture materials should be able to retain adequate strength under all possible physiological and pathological conditions. It is known that the pH of gastric juice in the stomach can go as low as 0.9 to 1.5 while pancreatic juice in the duodenum ranges from 7.5 to 8.2. Urinary pH often ranges from 4.5 to 8.0. Because the degradation mechanism of synthetic absorable suture materials is of a hydrolytic nature (refer to Section B.6 Biodegradation phenomenon), it must be affected by the pH of the environment in the same way as it is affected in the simple organic esters.

The pH dependence of the hydrolytic degradation of Dexon and Vicryl sutures are shown in Figure 9 [29]. The results obtained in this study have indicated that both Dexon and Vicryl sutures exhibit quite different hydrolytic degradation at various pH levels and immersion times. They degrade significantly faster in a high-alkaline buffer than in acidic and physiological buffers. Vicryl suture specimens at the physiological pH, however, retained the largest amount of tensile strength of the three buffers studied. Dexon suture specimens retained the best strength at the acidic condition. Vicryl sutures in general showed better hydrolytic resistance than Dexon within the studied pH range. The observed bell-shaped, pH-influenced, strength retention profiles associated with all Vicryl and some Dexon suture specimens suggest that hydrolysis of these suture materials is catalyzed by either hydrogen or hydroxy ions, as are many simple monomeric organic esters.

The reported pH dependent hydrolysis of Dexon and Vicryl sutres in this *in vitro* study probably deserve the attention of surgeons choosing between these absorbable suture materials. In the case of an acidic environment such as the stomach, there is very little difference in the hydrolysis rate between Dexon and Vicryl sutures; the latter is only slightly better than the former. In the case of an alkaline environment, such as physiological pH or a proteus-infected urinary tract, Vicryl sutures appear to retain much better tensile strength than Dexon sutures, and hence are the better choice in that circumstance. This difference in strength retention should be considered along with the capability of the suture materials to elicit the formation of urinary calculi in selecting proper suture materials for urological surgery. Other investigators, however, have recently reported that there is no significant difference in the degradation rate of PGA and Poly(glycolide-lactide) copolymers of compositions 50/50 and 70/30 mole % within the pH levels of 5.0 and 9.0 [30]. The reason for this discrepancy is not apparent. It might be attributed to the difference in the composition and physical form of the specimens.

B.4.4 Stiffness and Flexibility

The stiffness and flexibility of a suture material are very important to its handling property and knot security. Flexibility is particularly important for ligaturing small blood vessels and for sutures with small loops. Stiff sutures require larger loops and are more difficult to knot. In a continuous suturing technique with small loops, a stiff suture material, due to its tendency to relax from small loops, acts like a spring which pulls the wound edges apart rather than bringing them together. Thus, flexible suture materials are highly desirable.

There are several ways to evaluate the stiffness of a fiber: 1) the loop method, 2) the dynamical vibration method, and 3) torsional stiffness. The last method is the only one reported to date [31]. Suture specimens of identical length and size are placed on a fixed support and one end of the suture material is rotated until the other end starts to turn. The number of turns the specimen takes before the other end starts to turn is used as a relative measurement of the stiffness of the specimen to torsion. The resulting torsional stiffness is directly proportional to flexibility, but the reader should be aware that none of the current standard stiffness tests simulate the actual in vivo condition.

Holmlund's results indicate that 2-0 Prolene, catgut, and nylon (monofilament) sutures have the same order of stiffness and are the stiffest, while the same size of PGA and silk are the most flexible [31]. Polyester sutures (Mersilene) are in the middle. In general, suture materials have monofilament configurations are less flexible than multifilament sutures of the same size material. The flexibility of a suture also depends on its size; the flexibility increases as the size decreases. Thus, if a less flexible suture material must be used because of its other important properties, the suture of the smaller size can be used for better flexibility. Both physical configuration and size of suture materials should be considered together with stiffness data.

B.4.5 Knot Strength and Security

A knot is the weakest point in any suture material. The portion of the suture material immediately adjacent to the knot is the second weakest point. Numerous wound disruptions are due to either the breakdown of the knot or the slippage and untying of the knot. This problem is even more severe with the increasing availability of new synthetic suture materials. It has also been found that the strength of a suture material changes considerably with the knot type and suture technique, particularly a single loop suture [31]. The magnitude of this change sometimes reaches as much as ten times. Thus, knot strength and security play an important role in the successful use of suture materials in wound healing. Surgeons cannot use the same knot for every available suture material. The type of knot should depend on the kind of material selected.

Several studies of the suture's knot property have been reported [31-35]. One of the most limiting factors in these studies is personal; knots tied by different persons and even the same person on different occasions vary greatly. Thus, the data different investigators report do not always agree.

B.4.5.1 Definition and Classification

A surgical knot, as defined by Taylor, is the fastening made by entangling one or more cords, so that any tension on the fastening causes an increased contact pressure on the component parts of the knot. A knot stays tied due to the frictional force among filaments. Thus, the knot strength and security depend on the coefficient of friction of the suture materials as well as on how the knot is tied. An ideal surgical knot is one that requires the smallest

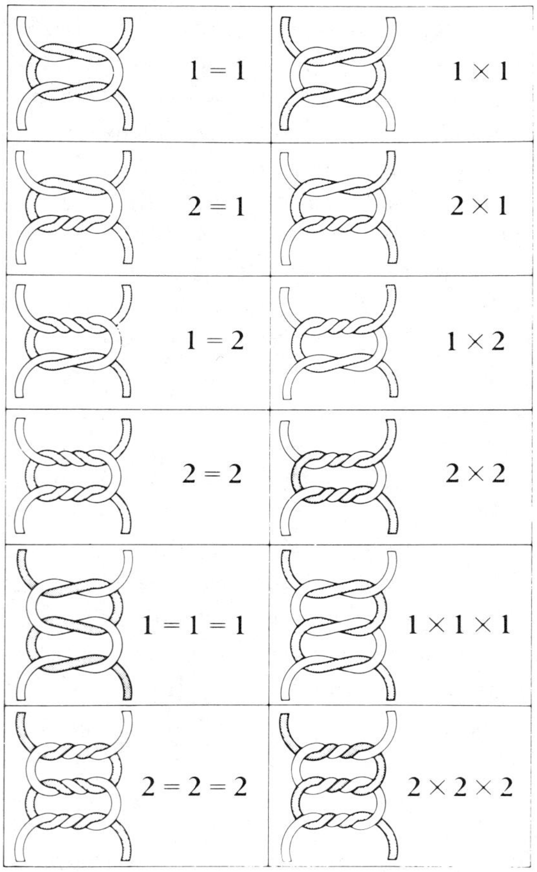

Figure 10. Tera's knot classification. (Courtesy Dr. Tera et al., Ref. 32).

amount of turn and throw to achieve high strength and security.

Due to the increasing availability of new suture materials and the various types of knot, a systematic classification and reproducible description of different knots is highly desirable. A better classification system has been proposed recently [32]. In that system, shown in Figure 10, the Arabic number stands for the number of times the thread ends are twisted about each other (called turn), while the symbols "crossed" (X) or "parallel" (=) indicate how the throws are combined. The symbol (=) shows that the threads enter and leave on the same side of the other thread, while the symbol (X) indicates that the two threads pass crosswise and not on the same side. According to this system, a square knot is 1 = 1, a granny knot is 1 × 1, and a surgeon's knot is 2 = 1. The results of twelve different types of suture materials on twelve different types of knot are shown in Table 4. The knot efficiency is defined as the percentage of the strength of a knotted suture with respect to the same but untied suture.

B.4.5.2 Knot Efficiency

The strength of a knot depends on numerous factors: 1) physical configuration (multifilament or monofilament); 2) the chemical nature of the suture material; 3) surface treatment; and 4) the type of knot. Both multi- and monofilament stainless steel sutures have the best average knot efficiency for all twelve types of knots, while silk (all types) and polyethylene sutures have the poorest. Catgut (plain and chromic), Dexon, Mersilene, and Prolene sutures are in the middle. Knot efficiency is independent of knot type for steel and catgut sutures (plain and chromic) only. Even though silk sutures show the poorest average knot efficiency, this does not mean that silk sutures are poor in all twelve types of knot. They may be very good in a few types of knot and poor in most other types of knot. Therefore, a high average knot efficiency for a suture means that the type of knot used is not important for the resulting knot efficiency of the suture. Any of the twelve knots will give the same order of knot efficiency. When dealing with a suture of low mean knot efficiency, surgeons should be more selective about the type of knot they use because the strength of the suture is highly dependent on the knot type.

Irrespective of the nature of the suture materials, an increase in both turn and throw increases the efficiency of the knot. For example, on the average (bottom row of Table 4), knot

Table 4. Comparison of Knot Efficiency of Suture Materials of Twelve Types of Knot. (Courtesy of Dr. Tera et al. Ref. 32)

Type of suture material; tensile strength of unknotted thread kp; and diameter, mm	Knot Strength in per cent of total tensile strength of the unknotted thread. Upper figure parallel knots, lower figure crossed knots							
	1 = 1 1 x 1	2 = 1 2 x 1	1 = 2 1 x 2	2 = 2 2 x 2	1 = 1 = 1 1 x 1 x 1	2 = 2 = 2 2 x 2 x 2	Mean	Mean for all knot types
Multifil steel	97	96	98	98	99	98	98	94
2.55 0.24	78	91	92	92	93	95	90	
Monofil steel	87	92	92	92	90	90	91	89
3.88 0.25	79	90	92	85	92	92	88	
Chromic catgut	59	61	60	65	58	61	61	63
2.76 0.31	60	72	54	72	57	75	65	
Plain catgut	65	54	65	67	61	63	63	61
2.74 0.31	60	54	52	68	62	65	60	
Dexon[R]	58	82	76	75	85	75	75	60
2.41 0.26	5	15	55	69	62	68	46	
Mersilene	70	79	87	75	74	79	77	70
2.22 0.23	23	42	61	95	70	88	63	
Supramid	18	21	45	34	44	75	40	39
3.07 0.24	19	23	18	65	57	54	39	
Nylon monofil	12	16	55	34	58	75	42	43
2.32 0.25	18	14	42	76	47	67	44	
Silky Polydek[R]	17	26	47	49	52	71	44	43
2.87 0.25	8	19	34	71	53	73	43	
Silk	21	25	38	48	53	63	41	43
1.88 0.25	13	37	33	60	45	63	42	
Polyethylene	17	12	31	48	51	65	37	38
2.76 0.25	13	9	33	72	32	77	39	
Prolene[R]	20	42	79	84	82	87	66	67
1.77 0.24	43	18	69	93	84	98	68	
Parallel knots, mean	45	50	64	64	67	75	61	59
Crossed knots, mean	35	40	53	77	63	76	57	
All knots, mean	40	45	59	70	65	76	59	

1 kp = 2.20 lb = 9.81 Newton

efficiency is almost doubled – from 40% to 70% – by increasing the number of turns from 2 (1 = 1 or 1 × 1) to 6 (2 = 2 = 2 or 2 × 2 × 2). In terms of knot type, parallel knots, on the average, are stronger than crossed knot (second bottom row). Again, this is a generalization based on average values.

Based on the above data, Holmlund has suggested the following selections of knots for various suture mateials [31]:

Suture Materials	**Type of Knot**
Catgut (plain and chromic)	1=1=1 or 2×2
Dexon	1=1=1
Steel wire	1=1
Silk and braided polyester	1=1=1 or 2×2
Coated polyester	2×2
Monofilament nylon, polyolefin	2×2

B.4.5.3 Knot Security

With regard to knot security, both chromic and plain catgut sutures exhibit no slippage, regardless of knot type. Multi- and monofilament stainless steel sutures rarely slip. Mersilene (uncoated Dacron) and Dexon sutures slip in slightly more than one quarter of all instances.

Silk, monofilament nylon, and polyethylene sutures slip in more than two-thirds of occasions. In the Magillian study, he concluded, however, that Prolene, Mersilene, and Polydek (Dacron with light Teflon coating) have the same knot security as silicone coated silk, while the silicone and heavily Teflon coated Dacron (Tri-Cron® , and Tevdek® , respectively) show significantly less knot security than their uncoated or lightly coated counterparts [35]. All investigators agree that coated suture materials are less knot secure than uncoated. This is believed to be due to a lower coefficient of friction, which allows the knot to slip easier. Knot security is also improved with an increase in the number of turns and throws [32]. Hence, 2 = 2 = 2 knot is far more secure than 1 = 1 knot. It is important that the number of throws and turns should not be overdone because the less bulk of foreign materials that remain inside the body, the better.

Knot security and strength also depend on several other factors, like the moisture absorption capability of the suture materials, suture uniformity, and the length of cut suture ends [34]. In general, increasing moisture absorption decreases knot security due to the tendency to swell the knot loose rather than a decrease in the frictional coefficient. Catgut suture is a typical example. Surface treatments alter the moisture absorption capability of the suture material and hence, change the knot security. The length of the cut ends is important for the tension of suture materials whose knots often slip slightly and then hold.

B.5 Biological Property of Suture Materials

All suture materials are foreign to the body and hence produce an inevitably wide range of biological responses in the living tissues which they sew together. These responses range from an inflammatory reaction due to the trauma of insertion to foreign body reaction because of the chemical, physical, and mechanical properties of the suture materials. A knowledge of tissue responses to suture materials is important because the wound healing process, its rate, and complications are greatly influenced by the tissue reactions to suture materials. An excessive tissue reaction around suture materials could result in 1) cutting out of sutures, 2) delay in healing, 3) granuloma and sinus formation, 4) predisposition to infection.

Suture materials which generate a marked tissue response are more liable to cut out and thus weaken wound strength. This is because an excessive inflammatory reaction may lead to the softening of the surrounding tissues with disruption of collagen fibers [36]. Cotton, nylon, polyester, and stainless steel sutures produce the strongest wounds while both plain and chromic catgut produce the weakest during the first five days [36]. Silk sutures are slightly better than catgut in the lag phase, but there is no appreciable difference between the two thereafter. Wound strength is greater when closed with PGA than with chromic catgut in the rectus muscle of rabbits.

It has been recognized that suture materials which enhance a marked exudative tissue reaction (edema) would delay wound healing. The onset of the fibroplasia phase also appears to depend on the suture material [36]. It has been reported that fibroblasts appear earlier around silk than catgut sutures. With certain suture materials, the delay in fibroplasia is purely a local phenomenon.

A granulomatous reaction around a buried suture material, particularly in the superficial layers of the skin, is a suture granuloma. Most granulomas are minor and consist of a layer of macrophages around the suture material, surrounded by a few fibroblast cells and a thin fibrous capsule encapsulating the suture. The formation of granuloma is related to the chronic inflammatory reaction caused by suture materials. Thus, non-absorbable suture materials are the worst offenders. Absorbable sutures, do not usually form suture granulomas except for catgut sutures, particularly chromic one [31].

With a more intense inflammatory reaction around a suture, or in a chronic suture granuloma, a discharging sinus can form, which clears up only when the suture is removed or extruded. This could be disastrous following herniorrhaphy. It is believed that the frequency of this complication is directly related to the degree of contamination, physical configuration and mechanical property (resulting in mechanical irritation) of suture materials. An infected wound is more liable to form a sinus than a clean wound is [36].

This dependence sometimes relates to the physical configuration of suture materials. Braided multifilament non-absorbable sutures have a greater incidence of sinus formation than monofilament suture materials. Suture materials made of natural fibers, silk, cotton, and catgut are worse than synthetic suture materials, particularly in the presence of infection. This may be due to a more marked tissue reaction in natural than in synthetic fibers. A sinus seldom forms with synthetic monofilament sutures even when the wound is infected. For example, the chance of sinus formation in an infected wound containing a silk suture is 80%, while the incidence is probably between 6 and 8% if a synthetic monofilament suture is used [36]. The incidence of sinus formation could also be reduced with a smaller gauge suture material with the ends buried or cut flush with the knot. This is particularly true in rigid suture materials placed directly beneath the skin.

Excessive tissue reactions from suture materials could also predispose infection. It is believed that the inflammatory as well as foreign body reactions due to the presence of any suture material in a wound may provide a favorable environment (e.g., exudate and lowered body natural defense) for bacterial growth. The physical configuration of suture materials may also relate to the incidence of wound infection. The exact mechanism by which suture materials facilitate infection is still unknown. This relationship will be discussed in more detail in the section on Wound Infection.

Because of the very important role of biological reaction to suture materials in wound healing, extensive studies have been conducted and vast amounts of data have been published [27,36,37]. Basically, the biological reaction can best be studied through both cellular morphologic observation and enzyme histochemistry. The former can be assessed according to the reaction degree and area size by microscopic observation of the type and population of the responding cells, as well as edema and necrosis. The latter is particularly useful in the evaluation of the in vivo absorption mechanism of absorbable suture materials.

The general picture of cellular response to both absorbable and nonabsorbable suture materials involves the formation of a band of fibrous connective tissue encapsulating the suture material, as shown in Figure 11. The width of the band and the amount of surrounding macrophage and giant cells are related to the severity of the tissue reaction. The more inert the suture material is, the narrower the fibrous connective tissue band with little cellular reaction appearing. If the suture material is of a multifilament nature, the filaments are widely separated and surrounded by invading cells (see Figure 11). In the case of absorbable sutures, the filaments are gradually eroded after implantation. The degree of tissue reaction depends

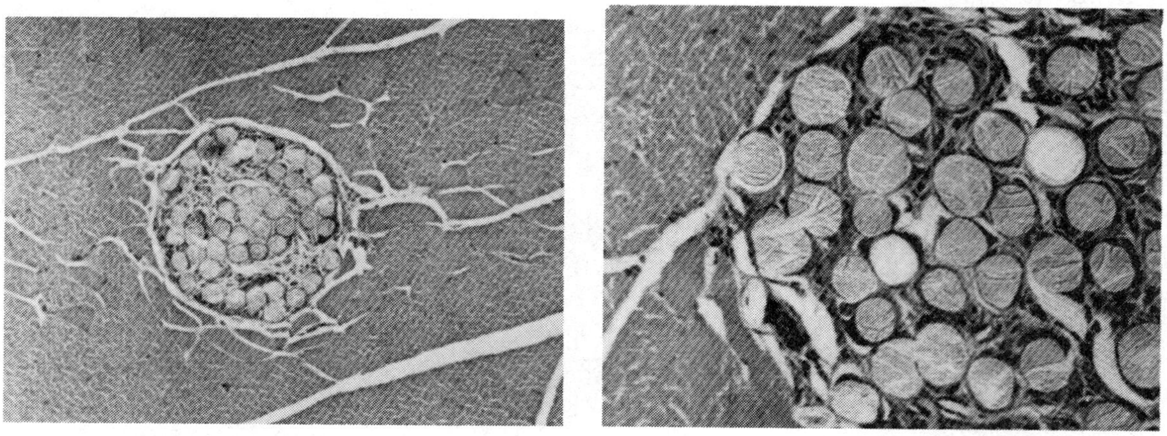

Figure 11a. Figure 11b.

Figure 11. Scanning electron micrographs of synthetic absorbable sutures in rat after 42 days implantation. (a) Size 4-0 PGA, ×85; (b) Size 4-0 Polyglactin 910, ×212. (Courtesy Dr. Craig et al., Ref. 38)

largely on the chemical nature but moderately on the physical configuration of suture materials. Suture materials of a protein and cellulose nature produce more marked tissue reactions than those of a synthetic nature, while a greater response is caused by multifilament sutures than by monofilament ones.

B.5.1 Absorbable Materials

Catgut Suture

Because of its foreign protein nature, catgut sutures elicit a far more intense tissue reaction than synthetic absorbable and most nonabsorbable sutures. Plain catgut produces the worst reaction associated with an early, prolonged and marked exudate with some tissue necrosis [36,37]. Chromic catgut causes a less pronounced but persistent tissue reaction. Areas of catgut suture degradation contain dense accumulations of macrophages and lymphocytes. The suture is packed with dense masses of chronic inflammatory cells with several large foreign body giant cells. After complete absorption, it is replaced by a dense mass of macrophages. This marked inflammatory reaction may cause the breakdown of collagen (and hence lower wound strength) and a predisposition to infection. Plain catgut sutures also swell to four times their size; chromic catgut swells double. Thus catgut sutures act as a large foreign body.

The rate of absorbability of a suture material is a primary factor in determining its tissue irritability. The prolonged existence of a foreign material like sutures in the tissue raises the question of long term adverse effects. Ideally, a suture should be quickly degraded and absorbed as soon as it serves its function. In vivo, catgut sutures (both plain and chromic) exhibit an irregular pattern of absorption. Although they are generally recognized to be absorbed at 40 days, many fragments are found after 50 to 60 days in rabbits [28]. The histologic study showed that catgut sutures had been entirely resorbed and replaced by a dense mass of macrophages at the 75 day interval. The absorption and degradation of catgut sutures involve mainly proteolytic enzymes of the phagocytes and other cells.

Polyglycolic Acid and Polyglaction 910

Both of these suture materials elicit minimal tissue reactions; the histologic grading of tissue response is shown in Table 5 [28,38]. Cellular reactions are mainly mononuclear in character and appear to be limited to the immediate surrounding of the suture strands. The close macrophage/suture interaction in the early period observed is not common with nonhydrolyzable suture materials. There is no acute vascular reaction. Infiltrating cellular elements disappear with almost no trace of the lesion following complete absorption. The tissue reaction to polyglycolic acid lasts substantially longer than that associated with its lactide copolymer (polyglactin 910). The latter is absorbed by 90 days, while considerable quantities of PGA remain at 120 days [38]. Upon wetting, PGA and Polyglactin 910 do not swell and hence act as a small foreign body.

Table 5. Sewell's Tissue Response Scores for 2-0 Polyglycolic Acid and Polyglactin 910 Sutures After Intramuscular Implantation Into Rats. (Courtesy of Dr. Craig et al. Ref. 38).

Post-implantation Days	Polyglycolic Acid*		Polyglactin 910*	
	Average	Range	Average	Range
4	21 (11)	16-27	25	14-33
14	12 (10)	10-16	17 (8)	14-24
42	17 (9)	13-22	18 (10)	16-23
49	18 (11)	14-25	18	13-26
56	14	12-18	14 (10)	10-19
63	14	12-16	14 (9)	10-16
70	14	10-22	11	9-15
90	11	9-14	10	9-14
120	12	9-26	9 (11)	0-14

* Scores are average of 12 sites except as noted in parentheses.

The biodegradation and absorption of these two synthetic suture materials is independent of cellular or enzyme activity; an aqueous environment is the only requirement for their degradation and absorption. Thus hydrolysis is apparently the chief mechanism of their degradation. The hydrolytic degradation products of these suture materials are actively metabolized by the cells in contact with the suture materials. Support for this hypothesis may be found in the observed increase in adenosine triphosphatase activity, which is known to be associated with oxidative phosphorylation and active transport processes in the cell. Recently, Williams demonstrated that certain enzymes such as esterase, ficin, and bacteria are able to influence the rate of hydrolysis of PGA under the appropriate conditions. The rate of degradation, both in vitro and in vivo is reduced in the presence of staph. aureus. The detailed degradation phenomena of synthetic absorbable sutures will be discussed under the section of "Biodegradation Phenomena."

B.5.2 Nonabsorbable Suture Materials

All nonabsorbable suture materials elicit less tissue reaction than catgut. In this group, nonsynthetic suture materials like silk, cotton, and flax induce somewhat stronger tissue reactions than synthetic ones, as shown in Table 6 [39]. Even after two years of implantation, histiocytes and some lymphocytes are still present around the silk sutures. The mononuclear response is fairly marked. Homsy demonstrated that this intense interaction of silk sutures is due to the combined effects of physical configuration (braid) and chemical constitutents (protein) of silk [37]. Treating the surface of silk sutures with silicone, wax, or protein reduces the tissue reaction with silicone having the best results. Silk sutures are also absorbed slowly, and a decrease in the amount of silk fibers is observed over two years [39]. The early tissue reaction to cotton sutures is similar to that of silk sutures, with a slightly greater overall cellular reaction due to the separation of individual fibers from the main mass. Cotton sutures show no evidence of disappearance.

Table 6. Sewell's Tissue Response Scores for Nonabsorbable Sutures After Intramuscular Implantation into Rabbits. (Courtesy of Dr. Postlethwait, Ref. 39).

	Silk	Cotton	Nylon	Polypropylene	Dacron	Polydek	Trevdek
Weeks							
1	43.9	47.9	37.5	38.2	39.9	40.6	39.9
2	44.1	48.6	32.8	33.3	31.6	32.2	39.4
4	44.9	45.7	28.8	32.2	29.9	37.8	40.6
Months							
3	38.1	38.6	24.4	19.3	25.4	29.0	40.2
6	35.0	38.9	17.6	20.3	24.6	36.5	35.4
12	32.7	32.6	12.6	22.3	22.2	27.7	22.7
18	31.7	34.5	13.5	15.8	18.8	30.6	30.5
24	33.1	35.4	13.4	21.3	20.2	33.1	25.5

(The lowest grade attainable is 9.)

Synthetic nonabsorbable suture materials elicit much less tissue reactions than do the corresponding natural suture materials. Among the synthetic materials, multifilament configurations cause more tissue response than monofilament ones. By comparison, the tissue response to polypropylene monofilament suture is minimal. This suture material contains no hydrolyzable linkages, is essentially inert, and no gross morphological distinction between suture site and normal tissue can be made. A proliferation of fibrous connective tissue which encapsulates the polypropylene suture occurs early and rapidly, and a narrow fibrous capsule persists. Monofilament nylon 66 and 6 sutures behave very much like polypropylene sutures. In the first week, the acute inflammatory reaction occurs, limited in degree and dominated by histocytes and fibroblasts, with a few lymphocytes and neutrophiles. The sutures are firmly encased in a thin, fibrous capsule. Multifilament nylon sutures induce a slightly greater tissue response than monofilament nylon. Presumably, physical factors become signifciant. It is ascribed partly to the large surface exposed to the tissue and partly to a certain remaining capillarity [31].

Uncoated braided polyester sutures exhibit a slightly wider connective tissue zone than monofilament nylon and polypropylene sutures. After two years, only a minimal number of histocytes are seen. Teflon-coated braided polyester sutures differ from uncoated polyester sutures after only about one month. Due to the detachment of teflon particles, they stimulate their own intense cellular reaction, mainly histocytes and lymphocytes. Finally, stainless steel sutures cause very little tissue response. The order of tissue reaction to nonabsorbable suture materials is summarized as follows:

> Cotton, silk > multifilament polyester (coated) > multifilament polyester (uncoated), multifilament nylon 66 and 6 > monofilament nylon, polypropylene, stainless steel

B.5.3 Wound Infection

The development of postoperative wound infection often retards normal wound healing. From the point of view of suture materials, it is important to know whether the presence of a suture material in a surgical wound increases the wound's susceptibility to infection and if so, how it varies with different suture materials. Numerous studies in this area have been reported, but unfortunately the results do not quite agree.

Alexander found no significant difference in the severity of infection by S. aureus among multifilament nonabsorbable sutures, silk (braided, uncoated, and coated), braided nylon, twisted cotton, and stainless steel [40]. Sutures in multifilament form resulted in higher wound infection than the same suture in monofilament form. Twisted silk sutures were associated with producing more infection than braided silk. This demonstrates that the physical structure of the nonabsorbable sutures is more important in inducing wound infection than the chemical constitutents (including coating materials). It has been postulated that due to the topology of the multifilament suture, it is difficult for inflammatory cells to reach the bacteria hiding deep in the interstices of the multifilament suture. Hence, phagocytic activity is difficult. It has also been suggested that multifilament sutures induce stronger tissue reactions and hence weaken the tissue's defense capability toward bacteria. Thus, the degree of enhancement of infection by a suture is parallel to the degree of inflammatory reaction caused by the suture. The superior resistance to infection of chromic and iodized catgut suture, compared to plain catgut sutures, demonstrates this point of view further.

Edlich observed that even the most inert nylon sutures tend to elicit significantly greater degrees of infection in tissues contaminated with either S. aureus or E. coli than the correspondingly contaminated needle puncture wound [41]. Thus, the use of surgical tape to close contaminated wounds was suggested. Among absorbable sutures, both plain and chromic catgut sutures induce higher incidences of gross infection than PGA, possibly due to the antibacterial activity of the degradation products of PGA. Among nonabsorbable sutures, braided nylon sutures have significantly lower infection rates in contaminated tissues than other multifilament nonabsorbable sutures, with polyester sutures second. Stainless steel sutures have a potentially greater incidence of gross infection than nylon and polyester sutures do, but significantly less than silk and cotton sutures, which are the worst in this group. When comparing the same sutures with different physical configurations, Edlich found that the physical structure of a suture is less important in enhancing infection than the chemical nature of the suture is. This conclusion is different from Alexander's and may be due to different experimental techniques. Alexander used knotted sutures, while Edlich used straight sutures. Knotted sutures may exaggerate the physical characteristics of both mono- and multifilament sutures and hence provoke different inflammatory reactions in tissues.

B.5.4 Carcinogenicity

It has been shown that suture materials can not only be vehicles for the mechanical transplantation of tumor cells, but also can interact biologically with the surrounding tissue and exert influence on cancer cells to determine the likelihood of their growth [42]. The degree of potentiation of tumor growth by a suture material appears to parallel its effect in wound infection.

In a recent study of the use of B16 Melanoma tumor model in mice, Pendergrast and his coworkers show that all tested suture types (chromic catgut, PGA, silk, nylon, and steel) potentiate earlier tumor occurrences and growth when the inoculating dose is 1×10^5 or above. With the normal subclinical cell dose, namely 1×10^3, only silk and steel sutures consistently increase the rapidity of onset and the total number of tumors. In comparison, chromic catgut and PGA do not increase tumor occurrence at this cell dose level. Monofilament nylon suture is the only one which does not cause earlier occurrence or a greater number of tumors.

This difference has been attributed to the different capability of suture materials in eliciting wound infection. The previous section indicated that silk sutures elicit the greatest incidence of wound infection among nonabsorbable suture materials, monofilament nylon and polypropylene the least. It is believed that the excessive inflammatory response of silk may impair the tissue's ability to resist both bacterial infection and tumor growth.

Stainless steel is the exception: Stainless sutures elicit minimal tissue reaction but cause a relatively significant incidence of wound infection and tumor occurrence. It has been proposed that the physical properties of the suture may be related to this paradoxical effect [41]. Because stainless steel sutures are stiff, they may cause additional tissue damage due to their inability to conform to the topology of the wound tissue. Such additional tissue damages renders tissue less resistant to either bacterial infection or tumor growth.

Surgeons thus should be aware of the fact that even the most inert suture material enhances tumor occurrence and growth at the tumor cell dosage levels of 10^4 and above. At this clinical level they should practice the best possible suture techniques to eliminate tumor seeding in the wound. When only a relatively small tumor cell level is present (10^3 and less), the type of suture material used in wound closure is important to the degree of facilitation of tumor growth. Different suture materials could cause various degrees of tumor occurrence and growth at the subclinical tumor cell dosage level.

B.5.5 Thrombogenicity

The success of cardiovascular surgery such as the anastomoses of arteries and veins and the anchorage of prosthetic heart valves partially depends on the thrombogenicity of suture materials. Due to the broad chemical, physical, and biological characteristics of currently available suture materials, a wide range of thrombogenicity of these suture materials would be expected. A recent study of five suture materials (Prolene, Mersilene, Vicryl, Silk, and Ethilon) using scanning electron microscopy has shown that polypropylene was the most blood compatible material, silk was the most thrombogenic [43]. Nylon 66 showed deposits of thrombocytes and fibrin on its surface during the first three postimplantation weeks. Uncoated polyester sutures exhibited a fairly satisfactory antithrombogenicity and displayed minimal traces of fibrin on the surface at fourteen days after implantation. Vicryl sutures showed a thrombogenicity similar to Mersilene's at three days, and were covered extensively by thrombocytes with slender extrusions and irregularly shrunken erythorcytes at seven days and thereafter. At fifty-six days, Vicryl sutures were entirely covered by neointima. It is believed that the degradation property and the chemical nature of the degradation products of Vicryl sutures could modify their thrombogenicity according to the length of implantation.

B.6 Biodegradation Phenomenon of Synthetic Absorbable Sutures

The main difference between natural and synthetic absorbable sutures in biodegradation is that the former depend on the proteolytic enzyme activity for the breakdown of peptide linkages, while the latter depend mainly on hydrolysis of aliphatic ester bonds by body fluids. Because of their hydrolytic instability, synthetic absorbable sutures lose their tensile strength as they biodegrade.

Very recently, the degradation mechanism of PGA in vitro has been proposed on the basis of a microfibrillar model of fiber structure [44]. This model is based on microfibrils in which alternative crystalline and amorphous regions arrange in the direction of the fiber axis. In each microfibril, some polymer chains will pass through several crystalline and amorphous regions along the fiber axis and other chains will return to the crystallite of the origin, but not necessarily in juxtaposition. The crystalline regions are composed of chain sequences in ordered or preferred conformation. The amorphous regions containing chain folds, chain ends, and tie-chain segments are in characteristically disordered conformations. In the microfibrillar model, two types of tie-chain segments can be formed: interfibrillar and intrafibrillar. Their major function is to tie crystalline blocks together and to support and transmit tensile loads to the crystalline regions.

On the basis of this model, it is believed that degradation proceeds through two main stages, with the first stage in the amorphous region, the second in the crystalline region. When the material is immersed in aqueous solution, the water molecules which diffuse through the polymer accommodate themselves readily in the amorphous zone, and not at all in the crystalline zone. The structure of the amorphous zone is the more open of the two: water penetrates easily. The crystalline region is highly packed, with a densely ordered crystalline structure; little or no water penetrates there.

Because of this difference, hydrolytic degradation starts in the amorphous regions, as the tie-chain segments, free chain ends, and chain folds in these regions degrade into fragments. As the degradation proceeds, the size of the fragments reaches the stage where they can be dissolved into the buffer medium. This dissolution removes the fragments from the amorphous regions, and a loss of materials results. As sufficient amounts of chain segments in these regions are removed, the spaces originally occupied by chain segments become vacant and large enough to be visible as cracks.

The cracks are believed to be initiated on the surface of the fiber and to grow circumferentially around and deeper into the interior of the fiber. This is because alkaline hydrolysis of a fiber has been reported to be a surface phenomenon. As microcracks form on the surface of fibers, more hydroxyl ions penetrate into these areas and microcracks propagate more deeply in the bulk of the fibers, until the cracks cut through the whole fibers and scissions result. Figure 12 illustrates this.

Along the degradation in the amorphous region, chain scission results in a lesser degree of entanglement of long-chain molecules located in the amorphous regions, as well as lower ax-

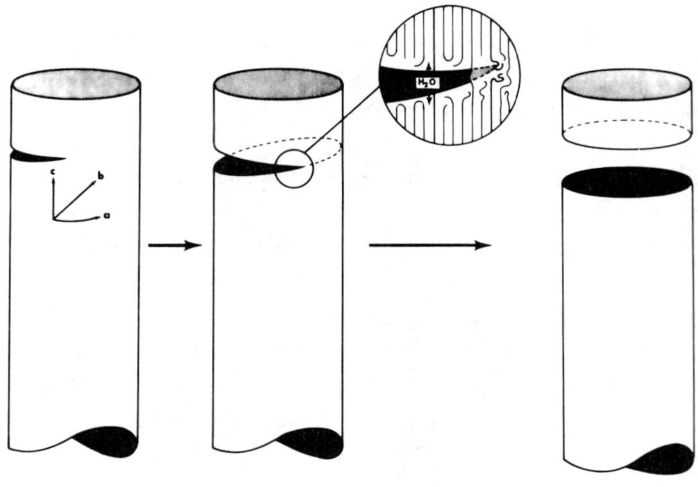

Figure 12. Schematic drawing of surface crack formation in PGA suture materials. A- Initiation; B - Propagation; C - Fragmentation.

ial elastic moduli and tensile strength. Therefore, the remaining undegraded chain segments in the amorphous regions obtain better chain mobility; they can move and reorganize themselves from a disordered to an ordered state. Further crystallization is induced and an increase in crystallinity thus observed.

When all the amorphous regions have been removed by hydrolysis, the second stage of degradation starts. The degree of crystallinity reaches a maximum at the end of the first-stage degradation, and starts to decrease as hydrolysis destroys the crystalline lattice. During this first perid, the loss of tensile strength is also the greatest due to the scission of tie-chain segments. When changes of the degree of crystallinity were observed, the first-stage degradation was predominant during the 21-day immersion period, while the second-stage degradation became important after the 21-day degradation period. The first-stage degradation still proceeded, but at a much lesser degree, until all the tie-chain segments located in the amorphous regions were degraded. The material then exhibited no tensile strength.

B.7 Sterilization of Suture Materials

Basically, suture manufacturers frequently use two sterilization methods: ionizing-radiation and ethylene oxide treatment. The former consists of high energy electrons and Co^{60} γ-irradiation. Usually, a dosage of 2.5 Megarads (1 RAD = 6.24×10^{23} eVg^{-1}, 1 MRAD = 10^6 RAD) has been used. The advantages of ionizing-radiation are speed, convenience, and reproducible control. The suture materials can be sterilized after packaging; hence, contamination after sterilization can be pretty well avoided. The disadvantage is the change of properties after irradiation. These include the degradation of polymer chains, cross-linking, evolution of gases, discoloration, and heat build-up. The change of mechanical properties due to either chain scission or crosslinking is the most important concern in suture use. Whether the reaction will be characterized predominantly by scission or by crosslinking depends on several factors, including the chemical structure of the suture materials, the amount of dosage, the rate of dosage, and the environment of the suture materials during irradiation. In reference to the last factor, irradiation in air has a more adverse effect on properties than in an inert environment. But sterilization is less effective in the absence of air [45]. The orientation of polymer chains has also been reported to have some influence on the direction of the overall radiation reaction, which is thought to be due to the difference in chain mobility.

The only absorbable suture materials that are sterilized by ionic radiation (i.e., high energy electrons) is catgut. It was reported that only 4 to 8% of tensile strength is lost. A loss of up to 15% was also observed by γ-irradiation. When PGA and its lactide copolymer are subjected to γ-irradiation, the predominant effect is chain scission. In a recent study, a steady and progressive decline in the mechanical properties of PGA sutures with increasing irradiation dosage was observed [46]. There was a sharp drop in breaking tensile strength (6.03 to 4.82 gpd) and elongation (38.7% to 33%) after a 2.5 MRAD dosage. The sensitivity of this polymeric material to both hydrolytic species and γ-irradiation provides us with a unique opportunity to examine the gross morphological changes resulting from γ-irradiation and hydrolytic degradation. The surface changes observed through a scanning electron microscope (SEM) provide direct visual evidence of how PGA degrades hydrolytically and how γ-irradiation alters the hydrolytic degradation phenomenon of PGA. This information could greatly aid in demonstrating the validity of the proposed degradation mechanism outlined in the biodegradation phenomenon section.

The most important gross morphological characteristic of PGA sutures that have been subjected to both hydrolytic and γ-irradiation degradation is the formation of surface cracks on the filaments, as shown in Figure 13. The filaments seem to be built up by laying a number of similarly sized chips one upon another. The distance between the two adjacent cracks was quite similar along the fiber axis (1u). The regularity in these surface cracks increases with an increase in either the dosage level or extent of hydrolysis, or both. Another unique characteristic of these surface cracks is that the circumferential propagation of the cracks goes in a perpendicular or nearly perpendicular direction to the fiber axis. No propagation of cracks at any other angles, particularly along the fiber axis, was observed. This characteristic is important for the degradation mechanism of fibrous materials. The arrangement of surface cracks, their orientation on the filaments, and the direction of crack propagation provide useful information for depicting the mechanism of hydrolytic degradation in this class of fibrous material.

All the synthetic nonabsorbable suture materials except polypropylene are also sterilized by Co^{60} γ-irradiation. They are expected to have some changes in properties, but no results of clinical significance have been reported. Nylon, polyester, and polypropylene sutures show minimal strength loss after γ-irradiation sterilization.

For those polymeric materials which are severely damaged by radiation sterilization, ethylene oxide gas is used for sterilization. The gas is often diluted with CO_2 or with freons. The lethal activity of ethylene oxide resides in its alkylating power of the various functional groups (−SH, −COOH, −OH, NH_2) of enzymes, proteins, and nucleic acids. The major disadvantages are the length of time required and the residual. The sterilization takes about 6 to 12 hours at 25 °C due to the slow uptake of gas. This length of time also depends on the thickness of specimens and temperature. Four hours are usually satisfactory at 50-60 °C. Sterilization is done in a relative humidity of 30 to 40%. A minimum concentration of 450 mg/l is recommended, and a higher concentration is desirable if sterilization time is shorter. Since the effectiveness of sterilization is reduced if moisture is not adjacent to the microorganisms, the moisture absorption capability of suture materials should be considered together with the

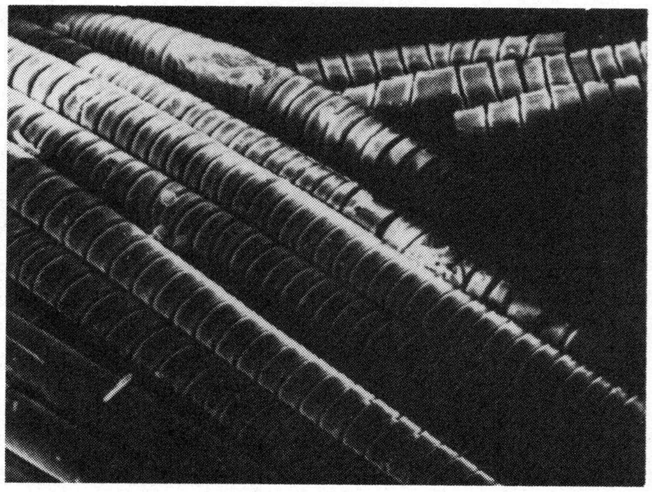

Figure 13. Scanning electron micrograph of 2-0 PGA suture γ-irradiated at 20 MRADs and 40 days immersion in physiological saline solution at 37°C. ×1000.

type of sterilization method. In addition, a period of "sitting" is required after exposure to th gas in order to remove the gas trapped inside the material. This lengthens the operation tir further. Since ethylene oxide is toxic to human beings, its residual amount is an important co cern. The FDA-recommended guideline is 250 ppm. PGA, polyglactin 910, polypropylene ar cotton are the suture materials which are sterilized by this gaseous method. When comparir ionizing radiation with ethylene oxide methods, it has been reported that the latter reduc tensile strength more than the former in nylon 66 sutures.

B.8 New Suture Materials

With the goal of developing suture materials that are more flexible yet strong, a ne biodegradable polymer, polydioxanone, has been recently reported to be a promising ne synthetic absorbable suture material [1]. The material is a homopolymer of p-dioxan-2-one (shown below), and is

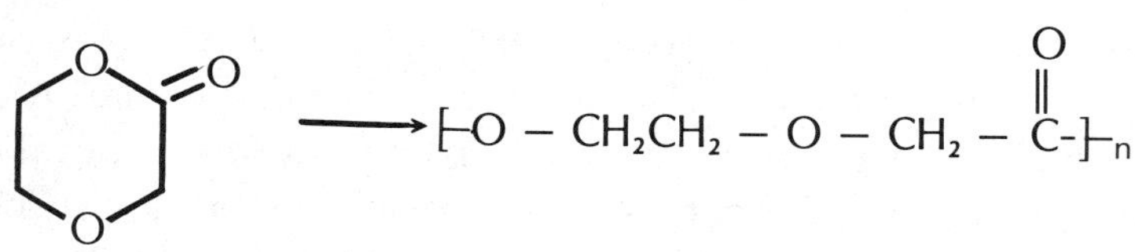

polymerized in the presence of Et_2Zn catalyst. The fiber is obtained from the melt-extrusion the polymer chips. The manufacturer has claimed the new absorbable suture material ma from poly(p-dioxanone) is flexible, soft, and easy to tie in a knot. It retains better and longer t sile strength in vivo than all other absorbable suture materials. It can be sterilized either by C or ethylene oxide. The tissue response of this polymer is on the same order of that of PGA and polyglactin 910, but it has better hydrolytic resistance. The absorption involves the breaking down of the monofilaments into hundreds of long, thin fragments and subsequent incorporation into single giant cells or macrophages.

C. TISSUE ADHESIVES

The idea of using sutureless methods to close surgical wounds can be found as early as 1791, when John Hunter concluded that, "The passage of needle and ligature must always produce suppuration through the whole passage and the use of a sticking plaster would be more general in its application." Since the late 1950s and early 1960s, there has been an increasing interest in and demand for using techniques and materials other than conventional sutures to close wounds in certain surgical problems arising from the narrowing of small vessel anastomoses, vascular repairs in heparinized patients, leakage from stump closure of the duodenum and bronchus, luminal narrowing of ductal repairs, and the closure of lacerated solid organs. Tissue adhesives have thus been developed and become an integral part of wound-closure management. Tissue adhesives are mainly used in those areas which do not lend themselves to sutures. Their advantages are: 1) rapidity of wound closure; 2) the ability of a complete closure to prevent seepage of blood and fluids (blood vessels and intestine); 3) the possibility of closing the wound without undue deformation of tissue (e.g., cosmetic surgery); 4) the successful closure of tissues which are too weakened or diseased to permit effective suture (liver, kidney, spleen); and 5) their success in organ transplantation, in which minimal occlusive time and vascular patency are extremely important.

An ideal tissue adhesive should: 1) be able to bond rapidly to moist living tissue; 2) have adequate bonding strength not affected by moisture; 3) be free from systemic and cellular toxicity; 4) be biodegradable; 5) be fairly flexible; 6) have wettability and spreadability; 7) have adequate polymerization time and low heat of polymerization; 8) lack of carcinogenicity and antigenicity; 9) have shelf stability and 10) be capable of sterilization. Efforts which have been devoted developing tissue adhesives with these ideal properties have resulted in numerous types of tissue adhesives which are available either commercially or experimentally. In general, they are classified into synthetic and natural origins.

In the synthetic tissue adhesive system, N-alkyl-α-cyanoacrylate is probably most important and has been subjected to the most extensive study [47,48]. Other polymers like rubber latex, epoxy resin, isocyanate-terminated polyesters, polyvinyl alcohol, and formaldehyde resins are also used, but to a lessor extent due to not bonding well to tissue or slow bond formation or both.

Among tissue adhesives of natural origin, formaldehyde cross-linked gelatins appear to be the most important and successful. They are the current leading contender with the alkyl-α-cyanoacrylates for the interest and attention of researchers [48,49]. The reason for the development of this system is that tissue fibers consist largely of polypeptide chains, and adhesives derived from materials of similar structure have properties closer to the ideal tissue adhesive. Other natural tissue adhesives include the plasma fractions (mainly fibrinogen).

C.1 Design Principles of Tissue Adhesives

The knowledge of the adhesion mechanism of tissue adhesives is the foundation of the development of new tissue adhesives. The common basic principles of adhesion operate in tissue adhesives. There are two general kinds of bonding involved in any type of adhesion: primary and secondary. The former includes covalent, metallic, and electrostatic bonds, whereas the latter includes hydrogen bonds, dipole-dipole attraction, van der Waal's force, and London dispersion force. Primary bonds are stronger than secondary bonds. Due to the highly polar nature of the tissue surfaces and the large volume of water in the tissue, the secondary bonding seems to be important. However, it often deteriorates because of the penetration of water into the tissue and adhesive interface, and the subsequent replacement of the scondary bond between tissue and adhesive by H-bonds. Thus, in order to achieve a permanent and strong bonding between tissue and adhesive, the formation of primary bonds through chemical reaction is highly desirable in the development of an ideal tissue adhesive.

A number of functional groups have been found in the tissue that are capable of reacting with adhesives. They are mainly $-OH$, $-NH_2$, and $-COOH$. In designing polymers for tissue adhesive use, the polymer should have the right reaction end groups which will form primary bonds with the tissue's functional groups. Thus, polymers containing aldehyde, isocyanate, or diazonium salt groups will react with the tissue's $-NH_2$ functional group to form covalent bonds, while polymers containing acyl halide or anhydride end groups will react with the tissue's $-OH$ functional group.

Another requirement of a tissue adhesive is that it must be fluid for easy handling and application, and solidify after application. The use of heat and pressure to facilitate solidification is highly improbable due to the possible damage of tissue. The appropriate means of solidification are: 1) rapid polymerization of liquid monomers; 2) the use of reactive prepolymers; 3) solvent removal; 4) breaking polymeric emulsions by pH change; and 5) precipitation of polymers by exposure to body environment.

C.2 Natural Tissue Adhesive Systems

The most successful tissue adhesives in this system are gelatin-resorcinol-formaldehyde (GRF). The molecular weight of gelatins ranges from 30,000 to 120,000. Gelatin is chemically somewhat similar to connective tissue. The framework of GRF is the polycondensation product of resorcinol (a phenol) and formaldehyde by releasing water. Gelatin then fills the spaces in the framework to form a glue with the consistency of hard rubber. The polycondensation reaction releases a small amount of heat and is pH-dependent. The reaction occurs preferably in an alkaline condition. A small amount of moisture is not detrimental to the formation of a satisfactory adhesion. The useful life of GRF at body temperature is about 30 seconds. Bond strength and resistance to exposure to Ringer's solution improves as the ratio of resorcinol to formaldehyde increases. One of the mechanisms responsible for the adhesive properties of GRF is believed to be the H-bonding between the cross-linked gelatin and the tissue.

Numerous investigators (mainly in Europe) have reported the successful use of GRF as a tissue adhesive and as a hemostatic agent in a vast number of applications. The GRF adhesive adheres well to dry as well as wet wound surfaces. It is elastic and has a good tensile strength. Due to its strong bactericidal effect, wound infection hardly ever occurs. Tissue irritability from GRF in the parenchymatous organs such as lung, heart, kidney, liver, and intestine is minimal and insignificant; GRF is best when used in repairing these organs. It has been postulated that the degree of tissue reaction of GRF appears to relate in part to the vascularity of the tissue to which GRF is applied. Apparently, the formaldehyde (a protein precipitant) can be carried away more rapidly in a highly circulated tissue; and less tissue damage will result from the local concentrated formaldehyde. This also illustrates why GRF adhesive results in more tissue response in cartilage, which is a tissue with poor circulation. The use of a pH-controlled system has been found to reduce undesirable tissue irritability [48]. Minimal foreign body reaction occurs on wounds closed by GRF and macrophages are the major inflammatory cells around GRF.

The tensile strength of incised skin wounds closed by GRF and linen suture has been compared [49]. Skin wounds closed by applying GRF on the wound surface exhibited wound tensile strength almost triple that of the sutured skin wound during the first postoperative week. In short, GRF tissue adhesive shows the best results in closing frail and highly vascularized tissue in order to minimize tissue irritation as well as utilize its hemostatic ability.

C.3 Synthetic Tissue Adhesive System

As mentioned earlier, there are numerous types of synthetic tissue adhesive. Alkyl-α-cyanoacrylate has received the most attention in research and use because of its hemostatic capability as well as its tissue bonding ability. Methyl-α-cyanoacrylate was the first in the series to be evaluated extensively. Although it has the advantage of rapid disappearance, it elicits severe local tissue response and has been virtually abandoned. Higher homologs have thus been developed and studied in the search for better tissue-tolerance materials. Clinical applications of tissue adhesives include the bonding of lacerated fragments of solid organs, anastomosis of tubular organs, approximation of severed nerves, placement of skin grafts, and repair of incised wounds.

The most common preparation of cyanoacrylate monomers involves the base-catalyzed Knoevenagel condensation of a cyanoacetate and formaldehyde, as illustrated below:

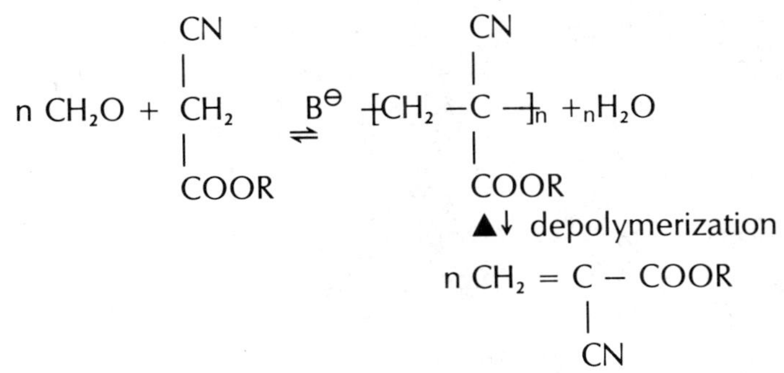

The use of a nonaqueous organic solvent for the azeotropic removal of H_2O could eliminate the water instability problem of the monomers. The depolymerization stage is the most difficult part of the preparation, and takes place by a free radical mechanism in the backbone chain. The rate of degradation decreases as the size of the R group increases. Anionic or free radical stabilizers (e.g., SO_2, hydroquinone) are frequently added to prevent the repolymerization of the monomer, and hence enhance its shelf life.

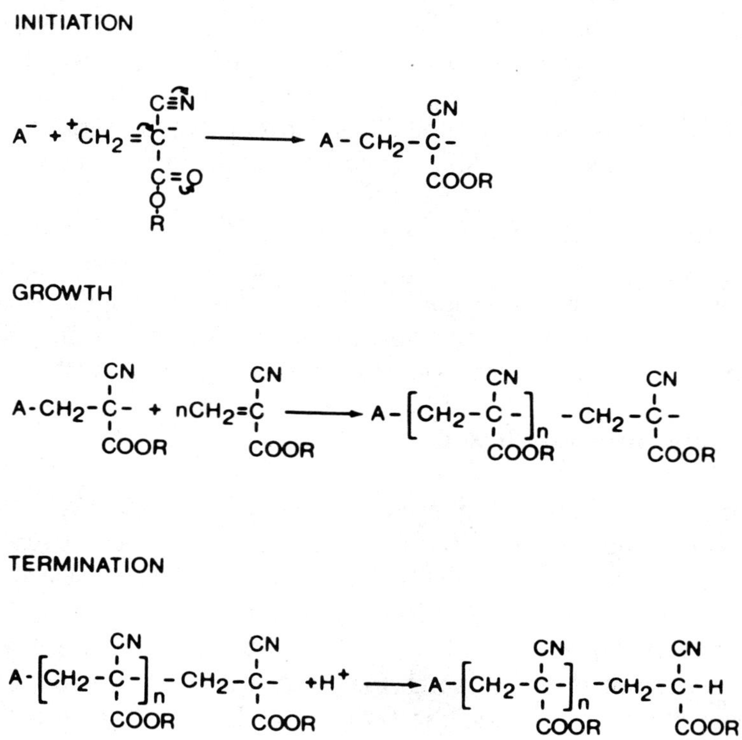

Figure 14a. Polymerization mechanism of alkyl α-cyanoacrylate tissue adhesives. (Courtesy of Dr. Refojo et al., Ref. 3).

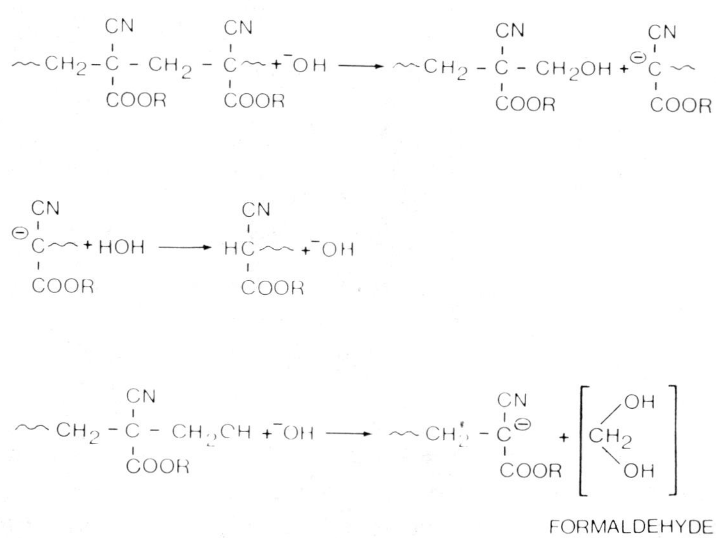

Figure 14b. Degradation mechanism of poly (alkyl α-cyanoacrylate) in aqueous medium. (Courtesy of Dr. Refojo et al., Ref. 3).

C.3.1 Preparation of Poly(alkyl α-cyanoacrylate)

The cyanoacrylate adhesive solidifies through an anionic polymerization mechanism initiated by water or another weak base (e.g., alcohol). As shown in Figure 14a, the polarization of the C—C double bond by the nucleophile initiates the polymerization. It has been suggested that hydroxy and amino groups of protein molecules in the tissue may possibly be involved in this initiation *in vivo*. Such initiation could lead to primary chemical bonding to the tissue. Propagation follows as the carbanion ion reacts with monomers. The reaction terminates as the growing polymer chain reacts with an acid. The problem that is commonly encountered in polymerization is shrinkage, which can result in voids in the system and hence weaker bonding strength. Whether this shrinkage will actually cause bonding problems in vivo has not been clinically reported.

The rate of polymerization of the homologous series of cyanoacrylate tissue adhesives depends on several factors, such as the environment of the polymerization and the number of carbons of the alkyl group. In water, increasing the number of carbons from methyl to n-heptyl increases the time of polymerization from ten seconds to 300 seconds (aqueous effect). The order of the polymerization rate is reversed: faster in higher homologs and slower in lower homologs in blood or *in vivo* (blood effect) [48]. This difference in polymerization rate may be due to the difference in wettability and spreadability of the homologous series. The higher homologous monomers wet and spread better on the tissue surface than the lower homologous monomers. As the monomers spread more on the tissue surface, more catalyst sites present on the tissue surface become available, and hence faster polymerization occurs. In addition, wettability and spreadability are very important in determining the effectiveness of α-cyanoacrylate adhesives in achieving hemostasis.

The lower homologs (methyl and ethyl α-cyanocrylates), which are more hydrophilic toward H_2O, form liquid lenses and do not spread on blood. Hence, the polymerization is limited to the surface of the droplet. The diffusion of nucleophiles through the already formed polymer film into the interior of the droplet is needed for further polymerization. Polymerization at a considerably slower rate (300 secs.) is thus observed in the tissue.

The medical implication of the polymerization rate is that instantaneous polymerization is not always an advantage, particularly in anastomosis or closure of tubular organs. It is desirable to have enough time to bring the wound surfaces together accurately. If the polymerization time is too long, as with the lower homologous α-cyanoacrylates, it is inappropriate for clinical use because of the difficulty in keeping the wound surface dry and in a steady position for a long time.

C.3.2 Physical and Mechanical Properties

The hardness and tensile breaking strength of these homologous polymers increases, whereas elongation at break decreases with the decrease in size of the alkyl group. The impact strength of the homologous series is generally low and brittleness decreases with an increase in the size of the alkyl group. Thus plasticizers are occasionally used to improve impact resistance. For medical use, higher homologs are more appropriate than lower ones because they are more compatible with the tissue.

C.3.3. Biodegradation Mechanism

The need for a biodegradable tissue adhesive is obvious. The presence of undegraded polymer fragments decreases the surface area available for collagenous union of the wound edges. Accordingly, the fibroplasia phase is mechanically impaired and occurs only after enough adhesive has degraded to permit bridging of the fibroblasts.

Poly(alkyl-α-cyanoacrylate) based tissue adhesives biodegrade inside the body. In the presence of an aqueous environment, the polymer gives rise to its degradation products, formaldehyde, and other breakdown products. The rate of degradation is the greatest for methyl α-cyanoacrylate, and diminishes as the size of the alkyl group increases at pH = 7.0 [47,48]. α-cyanoacrylates with branched alkyl groups also degrade faster than their straight chain homologs. The rate of degradation is higher in alkaline solution (pH = 8) for all homologous α-cyanoacrylates and differs only slightly from one to another. For example, the rate constants of both methyl and n-butyl α-cyanoacrylates at pH = 7.0 are 3.0×10^{-3} and 1.0×10^{-5}, respectively.

This alkaline-accelerated aqueous degradation suggests that the mechanism must involve the initial attack of hydroxyl ions on the chain methylene group and subsequent chain scission occurs as shown in Figure 14b. The degradation *in vitro* would reach an equilibrium at which the concentration of formaldehyde produced remains constant. In addition to the dependence of the degradation rate on the pH, and size of the alkyl group, Vezin has recently reported that polymer particle specific surface, particle size, molecular weight, and molecular weight distribution also affect the in vitro heterogeneous phase degradation rate of the poly(alkyl α-cyanoacrylate) [50]. The degradation occurs at the chain ends and travels along the polymer chain.

C.3.4 Toxicity

As a result of the degradation of tissue adhesives, their levels of toxicity depend in part on the chemical nature of the degradation products and the rate of degradation. Thus, higher homologs of alkyl α-cyanoacrylate are less toxic than their lower counterparts because of their slower rate of degradation. The order of tolerance levels of the most commonly used synthetic tissue adhesives are as follows: n-decyl, n-octyl, n-heptyl, n-butyl, and isobutyl α-cyanoacrylates are well-tolerated; methyl α-cyanoacrylate is least tolerated [3].

Both degradation products, formaldehyde and an alkyl α-cyanoacrylate, can elicit acute inflammatory responses. The fact that the higher homologs are tolerated better than the lower homologs implies that the rate of degradation is the critical factor in determining the level of tissue tolerance of these materials. A rapidly degraded polymer like poly(methyl α-cyanoacrylate) would result in a high local concentration of formaldehyde and alkyl α-cyanoacrylate in the tissue. If the degradation products are built up faster than the tissue's capability to metabolize them, the local concentration of degradation products increases and elicits a stronger tissue response. Since higher homologs degrade slowly, the tissue tolerates them better. The metabolites are eliminated through the normal excretory routes.

In ophthalmology, the tissue response is also found to depend on the amount of adhesive materials used [3]. The smaller the amount of adhesive used, the less the tissue reaction elicited. The fairly good tolerance reported in ocular surgery could be attributed to the small amount of adhesive used, ranging from half a microliter to several microliters per application.

This tissue response is obviously related to the rate of build-up of degradation products and the tissue's ability to metabolize them.

Other factors such as the orientation and crystallinity of the polymer could also affect its rate of degradation. A more oriented and crystallized polymer is expected to degrade more slowly and hence be less toxic. No data have been reported in this area.

Since the higher homologs degrade very slowly, their long-term effects, such as carcinogenicity or sterile abscess formation, have been a great concern. At present, they have disappeared from the shelves in the United States, but they will enjoy great popularity in Europe and Asia. In the author's opinion, these materials should be used strictly as a life-saving product in mass casuality situations like combat, where the number of patients makes time important, or in the control of hemorrhaging from lacerated solid organs like the liver and kidney.

D. SUMMARY

Because of the complications involved in wound healing, various types of wound closure biomaterials are needed. Wound closure biomaterials are generally classified into two major categories: suture materials and tissue adhesives. The former is still the major means of closing wounds, particularly in the United States. The chemical, physical, mechanical, and biological aspects of these materials have been reviewed. Among the absorbable sutures, polyglycolic acid and polyglactin 910 are considered to have the best balance of overall properties. They elicit minimal tissue reactions and have uniform and reproducible properties. Unlike catgut and collagen sutures, their biodegradation mechanism is believed to involve hydrolysis of ester bonds on the backbone chain. A microfibrillar model of fiber structure has been used as the basis for the proposed in vitro degradation mechanism of these suture materials. Among the nonabsorbable suture materials, those of natural origin like silk or cotton elicit much stronger tissue reactions than those of synthetic origin, but some of them have superior handling properties. Polypropylene and polyester sutures retain tensile strength best; whereas silk sutures lose half of their strength in 12 weeks. The ultimate solution of choosing suture materials with the right mechanical properties for closing specific wounds might be to select a suture whose stress-strain has the best match with the stress-strain data of the tissue to be sewed. Other properties such as tissue reactions, wound condition, knot strength and security, and degree of absorption should also be considered, along with the suture's mechanical properties. The final selection will likely be a compromise of these properties for optimum performance.

Tissue adhesives have an advantage over suture techniques in special clinical conditions. They close the wound, particularly lacerated solid organs, more readily and rapidly with hemostasis capability. The sutureless wound attains an immediate tensile strength approximately that of the sutured wound on days four to six. The gelatin-resorcinol-formaldehyde (GRF) adhesive seems to have better promise and potential than alkyl α-cyanoacrylates. The major disadvantage of the latter is their toxic tissue response and long term effects. However, they are frequently used in Europe and Asia. They should be reserved only for mass casualty situations like combat in which life saving is more important than anything else.

E. REFERENCES

1. Ray, J. A., Doddi, N., Regula, D., et al., "Polydioxanone (PDS), A Novel monofilament Synthe-

tic absorbable suture," Surg. Gynecol. Obst., 153: 497-507 (1981).
2. Gottlob, R. "Adhesives in Surgery," Proceedings of the International Symposium, Vienna Academy of Medicine, Vienna (1968).
3. Refojo, M. F., Dohlman, C. H. and Koliopoulos, J., "Adhesives in Ophthalmology: A Review." Survey of Ophthalm. *15(4)*, 217-236 (1971).
4. Frazza, E. J. and Schmitt, E. E. "A new absorbable suture," J. Biomed. Mater. Res. Symp., *1*, 43-58 (1971).
5. Filachione, E. M. and Fisher, C. H., "Lactic acid condensation polymers – preparation by batch and continuous methods," Ind. Eng. Chem. *36(3)*, 223-228 (1944).
6. Wise, D. L., Fellmann, T. D., Sanderson, J. E. and Wentworth, R. L., "Lactic/Glycolic Acid Polymers," in "Drug Carriers in Biology and Medicine," New York, Academic Press, p. 237-270 (1979).
7. Chujo, K., Kobayashi, H., Suzuki, J., Tokuhara, S. and Tanabe, M., "Ring-Opening Polymerization of Glycolide," Die Makromol. Chemie, 100, 262-266 (1967).
8. Cherdron, H., Ohse, H. and Korte, F., Homopolymerization of 4-, 6-, and 7-Membered Lactones with Cationic Initiators," Makromol. Chemie, *56*, 179-186 (1962).
9. Ethicon, Inc., New Jersey, U.S. Patent 1,332,505 (1973).
10. Kulkarni, R. K., Moore, E. G., Hegyeli, A. F. and Leonard, F., Biodegradable Poly(Lactic Acid) Polymers, J. Biomed. Mater. Res., *5*, 169-181 (1971).
11. Chatani, Y., Suehiro, K., Okita, Y., Tadokoro, H. and Chujo, K., "Structural Studies of Polyesters, I. Crystal Structure of Polyglycolide," Die Makromol. Chemie, *113*, 215-229 (1968).
12. Chujo, K., Kobayashi, H., Suzuki, J. and Tokuhara, S., "Physical and chemical characteristics of polyglycolide," Die Makromol. Chemie, *100*, 267-270 (1967).
13. Daubeny, R. P., Bunn, C. W. and Brown, C. J., "The Crystal Structure of Polyethylene Terephthalate," Proc. Roy. Soc., A226 (1167), 531-542 (1954).
14. Venkatesh, G. M., Bose, P. J. and Khan, A. H., "Vibrational spectroscopic study of poly(ethylene terephthalate) crystallized by annealing in the oriented state," J. Appl. Polym. Sci., *26*, 223-230 (1981).
15. Heuvel, H. M. and Huisman, R., "Effect of Winding Speed on the Physical Structure of As-Spun Poly(Ethylene Terephthalate) Fibers, Including Orientation-Induced Crystallization," J. Appl. Polym. Sci., *22*, 2229-2243 (1978).
16. Moncrieff, R. W. "Nylon" in the "Man-Made Fibres," New York, John Wiley and Son, p. 333-407 (1975).
17. Kohan, M. I., "Preparation and Chemistry of Nylon Plastics" in "Nylon Plastics" (Ed. Kohan, M. I.), New York, Wiley-Interscience, p. 13-81 (1973).
18. Bunn, C. W. and Garner, E. V., "The Crystal Structure of Two Polyamides (Nylons)," Proc. Roy. Soc., *A189*, 38-68 (1947).
19. Sbrolli, W., "Nylon 6" in "Man-Made Fibers Science and Technology" (Ed. Mark, Atlas and Cernia), Vol. 2. New York, Wiley-Interscience, p. 229-295 (1968).
20. Heuvel, H. M. and Huisman, R., "Effects of winding speed, drawing and heating on the crystalline structure of Nylon 6 yans," J. Appl. Polym. Sci., *26*, 713-732 (1981).
21. Goodman, M., "Topics in Stereochemistry," (Eds. Allinger, N. L. and Eliel, E. L.), Vol. 2, New York, Wiley-Interscience, p. 73 (1967).
22. Kaufman, H. S. and Falcetta, J. J., "Introduction to Polymer Science and Technology: An SPE Textbook," New York, Wiley-Interscience, p. 92-103 (1977).
23. Cossee, P., "The Stereochemistry of Macromolecules," (Ed. Ketley, A. D.), Vol. 1, New York, Dekker (1967).
24. Chu., C. C., "Mechanical Properties of Suture Materials: An Important Characterization," Annals of Surgery, *193*(3), 365-371 (1981).

25. Holmlund, E. W., "Physical properties of surgical suture materials: stress-strain relationship, stress-relaxation and irreversible elongation," Ann. Surg., *184*, 189-193 (1976).
26. Taylor, T. L. "Suture Materials: A comprehensive review of the literature," J. Am. Podiatry Assoc., *65(7)*, 649-661 (1975).
27. Winkle, W. V. and Salthouse, T. N. "Biological response to sutures and principles of suture selection," Ethicon, Inc. (1976).
28. Katz, A. R. and Turner, R. J. "Evaluation of Tensile and Absorption Properties of Polyglycolic Acid Sutures," Surg. Gynecol. and Obst., *131*, 701-716 (1970).
29. Chu, C., "A Comparison of the Effect of pH on the Biodegradation of Two Synthetic Absorbable Sutures," Annals of Surgery, 195: 55-59 (1982).
30. Reed, A. M. and Gilding, D. K., "Biodegradable Polymers for Use in Surgery – Poly(glycolic)/Poly(lactic acid) Homo and Copolymers: 2. In Vitro Degradation, Polymer, *22(4)*, 494-498 (1981).
31. Holmlund, D., Tera, H., Wiberg, Y., Zederfeldt, B. and Aberg, C., "Sutures and techniques for wound closure," New York, Naimark and Barba (1978).
32. Tera, H. and Aberg, C., "Tensile strength of 12 types of knot employed in surgery, using different suture materials," Acta Chir. Scand. *142(1)*, 1-7 (1976).
33. Herrmann, J. B., "Tensile Strength and Knot Security of Surgical Suture Materials," Am. Surg., *37*, 209-217 (1971).
34. Taylor, F. W., "Surgical knots and sutures," Surgery, *107*, 498-510 (1938).
35. Magilligan, D. J. and DeWeese, J. A., "Knot security and synthetic suture materials," The Am. J. Surg., *127* 355-358 (1974).
36. Everett, W. G., "Suture Materials in General Surgery," Progr. Surg., *8*, 14-37 (1970).
37. Homsy, C. A., McDonald, K. E. and Akers, W. W., "Surgical suture-canine tissue interaction for 6 common suture types," J. Biomed. Mater. Res., *2*, 215 (1968).
38. Craig, P. H., Williams, J. A., Davis, K. W., et al., "A biological comparision of polyglactin 910 and polyglycolic acid synthetic absorbable sutures," Surg. Gynecol. and Obst., *141*, 1-10, (1975).
39. Postlethwait, R. W., "Long-term comparative study of nonabsorbable sutures," Ann. Surg., *171(6)*, 892-898 (1970).
40. Alexander, J. W., Kaplan, J. Z. and Altemeier, W. A., "Role of suture materials in the development of wound infection," Ann. Surg., *165(2)*, 192-199 (1967).
41. Edlich, R. F., Panek, P. H., Rodeheaven, G. T., et al., "Physical and chemical configuration of sutures in the development of surgical infection," Ann. Surg. *177(6)*, 679-688 (1973).
42. Pendergast, W. J., Futrell, J. W. and Mardiney, M. R., "Differences in Potentiation of Melanoma Growth by Absorbable and Nonabsorbable Sutures," J. Surg. Oncol. *8*, 223-228 (1976).
43. Dahlke, H., Dociu, N. and Thurau, K., "Thrombogenicity of different suture materials as revealed by scanning electron microscopy," J. Biomed. Mater. Res., *14*, 251-268 (1980).
44. Chu, C. C., "Hydrolytic degradation of polyglycolic acid: Tensile strength and crystallinity study," J. Appl. Polym. Sci., *26*, 1727-1734 (1981).
45. Bloch, B. and Hastings, G. W., "Plastics Materials in Surgery," 2nd ed., Springfield, Charles C. Thomas, (1972).
46. Campbell, N. D. and Chu, C. C. "The effect of γ-irradiation on the in vitro degradation of polyglycolic synthetic sutures in physiological saline," Trans. of the 7th annual meeting of the Society for Biomaterials in conjunction with the 13th International Biomater. Symp. Vol. IV, p. 66, Troy, New York, May 28-31, (1981).
47. Leonard, F., Kulkarni, R. K., Brades, G., et al., "Synthesis and degradaton of Poly(alkyl α-cyanoacrylates), J. Appl. Polym. Sci., 10, 259-272 (1966).
48. Matsumoto, T., "Tissue Adhesives in Surgery," New York, Medical Examination Pub. (1972).
49. Vandor, E., Mozsary, P. and Reffy, A., "A critical study on the preparation and application of gelatinresorcinol tissue adhesive crosslinked by formaldehyde," Z. Exper. Chirurg. *13*, 43-51 (1980).
50. Vezin, W. R. and Florence, A. T. "In vitro heterogeneous degradation of Poly(n-alkyl α-cyanoacrylates), J. Biomed. Mater. Res. *14*, 93-106 (1980).

Chapter 23

Immobilization of Bioactive Components via Radiation-Induced Polymerization

Isao Kaetsu
Takasaki Radiation Chemistry Research Establishment
Japan Atomic Energy Research Institute
Takasaki, Gunma, Japan

ABSTRACT

Vinyl Polymers as carrier and radiation polymerization as mean were investigated for the physical immobilization of biocomponents. The glass-forming monomers having the stable supercooling property and the large polymerizability at low temperature were used as advantageous carrier. Characteristics of this method are its freedoms of selectivity in material and condition and its general applicability. Namely, these are freedom for carrier from hydrophobic to hydrophilic polymer freedom for biocomponent from molecules to organisms, freedom for shaping forms, freedom for biocomponents distribution from inner entrapment to surface adhesion and freedom for degree of immobilization from tight fixation for repeated use to loose entrapping for controlled release. Immobilized biomolecules such as immobilized enzyme and immuno globulin were used for the surface reactions such as enzymatic reaction and immuno reaction. Immobilization of physiologically active molecules was applied to controlled slow release. Various entrapping techniques for drugs were developed for design and control of widely ranged releases. The release technique was applied successfully to the local chemotherapy with immobilized anticancer capsules. The technique was also applied to the release of steroid hormones and gave the promising results. The technique for the stable immobilization of cells was developed. Some of the immobilized cells were used effectively as antigens for immunoassay. Some unstable tissue cells were stabilized by immobilization remarkably. The immobilized microorganisms showed the active growth in the optimum porous structure of the carrier, while the multiplication of immobilized tissue cells was accelerated on the optimum microsurface structure of the carrier polymer.

INTRODUCTION

It has become a research problem of more and more importance to develop a technique for utilization of various bioactive components such as enzymes, bioactive proteins, microbial cells, tissue cells, and physiologically active substances [1-5]. Development of two kinds of technique would be necessary for the artificial utilization of biocomponents. One is the technique for the improvement of biocomponent itself such as new discovery, mutation, cell fusion, and genetic technology. The other is the technique for the improvement of usage and engineering of biocomponent. For useful design and effective use of biocomponent as a device or system for bioreactors and artificial organs, it is inevitably necessary to modify the biocomponent with a suitable carrier. As well known, this kind of technique is called immobilization. Namely, immobilization means the modification of biocomponent into a solid system having the convenient size, form, shape, structure, and physical properties for the artificial uses [6-7]. The purpose of immobilization might be summarized as follows:

(1) Insolubilization, solidification for a repeated and a continuous use
(2) Distribution, composing for a controlled slow release
(3) Shaping, molding into a convenient size, form, and structure
(4) Improvement, useful attachment of physical and chemical properties with the carrier
(5) Stabilization, protection for a longer time under severer and more widely ranged conditions
(6) Acceleration, promotion of culture and growth
(7) Acceleration, control of cell fusion and mutation
(8) Control of specificities in substrate selectivity and immunological recognition

These purposes include those of various research stages and of various possibilities for realization. Purposes (1)-(3) have been proved experimentally to be realized [8-9]. Purposes (4)-(6) are now studying actively with a promising prospect [10-11]. Purposes (7) and (8) would be the important problems in the near future [12].

A number of immobilization methods has been studied and proposed by many workers [13-16]. The purpose of our studies is also to establish a new immobilization method having a wide freedom and a universal applicability to materials, objects and usages. Our research group made a basic research in the field of radiation-induced polymerization in the period from 1965-1973 [17-21]. The authors found and clarified the characteristic polymerization of glass-forming vinyl monomers in a supercooled state at low temperature with radiation. Since 1973, we have applied this polymerization technique to the immobilization of biocomponents [22-25]. A fundamental immobilization method has been developed until 1976, and since then applications of this technique has been done to the various objects and uses in the two fields of medical application and of energy and resource developments [26-29]. The present method has three key-point characteristics, that is:

(1) Use of synthetic high polymer for immobilization carrier
(2) Use of radiation for immobilization mean
(3) Physical adhesion or attachment through polymerization in the immobilization principle

All these points contribute to the very wide freedom of selectivity in the method and the product. The detailed characteristics are described in the following section as well as the detailed experimental method in relation to their merits and significance. In this article, the author reports and introduces the outlined feature of our immobilization technique and the recent results of its applications in the field of biomedical use.

Method and Characteristics of the Present Immobilization

1. Fundamental Method

Figure 1 shows the fundamental process of the present immobilization method [30]. As shown here at first, bioactive component mixed with polymerizable monomer to form a mixture. Sometimes, biocomponent is preliminarily mixed with suitable buffer solution of various pHs to form solution or suspension as in the case of enzyme, protein, and cell immobilization. In other cases such as immobilization of drug and a certain kind of microbial cell, biocomponent is often mixed with a monomer directly. The kind, combination (comonomer system for copolymerization), and concentration (composition ratio to buffer and biocomponent) of the monomer differ greatly depending on the kind of biocomponent and the purpose of immobilization. Then, the mixture (solution, slurry, suspension or emulsion) of biocomponent and monomer is shaped into a desirable form, cooled, and polymerized (hardened) by irradiation to give the product (biocomposite). The required size, shape, and structure of biocomposite are very multiple and variable according to the use especially for the controlled in vivo release and the artificial organ. The shaping methods in practical are as follows:

(a) Multiple Forms. It is possible to give any desired form at will to the biocomposite by pouring the above mixture into a mold of glass or metal designed to fit the required form and polymerizing it by irradiation. Many forms such as tablet (button), disk, sheet, fiber, pellet, ball, rod, nail, and needle can be obtained [9,13].

(b) Sphere and Microsphere. A simple way is to crush the polymerized biocomposite into fine powder. But, in order to obtain the microsphere, suspension techniques are used. A simple one is attained by the suspension polymerization of hydrophobic vinyl monomer in buffer solution (suspension mixture of biocomponent-buffer and hydrophobic monomer). Another one is that a mixture of biocomponent and monomer is dropped into a cooled dispersion medium (precipitating medium) to form microsphere and then polymerized by irradiation. For the purpose to obtain highly fine microsphere in the order of 0.1-10 microns, emulsion polymerization of biocomponent-buffer and monomer emulsion is used [32,33].

(c) Membrane. A simple way is a casting of biocomponent and monomer mixture into a film and polymerizing. Another way is to cut or slice the polymerized block biocomposite into thin membranes, for example, into 10-20 microns membrane by microtome slicing. Coating is also useful. In this case, the original mixture is coated on a surface of base material such as plastic film, fiber, tube, filter or bonded material and polymerized by irradiation.

(d) Composite of Multi-Layer or Multi-Dispersion Structures. Specific structures such as multi-phase or multi-dispersion phase give important effect on the property and function of carrier as well as its material and shape. If crystalline or crystallizable substance at low temperature is added to the biocomponent and monomer mixture before polymerization, a carrier matrix having porous structure is obtainable owing to the dissolution out of crystalline substance from the polymer after polymerization. Usually water in buffer solution becomes

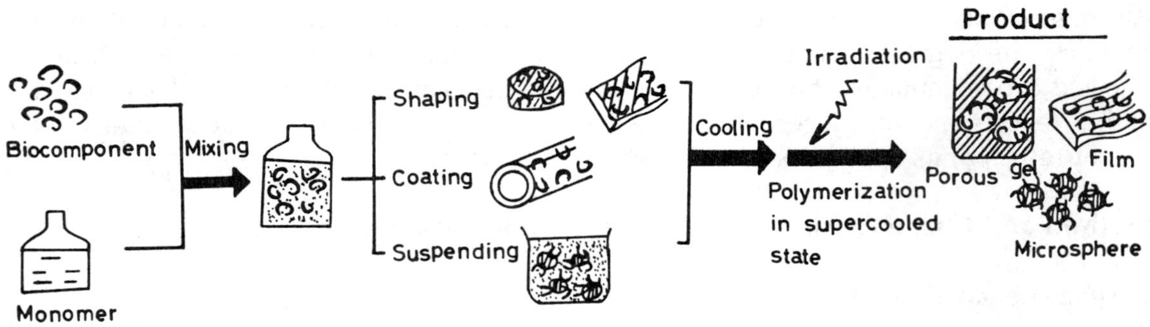

Figure 1. Process of immobilization with vinyl monomers by radiation polymerization method.

ice in low temperature polymerization and act as such kind of pore-making agent to give a porous biocomposite. Dioxane, polyethylene glycol, and many other crystallizable solvent are the typical pore-making agent. The porosity in the carrier changes depending on the concentration of the added pore-making agent. On the other hand, if an insoluble filler substance is added to the mixture, the resulted biocomposite has a filler-fixed structure. Various natural and synthetic polymers, inorganic adsorbent, filter material, and bonded material are the examples of filler. The filler density in the carrier is widely variable by the concentration ratio of monomer, biocomponent, and filler. In the cases of extremely large filler content, the density of polymer matrix decreases to an extremely small one and monomer (polymer) becomes a mere binder to adhere and connect between the filler and the biocomponent. These are examples of multi-dispersion composite. Furthermore, composites of multi-layer structures are obtainable as the following two means. The one mean consists of the repeated process of dispersing the divided composite into monomer mixture again and polymerizing it by irradiation. The other one consists of the repeated process of overlapped coating of monomer mixture on the composite surface and polymerizing it by irradiation. The multi-layer composites are useful for the controlled slow release [34,35,36].

In the present immobilization, the biocomponent-monomer mixture is shaped and composed before polymerization in the manner as described above, and then cooled to a low temperature usually 0°C and −80°C by immersing the glass ampoule or mold including the shaped mixture in a frozen coolant in Dewar vessel. Immobilization is completed by irradiation by the Dewar vessel to polymerize the monomer in it keeping the low temperature. Gamma-ray from a source such as cobalt 60 or cesium 137 is conveniently used because of its large penetrating power through Dewar vessel, while electron beam from an electron accelerator is also available for quick and large amount polymerization. In the fundamental method, biocomponent and monomer are mixed at the same time to form a mixture and then it is shaped for polymerization (Figure 2). Recently, it has been found that separative addition of biocomponent or monomer is also possible before radiation polymerization. For example, post addition of biocomponent to the shaped monomer or post addition of monomer to the shaped biocomponent followed by the radiation polymerization is now being studied. These variations will be especially effective for the surface immobilization and the surface reaction with the biocomposite.

2. Characteristics

Polymeric material is obviously one of the most preferable medium for a modification of

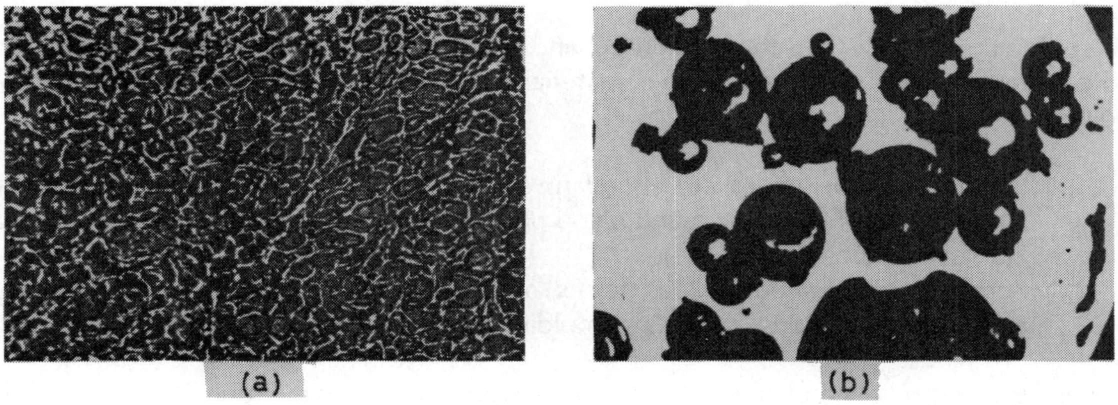

Figure 2a. *Figure 2b.*

Figure 2. Microphotographs of microbial cell immobilized by the polymerization of hydrophilic monomer (a, 2-hydroxyethyl methacrylate) and hydrophobic monomer (b, diethyleneglycol dimethacrylate.

other materials. However, synthetic high polymer has not been used so widely and generally as a carrier for physical immobilization. The reason might be that in the hitherto known physical immobilization method called entrapping method, enzyme was included inside a network structure of crosslinked hydrophilic polymer such as polyacrylamide and polyvinyl alcohol [37,38]. It was thought, in general, that only hydrophilic polymer was available as a carrier, because enzyme can dissolve only in water (buffer) and therefore homogeneous mixture to be immobilized can be obtained only by the hydrophilic components systems. The kind of hydrophilic synthetic polymer is rather limited in the narrow range for selection. This might be reason for the hitherto limited utilization of synthetic polymers for physical immobilization.

The author studied the use of vinyl polymers as carriers for the present immobilization and found that they are generally usable for the purpose. The utilizable material as a carrier in the present method is summarized as follows:

(1) Alkyl methacrylate, acrylate, and their analogues
$$CH_2{=}CXCOOR$$
(2) Hydroxyalkyl methacrylate and acrylate
$$CH_2{=}CXCOO(CH_2)_nOH$$
(3) Polyethylene glycol dimethacrylate and acrylate
$$CH_2{=}CXCOO(CH_2CH_2O)_mOCXC{=}H_2C$$
(4) Polyfunctional monomers
(ex) trimethylolpropane trimethacrylate and neopentyl glycol dimethacrylate
(5) Other vinyl monomers to be copolymerized with the above mentioned monomers
(ex) styrene, vinyl acetate, vinyl pyrrolidone, and acrylonitrile
(6) Natural polymers, monomer or oligomer for polyaddition and polycondensation to be mixed and polymerized in blend with the above mentioned vinyl monomers
(ex) collagen, albumin, epoxy compound, organosilane compound, and polypeptide

where X is the H or CH_3, R is the alkyl group, and n and m are the integer larger than one. The advantages of these synthetic polymer material can be summarized to the following two points:

(1) Its kinds and properties are abundant and widely ranged. Combinations are also usable by copolymerization and blend polymerization. In addition, molecular design and new synthesis are possible.
(2) Modification to various shapes, forms, and structures are easy and widely variable under mild conditions, by casting, molding, coating etc.

General use of synthetic polymer ranged both in hydrophobic and hydrophilic materials is the first characteristic of the method. The second remarked feature of the method is the physical immobilization by polymerization. It is almost impossible to mix or compose a biocomponent with polymeric materials through softening or melting of the latter by heat. Mixing of components in a monomeric state and then fixing its state and structure by polymerization are, of no doubt, one of the best ways to keep the original activity of biocomponent and also design and control the shape and structure of the system freely.

The author used the radiation as the mean of polymerization which had several conveniences. Principally, in physical immobilization, monomer or polymer carrier has the three contributions:

(1) Functions as a binder for biocomponent to form solid biocomposite
(2) Benefitable interaction with biocomponent such as stabilization and growth acceleration
(3) Addition of new properties to biocomposite such as convenient shape, mechanical strength, biocompatibility, and separative function

The weight of importance for the three factors differs by the case. Vinyl monomers are advantageous and fitable to (2) and (3) as well as to (1). But, other monomers such as those of polyaddition and polycondensation types can also be available for the purpose (1), so far as the hardening reaction can be carried out simply under a mild condition. Though numerous immobilization methods has been known, chemical binding with covalent bond and physical trapping including entrapping, adhesion (attachment), ionic adsorption, and mechanical adsorption are fundamental ones in principle.

As well known, immobilization by chemical binding has the merits in a firm and strong fixation as well as naked fixation on a carrier surface. But, it was not satisfactory in the simplicity of immobilization procedure and condition, in activity yield to the original activity of native biocomponent and in general applicability to biocomponents.

Physical immobilization seems to have more universal applicability to general biocomponent, though it has some ambiguity in mechanism and weakness in fixation. Moreover, physical method seems to be more fitted to the full use of synthetic polymer, because it is generally applicable to any kind of vinyl monomer for polymerization. Namely, the following five kinds of large freedom for wide selection can be gained as the result of (1) physical immobilzation and (2) general use of synthetic polymers. That is:

(1) Freedom of carrier selection over wide range from hydrophilic to hydrophobic ones or

from soft elastic to hard plastic, for example
(2) Freedom of biocomponent distribution in carrier from surface adhesion to inner entrapment
(3) Freedom in the degree of immobilization in carrier from tight fixation for continuous reaction to loose trapping for controlled release
(4) Freedom of shaping and structure organizing
(5) Freedom of biocomponent selection over wide range from molecular such as enzyme and protein to organism such as microbial cell and tissue cell.

As for the freedoms (1), (4) and (5), no more explanation will be necessary. Freedom means the relatively large range and capacity of selection for the most suitable combination of factors from (1) to (4) according to the need (5) and its uses. Freedoms (3) and (4) can be attained only by the physical immobilization. Both are controllable by design and control of mixing method and procedure of components and also by the selection of suitable carrier according to the kind and property of biocomponents. Surface adhesion is useful for surface reaction with the fixed biocatalysts and inner entrapping is useful for cell culture and for controlled slow release. Degree of immobilization from tight and strong fixation to gradual leakage and release is affected by various factors related to the immobilization conditions as summarized in Table 1. Finally, use of radiation as a mean of polymerization is also the characteristic of this method. Radiation produces chemical species such as ion and radical through its path to cause the subsequent chemical reactions such as polymerization and crosslinking or degradation. The most specific property of radiation different from other reaction means such as photo-irradiation, plasma-irradiation and laser-irradiation is its excellent penetrating power through the irradiated substances. Therefore, the most characteristics of irradiation effect are the fact that radicals of any desired concentration can be formed in the irradiated material at any temperatures at any pressures and in any reaction phases. Namely, the large freedoms of reaction condition and environment are permissible in radiation reaction. Especially, the most characteristic reactions induced by radiation are a solid reaction and low temperature reaction.

As well known, many kinds of solid reaction by irradiation are utilizing in the biological field, for example, in sterilization of medical instrument, in mutation of plants and organisms and in food irradiation. Radiation has also been used for plastic synthesis at low temperature and in solid state.

As reviewed in the introduction, the author developed the study and application of radiation-induced polymerization in a supercooled state using glass-forming monomers. This polymerization is specified for an extremely high viscosity of the supercooled monomer at low temperature near Tg (glass transition temperature). Therefore, it can be carried out only by radiation such as gamma-ray and electron beam. The author found based on the experiences in this field, that radiation is especially useful as a mean of stable modification of relatively unstable functional substances into a plastic by polymerization to give the functional composite. The typical example was the immobilization of biocomponents. The advantages of radiation for the immobilization can be summarized as follows:

(1) Original activity of biocomponent is kept without significant inactivation owing to the treatment and reaction at low temperature in addition to the mixing in a liquid state with monomer. Radiation damage on biocomponent can be retarded almost com-

Table 1. Uses of the Biocomposites Obtained by Physical Immobilization

Reaction	Biocomponent			Use
Surface reaction with fixed biocomponent	Molecule	Enzyme (for small substrate)	Glucose oxidase Cholesterol oxidase Urokinase Urease etc	Device and reactor for medical use
		Enzyme (for large substrate)	Cellulase Glucoamylase Lipase etc	Device and reactor for hydrolysis
	Cell	Microbial cell	Streptomyces phaechromegenes etc	Device and reactor for isomerization and fermentation
		Tissue cell	Chloroplast Erythrocyte antigen cell etc	Device and reactor for photo synthesis, artificial organ immunoassay, immunothrapy
Controlled slow release	Molecule	Anticancer	Mitomycin C 5-Fluorouracil Bleomycin hydrochloride	Local chemotherapy
		Hormone	Steroid hormones	Delivery chemotherapy
		Enzyme	Uricase	Delivery chemotherapy
Culture and product release with fixed biocomponent	Cell	Microbial cell	Trichoderma reesei Saccharomyces formosensis	Deliverv and reactor for cell culture and product release
		Tissue cell	C_6 cell (glinial cell) GH_3 cell	

pletely choosing the suitable irradiation conditions such as small dose less than 1×10^6 rad and low temperature below 0°C. Because, polymerization is a chain reaction and so it needs far much smaller dose than that necessary for an inactivation of biocomponent especially at low temperature region.

(2) Polymerization in multiple and complicate forms, shapes and structures are completed easily owing to the penetrating ability of radiation through the mold and the viscous monomer.

(3) No toxic component such as catalyst residue is included in the product. This is useful for medical uses.

Conclusively, the characteristics of the proposed method and the product are summarized to the three points:

(1) Simple and mild process
(2) General applicability to components and uses
(3) Large freedom for materials, methods and effect (functions)

These are the result of the three methodological characteristics: (1) physical immobilization, (2) use of vinyl polymers, and (3) use of radiation.

3. Uses

The resulted biocomposite can be used for the three types of functions:

(1) Fixation
(2) Release
(3) Fixation for culture and product release

As shown in Table 1, the fixation is mainly done on carrier surface physically for surface reactions, while immobilization for release is usually done inside carrier matrices. The uses can also be classified as (1) fixation and release of molecules and (2) fixation or combination of fixation, culture and release in cells. These uses are intended for the bioreactor for energy and resource utilization and development and also for artificial organs, in a broad sense, including drug delivery system and diagnosis material in the medical field. In the next section, some aspects of applications will be introduced with the practical examples.

Application to Enzyme Fixation for Medical Uses

1. Fixation of Enzyme on Plastic Surface for Medical Inspection

Immobilization of molecular level biocomponents such as enzyme, protein and physiologically active substance covers the application uses in the following three fields:

(1) Inner reaction with small substrate with an entrapped biomolecule inside hydrophilic or hydrophobic carrier matrix in aqueous or in organic solvent medium
(2) Release of biomolecule entrapped inside hydrophilic or hydrophobic carrier matrix
(3) Surface reaction with small or large substrate with adhered biomolecule on hydrophilic or hydrophobic carrier surface in aqueous or in organic solvent medium

Among them, the surface reactions by physically adhered biomolecules are the characteristic uses of the method different from those of hitherto known physically entrapping immobilization. According to the present method, biocomponent, both of molecular level and of cell level can be immobilized physically on carrier surface. The reason is attributed to the fact that in this method, phase separation occurs at low temperature between the supercooled monomer phase and the frozen aqueous phase and then the biocomponent is concentrated on the surface of monomer phase or inter facial region of the two phases to be dispersed and fixed by polymerization. Furthermore, phase separation between monomer and buffer is already done in the starting mixture in the case of hydrophobic monomer carrier. Sometimes, biocomponent is dispersed on monomer surface directly with little use of buffer solution and immobilized by polymerization. It can be said that the use of less hydrophilic or rather hydrophobic monomer makes it possible to immobilize the biocomponent on carrier surface physically. In other words, it is not necessary to start for immobilization from a homogenous aqueous mixture of monomer, buffer, and enzyme to form a homogeneous hydrophilic gel entrapping enzyme.

The surface immobilization of biocomponent has been proved by the following facts:

(1) Michaelis-Mentein value (Km) for the enzymatic reaction with the immobilized biocomponent is very close to that in the reaction with native biocomponent.
(2) Predominant surface distribution of biomolecule is observed by fluorescence caused by the fluorescence agent connected to the biomolecule.

(3) Surface concentration of cell and organism is observed in microscopic observation.
(4) Bioreactions with high molecular weight or solid substances occur effectively with the immobilized biocomponents.
(5) Bioreactions occur effectively in aqueous medium with the hydrophobic biocomposite.
(6) Cell growth proceeds in the immobilized composite.

Surface reactions are advantageous in their large reaction rates due to the reduced diffusion resistance of carrier for substrate and in their applicabilities for large substrates such as solid or high polymer in aqueous or organic medium. As surface reaction is directly affected by the surface area of carrier, carrier forms of large surface areas such as microsphere, porous gel and membrane are desirable. Immobilization in a thin layer or skin on a base material by coating technique is important for this purpose. It is also advantageous from the view point of utilization of useful base material in shapes and properties such as mechanical strength, flexibility, durability, transmissible or separative function, bioaffinity, optical quality, and economic availability. The authors investigated the immobilization of some enzymes on surfaces of plastic film and tube by coating [39]. As the base materials, films and tubes of polyethylene and of polyvinyl chloride were chosen, because they were used most generally in the field of medical inspection and cure. Film of 100 microns thick and tube of 3 mm inner diameter, were used for experiment. As the medically useful enzymes, glucose oxidase and peroxidase for blood sugar inspection, and phospholipse and cholesterol oxidase for blood component analysis were tried for immobilization. The fundamental method consists of coating of the monomer-enzyme mixture in buffer on a plastic surface, cooling to low temperatures and polymerizing it by irradiation. However, it was difficult to form a membrane well adhered to the relatively inert and non-polar base material such as polyethylene and polyvinyl chloride. If the adhesiveness between the two phases, base polymer and carrier polymer including biocomponent is poor, the coated membrane cracks and releases easily in the repeated uses. The authors solved this problem by trying two means. One is the double coating method. That is, first an undercoating with a suitable polymeric composition is done directly on the base plastic to form a membrane having sufficient adhesiveness to both base polymer and carrier polymer. Then, the main coating is done on the undercoat and cured by irradiation to form the film carrier membrane including biocomponent. Cellulosic derivatives and certain kinds of alkylsilane compound is the example of polymers for undercoating. Another mean is the improvement of base surface by grafting. For example, polyethylene and polyvinyl chloride have sufficient adhesiveness with other vinyl polymers by grafting polymethacrylate or polyacrylate such as methyl methacrylate with radiation. Then, the firm coating including biocomponent becomes possible on the grafted base polymers. The techniques for grafting using radiation have been studied extensively by numerous workers and the coating technique was studied by the author previously for the purpose of surface improvement of optical plastics [40,41].

These techniques are available also for surface immobilization. The coating method for film can be selective among several ones such as dipping, painting, and spraying. But, coating for very narrow tube is difficult by those means and it can be carried out by injecting the monomer-biocomponent mixture inside the tube. The additionally found advantage of radiation method at low temperature was that the coated membrane of monomeric mixture hardly flows owing to the large viscosity of supercooled monomer at low temperature and so a regular and uniform membrane formed inside the tube. On the other hand, only an irregular membrane spread almost to choke the hollow space of tube was obtained by catalytic polymerization of coated membrane.

The similar effect was obtained also in the case of radiation polymerization of monomeric microsphere at low temperature, in which no irregular transformation or mutual aggregation of microspheres occurred owing to the high viscosity of supercooled monomer [42]. Figures 3 and 4 are the examples of the enzyme immobilization by these means and the uses for medical analysis. Figure 3 is the case of immobilized glucose oxidase and glucose peroxidase on inner wall of narrow plastic tube obtained by the double coating method, while Figure 4 is the result of same immobilized enzymes on plastic film obtained using the grafting method. According to these results, the coated films and tubes can be used in the repeated long uses for surface reactions with constant and stable activity. These materials can be connected and used continuously as a unit flow path for blood sample in a circular line system for blood analysis. The similar results were obtained also in other immobilized enzymes for medical analysis of other substances in blood.

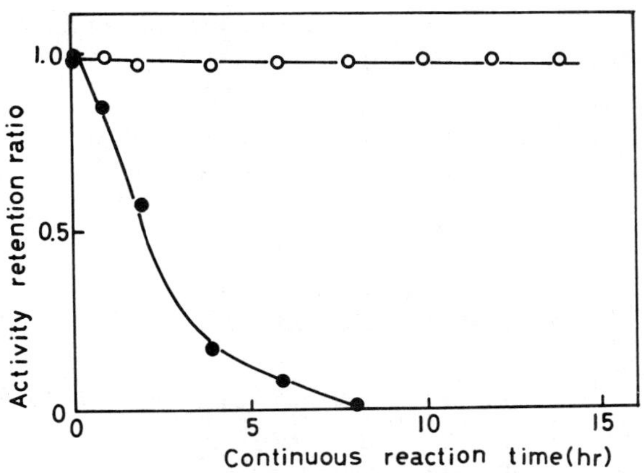

Figure 3. Activity retention with the continuous use of immobilized glucose oxidase membrane on the undercoated polyvinyl chloride tube for blood sugar analysis. (O) 2-hydroxyethyl methacrylate-tetraethyleneglycol dimethacrylate (1:1) polymer undercoated tube; (●) no undercoated tube. Monomer for immobilization: same as under coating composition; Irradiation: 5 × 10⁵r at −78°C; Enzyme reaction: 0.3ml/min flow of 1.0% glucose solution at 30°C.

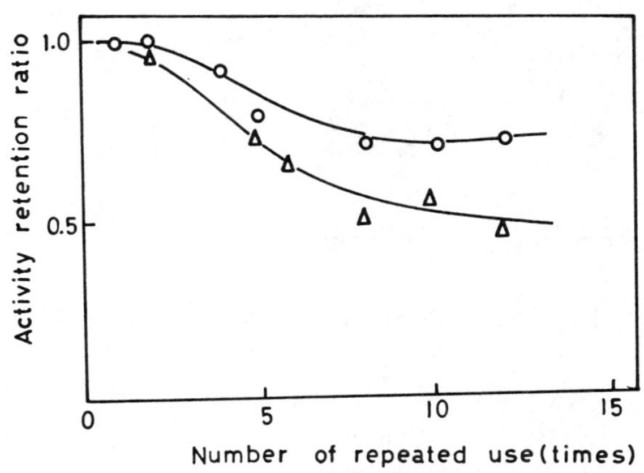

Figure 4. Activity retention with the repeated use of immobilized glucose oxidase membrane on the grafted polyethylene tube and film. (O) 30% methyl methacrylate grafted polyethylene tube (3mm diameter); (Δ) 30% methyl methacrylate grafted polyethylene film (0.5mm thickness). Monomer for immobilization: 2-hydroxyethyl methacrylatete-traethyleneglycol dimethacrylate-diethylaminoethyl methacrylate (2:2:1) 50% in buffer; Irradiation: 5 × 10⁵r at −78°C; Enzyme reaction: 30 min with 1% glucose oxidase at 30°C.

2. Fixation of Enzyme for Surface Modification of Medical Plastics

The same immobilization technique as used in the previous section was applied also to the enzymes for medical uses other than analysis. For example, urokinase was immobilized on the surface of polyethylene film in order to give thrombogenicity on the base material surface. The base film was grafted with methyl methacrylate by radiation-induced graft copolymerization and then the monomeric mixture including urokinase was coated and polymerized by irradiation. The product was tested for thrombogenecity test by immersing and incubating it in the blood and measuring the increase of coagulated blood content with the elapse of incubation time. The result is shown in Figure 5. As shown here, the film with the immobilized urokinase has the considerable thrombogenecity on the surface. Therefore, it is possible to improve the thrombogenecity of plastic surface used as medical instrument such as injector, tube for blood transport and other instrument or system to contact with blood by this kind of coating immobilization. The similar technique is available to other thrombogenetic substances such as heparin and also to other functional biomolecules such as asparaginae, uricase and urease in relation to the field of medical cure.

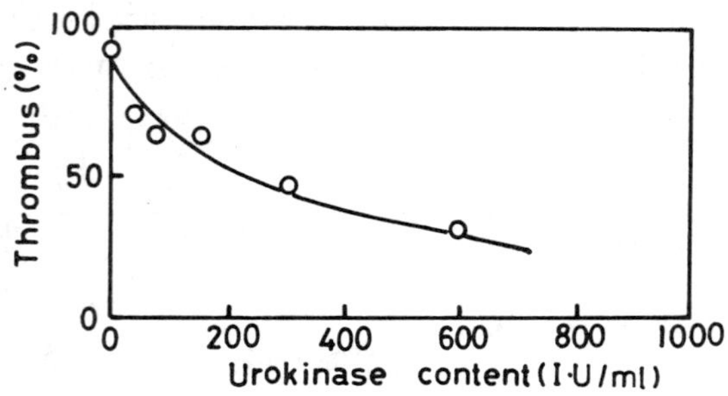

Figure 5. Relationship between the thrombus in immobilized urokinase membrane on grafted polyethylene film and the amount of urokinase added for immobilization. Monomer composition for immobilization: 50% 2-hydroxyethyl methacrylate-tetraethyleneglycol dimethacrylate-diethylaminoethyl methacrylate (2:2:1) in buffer solution. Base material: methyl methacrylate grafted polyethylene film. Polymerization: 5×10^5 at $-78°C$.

Application to Immunological Uses

1. Fixation of Antibody Molecules on Polymer Surface for Immuno-Diagnosis

Recently, with the progress of immunological researches, immuno-assay for medical diagnosis is studying actively. This field seems promising in the future possibility to cover a large scope of diseases including cancer, hereditary disease and other serious diseases. Radioimmuno assay is the most preceding technique in the immuno-diagnosis field. Enzyme immuno-assay has been studied in recent years. It is expected that more effective assay methods such as fluorescence and laser would be used in the near future. However, immobilization technique can be contributed to all immuno-assays, because the use of solid system is necessary to carry out the immuno-reaction and assay efficiently and conveniently. Immuno-reaction is the reaction of high molecular weight substance such as immuno-globulin and so it requires the surface reaction on the immobilized materials. The authors tried the application of radiation method to the immobilization of antibody, immunologbulin as the object of molecular level. The object for immobilization was anti-alpha pheto protein [12]. Two kinds of techniques were applied for the immobilization in membrane form. The one was the slicing method of radiation polymerized cylindrical block composite including antibody into thin porous membranes of 10-20 microns in thickness with a microtome. Another was the coating method on the small film connected with a plastic stick to handle by dropping a few drops of the monomer-antibody-buffer mixture with an injector and then polymerizing it with radiation. As the base film, paper or synthetic paper was used in this method. Then the products were used for immuno-reaction with a serum containing alpha pheto protein as antigen and assayed according to the conventional procedure for the enzyme immuno-assay, which consists of reaction with peroxidase labelled second antibody, enzyme reaction with the labelled peroxidase and this followed its colorimetrical assay. The optical density obtained from the enzymatic assay using the immobilized antibody increased with the concentration of antigen in the serum showing a well respondent relation. The results in the slicing and coating method membranes were shown in Figure 6. It was found that these membranes caught alpha pheto protein in the serum quantitatively in the order of ng/ml in concentration. The results were compared with those in radio-immunoassay for more than 900 serum samples of the patients. The correlation coefficient between the two methods was 0.98. The fact proved that surface reaction occurred effectively between the antigen and the immobilized immuno globulin. This might be the first case in which enzyme immuno assay was carried out effectively with the physically immobilized antibody in the thin membrane forms. The sensitivity of the material was comparable or rather superior to that of material obtained by chemical binding immobilization. One of the large merits of this physical method is its simplicity in the preparation process of the material. Slicing or coating can be done easily for mass production. Another advantage of this method is the convenience in reaction and assay operations such as washing to remove the unreacted second antibody.

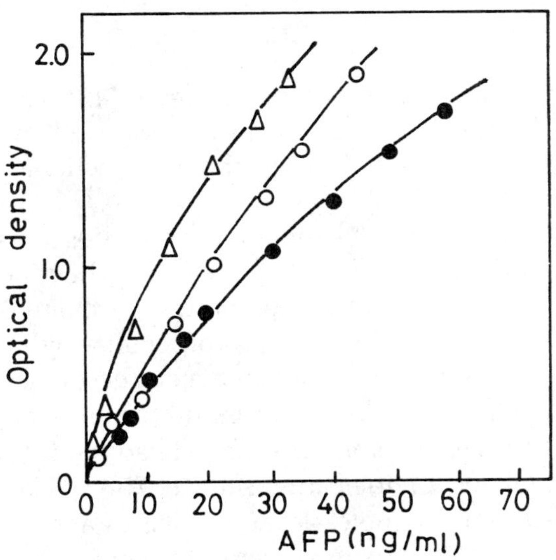

Figure 6. Relation between optical density and AFP content in enzyme immunoassay by the immobilized anti-AFP. (O) thin porous membrane of 2-hydroxyethyl methacrylate polymer sliced by microtome; (●) microsphere of neopentylglycol dimethacrylate polymer obtained by suspension polymerization; (Δ) thin membrane of 2-hydroxyethyl methacrylate polymer coated on a synthetic paper. Irrad.: 1×10⁶r at −78°C.

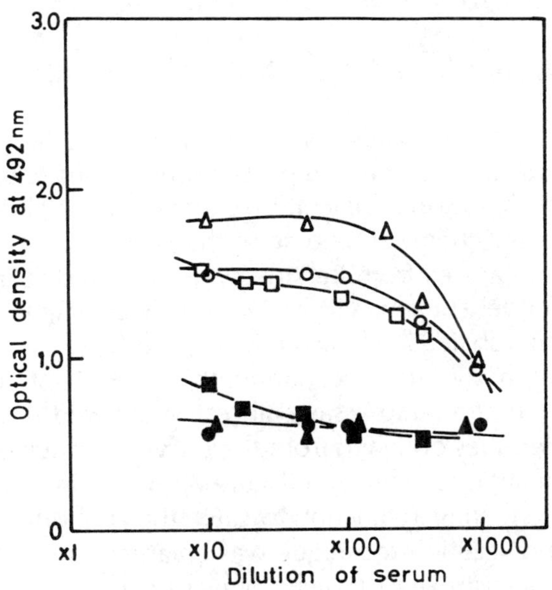

Figure 7. Enzyme immunoassay with the immobilized cells as antigens. (O) immobilized Raji cell; (Δ)immobilized Fujimaki cell; (□) immobilized Plasmodium berghei (antigen for mouse maralia); (●) intact Raji cell; (▲) intact Fujimaki cell; (■) intact Plasmodium berghei. Carrier: 2-hydroxyethyl methacrylate polymer sliced thin porous polymer; Irradiation: 1×10⁶r at −78°C; Immuno reaction: for 1 hr at 37°C.

Activity yield (generally expressed as a ratio of activity of the immobilized biocomponent to that of the originally used free biocomponent) of the immobilized antibody was not so high as that of the immobilized enzyme for the small substrate. This is due to the reaction with large substance such as antigen. However, in this case, the sensitivity for antigen in the assay is very high and the activity yield is enough to evaluate the specific adsorption of antigen for practical use. The activity yield can be variable controlling the hydrophilicity and hydrophobicity of the carrier by copolymerization. A maximum activity yield was attained at an optimum composition of hydrophilic monomer (for example, 2-hydroxyethyl methacrylate) and hydrophobic monomer (for example, polyethylene glycol #200 dimethacrylate). This result might be attributed to the maximum quantity of the bared and exposed antigen on the carrier in the optimum hydrophilicity or hydrophobicity, because the exposure degree of biocomponent on the carrier surface is the most important factors to affect the reactivity with the large substances such as antigen. The similar result concerning the optimum hydrophilicity was found also in the immobilized enzymes for hydrolysis of large substrates such as starch, cellulose, and protein. Conclusively, it is possible to apply the physical immobilization to molecular level antibody and carry out the immuno-reaction and the enzyme immuno assay effectively on the carrier surface.

2. Fixation of Antigen Cells on Polymer Surface for Immuno-Diagnosis

The authors applied the immobilization to the biocomponents of cell level [43]. Few research has been reported on the use of immobilized cell as antigen. Furthermore, cell immobilizaton is difficult by chemical immobilization owing to unstableness and less functionality for chemical binding of the cell.

Raji cell from Berkitte Lynphoma and Fujimaki cell from B cell lymphoma were chosen as model antigen cells and immobilized according to the slicing and coating methods. Then the immobilized cells were incubated in contact with the serum containing immuno-globulin as antibody. After incubation, the reacted antibody was analyzed by the usual procedure of enzyme immuno assay. All results showed the well respondent relations between the optical densities obtained from the enzyme immuno-assay of the immobilized cells and the amounts of antibody in serum (Figure 7). According to these results, the immobilized cell had the sufficient antigen function to catch the antibody, quantitatively on the carrier surface. The cell immobilization technique was enlarged to various cells. For example, as the models of antigen organism yeast (Saccharomyces cerevisiae) and E. Coli NIJ were investigated for immobilization. Those immobilized microorganism also showed the good correlationship between the result of enzyme immuno assay and the amount of antibody. It was also ascertained that the immobilized microorganisms reacted with their antibody with specific selectivity and had no cross-reactivity with other microorganism species. These can be utilizable not only for antibody assay but also for a quantitative count of cell numbers by the competitive immunoreaction between the immobilized cell and the free cell in serum.

Other investigations were made on the more practically useful objects. For example, Melozoit, Plasmodium malariae was immobilzed by the same method. The immobilized melozoit, showed the sufficient activity for the immuno-reaction with the anti-Plasmodium malariae and quantitative assay was possible. It was proved that the physical immobilization method by radiation polymerization is applicable to both of antigen and antibody for immobilizations and to both of organism or cell level and of molecular level. The immobilization technique will be available for the following purposes in the future.

(1) Immuno-diagnosis with immobilized antigen and antibody
(2) Immuno-therapy by means such as blood cleaning with the immobilized antigen and antibody, and controlled release of immuno-therapeutic substances
(3) Immunological prevention by means such as immunological recognition and prevention system to release antibody with the immobilized cell system
(4) Diagnosis cure and prevention system utilizing the selective adsorption of the immobilized antigen and antibody as a delivery guide

The progressive studies on the three regions are expected for those purposes:

(1) Progress in the finding of immunological relation between the diseases and the immunological mechanisms
(2) Progress in the production and treatment of antigen and antibody to improve the stableness, purity, and reactivity
(3) Progress in the immobilization and assay techniques to improve the reactivity, selectivity, and sensitivity

Application to Controlled Release of Drug

1. General Aspect of Immobilization Technique for Controlled Release

Controlled slow release is characteristic and successful uses of the physical immobilization. The authors studied the immobilization technique of biocomponent for the controlled release based on the same fundamental method as for the fixation [44]. The main differences between the two techniques for fixation and for release are as follows:

(1) Release requires inner distribution of biocomponent inside carrier matrix by entrapping, while fixation needs surface distribution on carrier by adhesion
(2) Release mainly concerns to molecular level biocomponent preferably of relatively low molecular weight except the case of the increased growth stage in cell culture
(3) Hydrophobic carrier system including no solvent such as buffer solution is used in general except for the release of high molecular weight compound fitted to hydrophilic system

However, it is obvious that the two immobilizations are the continuous technique and fixation and release are the continuous functions controllable by the firmness and tightness of immobilization. The degree of such firmness and tightness depends on the various factors listed in Table 2. As shown here, fixation and release functions can be controlled by desigining of the factors concerning carrier and immobilization condition according to the factors in drug and its usage condition. The immobilization technique for release can be divided into the two types: (1) general technique and (2) specific technique. The general technique, consists of three fundamental means:

(1) Design of hydrophilicity and crosslinking density of carrier polymer, to control the diffusion of drug through matrix

Table 2. Effect of Various Factors on Fixation and Release in Physical Immobilization

Factor		Effect on fixation	Effect on release
1. Factors relating to carrier			
(1) Hydrophilicity →	Increase	Loosen	Accelerate
(2) Crosslinking density →	Increase	Strengthen	Retard
(3) Affinity with drug →	Increase	Strengthen	Retard
(4) Biodegradativity →	Increase	Loosen	Accelerate
(5) Surface area →	Increase	Loosen	Accelerate
(6) Diffusion barrier (filler, multilayer etc) for drug →	Increase	Strengthen	Retard
(7) Diffusion promotor for drug (pore-making agent, swelling agent etc) →	Increase	Strengthen	Retard
2. Factors relating to biocomponent			
(1) Size, molecular weight →	Increase	Strengthen	Retard
(2) Solubility into medium →	Increase	Loosen	Accelerate
(3) Diffusivity in carrier →	Increase	Loosen	Accelerate
(4) Concentration in carrier →	Increase	Loosen	Accelerate
(5) Affinity with carrier →	Increase	Strengthen	Retard
3. Factors relating to use condition			
(1) Affinity of reaction medium with biocomponent →	Increase	Loosen	Accelerate
(2) Temperature →	Increase	Loosen	Accelerate
(3) Pressure →	Increase	Strengthen	Retard
(4) Speed of stirring and shaking →	Increase	Loosen	Accelerate

(2) Design of porous carrier structure to increase the inner surface area for drug dissolution
(3) Design of filler-filled structure or masked (coating) structure of carrier to increase the barrier or resistance for drug diffusion

Most of usual requirements for drug release can be satisfied by the application of the general technique to the real systems, according to the required drug to be immobilized, shape to be given and functions such as rate and period.

For example, release of water soluble and relatively low molecular weight drugs is controllable to any initial, stational, and final rates and durable period by the design of hydrophilicity (hydrophobicity) and crosslinking density of carrier. However, for the release of the following cases, designs of porous carrier become necessary: (1) release of high molecular weight substance and (2) release of substrate insoluble or poorly soluble in water. On the contrary, for the release of the following cases, filler-filled (or masked) structure of carrier is effective: (1) long period release of very low molecular weight drug and (2) long period release in the shape of the large surface area ratio to volume such as in microsphere and needle capsules. Some examples are shown in Figures 8, 9, 10, and 11.

Furthermore, the specific technique was developed to fill the following requirements:

(1) Release of a drug in the multiple stages to give the apparent overall linearity to the time-release curve (to give apparent constant release rate)
(2) Release of multi-component drugs from the same carrier with different induction periods to the beginning of release
(3) Release of multi-component drugs of different molecular weight at the same time in the same rate from the carrier
(4) Release with cycles in repetition of the interval pause and the interval release

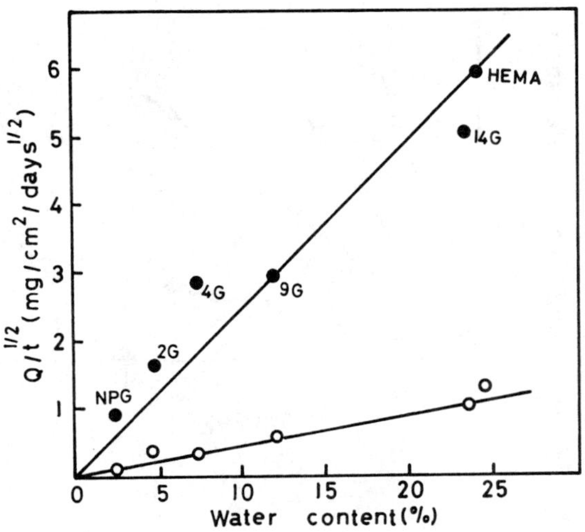

Figure 8. Effect of water content of vinyl polymer on the magnitude of biological active substance release from the capsules; biological substance-30mg, monomer-0.2ml, irradiation-1Mrad at −78°C in vacuo, capsule size-5mm in diameter flat circular type, dissolution test-borate buffer (pH 8.5) for uricase and saline for BLM at 37°C. (●) BLM (Mw is 1500-600), (O) Uricase (Mw is 1.2×10^5).

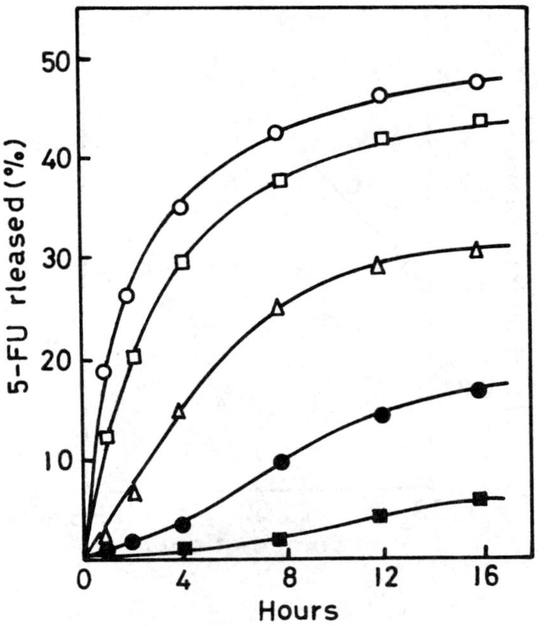

Figure 9. Drug release from 2-hydroxyethyl methacrylate polymer matrix containing 5-FU as a function of activated charcoal concentration in 2-hydroxyethyl methacrylate-drug-absorbent system. Activated charcoal concentration: (O) 0mg, (□) 10mg, (Δ) 50mg, (●) 100 mg; (■) 300mg.

(5) Release with on-off regulation mechanism

(6) Release with highly selective delivery and adsorption to the aimed organ

For the purposes from (1) to (4), multi-layers or multi-phases structure of composite consisting of various polymer-drug compositions from zero to 100% of each component was designed and tested. This kind of structure was proved to be effective for the purposes. Various practical requirements for release function can be satisfied by suitable combination of these general and specific techniques. Some examples are given in Figures 12, 13 and 14. Techniques for purposes mentioned (4), (5) and (6) are now under trial stage for the possibility and would be the important problems to be solved in the future.

Shape design of polymer-drug composite is another important technical problem for the release. It is especially important for the in vivo uses such as local and delivery chemotherapies. As already described, shaping is very free and easy in the low temperature radiation polymerization as well as multi-structure making and monomer-drug mixture can be shaped into various sizes and forms according to the requirement as shown in the typical examples of Figure 15. The design of the material polymer for carrier also has the large freedom of selection as described before. Some important factors such as hydrophilicity, (or hydropho-

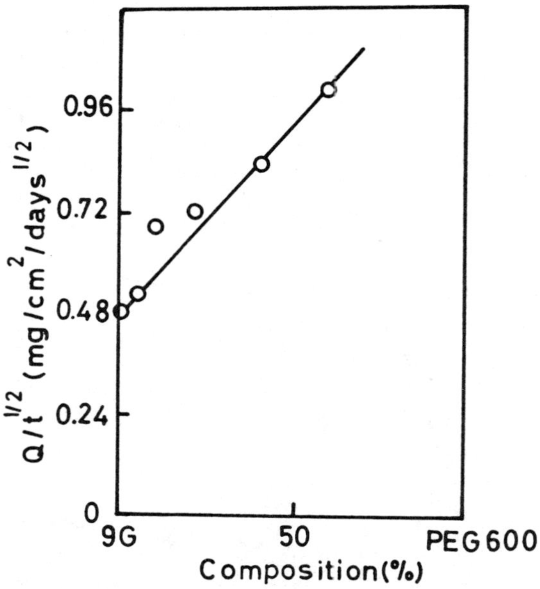

Figure 10. Effect of 9G-PEG 600 composition (porosity) on the magnitude of urokinase release from porous 9G polymer capsule; urokinase-30mg, 9G-PEG mixture-0.2ml, irradiation-1 Mrad at −78°C in vacuo, capsule size-5mm in diameter flat circular type, dissolution test-borate buffer (pH 8.5) at 37°C.

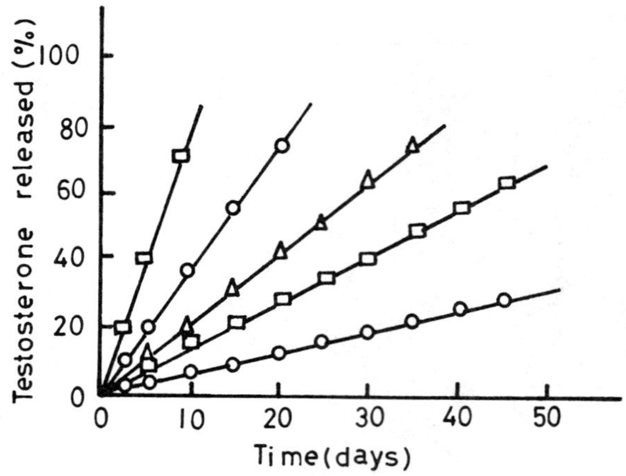

Figure 11. Release profile of hormone from tube-type capsule containing 5 mg of testosterone. Release rate: (■) 400 μg/day, (●) 190, (Δ) 110, (□) 70, (O) 25.

bicity), elasticity (or plasticity), and mechanical strength have already been proven for testing and satisfied the practical requirements to some degrees. But, some in vivo properties such as biocompatibility and biodegradativity should be proven further in the future. Vinyl polymers used in vivo implantation and local chemotherapy in the present showed no serious troubles such as inflammation and necrosis against the tissues surrounding. Thrombogenecity would be given in microspheres used for delivery type chemotherapy through blood circulation. Biodegradativity is the important problem, too. At present, use of carrier having large biodegradativity showed the general tendency to be inconsistent with long durability of release. Moreover, the hitherto known biodegradative materials are limited to a narrow scope of natural polymers. The authors found that thermally treated proteins such as denaturalized albumin gave the relatively long release period for a month as well as the good biodegradativity. The blend composite of vinyl polymer-denaturalized protein including drug was obtained by the polymerization of vinyl monomer-albumin mixture and the thermal treatment [45]. This composite showed the intermediate release period and enzyme digestivity according to the additional law of monomer-protein composition. The authors are trying to find the synthetic carrier materials such as polypeptide to fill the biodegradativity and long release consistently as well as desirable biocompatibility, shapability, and mechanical properties. It is expected that solution of these problems would be accelerated with the advance in the study of biomedical polymer for artificial organ and its intercourse with the study of biocomposite

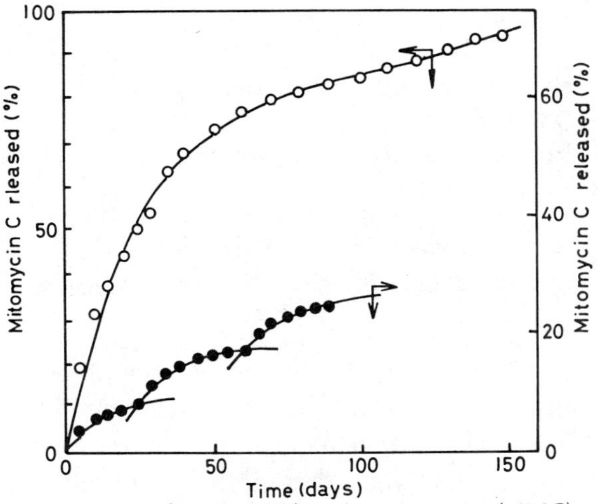

Figure 12. Release profile of mitomycin (MMC) from radiation polymerized capsules. (○) 200mg MMC was included in 20% polymethyl methacrylate (PMMA)-80% diethyleneglycol dimethacrylate (DGDA) polymer by irradiation 1×10⁶r at −78°C. (●) 20mg of MMC was included in 0.3g trimethylolpropane trimethacrylate (TMPT) polymer by irradiation. This was included again in 0.4g 10% PMMA-90% DGDA polymer by irradiation. Inclusions were repeated furthermore to obtain the final product.

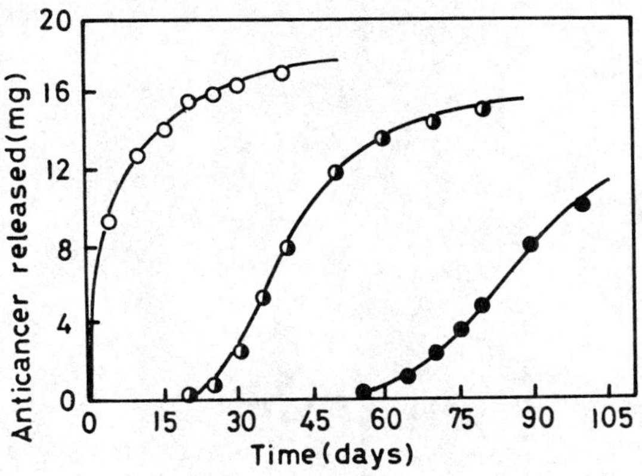

Figure 13. Release profiles of anticancers from single radiation polyemrized capsule containing various anticancers such as 20mg of MMC, 20mg of 5-FU and 20mg of ADM.

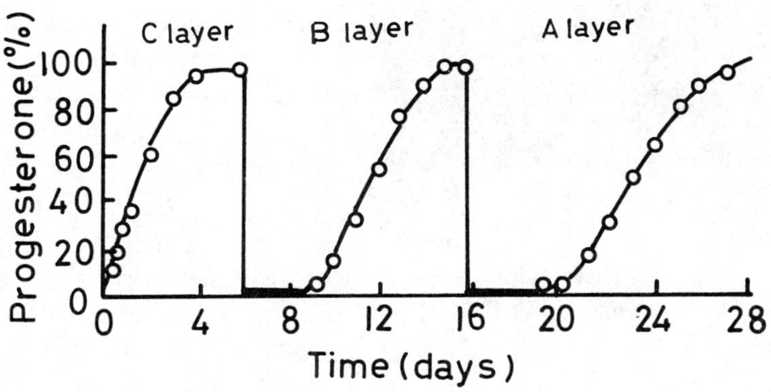

Figure 14. Cycle release profile of progesterone from a flat circular capsule consisting of multi-layer.

for in vivo release and chemotherapy. The use of these polymer-drug composites can be divided as follows:

(1) Local chemotherapy by direct implantation, injection or attachment to the aimed organ
(2) Drug delivery system through blood circulation by direct dosage to blood with chemotherapy in blood or in terminal blood vessel
(3) Local or general chemotherapy with drug delivery system through blood circulation

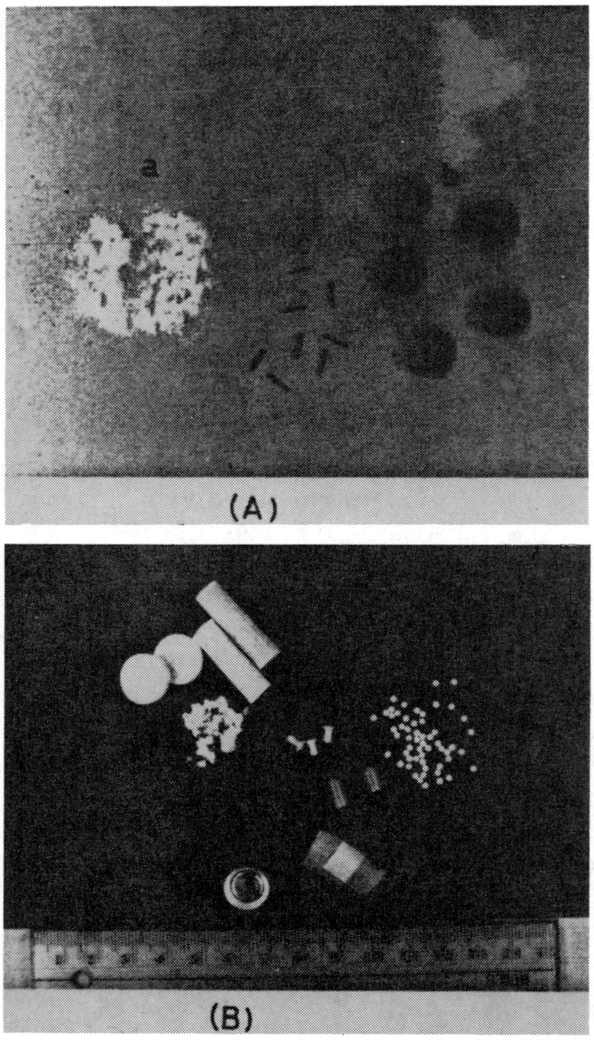

Figure 15. Photographs of various shaped polymer-anticancer capsules. (A) Capsules including MMC: (a) microsphere, (b) buttan, (c) needle. (B) Capsules including various anticancers.

by indirect dosage to the remote part other than the aimed one.

Some practical examples for these uses will be shown in the next sections.

2. Immobilization and Release of Anticancers for Local Chemotherapy

The first application of technique was done to the local chemotherapy with the immobilized anticancers. The reason for this application was that the prevention of secondary reaction and the efficient damage effect on cancer were expected by the direct local dosage and the gradual release of anticancer. Various anticancers such as mitomycin C, 5-fluorouracil, bleomycin hydrochloride, and adriamycin were tested for immobilization. Mitomycin C (MMC) was mainly investigated for animal and clinical experiments [46,47]. For example, the button-shape capsule containing 20 mg MMC was implanted in the cancered part of animal (Ehrlich ascites carioma, 5×10^{6}/0.2 ml, was innoculated into the abdomial cavity of females ICR mice). It was found that the MMC capsule of hydrophobic polydiethylene glycol dimethacrylate carrier was most effective to retard the tumor growth and the capsule implanted group showed the survivor ratio of about four times than that of control group including no capsule shown in Figure 16. In another experiment, the button capsule containing MMC was implanted to the sarcoms 180 tumored mouse. The effect in capsule group was compared to that of injection group injected with MMC. Both of the two groups showed the retardation effect for tumor growth. But, the result of blood component analysis proved no abnormal change in the capsule group mouse, while the serious decrease of the number of leucocytes to about one half of the normal value was observed in the injection group mouse. The animal test by beagle dog also proved the similar effect. According to the analysis on the distribution of MMC concentration in the surrounding tissue, diffusion out of MMC was limited within the very narrow range of about one cm around the capsule. Therefore, the action of the capsule is very local.

Based on the results of animal experiments, anticancer capsule was applied to clinical test

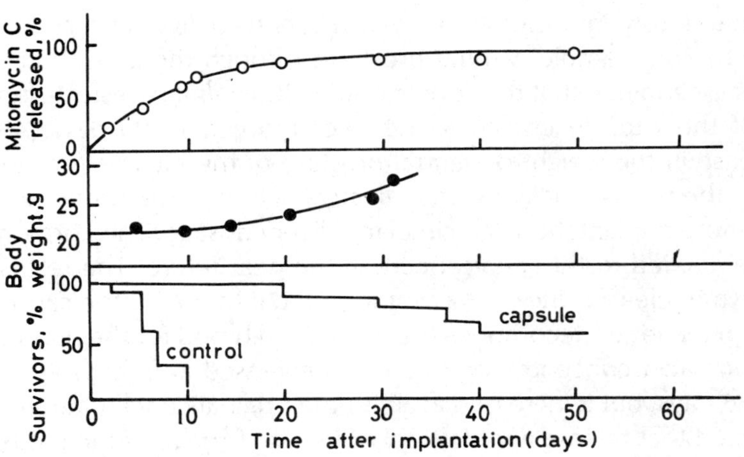

Figure 16. Relation between the in vitro release of MMC, the weight increase of ascites tumor mouse implanted MMC capsules and the survivor ratio with the time.

in the region of digestive system surgery and urology. Three kinds of shaped hydrophobic capsule button of 14 mm diameter and 4 mm thick, needle of 0.8 mm diameter and 7 mm long, and microsphere of 70-120 microns diameter were used. Four capsules of button containing 20 mg MMC in each capsule were sewed on the cancered part with yarn through the two holes of capsule center. Needles containing 5 mg MMC in each capsule were injected to the cancered part by injector and microspheres containing 20 mg MMC in total were inserted by cathertel without laparotomy operation, respectively. More than 110 patients such as gastric cancer, carcinoma of the esophagus, cancer of the gall bladder, cancer of colon, ovarian cancer, renal cancer, and testicular tumor have been applied to this local chemotherapy. The most remarkable effect was that of disappearance or improvement of pain due to the serious stage of cancer, though it appeared again after several months in some cases. Some of the patients recovered and returned to social life. No abnormal changes were observed with the elapse of time in the inspection values of blood pictures and blood contents. No other general appearances to show on suggest the secondary reaction were recognized too. The observed MMC concentration in blood was of very low level in the order of 5×10^{-3} μg/ml. These results proved the local action and distribution of MMC from the capsule. The effect on the long time range recovery and the complete cure can not be conclusive at the present stage. However, the plan has started this year to carry out the cinical applications more than 400 examples for the following two years by the project team consisting of Universities and Institutes in Japan to evaluate the clinical effect and merit in the region of digestive system surgery, urology, and other fields.

3. Immobilization and Release of Hormone and Enzyme

Hormone is also suitable for the controlled release by the reason that it essentially needs the release and action of long time, constant in very small concentration and furthermore often in cyclic style at intervals. These characeristics of hormone probably fit to the advantage of the capsule. Steroid hormones such as testosterone, progesterone, AA 560, and DHT were chosen as models. In the animal experiments, the hormone containing tablet capsules was implanted subcutaneously in the castrated wistar rats to deliver and make the action of released hormone to, for example, ventral prostrate through the general circulation of blood (Figure 17). It was ascertained that the concentration 300 ng/ml of testosterone was constantly kept in blood of the capsule implanted rat over more than 90 days [48]. Moreover the remarkable increase in the weight of ventral prostate of the rat was recognized. These facts proved obviously the release, delivery and effective action of the hormone from the capsule by this kind of remote implantation and circular delivery dosage. The hormone capsule and its technique will be applied to the medical cure in the near future. The release technique was used also for enzyme release. Uricase was immobilized into the button capsule and implanted intraperitoneally in the rat to decompose the uric acid in blood for the purpose of gout cure. It was found that uric acid concentration in blood decreased after capsule implantation soon with the time for 3 days, but it increased again to the original concentration level after 4 days. This result suggested that release and delivery of uricase from abdomen to blood occurred at first, and then the release or delivery was stopped by any reason such as the entrapping of capsule by the newly formed tissue cells around the capsule or the inactivation of the released uricase by protease or antibody. This problem might be the specific one to the remote circular type release of protein, polypeptide or high molecular weight substances from the implanted capsule and to be solved in the near future.

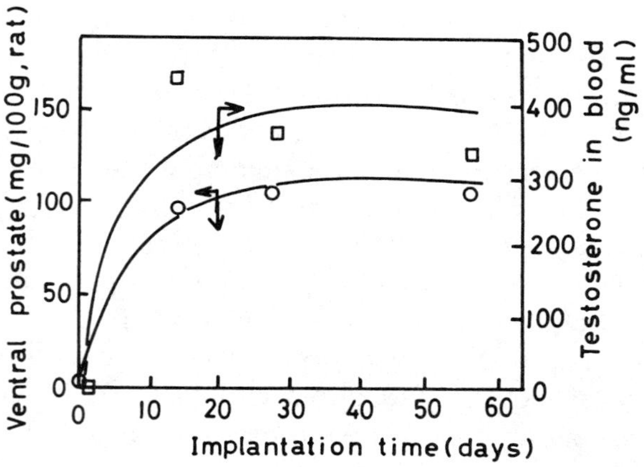

Figure 17. Relationship between the weight of ventral prostate per 100 of rat and the testosterone in blood as a function of implantation time using the castrated wistar rat (2 weeks); testosterone-50mg, 10% Pst-90% 2G mixture-0.2ml, Irradiation-1 Mrad at −78°C in vacuo, capsule size-8mm in diameter flat circular type.

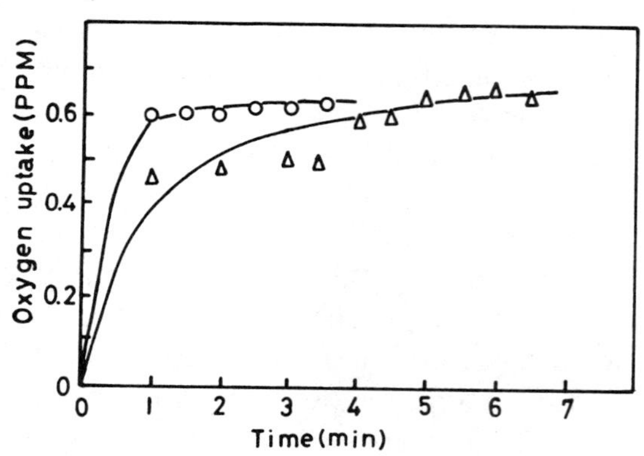

Figure 18. Oxygen uptake of hemoglobin in intact and immobilized erythrocytes. (O) intact erythrocyte, (Δ) immobilized erythrocyte. Monomer composition; M-23G 5%-14G 4.5%-GA 0.5%, Irradiation, 1×10⁵r at 4°C.

Application to Cell Technology

1. Fixation of Cells for Biological Reactions

Immobilization of tissue cell and microorganism such as microbial cell and organella can be carried out advantageously by the present method, because of the physical and mild immobilization. It was found that tissue cells are immobilized stably in whole cell state on the carrier by choosing the suitable conditions such as very small irradiation dose less than 10^5 rad and very low monomer concentration less than 10%.

At the first study, chloroplast from spinach was immobilized and used for the oxygen forming reaction of Hill reaction in the PS II process of photo-synthesis [49]. The immobilized chloroplast with carriers such as methoxypolyethylene glycol methacrylate and polyethylene glycol dimethacrylate polymers retained the oxygen formation activity of 30-50 percent of the original one after the storage (4°C) longer than 40 days, while the activity of intact cell was lost completely within one day. This was the example in which the stability of the tissue cell increased remarkably by the immobilization. The reason was not clear, but a certain kind of protective effect might be obtained by covering the naked cell with polymer matrix. However, the durabilty for the repeated uses for reactions is not sufficient yet. Then erythrocyte was immobilized stably with the same carriers in whole cell state without hemolysis. The immobilized erythrocyte was stabler for hemolysis than the intact one. The reversible adsorption and desorption of oxygen was observed in the immobilized erythrocyte with a little time delay to that in the intact erythrocyte as shown in Figure 18. Catalase actvity was also observed in the immobilized erythrocyte. These results showed that the immobilized tissue cells can be used for various biological reactions as bioreactor and artificial organ. The stability of the tissue cell increased remarkably in the immobilized enzyme, but its durability for long use should be improved further for the practical use. As shown in Figure 19, the immobilized cells was covered with carrier polymer in various degree of thickness. The technique for the control of optimum carrier thickness and optimum exposure of the immobilized cell will be studied in the future in relation to its reactivity and stability.

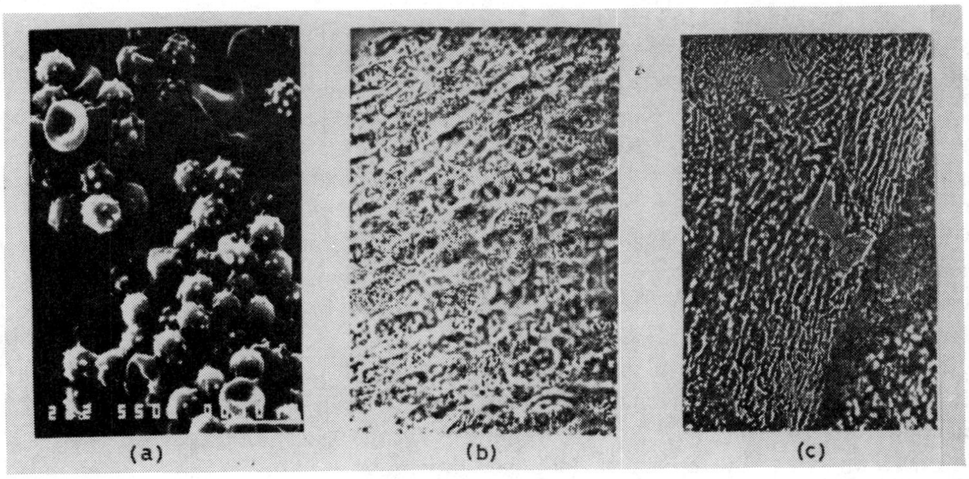

Figure 19. Photographs of immobilized cells. (a) erythrocyte, (b) liver, (c) yeast.

2. Fixation of Cells for Culture and Product Release

Some microorganisms such as enzyme productive cell and yeast were immobilized and cultured in the carrier matrix. For the optimum culture of immobilized microorganism it was necessary to minimize the irradiation dose and the monomer concentration as well as in the case of tissue cell immobilization. Moreover, certain suitable porous structure is also necessary for the effective culture. For example, Trichoderma reesei, a cellulase productive microbial cell was immobilized with various carriers such as polyethylene glycol dimethacrylate and 2-hydroxyethyl methacrylate polymers. The porous stucture was given by the addition of pore-making agent such as crystalline compounds or of bonded materials such as gauze and filter. The immobilized Trichoderma cell carried out growth in the carrier and showed considerable cellulase activity due to the released cellulase [50].

Yeasts could be multiplied effectively in the carrier consisting of methoxy polyethylene glycol methacrylate polymer and gauze. Study on the optimum property, density and porosity of carrier polymer for the culture and productive function of various microorganisms will be one of the most interesting future problems. For the purpose of tissue cell culture, the adsorption or attachment of cell on the carrier surface is essentially necessary. In this case, three dimensional space is not necessary, but two dimensional plane space is needed for the adsorption and growth of cell. For examples, C_6 cell and glial cell were cultured on various carrier membranes. Some carriers showed the accelerating effect on tissue cell growth more than the commercially available material such as falcon. The optimum property and the microsurface structure of carrier will be the future problem. The immobilization technique for the repeated and continuous use, stabilization, culture and productive release will be able to apply in the future to the new species obtained by the biotechnology such as mutation, genetic engineering and cell fusion. It is one of our purposes to clarify and find the positive effect of polymeric material and polymer modification on the cell technology.

REFERENCES

1. Kao, K. N. and Michayluk, M. R., "A method for high-frequency intergeneric fusion of plant protoplasts," Planta, *115,* 355-367 (1974).
2. Rajaraman, R., Rounds, D. E., Yen, S. P. S. and Rembaum, A., "A scanning electron microscope study of cell adhesion and spreading in vitro," Experimental Cell Research, *88,* 327-339 (1974).
3. Strandberg, G. W. and Smiley, K. L., "Free and immobilized glucose isomerase from Streptomyces phaeochromogenes," Appl. Microbio., *21,* 588-593 (1971).
4. Langer, R. and Forkman, J., "Polymers for the sustained release of proteins and other macromolecules," Nature, *263,* 797-800 (1976).
5. Gearhart, J. P., Witherington, R. and Coleman, C. H., "Subcutaneous estradiol pellet implantation in management of advanced prostatic carcinoma," Urology, *17,* 44-48 (1981).
6. Kaetsu, I., Kumakura, M., Yamada, A. and Sakurai, Y., "Immobilization of enzymes for medical use by radiation polymerization at low temperature," Artificial Organs (Japan) *8,* 226-228 (1979).
7. Kaetsu, I., Kumakura, M., Yoshida, M., Asano, M., Himei, M., Tamura, M. and Hayashi, K., "Immobilization of enzymes by radiation," Radiat. Phys. Chem., *14,* 595-602 (1979).
8. Kumakura, M., Yoshida, M., Asano, M. and Kaetsu, I., "Immobilization of Streptomyces phaerochromogenes by radiation induced polymerization of glass-forming monomers," Biotechnol. Bioeng., *21,* 679-688 (1977).
9. Kaetsu, I., Yoshida, M. and Yamada, A., "Controlled slow release of chemotherapeutic drugs for cancer from matrices prepared by radiation polymerization at low temperatures," J. Biomed. Mater. Res., *14,* 185-197 (1980).
10. Fujimura, T., Yoshii, F., Kaetsu, I., Inoue, Y. and Shibata, K., "Effect of irradiation and immobilization on spinach chloroplast activities," Z. Naturforsch., *35c,* 477-481 (1980).
11. Kaetsu, I. and Yoshii, F., "Immobilzation of cells by polymerizing adhesion method and effects of viscous solvents and monomers on it," Polymer Preprints, Japan, *29,* 1059-1062 (1980).

12. Kaetsu, I., Kumakura, M., Suzuki, M., Waki, S., Suzuki, M., Kikuchi, S., Seido, T. and Adachi, S., "Application of immobilized materials prepared by polymerizing adhesion method to the field of immunoassay," Polymer Preprints, Japan, *29,* 1067-1070 (1980).
13. Melrose, J. H., "Insolubilized enzymes; Biochemical applications of synthetic polymers," Rev. Pure and Appl. Chem., *21,* 83-119 (1971).
14. Linko, Y., Saarinen, P. and Linko, M., "Starch conversion by soluble and immobilized α-amylase," Biotechnol. Bioeng., *17,* 153-165 (1975).
15. Gregor, H. P. and Rauf, R. W., "Enzyme-coupled ultrafiltration membrane," Biotechnol. Bioeng., *17,* 445-449 (1975).
16. Deutsch, D. G. and Mertz, E. T., "Activation of plasminogen with insoluble derivatives of urokinase," J. Med., *3,* 224-230 (1972).
17. Kaetsu, I., Yoshii, F. and Watanabe, Y., "Radiation-induced polymerization of glass-forming monomers VII. Polymerization in supercooled state under high pressure," J. Polymer Sci.; Polymer Chem. Edn., *16,* 2645-2650 (1978).
18. Kaetsu, I., Ito, A. and Hayashi, K., "Radiation-induced solid-state polymerization in binary systems. IX. Polymerization and forming of multicompounds systems including inorganic acid and acrylic monomers," J. Appl. Polymer Sci., *17,* 2753-2759 (1973).
19. Kaetsu, I. and Watanabe, Y., "Temperature dependence of initial polymerization rate in radiation-induced polymerization of polyfunctional glass-forming monomers," Polymer Letters, *15,* 235-238 (1977).
20. Kaetsu, I. and Yoshida, M., "New coating materials and their preparation by radiation polymerization III. Antifogging coating composition," J. Appl. Polymer Sci., *24,* 235-247 (1979).
21. Okubo, H., Honda, S., Yoshii, F., Morita, Y. and Kaetsu, I., "Casting of organic glass by radiation-induced polymerization of glass-forming monomers at low temperatures VII. Casting polymerization of methyl methacrylate prepolymer by irradiation," J. Appl. Polymer Sci., *22,* 45-52 (1978).
22. Kumakura, M., Yoshida, M. and Kaetsu, I., "Immobilization of Streptomyces phaeochromogenes cells at a high concentration by radiation-induced polymerization of glass-forming monomers," European J. Appl. Microbiol. Biotechnol., *6,* 13-22 (1978).
23. Kumakura, M., Yoshida, M., Asano, M. and Kaetsu, I., "Immobilization of enzymes by radiation-induced polymerization of glass-forming monomers. Double entrapping of enzymes in the presence of various additives," J. Solid Phase Biochem., *2,* 279-288 (1977).
24. Kaetsu, I., Kumakura, M. and Yoshida, M., "Enzyme immobilization by radiation-induced polymerization of 2-hydroxyethyl methacrylate at low temperatures," Biotechnol. Bioeng., *21,* 847-861 (1979).
25. Kaetsu, I., Kumakura, M. and Yoshida, M., "Enzyme immobilization by radiation-induced polymerization of hydrophobic glass-forming monomers at low temperatures," Biotechnol. Bioeng., *21,* 863-873 (1979)
26. Yoshida, M., Kumakura, M. and Kaetsu, I., "Preparation and its drug release property of radiation polymerized poly(methyl methacrylate) capsules including potasium chloride," Kobunshi Ronbunshu, *36,* 35-40 (1979).
27. Yoshida, M., Kumakura, M. and Kaetsu, I., "Controlled drug dissolution by radiation-induced polymerization in the presence of dimethylaminoethyl methacrylate-methyl methacrylate copolymer or methacrylic acid-methyl acrylate copolymer," J. Pharm. Sci., *68,* 860-862 (1979).
28. Kumakura, M. and Kaetsu, I., "Radiation-induced degradation and subsequent hydrolysis of waste cellulose materials," Internat. J. Appl. Radiat. and Isotopes, *30,* 139-141 (1979).
29. Kaetsu, I., Kumakura, M., Fujimura, T., Kojima, T. and Tamada, M., "Hydrolysis of high molecular weight or solid substrates with the immobilized enzymes and microbial cells prepared by polymerizing adhesion method," Polymer Preprints, Japan, *29,* 1063-1066 (1980).
30. Yoshida, M., Kumakura, M. and Kaetsu, I., "Mechanism of immobilization of enzymes by radiation-induced polymerization of glass-forming monomers," J. Macromol. Sci.-Chem., *A14,* 541-544 (1980).

31. Kaetsu, I., Yoshida, M., Yamada, A., Sakurai, Y., Nakamura, K., Hanyu, F., Yasui, H., Takara, M. and Sakatoku, J., "Effect of shapes and structures of chemotherapeutic anticancers. Polymer composites on release functions," Artificial Organs (Japan), *9,* 1128-1131 (1980).
32. Yoshida, M., Kumakura, M. and Kaetsu, I., "Immobilization of cellulase in the swollen microsphere by radiation polymerization," Polymer J., *11,* 915-919 (1979).
33. Kumakura, M., Yoshida, M. and Kaetsu, I., "Immobilization of glucose isomerase containing Streptomyces phaeochromogenes cells fine-particle form," Appl. Environment. Microbiol., *37,* 310-315 (1979).
34. Yoshida, M., Kumakura, M. and Kaetsu, I., "Immobilization of enzymes by radiation-induced polymerization of glass-forming monomers. 1. Immobilization of some enzymes by poly(2-hydoxyethyl methacrylate)," Polymer, *20,* 3-8 (1979).
35. Yoshida, M., Kumakura, M. and Kaetsu, I., "Immobilization of enzymes by radiation-induced polymerization of glass-forming monomers. II. Effects of cooling rate and solvent on porosity and activity of immobilized enzymes," Polymer, *20,* 9-12 (1979).
36. Kaetsu, I., Kumakura, M., Yoshida, M., Yamada, A. and Sakurai, Y., "Study on anticancer capsules having slow release function. Capsulation technique by radiation," Artificial Organs (Japan), *8,* 797-799 (1979).
37. Kawashima, K. and Umeda, K., "Immobilization of enzymes by radiopolymerization of acrylamide," Biotechnol. Bioeng., *16,* 609-621 (1974).
38. Maeda, H., Suzuki, H. and Yamauchi, A., "Preparation of immobilized enzymes using poly(vinyl alcohol)," Biotechnol. Bioeng., *15,* 607-610 (1973).
39. Kaetsu, I., Kumakura, M., Asano, M., Yamada, A. and Sakurai, Y., "Immobilization of enzymes for medical uses on plastics surfaces by radiation-induced polymerization at low temperatures," J. Biomed. Mater. Res., *14,* 199-210 (1980).
40. Okubo, H., Kato, M., Yoshida, M., Ito, A. and Hayashi, K., "New coating materials prepared by radiation-induced polymerization. I. Mar-resistant coating composition and properties," J. Appl. Polymer Sci., *22,* 487-496 (1978).
41. Yoshida, M., Okubo, H. and Kaetsu, I., "New coating materials prepared by radiation-induced polymerization. II. Study on the polymerization mechanism of mar-resistant coating composition," J. Appl.Polymer Sci., *22,* 823-832 (1978).
42. Yoshida, M., Kumakura, M. and Kaetsu, I., "Drug entrapment for controlled release in radiation-polymerized beads," J. Pharm. Sci., *68,* 628-631 (1979).
43. Kaetsu, I., Kumakura, M., Kikuchi, S., Adachi, S. and Suzuki, M., "Immobilization of E. Coli as an antigen by radiation polymerization," Biomaterials, in press.
44. Yoshida, M., Kumakura, M. and Kaetsu, I., "Controlled release of biofunctional substances by radiation-induced polymerization. 1. Release of potassium chloride by polymerization of various vinyl monomers," Polymer, *19,* 1375-1378 (1978).
45. Yoshida, M., Asano, M., Kaetsu, I., Nakai, K., Yamanaka, H., Suzuki, T., Shida, K. and Suzuki, K., "Release of testosterone from protein-vinyl polymer composite matrices," Biomaterials, in press.
46. Nakamura, M., Takada, T., Takasaki, T., Kobayashi, S., Hanyu, F., Yamada, A., Sakurai, Y., Okawa, T., Kaetsu, I. and Yoshida, M., "Clinical study on controlled release capsule of mitocycin C for the treatment of inoperable pancreatic cancer," Gan to Kagakuryoho, *7,* 1824-1831 (1980).
47. Yamada, A., Machiyama, E., Kabei, N., Kikuchi, M., Sakurai, Y., Hanyu, F., Yoshida, M., Kumakura, M. and Kaetsu, I., "Study on controlled release from anticancer drug capsule made by radiation-induced polymerization at low temperature," J. Tokyo Wom. Med. Coll., *49,* 481-490 (1979).
48. Yoshida, M., Asano, M., Kaetsu, I., Nakai, K., Yamanaka, H., Suzuki, T., Shida, K. and Suzuki, K., "In vitro and in vivo release of testosterone from vinyl polymer matrices," Biomaterials, in press.
49. Kaetsu, I., Yoshii, F. and Fujimura, T., "Effect of viscous solvents and monomer on conversion of intact and immobilized chloroplasts," Z. Naturforsch., *35c,* 1052-1056 (1980).
50. Yoshii, F., Fujimura, T. and Kaetsu, I., "Stabilization of chloroplast by radiation-induced immobilization with various glass-forming monomers," Biotechnol. Bioeng., *23,* 833-841 (1981).

Chapter 24

Use of Polymers in Controlled Drug Release

J. Heller
Director, Polymer Sciences Department
SRI International
333 Ravenswood Avenue
Menlo Park, CA 94025

ABSTRACT

Three methodologies for the controlled release of therapeutic agents are described. These are diffusional, osmotic, and erosional. In diffusional devices a therapeutic agent is either dispersed in a polymer matrix or is placed in a core that is surrounded by a polymer membrane and release occurs by diffusion through the matrix or the polymer membrane. Devices where a volatile agent is placed in a hollow fiber and is allowed to evaporate through the open end are also described. In osmotic devices a therapeutic agent is contained in a rigid housing and is pumped through a small orifice in the housing as a consequence of water penetration into the device through a semipermeable membrane driven by an osmotically active agent. In erosional devices the active agent can be chemically attached to a polymer backbone and released as its attachment to the polymer backbone cleaves by a hydrolysis reaction. The active agent can also be placed in a core and released by diffusion through a bioerodible polymer membrane or dispersed in a bioerodible matrix and released by diffusion from the matrix. Devices where drug release is controlled by polymer erosion are also described. Each methodology is illustrated with specific examples chosen whenever possible from commercial products.

INTRODUCTION

The need for devices that can deliver specific therapeutic agents to selected body sites at precisely controlled rates is best described by referring to Figure 1 which shows plasma drug concentration following the absorption of a therapeutic agent. Also shown are drug concentration levels above which a specific drug is toxic and below which it is not therapeutically effective. The difference between the two levels is known as the therapeutic index.

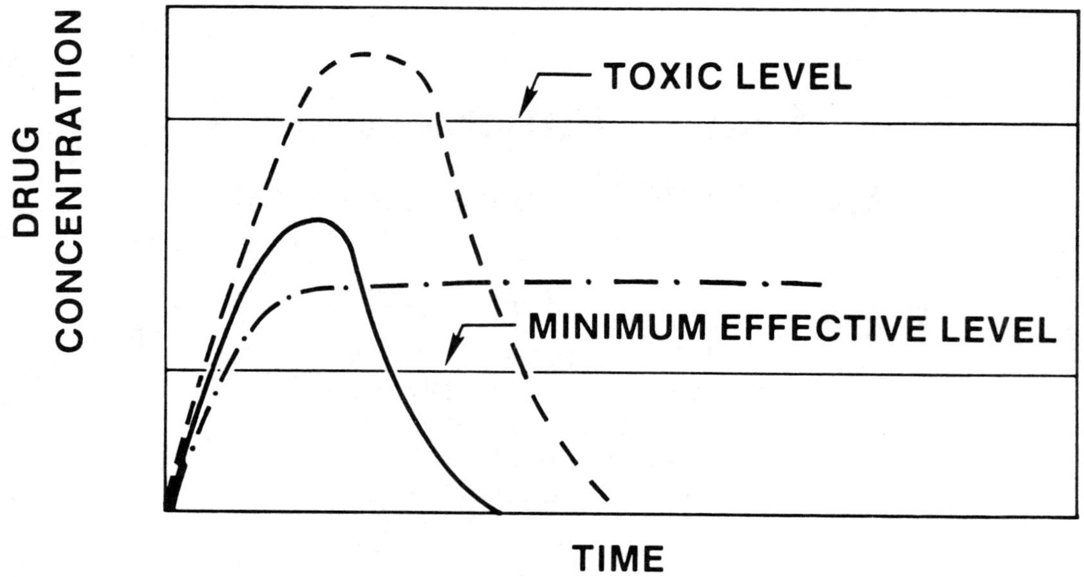

Figure 1. Drug concentration following absorption of therapeutic agent as a function of time. —— safe dose; -- unsafe dose; ● —— ● controlled release. (Reprinted with permission from Roseman, T. J., and Yalkowsky, S., H., in Controlled Release Polymeric Formulations, *Paul, D. R., and Harris, F. W., Eds., ACS Symposium Series 33, American Chemical Society, Washington, DC, 1976, p. 35).*

Drug plasma concentration after a single dose administration rapidly increases, then exponentially decays as the drug is excreted and/or metabolized. The drug is therapeutically effective only while the plasma concentration is above the minimum effective level, at which point another dose must be administered. The only way to increase length of therapeutic effectiveness is to increase initial loading. However, plasma drug concentration then exceeds the toxic level. Therefore, a methodology that allows the plasma drug concentration to be maintained at any desired level for long periods of time while never approaching the toxic level clearly represents a significant advance in drug therapy.

In the following sections, we review available controlled release methodologies that involve polymers in the rate control mechanism. These methodologies are divided into three categories: (1) diffusion controlled, (2) osmotically controlled, and (3) erosion controlled. A general discussion of each methodology is first presented, followed by selected examples of various applications. These have been selected to illustrate the methodology, and no attempt to tabulate all known applications has been made. Whenever possible, examples used in commercial production have been selected.

DIFFUSION CONTROLLED DEVICES

Three types of diffusion controlled devices are considered: (1) reservoir devices surrounded by a rate-controlling membrane, (2) monolithic devices, and (3) hollow fibers.

Reservoir Devices Surrounded by a Rate-Controlling Membrane

General Considerations

Transport of a permeant through a nonporous, homogeneous polymer film occurs by dissolution at one interface of the membrane and then diffusion down a gradient in thermodynamic activity [1]. It can be described by Fick's first law

$$J = -D \frac{dC_m}{dx} \tag{1}$$

where J is the flux in g/cm²-sec, C_m is the concentration of the permeant in the membrane in g/cm³, dC_m/dx is the concentration gradient, and D is the diffusion coefficient of the permeant in the membrane in cm²/sec.

Because the concentration of the permeant just inside the membrane is not known, it is related to the concentration in the medium surrounding the membrane by

$$\begin{aligned} C_{m(o)} &= KC_o \text{ at the upstream side } (x = 0) \\ C_{m(\ell)} &= KC_\ell \text{ at the downstream side } (x = \ell) \end{aligned} \tag{2}$$

where K is a distribution coefficient analogous to a liquid-liquid partition coefficient.

The diffusion process is schematically represented in Figure 2. At steady state, equation (1) can be integrated to give

$$J = D \frac{C_{m(o)} - C_{m(\ell)}}{\ell} = D \frac{\Delta C_m}{\ell} \tag{3}$$

Using equation (2), equation (3) can be rewritten as

$$J = \frac{DK\Delta C}{\ell} \tag{4}$$

where ΔC is the difference in concentration between the solutions on either side of the membrane.

If the thermodynamic activity of the drug in the reservoir remains constant, if there is no change in the rate-limiting membrane characteristics, and if infinite sink conditions are maintained at the downstream side of the membrane, rate of drug release will be constant and can be predicted from a knowledge of membrane permeability and device configuration.

Thus for a slab having a total surface area A, Fick's law can be restated as follows:

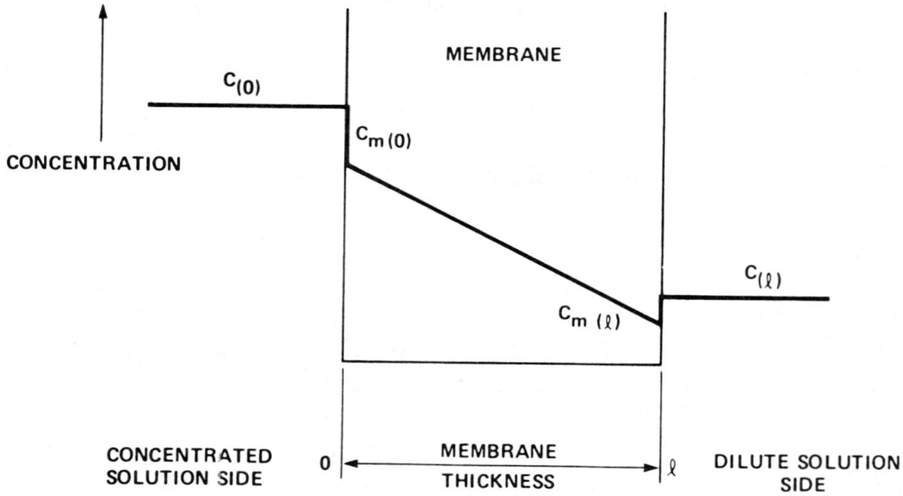

Figure 2. Schematic representation of the concentration gradient across a membrane. (Reprinted with permission from Baker, R. W., and Lonsdale, H. K., in Controlled Release of Biologically Active Materials, *Tanquary, A. C., and Lacy, R. E., Eds., Plenum Press, New York, 1974, p. 19).*

$$\frac{dM_t}{dt} = \frac{ADK\Delta C}{\ell} \tag{5}$$

where M_t is the amount of drug released and dM_t/dt is the release rate at time t.

Similarly, for a cylinder of inside and outside radii r_o and r_1 and height h, Fick's law is rewritten as

$$\frac{dM_t}{dt} = \frac{2\pi hDK\Delta C}{\ln(r_o - r_1)} \tag{6}$$

Finally, for a sphere of inside and outside radii r_o and r_1, the corresponding expression is

$$\frac{dM_t}{dt} = 4\pi DK\Delta C \frac{r_o r_1}{r_o - r_1} \tag{7}$$

In certain applications it may be desirable to replace the dense membrane structure with a microporous, hydrophobic structure. Such membranes have well-defined pores connecting the two sides of the membrane; these pores can be used to immobilize a liquid that is different from the external environment. Diffusion of a permeant then occurs principally by diffusion through the liquid-filled pores.

The flux through such a membrane can be expressed as

$$J = \frac{EDK\Delta C}{\tau\ell} \tag{8}$$

where E is the porosity of the membrane and τ the tortuosity [2].

Even though devices consisting of a reservoir surrounded by a barrier membrane should theoretically be capable of delivering therapeutic agents at a constant rate, also referred to as zero-order kinetics, in practice several factors contribute to deviations from zero-order kinetics. The two most important factors are boundary layer effects and the burst effect.

Boundary layer problems arise in applications in which the rate of removal of the drug from the membrane is slow so that the concentration of the drug at the membrane surface increases with time. Then, as predicted by equation (4), the term ΔC decreases and consequently the flux J also decreases. In the extreme case of drugs having very low water solubility, the concentration of the drug at the membrane surface can reach saturation value, at which point diffusion will stop and rate of drug delivery is completely governed by the rate at which the drug diffuses from the device. The problem has been treated theoretically and is shown in Figure 3 [1].

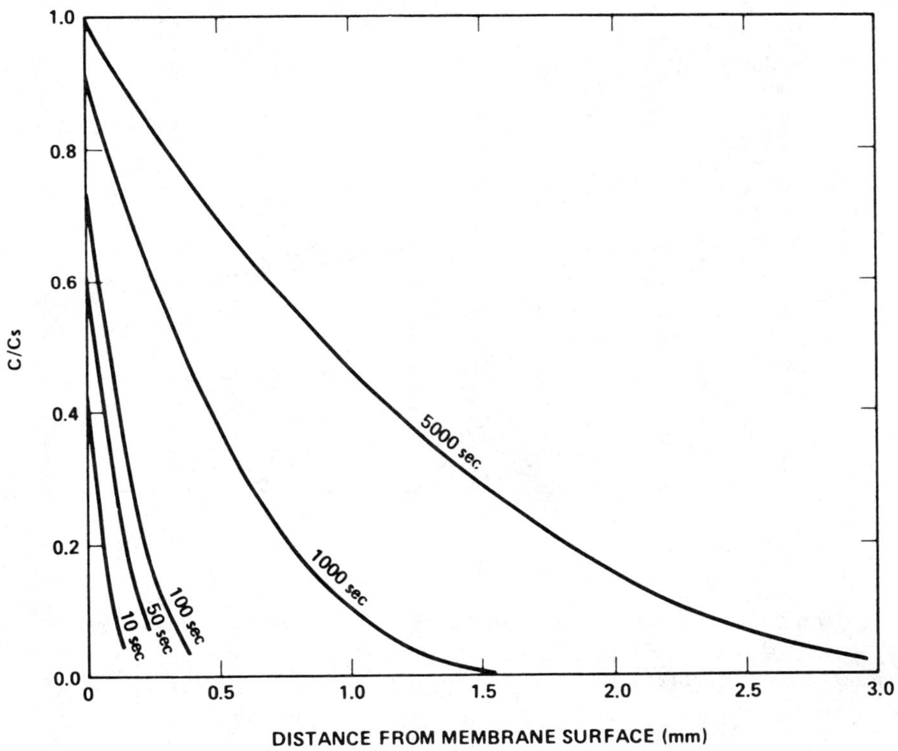

Figure 3. Drug concentration near the surface of a membrane releasing drug into an unstirred fluid. Drug diffusion coefficient = 2×10^6 cm²/sec and ratio of J_{max} to $C_s = 1$. (Reprinted with permission from Baker, R. W., and Lonsdale, H. K., in Controlled Release of Biologically Active Materials, *Tanquary, A. C., and Lacey, R. E., Ed. Plenum Press, New York, 1973, p. 59).*

While the drug-release device is in storage, the drug contained in the core will saturate the membrane surrounding the core; then, when the device is placed in a desorbing medium, the drug will rapidly desorb from the membrane. This rapid rate of drug release, which precedes the steady-state release, is known as the burst effect. The magnitude of the burst effect is determined by the diffusion coefficient of the drug in the membrane, membrane thickness, and length of storage of the device. The effect of storage on rate of delivery of estriol from Estane 5714 polyurethane cylindrical devices is shown in Figure 4 [3].

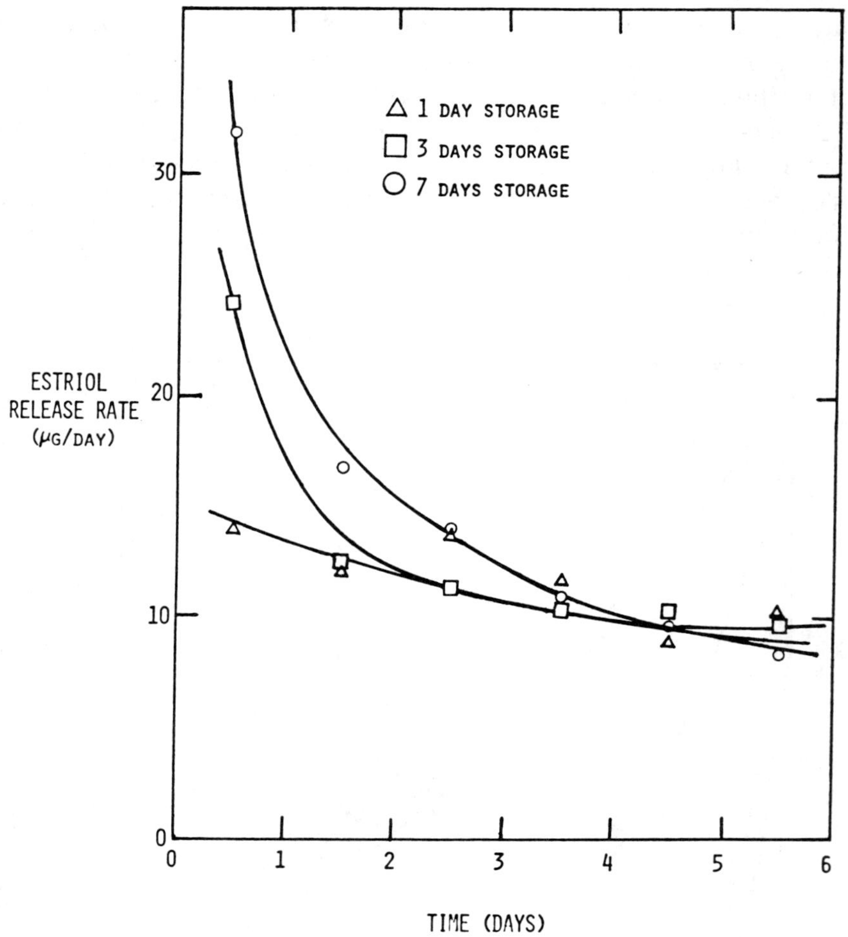

Figure 4. Release rate versus time from estriol-containing devices stored in air at 37°C for varying time periods (from Baker, R. W., Lonsdale, H. K., Tuttle, M. E., and Ayres, J. W., in Drug Delivery Systems, Proceedings, *Gabelnick, H. L., Ed., DHEW Publication No. (NIH) 77-1238 1976, p. 70).*

Applications

Several devices using rate-limiting membranes surrounding a reservoir that contains an active agent have reached commercial production. One such a device, developed by the Alza Corporation, is the Ocusert® (Figure 5) designed for treatment of open-angle glaucoma [4]. The drug reservoir is a film of pilocarpine in alginic acid and is surrounded by an annular ring with incorporated titanium dioxide pigment, which provides visibility for the otherwise transparent system. The ethylene-vinyl acetate copolymer rate-controlling membranes are laminated onto the annular ring, and the device is sterilized by irradiation.

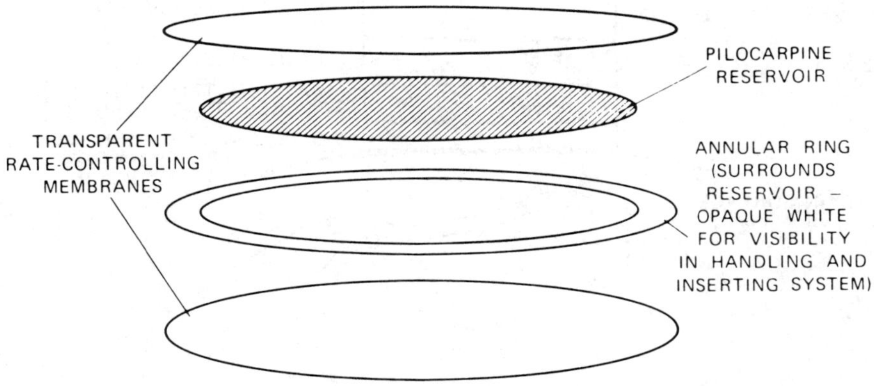

Figure 5. Schematic diagram of ocular therapeutic system. (Reprinted with permission from Chandrasekaran, S. K., Benson, H., and Urquhart, J., in Sustained and Controlled Release Drug Delivery Systems, *Robinson, J. R., Ed., Marcel Dekker, New York, 1978, p. 571).*

In vitro release rate of pilocarpine is shown in Figure 6 [4]. After an initial burst caused by diffusion of drug from the core into the rate-limiting membrane, the release rate is relatively constant over a seven-day period.

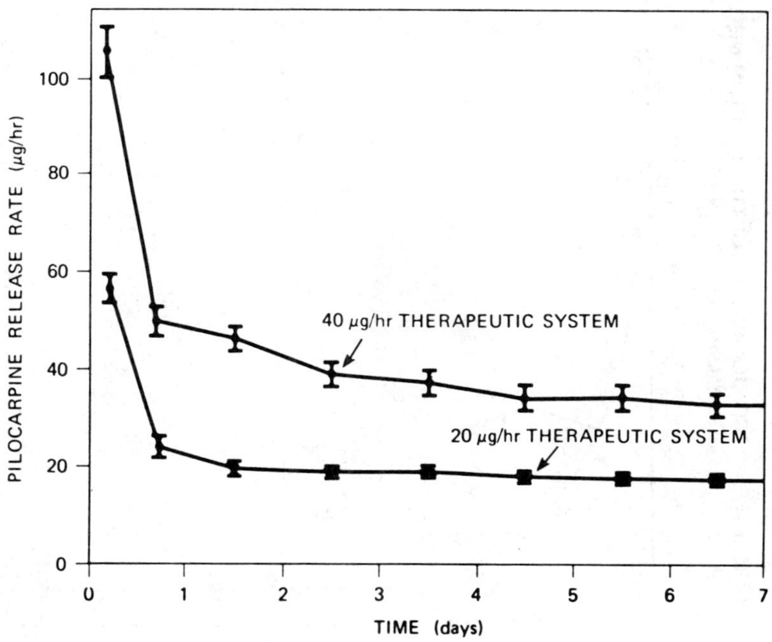

Figure 6. In vitro *release rates for the pilocarpine ocular therapeutic systems. (Reprinted with permission from Chandrasekaran, S. K., Benson, H., and Urquhart, J., in* Sustained and Controlled Release Drug Delivery Systems, *Robinson, J. R., Ed., Marcel Dekker, New York, 1978, p. 572).*

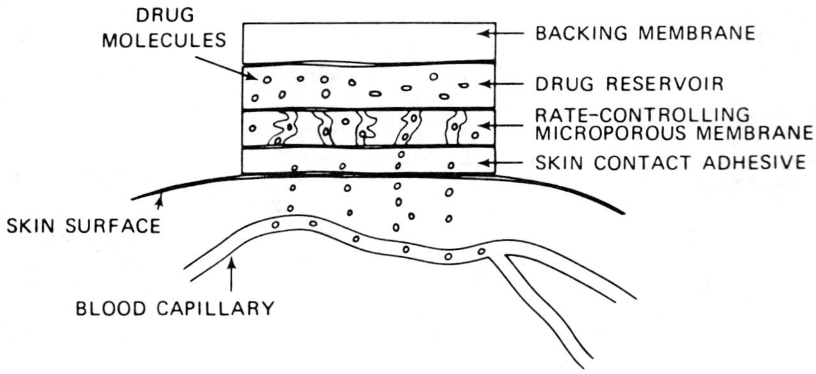

Figure 7. Schematic diagram of a transdermal therapeutic system. (Reprinted with permission from Chandrasekaran, S. K., Benson, H., and Urquhart, J., in Sustained and Controlled Release Drug Delivery Systems, *Robinson, J. R., Ed., Marcel Dekker, New York, 1978, p. 581).*

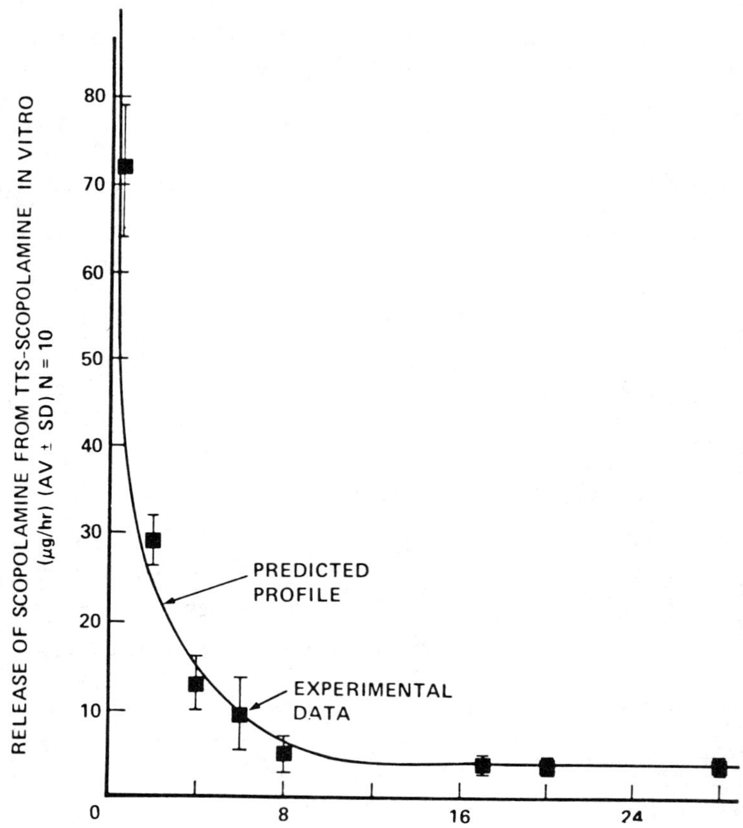

Figure 8. In vitro *release rate for a transdermal therapeutic system (scopolamine). (Reprinted with permission from Chandrasekaran, S., K., Benson, H., and Urquhart, J., in* Sustained and Controlled Release Drug Delivery Systems, *Robinson, J. R., Ed., Marcel Dekker, New York, 1978, p. 582).*

Another device, also developed by Alza Corporation, is designed to administer scopolamine across the intact skin. Because the intact human skin is sufficiently permeable to scopolamine, the use of adjuvants is not necessary, and the flux of the drug contained in a reservoir is controlled by a microporous membrane with fluid-filled pores. The nature of the microporous membrane or the fluid has not been disclosed. Figures 7 and 8 show how the device is constructed and the *in vitro* release rate of scopolamine, respectively [4].

Another device, developed by the Health Chem Corporation, is shown in Figure 9. The device is designed for the controlled release of chemical agents for pest control management. As with all systems described in this section, the active agent is contained in a core, and its release to the outside environment is controlled with a rate-limiting membrane. The rate of release of a fly-repellent from a typical device is shown in Figure 10 [5].

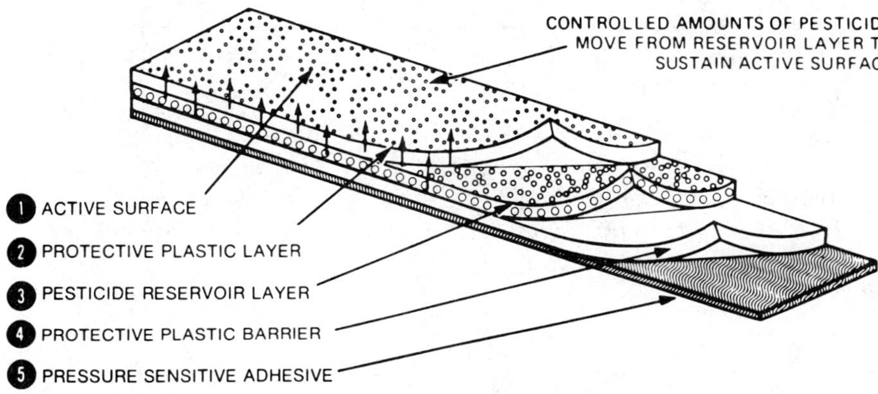

Figure 9. Schematic of Hercon®, a laminated controlled release structure. (Reprinted with permission from Kydonieus, A. F., in Controlled Release Pesticides, *Scher, H. B., Ed., ACS Symposium Series 53, American Chemical Society, Washington, DC, 1977, p. 154).*

Monolithic Devices

General Considerations

In a monolithic device the therapeutic agent is intimately mixed in the rate-controlling polymer, and release occurs by diffusion of the agent from the device. It is necessary to consider two types of devices. In one, the drug is dissolved in the polymer, whereas in the other, the drug is dispersed in the polymer.

For a drug dissolved in the matrix, release kinetics can be calculated by two equations [1]. One, known as the early time approximation [equation (9)] holds true for the first 60% of the release rate, after which it is calculated from equation (10), which is known as the late time approximation.

$$\frac{dM_t}{dt} = 2M_x \left(\frac{D}{\pi \ell^2 t}\right)^{1/2} \qquad (9)$$

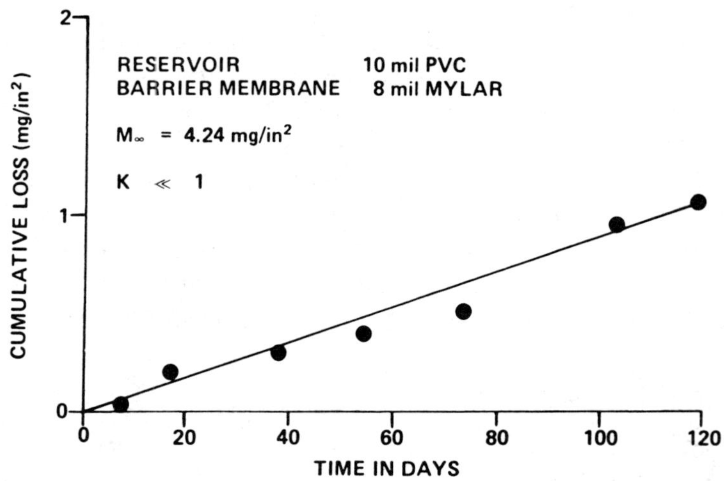

Figure 10. Release of MGK R-874 fly-repellent from a Hercon® multilayered dispenser. (Reprinted with permission from Kydonieus, A. F., in Controlled Release Pesticides, *Scher, H. B., Ed., ACS Symposium Series 53, American Chemical Society, Washington, DC, 1977, p. 156).*

$$\frac{dM_t}{dt} = \frac{8DM_x}{\ell^2}\exp\left(-\frac{\pi^2 Dt}{\ell^2}\right) \tag{10}$$

These equations predict drug release rate from a slab of thickness ℓ where M_x is the total amount of drug dissolved in the polymer and M_t is the amount released at time t. As equation (9) shows, the drug release rate decreases as $t^{-1/2}$ over the first 60% of the release; over the remainder of the release the rate decays exponentially according to equation (10). Plots of these two approximations are shown in Figure 11.

When the drug is dispersed in the polymer, release kinetics have been derived by Higuchi

$$\frac{dM_t}{dt} = \frac{A}{2}\left[\frac{2DC_sC_o}{t}\right]^{1/2} \tag{11}$$

where C_s is the solubility of the drug in the matrix and C_o is total concentration of drug in the matrix (dissolved plus dispersed) [6].

Unlike the slab with dissolved drug in which the rate is proportional to $t^{-1/2}$ only during the early portion of the release curve, slabs with dispersed drug maintain a $t^{-1/2}$ dependence over the major portion of the release curve and deviate from this dependence only when the concentration of the drug remaining in the matrix falls below the saturation value.

Because of the $t^{-1/2}$ dependence, a plot of cumulative drug release versus $t^{-1/2}$ will yield a straight line. Furthermore, according to equation (11), drug release rate is proportional to the square root of the drug loading. Plots of cumulative drug release versus $t^{-1/2}$ for various concentrations are shown in Figure 12 [7].

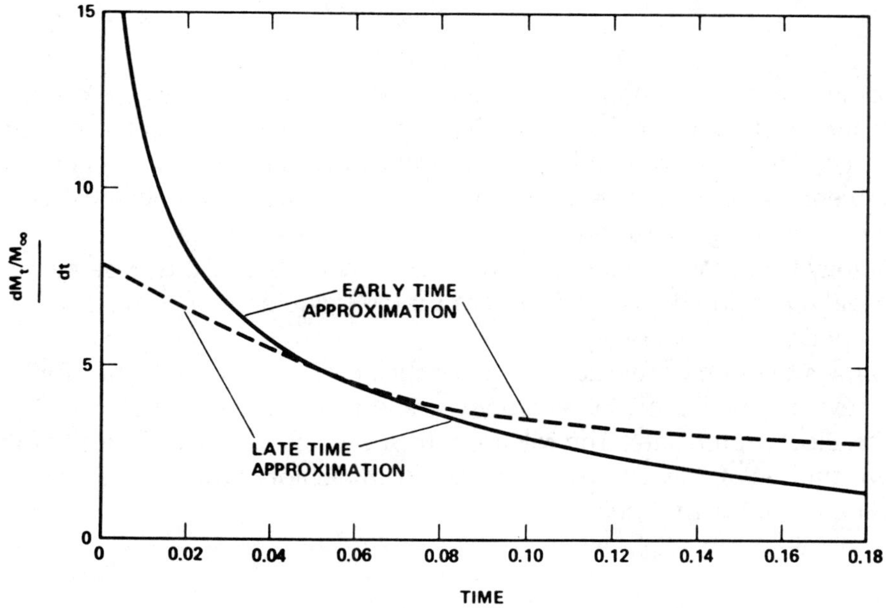

Figure 11. Release rate of drug initially dissolved in a slab as a function of time. (Reprinted with permission from Baker, R. W., and Lonsdale, H. K., in Controlled Release of Biologically Active Materials, *Tanquary, A. C., and Lacy, R. E., Eds., Plenum Press, New York, 1974, p. 43).*

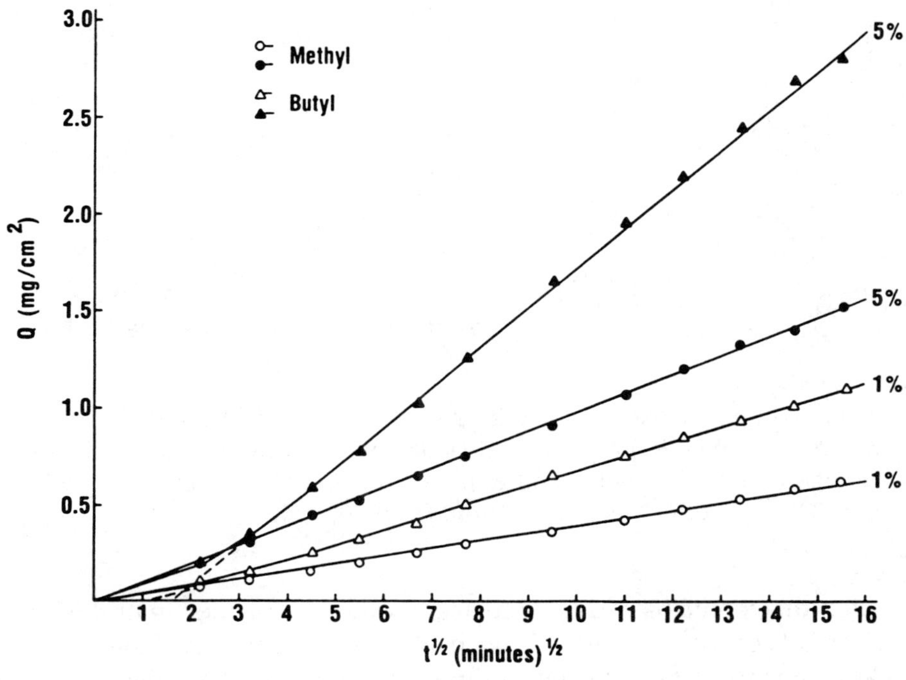

Figure 12. Plots of cumulative drug released (Q) versus $t^{1/2}$ for the methyl and butyl esters of p-aminobenzoic acid from silicone rubber disks at two loading doses (Reprinted with permission from Roseman, T. J., and Yalkowsky, S. H., in Controlled Release Polymeric Formulations, *Paul, D. R., and Harris, F. W., Ed., ACS Symposium Series 33, American Chemical Society, Washington, DC, 1976, p. 46).*

Applications

Although drug release from monolithic systems does not proceed by zero-order kinetics, it is the simplest and most convenient way to achieve prolonged release of an active agent. Such devices can be conveniently prepared by using simple polymer fabrication techniques involving a physical blending of the active agent with a polymer matrix, followed by compression molding, injection molding, extrusion, calendering, or solvent casting.

This technology is used in numerous products. However, because release rate is not constant, commercial utilization has been limited to prolonged release of pesticides, fertilizers, or antifouling compounds for marine applications.

Figure 13 shows the rate of release of the insecticide dichlorvos from the Shell No-Pest® strip [8]. The device contains ∼20% dichlorvos dispersed in poly(vinyl chloride) plasticized with about 30% dioctyl phthalate. The release rate shown as total weight loss of the device represents a weight loss of only 6% which includes both dichlorvos and plasticizer and follows the usual decline of rate with time.

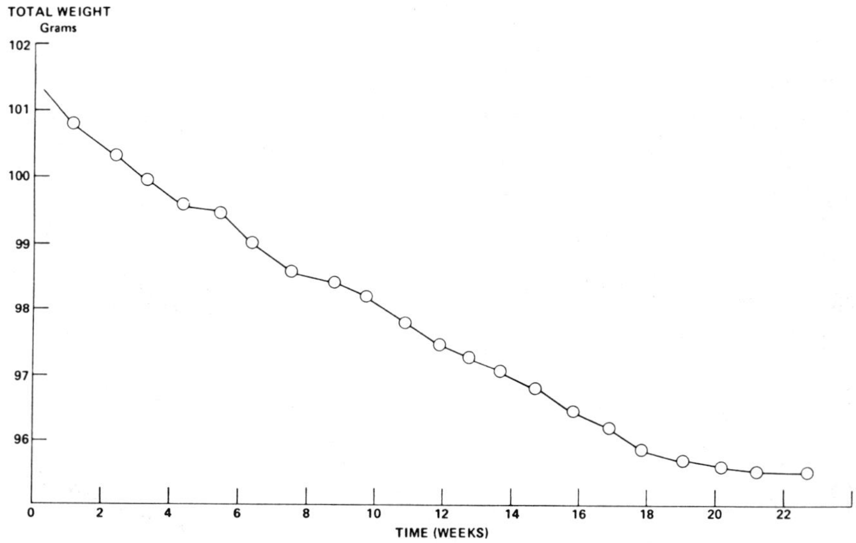

Figure 13. Weight loss: No-Pest® Strip, 20% dichlorvos and related products. (Reprinted with permission from Cardarelli, N. F., in Controlled Release Technologies: Methods, Theory and Applications, *Vol. I, Kydonieus, A. F., Ed., CRC Press, Boca Raton, FL, 1980, p. 59).*

Another device that contains a drug dispersed within a polymer matrix without incorporated plasticizer is Ecopro™ developed by Environmental Chemicals, Inc. [8]. The device manufactured as an anchored floating chip is shown in Figure 14. These devices are intended to control a range of aquatic species such as mosquito larvae or the snail host of schistosomiasis.

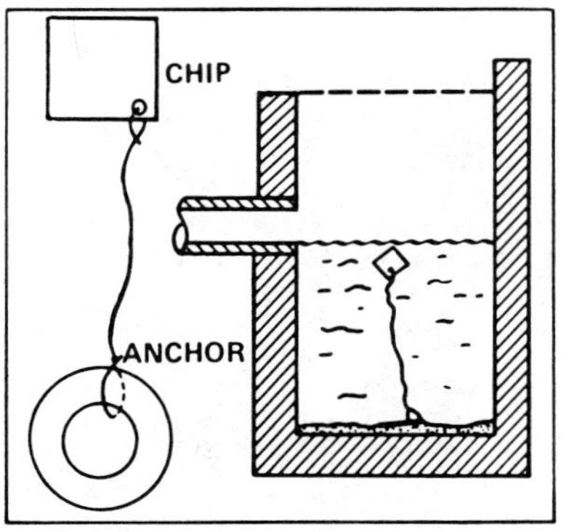

Figure 14. Floating larvicide (Ecopro 1700). (Reprinted with permission from Cardarelli, N. F., in Controlled Release Technologies Methods, Theory and Applications, *Vol. I, Kydonieus, A. F., Ed., CRC Press, Boca Raton, FL, 1980, p. 63).*

Hollow Fibers

General Considerations

Hollow fiber devices differ from the diffusional devices considered in the two previous sections in that release of the active agent is not moderated by a rate-controlling membrane. Instead, the active agent, which must be a relatively volatile liquid, is placed in a hollow fiber sealed at one end and is allowed to evaporate.

The mechanism of release thus consists of the following three steps [9]:

(1) Evaporation at the liquid-vapor interface.
(2) Diffusion from the liquid-vapor interface to the open end of the lumen.
(3) Convection away from the open end.

These three steps are illustrated in Figure 15.

The rate-controlling step will generally be step (2), and the diffusive process has been likened to membrane release systems by considering the stagnant vapor column in the lumen of the hollow fiber as a gaseous membrane through which the active agent must permeate.

The release from hollow fibers has been described mathematically by the following relationship [9]:

$$\frac{d\ell}{dt} = \left[\frac{McD}{2p}\frac{P_a^{vap}}{P}\right]^{1/2} t^{-1/2} \qquad (12)$$

where $d\ell/dt$ is the rate of change of the meniscus level and is directly related to the release of the active agent, M is the molecular weight, p is the densityP_a^{vap} is the vapor pressure, c is the molar density, D is the diffusion coefficient, and t is the time. The vapor pressure in equation (12) is not a true equilibrium vapor pressure but a reduced value because of the curved meniscus of the liquid in the capillary. Because the meniscus is dependent on the diameter of the capillary and capillary material, release rate depends on the size and the construction material of the hollow fiber.

Applications

Although hollow fiber technology is a method applicable to any volatile material, cost

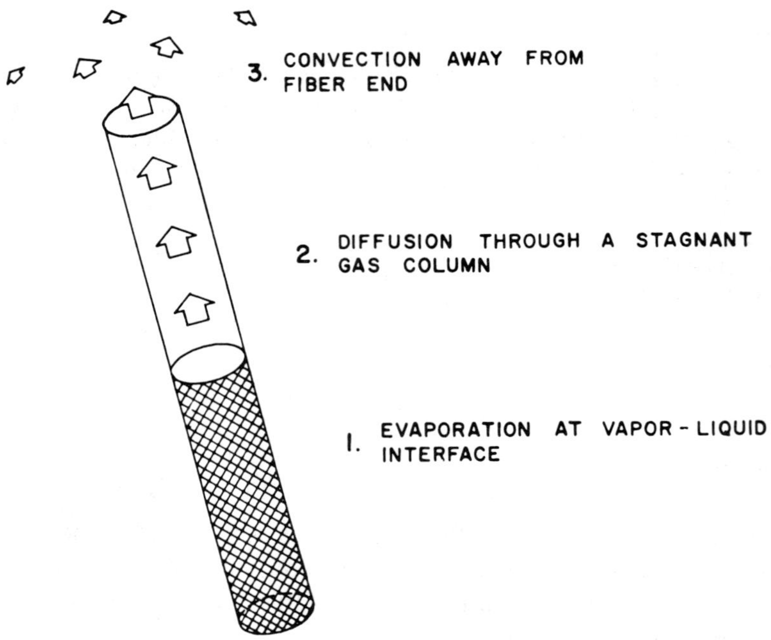

Figure 15. Mechanism of vapor release from hollow fibers (one end sealed). (Reprinted with permission from Brooks, T. W., in Controlled Release Technologies: Methods, Theory and Applications, *Vol. II, Kydonieus, A. F., Ed., CRC Press, Boca Raton, FL, 1980, p. 167).*

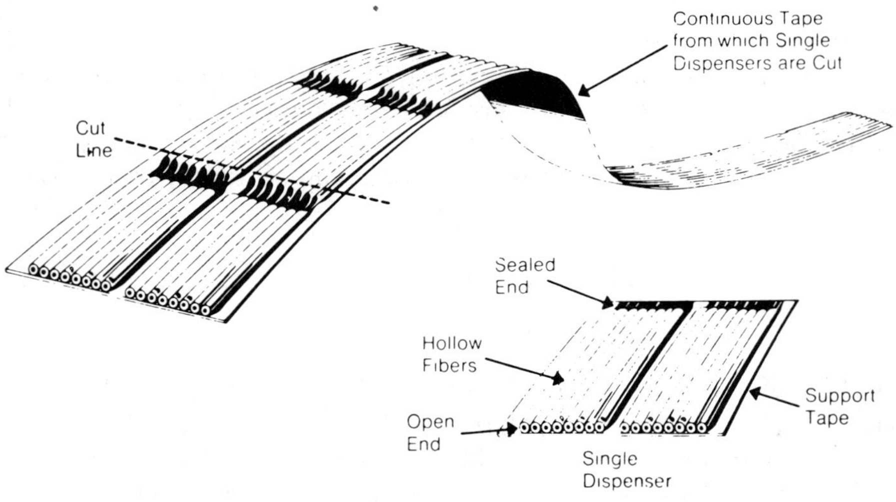

Figure 16. Tape form of hollow fiber vapor dispenser. (Reprinted with permission from Brooks, T. W., in Controlled Release Technologies: Methods, Theory and Applications, *Vol. II, Kydonieus, A. F., Ed., CRC Press, Boca Raton, FL, 1980, p. 173).*

considerations limit this technology to materials active at extremely low concentrations. Consequently, this technology has been applied exclusively to controlled delivery of insect pheromones.

Hollow fiber formulations are available as parallel arrays of fibers fixed to an adhesive tape or as chopped fibers. A parallel array dispenser is shown in Figure 16 [9]. In this dispenser the fibers are pressure-filled with the active material, then sealed ultrasonically at regular intervals. Release is activated by cutting the tape, thus opening the fibers. In chopped fibers the filled individual fibers are sealed at regular intervals and then chopped at a predetermined distance from the seal. The chopped fibers are stored in hermetically sealed containers, and release is activated when the container is opened.

A typical plot of amount of compound dispensed from hollow fibers as a function of time is shown in Figure 17 [10]. The high initial rate is considered to be due to the liquid meniscus being near the open end of the tube.

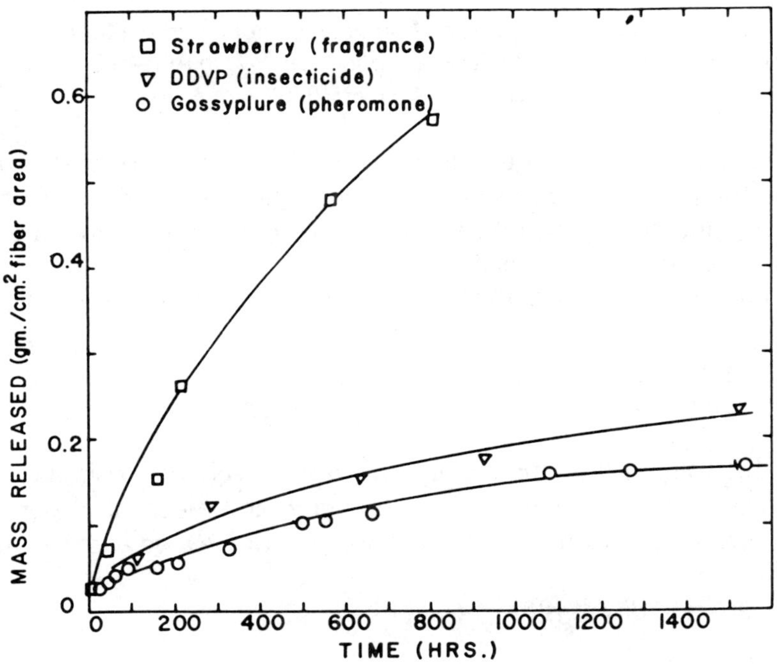

Figure 17. Vapor release curves for various materials from hollow fibers. (Reprinted with permission from Ashare, E., Brooks, T. W., and Swenson, D. W., in Controlled Release Polymeric Formulations, *Paul, D. R., and Harris, F. W., Eds. ACS Symposium Series 33, American Chemical Society, Washington, DC, 1976, p. 278).*

OSMOTICALLY CONTROLLED DEVICES

General Considerations

The operation of an osmotic pump can be described by referring to Figure 18 [11]. In this device an osmotic agent is contained within a rigid housing and is separated from a drug com-

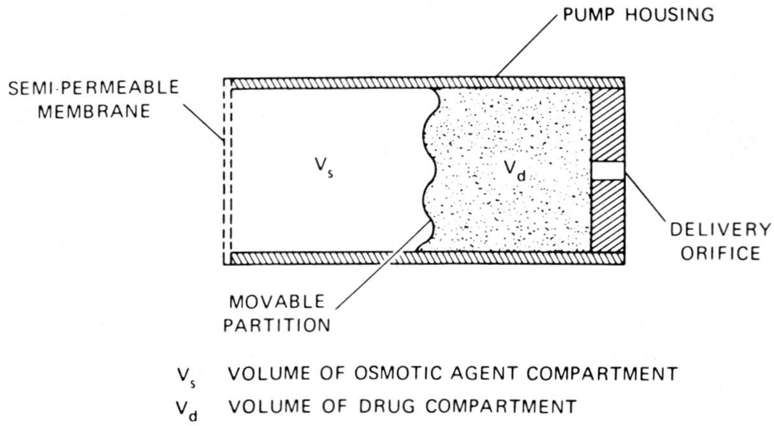

Figure 18. Schematic representation of an osmotic pump. (Reprinted with permission from Theeuwes, F. and Yum, S. I., in Ann. of Biomed. Eng. 4, *343-353 (1976).*

partment by a movable partition. One wall of the rigid housing is a semipermeable membrane so that when the pump is exposed to an aqueous environment water will be driven osmotically across the membrane; the increased volume within the osmotic compartment will force the drug out of the device through the delivery orifice.

The volume flux of water across the semipermeable membrane is given by

$$\frac{dV}{dt} = \frac{A}{\ell} L_p (\sigma \Delta\pi - \Delta P) \tag{13}$$

where dV/dt is the volume flux, $\Delta\pi$ and ΔP are, respectively, the osmotic and hydrostatic pressure difference across the membrane, L_p is membrane mechanical permeability coefficient, σ is the reflection coefficient, and A and ℓ are membrane area and thickness, respectively.

The drug delivery rate dM/dt is then given by

$$\frac{dM}{dt} = \frac{dV}{dt} C \tag{14}$$

where C is the concentration of the drug in the solution pumped out of the orifice.

Devices using osmotic energy to control delivery of therapeutic agents have important benefits, including

(1) The devices are generic in that they operate independent of agent properties.
(2) The devices are able to deliver macromolecules that cannot be delivered at constant rates from diffusional devices.
(3) Constant delivery rates much higher than those available from diffusional devices can be realized.

Applications

Two osmotic drug delivery devices have reached commercial production. One of these, shown in Figure 19, is manufactured by the Alza Corporation under the trade name of Alzet® [11]. The device is a capsule approximately 2.5 cm long and 0.6 cm in diameter. The drug is contained in an innermost impermeable flexible reservoir surrounded with an osmotic agent, which in turn is surrounded and sealed within a rigid cellulose acetate semipermeable membrane.

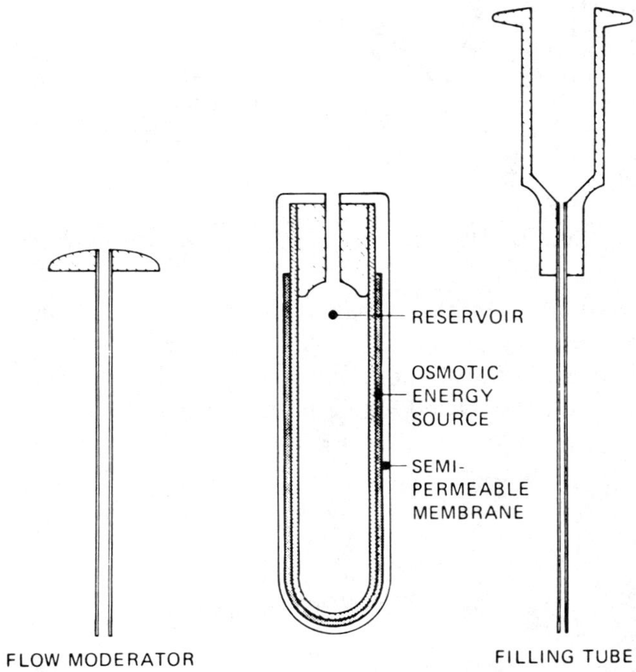

Figure 19. Osmotic pump and components (Reprinted with permission from Theeuwes, F. and Yum, S. I., in Ann. of Biomed. Eng. 4, *343-353 (1976).*

When the device is placed in an aqueous environment, water is osmotically imbibed across the semipermeable membrane, and the drug contained within the flexible reservoir is pumped out of the device. Because the driving force is the osmotic transport of water across the membrane, performance of the device is essentially independent of the environment within which the pump operates. Thus, as shown in Figure 20, about the same drug release rate is observed in isotonic saline at 37 °C and from subcutaneous implants in rats or mice [12].

Another device, also manufactured by the Alza Corporation is the Osmet™ delivery system shown in Figure 21 [13]. This device differs from that previously described in that the drug serves as the osmotic agent, which is surrounded by the rigid semipermeable membrane containing a delivery orifice. Major application is for gastrointestinal drug deliveries because delivery rate is pH-independent as shown in Figure 22 [13].

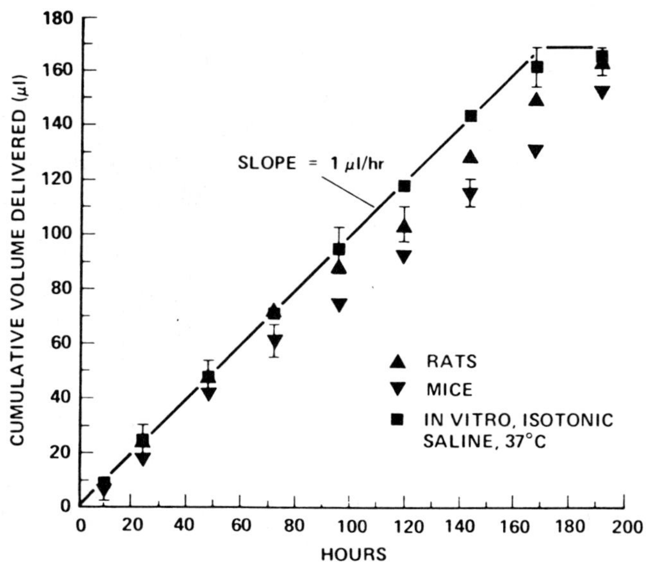

Figure 20. Cumulative volume delivered from miniaturized osmotic pump. (Reprinted with permission from Theeuwes, F., in Controlled Release Technologies: Methods, Theory and Applications, *Vol. II, Kydonieus, A. F., Ed., CRC Press, Boca Raton, FL, 1980, p. 201).*

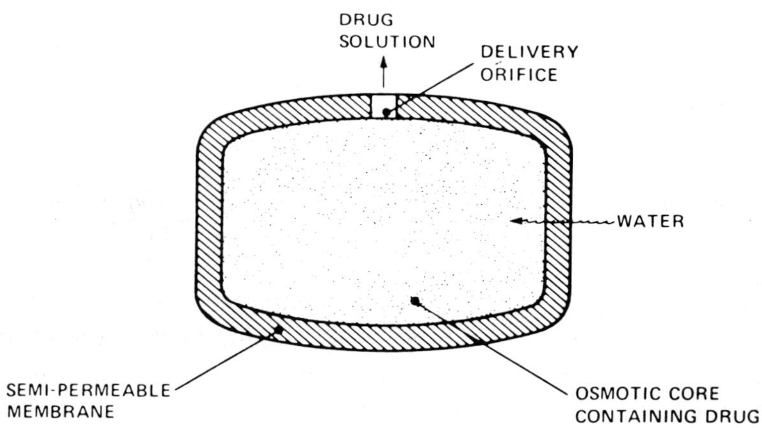

Figure 21. Elementary osmotic pump cross section. (Reprinted with permission from Theeuwes, F., J. Pharm. Sci., 64, *1987-1991 (1975).*

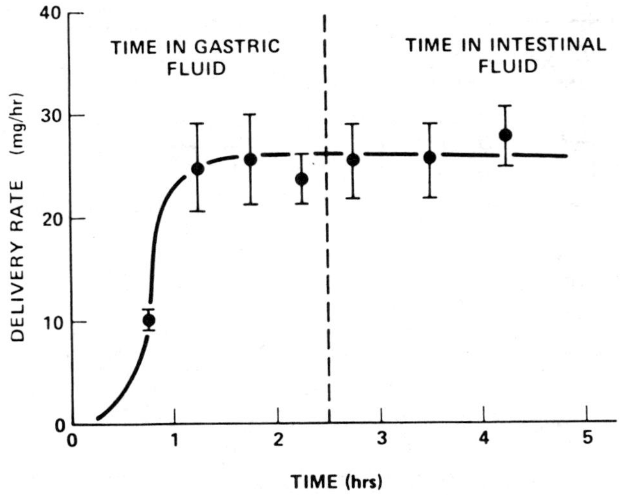

Figure 22. In vitro *release rate of sodium phenobarbital from elementary osmotic pump systems. (Reprinted with permission from Theeuwes, F. in* J. Pharm. Sci., 64, *1987-1991 (1975).*

EROSION CONTROLLED DEVICES

General Considerations

The principal rationale for constructing bioerodible devices is that expended devices need not be removed from their site of application. In some uses, such as topical applications at readily accessible body sites, bioerosion may simply be a convenience, whereas in other applications, such as implants, bioerosion eliminates the necessity for surgical removal.

Polymer bioerosion can be defined as the conversion of an initially water-insoluble material to a water-soluble material and does not necessarily signify a major chemical degradation. The various bioerosion mechanisms can be systematized into the three distinct types shown in Figure 23 [14].

In general terms, Type I erosion encompasses water-soluble polymers that have been insolubilized by hydrolytically unstable crosslinks. Type II erosion includes polymers that are initially water-insoluble and are solubilized by hydrolysis, ionization, or protonation of a pendant group. Type III erosion includes hydrophobic polymers that are converted to small water-soluble molecules by backbone cleavage.

Clearly, these three types represent extreme cases, and actual erosion can be a combination of these types. Thus, it is possible to develop a combination of Type I and Type III erosion in which initial hydrolysis involves crosslink cleavage with subsequent backbone cleavage of the high-molecular-weight, water-soluble polymer. Similarly, a Type II and Type III erosion can be developed in which initial solubilization is by ionization, protonation, or hydrolysis, followed by backbone cleavage of the soluble polymer.

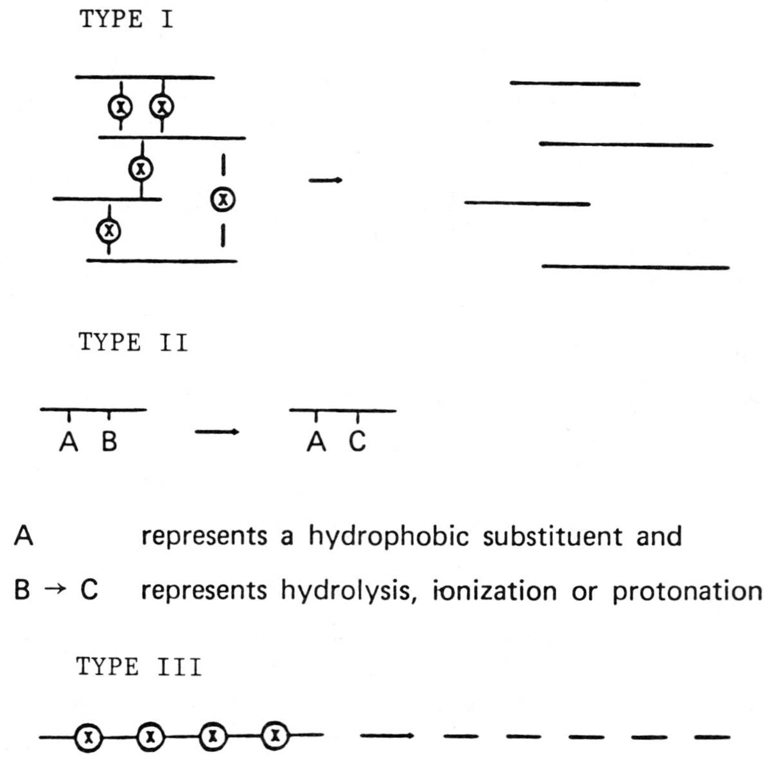

Figure 23. Schematic representation of bioerosion mechanisms. [(Reprinted with permission from Heller, J., Biomaterials, 1, *51-57 (1980)]*

Each type of polymer erosion has certain advantages and limitations, and the choice of a particular erosion mechanism is dictated by the specific application.

Type I Erosion

In systems based on Type I erosion, water-soluble macromolecules are converted to a three-dimensional network by means of hydrolytically labile crosslinks. As long as the crosslinks remain intact, the network is insoluble, and, when the network is placed in an aqueous environment, it can swell only to the extent allowed by the crosslink density. As the crosslinks cleave, crosslink density decreases, and the matrix will begin to swell until ultimately, with the majority of crosslinks cleaved, the matrix will dissolve.

Such a system has two inherent limitations. First, the progressive swelling of the matrix before dissolution will limit its use to applications where dimensional stability is of little importance. Second, because a system consisting of crosslinked water-soluble polymers is a hydrogel, it is completely permeated by water; therefore, the water solubility of the incorporated therapeutic agent becomes a very important consideration. Clearly, low-molecular-weight compounds with appreciable water solubility will be rapidly leached, independent of the matrix erosion rate.

Type II Erosion

In systems based on Type II erosion, water-insoluble macromolecules are converted to water-soluble macromolecules by hydrolysis, ionization, or protonation of a pendant group. Because no backbone cleavage takes place, the solubilization does not result in any significant change in molecular weight. However, unless the backbone is also degradable, polymers in this category are only useful in topical applications in which elimination of high-molecular-weight, water-soluble macromolecules proceeds with no difficulty.

Two classes of devices that uses Type II erosion have been developed. In one class the therapeutic agent is dispersed within or surrounded by the polymer matrix and is released as solubilization takes place. The other class contains the active agent covalently bonded to the polymer chain by a hydrolytically unstable bond and is released to the surrounding medium as the bond cleaves.

Type III Erosion

In systems based on Type III erosion, high-molecular-weight, water-insoluble macromolecules are converted to small, water-soluble molecules by a hydrolytic cleavage of labile bonds in the polymer backbone. Because these polymers are converted to small, water-soluble molecules, the principal application of these systems is for the systemic administration of therapeutic agents from subcutaneous, intramuscular, or intraperitoneal implantation sites. Clearly, the development of a useful system mandates that all degradation products be completely nontoxic.

Mechanism of Drug Release

Bioerodible devices can be grouped into two broad categories, depending on the drug release mechanism: devices in which a drug is surrounded by a rate-controlling bioerodible membrane and monolithic bioerodible devices in which drug release is controlled by diffusion or erosion.

The rate of drug delivery from devices that have a rate-controlling bioerodible membrane surrounding a drug core is constant and predictable as long as the membrane remains intact until drug delivery has been completed. Clearly, if the rate-controlling membrane erodes significantly during drug delivery, changes in membrane thickness or physical properties would be reflected in changes in drug delivery rate. In an extreme case, the membrane could rupture, and the drug contained in the core would be abruptly released. Thus, in this type of device the rate of drug release can be usefully controlled only by changing the nature of the bioerodible membrane; bioerosion simply removes the expended device.

Drug release from monolithic devices can be usefully controlled by either diffusion or erosion. If erosion of the matrix is very much slower than drug diffusion, the release kinetics follow the Higuchi model, as described under monolithic diffusional systems.

If erosion is relatively fast and the drug is well immobilized in the solid matrix so that diffusional release is minimal, matrix erosion determines rate of drug release. However, it is important to distinguish two types of hydrolytic erosion of a solid, hydrophobic polymer. In one, referred to as homogeneous erosion, the hydrolysis occurs at a uniform rate throughout the matrix. In the other, called heterogeneous erosion, the process is confined to the surface of the device and is, for that reason, commonly referred to as surface erosion.

Consequently, in a pure homogeneous process, the matrix will remain physically intact until all parts reach some critical degree of reaction, at which point the matrix disintegrates. In a pure heterogeneous process, however, only the outer surface layers dissolve while the interior remains intact.

A detailed understanding of drug release from a matrix that is undergoing a homogeneous erosion process is complex because it will be a combination of diffusion and erosion [15]. Because the matrix changes due to the bulk erosion process, permeability of the polymer to the drug will increase with time. Consequently, the rate of drug release may at first show the normal decline predicted by the Higuchi equation, but as the increasing polymer permeability gradually offsets this decline, the rate of drug release may eventually accelerate. Furthermore, if the matrix disintegrates before drug depletion, a large burst in rate of drug delivery will be noted.

Clearly, a heterogeneous or surface erosion, process is much more desirable because it can lead to zero-order drug release provided diffusional release of the drug is minimal and the overall surface area of the device remains constant. Furthermore, such a process avoids deterioration of mechanical properties, which can take place when random chain scission occurs within the bulk of a solid device.

Even with devices that do not maintain constant surface area, the rate of drug release is predictable and can be calculated from theoretical considerations by the following relationship [16]:

$$M_t/M_\infty = 1 - [1 - k_o t/C_o a]^n \qquad (15)$$

where

M_t = drug released at time t
M_∞ = drug released at device exhaustion
k_o = erosion constant
C_o = uniform initial drug concentration in matrix
a = radius of sphere or cylinder, or half thickness of slab
n = 1 for a slab, 2 for a cylinder, 3 for a sphere

Applications

Type I Erosion

Because Type I materials are completely permeated by water, they are clearly unable to immobilize small molecules having appreciable water solubility. Consequently, usefulness of these materials is limited to molecules having extremely low water solubility or to macromolecules that can be physically entangled in the hydrogel so that they can not diffuse out of the matrix even though they are freely soluble in water.

As an example of the first application, Figure 24 shows the rate of release of the highly water-insoluble hydrocortisone acetate from a gelatin matrix crosslinked with formaldehyde [14]. As indicated by the first-order dependence, the drug is released by a simple diffusional process, and the crosslinked gelatin matrix simply provides cohesiveness for the drug particles. Even though the release kinetics are not constant, useful release over many days is achieved.

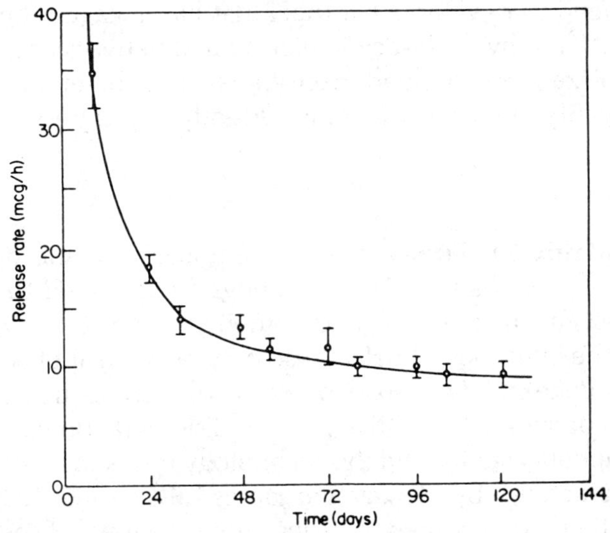

Figure 24. Release of hydrocortisone acetate from a crosslinked gelatin matrix. [Reprinted with permission from Heller, J., Biomaterials, 1, *51-57 (1980)].*

The first-order drug release also indicates that matrix erosion makes little or no contribution to drug release, and, because erosion of a formaldehyde-crosslinked gelatin is slow, drug depletion can occur before significant matrix erosion is noted. Such a device may be useful in applications where zero-order kinetics are not important and removal of the expended device is not convenient or desirable.

The entanglement of water-soluble macromolecules in hydrogels has been intensively investigated as a means of immobilizing enzymes or antigens and only limited attention has been devoted to methods in which bioerosion of these hydrogels is used as a means to control the release of the entrapped macromolecule [17].

One such example is the release of α-chymotripsin entangled in a hydrogel prepared from N-vinylpyrrolidone and N,N′-methylenebisacrylamide [18]. Although such hydrogels are generally not regarded as bioerodible, the crosslinks can nevertheless cleave as follows:

$$\text{R}-\overset{\text{O}}{\overset{\|}{\text{C}}}-\text{NH}-\text{CH}_2-\text{NH}-\overset{\text{O}}{\overset{\|}{\text{C}}}-\text{R} \xrightarrow{\text{H}_2\text{O}} 2\text{R}-\overset{\text{O}}{\overset{\|}{\text{C}}}-\text{NH}_2 + \text{H}-\overset{\text{O}}{\overset{\|}{\text{C}}}-\text{H}$$

where R represents a polymer chain. However, the rate of the cleavage reaction is very slow, and complete solubilization of a hydrogel prepared with an N,N′-methylenebisacrylamide crosslinker is achieved only at very low concentrations of the crosslinking agent. Thus, when α-chymotripsin was immobilized in a hydrogel prepared from N-vinylpyrrolidone and N,N′-methylenebisacrylamide, it was found that, when the N,N′-methylenebisacrylamide concentration was varied from 0.1 to 1.0 wt% with respect to N-vinylpyrrolidone, hydrogels could be prepared that would dissolve in several days or that were practically insoluble. However, even with the insoluble systems, a large portion of the enzyme diffused out of the hydrogel in 50 hours.

Clearly, there is a need to develop a hydrogel that has linkages considerably more labile than those based on N,N′-methylenebisacrylamide so that networks can be prepared that are tight enough to immobilize the entrapped macromolecule and yet are labile enough for erosion to occur at reasonable rates. Such work is currently in progress [19].

Type II Erosion

Agent Release by Matrix Solubilization. Major emphasis for the development of these materials has been on enteric coatings. These coatings are designed to be insoluble in a certain pH environment, usually the stomach, and to then dissolve abruptly in an environment of a different pH, such as the intestines. Usually these polymers are applied to pills as protective coatings and do not produce steady, sustained release of therapeutic agents. However, by using mixtures of enteric coatings, each with a different disintegration time, it is possible to prolong the action of therapeutic agents, and this technology forms the basis for products such as Contac Capsules manufactured by Menley and James Laboratories [20].

Because enteric coatings are designed to be insoluble at a low pH and soluble at a high pH, solubilization of the polymer can be accomplished by ionization of a carboxylic acid function. The most widely used enteric coatings are based on cellulose acetate phthalate [21], but enteric coatings based on partially esterified copolymers of methyl vinyl ether and maleic anhydride [22-24] or cellulose acetate succinate have also been described [25].

Although these polymers were originally designed to dissolve abruptly with a significant increase in external pH, in a constant pH environment they undergo a controlled dissolution process and are therefore useful materials for the controlled release of therapeutic agents dispersed within them.

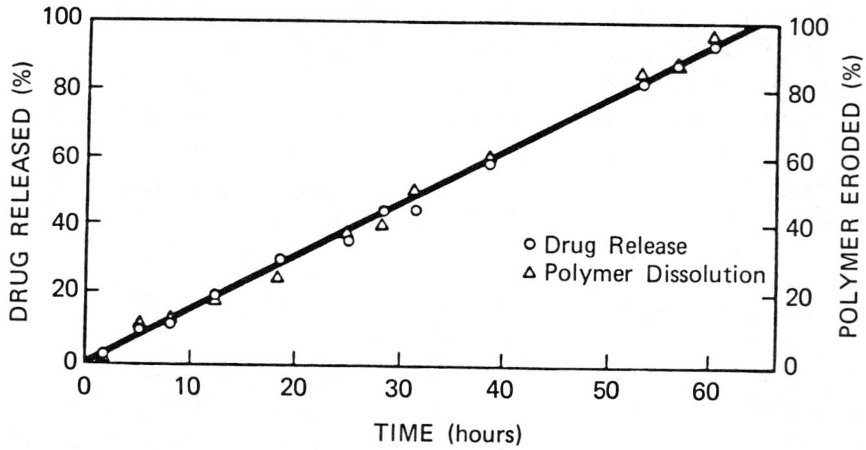

Figure 25. Rate of polymer dissolution and hydrocortisone release from n-butyl half-ester of methyl vinyl ether-maleic anhydride copolymer containing 10 wt% drug. [Reprinted with permission from Heller, J., Baker, R. W., Gale, R. M., and Rodin. J. O., J. Appl. Polymer Sci., *22, 1991-2009 (1978]).*

Figure 25 shows polymer dissolution rate and the rate of hydrocortisone release for an n-butyl half-ester of a methyl vinyl ether-maleic anhydride copolymer film containing the dispersed drug [26]. Each pair of points represents a separate device in which the amount of drug released by the device into the wash solution was determined by uv measurements and the amount of polymer dissolved was calculated from the total weight loss of the device. The excellent linearity of both polymer erosion and drug release over the lifetime of the device provides strong evidence for a surface-erosion mechanism and for negligible diffusional release of the drug. The latter result was independently verified by placing a drug-containing film in water at a pH low enough that no dissolution of the matrix took place and periodically analyzing the aqueous solution for hydrocortisone. None was found over several days.

In certain applications it may be desirable to develop materials that are stable at a high pH and dissolve at a low pH. This can be readily accomplished by using as the solubilization mechanism protonation of amine functions. A material typical of this group is cellulose acetate N,N-diethylaminoacetate, prepared by the amination of cellulose acetate chloroacetate with diethylamine [27]. Another material can be prepared by the addition of amines to crotonic acid esters of cellulose [28].

Agent Released by Hydrolysis of Covalent Link. This methodology allows the preparation of systems in which the polymer containing bound therapeutic agent can act either as a depot or as a carrier. In the depot mode the polymer is localized at a certain body site, and the drug is released by gradual cleavage of its atachment to the polymeric backbone. Clearly, the backbone polymer must also undergo a cleavage reaction so that no high-molecular-weight residues remain in the tissue after all the drug has been released.

One example of a depot system is norethindrone coupled to the water-soluble poly(N^5-hydroxypropyl-L-glutamine) by reaction with phosgene [29].

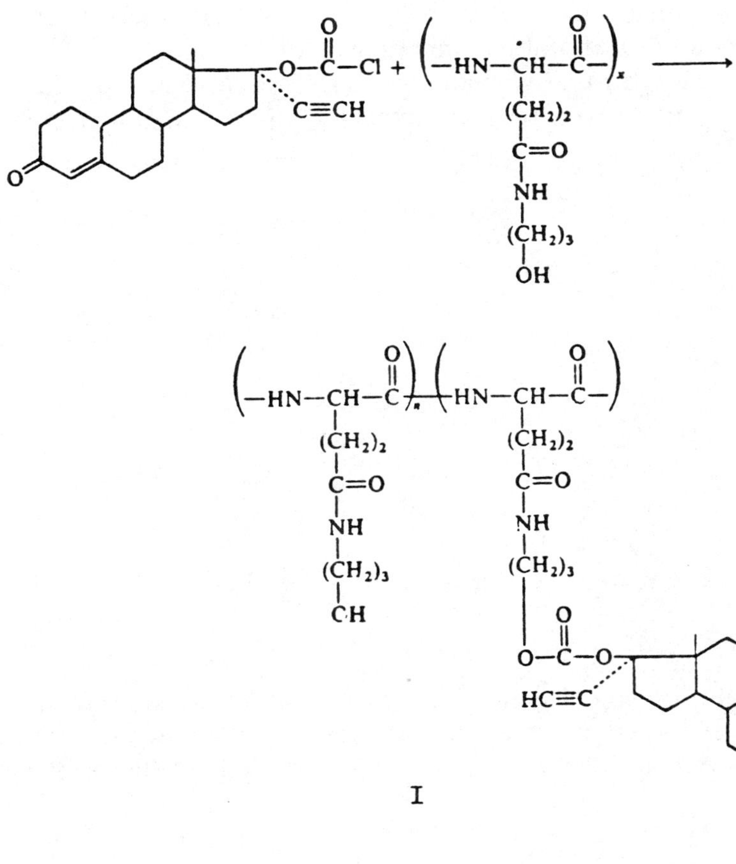

I

Reaction of the polypeptide hydroxyl group with the hydrophobic steroid produces a water-insoluble material that gradually solubilizes as hydrolysis of the carbonate linkage removes the steroid. *In vivo* release of tritiated norethindrone shown in Figure 26 reveals that the drug is released at a fairly constant rate for 144 days [29].

However, it is in the carrier mode that this methodology offers the unique possibility of carrying the drug to specific body sites. To achieve this specificity the water-soluble polymer carries, in addition to the bound therapeutic agent, a homing group. One example of such a polymer contains as the bioactive agent a p-phenylenediamine mustard and as the homing group immunoglobulin from rabbit antisera against mouse lymphoma cells.

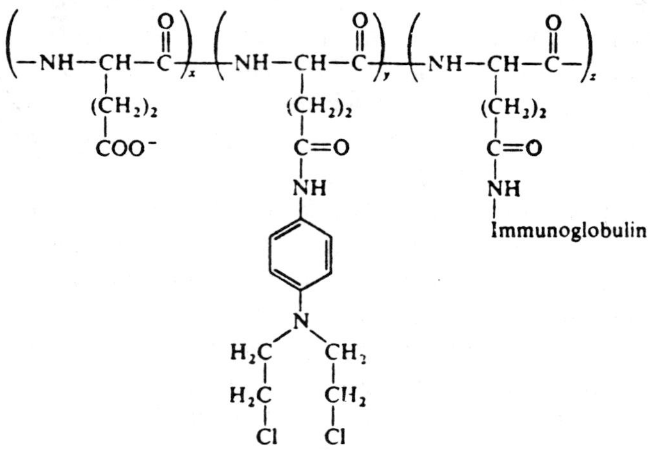

In vivo tests with this material showed that the polymer is much more effective than the polymer components or a mixture of the components [30].

This methodology has also been used in controlled release pesticide applications in which a pesticide is first made part of an acrylic or methacrylic ester that is then polymerized or copolymerized [31].

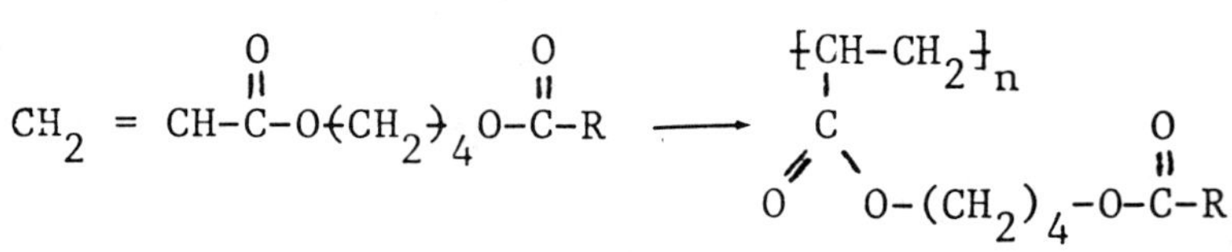

where R is

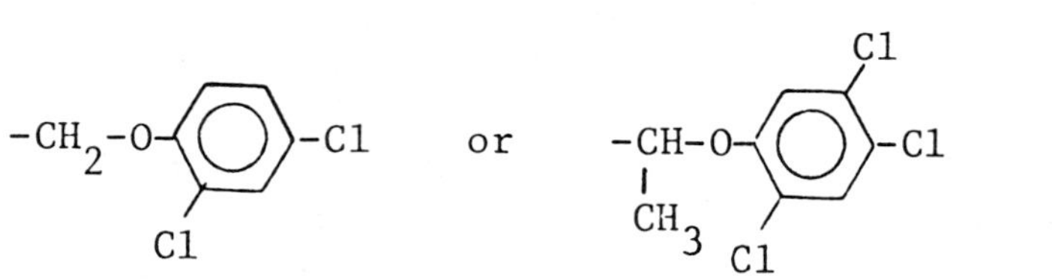

Pesticide release rates are shown in Figure 27. No hydrolysis occurs at pH 8 and 30°C when the hydrophobic polymer shown above is used. However, when a hydrophilic comonomer such as trimethylamine methacrylimide is used, slow hydrolysis of the ester groups takes place.

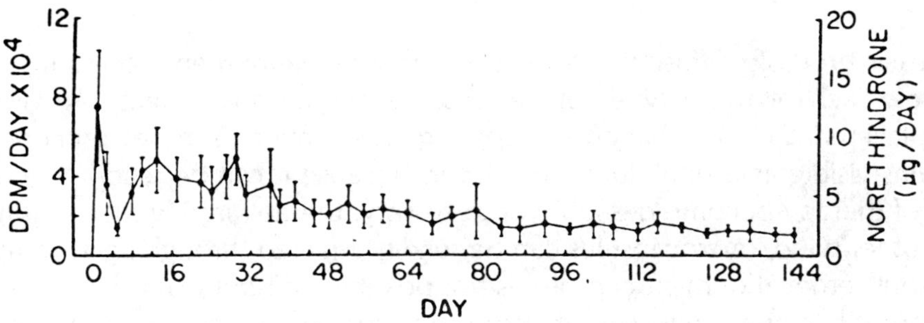

Figure 26. In vivo release of norethindrone from Polymer I. 10 mg Polymer I (4.9 mg norethindrone/2.92 × 10⁷ dpm), 5 rats average ± S. D. (Reprinted with permission from Petersen, R. V., Anderson, C. G., Fang, S. M., Gregonis, D. E., Kim, S. W., Feijen, J., Anderson, J. M. and Mitra, S., in Controlled Release of Bioactive Materials, *Baker, R. W., Ed., Academic Press, New York, 1980, p. 57).*

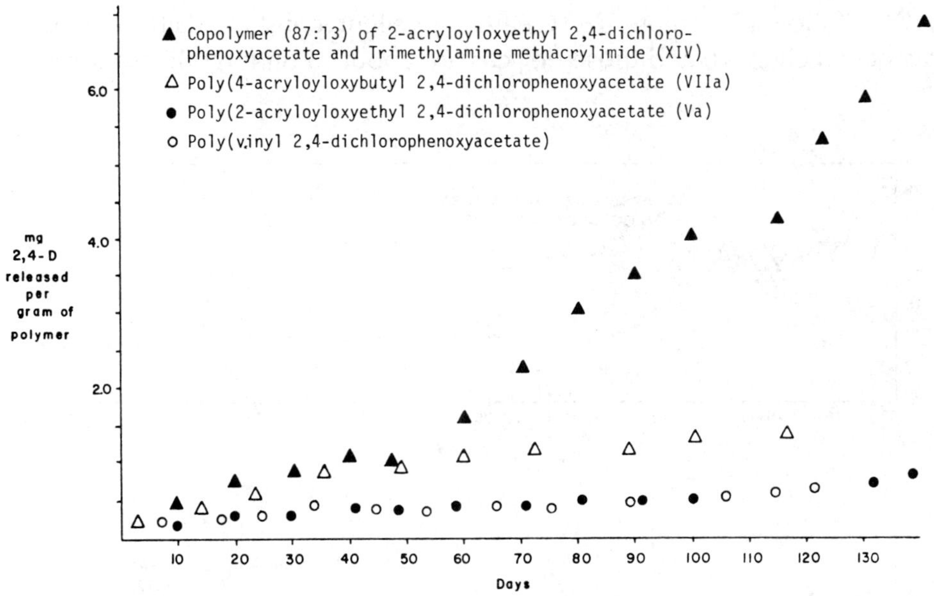

Figure 27. Hydrolysis data for pendant herbicides. (Reprinted with permission from Harris, F. W., Anlabaugh, A. E., Case, R. D., Dykes, M. K., and Feld, W. A., in Controlled Release Polymeric Formulations, *Paul, D. R., and Harris, F. W., Eds., ACS Symposium Series 33, American Chemical Society, Washington, DC, 1976, p. 226).*

Type III Erosion

Diffusional Devices. Erodible diffusional systems combine the attributes of a rate-controlling polymer membrane, which provides a constant rate of drug release from a reservoir-type device, with erodibility, which results in bioerosion and makes surgical removal of the drug-depleted device unnecessary. Because constancy of drug release demands that the bioerodible polymer membrane remain essentially unchanged during the delivery regime, significant bioerosion must not occur until after drug delivery has been completed. Thus polymer capsules will remain in the tissue for varying lengths of time after completion of therapy.

Two types of erodible diffusional devices are under development: rod-shaped inserts and microcapsules. Each of these types of devices has certain advantages and disadvantages. Subdermal placement of rod-shaped devices requires a minor surgical procedure, and the device remains visible as a small lump. However, because it can be readily removed should termination of therapy become desirable or necessary, therapy lasting many months is possible. On the other hand, microcapsules can be readily injected through an 18-gauge hypodermic needle, but retrieval of microcapsules is not possible without extensive surgical intervention. Therefore it has been suggested that the capsules be designed for relatively short term release, such as three months [32].

Major emphasis for the development of these erodible diffusional systems has been on devices that release contraceptive steroids or narcotic antagonists. The polymer systems most extensively investigated as a subdermal capsule for the release of levonorgestrel were various aliphatic polyesters and in particular poly(ε-caprolactone) [33]. The rate of release of levonorgestrel from such a device, developed by the Research Triangle Institute and named Capromor™, is shown in Figure 28. Clearly, excellent constant daily release over many months has been achieved, and those devices are about to undergo Phase II clinical testing.

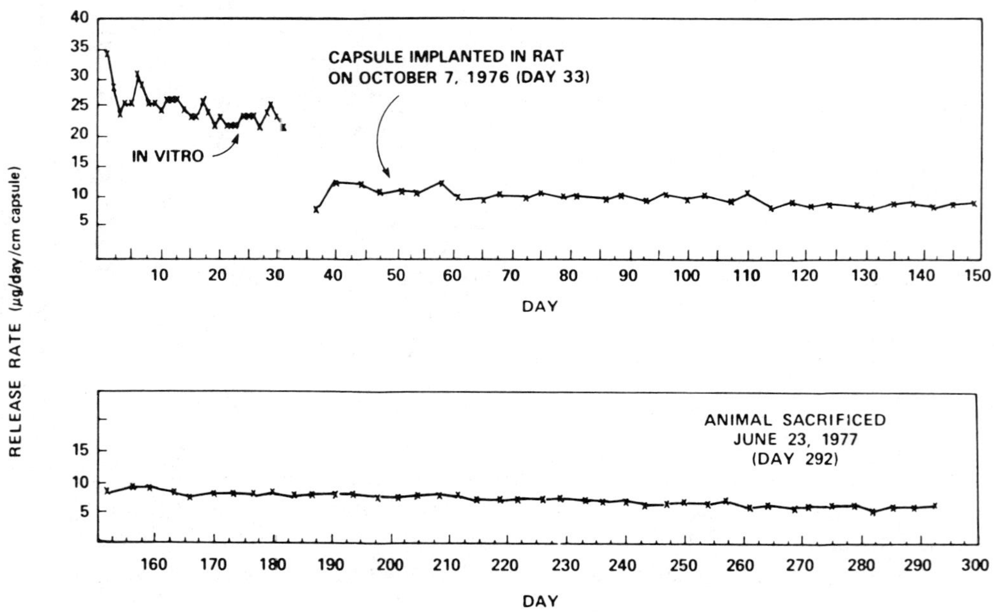

Figure 28. Daily rate of release of norgestrel from poly(ε-caprolactone) capsule implanted in rat after 32 days in vitro. *(Reprinted with permission from Pitt, C. G., Marks, T. A., and Schindler, A., in* Controlled Release of Bioactive Materials, *Baker, R. W., Ed., Academic Press, New York, 1980, p. 36).*

The polymer most actively investigated in microcapsular delivery systems is poly(DL-lactic acid), and release rate of norethindrone, measured as blood plasma level, from such microcapsules is shown in Figure 29 [34]. These data show reasonably constant blood levels

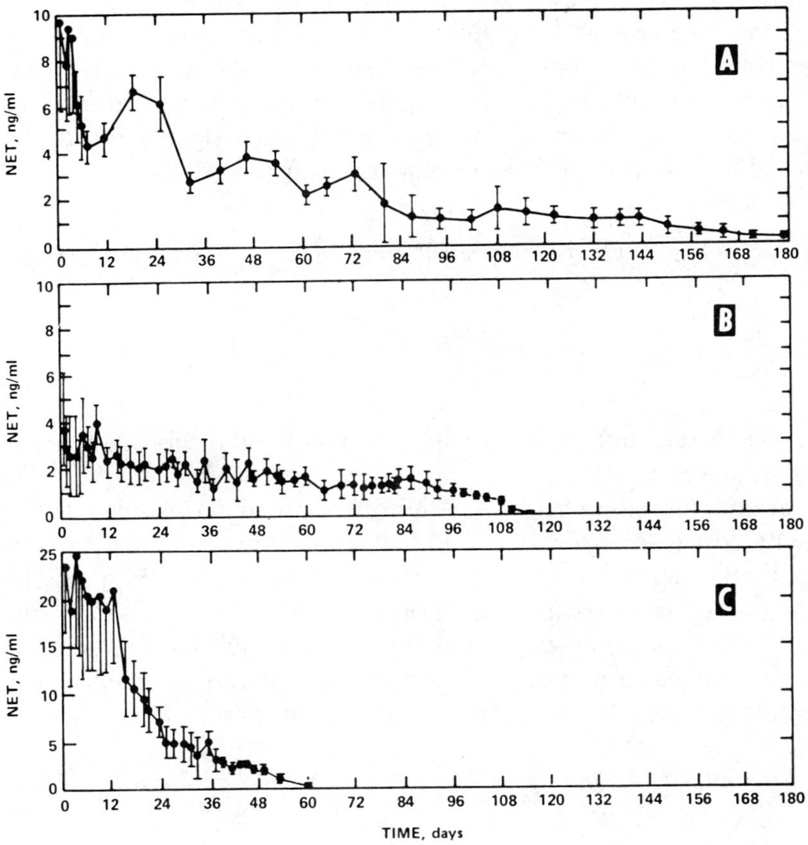

Figure 29. Baboon peripheral serum levels of immune-reactive norethisterone after intramuscular injection of 300 mg of poly(DL-lactic acid) microcapsules containing 75 mg of drug. Size of capsules are A = 10 to 240 μm, B = 65 to 124 μm, and C = 10 to 40 μm. (Reprinted with permission from Beck, L. R., Cowsar, D. R. and Lewis, D. H., in Biodegradables and Delivery Systems for Contraception, *Hafez, E. S. E., and van Os, W. A. A., Ed., G. K. Hall Medical Publishers, Boston, 1980, p. 75).*

and demonstrate that for a fixed total weight of microcapsules, rate of drug release and duration of therapy can be regulated by capsule size. Furthermore, because each capsule functions as an independent drug delivery system, the rate of drug delivery can also be regulated by variation in the total number of injected microcapsules.

Monolithic Devices. Drug release from bioerodible monolithic devices has been studied a great deal, and the majority of these studies used poly(lactic acid) or copolymers of lactic and glycolic acids [35,36]. Because these polymers undergo a bulk degradation process, drug release is controlled by a combination of diffusion and erosion. However, the relative contribution of these two factors is difficult to ascertain and varies with each particular system, so that drug release kinetics are usually not predictable or amenable to a detailed mechanistic interpretation. Nevertheless, several systems having potential for the prolonged release of various therapeutic agents, such as contraceptive steroids, narcotic antagonists, anticancer agents, and antimalarial agents, have been demonstrated [14,37].

Because poly(lactic acid) and poly(glycolic acid) were originally developed as biodegradable surgical sutures and were not intended to be used as bioerodible monolithic devices for controlled drug release, another class of polymers, poly(ortho esters), was specifically designed as monolithic matrices capable of undergoing a surface erosion process. Poly(ortho esters) were first disclosed in a series of patents assigned to the Alza Corporation and were prepared by a transesterification reaction as follows [38]:

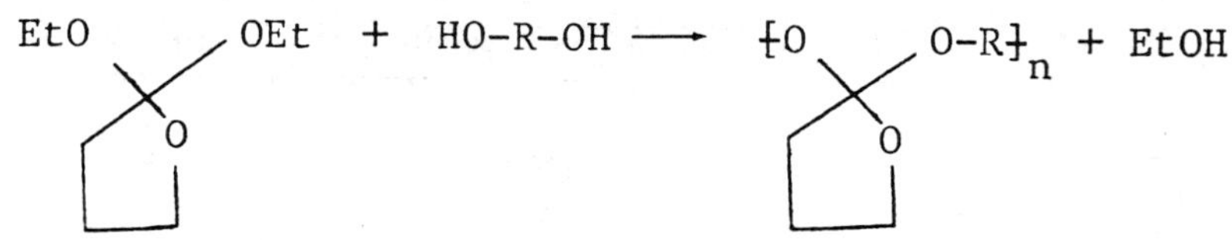

The poly(ortho ester) has not been structurally identified other than by its tradename Chronomer and later Alzamer™.

The release rate of naltrexone from an Alzamer™ polymer containing 10 wt% sodium carbonate and 20 wt% drug is shown in Figure 30 [39]. The *in vitro* release rate data show a linear release for 10 days after which the rate significantly accelerates and then rapidly declines. This behavior is not expected from a surface erosion process.

Poly(ortho esters) have also been produced by adding diols to diketene acetals [40]. Principally because of ease of monomer synthesis, polymers were prepared by adding various diols to 3,9-bis(methylene 2,4,8,10-tetraoxaspiro[5,5]undecane.

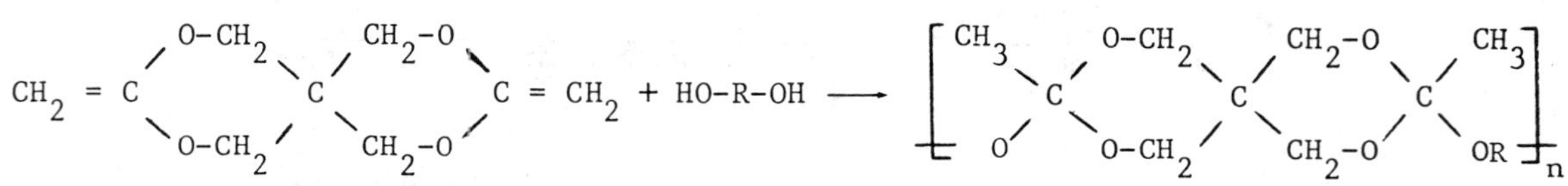

In view of the stability of poly(ortho esters) in alkaline environments, initial attempts to develop a surface-eroding system were based on the incorporation of sodium carbonate into the bulk material because of the expectation that polymer erosion would take place only at the outer surface of a solid device in which the incorporated basic salt is neutralized by the external buffer [41]. However, it was found that as a consequence of an osmotic imbibing of water caused by the incorporated water soluble salt, a swelling front develops and drug is released from the matrix by diffusion from the swollen polymer. Because poly(ortho esters) are stable in base, no erosion takes place. Nevertheless, as shown in Figure 31, a constant drug release is achieved.

The use of osmotically active neutral salts, such as sodium sulfate (also shown in Figure 31), produces a constant rate of drug release for about 60 days, after which drug release rate accelerates up to drug depletion. The number below the arrow indicates weight loss at 160 days. Clearly, polymer erosion significantly lags drug release [42]. Furthermore, the rate of drug release observed with sodium sulfate is not that expected from a simple movement of a swelling front but instead indicates that the active surface increases with time. This has been verified by noting a substantial increase in size and by scanning electron microscopy, which revealed a foam-type interior and heavy surface cratering [42].

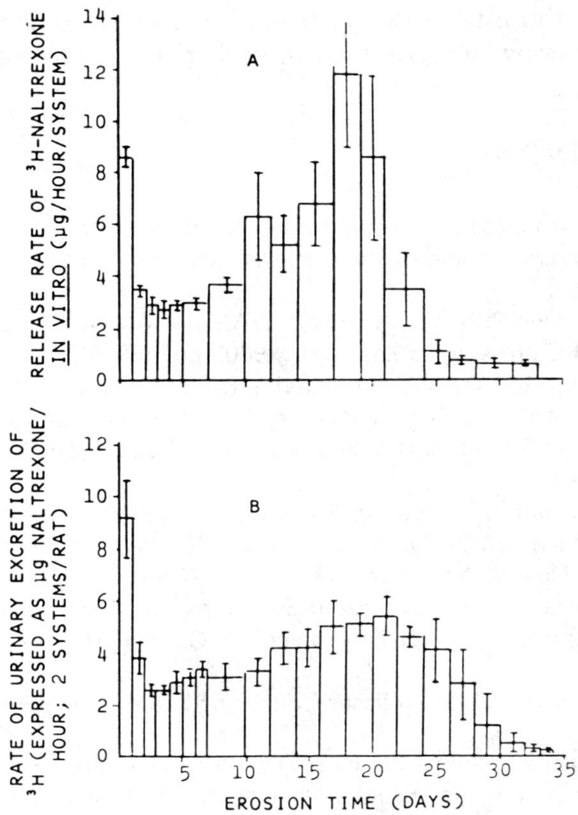

Figure 30. Rate of release of ³H-naltrexone in vitro (A) and urinary excretion of ³H in rats (B). Polymer/³H-naltrexone (20 wt%) system, rods 1 × 1 × 14 mm. (Reprinted with permission from Capozza, R. C., Sandelbeck, L., and Balkenhol, W. J., in Polymeric Delivery Systems, *Kostelnik, R. J., Eds., Gordon and Breach Science Publishers, New York, 1978, p. 65).*

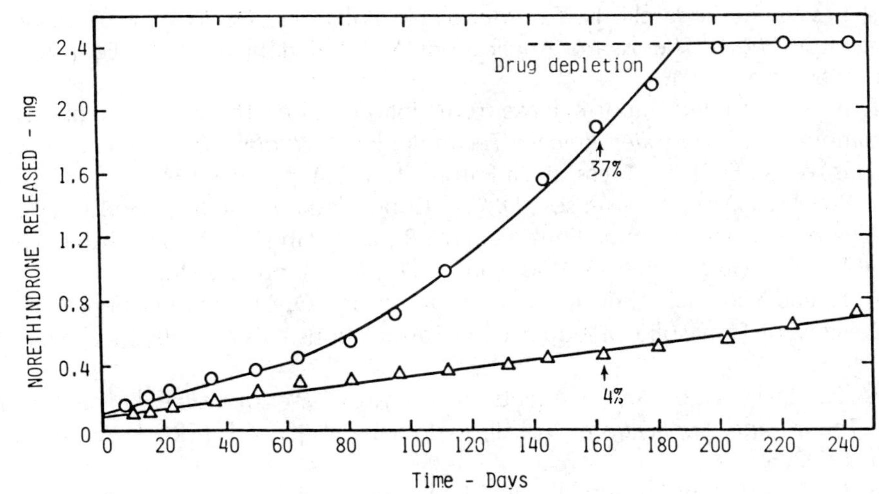

Figure 31. Norethindrone (NE) release from 3,9-bis(methylene 2,4,8,10-tetraoxaspiro[5,5]undecane)/1,6-hexane diol poly(ortho ester), 6.3-mm-diameter disks at pH 7.4 and 37°C. ○ - 10 wt% NE, 10 wt% Na_2SO_4 disk thickness 0.6 mm, total drug content 2.4 mg; Δ - 10 wt% NE, 10 wt% Na_2CO_3 disk thickness 1.2 mm, total drug content 4.0 mg.

Current work is aimed at producing poly(ortho ester) systems in which drug release and polymer erosion takes place concomitantly by using incorporated agents that are capable of lowering the pH at the polymer-water interface.

REFERENCES

1. Baker, R. W. and Lonsdale, H. K., "Controlled Release: Mechanism and Rates," in *Controlled Release of Biologically Active Agents,* Tanquary, A., C., and Lacey, R. E., Eds., (Plenum Press, New York, 1974), pp. 15-71.
2. O'Neill, W. P., "Membrane Systems," in *Controlled Release Technologies: Methods, Theory and Applications,* Vol. I, Kydonieus, A. G., Ed., (CRC Press, Boca Raton, FL, 1980), pp. 129-182.
3. Baker, R. W., Lonsdale, H. K., Tuttle, M. E., and Ayres, J. W., "Intrauterine Release of Estriol for Contraception, Part II. Device Fabrication and *In Vitro* Release Rates," in *Drug Delivery Systems, Proceedings,* Gabelnick, H. L., Ed. [U.S. Department of Health, Education and Welfare, DHEW Publication No. (NIH) 77-1238, 1976], pp. 49-78.
4. Chandrasekaran, S. K., Benson, H., and Urquhart, J., "Methods to Achieve Controlled Drug Delivery. The Biomedical Engineering Approach," in *Sustained and Controlled Release Drug Delivery Systems,* Robinson, J. R., Ed. (Marcel Dekker, New York, 1978), pp. 557-593.
5. Kydonieus, A. G., and Quisumbing, A. R., "Multilayered Laminated Structures," in *Controlled Release Technologies: Methods, Theory and Applications,* Vol. I, Kydonieus, A. G., Ed. (CRC Press, Boca Raton, FL, 1980), pp. 183-238.
6. Higuchi, T., "Rates of Release of Medicaments from Ointment Bases Containing Drugs in Suspension," *J. Pharm. Sci., 50,* 874-875 (1961).
7. Roseman, T. J., and Yalkowsky, S. H., "Importance of Solute Partitioning on the Kinetics of Drug Release from Matrix Systems," in *Controlled Release Polymeric Formulations,* Paul, D. R., and Harris, S. W., Eds. (American Chemical Society, ACS Symposium Series 33, Washington, DC, 1976), pp. 33-52.
8. Roseman, T. J., and Cardarelli, N. F., "Monolithic Polymeric Devices," in *Controlled Release Technologies: Methods, Theory and Applications,* Vol. I, Kydonieus, A. G., Ed. (CRC Press, Boca Raton, FL, 1980), pp. 21-71.
9. Brooks, T. W., "Controlled Vapor Release from Hollow Fibers: Theory and Applications with Insect Pheromones," in *Controlled Release Technologies: Methods, Theory and Applications,* Vol. II, Kydoneius, A. G., Ed. (CRC Press, Boca Raton, FL, 1980), pp. 165-193.
10. Ashare, E., Brooks, T. W., and Swenson, D. W., "Controlled Release from Hollow Fibers," in *Controlled Release Polymeric Formulations,* Paul, D. R., and Harris, F. W., Eds. (American Chemical Society, ACS Symposium Series 33, Washington, DC, 1976), pp. 273-282.
11. Theeuwes, F., and Yum, S. I., "Principles of the Design and Operation of Generic Osmotic Pumps for the Delivery of Semi-solid or Liquid Drug Formulations," *Ann. of Biomed. Eng. 4,* 343-353 (1976).
12. Theeuwes, F., "Delivery of Active Agents by Osmosis," in *Controlled Release Technologies: Methods, Theory and Applications,* Vol. II, Kydonieus, A. G., Ed. (CRC Press, Boca Raton, FL, 1980), pp. 195-205.
13. Theeuwes, F., "Elementary Osmotic Pump," *J. Pharm. Sci., 64,* 1987-1991 (1975).
14. Heller, J., "Controlled Release of Biologically Active Compounds from Bioerodible Polymers," *Biomaterials, 1,* 51-57 (1980).
15. Heller, J., and Baker, R. W., "Theory and Practice of Controlled Drug Delivery from Bioerodible Polymers," in *Controlled Release of Bioactive Materials,* Baker, R. W., Ed. (Academic Press, New York, 1980), pp. 1-17.
16. Hopfenberg, H. B., "Controlled Release from Erodible Slabs, Cylinders and Spheres," in *Controlled Release Polymeric Formulations,)* Paul, D. R., and Harris, F. W., Ed. (ACS Symposium Series 33, American Chemical Society, Washington, DC, 1976), pp. 26-32.

17. Goldman, R., Goldstein, L. and Katchalski, E., "Water Insoluble Enzyme Derivatives and Artificial Enzyme Membranes," in *Biochemical Aspects of Reactions on Solid Supports,* Stark, G. R., Ed., (Academic Press, New York, 1971), pp. 1-77.
18. Torchilin, V. P., Tishenko, E. G., Smirnov, V. N., and Chazov, E. I., "Immobilization of Enzymes in Slowly Soluble Carriers," *J. Biomed Mat. Res., 11,* 223-235 (1977).
19. Heller, J., Baker, R. W., Helwing, R. F. and Tuttle, M. E., "Controlled Release of Water-Soluble Macromolecules from Bioerodible Hydrogels," in preparation.
20. Ballard, B. E., and Nelson, E., "Prolonged-Action Pharmaceuticals," in *Remington's Pharmaceutical Science,* 15th Edition (Mack Publishing Co., Easton, PA, 1975), pp. 1618-1643.
21. Wagner, J. G., and Long, S., "Enteric Coatings III. An Improved Enteric Coating and Its In Vitro Evaluation," *J. Pharm. Sci., 49,* 121-127 (1960).
22. Lappas, L. C., and McKeehan, W., "Synthetic Polymers as Potential Enteric and Sustained-Release Coatings," *J. Pharm. Sci., 51,* 808 (1962).
23. Lappas, L. C., and McKeehan, W., "Polymeric Pharmaceutical Coatings Materials I. Preparation and Properties," *J. Pharm. Sci., 54,* 176-181 (1965)
24. Lappas, L. C., and McKeehan, W., "Polymeric Pharmaceutical Coatings Materials II. In Vivo Evaluation as Enteric Coatings," *J. Pharm. Sci., 56,* 1257-1261 (1967).
25. Wilkens, L. O., Jr., Kochhar, M. M., Bennett, D. P., and Cosgrove, E. P., "Cellulose Acetate Succinate as an Enteric Coating for Some Compressed Tablets," *J. Pharm. Sci., 51,* 484-490 (1962).
26. Heller, J., Baker, R. W., Gale, R. M., and Rodin, J. O., "Controlled Drug Release by Polymer Dissolution. I. Partial Esters of Maleic Anhydride Copolymers – Properties and Theory," *J. Appl. Polymer Sci., 22,* 1991-2009 (1978).
27. Hiatt, G. D., Mench, J. W., and Fulkerson, B., "Amination of Cellulose Acetate Chloroacetate," *Ind. Eng. Chem. Prod. Res. Develop., 3,* 295-299, (1964).
28. Mench, J. W., and Fulkerson, B., "Addition of Amines to Crotonic Acid Esters of Cellulose," *Ind. Eng. Chem. Prod. Res. Develop. 7,* 2-7 (1968).
29 Peterson, R. V., Anderson, J. M., Fang, S. M., Feijen, J., Gregonis, D. E., and Kim, S. W., "Studies of Norethindrone Covalently Bonded to Poly-N^5-(3-Hydroxypropyl)-L-Glutamine," *Polymer Preprints, 20*(2), 20-23 (1979).
30. Rowland, G. R., O'Neill, G. J., and Davies, D. A. L., "Suppression of Tumour Growth in Mice by a Drug-Antibody Conjuate Using a Novel Approach to Linkage," *Nature (London), 255,* 487-488 (1975).
31. Harris, F. W., Aulabaugh, A. E., Case, R. D., Dykes, M. K., and Feld, W. A., "Polymers Containing Pendent Herbicide Substituents: Preliminary Hydrolysis Studies," in *Controlled Release Polymeric Formuations,* Paul, D. R., and Harris, S. W., Eds. (American Chemical Society, ACS Symposium Series 33, Washington, DC, 1976), pp. 222-230.
32. Beck, L. R., Pope, V. Z., Cowsar, D. R., Lewis, D. H., and Tice, T. R., "Evaluation of a New Three-Month Injectable Contraceptive Microsphere System in Primates (Baboon)," *Contraceptive Deliv. Syst., 1,* 79-86 (1980).
33. Pitt, C. G., Marks, T. A., and Schindler, A., "Biodegradable Drug Delivery Systems Based on Aliphatic Polyesters: Application to Contraceptives and Narcotic Antagonists," in *Controlled Release of Bioactive Materials,* Baker, R. W., Ed. (Academic Press, New York, 1980), pp. 19-43.
34. Beck, L. R., Cowsar, D. R., and Lewis, D. H., "Systemic and Local Delivery of Contraceptive Steroids Using Biodegradable Microcapsules," in *Biodegradables and Delivery Systems for Contraception,* Hafez, E. S. E., and van Os, W. A. A., Eds. (G. K. Hall Medical Publishers, Boston, 1980), pp. 63-81.
35. Yolles, S., and Sartori, M. F., "Degradable Polymers for Sustained Drug Release," in *Drug Delivery Systems,* Juliano, R. L., Ed. (Oxford University Press, New York, 1980), pp. 84-111.
36. Wise, D. L., Gregory, J. B., Newberne, P. M., Bartholow, L. C., and Stanbury, J. B., "Results on Biodegradable Cylindrical Subdermal Implants for Fertility Control," in *Polymeric Delivery Systems,* Kostelnik, R. J., Ed. (Gordon and Breach Science Publishers, New York 1978), pp. 121-136.

37. Heller, J., "Drug Release from Bioerodible Systems," in *Pharmaceutical Applications of Controlled Release Drug Delivery Systems,* Langer, R. S., and Wise, D. L., Eds. (CRC Press, Boca Raton, FL), in press.
38. Choi, N. S., and Heller, J., "Drug Delivery Devices Manufactured from Poly(ortho esters) and Poly(ortho carbonates)," U.S. Patent 4,093,709 (June 6, 1978).
39. Capozza, R. W., Sendelbeck, L., and Balkenhol, J., "Preparation and Evaluation of a Bioerodible Naltrexone Delivery System," in *Polymeric Delivery Systems,* Kostelnick, J. R., Ed. (Gordon and Breach Science Publishers, New York, 1978), pp. 59-70.
40. Heller, J., Penhale, D. W. H., and Helwing, R. F., "Preparation of Poly(ortho esters) by the Reaction of Ketene Acetals and Polyols," *J. Polymer Sci., Polym. Lett., 18,* 619-624 (1980).
41. Heller, J., Penhale, D. W. H., Helwing, R. F., and Fritzinger, B. K., "Controlled Release of Steroids from Poly(ortho esters), in *Controlled Release Delivery Systems,* Roseman, T. J., and Mansdorf, S. Z., Eds. (Marcel Dekker, New York), in press.
42. Heller, J., Penhale, D. W. H., Fritzinger, B. K., Rose, J. E., and Helwing, R. F., "Controlled Release of Contraceptive Steroids from Biodegradable Poly(ortho esters)," *Contraceptive Deliv. Syst.,* in press.

Chapter 25

Magnetically Controlled Polymeric Delivery Systems

Robert Langer*†, Elazer Edelman‡ and Dean S. T. Hsieh*
**Department of Nutrition and Food Science*
Massachusetts Institute of Technology
Cambridge, Massachusetts
†Department of Surgery
Children's Hospital Medical Center
Boston, Massachusetts
‡Harvard Medical School
Boston, Massachusetts

ABSTRACT

Sustained release systems were made by incorporating powdered drug and magnetic steel beads within a polymer matrix. When exposed to aqueous medium, these polymers released the drug slowly and continuously. Application of an oscillating magnetic field caused the drug release rate to increase by as much as 30-fold. Different experimental methods of producing these matrices and of applying the magnetic fields are discussed.

Although numerous methods exist for delivery drugs from polymeric vehicles [1], all of them release these drugs at decreasing or, at best, constant rates. In the present communication, we report the development of a polymeric system capable of delivering macromolecules at increased rates on demand. By the simple technique of embedding small magnetic steel beads in the polymer along with the drug, release rates can be controlled by an oscillating external bar magnet. In this paper we discuss methods for fabricating i) polymeric slabs containing magnetic beads and ii) a hemispheric-shaped polymeric system containing an embedded magnetic ring. The former system is simpler to produce and more amenable to study. The latter system has the advantage that a nearly constant background release rate is obtained. We also report two methods of inducing an appropriate oscillating magnetic field.

METHODS OF PRODUCING MAGNETIC POLYMERIC SYSTEMS

1. Preparation of Magnetic Sustained Release Polymer Slabs

The procedure for preparing magnetic sustained release polymers was modified from our earlier methods of preparing nonmagnetic sustained release implants [2], and is shown in Figure 1. Polymer casting solution was made by dissolving ethylene-vinyl acetate copolymer [2] in methylene chloride to achieve a 10% (w/v) solution. One-half gram of powdered drug (bovine serum albumin; Sigma Chemical Co., St. Louis, MO) which had been sieved to contain particles between 149 and 210 μm, was mixed with 10 ml casting solution. The suspension was poured quickly onto a leveled glass mold (7 × 7 × 0.5 cm) which had been previously cooled by placing it on dry ice for 5 minutes. The mold remained on the dry ice throughout the procedure. Immediately following the pouring of the polymer-drug-mixture, magnetic steel beads (79.17% iron, 17% chromium, 1% carbon, 1% manganese, 1% silicone, 0.4% phosphorus, 0.4% sulfur, and 0.75% molybdenum; 1.4 mm diameter; from Ultraspherics, Inc., Marie, MI) were placed onto the mixture using a loading device.

The loading device was made of one bacterial culture petri dish (Falcon 1001, Oxnard, CA) with the bottom sitting inside the inverted lid (Figure 2a). (A rectangular-shaped device has also been used and often facilitates the bead dropping procedure). Both the bottom and the lid have an identical arrangement of 263 holes (1.8 mm diameter) with 3 mm spacing. While the plates were shifted with respect to each other such that the upper and lower holes were off-set, the upper holes were filled with magnetic steel beads (Figure 2b). The plates with magnetic beads were positioned over the polymer slab in the mold. When the plates were shifted back so that all the holes were aligned, the magnetic steel beads dropped onto the polymer in a uniform array (Figure 2c).

Two minutes after the magnetic beads were added, a top layer of polymer-drug mixture identical to the bottom layer was cast over the beads. After the entire mixture had solidified (approximately 10 minutes), the slab was transferred to a −20 °C freezer for 48 hours followed by further drying at 20 °C under a houseline vacuum (600 millitorrs) for an additional 24 hours.

The dried magnetic polymer slab was photographed to show its appearance (Figure 3a) and also exposed to x-ray to reveal the magnetic beads contained in the polymer slab (Figure 3b).

The use of low temperature casting and drying prevents migration of the drug powder [2]. The use of a 3-step procedure to embed the beads between two layers of partially fluid polymer-drug mixture provides vertical homogeneity of the beads while the device used to place the beads between polymer layers provides horizontal uniformity.

In preliminary experiments, various sizes of magnetic steel beads were embedded in the polymer slabs ranging in diameter from 0.5 to 1.4 mm. The polymer slabs containing 1.4 mm beads gave the maximum release rates of albumin. However, we do not know if this bead size will be optimal for other molecules.

2. Preparation of Magnetic Polymeric Hemispheric Devices

To achieve constant release from diffusion-controlled matrix devices, we have previously proposed that optimal results can be obtained with a hemisphere-shaped system that is laminated with an impermeable coating except for a small cavity in the center face [3]. Since

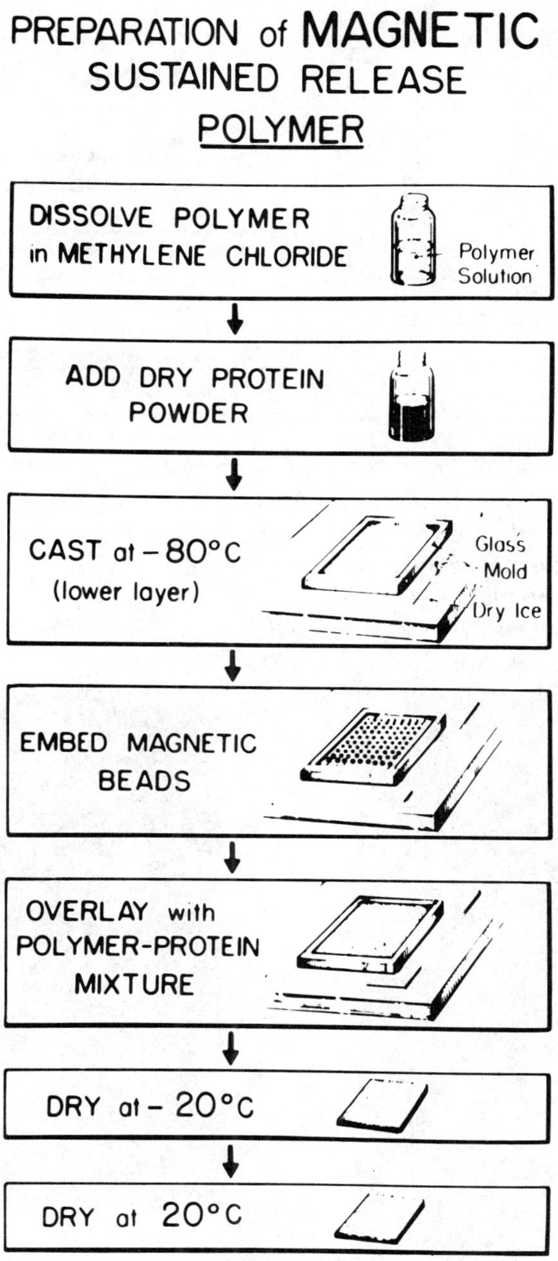

Figure 1. Flow diagram of the procedure for preparing magnetic sustained release polymers [5].

the release rate is inversely proportional to the drug diffusion distance from the release surface, the principle of altering matrix geometry is to increase the available area of drug to compensate for the increase in the drug diffusion distance. Experiments were further designed to prove the theoretical analysis and to develop simple fabrication procedures for releasing high molecular weight drugs at a constant rate [4]. This procedure was adapted as discussed below to produce a hemispheric magnetic device with a constant background release rate.

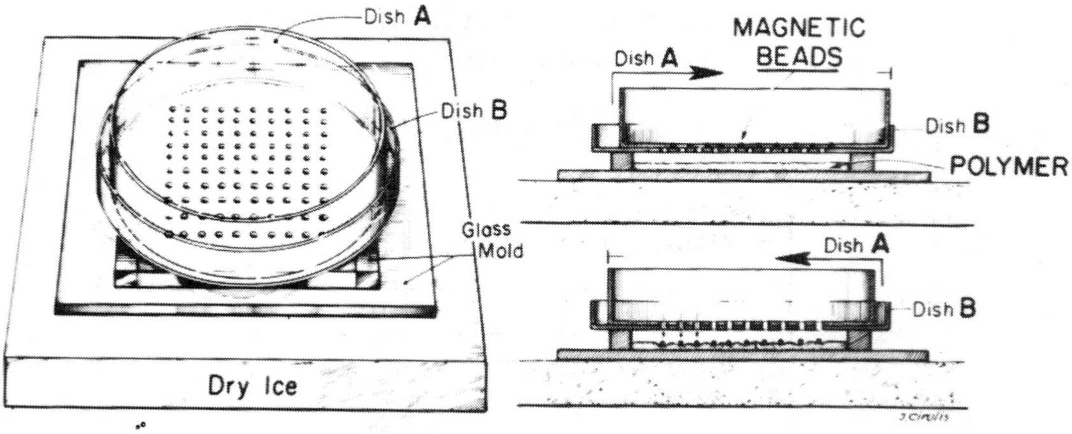

Figure 2. Diagram of a loading device and the procedures of loading magnetic beads [5]. a) Assembly of the petri dish (top and bottom) loading device, the glass mold, and dry ice. b) To load beads onto the device, the top and bottom lids are offset with respect to each other. The holes are filled with magnetic beads. As long as the lids are offset, the beads will remain in the loading device. c) To place beads onto the polymer mixture, the holes of the top and bottom lids are aligned. The magnetic beads now drop onto the polymer mixture.

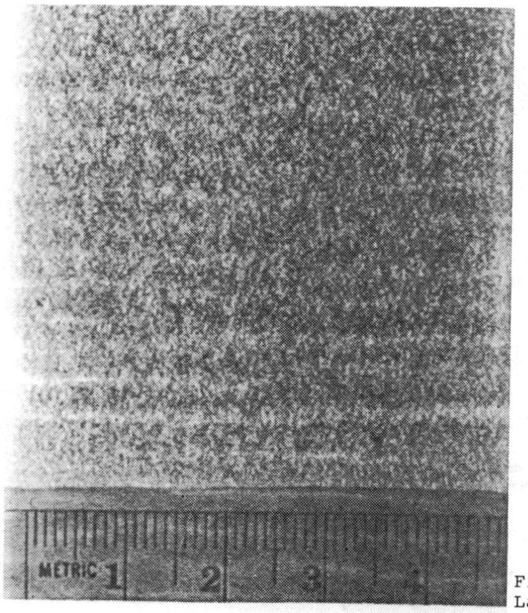

Figure 3a
Langer et al.

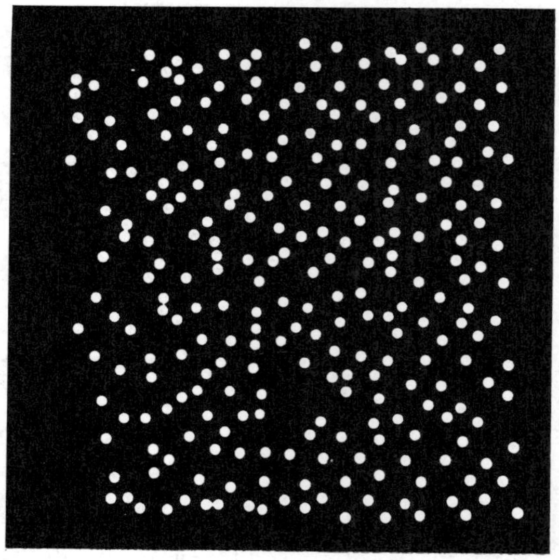

Figure 3b
Langer et al.

Figure 3. a) Photograph of a magnetic polymer slab. (magnification, 1.8×) [5]. b) X-ray photograph of a magnetic polymer slab. (magnification, 2.2×) [5].

The molds used for fabricating hemispheric magnetic devices were composed of glass and had a hemispheric bottom (13 mm diameter × 11 mm height). These molds were made from glass test tubes by cutting off the bottoms. To prevent these molds from falling over, an embedding platform was made. This platform was constructed by pouring 15 ml of molten paraffin into a bacterial petri dish, and then placing empty glass molds into the paraffin so that they touched bottom. After allowing the paraffin to harden, the molds were removed and the indentations left behind in the paraffin could be used to subsequently support the molds.

The procedure for preparing the hemispheric magnetic system was adapted from earlier procedures [2,5] and consists of four stages; (i) casting, (ii) drying, (iii) coating, and (iv) opening a cavity. The rationale for the precise procedures used (e.g., the temperatures used in the drying steps) can be found in earlier papers [2-5]. The procedure is shown schematically in Figure 4 and described in detail below.

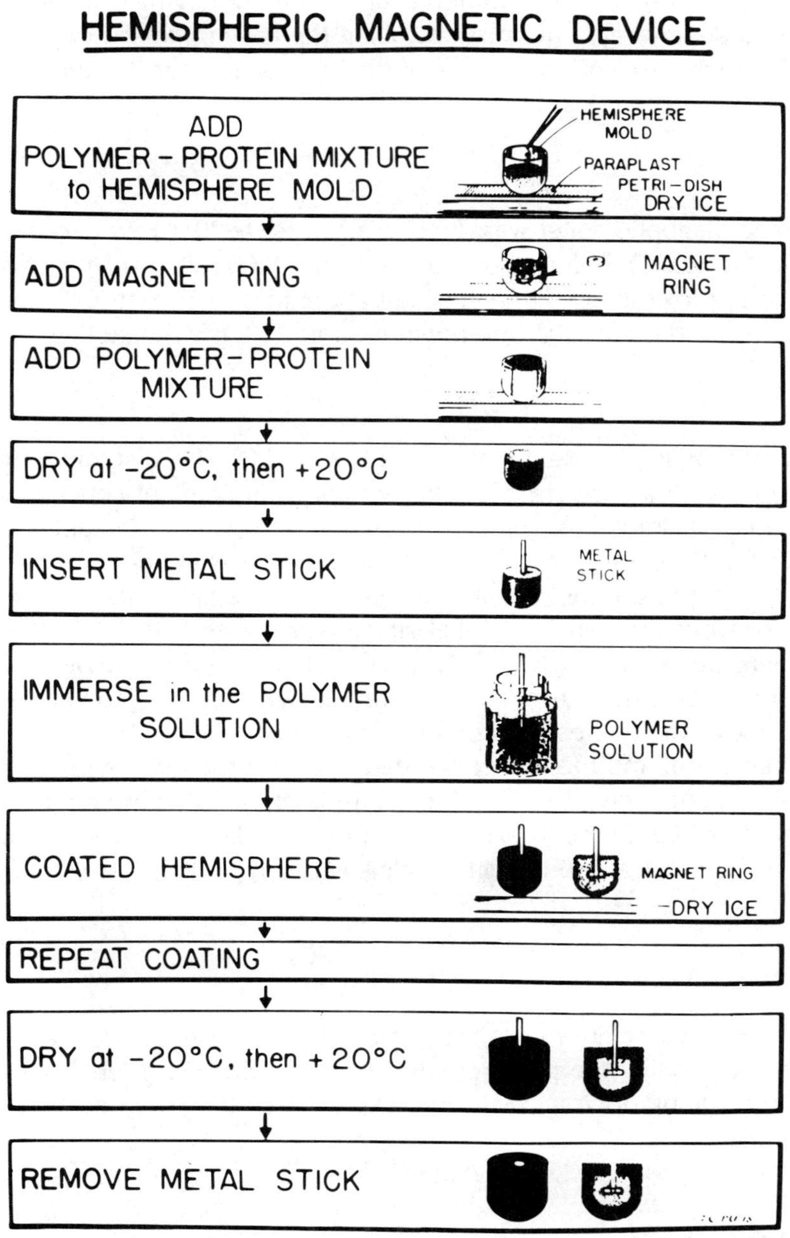

Figure 4. Procedures for making hemispheric magnetic pellets [6].

Casting

A layer of protein-polymer mixture was cast in a glass mold with a hemispheric bottom (13 mm O.D. × 11 mm I.D. × 11 mm height) placed on a block of dry-ice. The protein loading was one-third of the mixture (w/w). A single hollow cylinder magnet (3 mm O.D. × 1.5 mm I.D. × 1.5 mm height, obtained from Permag Northeast Co., Billerica, MA) was then placed in the center after waiting for one minute. Another layer of protein-polymer mixture identical to the first layer was immediately cast onto it. Controlling the casting time is important to prevent the magnet from settling out, and to assure that the two layers of protein-polymer mixture will adhere tightly.

Drying

The hemispheric magnetic pellet was dried in a freezer (−20°C) for two days followed by drying in a dessicator (20°C) under a houseline vacuum (600 millitorrs) for two days [2]. The finished pellet was approximately 6 mm in height and 8 mm in diameter. Its composition was approximately 51.5 mg protein, 103. mg polymer, and 71.6 mg magnet.

Coating

The hemispheric pellets were twice coated with 20% EVA solution (containing no macromolecules) to form an impermeable barrier. (Several coats of concentrated EVA solutions containing *no* macromolecules have been shown to form impermeable barriers [4]). The coating procedure is described as follows: (i) the tip of a cylindrical metal stick (1.8 mm diameter × 30 mm length) was inserted into the center of the flat surface of each hemisphere pellet to a depth of approximately 3 mm. (ii) Using the uninserted portion of the stick as a handle, the hemisphere pellets were placed directly on the surface of a block of dry ice for 10 minutes. (The round bottoms of the pellets were touching the dry ice.) (iii) Again using the metal stick as a handle, the cooled hemisphere was immersed into 20% EVA solution at 20°C for 10 seconds, removed, and then placed immediately on the dry ice for 10 minutes. (iv) A second layer of coating was done in the same manner as described above. (v) The hemispheres were then put in the freezer (−20°C) for two days followed by further drying at 20°C for two days in a dessicator under a houseline vacuum (600 millitorrs) to remove residual solvent [2].

Opening a Cavity

To create the exposed cavity in the face of the hemisphere pellet, the metal stick was removed by gently encircling the polymer surface immediately surrounding the stick with a scalpel-blade. The resulting polymer pellet now appears as shown schematically in Figure 5.

TRIGGERING DEVICES

Our original triggering device was modified from a commercial speed-controlled rocker (Minarik Electric Co., Los Angeles, CA) by placing a permanent magnet bar (Crucore Magnet Bar, No. RE80108, Permag Northeast Co.) on one end of the rocker and a balanced weight on the other end (Figure 6). The frequency of the motion was 18 cycles/minute. Thus,

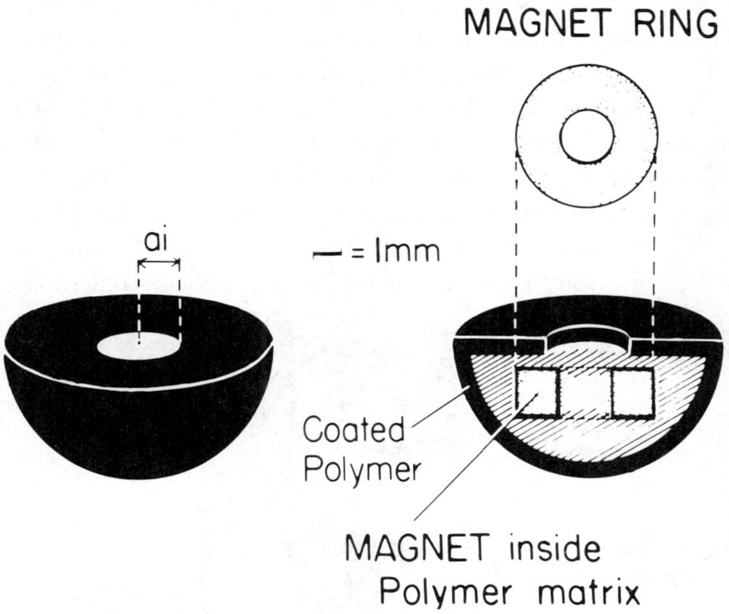

Figure 5. A schematic diagram of a hemispheric magnetic pellet. The polymer matrix was made of ethylene-vinyl acetate copolymer (Elvax® 40). All sides were coated with pure polymer except the cavity on the flat surface. Drugs were forced to release from this cavity [6].

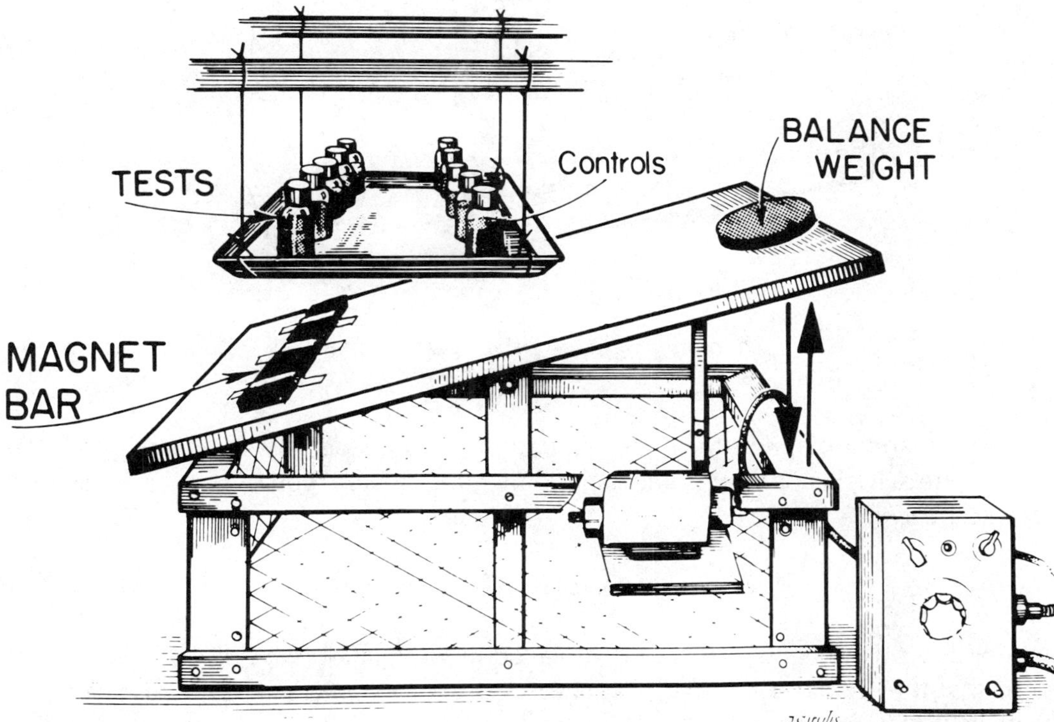

Figure 6. Diagram of a motor-driven seesaw rocker used as a triggering device [5].

an oscillating magnetic field ranging from ½ gauss (the magnetic field strength on the surface of the earth) to approximately 1,000 gauss was created for triggering.

However, this system had limitations such as limited oscillation frequency and it could only test a few samples at a time. A modified device was therefore built (Figure 7). In this device, vials were securely held in holes drilled through a ¼″ plexiglass plate below which a second plate rotated as it was driven by direct motor drive. Stronger magnets with surface field strength of 25 kilograms were employed. A motor (hp +70, 8 lb, torque 24 rpm) was used to rotate the bottom disc containing the magnets (Figure 7). Frequency was adjustable by means of a speed regulator. This system could easily accommodate 24 test vials.

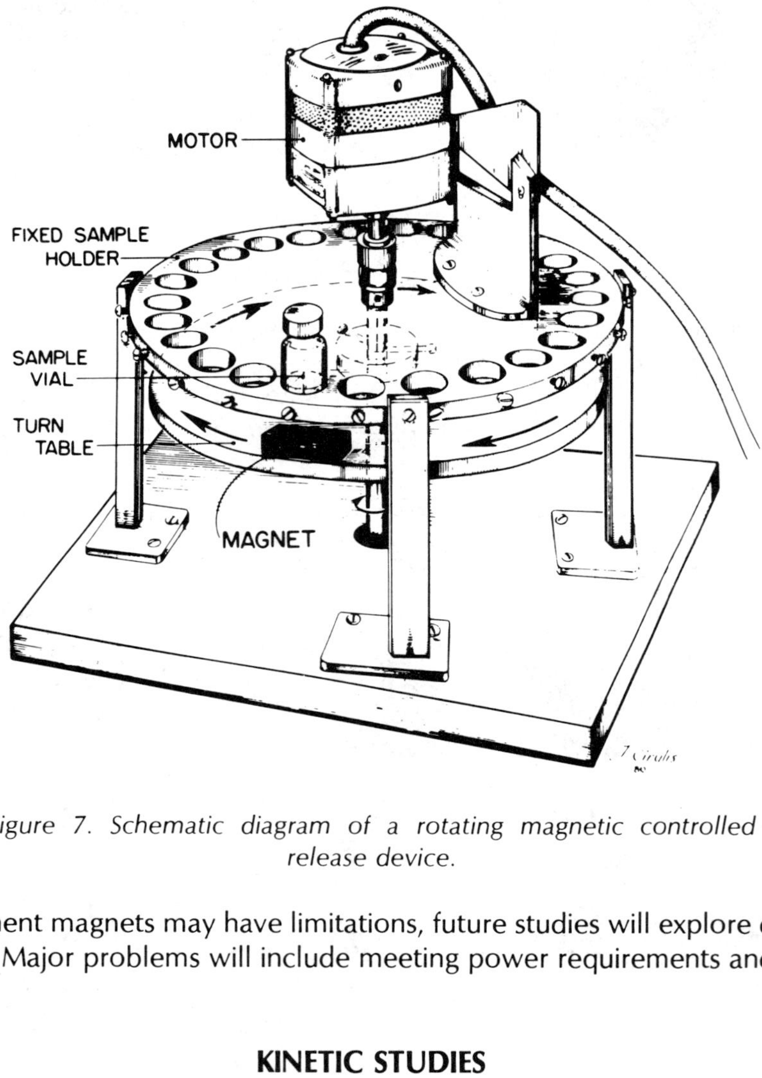

Figure 7. Schematic diagram of a rotating magnetic controlled release device.

Since permanent magnets may have limitations, future studies will explore degaussers and electromagnets. Major problems will include meeting power requirements and dissipation of generated heat.

KINETIC STUDIES

In kinetic studies, samples have been placed in scintillation vials directly [5] or they were fixed so that they could not move. The latter was accomplished by suspending a pipet [6] or polyvinyl chloride rod from the top of a scintillation vial cap and glueing the polymeric system to the base of the pipet or rod. Samples were then exposed to alternating periods of triggering and non-triggering. After each time point, the polymer system was transferred into fresh release media and the absorbance of the released solution determined spectrophotometrically [2].

RESULTS

When exposed to the oscillating magnetic field, (Figure 6) polymer slabs released up to 100% more drug than when the magnetic field was discontinued (Figure 8). For example, the first 6-hour exposure period showed an average release rate of 125 μg/hour compared to 40 μg/hour in the following 6 hours of no exposure. The differential decreased with increasing time, but was still significant at the end of the experiment (37 μg/hour versus 25 μg/hour). Numerous controls were conducted and in no case was magnetic modulation observed, including a control in which a constant 1,000 gauss magnetic field was maintained throughout the entire triggering interval [5].

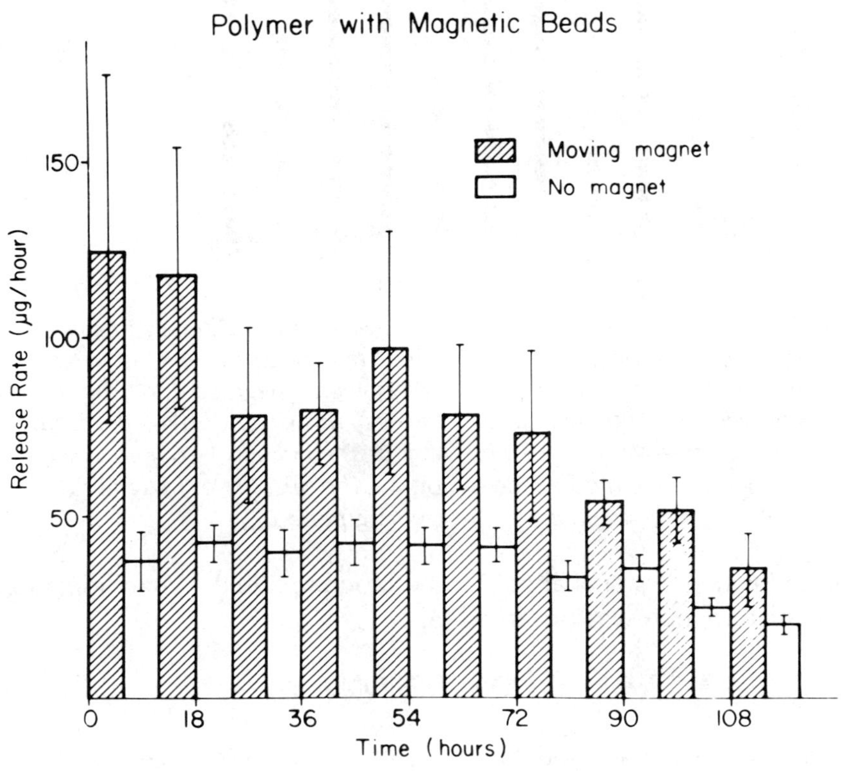

Figure 8. Modulated sustained release of bovine serum albumin (BSA) from polymeric vehicles by magnetism. Each histogram represents the average release rate of BSA from 8 polymer squares (1 cm × 1 cm) [5]. There was a 72-hour prerelease period in this experiment.

The hemispheric systems were exposed to the magnetic field (Figure 7). Bovine serum albumin was used as a model compound to demonstrate the feasibility of magnetic modulation with this design. The results showed that the average baseline release rate was 14.8

μg/hour, and the average burst of modulated release was 424.1 μg/hour (Figure 9). This represents a 29-fold increase. The systems could deliver drugs for one month and the burst of release could be repeatedly modulated when desired. Other simulated test drugs such as pepsin and insulin also showed modulated release when exposed to the magnetic field. Control hemisphere pellets which were not exposed to the magnetic field delivered drugs at a constant baseline level release rate without significant fluctuation (Figure 10).

MODULATED RELEASE OF BSA BY MAGNETISM

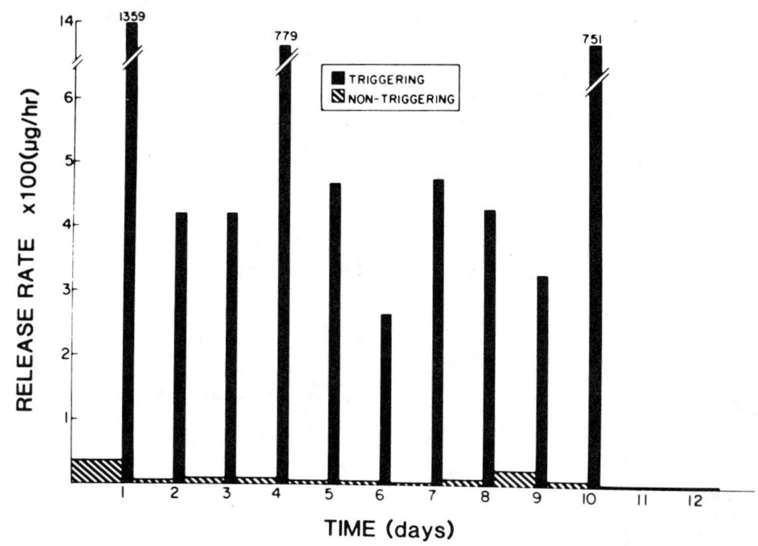

Figure 9. Magnetic modulation of bovine serum albumin released from a hemisphere pellet. Before triggering, the pellets were prereleased for one day. The pellets were triggered for 5 hours, followed by nontriggering for 19 hours. This cycle of triggering and nontriggering was repeated daily [6]. ■ The quantity of BSA released during magnetic modulation period. □ The quantity of BSA released during nontriggering period.

The magnetic polymer systems appear to be biocompatible. When implanted into rabbit corneas [7], no inflammation was observed [5].

DISCUSSION

The mechanism of magnetic modulation is not known. We have previously shown that embedded proteins form microchannels in the polymers [8]. These channels are large enough to permit macromolecular diffusion. One might speculate that the beads cause alternating compression and expansion of the channels, thereby squeezing more drug out in the presence of the magnetic field.

The major problem encountered thus far is irreproducibility both with respect to differences in release rates among different pellets within a given triggering period and among the same pellets within different triggering periods. These irreproducibilities are particularly

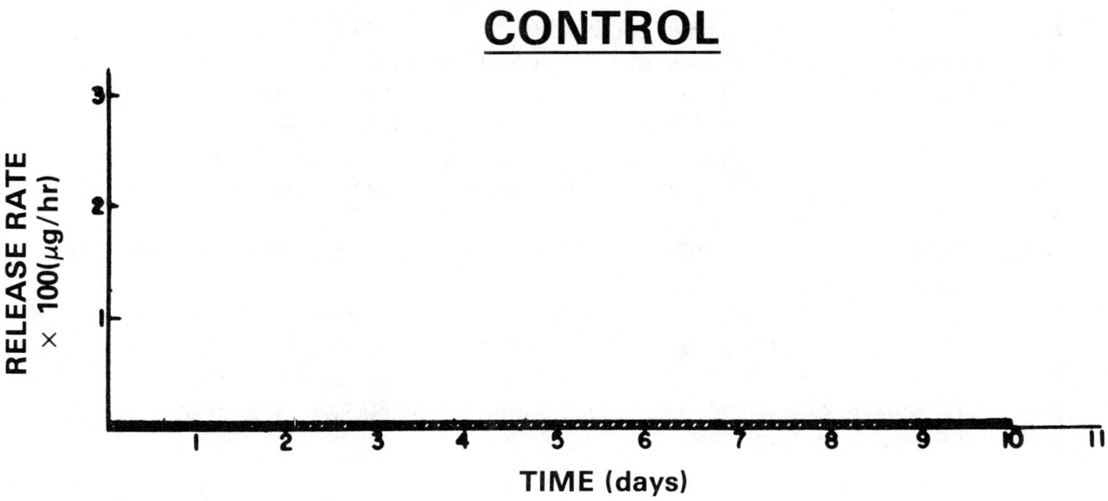

Figure 10. Control experiments for hemispheric magnetic pellets. The pellets containing BSA were prepared in the same manner as those in Figure 9. They were not exposed to magnetic triggering at all. The samples were transferred into fresh saline solution in the same intervals as those shown in Figure 9 [6].

significant in the case of the hemisphere. Possible causes leading to these irreproducibilities may result from the techniques used to open the cavity on the flat surface of the hemispheric magnetic pellets and from the inconsistencies in manipulations conducted during the magnetic modulation. Improved techniques such as computer-aided drilling may prove useful in opening the cavity; to improve the consistency of magnetic modulation, the use of a degausser may be helpful.

Modulated delivery systems controlled by external means may ultimately improve the release pattern of certain drugs such as insulin. For example, studies have shown that excellent control of blood glucose can be achieved using large pumps that infuse insulin at a constant rate, but are capable of increasing the rate before meals. We have recently shown that a pellet of ethylene-vinyl acetate copolymer containing insulin, without magnetic beads, will bring about normoglycemia in diabetic rats for one month after a single implant [9]. These pellets, though at a much earlier stage of development than pumps, contain 100-fold greater quantities of insulin per unit volume (at 50% loading by weight a 10 cc pellet contains a 10-year supply of insulin for a human) and contain no moving parts. One might speculate that with further development, insulin pellets might be implanted subcutaneously (e.g. wrist area) and triggered to release more drug by a watch-like device worn on the wrist. Modulated release systems triggered by magnetism or other means may also be useful for delivering hormones for birth control and other therapies.

REFERENCES

1. Langer, R., Controlled Drug Release Via Polymeric Delivery Systems. Chem. Eng. Commun., 6:1-48, 1980.
2. Rhine, W., Hsieh, D. S. T., and Langer, R., Polymers for Sustained Macromolecule Release: Procedures to Fabricate Reproducible Delivery Systems and Control Release Kinetics. J. Pharm. Sci., 69:265-270, 1980.
3. Rhine, W., Sukhatme, V., Hsieh, D., and Langer, R., A New Approach to Achieve Zero-Order Release Kinetics from Diffusion-Controlled Polymer Matrix Systems, in *Controlled Release of Bioactive Materials*. R. Baker Ed., New York, Academic Press, pp. 177-188, 1980.

4. Hsieh, D., Rhine, W., and Langer, R., Zero-Order Controlled Release Polymer Matrices for Micromolecules and Macromolecules. J. Pharm. Sci., in press.
5. Hsieh, D. S. T., Langer, R., and Folkman, J., Magnetic Modulation of Release of Macromolecules from Polymers. Proc. Natl. Acad. Sci. USA, 78:1863-1867, 1981.
6. Hsieh, D. S. T., and Langer, R., Zero-Order Drug Delivery Systems with Magnetic Control, in *8th International Symposium on the Controlled Release of Bioactive Materials.* Z. Mansdorf and T. J. Roseman, eds., New York, Marcel Dekker, in press.
7. Langer, R., Brem, H., and Tapper, D., Biocompatibilty of Polymeric Delivery Systems for Macromolecules. J. Biomed. Mat. Res., 15:267-277, 1981.
8. Langer, R., Rhine, W., Hsieh, D. S. T., and Bawa, R., Polymeric Delivery Systems for Macromolecules: Applications and Factors Controlling Release Kinetics in *Controlled Release of Bioactive Materials,* R. Baker, ed., New York, Academic Press, pp. 83-98, 1980.
9. Creque, H., Langer, R., and Folkman, J., One Month Sustained Release of Insulin from a Polymer Implant. Diabetes, 29:37-41, 1980

Chapter 26

Controlled Release of Bioactive Agents for The Design of Blood Compatible Polymers

James C. McRea
Research Assistant Professor of Pharmaceutics and Research Instructor of Surgery
Department of Pharmaceutics and Division of Artificial Organs

and

Sung Wan Kim
Professor of Pharmaceutics
Department of Pharmaceutics
University of Utah
Salt Lake City, Utah 84112

ABSTRACT

The ability to prevent thrombus formation on foreign surface and yet maintain normal hemostasis within the body presents a tremendous challenge. Controlled release of bioactive agents from commercially available polymers provides a novel approach towards the improvement of polymer biocompatibility. This approach allows for the design of a monolithically dispersed polymer matrix containing pharmacologically active agents which accomplishes two major goals of controlled drug delivery systems; 1) that predictable sustained release of an active agent can be maintained and, 2) that the active agent can be released at the desired site of activity at therapeutic levels while minimizing unwanted systemic effects. This chapter describes the procedures and methods for the development and evaluation of prostaglandins (PGE_1, PGD_2 and PGI_2) monolithically dispersed inhydrophobic biomedical polymers. These techniques include diffusion studies, tensile testing, thermal analysis, and infrared spectroscopy for quantitative and qualitative analyses for characterization of prostaglandin stability. Also a series of ex vivo procedures are described which evaluate biological activity.

I. INTRODUCTION

Blood bags, transfusion sets, blood filters, vascular grafts, hemodialysis and cardiopulmonary bypass circuits, extracorporeal membrane oxygenation and cardiac assist systems are prime examples of the ever-increasing use and development of devices and materials that constitute methods by which failing organ systems can be augmented or supplanted. Paradoxically, these life-saving tools can and do pose a potentially life-threatening condition of foreign-surface-induced thrombosis. Current methods of systemic anticoagulation that are used to minimize the effects of surface-induced thrombosis create an equally precarious condition, resulting in the loss of normal hemostasis.

The concept of controlled drug delivery primarily embodies two major ideas: 1) predictable, sustained release of an active agent from a properly selected polymeric material, to act as a rate-controlling device, container, or carrier, and 2) release of the active agent will occur at or near the desired site of activity [1]. Polymeric controlled release devices can be categorized into three major groups. The first group consists of those devices in which the active agent forms a core surrounded by an inert diffusional barrier (i.e., a reservoir device). The second group consists of those in which the active agent is either dissolved or dispersed within an inert diffusionable matrix (i.e., monolithic device). The third group consists of those devices in which the active agent is covalently bound to a polymeric backbone, and is released through degradation of the covalent bond, or degradation of the polymer backbone (i.e., biodegradable device), or a combination of both [2].

A dispersed monolithic system contains both dissolved and undissolved active agent within the polymer matrix. The demonstrated effectiveness of controlled release of active agents [3-5] affords several main advantages towards the problem of surface-induced thrombosis. Primarily, the active agent is released at the desired site of activity, the blood-polymer interface. Secondly, with proper design, optimum levels of agent can be released at the target site, and undesirable or toxic general systemic effects can be significantly reduced or eliminated. Finally and perhaps most importantly in the development of biocompatible polymers, a monolithically dispersed system can provide "protection" for the chemically labile structure of the bioactive agent. This is an important consideration in the use of bioactive agents such as prostaglandins.

Prostaglandins are capable of stimulating the membrane-bound adenyl cyclase of the platelet [6,7], which in turn increases intracellular levels of adenosine 3′,5′-cyclic monophosphate (cAMP). This increase in cAMP levels of the platelet has been associated with a marked decrease in platelet aggregation [8] and in the presence of higher prostaglandin concentration, inhibition of adhesion results [9]. The vessel walls of the circulatory system can synthesize PGI_2 from its own endogenous production of endoperoxide as well as from endoperoxides produced by the platelets. Thus, when an approaching platelet encountered by the endothelial surface of the vessel, prostaglandin synthetase can convert the platelet endoperoxides to PGI_2 [9]. Figure 1 schematically illustrates how this hormonal interplay between porstaglandins and the membrane-bound enzymes of the platelets can be duplicated by a monolithic, controlled release polymer at the blood-polymer interface.

Based on this rationale the three major objectives in the development of controlled release of bioactive agents (in this case, prostaglandin) for the design of a biocompatible polymer are:

1. To determine if prostaglandins can be physically combined with commercially available hydrophobic biomedical polymers, to provide a sustained release monolithic polymer system.

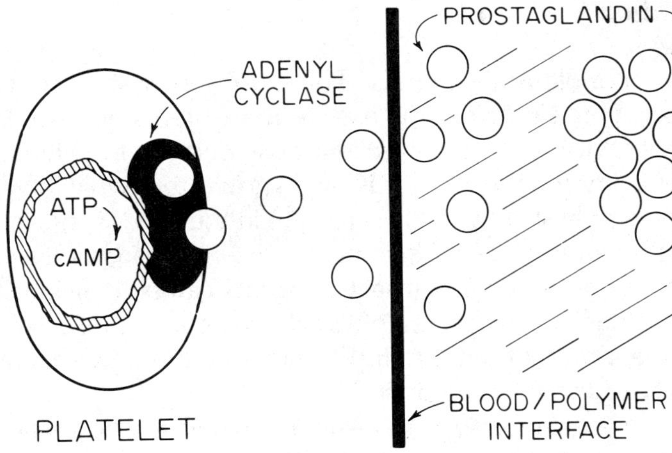

Figure 1. Controlled drug delivery at the blood-polymer interface.

2. To determine if prostaglandin chemical structure and resultant biological activity can be sufficiently stabilized in a monolithic polymer system to provide the release of a pharmacologically active agent at the blood-polymer interface.

3. Finally, to determine if monolithic prostaglandin-releasing polymer system can be utilized for the prevention of foreign-surface-induced thrombus formation.

II. MATERIALS AND METHODS

A. Materials

The hydrophobic polymers in the fabrication of the monolithic controlled release systems are poly(ether urethane), Biomer (Ethicon, Somerville, New Jersey), and a plasticized poly(vinyl chloride) (PVC), Tygon (Norton Plastics, Inc., Akron, Ohio). Biomer is received as a 30% by weight solution in N,N-dimethyl acetamide (DMAC). The Biomer solution is diluted to a 15% by weight solution in DMAC (Baker Chemical, Phillipsburg, New Jersey) and precipitated in distilled water. The precipitate can be thoroughly rinsed, patted dry, and vacuum desiccated for 12 hours at room temperature. The dried polymer precipitate can then be stored in a dry glass container and refrigerated. PVC, received as extruded tubing, can be granulated and stored in glass containers at room temperature.

Prostaglandin E, (PGE_1), prostaglandin D_2 (PGD_2), and prostaglandin I_2 (PGI_2) (The Upjohn Company, Kalamazoo, Michigan) are used as received with no attempt at further purification. Both PGE_1 and PGD_2 are provided in the acid form as a crystalline powder. PGI_2 is received as a sodium salt. All samples are best stored at −20°C in the crystalline form. Nonspecific tritiated prostaglandins (New England Nuclear, Boston, Massachusetts) were received in a water:ethanol solution. The cyclic adenosine monophosphate (cAMP) (Sigma Chemical Co., St. Louis, Missouri) is obtained in an acid form, an ammonium salt of this compound is prepared by titration with 30% ammonium hydroxide to a pH of 7.40.

B. Monolith Fabrication

As stated earlier, a monolithically dispersed drug polymer system contains an active agent physically combined within a polymer matrix. For the systems discussed, it has been established that the solvent DMAC provides excellent dissolution of the Biomer and the same apparent degree of solubility for the PVC. It is also known that while both cAMP, as well as prostaglandins, dissolve only slightly (<1 mg/100 ml) in the DMAC solvent, the use of sonication for less than five minutes (to avoid heating) results in a moderately stable suspension. In this way, dry amounts of both polymer or active agents can be individually weighed, DMAC added, and the two solutions can then be physically mixed. The mixing of the polymer solution with the active agent present tends to further stabilize the active agent suspension due to the increased viscosity of the final solution.

The mixing of an active agent suspension with a polymer solution requires care to prevent the introduction of large air bubbles into the final casting mixture. This can be accomplished by mixing with magnetic stir bars so that the surface of the suspension does not entrap air upon agitation.

Once the mixtures are thoroughly combined, they can be cast into appropriate molds. In this case, several materials may be used as mold surfaces: glass, polypropylene or polydimethyl siloxane. Since all of the active agents such as prostaglandins are heat labile, solvent extraction requires two steps. The first procedure requires placement in a circulating air oven for 6 to 10 hours at a temperature of less than 30°C. Once the polymer is properly "set," tacky though no longer fluid, it may be placed in a vacuum chamber at room temperature at 50 μm of mercury for 10 hours. Once fabricated, monoliths should be stored in sealed glass containers at room temperature.

C. Release Studies

The PGE_1, cAMP acid and cAMP as an ammonium salt have each been combined with Biomer and PVC to form monolithic polymer films. Each system contains a 10% by weight drug to polymer loading dose and is solvent cast. All samples should be handled with gloved hands or clean metal forceps, measured, weighed and placed into the release chambers.

The total volume of the elution media, 0.15 M phosphate-buffered saline (PBS), pH 7.4, is maintained for each chamber throughout the releasing period. Constant stirring at approximately 1500 rpm is used to minimize boundary layer effects at the surface of the releasing monoliths. At prescribed intervals over a test period, 50 μl samples are taken, weighed, and mixed with 10 ml of scintillation fluid and counted on a scintillation spectrometer.

Based on the known amount of radioactivity of the labeled prostaglandin within the monolith, counts of disintegrations per minute (dpm) give the amount of prostaglandin released as a function of time. Data can then be plotted as total amount released per root time, and as rate of release (mass per unit time per surface area of the monolith) as a function of root time.

D. Physical-Mechanical Properties

Mechanical properties of monolithic polymer films may be measured by means of simple tensile strength testing. Young's modulus, Y, or the elastic modulus of polymers, can be measured by the relationship Y = stress/strain, where stress is the applied force per unit area and strain is the percent elongation of the polymer sample.

E. Differential Scanning Calorimetry

This technique of thermal analysis (DuPont DTA 990 Scanning Calorimeter, DuPont, Wilmington, Delaware) may be used to determine the concentration of PGE_1 dispersed within the polymer and to further determine the solubility of PGE_1 in the polymer matrix.

Hermetically sealable pans and lids are tare weighed and partially filled with equal volumes of polymer solutions and reweighed. Varying amounts of PGE_1 are then added to the polymer solution directly, and stirred and again reweighed. The solvent is then removed, as described above and the samples are again weighed. By using this procedure, a precise percent of loading dose of the monoliths can be made. During the entire casting procedure, special care must be taken not to touch or contaminate the aluminum pans, since body oils can affect the relative heat capacity of the test samples.

At the same time that test samples are prepared, "pure" polymer and PGE_1 standards are made to provide thermographs of individual components of the monoliths to be later tested. Once all samples were prepared, the pans are hermetically sealed. A pan (containing the material to be tested) is placed on the heating element of the calorimeter adjacent to, but not touching, a similar but empty pan. The heating element was then cooled with liquid nitrogen to a temperature of $-80°C$. The element is then heated to maintain a constant temperature increase per unit time; this is plotted against changes in the amount of heat or calories required to maintain a constant temperature increase. The resultant graph indicates the relative change in the heat capacity of the material in the pan, and can indicate whether the phase transition which the material is undergoing is endothermic or exothermic, and at what temperature the transition occurs. The shape, direction, and position of endotherms describe the glass, melting, and degradation transitions of the material tested.

Once the characteristic endotherm of the "pure" standards are verified, the test samples containing various amounts of dispersed PGE_1 in polymer are tested. By plotting the known concentration of the dispersed PGE_1-polymer samples with respect to peak height change of the prostaglandin melting transition, a straight line plot can be made. The intercept of this line on the y axis (concentration of PGE_1 in the polymer) indicates the amounts of PGE_1 actually dissolved in the polymer matrix.

F. Infrared Spectroscopy

Infrared spectroscopy (Beckman Microlab™ MX620, Beckman Instruments, Inc., Irvine, California) was also used to determine the concentration of the prostaglandins within the polymer matrix. Moreover, this technique also provides structural information about the prostaglandins, which in turn can be related to activity and stability of the prostaglandins within the polymer.

Sample preparation for IR analysis is slightly modified from previous methods described. In the development of procedures to perform quantitative multicomponent IR analysis, it is important to first prepare "pure" individual component standards. This must include the polymers as well as each of the bioactive agents used.

The preparation of the polymer samples is similar to the techniques described previously;

however, since transmission IR was being used, the final films must be thinner than those used in previous analyses.

The preparation of the prostaglandin standards is accomplished by weighing out a small amount of each prostaglandin onto the NaCl disk, then adding a drop of absolute ethanol to dissolve the prostaglandin over the surface of the NaCl crystal. The high solubility (greater than 5 mg/ml) of the prostaglandin in ethanol, and the higher vapor pressure of ethanol, result in the production of a uniform glaze of prostaglandin to recrystallize over the surface of the NaCl disk. These samples are further vacuum desiccated to remove any residual ethanol from the surface.

Once the sample standards of each component of the monolithic systems are prepared, a high resolution IR scan in the range of 4000 cm^{-1} to 600 cm^{-1} may be performed on each prostaglandin and each polymer. The microprocessor controlled IR is capable of storing an entire spectrogram of each component onto a floppy disk for later spectral manipulation.

Overlays of each prostaglandin spectrogram can then be placed onto the spectrogram of each polymer to determine peaks of unique and isolated character. These peaks are then rescanned in their respective ranges from each of the "pure" standards, one wave number at a time, to determine the frequency (actual wave number) of minimum IR transmission. This is possible with the microprocessor-controlled monochrometer, which gives a digital reading of percent transmission at each wave number. Once the exact wave number of minimum transmission for each standard is established, this then becomes the "analytical frequency" for the quantitative analysis. At the same time that the analytical frequencies are determined, it is necessary to define three background frequencies. These are regions common to all spectra to be analyzed which result in IR transmission of nearly 100%. These background frequencies provide a baseline for the quantitative analysis.

It is also important to consider the linearity of the relationship between the adsorption and concentration of the components before attempting quantitative analysis. The programming of this IR system is designed to compensate for regions of nonlinearity within any absorbance versus concentration plot, by means of a zero-intercept slope-correction routine incorporated into the quantitative analysis program.

To verify the "discreteness" of the analytical frequencies of each of the individual components, a technique of computerized spectral manipulation has been employed. Even though the analytical frequencies appear at unique positions for each of the components on individual spectrograms, there was no certain method for predicting the effects of molecular interaction of the combined systems, and how they may shift or influence the analytical frequencies beyond the normal, additive effect that would be expected. To this end, a "theoretical" monolithic spectrogram was created by means of computerized spectral addition (in the appropriate portion) of the various individual spectra of the previously stored standards. These theoretical spectra result in spectra accounting for only the additive effects of absorption with no effects of molecular interaction, such as ionic interaction or hydrogen bonding. The "theoretical" spectra can then be compared to "actual" spectra of real monolithic systems, physically prepared in the same proportions as the "theoretical" spectra. This procedure verifies the uniqueness of the analytic frequencies used.

G. Monolithic Activity and Stablity Biological Assay

Inhibition of platelet aggregation, a simple procedure has been developed to assay biological activity of the prostaglandins and determine if the conditions of monolith fabrication result in degradation of the active agents.

In this procedure, Biomer and PVC monoliths dispersed PGE_1 are solvent cast directly to polydimethyl siloxane gaskets. The gaskets are then attached via pressure plates to 5.0 ml volume polycarbonate chambers, similar to a Mason cell [10]. An identical series of chambers containing prostaglandin-free polymer can be similarly prepared to serve as controls. Both sets of chambers are presoaked in PBS buffer for 2 hours at 37 °C under mild rocking agitation. Phosphate-buffered saline buffer samples are then taken from each chamber and aggregation tests performed as described by Born [11]. A 100 μl volume of the buffer is preincubated with PRP, then ADP induced to determine the activity of PGE_1 released into the buffer solution. The same procedure is performed on buffer from the control chambers.

The chambers are then filled with fresh PRP and mildly agitated for 20 minutes at 37 °C. Aliquots of PRP can be removed from the respective chambers and induced to aggregation with ADP. In this way, the extent of inhibition of aggregation imparted directly to the PRP is also measured. This technique can be used further to determine the stability of all three prostaglandins in both polymer systems as a function of storage time, when stored as monoliths in desiccated glass containers. For this evaluation all samples to be tested during the one-month period are cast and extracted at the same time. Tests should be conducted 24 hours after casting and solvent extraction, and thereafter at approximately one-week intervals, as in the tests described above.

Maximum aggregation may be determined by the increased addition of ADP to provide sustained, irreversible aggregation, whereas minimum aggregation (or maximum inhibition) is determined by preincubation of an appropriate prostaglandin solution (freshly prepared), both must be tested on the same batch of PRP, a fraction of which can be later exposed to test chambers which serve as external controls. The PRP, which is exposed to test chambers of prostaglandin-free polymers, serve as internal controls.

H. Prolongation Whole Blood Clotting Times

An evaluation of whole blood clotting time has been performed to evaluate the effect prostaglandin releasing polymers have on the formation of thrombus when exposed to bovine whole blood. This test is a modified version of the Lee-White whole blood clotting test [12].

The casting procedure for this type of study is similar to that described previously. However, during the initial solvent extraction, rotational casting must be used to provide a uniform film coating of the monoliths on the inside of the 12 × 75 mm borosilicate tubes. Tubes containing only Biomer and PVC coatings should also be prepared as controls, while uncoated glass tubes are used as standard references.

Sample tubes may be prepared 24 hours prior to testing. Each surface to be evaluated is prepared in triplicate; this includes glass references and polymer controls. All tubes are then presoaked for 20 minutes with normal saline. Bovine whole blood, collected by double syringe technique from the jugular vein is used. The soaking solution is shaken out of all tubes, 1.0 ml aliquots of blood are dispensed into each tube beginning with the glass reference, the controls, and the six monolith-coated tubes; a timer is begun upon the introduction of blood to the glass reference. A second parallel set of tubes are then filled in the same sequence as will be a third set. After five minutes, the first set of tubes are sequentially tilted (in the order of filling) at one-minute intervals. The time at which blood will no longer flow upon inversion of tube is noted and the corresponding tube of the second set is then tilted at the next one-minute interval. The entire process, noting each time at which clot formation occurs is repeated until all tubes clot.

The final clot times recorded, are by the final time of the glass reference tube. The "clotting index" thus expressed may be compared with blood tested on different days from different animals.

A useful statistical treatment of this data consists of a two-way, multi-analysis of variance [13], which indicates the significance of contribution of the prostaglandins and the polymers to changes in clot time, individually and in combination.

I. Evaluation of Adhesion Versus Aggregation Effects

The effects of prostaglandin E_1 and I_2 released from a PVC monolith on platelet adhesion and aggregation, have been evaluated in bovine whole blood by exposure to releasing monolithic polymers and their respective control surfaces.

To evaluate the effects of releasing monoliths at the blood-polymer surface interface (interfacial dosing effects), the test cell and method of Olijslager [14] have been used. This test cell consists of two polymer coated glass slides positioned between a silicone rubber gasket to provide a uniform blood-flow channel with both polymer surfaces exposed to blood perfusing under controlled hemodynamic conditions. A single prostaglandin-releasing test cell consists of two coated slides juxtapositioned to form a blood channel (1 mm $\times$ 3 mm) while an identical control test cell consists of two nonreleasing PVC surfaces.

The PGE_1 test cells with their respective controls are assembled and primed with isotonic phosphate buffer (pH 7.4) solution and allowed to hydrate for 10 minutes prior to whole-blood perfusion. The PGI_2 test cells with respective controls were allowed to hydrate in Tris-buffer with 5% dextrose (pH 8.69 at 25 °C) to insure the stability of the released prostaglandin I_2 for further assaying.

Blood is perfused through the test cells with a Harvard infusion syringe pump at room temperature and at a flow rate of 2.5 ml/min. All fractions of the isotonic buffers used to hydrate the test cells are collected and tested via ADP induced aggregation on PRP to verify the antiaggregatory activity of any released prostaglandins. Sequential 10 ml whole blood samples, perfused through the test cels, are also collected upon exiting the test cells from which PRP and PPP fractions are also prepared for determination of any inhibitory activity of aggregation imparted directly to the platelets.

Following a 20 ml volume of whole blood perfusion, the cells are immediately flushed with 20 ml of the appropriate buffer, of which the last 1.0 ml is collected and evaluated for prostaglandin activity by aggregation of PRP. The cells are then perfused with 10 ml of 2.0% glutaraldehyde in PBS (pH 7.4) for one hour, to fix adhering platelets. The test cells are alternately rinsed with fresh glutaraldehyde solution and distilled water. The test cells can then be disassembled and the blood-contacting surfaces air-dried and stained with 0.2% cresyl violet acetate. The number of adhering platelets per unit surface area are then counted over predesignated sites throughout the entire area of the exposed surface of each slide. Platelets are easily counted via visible light microscopy at 600$\times$ magnification.

III. RESULTS AND DISCUSSION

A. Release from Monolithic Systems

The plotting of release rates (Figure 2), rate of release per unit area against time in days, discerns the burst effect typical of monolithic systems. It can be seen in Figure 2, that while PVC-cAMP acid and Biomer-PGE_1 systems demonstrate release rates of 201.0 and 67.0 μg/hr/cm², respectively, the three remaining monoliths also indicate initial high rates of release, though for shorter duration. However, all systems eventually achieve steady state release conditions of approximately the same order of magnitude, 1.50 to 8.50 μg/hr/cm² by the end of the first 48-hour period.

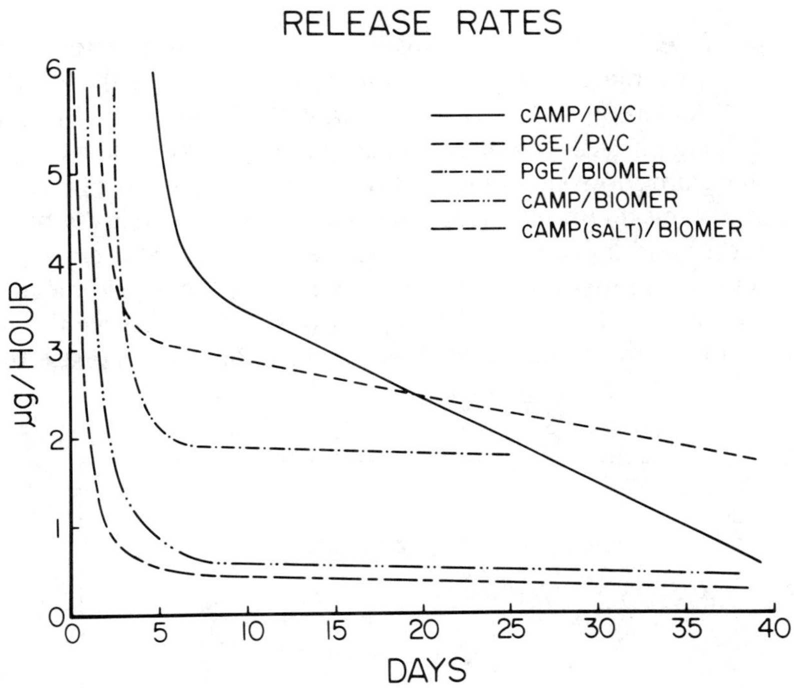

Figure 2. Rate of release of active agents versus time.

On the basis of a gross visual examination, the only samples to show an obvious physical difference (a higher degree of opacity) from control samples of agent-free polymer disks have been the PVC-cAMP acid and the Biomer-PGE_1 monolith systems, both of which demonstrate greater burst effect release character. The remaining monolithic systems of PVC-PGE_1, Biomer-cAMP acid, and Biomer-cAMP salt, show no gross change in physical appearance in comparison to polymer controls. This suggests that the dispersed agents in these latter three monolithic systems may achieve a greater degree of dissolution within the polymer matrix, thus supporting the tenet that the release mechanism of these monoliths is more diffusionally controlled at an earlier period, rather than by a dissolutional process of dispersed particles at the surface, as would be evidenced by a large burst effect.

B. Differential Scanning Calorimetry

The determination of the solubility of a dispersed agent in the polymer matrix, can be empirically determined by a separate experiment. This procedure involves placing an agent-free sample of the polymer matrix into a supersaturated solution of the agent and allowing the polymer to equilibrate absorption of the agent from the saturated aqueous solution. However, in the case of prostaglandin releasing polymers this procedure is prohibitive for two major reasons, the first being that the stability of the prostaglandins in aqueous solution at the temperatures required for equilibrium to be established is too low. The possibility of measuring the solubility of the PGE_1 degradation product rather than that of PGE_1 itself was more likely. Secondly, the availability of adequate amounts of PGE_1 required to create the necessary saturated solutions is cost prohibitive. For these reasons, the use of differential scanning calorimetry has been used as a method for determining the solubility of PGE_1 in the polymer matrix.

With the use of DSC, it is not only possible to determine the solubility of a drug in a polymer; it is also possible to obtain the total concentration of the dispersed drug in the polymer matrix [15], determine the purity of drugs to be dispersed [16] as well as make assessments regarding physical-chemical changes in the polymer matrix itself [16,17]. A composite DSC thermogram shown in Figure 3 provides an example of how this method has been applied. The y axis of this thermogram represents the relative heat flow where downward is an endothermic process and upward along this axis describes an exothermic process, both with respect to the rate of temperature change shown along the x axis. Since the temperature change is held at a constant rate (20°C/min.), it is possible to observe the relative change in the heat capacity of the material heated. This indicates the various phase transitions that occur.

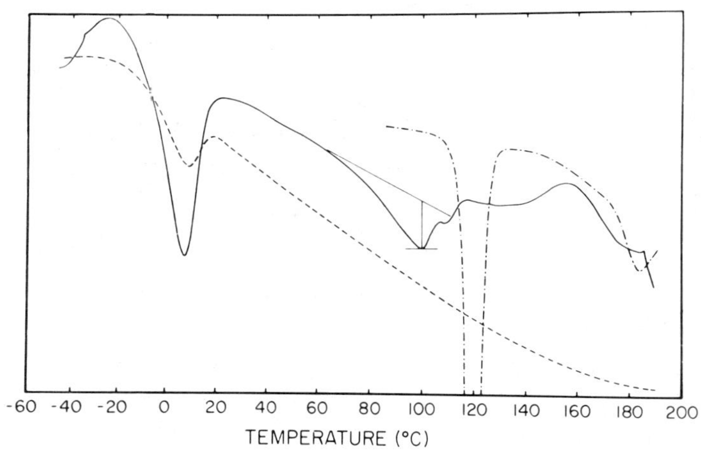

Figure 3. Differential scanning calorimetry (DSC) for determining solubility of prostaglandin E_1 in Biomer by phase transition changes of active agent within polymer.

The dashed and dotted lines indicate the melting transition of PGE_1 when tested alone. This is verified by data on the melting point of PGE_1 (115-116°F) provided by the manufacturer [18].

The steepness of the endotherm (the abrupt change from baseline to the downward descent of the endotherm) is an indication of the purity of the compound being tested [19]. The endotherm ideally should be a single, straight line perpendicular to the x axis. In the case of the Biomer thermogram represented by the dashed line, the endotherm is broader and is not as steep in its descent of the Tg (glass transition) endotherm. This would be expected of a block copolymer since its Tg value becomes an intermediate value of the individual block copolymer segments present [17]. However, this Tg can still be determined and will be discussed below.

Once the individual components of the monolith are characterized, a series of monoliths of known concentrations ranging from 5% to 25% by weight of prostaglandin-Biomer, are evaluated by scanning calorimetry. The results of a monolith thermogram are shown in Figure 3 by the solid line. The major characteristics of this thermogram are the enhanced Tg endotherm of the Biomer and the greatly reduced and left shift of the PGE_1 T_m endotherm. The Biomer Tg endotherm can be explained in a relatively straightforward way from the free-volume concept described by Struik [16]. This basically states that the free volume is reduced when the internal energy of the polymer is lost. The presence of the dispersed prostaglandin within the polymer matrix could result in the loss of free volume, requiring an absorption of energy (endothermic) to achieve the glass transition at the same temperature. Though this effect has been noted at all concentrations of monoliths, no apparent relationship between the Tg peak height change and the concentration of PGE_1 in Biomer has been developed.

In the case of PGE_1 and T_m endotherm, a reliable and linear relationship can be made between the concentration of PGE_1 in Biomer and peak height of the new PGE_1 T_m endotherm, as seen on the solid line thermogram of Figure 3. Peak height was simply measured by extending the baseline portion of the thermogram beyond the T_m endotherm and drawing a perpendicular at the endotherm minimum. The point at which the extended baseline and the perpendicular intersect at the point of the minimum defines the peak height.

By varying the concentration of the monoliths tested and measuring the peak height of the PGE_1 T_m endotherm, as described above, a calibration curve can be made (Figure 4). A least-mean squares linear regression treatment of the data describes a slope of 0.76, with a coefficient of determination, $r_2 = 0.97$. The intercept of the plot represents the solubility of the PGE_1 in Biomer, C_s, where C_s = 0.80% by weight PGE_1-Biomer.

As mentioned above, the purity of the individual monolith components can be determined from the steepness of the respective endotherm on any particular thermogram. An example of the usefulness of this knowledge is seen in Figure 5. This shows the thermogram of a "pure" PGI_2 sample as received from the manufacturer. The PGI_2 is the most labile of the prostaglandins used. The melting point of this compound is reported by the manufacturer as 163-166°C. By examining the thermogram in Figure 5, a broad, small endothermic peak is seen in this approximate region. However, a more apparent endotherm is observed somewhat left of the expected PGI_2 T_m endotherm. This larger endotherm, when properly measured (as indicated by the dashed line extended from the baseline of the thermogram and another from the slope of the endotherm, with a perpendicular drawn at the intersection to the temperature on the x axis), indicates a transition temperature which corresponds to the upper melting point range of 6-keto-$PGF_{1\alpha}$, (60-105°C), the known degradation product of PGI_2. The wide ranging melting point is attributed to the hemiketal hydroxy ketone equilibrum expected for 1,4-hydroxy ketones [20]. This result indicates the need for alternate methods for determining activity of prostaglandin (and relative purity) and are discussed below.

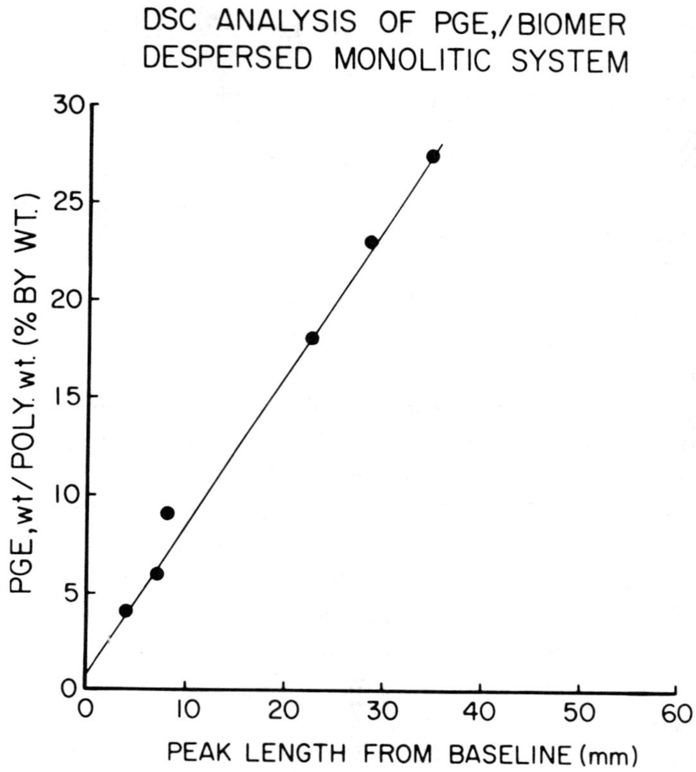

Figure 4. Linear regression plot of differential scanning calorimetry data; weight percent (drug-polymer) versus peak height change in melting point transition of prostaglandin E_1 endotherm.

C. Tensile Testing

Another method used to determine the effect that a dispersed prostaglandin may have on the polymer matrix is tensile testing. Table 1 gives a summary of the results of this study. It can be seen that the Biomer monoliths are not significantly different from the control values of the Young's modulus.

Table 1. Moduli of Dispersed Monolithic Polymers

	Biomer (polyether urethane)	Tygon (polyvinyl chloride)
With PGE_1 before release	4.33 ± 0.25	5.25 ± 0.51
Control PGE_1 free	4.20 ± 0.41	5.32 ± 0.25

Units 10^5 dynes/cm^2
N = 6 for each value

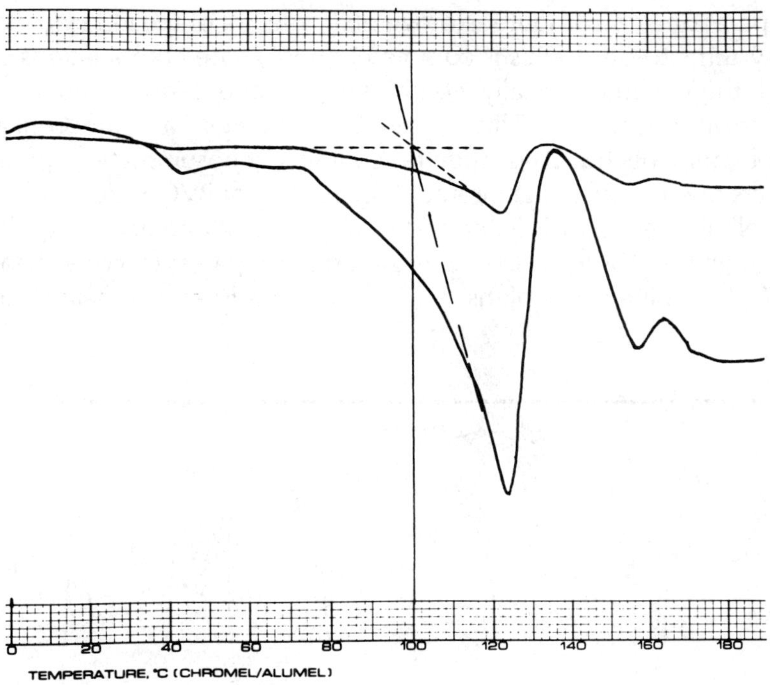

Figure 5. Example of prostaglandin I_2 impurity determined by differential scanning calorimetry from broad endothermic peak at melting point transition. Solid perpendicular line at approximately 100°C indicates true melting point as determined by intercept of dashed lines.

At best, this type of information gives only a gross comparison of mechanical strength changes. Also, as with the case of DSC, both analytical techniques are destructive. Further, the application of DSC does not prove useful when determining the concentration of dispersed agents in polymers such as PVC, due to the high plasticizer concentration. This indicates the use of other, more direct and nondestructive analytical procedures.

D. Infrared Spectroscopy

Multicomponent IR analysis has been attempted as a nondestructive analytical method for the study of molecular interactions of the monolithic prostaglandin-polymer systems, as well as determination of the prostaglandin's biological stability within the polymer matrix. These studies are now possible with the use of a computer-controlled IR spectrophotometers which afford spectral data storage and manipulation capacities.

Qualitative analysis is conducted to substantiate the indications from release study results which suggest that PVC-prostaglandin monolithic systems may have greater molecular interaction between individual components, than do those of the Biomer-prostaglandin monoliths. A simple procedure to test this hypothesis, based on Beers Law of Additivity of Absorbances [21], may be used. Essentially, this law states that given that no molecular interactions exist between two molecular species within the observed system, their respective absorbances should be the simple sum of the individual components, or simply additive.

After the preparation and computer storage of all spectra of the individual components for the monolithic systems to be studies is complete, appropriate combinations can be recalled, normalized, and then mathematically combined [22] and reproduced by the computer-controlled spectrophotometer. This process produces a "theoretical" monolithic prostaglandin-polymer spectra. This spectra contains the summation of all absorbances without any effects due to molecular interactions. Spectra of PVC added with PGE_1 alone, and PGI_2 alone, as well as spectra of Biomer added with PGE_1 alone and PGI_2 alone, have been "created" in this manner. These spectra can then be compared to corresponding spectra of "actual" physically combined monoliths which have also been normalized for comparative reasons.

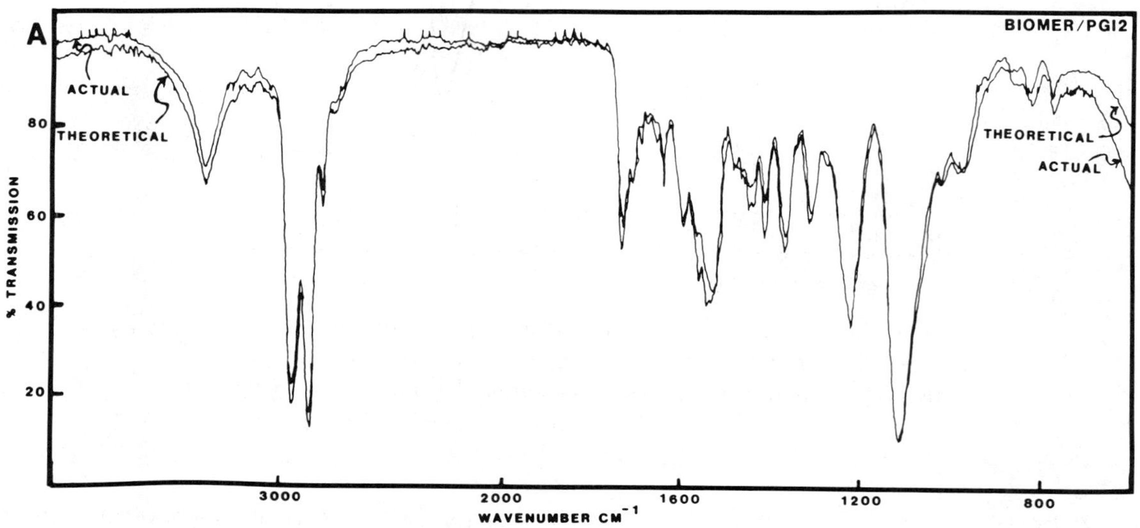

Figure 6A. Infrared spectroscopy of Biomer-prostaglandin I_2 monolithic system, both actual spectra and computer predicted theoretical spectra.

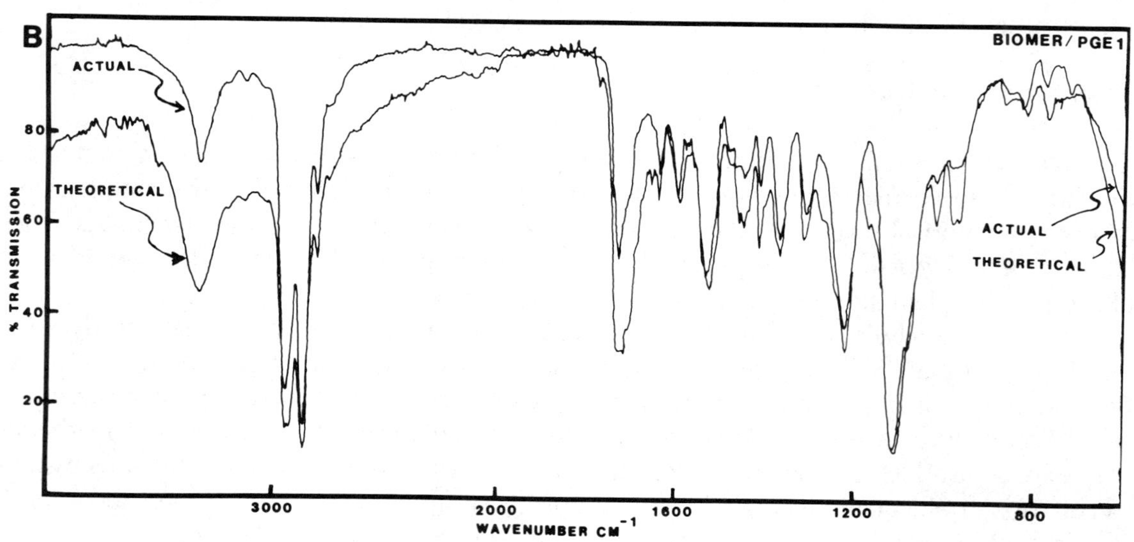

Figure 6B. Infrared spectrascopy of Biomer-prostaglandin E_1 monolithic system, both actual spectra and computer predicted theoretical spectra.

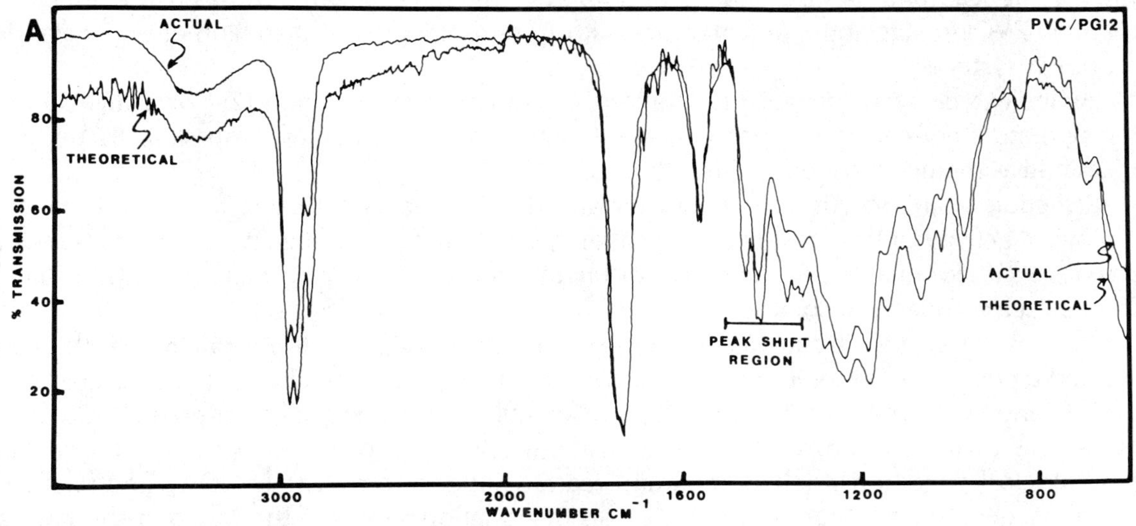

Figure 7A. Infrared spectroscopy of polyvinyl chloride-prostaglandin I_2 monolithic system, both actual spectra and computer predicted theoretical.

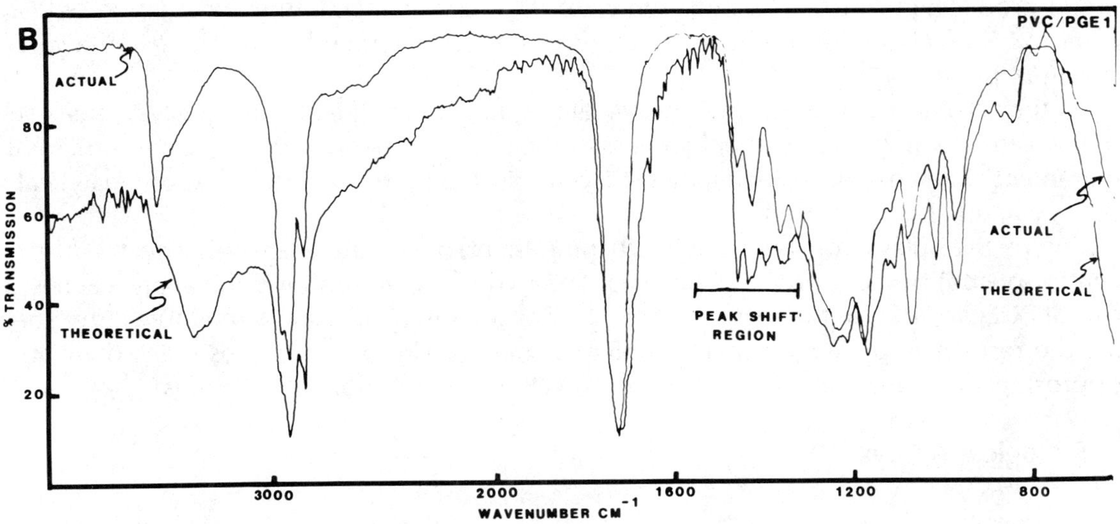

Figure 7B. Infrared spectroscopy of polyvinyl chloride-prostaglandin E_1 monolithic system, both actual spectra and computer predicted theoretical spectra.

The results of comparing the "theoretical" monolithic spectra to the "actual" monolithic spectra are shown in Figure 6 and 7. Figure 6A shows the "actual" and "theoretical" spectra of the PGE_1-Biomer monolith. Figure 6B shows the same for the PGI_2-Biomer monolith. It can be seen that even though the spectra does not fit exactly (due to effects of the normalization of spectra), all peaks occur at the same wave number, and all peaks achieve the same peak height relative to those of the same spectra. However, in Figures 7A and 7B, (the PVC monolith counterparts to the Biomer monoliths) there is much greater discrepancy between the "theoretical" and "actual" spectra of both systems, suggesting that molecular interactions found in PVC-prostaglandin polymer monolith systems are greater than Biomer-prostaglandin monolith systems.

As indicated above proper preparation [23,24] and determination [25] of analytical and background frequencies of appropriate reference standards makes it possible to perform quantitative multicomponent analysis [26].

Selection of an analytical frequency produced by molecular structure associated with the biological activity of the prostaglandins studied, is helpful for determination of stability, but is not necessary for quantitative analysis. Fortunately, in this case analytical frequencies resulting from structure related to biological activity have been found and used.

The loss of an OH group on the number 11 carbon [27] and the formation of the conjugated diene of the 5 member ring, describes the major structural change in the degradation of PGE_1 and PGB_1. The sensitivity of PGE_1 to even mildly acidic or alkaline conditions or oxidizing agents (even air) can result in isomerization, epimerization, or primarily in the case of physiological conditions, dehydration and rearrangement from PGE_1 to PGA_1, and finally to the more energetically stable PGB_1 [27]. This degradation results in the loss of a shoulder at 3522 cm^{-1} on the IR spectra, and is used as the analytical frequency of PGE_1.

Structural changes resulting in the loss of antiaggregatory activity of PGI_2 occur during acid catalyzed hydrolysis of the cyclopentanone ring and tautomerization of the 6-carbon hydroxy group producing 6-keto $PGF_{1\alpha}$ [28]. The chief structural change in the degradation of PGI_2 to 6-keto $PGF_{1\alpha}$ is characterized by the opening of the cyclic enol ether, resulting in the loss of a strong IR peak at 1563 cm^{-1}.

In the selection of the polymer analytical frequencies for quantitative analysis, peak selection was made on the basis of uniqueness of the peak's position and not on any structural requirement. The analytical frequency for Biomer is 1117 cm^{-1}, and for PVC an analytical frequency at 1429 cm^{-1} is used.

Figure 8 displays the resultant multicomponent quantitative analysis spectra (the four center spectra) of the monolithic systems. The two top spectra shows the analytical frequencies of PGE_1 and PGI_2 in the regions where they occur. On either side of the four center spectra are the respective prostaglandin-free polymer spectra. This demonstrates the "isolate-ability" of prostaglandin analytical frequencies in multicomponent monolith systems.

E. Biological Assays

The results of direct biological assays have been evaluated on a similar series of polymers as described in the IR analysis.

Part A of Figure 9 shows the stability of PGE_1, PGD_2, and PGI_2 dispersed in Biomer during a one-month period. It can be seen that the same level of activity is maintained, 75% to 80% inhibition of ADP-induced aggregation of the PRP that was exposed directly to the test monoliths. The control polymer demonstrates an inexplicably high inhibitory activity on the first day of testing, dropping rapidly, however, by the second test day. However, when a 50-μl aliquot of the presoaking buffer is taken and added to an external PRP control (PRP not exposed to the monoliths), as can be seen in Figure 9C, it is evident that the PGI_2 in Biomer begins to lose activity after the second week (approximately 40% inhibition) and is comparable to the control value by the last week. The differences seen between Figure 9A and 9C occur because the amount of prostaglandin that is being tested when going from the directly ex-

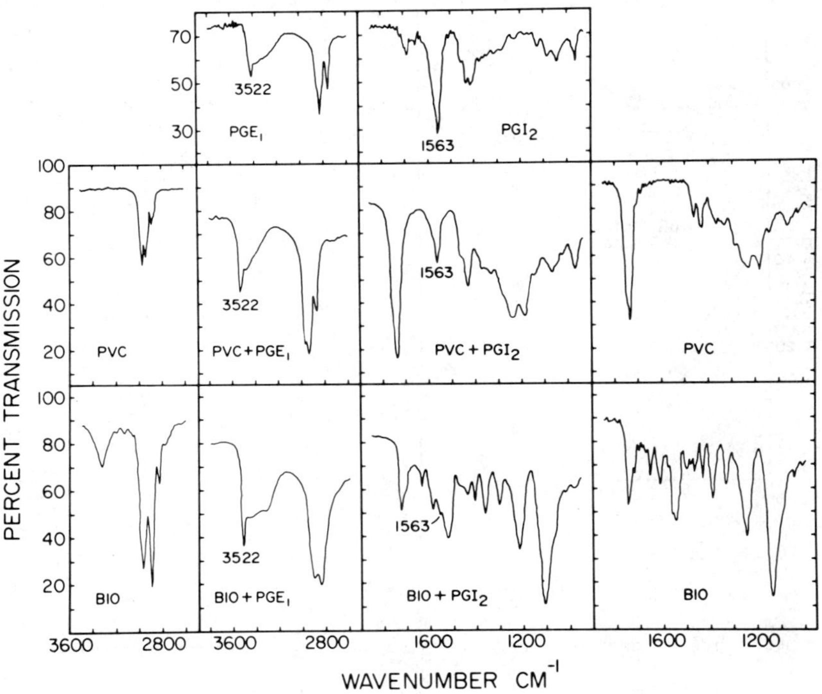

Figure 8. Quantitative analysis matrix of infrared spectra with analytical frequencies of individual components and multicomponent spectra.

posed PRP system to the testing of buffer in unexposed PRP is greatly reduced to provide some sensitivity as to the level of release in the testing procedure. Even so, this reduced amount of prostaglandin that is available in the 50-μl aliquot and added to fresh PRP should be in excess (10^{-5} to 10^{-6} M) of the amount required that was previously determined to achieve maximum inhibition of aggregation. These estimates of amounts are based on release rate studies described previously.

A similar effect on stability is observed in the testing of the PVC monolithic system. However, in Figure 9B, where PRP is in direct contact, it is seen that PGI_2, released from this monolith system begins to lose activity (only 50% inhibition) within the second week, remaining at this approximate level of activity through to the fourth week. Taking a 50-μl aliquot of the presoaking buffer magnifies the effect seen in the exposed PRP test, and shows a complete loss of activity of PGI_2 released from PVC by the end of the second week and throughout the test period.

When comparing the two monolithic polymer systems, Biomer and PVC, under comparable conditions (parts A and B of Figure 9), only PGI_2 exhibits a decrease in inhibitory activity. This indicates an inability of the PVC to "protect" the labile structure of PGI_2 as effectively as does Biomer. Both control polymers shown in Figure 9A and 9B demonstrated enhanced aggregation during the testing period. This is possible since the zero level is established by the ADP-induced aggregation of external PRP control, which is not exposed to any polymeric test surfaces, thus the negative inhibition of the control polymers may be a result of the endogenous ADP release effect of the platelets [29].

Recent reports provide some insight into the concept that the presence of certain

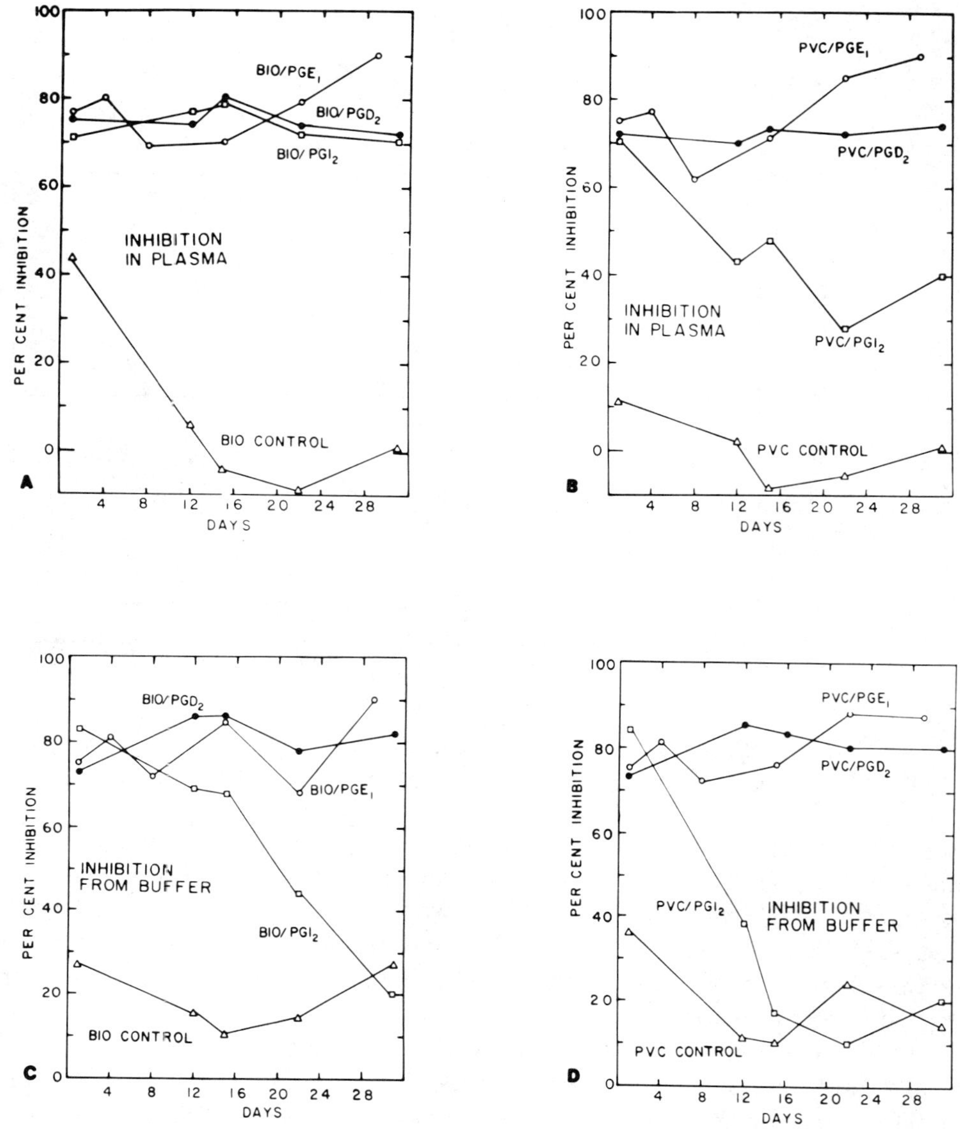

Figure 9. Stability testing of prostaglandin releasing monolithic polymers after storage.

molecular interaction or microenvironmental changes of PGI_2 will "protect" or stabilize its labile chemical structure, increasing its biological half life. One such study by Pifer [30] has found that PGI_2 exhibits a longer half life of activity in human blood than occurs in *in vitro* buffers. This protective effect has been attributed to the binding of PGI_2 to serum albumin. It is proposed that the binding of PGI_2 to albumin may result in stabilization by immobilizing carboxyl group or through limiting the access of solvent. The effects of pH, as reported previously [28], are also supportive of this rationale, since the protective effect of albumin in plasma (pH 7.85) is greater than is found in whole blood (pH 7.55) when incubated at the same rate [30].

Wynalda's work [31] reinforces this concept of PGI_2 stabilization. This study reports that while albumin contains twice as many basic amino acid residues as do other proteins, the stabilizing effect may be due to the location and type of residues present rather than total amino acid content. Wynalda has also shown that increased fatty acid concentration beyond physiological range reverses the stabilizing effect on PGI_2 by albumin, implying a competitive displacement mechanism; this is consistent with known fatty acid-albumin binding phenomena [32].

It is interesting to note that poly(ether) urethanes such as Biomer demonstrate a greater albumin adsorption isotherm than do other polymers [33]. It may be possible that the same interactions that result in a greater albumin adsorption of Biomer contribute to the stabilization of PGI_2 when monolithically dispersed in Biomer. It has also been found that monolithic systems of Biomer demonstrate less water uptake (2% by weight, during diffusion studies) than do PVC (14 to 18% by weight) indicating protection against hydrolytic attack.

F. Whole Blood Clotting Activity of Prostaglandin Monoliths

Platelets are intimately involved in the intrinsic coagulation pathway, both as mediator [34] and at times as initiators [35]. The effect that a prostaglandin-polymer monolith will have on whole blood clotting times (WBCT) provide useful information of efficacy. Figure 10 gives the results of WBCT for the Biomer monolithic systems. The relative change in the WBCT is expressed as a ratio with respect to the glass reference (polymer or monolith WBCT over glass WBCT). It can be seen that all monolithic systems show a relative increase over the control, though this is not found to be statistically significant. In Figure 11, results are given for the PVC monolithic systems. In this series it has been found that only PGD_2 in PVC increases the WBCT to any level of significance ($p < 0.025$). Table 2 summarizes the statistical treatment of this study. These results may suggest that with respect to WBCT tests, the presence of prostaglandin in Biomer may not be discernable from the effect that Biomer alone will exhibit. However, in the case of PVC, one explanation may be that PGE_1 is not as active as PGD_2 at equal concentrations (assuming the release of each is approximately equal) and that PGI_2 is less stable within the PVC matrix than is PGD_2, accounting for the PGD_2-PVC monoliths prolongation of WBCT. The equivocal nature of these data may be more indicative of inappropriate test selection than effectiveness of the prostaglandin monoliths to affect whole blood clotting. For example, the WBCT is a static test. "Stasis thrombus" is a term used to describe the type of thrombosis which occurs primarily in the venous sytem and can occur via the intrinsic clotting system [34]. The presence of activated factor XII (XIIa) generated during collection of the blood, can initiate the intrinsic system under these static conditions; and while platelets certainly mediate [35,36] and may even initiate [37,38] intrinsic coagulation, the result of the inhibition of platelet activity under these conditions is one of rate and not of outcome; thrombus will eventually form. It has been shown that typically, platelet-active agents do not reduce the incidence of venous thrombosis *in vivo* [34], whereas anticoagulants (such as heparin, coumadin) have had considerable therapeutic effect.

G. Adhesion-Aggregation Effects on Monoliths

The results of the extent of adhered platelets found on monolithic prostaglandin-PVC surfaces and the corresponding values of percent inhibition achieved by various fractions of either whole blood or buffer, are presented in Table 3. As indicated from this table, both monolith systems exhibit antiaggregatory activation, as measured in the fractions tested after perfusion. However, only the PGE_1-PVC surface demonstrated significantly reduced platelet adhesion.

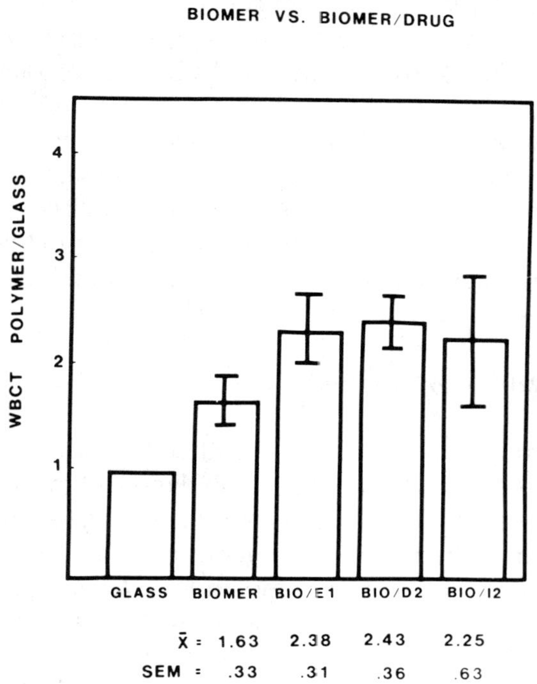

Figure 10. Whole blood clotting time (WBCT) tests of prostaglandin monolithically dispersed in Biomer.

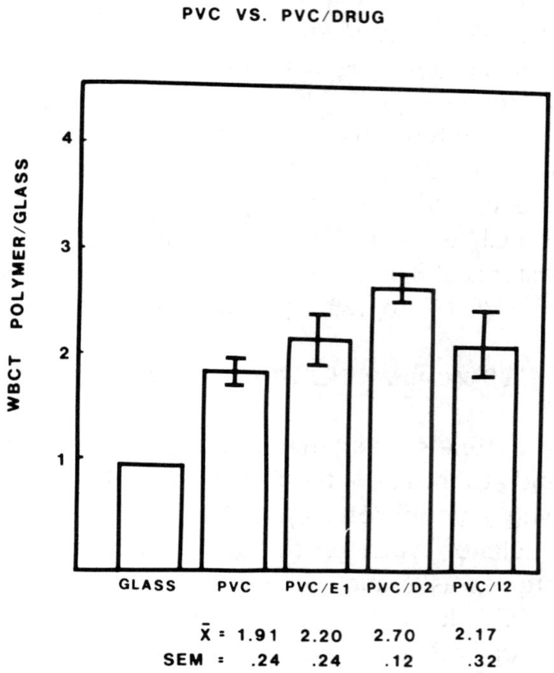

Figure 11. Whole blood clotting time (WBCT) tests of prostaglandin monolithically dispersed in polyvinyl chloride.

As has been developed throughout this discussion the role of the platelet in the intricate feedback and modulating mechanisms of coagulation, cannot be strictly differentiated into initiating or mediating events. It is, however, generally accepted that there is a basic platelet phenomenon that occurs at least with respect to its contact interaction with a surface [39], providing interaction times are adequate. It has been stated by Salzman that if there is no platelet adhesion, there is no release or aggregation [29], and within the context of the preceding statement this is basically true. Yet Salzman goes on to state, however, that release is not necessary for aggregation in response to platelet surface interactions, and that release is not a prerequisite for aggregation to occur. In this same study, it was also pointed out that while PGE_1 was capable of preventing platelet release and platelet thrombi, single platelet adhesion persisted.

In a more recent work on platelet adhesion and release, studying interfacial concentration of released materials [40], it was found that at a site of injury ADP release would be high enough to induce shape changes in adherent platelets, but there was no corresponding platelet aggregation, though trace amounts of collagen would act synergistically to result in aggregation. This synergism could ultimately result in the formation of thrombus. However, before activity proceeds this far, one other consideration must be made, the effects of shear stress. The force of moving blood at the surface, according to Grabowski [41] can, at high shear rates found arterially, cause a dilution of ADP levels and reduce platelet-ADP interaction time, thus reducing the formation of subsequent aggregate growth as well as reduce the interaction time of a platelet with a surface of potential contact.

Table 2. Two-Way ANOVA Analysis of Whole Blood Clotting Times

Polymer (rows)	Control	Prostaglandins (columns)		
		PGE_1	PGD_2	PGI_2
Biomer	1.63 ± 0.33	2.38 ± 0.31	2.43 ± 0.36	2.25 ± 0.63
PVC	1.91 ± 0.11	2.20 ± 0.24	2.70 ± 0.12	2.17 ± 0.32

n = 4 for all values.
Clotting times shown in minutes.

	df	SS	MS	FS	P
Subgroup	7	2.98	0.43		
Column	3	2.60	0.87	1.93	$F_{(3,24)[0.025]}$
Row	1	0.04	0.04	0.09	NS
Interactions	3	0.34	0.11	0.24	NS
Within Subgroups	24	10.84	0.45		
TOTALS	32	13.82			

Table 3. Adhesion Versus Aggregation Effects on Prostaglandin-Dispersed Polymer Surfaces

Platelet Adhesion		Percent Inhibition of Aggregation			
Polymer System	Plt/mm^2	Soak Buffer	1st Blood Fraction	2nd Blood Fraction	Rinse Buffer
PGE_1-PVC	11.25 ± 3.68	90%	90%	95%	50%
PVC (Control)	50.65 ± 8.87	<5%	<5%	<5%	<5%
PGI_2-PVC	25.00 ± 18.61	95%	75%	75%	30%
PVC (Control)	30.43 ± 7.62	<5%	<10%	<5%	0%

It has also been found that the inhibition of PGI_2 production, via administration of aspirin, by the endothelial cells, does not affect platelet adhesion either *in vitro* or *in vivo* [42], and while it appears that PGI_2 does not inhibit platelet adhesion any better than shear stress [40,41], PGI_2 is extremely effective in preventing aggregation and subsequent platelet thrombi. This has been shown by several researchers [43-45].

It appears that the effectiveness of prostaglandins released at a surface cannot be adequately evaluated on the basis of platelet adhesion alone. Even at normal physiological conditions, the systemic concentration of PGI_2 is not high enough to prevent platelet adhesion, but can prevent aggregate and thrombi formation at the surface [45,46].

REFERENCES

1. Paul, D. R., "Polymers in Controlled Release Technology," *Controlled Released Polymeric Formulation,* D. R. Paul and F. W. Harris (Eds.) A.C.S. Symposium Series 33, Washington, D.C., American Chemical Society, p. 1, 1965.
2. Kim, S. W., "Polymers for medical and drug delivery applications," J. Korean Soc. Med. Biol. Eng., 1(1):85-90, 1980.
3. Kostelnik, R. J., "Controlled Release of Effectors from Polymers and Microcapsules," *Polymeric Delivery Systems,* New York, Gordon and Breach Science Publishers, 1976.
4. Baker, R., "Controlled Release of Antithrombotic Agents from Polymer Matrices," *Controlled Release of Bioactive Materials,* New York, Academic Press, p. 107, 1980.
5. Juliano, R. L., "Controlled Drug Release from Polymeric Delivery Systems: Biomedical Applications and Physicochemical Principles," *Drug Delivery Systems: Characteristics and Biomedical Applications,* New York, Oxford University Press, 1980.
6. Salzman, E. W., Keusler, P. C., and Levine, L., "Cyclic 3′,5′-adenosine monophosphate in human blood platelets," Ann. N.Y. Acad. Sci., *201*:61-71, 1972.
7. Salzman, E. W., "Cyclic-AMP and platelet function," N. Engl. J. Med., *286*:358-363, 1972.
8. Salzman, E. W., and Levine, L., "Cyclic 3′,5′-adenosine monophosphate in human blood platelets II: Effect of N6-2′-O-dibutyryl cyclic 3′,5′-adenosine monophosphate on platelet function," J. Clin. Invest., *50*:131-141, 1971.
9. Ts'ao, C., Holly, C., and Serieno, M., "Generation of a Platelet Aggregation Inhibiting Acivity by Deendothelialized Rat Aorta," Abstract presented at the American Society for Pharmacology and Experimental Therapeutics Symposium, 62nd Annual Meeting of Federation of American Society for Experimental Biology, Atlantic City, New Jersey, April 1978.
10. Mason, R. G., Shermer, R. W., and Zucker, W. H., "Effects of certain purified plasma proteins on the compatibility of glass with blood," Amer. J. Pathol., *73*:181-200, 1973.
11. Born, G. V., "Aggregation of blood platelets by adenosine diphosphate and its reversal," Nature, London, *194*:927-929, 1962.
12. Coleman, D. L., "In vitro blood materials interaction: Experimental procedures," Ph.D. Dissertation, University of Utah, Salt Lake City, Utah, 1980.
13. Sokal, R. P., and Rohlff, F. J., "Two-Way Analysis of Variance," *Biometry, Principles and Practices of Statistics in Biological Research,* San Francisco, W. H. Freeman Company, Chapt. 7, 1969.
14. Olyslager, J., Kim, S. W., Ebert, C. D., McRea, J. C., and Feijen, J., "Comparison of two platelet adhesion test cells — Hemodynamics and materials discrimination," Proceedings of the 3rd International Society of Artificial Organs, Artif. Organs, *5,* 1981, in press.
15. Theeuwes, F., Hussain, A., and Higuchi, T., "Quantitative analytical method for determination of drugs dispersed in polymers using differential scanning calorimetry," J. Pharm. Sci., *63*(3):427-429, 1974.
16. Juijn, J. A., "Crystallinity in Atactic Polyvinyl Chloride," *Physical Aging in Amorphous Polymers and Other Materials,* L. C. E. Struik (Ed.), Delt, The Netherlands, TNO Central Laboratorium, Communication No. 565, 1977.
17. Billmeyer, F. W. Jr., *Textbook of Polymer Chemistry,* 2nd Edition, New York, Wiley-Interscience, p. 208, 1971.
18. Pike, J. E., "Physical-Chemical Properties of Prostacyclin (PGI_2)," The Upjohn Company Technical Bulletin, Kalamazoo, Michigan, June 1974.
19. Barall, E. M., and Rogers, L. B., "Differential thermal analysis of organic samples - Effects of

geometry and operating variables," Anal. Chem., *34*(9):1101-1106, 1962.
20. Johnson, R. A., Lincoln, F. H., and Thompson, J. L., "Synthesis and sterochemistry of prostacyclin and synthesis of 6-keto $PGF_{1\alpha}$," J. Amer. Chem. Soc., *99*(12):4182-4184, 1977.
21. Sloane, H. J., and Galloway, W. S., "Spectrophotometric accuracy, linearity and adherence to Beer's Law," Appl. Spectrosc., *31*(1):25-30, 1977.
22. Bernard, J. L., and Sims, L. G., "Total Chemical Analysis with the Beckman Microlab MX Series of Computer Controlled IR Spectrophotometers: Part III Characterization of High Polymers," Beckman Company Technical Information Bulletin, T1502-IR-80-3, Irvine, California, March 1980.
23. Perry, J. A., and Bain, G. H., "General procedure for setting-up infrared differential analyses of multicomponents mixtures," Anal. Chem., *29*(8):1123-1127, 1957.
24. Wei, P. E., "Determination of ethylene-propylene copolymer composition by infrared analysis," Anal. Chem., *33*(2):215-217, 1961.
25. Pattacini, S. C., and Norwalk, C. T., "Infrared Spectroscopy and Computer Separation of Drug Mixtures," Perkin-Elmer Technical Information Bulletin IRB-61, September 1977.
26. Bernard, J. L., and Sheppard, H. J. L., "Total Chemical Analyses with Beckman's Microlab 600 Computing IR Spectrophotometer: Part III Quantitative Analysis of a Six Component Sample System," Beckman Company Technical Information Bulletin T1284-IR-78-20, Irvine, California, 1980.
27. Oesterling, T. O., Morozowich, W., and Roseman, T. J., "Kinetics of alkaline isomerization and hydrolysis of lincomycin monesters," J. Pharm. Sci., *61*:1861-1895, 1972.
28. Cho, M. J., and Allen, M. A., "Chemical stability of PGI_2 in aqueous solutions," Prostaglandins, *15*:943-954, 1978.
29. Salzman, E. W., Lindon, J., Brier, D., and Merrill, E. W., "Surface-induced platelet adhesion, aggregation and release," Ann. N.Y. Acad. Sci., *283*:114-127, 1977.
30. Pifer, D. D., Cagen, L. M., and Chesney, C. M., "Stability of prostaglandin I_2 in human blood," Prostaglandins, *21*(2):165-175, 1981.
31. Wynalda, M. A., and Fitzpatrick, F. A., "Albumins stabilize prostaglandin I_2," Prostaglandins, *20*(5):853-861, 1980.
32. Spector, A. A., Santos, E., Ashbrook, J., and Fletcher, J. E., "Influence of free fatty acid concentration on drug binding to plasma albumin," Ann. N.Y. Acad. Sci., *226*:247-258, 1970.
33. Kim, S. W., and Lee, R. G., "Adsorption of Blood Proteins onto Polymer Surfaces," *Advances in Chemistry,* Vol. 145, pp. 218-299, 1975.
34. Thomas, D. R., "Role of Platelets in Arterial and Venous Thrombosis," *Advances in Experimental Medicine and Biology,* Vol. 34, P. M. Mannucci and S. Gorini (Eds.), New York, Plenum Press, 1972.
35. Feijen, J., "Thrombogensis Caused by Blood-Foreign Surface Interaction," *Artificial Organs,* R. M. Kenedi, J. Courtney, J. D. S. Gaylord and T. Gilchrist (Eds.), London, MacMillan Press Ltd., Chapt. 4, 1977.
36. Walsh, P. N., "The role of platelets in the contact phase of blood coagulation," Brit. J. Haemat., *22*:237-254, 1972.
37. Walsh, P. N., "The effects of collagen and kaolin on the intrinsic coagulant activity of platelets. Evidence for an alternative pathway in intrinsic coagulation not requiring factor XII," Brit. J. Haemat., *22*:393-405, 1972.
38. Walsh, P. N., and Griffin, J. H., "The role of human platelets in the contact phase of blood coagulation," Clin. Res., *26*:509, 1978.
39. Holmsen, H., "Are Platelet Shape Change, Aggregation,and Release Reaction Tangible Manifestations of One Basic Platelet Function?" *Platelets: Production, Function, Transfusion and Storage,* M. Baldini, S. Ebbe (Eds.) New York, Grune and Stratten, 207-220, 1974.
40. Adams, G. Z., and Fenerstein, I. A., "Platelet adhesion and release: Interfacial concentration of released materials," Am. J. Physiol., *9*:240, H99-H108, 1981.
41. Grabowski, E. F., Franta, J. T., and Didisheim, P., "Platelet aggregation in flowing blood *in vitro* II. Dependence of aggregate growth rate on ADP concentration and shear rate," Microvasc. Res., *16*:183-195, 1978.

42. Dejana, E., Cazenave, J. P., Groves, H. M., Kinlough-Rathbone, R. L., Richardson, M., Packham, M. A., and Mustard, J. F., "The effect of aspirin inhibition of PGI_2 production on platelet adherence to normal and damaged rabbit aorta," Thromb. Res., *17*:453-464, 1980.
43. Fesus, L., Harsfalvi, J., Kovacs, E., Muszbek, L., and Sladler, I., "Effect of prostaglandin I_2 on platelet adhesion," Biomater., *2*:53-54, 1981.
44. Weiss, H. J., and Turitto, U. T., "Prostacyclin (prostaglandin I_2 PGI_2) inhibits platelet adhesion and thrombus formation on subendothelium," Blood, *53*(2):244-250, 1972.
45. Cazenave, J. P., Dejana, E., Kinlough-Rathbone, R. L., Richardson, M., Packham, M. A., and Mustard, J. F., "Prostaglandins I_2 and E_1 reduce rabbit and human platelet adherence without inhibiting serotonin release from adherent platelets," Throm. Res., *15*:273-279, 1979.
46. Van der Welder, A. J., Van den Dungen, J. J. A. M., Westerhof, N. J. W., and Weldevuur, C. R. H., "Platelet damage by protamine administration; protection by reducing protamine or by prostacyclin (PGI_2) treatment," Abstract, Europ. Soc. Artif. Organs, 6:194-201, 1979.

This work was supported by NIH grant HL-20251.

Chapter 27

The Use of Biological Processes in the Development of a Long-Term Percutaneous Energy Transmission System

Frizell L. Vaughan, Ph.D.[1], Isadore S. Bernstein, Ph.D.[2], Paul Freed, M.S., Bio. Eng.[3], and Adrian Kantrowitz, M.D.[4]

ABSTRACT

A percutaneous access device (PAD) for long-term implantation must meet complex requirements. It must control epidermal proliferation and migration and attenuate strain at the skin-device interface. We cultivate autologous fibroblasts in vitro *onto the neck of the device, expecting that after implantation the cells will merge with the dermis, forming a bond that provides both a biological and a physical barrier to downward migration of epidermal cells. A subcutaneous flange shields the skin-device interface.*

The results to date confirm the feasibility of this approach. Rats and pigs have been used to observe the behavior of PAD's constructed as described. In both species epidermal migration was inhibited by autologous fibroblast-coated PAD implants, but not by cell-free controls.

[1]Associate Professor, Department of Environmental and Industrial Health, School of Public Health, the University of Michigan.

[2]Professor, Department of Biological Chemistry and Department of Environmental and Industrial Health, The University of Michigan.

[3]Senior Research Associate, Surgical Research Laboratory, Sinai Hospital of Detroit.

[4]Chief, Division of Cardiovascular Surgery, Sinai Hospital of Detroit and Professor, Department of Surgery, School of Medicine, Wayne State University.

The work described in this Chapter was supported by Contract NO1-HV-8-2921 from the Devices and Technology Branch, Division of Heart and Vascular Diseases, National Heart, Lung and Blood Institute and by grants from the James and Lynelle Holden Fund, the Education Corporation and the General Research Fund of Sinai Hospital of Detroit.

INTRODUCTION

Percutaneous access devices (PADs) are artificially created discontinuities of the skin intended to establish a permanent passageway between the inside and the outside of the body without interfering with the host's normal physiologic responses. Given the tendency of epithelium to repair breaks in its continuity, the use of biomaterials in maintaining a surgically created opening and shielding surrounding tissue from forces applied by conduits that pass through a PAD is inherent in the very concept.

PADs have multiple uses in research as well as in clinical medicine but have been studied perhaps most extensively in relation to permanently implanted prostheses that augment the action of the failing heart. In such applications, infection and extrusion, probably the major causes of failure of PADs of any type, are of paramount importance, for the candidate for long-term mechanical ventricular support is likely to have diminished resistance to infection and be unable to tolerate repeated PAD replacement.

In this chapter we describe the concept of a novel PAD which in principle will overcome the limitations of earlier designs; review the practical measures required to translate our concept into an operational system; and present the data obtained to date in experiments performed to test the hypotheses on which the new design is based.

BACKGROUND

Throughout the long history of PADs, a fundamental problem has compromised attempts to implant a foreign body through the skin, i.e., the propensity of epidermal cells to seal off unnatural openings by proliferating until continuity has been restored. When the epithelium grows in this manner in proximity to an implant of inert foreign material, a sinus tract forms. Because the sinus tract is moist and warm, it provides conditions favoring the growth of many species of bacteria. If, on the other hand, epithelial proliferation around an implant continues to its natural end point, the implant is marsupialized [1,2].

In many research studies on experimental animals, the long-term stability of a PAD is not essential. In our own research, which extends over an 18-year period, it has been possible to maintain the PADs of dogs undergoing long-term studies for several months. Careful attention to hygiene appears to retard the onset of infection; and when bacteria do gain a strong foothold, it has been a relatively simple matter to implant another PAD in a different location [3]. In our own clinical studies, which include 5 implantations of mechanical auxiliary ventricles, the earlier PAD configuration utilized was a limiting factor [4]. Nevertheless, in these studies we obtained evidence that PAD failure might have become a problem had the patients lived beyond three months. PAD replacement every several months would obviously be unacceptable in clinical studies. This unacceptability has spurred the efforts of many different groups to find a permanent solution to the problem of PAD design.

Such efforts have in the main two distinguishing features: implant location, and choice of the characteristics of the biomaterial placed in apposition to the skin.

PAD Location

A number of investigators have suggested that anchoring a PAD to bone [5,6] is superior to fixation in soft tissue. Although this approach shields the PAD-tissue interface from forces applied directly to the PAD, forces directed toward the skin in the region surrounding the PAD are not attenuated. There are, moreover, problems specific to fixation to bone. Attachment of a PAD to such sites, for example, can lead to pseudoarthrosis through lysis of bone tissue, fracture, rarification, and bone cysts [5]. According to Pae [6] many dogs mutilated PADs implanted between two ribs, suggesting that PADs in this location can cause pain.

The only instances in which attachment of a pyrolitic carbon PAD to bone has led to seemingly unqualified success seem to be those of artificial hearing [7,8] and stimulation of the central nervous system. These are special cases, in the sense that the site behind the ear normally involves no movement of the skin. Also, because of the rich blood supply of the skull the host defense mechanisms are enhanced. On the thorax, the only comparable location is the sternum, where skin motion with respect to bone is an order of magnitude greater than behind the ear. The sternum provides no alternate site for a PAD that has to be relocated. Furthermore, an infection that originates here can be transmitted directly to the pericardium because of the proximity of the heart.

For these reasons, the PADs for cardiac assist prostheses utilized by many investigators have been designed for implantation in soft tissue.

Biomaterial—Skin Interaction

The second, and more important, approach to the problem of migration of epithelium has been the use of materials intended to "deceive" the basal cells into accepting them as a natural boundary to their migration. So far as we can determine, none of the materials tested prior to the research described in this report has been effective in this application. Such materials as vitreous carbon [9], Teflon [5], Nylon and Dacron velour [1,6,10], Dacron felt [11], polycarbonate [6], expanded polytetrafluoroethylene [12] and polyhydroxyethylmethacrylate [12] have been found unsatisfactory.

A number of impressions with implications for PAD design can be derived from related investigations:

1. The implant must form a strong bond with living skin components in order to prevent sinus-tract development with ensuing microbial infection.
2. Materials with smooth nonreactive surfaces are unsuitable because adequate bonds fail to develop and the material is eventually marsupialized, or the surrounding tissue is infected.
3. Modest success, as measured by useful life, has been obtained with materials, such as velour, which present a textured surface to the basal cells [10,11]. However, a serious drawback to use of velour was identified by one group of investigators. They found that because attachment to the basal layer of the skin was firm, the differentiating cells tended to carry the attached velour up to the surface as they matured to form the stratum corneum [1]. The result was a persistent tendency slowly to extrude the implant.
4. Dacron and nylon felts have also led to infection, presumably because tissue cannot completely fill the interstices of the material. "...[V]oids beyond the tissue's grasp probably serve as a wick, bringing nutrient tissue juices to the surface where hungry microbes abide" [1]. Grosse-Siestrup [13], however, reported good results using Dacron velour mounted on a flexible substrate.

A comparatively recent approach which seemed to provide a PAD whose design was compatible with these impressions was developed by Robinson et al. [14]. They developed a polyurethane membrane coating for implants, the "Microporous Tissue Interface" (MTI). It possesses a uniform distribution of noncommunicating microcavities of 50-150 μm diameter and less than 200 μm in depth. Robinson et al. observed strong tissue bonding, attributing it both to the firm cellular adhesion to the polyurethane and to the interlocking of tissue with micropores [14]. We believe that the MTI may indeed slow the inward proliferation of the basal cells, but no mechanism has been suggested by which MTI can prevent inward proliferation.

In brief, whereas some of the biological attributes of an effective PAD have been identified and a range of materials defined that might lend themselves to incorporation in a PAD, as of 1979 no system suitable for use in connection with long-term implantation of cardiac assist systems had demonstrated adequate reliability. Upon reflecting on our own observations and reports in the literature, it occurred to us that another type of tissue-implant bond may be more effective and thus biologically more significant than those upon which earlier PAD designs were based. That bond would be between the implant and the dermis. As pointed out by Winter [12], basal cells of the epidermis do not invade the dermis under normal conditions and are probably prevented from doing so by structures in the dermis, perhaps collagenous in nature. An example of a natural permanent breech in the epithelial membrane is the teeth [12]. It may be the periodontal membrane, composed of collagen fibers embedded in the tooth and surrounding areas, that blocks epithelial migration around the dentition. It is possible that basal cells may not migrate through a healthy, intact dermis composed of active fibroblasts and polymerized collagen.

We hypothesized that the conditions for such inhibition would be provided by a percutaneous implant with a porous surface precoated with autologous dermal elements which form a collagenous matrix; the dermal elements would be expected to interlock firmly with the implant surface.

We further hypothesized that an implant of this type would allow firm attachment of the PAD to the surrounding tissue. And since the PAD would be subject to varying loads (e.g., those due to the patient's movements, attachment and disconnection of the coupling to an external power source) which tend to produce mechanical separation of the tissue-implant bond, it would also be necessary to stabilize the PAD and protect the PAD-tissue interface from loads which exceed the strength of the tissue-implant bond.

In the next section we describe the manner in which these rather general considerations were translated into a program of research.

CONSIDERATIONS IN THE DESIGN OF AN IMPROVED PAD

The overall objective of our research on PADs, like that of others in this field, has been the development of a validated design which satisfies long-term performance criteria, including freedom from infection, extrusion and marsupialization. By meeting two requirements beyond those applicable to any implant, we hypothesize, a PAD with the desired characteristics can be constructed. As summarized in the preceding section, these requirements comprise control of epidermal migration and protection of the tissue-implant seal from mechanical stresses (see Figure 1, which defines the terminology used in this report).

The techniques required to mount an investigation of a PAD meeting such requirements

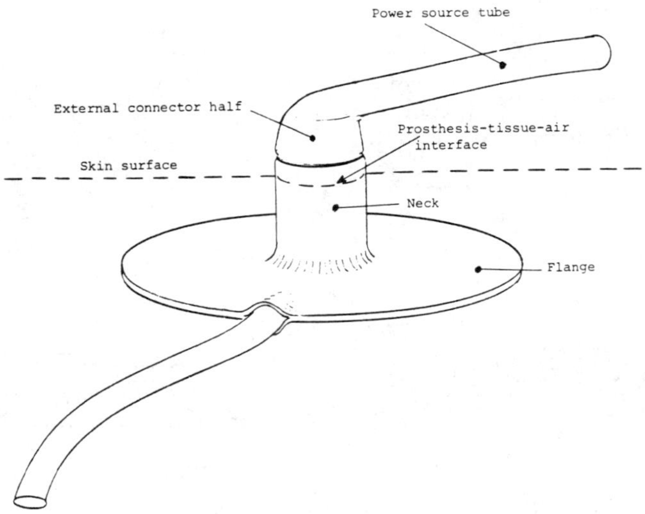

Figure 1. Schematic representation of percutaneous access device (PAD) defining terms used in the text.

fall chiefly into their several disciplines, including investigative dermatology, cell biology, biomedical engineering, and experimental surgery. Accordingly, a program of collaboration was established between investigative dermatologists of the University of Michigan School of Public Health and the staff of the Surgical Research Laboratory of the Sinai Hospital of Detroit.

From the outset we recognized the need to develop three principal techniques in order to implement the proposed PAD concept.

1. Coating the PAD with Autologous Cells. Under normal conditions basal cells do not proliferate through the intact dermis, probably because of inhibition by the dense fibroblast-collagen network within the dermis. Accordingly, if the PAD neck were covered with autologous fibroblasts and collagen that formed a permanent attachment with the *in situ* dermis upon implantation of the PAD, the resulting continuous fibroblast-collagen network would be expected to act as a barrier to epidermal cell migration inward along the PAD neck. Attachment of dermal elements to the biomaterial used as the PAD neck would be optimized by creating pores of micrometer size in the surface of the material prior to the *in vitro* proliferation of autologous fibroblasts. We have elected to describe the eventual surface that results from these steps as the autologous "living" collagen-coated nanoporous surface, or, in brief, as the "ALCON" surface.

2. Surgical Excision of Surrounding Epidermis. In order to prevent epidermal downgrowth before a continuum between the *in situ* dermis and the coated PAD has formed, a uniform diameter of the epidermis is excised that is concentric with, and adjacent to, the opening in the skin through which the PAD neck protrudes.

3. Alteration of Skin Stress-Strain Characteristic. To ensure that mechanical stresses do not disrupt the ALCON surface-tissue interface, the stress-strain characteristic of the skin in the region of the PAD is altered. This is accomplished by incorporating in the PAD design a relatively stiff Dacron velour-covered flange which is placed directly beneath the dermis. As a result, the PAD implantation site moves as a unit in response to applied forces, and relative motion between the skin and the PAD neck is thereby prevented (Figures 2 and 3).

Thus, the investigation of the construction of a PAD capable of long-term implantation

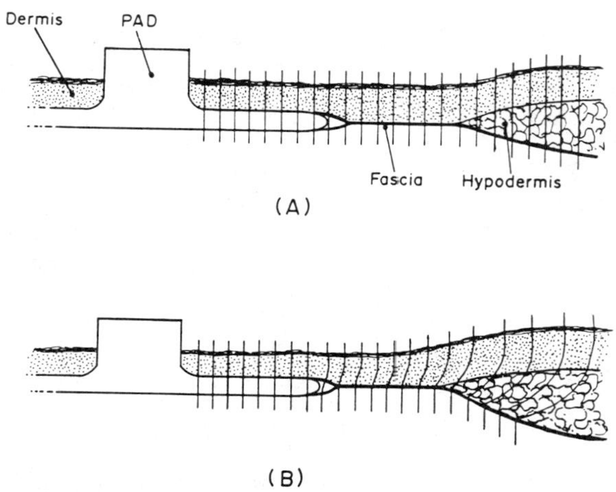

Figure 2. Schematic diagram of PAD implanted according to proposed technique. (A) Resting state. (B) When force is applied, strain is maximal at outer margin of PAD and beyond but remains minimal in region of PAD neck, as in A.

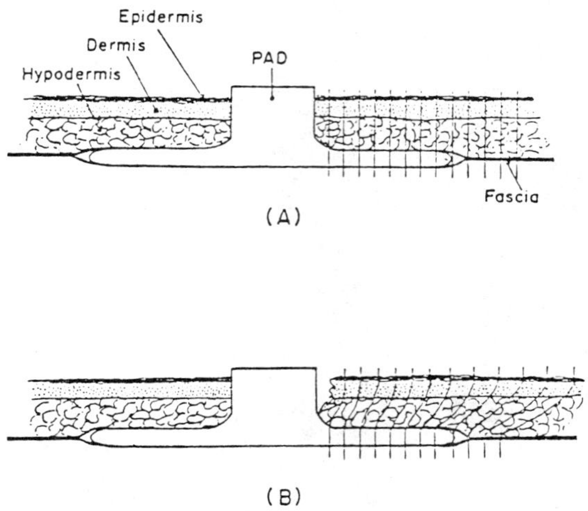

Figure 3. Schematic view of a PAD with large flange implanted in soft tissue according to conventional technique. (A) Resting state. Imaginary grid marks are vertical, indicating that no forces are being applied to the region containing the PAD. (B) Force has been applied. Grid marks indicate displacement pattern. Because of fixation technique displacement is maximal in vicinity of PAD neck, and tear results. The implantation technique we use presently is shown in Figure 2.

presented several problem-solving areas, of which the chief ones are as follows:

- Selection of a material or materials demonstrated to be essentially inert and nontoxic to mammalian fibroblasts.
- Demonstration that such materials retain structural stability despite exposure to chemical and physical treatments in cleaning, etching, and sterilization.
- Development of techniques for isolating fibroblasts from experimental animals to produce autologous, immunologically acceptable cells.
- Selection of a basal medium plus chemical and biological additives to promote maximal proliferation of, and collagen production by, fibroblasts *in vitro.*
- Development of pretreatment procedures to improve attachment and proliferation of fibroblasts on the selected test materials.
- Investigation of physical and chemical procedures for producing nanopores of appropriate size and density in the selected materials.
- Development of histological methods suited to observation and evaluation of the interaction of cultured biological materials with the device surface and with *in situ* host tissues using light or electron microscopy, or both.
- Development of appropriate procedures for coating the cylindrical neck portion of the PAD with fibroblasts *in vitro.*
- Development of surgical procedures for proper subcutaneous placement of the flange portion of the PAD so as to obtain maximal strain relief.

- Development of techniques for quantitating stress-strain in the skin.
- Development of a mechanical design for the PAD that is compatible with both the conduit-carrying requirements and the material chosen.
- Development of surgical implantation techniques used both for sealed-down and full scale implants.
- Development of appropriate surgical procedures to ensure uniform removal of the epidermis immediately surrounding the implant opening and proper placement of the device without disturbing the fibroblast-collagen coat on the neck.
- Development of appropriate postoperative procedures to protect the implant from physical damage and contamination by the test animal.

Additional important factors in the design of a PAD are protection of the implant from large forces of external origin (tension or torsion on the external power source tube, for example) and human-factors requirements. Consideration of the above factors has not been the primary focus of the work described here, in part because that design has been brought to a provisionally satisfactory level in our earlier work [15]. The essential feature in providing protection against external forces is the incorporation of a mechanical fuse in the PAD. The implantable and external halves separate at the prosthesis-tissue-air interface without damage if excessive force is applied from any direction (Figure 4). Figure 5 shows details of construction. Three magnets in each half of the connector are so arranged that the halves fit together in only one way and align themselves properly when brought into proximity. The magnets also serve as contacts for electrocardiograph leads, which pass from the magnets through circuitry that limits the current to 10 μA to a standard pacemaker connector to which leads from the myocardium are joined. When the power source tube is disconnected, a magnetic stainless steel cap fits over the external surface of the PAD to keep foreign matter out.

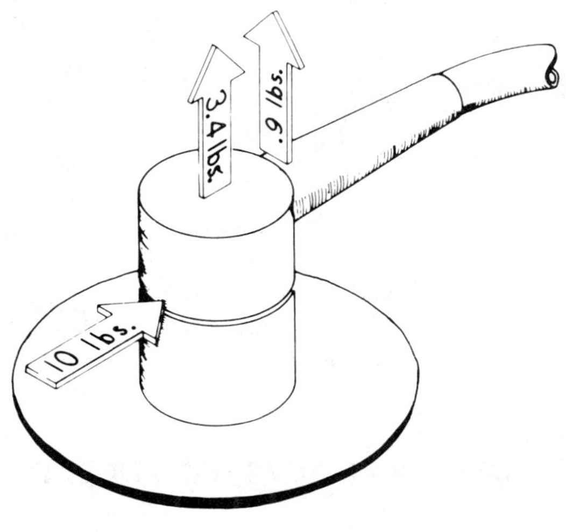

Figure 4. Schematic representation of magnetic connector which functions as a mechanical fuse. Connector halves are shown mated. Arrows indicate force vectors required to cause separation of the halves.

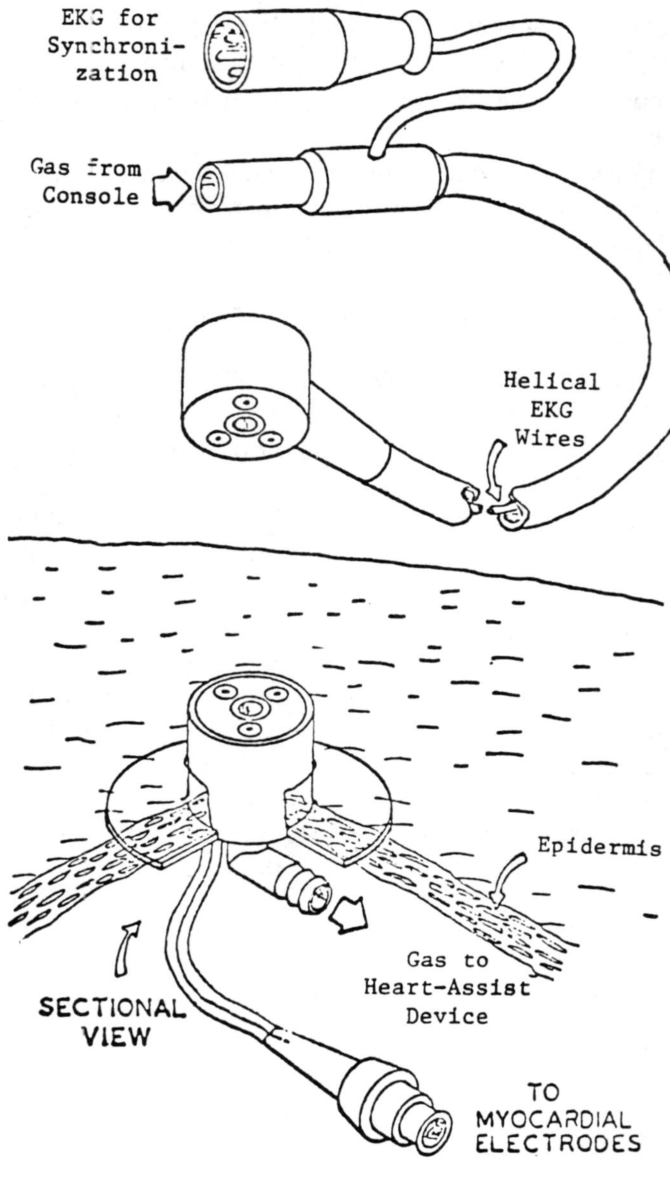

Figure 5. Overall concept of magnetic PAD.

In the remainder of this chapter, we describe our progress to date in relation to the above-listed problem areas.

SELECTION OF MATERIALS FOR THE PAD NECK

Critical to the development of an effective ALCON surface is the selection of an inert biomedical material that will support the *in vitro* proliferation of mammalian fibroblasts. The material of choice must not only be nontoxic but must demonstrate structural stability after exposure to various chemical and physical treatments used for cleaning, creation of pores, and sterilization. Table 1 lists the materials initially examined in this investigation. All are plastics that have been employed by various investigators as biomedical materials.

Table 1. Materials Evaluated for Task I

1.	Hytrel* polyesther elastomer[1]	4056	pellets
2,		5556	pellets
3,		6346	pellets
4,		7246	pellets
5,	Copel* silicone polycarbonate[2]	4330	powder
6,		3320	powder
7,		4020	cast sheet
8.		3320	cast sheet
9.		3320	extruded sheet
10,		MEM-213	cast sheet
11.		4020	extruded rod 2 m
12,		3320	extruded rod 2 mmD
13.	Lexan* polycarbonate[3]	104	sheet
14,		104	extruded rod
15.	Mylar*		sheet

*Reg. U.S. Pat. and TM Office
[1]Block copolymers of short-chain dial terephthalate and long-chain polyether dial terephthalate, Dupont.
[2]Poly (dimethyl siloxane) - bisphenol - a carbonate block copolymer, G.E.
[3]G.E.

Polyester elastomer (Hytrel, du Pont) was obtained as pellets which were formed into thin sheets by heating at 200°C for 15 minutes while pressed between two thick glass plates. This method resulted in a relatively transparent film which could be cleaned, sterilized, and seeded with mammalian cells; its surface could be observed with light or scanning electron microscopy.

Silicone polycarbonates (Copel, General Electric) with four different copolymer structures were studied, i.e. 3320, 4020, 4320 and MEM-213. They were obtained as powder, precast sheets, extruded sheets, or extruded rods 2 mm in diameter. The powder forms were used to cast sheets of desired dimensions. The powder was dissolved in a appropriate volume of methylene chloride (reagent grade). The resulting solution was poured into a selected casting vessel and slowly evaporated in a desiccator jar so as to result in a transparent, smooth sheet.

The precast and extruded sheets and rods were smooth and transparent and thus were used as received. All Copel materials could be sterilized and cleaned, and the resulting surfaces could be observed with light and electron microscopy.

Polycarbonate (Lexan 104, General Electric) was obtained as extruded rods and sheets which were smooth and transparent. In exploratory investigations the sheets and rods (2 mm) were used as obtained. In order to construct a PAD neck of the size to be implanted into the selected test animal, i.e., 1.1 cm in diameter and 1.1 cm in length, a special procedure was developed. This involved machining 1.1-cm-long solid pieces of Lexan 104 to the necessary dimensions and vapor polishing them.

Mylar was obtained as sheets and used as such. The sheets were semitransparent and after cleaning and sterilization did not allow clear observation of activity on the surface under the microscope. This material was eliminated early in this study.

Of the various materials screened, Lexan 104, Copel 3320, Copel 4330, and Copel 4020 were selected for further investigation. Copel 4330 was later arbitrarily eliminated in favor of Copel 3320 because of the similarity of the two in texture and response to physical and chemical treatments.

EFFECTS OF CLEANING AND STERILIZATION PROCEDURES ON PAD MATERIALS

All materials were effectively cleaned using Haemosol (Haemo-sol Inc., Baltimore, MD) at 0.5 oz/gal of warm water or Micro (International Products Corp., Trenton, NJ) at 2.5 oz/gal. Materials with nanoporous surfaces (see below) were also sonicated in one of these cleaning solutions. Final multiple rinsing in glass-distilled water, followed by drying at room temperature in a dust-free environment, completed the cleaning process.

The effects of various sterilization procedures on surface structure were subsequently examined, as was the ability of the resulting substrates to support the growth of rat fibroblasts *in vitro*. The sterilization procedures studied in addition to autoclaving were ultraviolet irradiation by means of exposure to UV from a bactericidal lamp (Sylvania G 15T8) at a distance of 6 in. for 15 min, and treatment of materials with 70% ethanol for 30 min followed by multiple washings with sterile water or balanced salt solution.

To assess the ability of substrates subjected to various cleaning and sterilization procedures to support mammalian cell growth, actively growing rat fibroblasts were harvested in the log phase of growth for seeding on to the selected substrates. The cells were seeded at a density of 10^5 cells/ml of culture medium (described below) directly on the test substrates contained in glass petri dishes (60 mm). After 7 days of incubation at 35 °C in a humidified atmosphere containing 5% CO_2, the resulting cell growth was harvested by thoroughly scraping the growth surface with a silicone policeman to remove attached cells. The suspended cells were then centrifuged and resuspended in a measured solution containing ethylene diaminetetraacetic acid (EDTA) and bovine serum albumin (BSA), agitated in order to produce a single cell suspension, and counted electronically after preparation of an appropriate dilution using a Coulter Model Z counter.

Sterilization procedures affected the four materials differently. Autoclaving (121 °C, 18 lb pressure, 15 min) caused some minor changes in surface characteristics of all materials but to different degrees, as observed by means of scanning electron microscopy. The more pliable Copel materials melted slightly at high temperatures and pressures. The results of 7 days of cell growth on materials which were sterilized by autoclaving, UV irradiation, and alcohol

Table 2. Seven Day Fibroblast Cell Growth on Selected Substrates Following Sterilization and Pretreatment Procedures

	Substrates											
Pre-Treatment	Commercial Plastic Petri Dishes			Copel 4330			Copel 4020[4]			Lexan 104		
	UV[1]	ETOH[2]	Auto[3]	UV	ETOH	Auto	UV	ETOH	Auto	UV	ETOH	Auto
None	100%[5]	-	-	70%	40%	70%	90%	50%	90%	100%	80%	100%
Serum	100%	-	-	90%	70%	80%	100%	50%	70%	100%	60%	100%
HFN	180%	-	-	160%	80%	180%	180%	90%	90%	170%	90%	180%
HFN + FGF	200%	-	-	180%	80%	180%	190%	180%	90%	200%	90%	200%

[1]Sterilized by ultraviolet irradiation
[2]Ethyl alcohol sterilization
[3]Autoclave sterilization
[4]Surface of plastic damaged by treatment with hot detergent used for cleaning
[5]Untreated commercial plastic petri dishes were used as control
Materials were cleaned by soaking in Haemo-Sol (microbiological cleaner) at 70°C for one hour followed by extensive rinsing with distilled water.

treatment (70% ethanol) are summarized in Table 2. Cell growth on materials which were UV sterilized or autoclaved compared favorably with that on commercially obtained culture dishes with no pretreatment. Some surface distortions also resulted from UV sterilization of Copel 4020 but did not affect growth. Growth on all surfaces sterilized with ethanol was substantially lesser than on control surfaces.

The results of pretreatment of the surfaces of sterilized materials with factors selected to improve cellular attachment and proliferation are also summarized in Table 2. When cellular attachment and proliferation were determined after 7 days of incubation, only Lexan 104 compared favorably with commercial culture surfaces in the absence of pretreatment. Slight improvement resulted when the Copel materials were pretreated with fetal calf serum (FCS). However, substantial improvement in attachment and growth resulted when these materials were pretreated with Human Fibronectin (HFN). Total growth after 7 days on commercial substrates pretreated with HFN increased nearly two-fold. Similar results were observed following pretreatment of the test materials. These studies clearly demonstrated the ability of this human protein to enhance the surface properties of these materials causing improved fibroblast attachment and proliferation. The addition of Fibroblast Growth Factor (FGF) further enhanced proliferation of the HFN-stimulated fibroblasts (FGF studies are discussed below).

DEVELOPMENT OF POROUS SURFACES ON PAD NECK MATERIALS

The purpose of making a surface nanoporous is to enhance attachment of cells or of collagen to the substrate while discouraging complete penetration by cells and invasive bacteria. The desired outcome is a firm bond between the *in vitro*-developed dermal elements and the PAD neck material that will resist both physical and biological disruption.

Three methods of nuclear bombardment that cause damage tracks in plastic substrates were examined. Pores in such substrates would then be expected to result from etching with an appropriate solvent. The three methods investigated were these:

1. Bombardment with deuteron particles (5 MeV) generated by a cyclotron (Michigan State University), followed by etching with NaOH.
2. Bombardment of materials with Alpha particles (8 MeV) generated from Americium-241, followed by etching with NaOH.
3. Bombardment with fission fragments from Californium-252, followed by etching with NaOH.

Of the three methods attempted, only the third, i.e., bombardment with Californium-252, produced satisfactory results. To produce a nanoporous surface using this method, each substrate was exposed to a 0.05-μg Californium-252 spontaneous fission source at a distance of approximately 3.9 cm. Californium-252 spontaneously produces 3.07×10^4 fission fragment particles per second. Because the range of the fragments in air at atmospheric pressures is less than 2 cm, it was necessary to expose the materials to the source in a vacuum chamber. Such a chamber was designed for this purpose and is shown in Figures 6 (diagrammatic cross section) and 7 (photograph of the two main parts); it serves as a permanent storage chamber for the radioactive source as well. A protective shield covers the source when not in use and can be manipulated from the outside. An adjustable sample stage (Figure 6) allows the operator to choose the sample-source distance.

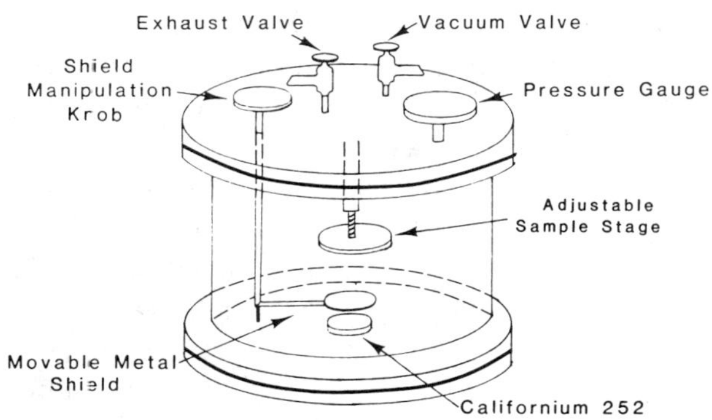

Figure 6. Schematic diagram of vacuum chamber for nuclear particle bombardment of substrates.

The density of the damage track that results from bombardment with fission fragments generated by Californium-252 is controlled by two factors, source-to-source sample distance and duration of exposure (Figure 8). Pore dimensions (diameter and depth) are controlled by etching time and temperature. The etching solution used was 6.25N NaOH prepared fresh. Etching temperatures ranged from 45-55°C to 68-72°C. As suggested by Fleischer [16], decreasing the etching temperature decreases the pore-diameter etching rate without correspondingly decreasing the pore-depth etching rate. Thus, lower temperatures favor the development of a pore that is longer than wide, a preferred feature in our application. The procedures we developed allow production of pores in Lexan and Copel 0.05-5 μm in diameter and 10-15 μm in length. Figure 9 shows scanning electron micrographs of Lexan 104

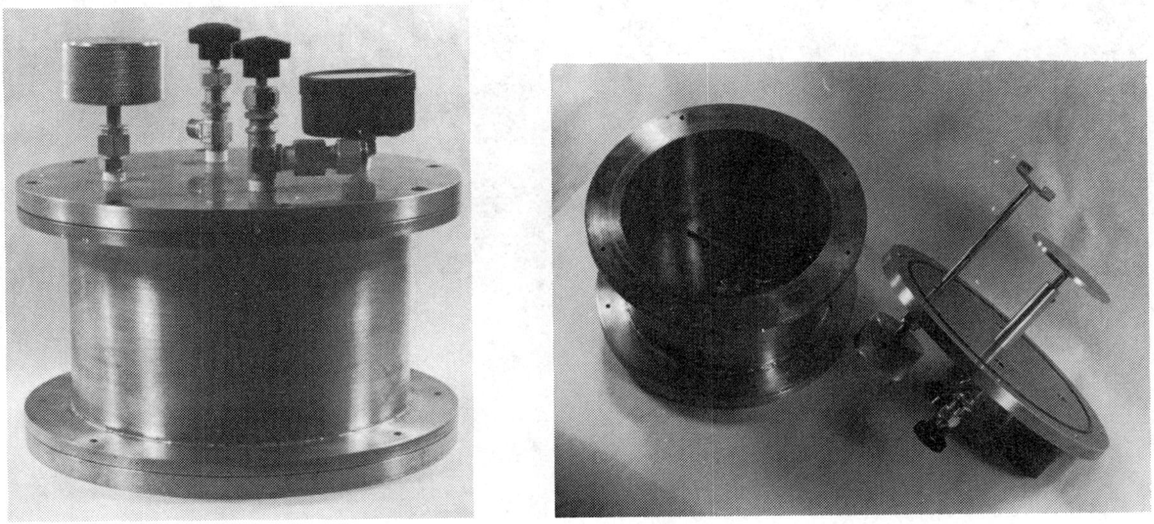

Figure 7. Photograph of (A) assembled and (B) unassembled vacuum chamber for nuclear particle bombardment.

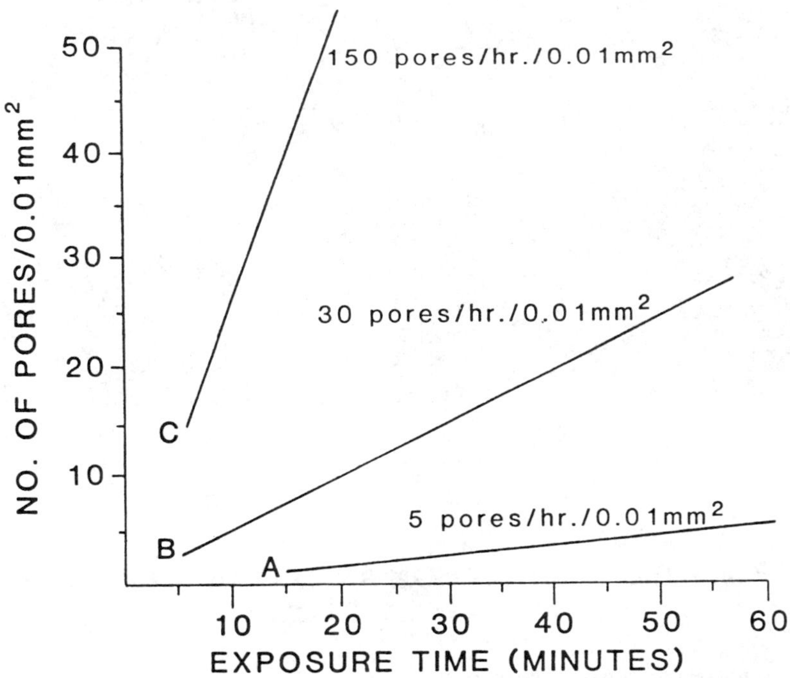

Figure 8. Pore production rates by Californium-252 at various distances from the source under vacuum, A - 10 cm, B - 6.25 cm, C - 1.25 cm.

containing pores that resulted from irradiation with Californium-252 followed by etching with 6.25N NaOH.

Two pore densities were selected for investigation, 15,000/mm² and 30,000/mm².

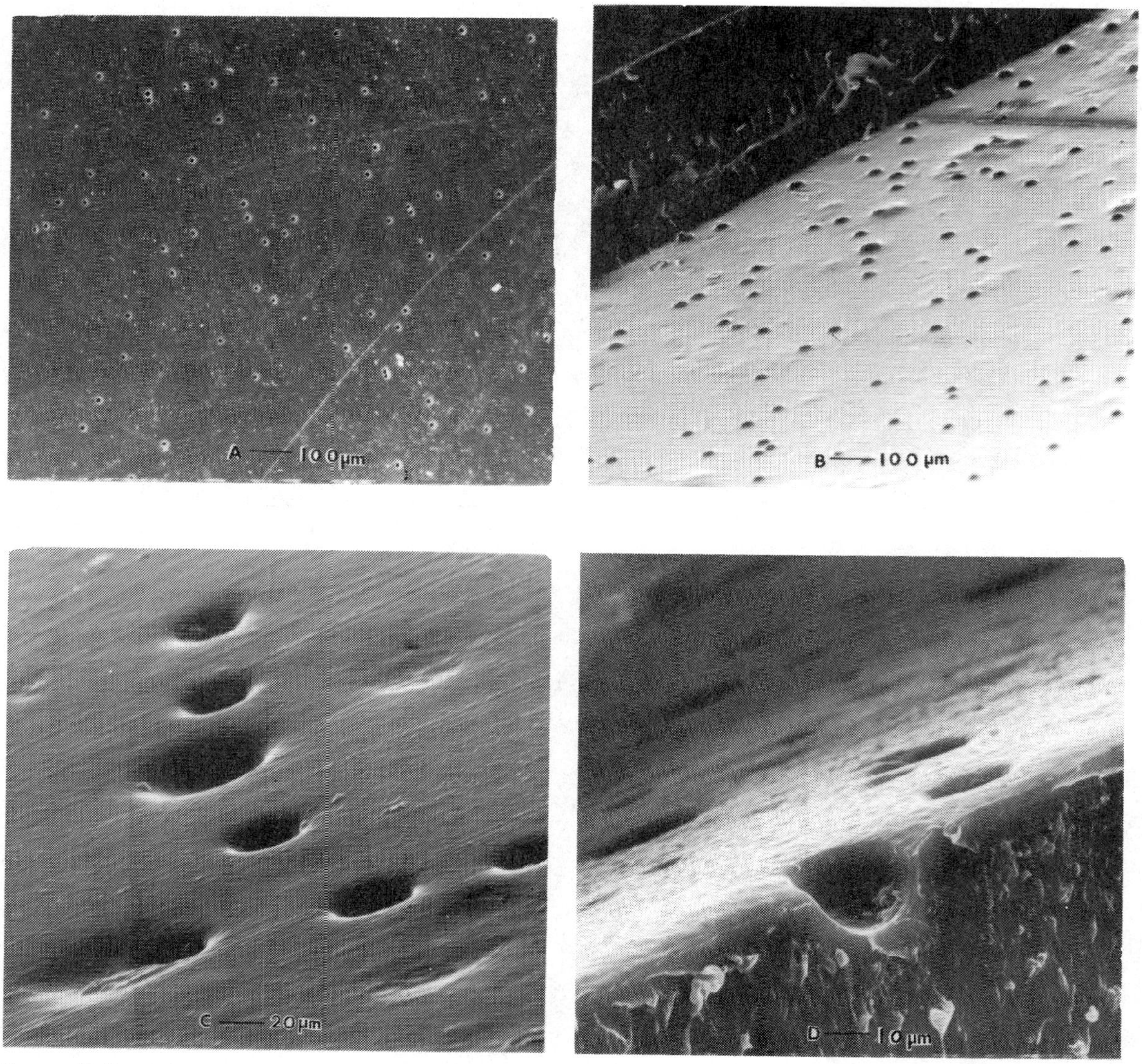

Figure 9. Scanning electron micrographs showing pores in test materials. Damage tracts produced by fission fragments were then etched for various periods. (A) Lexan etched 3 hrs. (B) 4020 etched 2 hrs. (C) 4020 etched 2 hrs. (D) 4330 etched 1 hr.

OPTIMIZING PROLIFERATION AND COLLAGEN PRODUCTION BY FIBROBLAST CULTURES

Isolation of Fibroblasts from Newborn Rats

Fibroblasts were obtained from the skin of newborn CFN rats using a procedure developed by those of us at the University of Michigan [17]. A flow diagram is outlined in Figure 10. This procedure results in a single-cell suspension which when seeded onto plastic culture vessels (Corning) at a density of 10^5 cells/ml results in a monolayer after 7-10 days incubation at 35°C

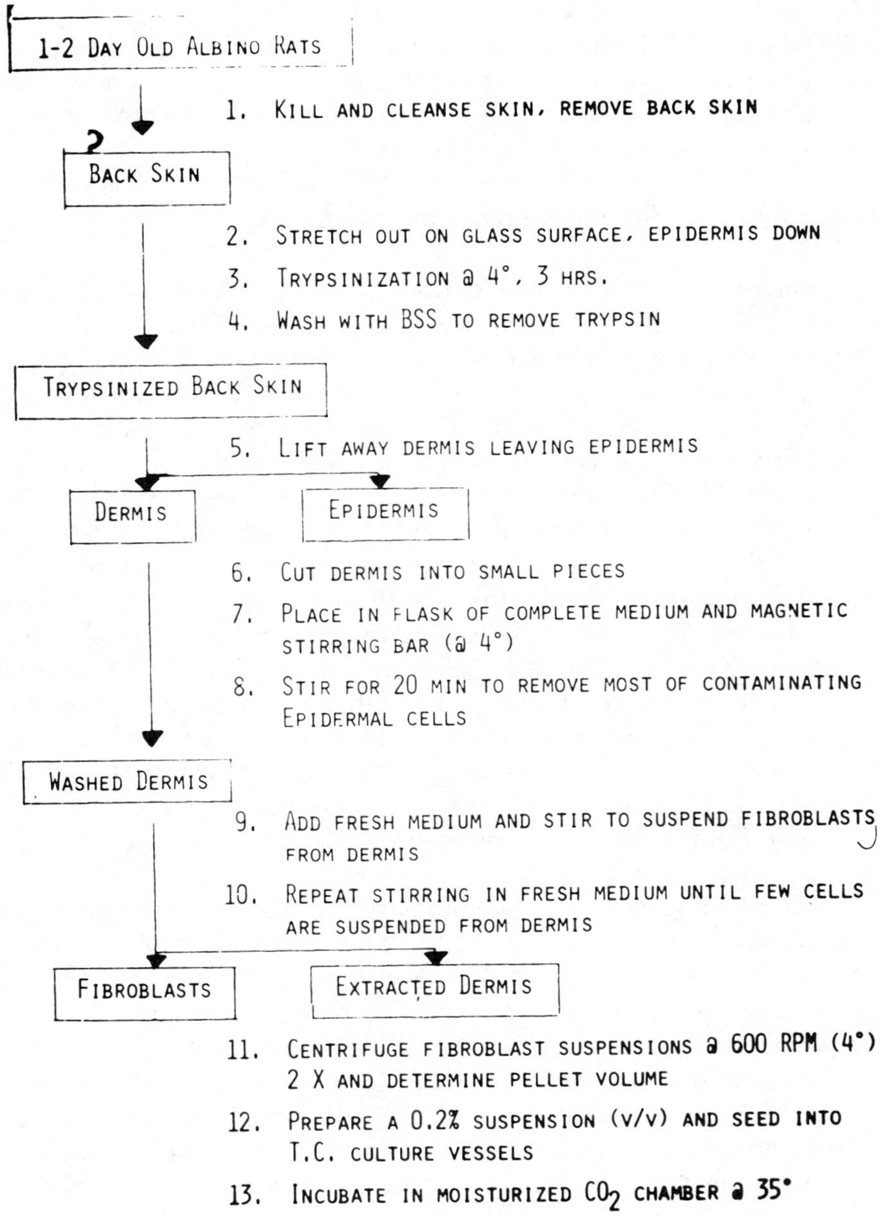

Figure 10. Flow diagram of rat fibroblast isolation technique.

in a humidified atmosphere of 95% air and 5% CO_2. These cells were harvested and seeded onto selected biomaterials to be used as PAD necks.

Isolation of Fibroblasts from Adult Swine

Skin biopsy specimens were obtained from miniature swine after sterilizing the area with iodine and 70% ethyl alcohol. The specimens were placed in a balanced salt solution and taken to a sterile transfer hood. The dermis was cut away from the epidermis and then into

2-mm pieces. These pieces were then placed in petri dishes (approximately 20 per 100-mm dish), allowed to attach, fed with complete medium (as described below), and incubated. Such explants produced outgrowths of fibroblasts in 3-4 weeks and a monolayer in approximately one month. After removal of the original explants and subcultivation, the resulting fibroblasts were used to seed PAD neck materials.

Culture Medium and Additional Medium Supplements

The basic medium selected for growth of both rat and pig fibroblasts was Eagle's Minimum Essential Medium (MEM) (K.C. Biological). This was supplemented with 10% fetal calf serum (FCS) to prepare complete medium (CM). CM also contained insulin (10.0 μg/ml) and hydrocortisone (10.0 μg/ml) as growth stimulants. The antibiotics penicillin (100 μg/ml), streptomycin (100 μg/ml), and fungizone (0.05 μg/ml) were routinely added to CM.

Special additional supplements were added for specific purposes: (1) stimulation of rapid cell proliferation, and (2) stimulation of maximum collagen production *in vitro*. Numerous additives have been tested which have been found to stimulate the proliferation of certain cell types and increase the rate of growth. Mammalian fibroblasts ordinarily proliferate until they form a confluent monolayer, at which time growth ceases because of contact inhibition. Additives were employed in the attempt to decrease the time necessary to achieve cell confluency and to overcome the effects of contact inhibition, allowing multilayers to form. The tissue culture medium additives tested (all from Collaborative Research, Inc., Waltham, MA) included the following: histamine, epidermal growth factor (EGF, isolated from male mouse submaxillary glands), fibroblast growth factor (isolated from bovine pituitary glands), endothelial cell growth supplement (ECGS, isolated from bovine neural tissue), multiplication stimulating activity (MSA, isolated from rat liver), and increased serum (FCS) concentration. Additives were tested in various concentrations and combinations.

The production of collagen *in vitro* by fibroblasts has been found to be highly dependent upon the use of several additives supplied to the basic medium. Ascorbic acid has been demonstrated to be necessary for the production of properly cross-linked hydroxylated collagen in tissue culture [18-19]. Confluent fibroblast cultures were treated with ascorbic acid (50 μg/ml) for 2 weeks. It has been demonstrated, here and elsewhere, that nonconfluent fibroblasts do not produce collagen *in vitro*. Following the 2-week treatment period, cell cultures were examined for the presence of collagen by both light and transmission electron microscopy. Two other additives, α-ketoglutaric acid at 100 μg/ml and ferrous ion ($FeSO_4$, 0.25 μM) were also investigated as important co-factors of collagen hydroxylation and polymerization [18,20].

As shown in Tables 3 and 4, significant increases in fibroblast proliferation resulted when the cells were incubated in medium supplemented with various additives. The most effective stimulant to cell proliferation was FGF. The lowest concentration tested, 12.1 mg/ml, led to a greater than twofold increase in cell growth, and a sixfold increase was observed with the highest concentration tested, 100 mg/ml (Table 3). ECGS also stimulated fibroblast proliferation. It caused a more than fourfold increase in cell growth, as compared with controls, after one week and reduced the time necessary to reach confluency by 17-18 days (Table 4).

Only marginal stimulation was achieved with the other additives tested. MSA proved to be only mildly stimulatory in the early stages of cell culture (Table 4). The effects of FGF and increased serum concentration on growth rate was negligible. Histamine actually inhibited fibro-

Table 3. Comparative Growth of Rat Fibroblasts in Medium Supplemented with Various Additives[1]

ADDITIVE	CONCENTRATION	% GROWTH[2] (1 WEEK)	% GROWTH (3 WEEKS)
FGF	100 ng/ml	600%	—
	50 ng/ml	500%	100%
	25 ng/ml	350%	100%
	12.5 ng/ml	225%	—
EGF	20 ng/ml	90%	—
	10 ng/ml	110%	100%
	5 ng/ml	105%	100%
	1 ng/ml	100%	—
FCS	20%	125%	100%
	30%	60%	80%
Histamine	3.0 mg/ml	50%	60%
	1.5 mg/ml	70%	95%
	.75 mg/ml	110%	100%

[1]All cultures were originally plated with 80,000 CFN Rat Fibroblasts (S_2 generation) in 60 mm^2 tissue culture dishes.
[2]% growth compared to the control culture containing no additives. At three weeks the cells in the control culture are confluent.

blast growth at higher concentrations and was only moderately stimulatory at concentrations below 0.75 mg/ml (Table 4).

When combinations of additives were tested, FGF and ECGS together were more stimulatory than either alone, causing cultures to reach confluency in one quarter the time necessary for controls with no additives. Using transmission electron microscopy, we demonstrated that multiple cell layers developed in cultures receiving this combination (Figure 11).

Our studies showed that collagen production in cultures not supplemented with ascorbic acid was minimal. However, when ascorbic acid (50 g/ml) was added to the medium (in which FGF and ECGS had also been included) and the resulting growth examined by transmission electron microscopy, large amounts of collagen were observed filling the interstitial spaces between fibroblast multilayers (Figure 11). No collagen was visible in control cultures. Experimental and control cultures were also examined by means of light microscopy after staining with Tibor-Pap silver impregnation, and under polarized light. Collagen fibers were dramatically highlighted by both procedures, as shown in Figure 12. A dense network of collagenous material was observed in the cultures supplemented with ascorbic acid for 2 weeks, whereas control cultures gave little evidence of collagen formation. α-Ketoglutaric acid and ferrous ion did not stimulate collagen production when employed individually. However, a combination of α-ketoglutaric acid and ascorbic acid resulted in greater stimulation than ascorbic acid alone. Ferrous ions added to the medium did not result in any collagen

Table 4. Comparative Growth of Rat Fibroblasts in Medium Supplemented with Various Additives[1]

ADDITIVE	CONCENTRATION	% GROWTH[2] (1 WEEK)	AVERAGE NUMBER OF DAYS GROWTH UNTIL CONFLUENCY
Control	---	100%	29
FGF	50 ng/ml	540%	10
ECGS	100 µg/ml 200 µg/ml	375% 450%	12 11
MSA	67 ng/ml	200%	31
FGF +ECGS	50 ng/ml 100 µg/ml	610%	8
FGF +MSA	50 ng/ml 67 ng/ml	550%	10
FGF +ECGS +MSA	50 ng/ml 100 µg/ml 67 ng/ml	620%	8

[1]Originally plated with 50,C00 CFN rat fibroblasts (S_2 generation) in 60 mm² tissue culture dishes.
[2]% growth compared to the control cultures containing no additives.

production even when combined with ascorbic acid and α-ketoglutaric acid.

In addition to stimulating collagen production by fibroblasts, ascorbic acid also caused an increase in cell proliferation and growth rate. Transmission electron microscopy of cultures supplemented with ascorbic acid alone showed a significant multiple layer development which was not present in control cultures. On the other hand, α-ketoglutaric acid inhibited proliferation in nonconfluent cultures and as a result prevented collagen formation.

OPTIMIZING CELL ATTACHMENT TO, AND PROLIFERATION ON, BIOMATERIAL SURFACES

A number of studies were performed to examine the nature of the relationship between fibroblast and collagen layers and the biomaterial substrate. Five different groups were studied, as outlined in Table 5. The groups varied in the additives used and in the pretreatment of the substrates. The effects of pretreatment were examined because fibroblasts obtained from fresh tissue (primary cultures) usually did not attach to, and proliferate on, the selected PAD neck materials as they did on commercially obtained culture plastics. The effects of pretreatment of the surfaces with fibronectin, 1N NaOH and undiluted FCS on cellular attachment and proliferation were therefore studied. Fibronectin (Collaborative Research) was

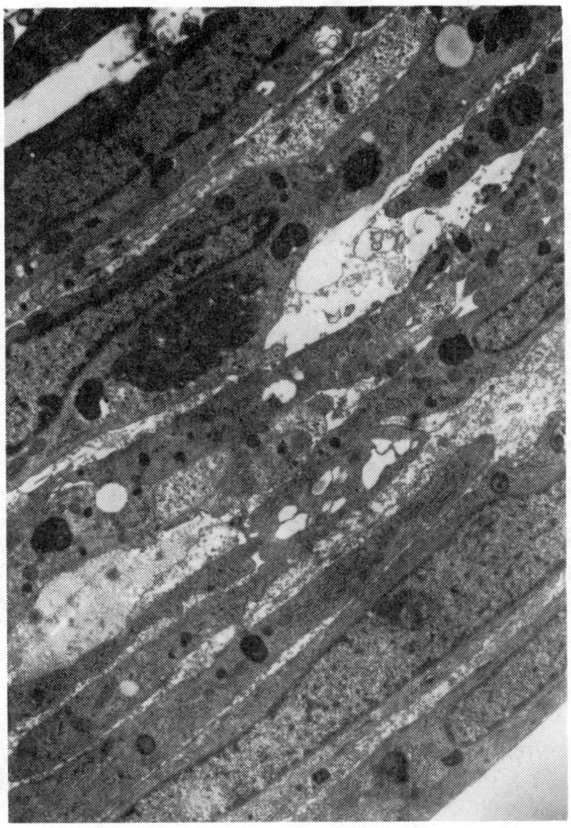

Figure 11. Transmission electron micrograph of rat fibroblast cell layers developed in vitro. *Cell cultures were treated with fibroblast growth factor (FGF) and ascorbic acid causing multilayers. Collagen fibers can be seen filling the intercellular spaces.*

dissolved in MEM and applied to the plastic at 4 ng/cm² of surface for one hour prior to seeding with cells. Plastics were also soaked in FCS for one hour prior to use. Pretreatment of plastics with IN NaOH lasted for 18 hours. In all of these studies the nanoporous plastic materials contained 15,000 pores/mm²; the pores were 1 μm in diameter and 15-20 μm in depth.

Transmission electron microscopy studies were performed on both smooth and nanoporous substrates coated *in vitro* with rat fibroblasts. The results were as follows: In Group 1 samples, grown in the absence of FGF, a fibroblast monolayer formed on the substrate after 3 weeks. Longer periods of cultivation did not alter these results. In all other groups FGF was used, and multiple layers of fibroblasts formed. These results indicated that contact inhibition, a phenomenon which causes proliferation in fibroblast cultures to stop once a monolayer of cells is confluent, was overcome by the use of FGF, allowing a fibroblast multilayer to form, a highly desirable result.

Group 1 and Group 2 samples contained no collagen at the end of the 3-week cultivation period. Group 3-5 samples, on the other hand, produced abundant collagen as a result of the use of ascorbic acid. A difference in the amount and distribution of collagen in the latter three groups was noted. Group 3 and 4 samples, treated with ascorbic acid daily starting 1.5 weeks

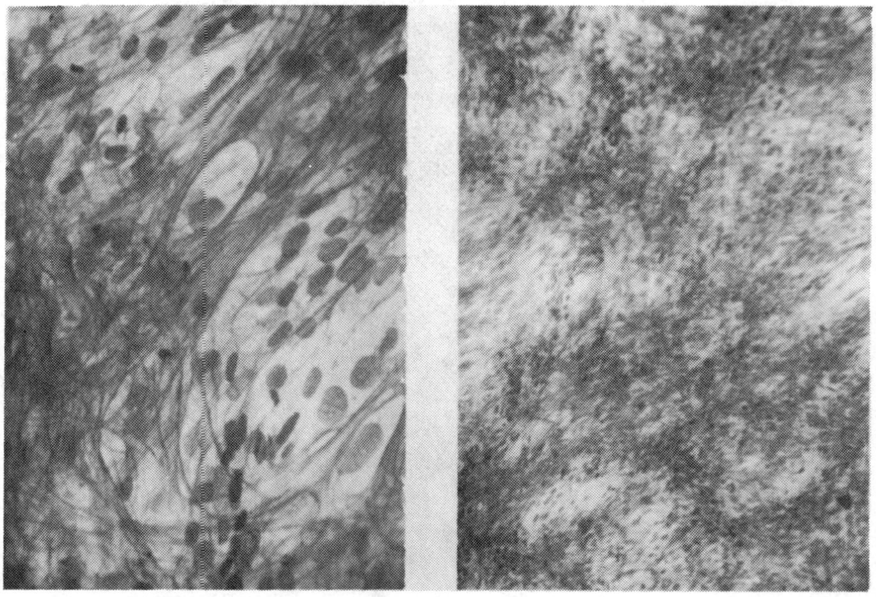

Figure 12. The left photograph shows collagen bundles overlying a dense rat fibroblast cell layer. The oval-shaped nuclei of the cells are seen. On the right, a similar cell layer is visualized under partially polarized light. The collagen fibers in one plane are highlighted as a result of their birefringence. These cell layers resulted from cultivation in vitro for two weeks with ascorbic acid-supplemented medium.

Table 5. Transmission Electron Microscopy Studies

Material and No. of samples	Nanoporous	Pretreatment	Age of Culture	Additives to Medium	Observations
Group 1 (Lexan) 6	No	None	3 weeks	None	Fibroblast monolayer. No collagen.
Group 2 (Lexan) 6	No	None	3 weeks	FGF	Multiple layers of fibroblasts. No collagen.
Group 3 (Lexan) 6	No	None	3 weeks	FGF Ascorbic Acid added daily after 1½ weeks of growth	Multiple layers of fibroblasts. Abundant collagen distributed between tightly packed cell layers. Cells tightly fused to surface of substrate.
Group 4 (Lexan) 10	Yes	HFN	3 weeks	FGF Ascorbic Acid added daily after 1½ weeks of growth	Multiple layers of fibroblasts. Abundant collagen distributed between fibroblast cell layers. Cells not tightly fused to surface of substrate. Many large gaps visible between cells and HFN surface coating. No cellular material in pores.
Group 5 (Lexan) 12	Yes	None	3 weeks	FGF Ascorbic Acid added daily starting day 1	Multiple layers of fibroblasts. Considerably more collagen than in Groups 3 and 4. Large bands containing only dense bundles of collagen were frequently observed. Cells tightly adherent to the surface of the substrate. Cell processes entered the pores and in many instances filled them entirely.

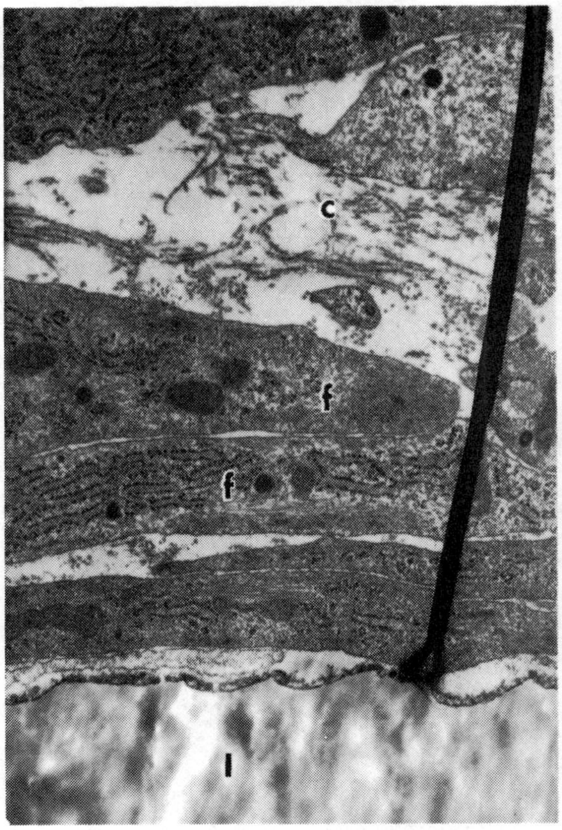

Figure 13. Transmission electron micrograph of rat fibroblasts on nanoporous Lexan substrate (L) pretreated with Human Fibronectin (HFN). No pores are visible in this section. The cell culture was treated with FGF and daily doses of ascorbic acid beginning 1½ weeks after subculturing. Note the formation of multiple fibroblast layers (F) and collagen (C) and the large gaps between the lower fibroblast layer and the HFN-coated Lexan. (3 weeks after start of subculturing, ×25,000).

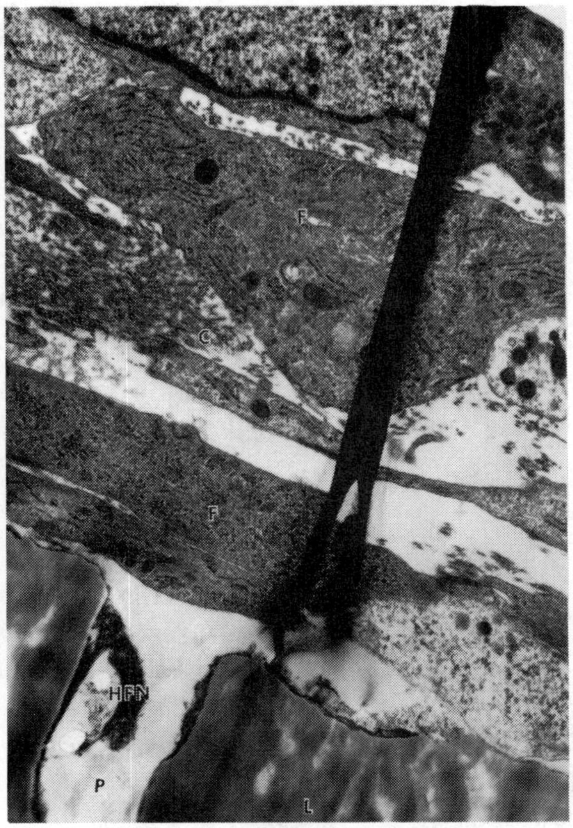

Figure 14. Transmission electron micrograph of rat fibroblasts on nanoporous Lexan substrate (L) pretreated with Human Fibronectin (HFN). The fibroblast and collagen layer is seen overlying a 1 μ pore (P). The cell culture was treated with FGF and daily doses of ascorbic acid beginning 1½ weeks after subculturing. Multiple fibroblast layers (F) and collagen (C) have formed. Note the large gaps between the fibroblast layer and the HFN-coated Lexan. (3 weeks after start of subculturing, ×25,000).

after subculturing, had moderate amounts of collagen distributed between the tightly packed fibroblast layers (Figures 13, 14). Group 5 samples, treated daily with collagen starting on the first day of subculturing, contained considerably more collagen than did the previous two groups. This collagen was organized in thicker bundles than in Group 3 and 4 samples and frequently appeared as a wide band between cell layers (Figure 15). We do not know which collagen arrangement will be more beneficial in relation to PAD function, but it does appear that by using different ascorbic acid initiation schedules, we have some control over the distribution of the collagen.

Group 4 samples, unlike those in all other groups, were treated with Human Fibronectin (HFN) prior to fibroblast coating. In these samples the fibroblasts usually did not appear to be

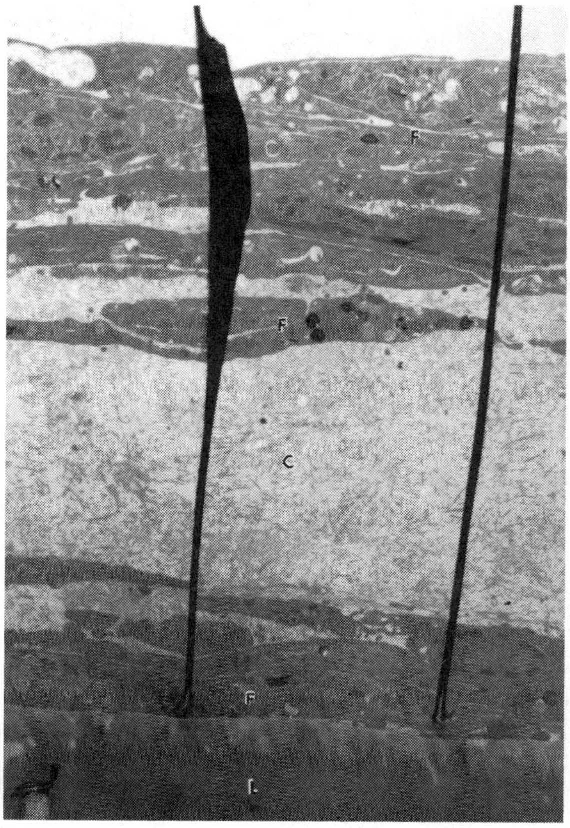

Figure 15. Transmission electron micrograph of rat fibroblasts on a nanoporous Lexan substrate (L). No pores are visible. Numerous fibroblast layers are apparent (F) as well as abundant amounts of collagen (C). This culture was treated with FGF and received daily doses of ascorbic acid starting immediately after subculturing. Note the wide band of collagen; similar bands were not seen when ascorbic acid treatment was started later in relation to the time of subculturing. The lowest fibroblast layer appears to be tightly bonded to the substrate, and a fibroblast process has filled the surface irregularity at the left-center of the micrograph (I). (3 weeks after start of subculturing, ×7,500).

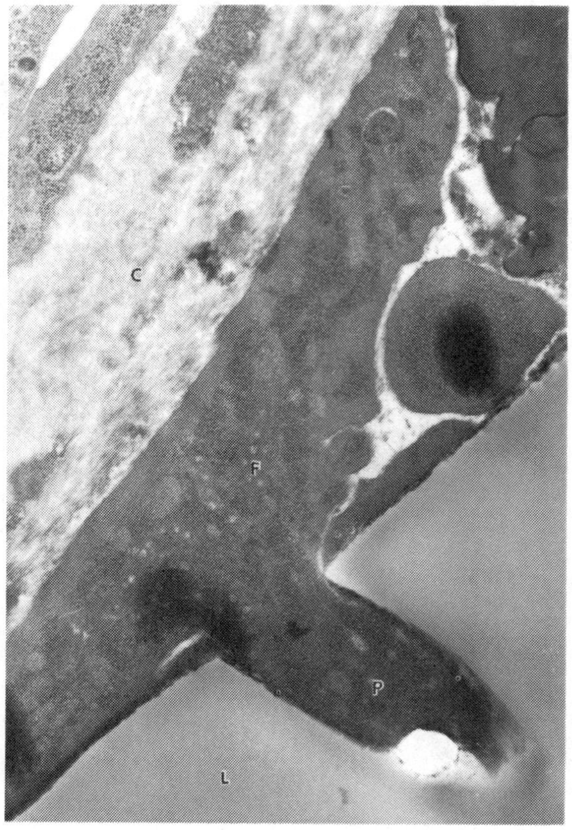

Figure 16. Transmission electron micrograph of rat fibroblasts (F) on a nanoporous Lexan substrate (L). This culture was treated with FGF and received daily doses of ascorbic acid starting immediately after subculturing. A process from the fibroblast is seen extending into a pore (P). Collagen fibers (C) are visible above the cells. Note the close association between the fibroblasts and the Lexan surface. The pore diameter is approximately 1 μm. The white area at the base of the pore is a section preparation artifact. (3 weeks after start of subculturing, ×35,000).

firmly attached to the surface of the substrate. Large gaps were usually present between cells and the HFN-coated substrate (Figures 13 and 14). Furthermore, no cellular material was ever seen entering the pores. In samples from other groups, the cells were tightly fused to the growth substrate with no noticeable gaps (Figures 11, 16, 17). In Group 5, the fibroblasts in direct contact with the substrate sent cellular processes into the pores, providing what was believed to be an excellent mechanical bond between cell and substrate (Figure 16). In many

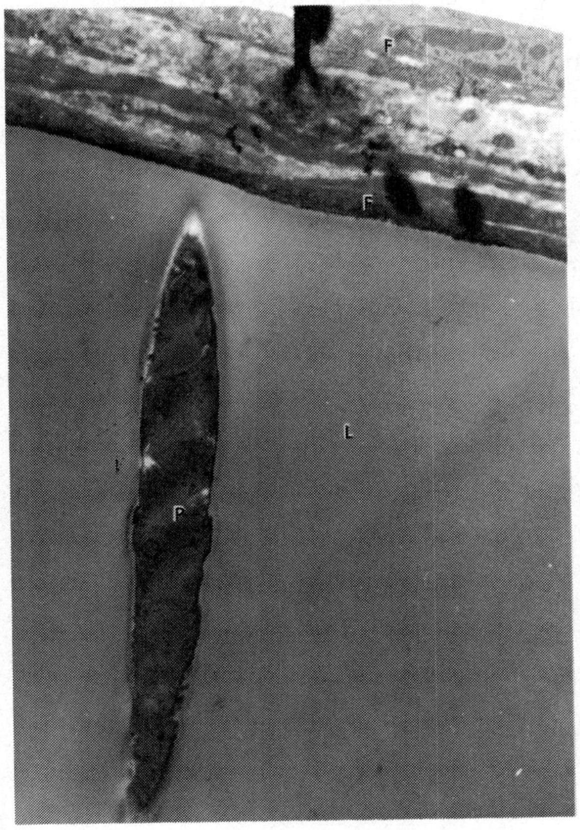

Figure 17. Transmission electron micrograph of rat fibroblasts (F) on a nanoporous Lexan substrate (L). This culture was treated with FGF and received daily doses of ascorbic acid starting immediately after subculturing. A very deep pore is seen here, completely filled by a process from a fibroblast on the Lexan surface. The pore does not extend to the surface because of the angle of the section. Note the close association between the fibroblasts and the Lexan surface. The pore diameter is approximately 1μm (3 weeks after start of subculturing, ×10,000).

cases cell processes filled the entire pore even when the pores were extremely deep (Figure 17). Because of these observations, it was hypothesized that the use of HFN in Group 4 samples was somehow responsible for both absence of cellular processes in the pores and the incomplete attachment of the cells to the growth substrate. No collagen was ever observed within the pores from any of these groups.

DEVELOPMENT OF PAD COMPONENTS FOR IMPLANTATION INTO LABORATORY ANIMALS

Development and In-Vivo Positioning of the Full-Scale PAD Flange

The technique of protecting the tissue-implant seal from mechanical stresses was investigated. The primary feature of this technique depends on the flange's implantation beneath, and in contact with, the dermis. The flange was 85 mm in diameter and composed of several layers of Dacron cloth and Dacron velour bonded by means of silicone adhesive, with a stainless-steel insert 38.5 mm in diameter in the center (Figure 18). Following implantation, the dermis was expected to interlock with the Dacron velour covering the flange. As a result, the PAD, its flange, and the dermis over the flange would move as one in response to external forces, transferring strain from the neck of the device to the outer edge of the flange (see Figure 2).

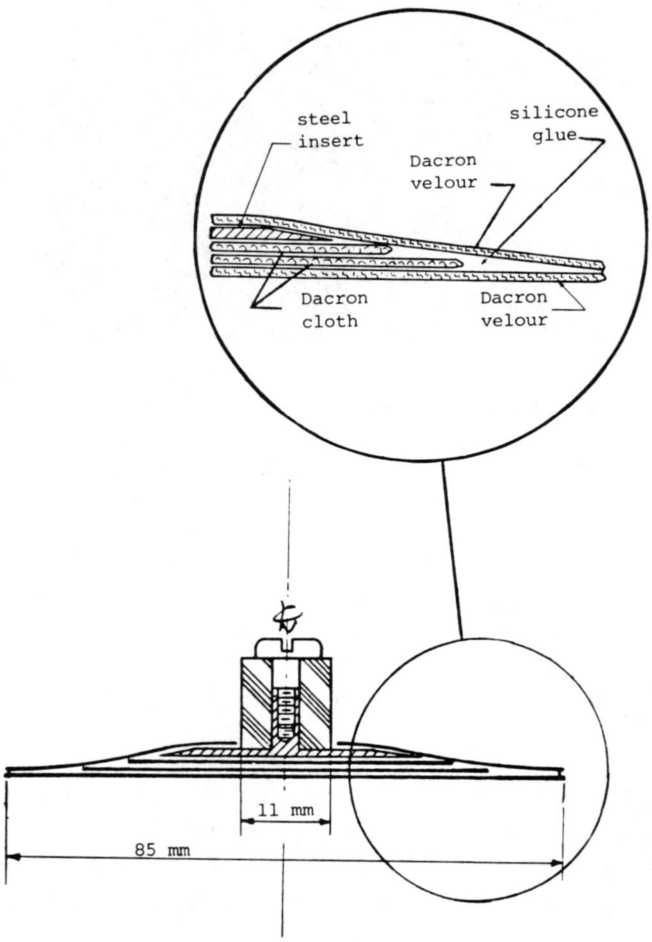

Figure 18. Simplified section of the full-scale PAD. Insert shows internal construction detail. Vertical dimensions of flange are out of scale.

Pigs were selected as the animal model because of the reported close resemblance of their skin to human skin [21]. Compared to most other species, the pig has a very thin hair covering. The skin of both man and pig participates in the dissipation of heat, and therefore each is well supplied with vascular plexuses and corium close to the epidermis [22,23]. However, there are also significant differences between pig and human skin. First, the overall thickness of the subcutaneous layer of the pig's adipose tissue is much greater than that in man. Second, the degree of tension in the skin is different. The skin along the spine is very taut in the pig whereas the ventral skin is somewhat loose and pliable. Therefore, it is only in the ventral area that the pig skin has a mobility which resembles that of man.

Several discs, surrogates for flanges, varying in diameter from 55 to 100 mm were placed subcutaneously in pigs. On the basis of *in vivo* and postmortem examinations, the initial surgical technique consisted of removal of most of the hypodermis and placement of the flange between the remaining hypodermis and fascia. Using this technique, flanges were implanted and stress-strain characteristics measured.

In order to enable measurement of strain, a grid was tattooed over the implant area prior to the surgical procedure. After the wound healed, a pneumatically operated device was temporarily glued to the skin over the implants at weekly intervals and was used to stretch as well as compress the skin up to 15%. The actual compression or stretch frequently was less than 15% since the maximal force the device could exert on the skin was limited to 90 newtons. Photographs were taken in all these positions (Figures 19-21). From these, the positions of the tattoo marks were digitized and fed into a computer, which calculated and plotted the strain versus position curve for each implant and control. The shape of this curve indicates how an external force is transmitted through the skin. Without an implanted flange, a straight line, indicating that the strain is equally distributed throughout the skin, would be expected. If the flange has been properly implanted, the strain-versus-position curve would be expected to deviate markedly from a straight line in the region corresponding to the center of the flange, indicating reduced skin stress in that location. Figure 22 shows a plot of the strain field, averaged for five weekly measurements, over a sham implantation (subcutaneous pocket is created surgically but no flange is implanted). Note that the strain is nearly uniform in distribution. It does depart slightly from the horizontal in the center. This is probably due to skin reinforcement by scar tissue resulting from the surgery. Points at either end of the curve usually had very large standard deviations. Figure 23 shows the strain field over a 100-mm implant. Strain was substantially reduced near the center of the plot (from +20 to −50 mm on the position scale). In order for strain to be redistributed effectively, the flange must be placed in direct contact with the dermis, with no hypodermis in between.

Assembly of the Full-Scale PAD

The neck of the PAD (described above), 11 mm in height and 11 mm in diameter, was coated with fibroblasts obtained from the recipient animal and assembled to the flange just prior to implantation. Attachment was accomplished by means of a screw introduced through the central conduit of the neck and fastened to the metal core of the flange (Figure 18).

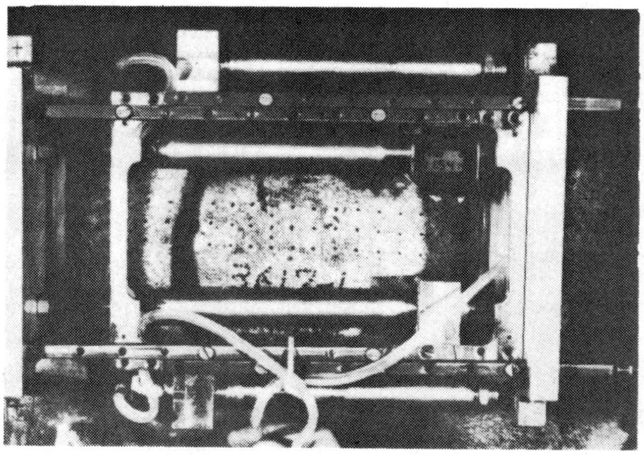

Figure 19. Device in its resting state attached to pig.

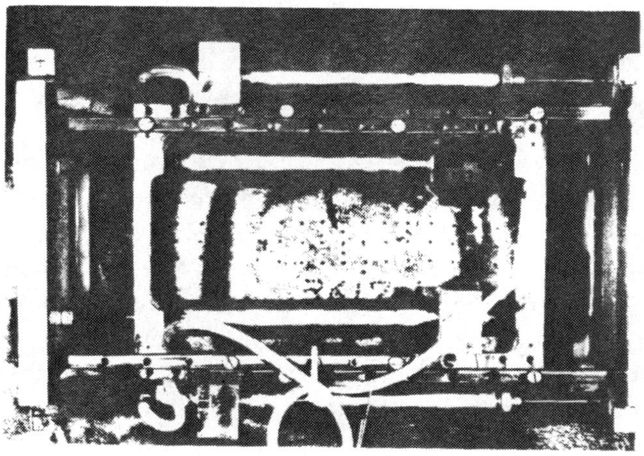

Figure 20. Device stretching pig skin by 15%.

IN VIVO EVALUATION OF SCALED-DOWN AND FULL-SCALE PADs

Rats

Thirty-four scaled-down PADs (half Lexan and half Copel 3320) were implanted in seven CFN rats. These implants were constructed by joining 10-mm lengths of extruded rods (2 mm in diameter) to a disk 6 mm in diameter (which serves as an anchor). The implantation technique in each case included removal of epidermis (4-mm diameter) from the area surrounding each implant site. A full-thickness skin incision was made along the center of the back, the skin lifted, and the implant inserted through the site from underneath. Six of the implants were smooth-surfaced controls (no pores), six were nanoporous controls (no cells), and 22 had ALCON surfaces, i.e., surfaces nanoporous coated with fibroblasts via cell culture. After 72 days,

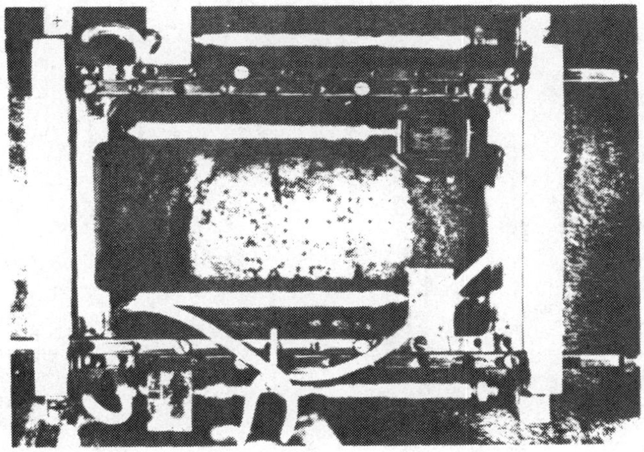

Figure 21. Device compressing pig skin by 15%.

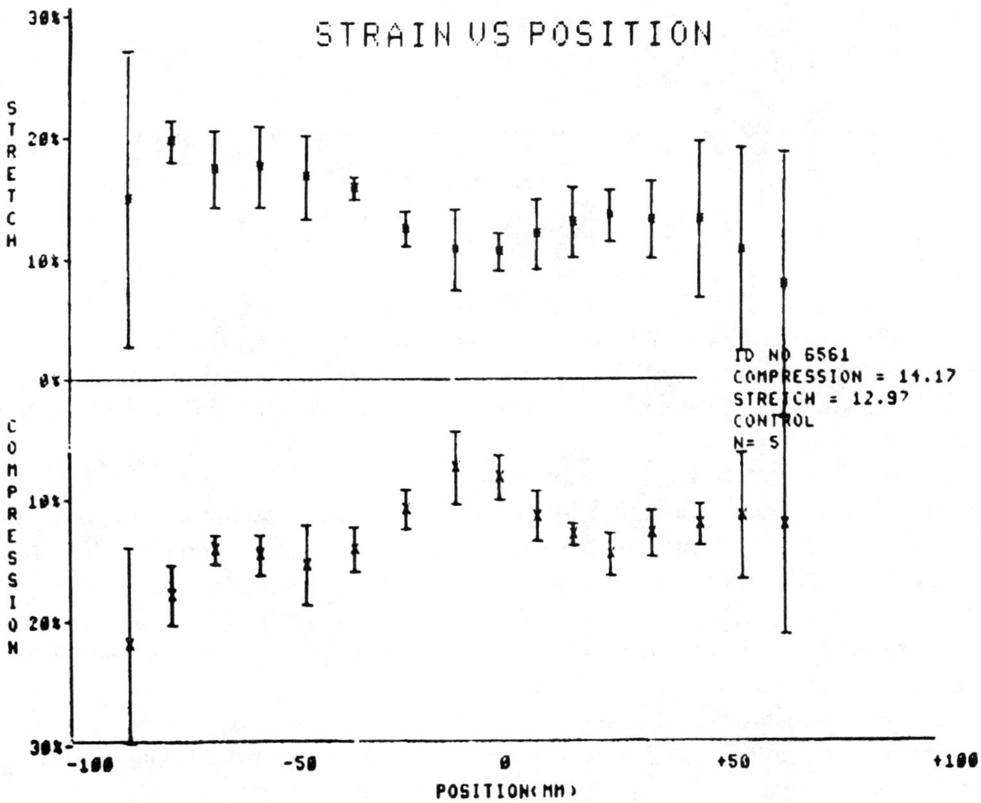

Figure 22. Average of strain field for five weekly measurements over a sham implantation site is shown. Bars are standard deviation.

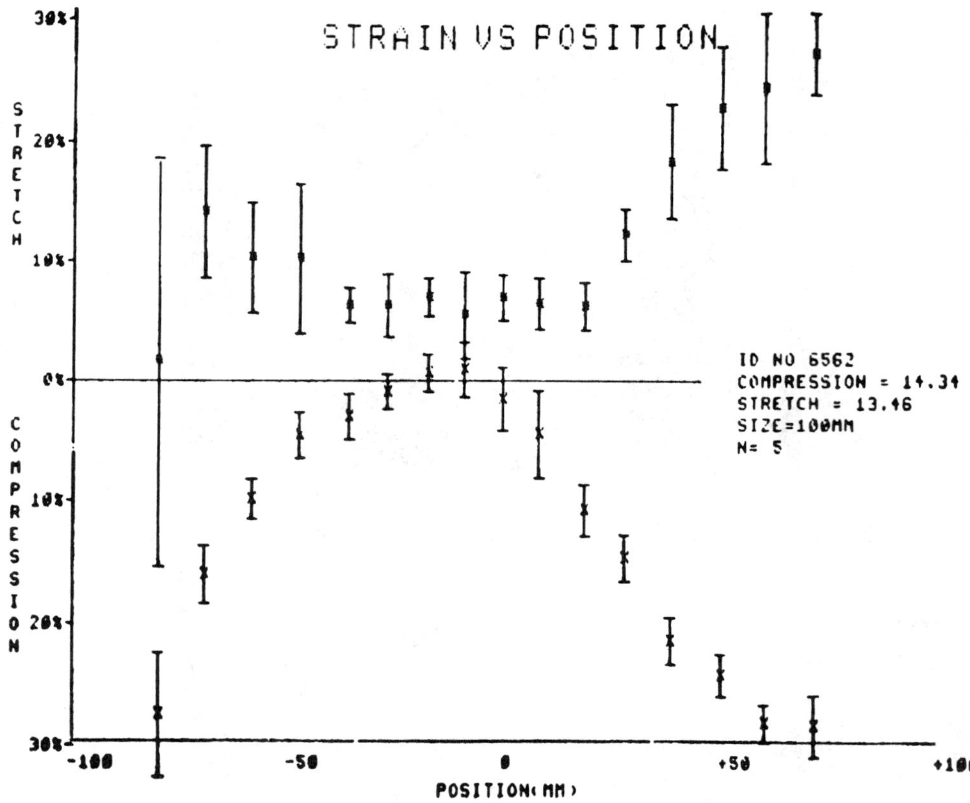

Figure 23. Strain field over a 100 mm implant. Note substantial strain reduction in center.

three rats were sacrificed and their 18 implants removed for examination. After 187 days another rat with two ALCON implants of Lexan and two of Copel 3320 was also sacrificed. At this writing, six implants remain *in situ*. Six were lost due to the death of one rat. All samples (implant and surrounding tissue) were sectioned using a cryostat and stained with Mayer's hematoxylin and eosin.

All implants examined showed signs of normal wound healing. No infection was detected in any of the tissue samples. The tissue surface immediately surrounding the implants showed hyperepithelialization, numerous neutrophils in the dermis, and remnants of scabs. This is seen in Figures 24-27 which are photomicrographs of cross-sections of devices and surrounding tissue 72 days after implantation. The epidermis on the control samples (uncoated, smooth) appeared to be moving down the wound opening, as seen in Figure 24. The epidermis on implants with ALCON surfaces, on the other hand, appeared to have stopped well short of the implantation site and a large scab was usually seen between the furthest point of epidermal migration and the site (Figure 25). Histological sections from implantation sites after 187 days are shown, respectively, in Figure 26 in which Lexan is the PAD neck material and in Figure 27 in which Copel 3320 was used. Both implants had ALCON surfaces and the epidermis appeared to have migrated up to the device-dermis junction and stopped in both cross sections. However, removal of the epidermis and a significant amount of dermis in the process caused a large wound, and healing was still incomplete more than six months after surgery.

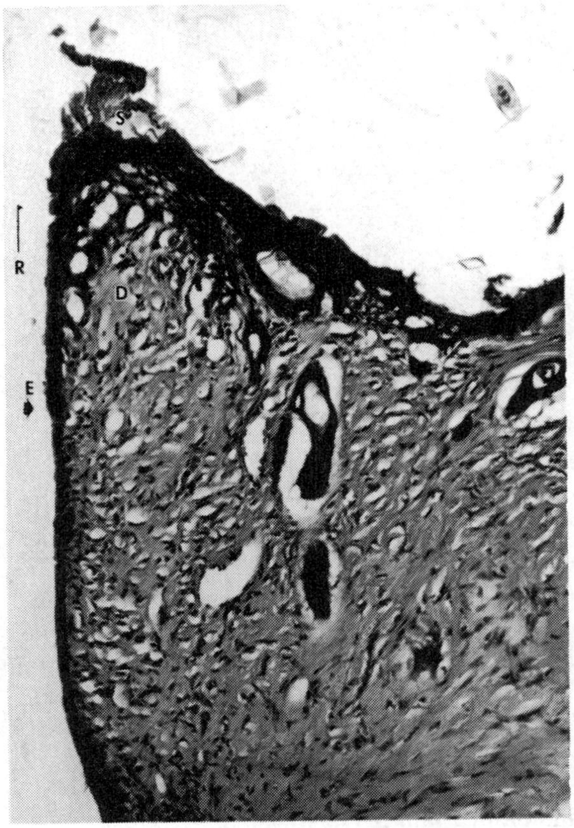

Figure 24. Control. Lexan rod (L) is nonporous and uncoated with fibroblasts. The remnants of a scab may be seen (S) and a large number of neutrophils is present in the dermis (D). E - marks furthest point of epidermal migration. Notice that the epidermis has started to move down the wound opening. Most likely, this will eventually lead to sinus-tract formation and marsupialization. (72 days after implantation, Hematoxylin and eosin, ×240).

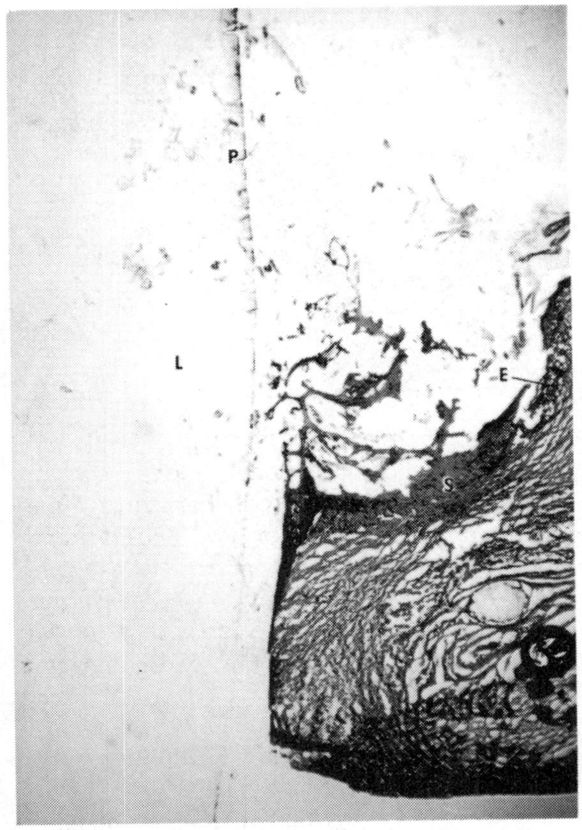

Figure 25. Nanoporous Lexan rod (L) precoated in vitro with autologous fibroblasts prior to implantation. Pores are visible in the rod (P). A large scab is still present (S), and the epidermis has not migrated beyond the scab as yet. E - marks the furthest point of epidermal migration. D - Dermis. (72 days after implantation, Hematoxylin and eosin, ×60).

It was decided that the material of choice for further study is Lexan, which consequently will be the only material used in future full-scale and scaled-down devices. A concentrated study of the biological processes involved in the interaction of PAD materials with host tissue has been initiated in the CFN rat. The influence of pores versus smooth surface, pore density, and pore size on tissue reaction and longevity of the implant is being studied. Parameters under study are summarized in Table 6.

Swine

Several technical considerations had to be addressed before implantations of full-scale PADs could proceed. The choice of a site for PAD implantation is an important determinant

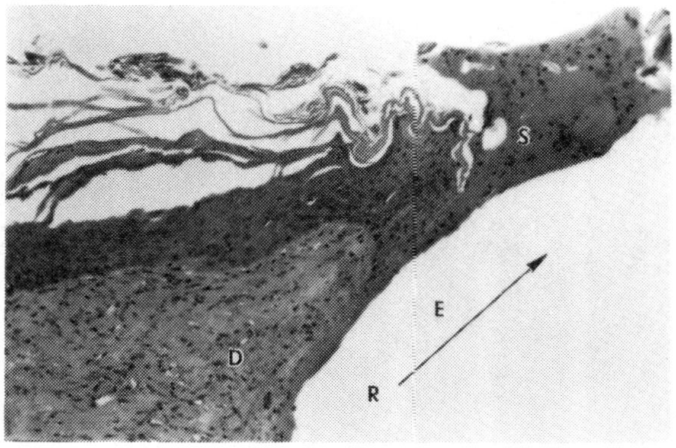

Figure 26. Photograph of histological section of ALCON surfaced polycarbonate implanted into a rat for 187 days. Epidermis appears to have migrated up to the rod-dermis junction and stopped. Although healing appears to be incomplete, there is still scab left as well as chronic fibrosis and inflammation as indicated by the presence of significant number of macrophages.

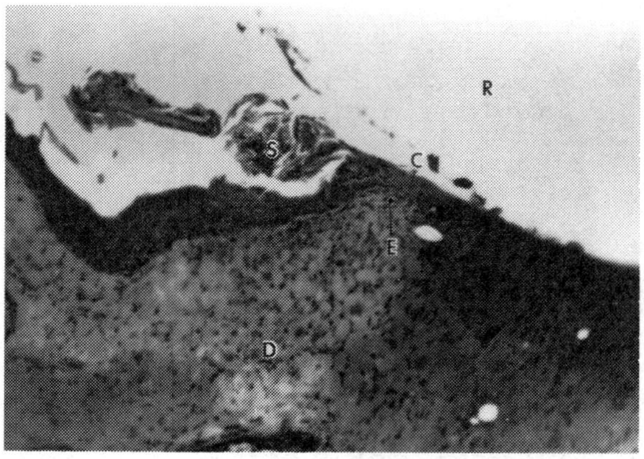

Figure 27. Photograph of histological section of ALCON surfaced Copel 3320 implanted into a rat for 187 days. Epidermis has migrated up to rod-dermis interface. Scab formation remains over the migrated epidermis. There is some ulceration overlayed by inflammatory exudate. Also, granulation tissue is evident. E - epidermis (↑ indicates furthest point of epidermal migration); R - implanted rod (↑ indicates rod direction as it protrudes through the skin); D - dermis; S -scab; Stained with H & E, 140×).

Table 6. Preimplantation Preparation of 2 mm Lexan 104 Rods for Use as Scaled-Down PAD Implants in CFN Rats

Category	Dia (m)	Pore Density $(x10^3)$	Cells
I	0	0	-
II	0	0	+
III	1,0	15	-
IV	1.0	15	+
V	1,0	30	-
VI	1.0	30	+
VII	0,5	15	-
VIII	0,5	15	+
IX	5,0	15	-
X	5,0	15	+

+ = fibroblast-coated *in vitro*.
− = no addition of cells *in vitro*.

of the success with which the device is used. This holds especially for experimental animals (swine, in this case) whose hygienic care is difficult and in which the extent of trauma to the implant that is due to the animal's actions can be influenced by the placement of the device. Swine tend to sleep on their sides. To reduce the animal's discomfort and thus minimize the likelihood of PAD damage, implantations are restricted to one side of the animal. Two sites can be used, one on the side of the abdomen and one over the ribs (Figure 28).

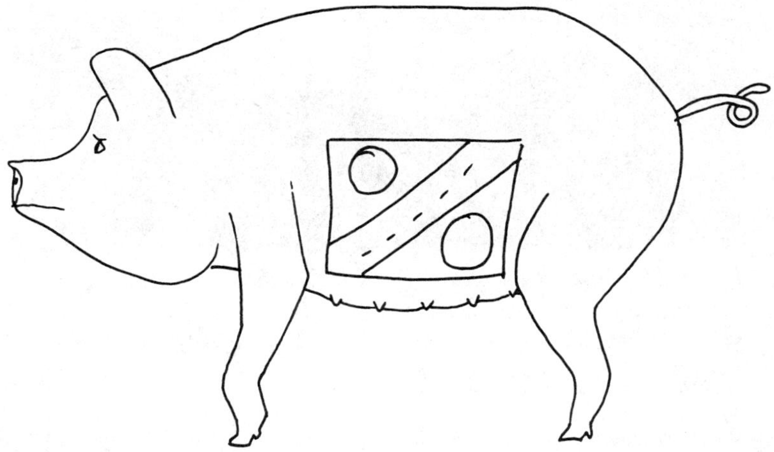

Figure 28. Considerations limiting the choice of implant site in miniature swine. Sites anterior or posterior to the rectangular area are unsuitable because of excessive movement of the skin in proximity to the animal's limbs and because of interference with limb motion; sites beneath the rectangle are unsuited because the animal may lie down on them; and those above the rectangle impinge on a region of thickened skin which poorly models the human integument. Within the rectangular area, the diagonal swath indicated is inappropriate because it lies over the edge of the rib cage. Of the remaining two regions within the rectangle, that in the lower posterior portion of the rectangle has the advantage of being a relatively compliant location overlying soft tissue.

To reduce the chances of contamination of the implantation site by fecal matter or as a result of savaging by the animal, a restraint system was devised that prevents it from lying down on the implanted side or from rubbing that side against the walls of the cage. The system consisted of a well-fitted body suit to which four straps were attached (Figure 29). For an implant on the swine's right side, the straps on the right were attached to the top of the cage and the straps on the left side were attached to the left wall of the cage, level with the animal's shoulder. Enough slack was left in the straps so as to restrict the animal's motion as little as possible consistent with the above requirements.

After various technical problems had been solved, a prototype of this arrangement worked as planned for 2 months. The animal then formed the habit of sleeping in a position that put all its weight against the restraining straps. This led to pressure necrosis at the edges of the body suit.

The system we now use is to apply a layer of bandages around the implant sufficiently thick

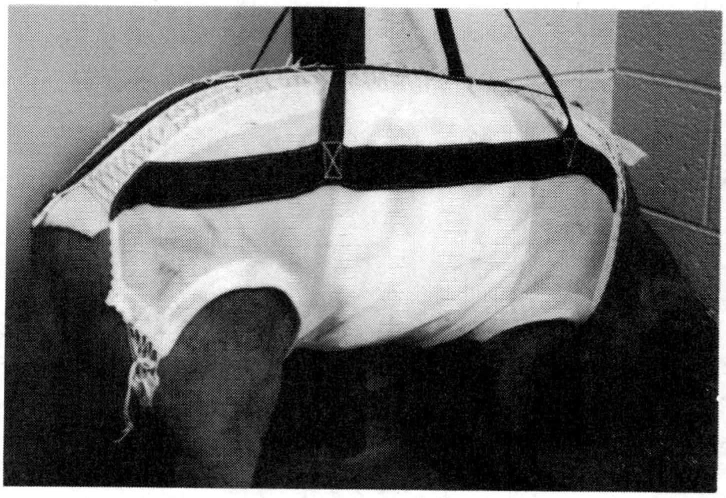

Figure 29. Restraint system consisting of body suit and straps for miniature swine used in initial studies. Slack was left in the straps to restrict animal's motion as little as possible consistent with protection of implant sites.

to cushion it. An elastic stocking with holes cut in it for the four legs is placed over the bandages covering the pig from neck to tail. This prevents the unraveling of the bandages. Bandages are changed every second day. To date this approach has worked well.

Continuous contact of the native dermis with the ALCON surface during the initial healing period is a necessary condition for successful PAD implantation. To make possible such apposition, a technique had to be developed for excising a circular area of skin of precisely specified diameter. After a number of false starts a trephine was developed for this purpose. In its first version, this instrument was made of steel. It outlined but could not completely cut a block of tissue of the appropriate diameter; a scalpel had to be used to complete the incision. The precision was insufficient and an oversize hole resulted. The next version of the trephine, made of carbide (Figure 30), was able to hold a much sharper edge. The use of this instrument appears to result in openings of the correct size.

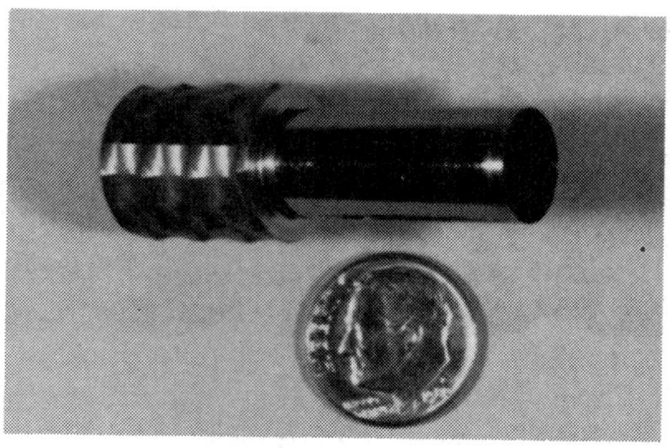

Figure 30. Photograph of carbide trephine.

The protocol for PAD implantation in miniature swine was as follows:

Recipient:	Adult female Yucatan miniature swine weighing 70-90 kg
Preoperative preparation:	NPO 12 hours preoperatively
Anesthesia:	Innovar-Vet 1 ml/14.6 kg, atropine sulfate 0.4 mg/kg, ketamine hydrochloride 11 mg/kg
Position:	Lateral recumbency
Skin preparation:	Shave, Betadyne scrub followed by 70% ethyl alcohol in three alternating sets, Betadyne as a final coating

Operative Procedure. The exact dimensions of the PAD are drawn on the skin surface with the aid of a nonfunctional device as a pattern. A 10- to 12-cm lateral skin incision, 2 cm cephalad from the edge of the desired pocket, is made down to the level of the hypodermis. A 10-cm diameter pocket immediately deep to the dermis and superficial to the underlying hypodermis is made by sharp dissection. Hemostasis is achieved by local pressure only. An effort is made to preserve all visible blood vessels.

After the pocket has been formed and hemostasis has been achieved, the epidermis is removed from a circular region 4 mm larger in diameter than the intended PAD neck by means of a dermatome. The skin is stretched, a block of reinforced silicone is temporarily inserted into the pocket, and a circular hole to accommodate the neck of the PAD is cut using the carbide trephine. The PAD neck is removed from the culture medium and assembled to the flange. It is inserted into the pocket and the neck of the device guided carefully through the circular access so as not to shear the fibroblast culture. The incision is closed by interrupted sutures using 2-0 nylon monofilament sutures. Hydron burn dressing is applied to the wounds.

Several full-scale PADs have been implanted in pigs. They include (1) smooth Lexan controls, without fibroblasts and (2) with fibroblasts, (3) Lexan implants with pores but without fibroblasts and (4) Lexan with pores and coated with fibroblasts, i.e., with ALCON surfaces. All implants appear free of infection and would be clinically accepted if used with an actual assist device. However, on the controls, a gap has opened between the skin and the neck of the implant which we believe is likely to become infected eventually. On the ALCON-coated necks there appears to be good adhesion between the skin and the implant, as indicated by the fact that even when one attempts to retract the skin from the device no gap opens. Figure 31 shows a photograph of a control PAD 22 days after implantation. Note the gap that has developed between the implant and surrounding skin. No such break is seen in an ALCON-surfaced PAD neck, as seen in Figure 32, which is a photograph of such a device 30 days after implantation.

CONCLUSIONS

Early results indicate that Lexan and Copel materials precoated with fibroblasts and collagen to result in the ALCON surface described will resist epidermal downgrowth along an

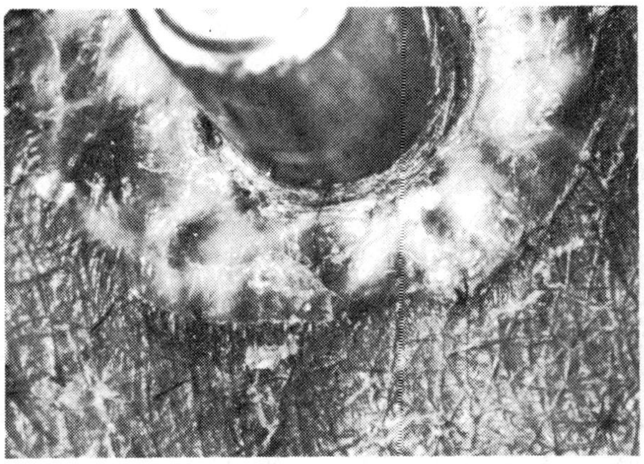

Figure 31. Photograph of control PAD twenty-two days post implantation. Note gap between skin and implant. The light areas of skin are newly formed and are lacking in pigmentation.

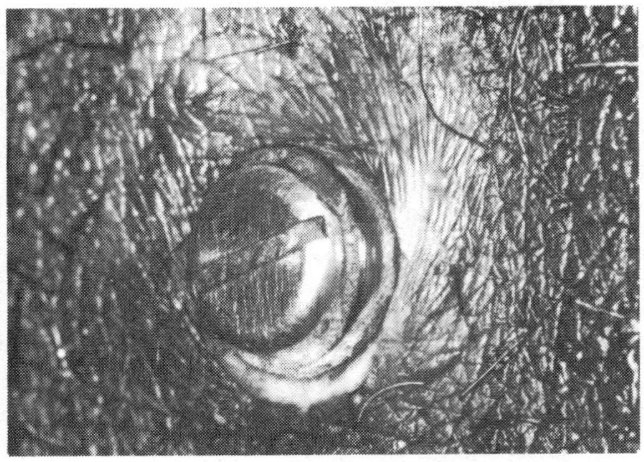

Figure 32. Photograph of ALCON surfaced PAD fifteen days post implantation.

implanted PAD more effectively than uncoated materials. The data are as yet insufficient to allow a prediction as to the length of time this inhibition of epidermal migration will last, preventing sinus-tract formation, infection, and other conditions which have been shown to contribute to PAD failure. The influence different pore sizes and densities have on the effectiveness of fibroblast and collagen attachment to the PAD surface has not been determined. We are currently investigating these relationships in rats using scaled-down PAD implants.

Proper placement of the flange portion of the PAD is essential. When even a thin layer of adipose tissue is present between the dermis and the implant as a result of unintentional variations in implantation technique, relative motion between skin and implant is possible, and local skin reinforcement and strain redistribution are diminished or even abolished. Where the implant is in direct, firm contact with the dermis, local reinforcement and strain redistribution do take place. Observations on pigs with full-scale PADs indicate that flange placement contributes to the stability of the complete device.

None of the data obtained thus far invalidates the concept of the proposed PAD.

REFERENCES

1. Hall, C. W.; Adams, L. M.; Chidoni, J. J.: Development of skin interfacing cannula. Trans. Am. Soc. Artif. Intern. Organs 21:281-288 (1975).
2. Mooney, V.; Hartmann, D. G.: Percutaneous passage, in *Biomedical Electrode Technology,* Miller, H. A. and Harrison, D. C., eds., Academic Press, Inc., New York (1974).
3. Schraut, W.; Kiso, I.; Freed, P.; Baechler, C.; Barnhart, M.; Riddle, J.; Mammen, E.; Mandell, G.; Kantrowitz, A.: Permanent in-series cardiac assistance with the dynamic aortic patch: blood-prosthesis interaction in long-term canine experiments. Surgery 79:193 (1976).
4. Kantrowitz, A.; Freed, P. S.; Hamada, O.; Kerin, N.; Rubenfire, M.; Wajszczuk, W.: Permanent in-series LV assistance: clinical experience in five cases. (Abstract) Proceedings of the 14th Annual Meeting, Association for the Advancement of Medical Instrumentation, Las Vegas, Nevada, April 1979, p. 142.
5. Al-Nakeeb, S.; Pearson, P. T.; Cholvin, N. R.: A thoracic percutaneous lead system: development and evaluation. J. Biomed. Mater. Res. 6:245 (1972).

6. Pae, W., Jr.; O'Bannon, W.; Prophet, G. A.; Donachy, J. H.; Abt, A.; Pierce, W. S.: Design and evaluation of a percutaneous transthoracic cannula. Trans. Am. Soc. Artif. Intern. Organs 22:135-148 (1976).
7. Mladejovsky, M. G.; Eddington, D. K.; Dobelle, W. H.; Brachman, D. E.: Artificial hearing for the deaf by cochlear stimulation: pitch modulation and some parametric thresholds. Trans. Am. Soc. Artif. Intern. Organs 21:1 (1975).
8. House, W. F.; Urban, J.: Long-term results of electrode implantation and electronic stimulation of the cochlea in man. Ann. Otol. 82:804 (1973).
9. Benson, J.: Carbon implant research. Proc. 18th National SAMPE Symposium (April 1973).
10. Grosse-Siestrup, C.; Affeld, K.; Weidermann, H.; Bucherl, E. S.: Artificial percutaneous leads allowing permanent epithelial ingrowth. Second International Symposium for Artificial Internal Organs, Tokyo, Japan (1977).
11. Rogers, A.; Morris, L. B.: Percutaneous leads for power and control of artificial hearts. Trans. Am. Soc. Artif. Intern. Organs 13:146-150 (1967).
12. Winter, G. D.: Transcutaneous implants: reactions of the skin-implant interface. J. Biomed. Mater. Res. Symposium 5:99-113 (1974).
13. Grosse-Siestrup, C.; Krautzberger, W.; Bucherl, E. S.: Arterio-venous shunt with percutaneous leads in calves for long-term in vivo testing of blood-contact materials. J. Biomed. Mater. Res. 13:15 (1979).
14. Robinson, T. C.: Clinical evaluation of microporous tissue interface dialysis shunts and catheters. Final report to Artificial Kidney Chronic Uremia Program, NIAMD, NIH (January 1976).
15. Freed, P. S.; Taro, G.: A transcutaneous safety release. Proc. 27th ACEMB 16:54 (1974).
16. Fleischer, R. L.; Price, P. B.; Walker, R. M.: *Nuclear Tracks in Solids,* University of California Press, Berkeley, CA (1975).
17. Vaughan, F. L.; Bernstein, I.A.: Studies of proliferative capabilities in isolated epidermal basal and differentiated cells. J. Invest. Dermatol. 56:454-466 (1971).
18. Barnes, M. J.: Function of ascorbic acid in collagen metabolism. Ann. NY Acad. Sci. 258:264 (1975).
19. Levene, C. I.; Bates, C.J.: Ascorbic acid and collagen synthesis in cultured fibroblasts. Ann. NY Acad. Sci. 258:288 (1975).
20. Switzer, B. R.; Summer, G. K.: Collagen synthesis in human skin fibroblasts: effects of ascorbate, α-Ketoglutarate and ferrous ion on proline hydroxylation. J. Nutr. 102:721 (1972).
21. Hartwell, S. W.: The mechanism of healing in human wounds. Charles Thomas, Publisher, Springfield, Illinois (1955).
22. Nickel, R.; Schummer, A.; Seiferle, E.: Lehrbuch der Anatomie der Haustiere. Wol. 1, Paul Parey, Berlin (1954).
23. Winter, G. D.: Epidermal regeneration studied in the domestic pig, in Epidermal Wound Healing, Maibach, H. I. and Rovee, D. T., eds., Yearbook Medical Publ., Inc., Chicago (1972).

Chapter 28

Interfacial Shear Strength of Implant/Intramedullary Bone in Geese

J. B. Park
Department of Biomedical Engineering
School of Engineering
Tulane University
New Orleans, LA 70118

AND

K. Markgraf
Department of Interdisciplinary Studies
College of Engineering
Clemson University
Clemson, SC 29631

ABSTRACT

Arthritis is among the commonest diseases affecting mankind. Of the 16.8 million arthritis sufferers in the United States, more than 3 million are completely disabled by the two major forms of arthritis, rheumatoid arthritis or osteoarthritis.

One method of relieving the disabling effects of arthritis is by the use of artificial finger joints. Artificial finger joints, such as the Swansom prosthesis, are used in those cases in which irreparable damage is sustained in the hand digits. The Swanson prosthesis, made of Silicone rubber, is widely used as an alternative to amputation or joint fusion.

In spite of its widespread use, Silicone finger joints exhibit relatively low resistance to tear propagation; in addition, Silicone rubber has a low modulus of elasticity, thus lacking optimum support to the finger joint. In this chapter we report the progress of our research and development of a grommet to be used in conjunction with the Swanson Silicone rubber finger prosthesis, to protect the Silicone rubber from cuts, and thus lower the incidence of tear failures.

INTRODUCTION

According to a survey conducted by the United States Public Health Service's National Center for Health Statistics between 1966 and 1967, approximately 16.8 million people in the United States suffer from some form of arthritis. It is estimated that at any one time 3.4 million people are completely disabled by arthritis. There are two major forms of arthritis. Rheumatoid arthritis is a generalized disease that affects the soft tissues of the joint capsule, the synovium; it is believed to be an immunological response within the synovial tissues. Osteoarthritis is a disease of the articular cartilage. The degradation of the articular cartilage could be due to a variety of mechanical (e.g., wear) or physiological reasons. Osteoarthritis accounts for approximately three-fourths of arthritis patients requiring treatment, although rheumatoid arthritis can often be the severest crippler of the two.

Also to be considered are those injuries to the joints due to trauma. The National Safety Council determined that in 1970, 2.2 million people received disabling work injuries. Disablement of the extremities accounted for 33% of these injuries; the digits of the hand were involved in 17% of these cases.

Whatever the cause, the functional loss of a joint can have severe physical as well as emotional consequences. This report deals with the research and development of a grommet to be used in conjunction with the Swanson silicone rubber finger prosthesis. The feasibility of the use of the grommet will be studied, but also of major consideration is whether a smooth or a textured surface metal of two alloys will provide for better appositional bone growth. The two alloys are cobalt chrome and titanium-6% aluminum-4% vanadium, both of which are widely used as implant materials.

HISTORY AND BACKGROUND

Finger Joint Prosthesis

One of the first recorded efforts of functional restoration of a joint by simple resection of the soft tissues was by Ambroise Pare in the sixteenth century. Resection arthroplasty is a surgical procedure involving the removal or resection of diseased tissues (e.g., synovium, tendon, bone) and reconstruction to produce a stable, functioning joint. With regards to rheumatoid arthritis, clinical studies have shown that the number of joints showing improvement diminishes as one advances from resection arthroplasty alone to complete arthroplastic reconstruction (i.e., prosthetic reconstruction). If the rheumatoid process is sufficiently advanced though, simple resection techniques become less effective than if done early in the course of the disease. Before the introduction of prosthetic replacement of the joints of the finger, the clinical alternatives to surgical reconstruction were amputation or joint fusion.

Brannon and Klein [1] reported on the development of the first finger prosthesis in 1959. The prosthesis was applied to those cases in which irreparable damage was sustained to the digits of the hand. The prosthesis was an all metal simple hinge design. Stainless steel was used in the original prosthesis but was changed to titanium due to its high corrosion resistance. The two metal stems are inserted into the intramedullary canal and are of a triangular configuration, a design feature to prevent rotation. The major complication of this technique is bone resorption due to the extreme differences in the elastic properties of the metal and bone. As the bone resorbs, the prosthesis settles into the phalanges resulting in reduced range of motion and stem rotation.

Flatt redesigned the Brannon-Klein prosthesis in 1961 in an attempt to alleviate this problem of stem rotation following bone resorption [2]; the single squared stem was replaced by two prongs. This prosthesis can be inserted easily as the prongs can be pressed together and thus locked into place by spring-back. In the long term, this compression and springback reaction lead to complications: bone erosion and possible metal fatigue.

In a 1963 follow-up study, Flatt noted that absorption had occurred but as yet there had been no mechanical obstruction to movement [3]. Flatt points out in both his 1961 and 1963 reports that prosthetic replacement should not be used to the exclusion of the more commonly practiced surgical techniques and only in limited applications. At the time of the 1963 report, the incidence of the use of the prosthesis versus surgery was only 8.2% for the proximal interphalangeal joint (PIP) and 18.7% for the metacarpophalangeal (MCP) joint. Similar observations and conclusions were noted by Girzadas in his study of Flatt's prosthesis [4].

Flatt later changed the original prosthetic design to improve the overall range of motion in MCP joint replacement; an enlarged version of the PIP joint prosthesis which had been used previously [5]. The axis of rotation was lowered, or offset volarly, from the prong level of the prosthesis. The hinge design was changed to alleviate the problems encountered due to what Flatt terms "Reciprocal Action Between Digital Joints." When the MCP joint was reconstructed with the old prosthetic design, a resultant poor range of motion at the PIP joint was associated with good range of motion at the MCP joint. Conversely, if the range of motion at the MCP joint was decreased, good range of motion was experienced at the PIP joint. It should be pointed out that prosthetic replacement of the MCP joint is generally more successful and that the studies dealt with in this paper are primarily concerned with MCP joint replacement.

What might be termed the second stage in the development of finger prostheses was initiated by the advent of medical-grade synthetic polymers. These polymers are characterized by a low elastic modulus and do not stress the bone as severely as the allmetal prosthesis, thus reducing the high incidence of bone resorption. In 1966, Swanson reported on the clinical trials of a flexible silicone rubber intramedullary stemmed finger-joint implant [6]. In 1968, Niebauer reported on the use of a silicone-covered Dacron hinge [7]; also, Calnan and Reis reported on their experiences with a polypropylene hinge [8]. A major distinction between the metal and polymer designs is that the metal prosthesis involves complete joint reconstruction (i.e., the prosthesis totally replaces the joint), whereas the polymer prostheses are used in conjunction to resection arthroplasty, resulting in a more natural joint system.

Resection arthroplasty alone can often have unpredictable results. This technique requires that the hand be immobilized for relatively long periods of time while the joint redevelops. Frequently this results in fibrosis of the soft tissues, compromising the joint's range of motion. Also a significant number of arthroplasties eventually dislocated. When good results were obtained, it was due to the satisfactory development of a collagen-rich mesothelial capsule, forming a pseudosynovium. Swanson proposed the use of a two-stemmed silicone rubber prosthesis to improve the success rate of finger-joint resection arthroplasty [9].

Swanson designed his prosthesis to aid resection arthroplasty with respect to certain considerations. Silicone rubber is a highly biologically inert material thus providing a noninflammatory implant surface and allowing no tissue ingrowth or adherence. Rather the encapsulation process already mentioned is oriented about the implant. The implant itself serves as an internal support for the new joint capsule. The Swanson implant has an extremely long flex life, having been machine flexed over 600 million cycles with no observable changes. Also the prosthesis serves to maintain proper bone alignment both vertically and laterally, while the flexible midsection maintains the proper width of the joint space.

Another important design feature of the Swanson prosthesis is the maintenance of the "gliding principle." As the silicone rubber prosthesis is stabilized by a fibrous encapsulation rather than mechanical means, a slight 1-2 mm piston-like movement within the intramedullary cavity occurs during flexion and extension of the joint. Rigid fixation is not desirable for a flexible implant as it would put intolerable strains on the implants. Also, the joint is allowed to find its own center of rotation; the implant does not interfere.

The use of the Swanson implant with resection arthroplasty alleviates the variable encapsulation process encountered in resection arthroplasty alone. Due to the internal support of the prosthesis, the hand is not required to be immobilized for as long a period of time allowing early physical therapy. Extensive clinical trials have shown that the use of the Swanson prosthesis improves the success rate and overall range of motion of the reconstructed joint versus simple resection arthroplasty [10-12].

Several problems are encountered, though, with the use of silicone rubber that are inherent to the material. Silicone rubber can undergo extensive elastic deformation – over 400% elongation, but it allows no plastic deformation. Silicone rubber has relatively poor resistance to tear propagation. Excessive stress concentrations may occur at nicks or abrasions of the surface – rough bone edges, handling. Thus when the implant is strained due to the material's inability to deform plastically it will result in propagation of the tear. Also, as silicone rubber has a very low modulus of elasticity, optimum support to the joint is not provided; the implant will deform elastically under normal finger tip forces.

In 1972, Swanson reported a 2% fracture rate of his silicone rubber prosthesis [13]. Several other researchers have noted a much higher fracture rate through roentgenographic studies. Beckenbaugh reported a fracture rate of 26.2% [10], while Hagert reported a failure rate of 25% [14]. The difference in the failure rates may possibly be attributed to the fact that in the roentgenographic studies any fractures, cracks, or fragmentations were considered failures although observable joint function may not have diminished.

Hagert proposed that the failure of the Swanson prosthesis is generally initiated by lateral loading causing deformation of the implant. "Pinching" of the hinge portion during extension has also been noted as a possible cause of failure. Swanson feels this is due to inadequate release of the joint deformity which results in the increased stresses on the implant. Gillespie, using fresh cadaver rays, also noted the poor lateral support; radial-ulnar drift was unpredictable and increased in proportion to the force applied – up to 90° RUD at 90° of flexion [15].

Although the joint can choose its own axis of rotation with the Swanson prosthesis, the axis may not necessarily be located in the hinge portion of the implant. Gillespie noted that the center of rotation was erratic. Maximum motion occurred at the bone-stem interface and most frequently at the proximal phalanx-distal stem junction. Motion at the hinge of the implant was also noted, particularly from 60° to full flexion. Buckling of the Swanson implant had also been observed roentogenographically by Hagert; buckling occurred in 15% of the cases post-operatively. The incidence of buckling may be less when the encapsulation process is complete. The implant may buckle at either stem or at both resulting in a s-shaped configuration; buckling generally reduces the joint's extensor forces. When buckling occurs, pressure is exerted on the dorsal portion of the metacarpal bone and the volar portion of the proximal phalanx. Hagert confirmed this as bone resorption was noted at these areas with resultant bone spur formation. The bone spur restricts flexion somewhat and is a site of possible implant damage.

The Niebauer silicone rubber prosthesis differs from the Swanson in that it is designed to be anchored within the intramedullary canal. The stems are surrounded by a Dacron mesh sutured in place by Dacron thread. The mesh allows for tissue ingrowth locking the prosthesis in place.

Many of the same problems encountered with the Swanson prosthesis also occurred with the Niebauer design: buckling post-operatively, failure by cracking, fracturing, and fragmentation. The Niebauer prosthesis has a higher failure rate than the Swanson prosthesis though. Beckenbaugh reported damage to 32.8% of the Niebauer prostheses [10] while Hagert noted a 50% failure rate [14]. The higher failure rate of the Niebauer prosthesis is due to the elastic property difference between Dacron and the silicone rubber. As the implant is flexed, the Dacron stresses the silicone rubber reducing the life span of the implant since the former is a much stiffer material.

During the 1970's, various metal-plastic total joint prosthetic designs were introduced: Strickland, Steffeell, St. George-Buchholz, Schultz. These prostheses are two-piece articulating implants made of dissimilar materials; the implants are set in the intramedullary canal with polymethyl methacrylate, a bone cement. Gillespie evaluated the biomechanical behavior of these implants at the MCP joint in his study using cadaver phalanxes [15].

The Strickland prosthesis has a fixed center of rotation and allows 5° of extension and 90° of flexion. A design of this prosthesis is the restriction of radial-ulnar drift −15° RUD in extension, 0° RUD in full flexion. The RUD was unaffected by the amount of force applied by the examiner. At the time of Gillespie's study, the Strickland prosthesis was unavailable for clinical use. Varied positioning of the center of rotation in relation to finger tip forces were being tested. The Steffee II prosthesis has a passive arc of motion from 15° of extension to 90° of flexion. As designed, the RUD was 25° at the neutral position decreasing to 0° RUD at full flexion. The Steffee II prosthesis has a fixed center of rotation that is set volarly to normal. This volar center was reflected in the finger tip force study. The extensor forces were higher than at preimplantation, or baseline, while the flexor forces were less than baseline in extension, approaching baseline with increasing flexion of the MCP joint.

The range of motion of the St. George-Buchholz prosthesis is limited by the soft tissues. This prosthesis allows 45° extension and 160° of flexion. The articulating stem is designed in two configurations to either restrict or allow a small arc of RUD; RUD was 5° and 15° for the two stem configurations. Regardless of the stem configurations, RUD was increased to 45° by an increased application of lateral force. The metal stem articulates through a slot of a bihemispherical plastic metacarpal component; these hemispheres separate under sufficient lateral force. Gillespie determined that cold flow or permanent deformation of the plastic occurs at a lateral load of 0.45 kg. The St. George-Buckholz prosthesis has a fixed center of rotation. No correlation to finger tip forces could be discerned when the center of rotation was surgically set dorsally or volarly to normal.

The Schultz prosthesis allows 0°-90° of flexion; no extension is allowed beyond neutral. It has an 8° arc of RUD in extension and 0° RUD at full flexion. The Schultz prosthesis is designed with a changing center of rotation. The distal metal component slides freely in an oblique dorsal-volar direction within a slot of the plastic metacarpal component. The center of rotation was found to vary unpredictably. Likewise, the finger tip force data was inconsistent. The Schultz prosthesis dislocated dorsally beyond 32° of forced RUD or at a 0.4 kg load.

Although the Swanson prosthesis cannot be considered the final word in finger joint replacement, it is presently the most widely used technique of prosthetic replacement. As the

Swanson prosthesis is used in conjunction with resection arthroplasty, there will be circumstances in which a total joint replacement is more appropriate (i.e., degradation of soft tissues beyond reconstructive restoration). If an option is available though, the Swanson prosthesis is generally the preferred choice. This is due in part to the simplicity of the surgical implantation of the Swanson prosthesis. If the proximal stem of the St. George-Buchholz is set 10°-20° rotated from normal, the plastic hemispheres were observed to separate approximately 2-3 mm. The design features of the Steffee II prosthesis could be totally offset by implantation dorsal to normal. Whereas, the Swanson prosthesis can actually be inserted upside down with little difference in its mechanical function; the prosthesis is surgically forgiving. Also the Swanson prosthesis is a less severe technique in that the natural joint is better preserved than with a total joint replacement. It should be emphasized that only those finger joints that are destroyed so extensively that soft tissue reconstruction alone would not re-establish function or relieve pain should be considered for prosthetic replacement.

The major problem encountered with the Swanson prosthesis is the high incidence of failure due to silicone rubber's poor resistance to tear propagation. Silicone rubber composites were tested as with the Niebauer prosthesis, the elastic differences of the materials reduced the life span of the prosthesis. In the early 1970's, new synthetic techniques were developed by Dow Corning to improve the cross-linking of silicone rubber. This reduced somewhat the incidence of cracks and fractures, but tear sensitivity remains as a major cause of failure.

What has been proposed is the use of a grommet or metal skirt to protect the implant from being cut by the edges of old or newly calcifying bone. The present study is being undertaken to elucidate the feasibility and possibility of firm fixation of the grommet stems in the intramedullary cavity by direct apposition of bone on the textured outer surfaces.

Porous Implants

At present, the expected lifespan of a prosthetic hip replacement is approximately 10-15 years. The limiting factor is the fixation of the prosthesis. The method of fixation most commonly practiced is the interposing of bone cement, polymethylmethacrylate, between the prosthesis and bone. Upon polymerization, the cement hardens serving as a grouting material locking the prosthesis in place. As the mechanical properties between the bone and cement are significantly different, the bone resorbs at areas of stress concentrations. Bone resorption aggravates the situation by increasing the stress concentrations on the remaining points of bone contact and also of the cement further degrading the bone-cement interface. Research of fixation by bone ingrowth into porous structures was initiated in an attempt to develop a stable long-term bone-prosthesis interface. The early attempts at prosthetic fixation by direct mechanical interaction between implant and tissue involve dental implants with threaded stems (i.e., screw). A screw provides an increased area for interlocking to occur between the bone and prosthesis. Moore designed his hip prosthesis with large fenestrations in the femoral stem to enhance prosthetic fixation [16]; the Moore prosthesis is stabilized by appositional bone growth rather than bone cement.

Surface macro-irregularities and macroperforations are limited in effecting implant-host stabilization. This is suggested by the unpredictability of sub-periosteal and endosseous dental implants [17]. Also toggle-type motion of orthopedic implants has been observed radiographically in spite of apparent bone growth through stem perforations [18]. A microporous surface has several advantages: (1) a greater area of mechanical interaction over which more positive and uniform interlocking may be obtained, (2) improved vascularity of tissue immediately apposed to the implant [19], (3) more rapid fixation.

In 1941, Cohen reported the effects of surface finish on removal torque of screws from bone and other materials [20]. At the time, clinical experience showed Co-Cr screws to be more firmly embedded in bone than S.S. screws. The question was whether there was a different tissue reaction to the two alloys, or whether the difference in removal torque was due to differences in the surface finishes. The standard surface finish of Co-Cr screws is dull- vapor-blasted, as opposed to stainless steel screws which are electropolished. Three surface types were tested: sand-blasted, sand-blasted followed by vapor blasting, electropolishing. Histologically no correlation of the tissue reaction to surface finish or alloy type was observed. Mechanically, the sand-blasted or coarser surface resulted in a higher removal torque; after 4 months *in vivo*, the removal torque for the sand-blasted finished screw was twice that of the electrolytically polished screw. The apposition of repairing fibrous tissue and bone was so close that an increase in 20 micro-inches in surface deviation from the reference plane of the surface resulted in a significant increase in removal torque.

Polymeric sponges were the first materials designed to allow bone ingrowth. In 1955, Struthers reported on the implantation of porous polyvinyl sponge in the ribs and sternum of dogs [21]. In 1968, Henefer reported on the use of an acrylate-amide sponge for the repair of alveolar bone defects [22]. In both cases, bone ingrowth was observed with no adverse inflammatory response or foreign body reaction. Neither report mentioned the pore size or percent porosity of the implanted sponge material.

Struthers noted the limitations of polymeric sponges as a replacement material for skeletal structures due to its poor mechanical properties. Smith developed a porous ceramic composite material, Cerosium, in order to provide a mechanically stronger bone substitute [23]. The pores of the ceramic material were impregnated with an epoxy-like resin. The composite surface was designed to have mechanical properties similar to bone to enhance bone ingrowth. The clinical results were generally poor for several reasons [24]. The epoxy resin degraded *in vivo* resulting in a loss of "ideal" physical properties. Also the small average pore size of 18 μm — maximum pore size 25 μm — was not conducive to bone ingrowth.

Extensive work has been done with porous metallic implants. Generally, there are two methods of preparation of porous surfaces: use of metallic powders sintered or sprayed upon a solid metal core, molding of metal fibers about and sintered to a solid metal core. As with Cerosium, the porous surface can be designed to have mechanical properties similar to bone. The modulus of elasticity and damping capacity, both dependent upon density, of the porous surface can approach values characteristic of natural bone. Similar moduli would reduce stress concentrations and subsequent bone resorption. The fact that the bone-implant interface is supported over an increased area, distributing or damping applied loads, also reduces stress concentrations. The solid metal core is the major load bearing component.

In 1971, Hirschhorn reported on a porous implant of sintered titanium powder [25]. Titanium was chosen because of its excellent biocompatibility. Also titanium has a relatively low modulus of elasticity (approximately 15×10^6 psi) and density (4.5 g/cc), thus proper porosity with respect to implant strength and tissue ingrowth could ensure a modulus approaching that of natural bone, 1-3 $\times 10^6$ psi. Hirschhorn studied implants of various particle sizes; the most favorable results were obtained from those implants with particle size, +40 mesh, pore sizes up to 200 μm at 75% porosity. Although there is a significant loss in strength, the tensile strength of the porous material approximated that of human bone – 7.8 × 10^3 psi. The samples were implanted in the femur of dogs for 49 days. Invasion by trabecular bone was noted with little if any interposed fibrous tissue. No signs of inflammation were observed.

In an earlier study, Lueck used an open pore metallic implant formed from molded titanium wire [26]. Implants of 45% and 65% porosity were tested in the dog; bone penetration was found to be greater for those implants with 45% porosity. Pore size was not mentioned. The strength of the bond increased up to three weeks at which it stabilized. The strength of the bond approximated that of normal trabecular bone. For porous implants, failure by shear generally occurs at the coating-bone substrate interface rather than through the porous layer.

As mentioned earlier, excessively high percent porosity results in insufficient implant strength. Also, too small a pore size inhibits bone ingrowth; rather fibrous tissue ingrowth occurs. Klawitter and Hulbert tested ceramic implants with pore sizes ranging from 50 to 200 μm to determine the optimum pore size [27]. They determined that a minimum interconnection pore size of 100 μm was required for mineralized bone ingrowth. Fibrous tissue ingrowth occurred with a minimum interconnection pore size of approximately 5 to 15 μm.

In the majority of the tests of bone ingrowth into porous implants, the implants were not directly loaded; the implants were inserted in a loaded intact bone. Several studies have been conducted to determine if bone ingrowth into a porous prosthesis will occur while being subjected directly to functional loading – dynamic loading. It is possible for slight or gross movement at the bone-porous implant to inhibit bone ingrowth.

Galante and Rostoker tested a porous femoral prosthesis of molded and sintered fibers of titanium [28]. Powder metallurgy techniques were not chosen for several reasons. Sintering of powdered metal particles closes many of the interconnecting pores, limiting bone ingrowth. For porous ceramics as well as sintered metal powders, the compliance (increment of strain per increment of stress) is only twice that of the dense material and smaller than that of bone. Consolidated metal powders are stronger than ceramics but are still brittle with poor toughness. For sintered fibers, the points of fiber contacts become metallurgical bonds providing considerable mechanical strength, completely interconnecting pores, and excellent resistance to crack propagation. The compliance of sintered fibers is also larger than bone due to the excellent energy absorbing interface.

The fiber coating had a pore size of 190 μm for 50% porosity. In a stress range of 35 to 127 kg/cm^2, the compliance of the porous coat was approximately 0.3-0.43% strain per 10 kg/cm^2. In the same stress range, the compliance of cortical bone is 11.36 × 11^{-4}% strain per 10 kg/cm^2 [29] while that of trabecular bone is 0.74% strain per 10 kg/cm^2 [30]. Square as well as round-shafted stems were tested. With a proper surgical fit, a square shaft could temporarily stabilize the prosthesis.

The prostheses were implanted in dogs and were evaluated at 3 months, 6 months, and 1 year; the animals appeared to bear their full weight on the prostheses during the experimental period. All the prostheses remained securely attached throughout the one year period. There was no evidence of disruption of the bone-prosthesis interface or formation of a fibrous capsule. The bone penetration was shown to be trabecular. Although bone ingrowth occurred only at the corners of the distal end of the square-stemmed prostheses, the tissue ingrowth was histologically the same for the two types of prostheses tested. Weight-bearing and the consequential slight motion in this experimental situation (i.e., loading in a human subject would be more severe) did not interfere with bone ingrowth.

Ducheyne also tested a porous prosthesis under dynamic loading conditions [31]. Pore sizes of 87 and 110 μm were tested. The mechanical strength of the interface corresponded to fibrous tissue ingrowth rather than infiltration of trabecular bone. Ducheyne notes two possible causes for lack of bone ingrowth. Movement at the interface may have been sufficient to inhibit penetration of bone into the pores. Also, the critical mean pore size for bone ingrowth with dynamic loading may be larger than for static loading and was not reached in this study.

Homsy developed a porous femoral prosthesis with a low modulus polymer coating, Proplast on a cobalt stem. Proplast is a composite of polytetrafluoroethylene and pyrolytic carbon [19]. Porosities between 70-90% with pore sizes ranging from 100-500μm were tested. The prosthesis were implanted in dogs and therefore dynamically loaded. It is Homsy's contention that "although tensile strength and modulus of elasticity of these porous structures [high modulus-metal coatings] can be made to approach the values for cortical bone, the more appropriate mechanical properties should approximate that of granulation and fibrous tissue (i.e., low modulus), the development of which within the implant must proceed prior to any bone formation."

The dogs were observed to ambulate freely after 2 weeks post-operatively, with only a slight limp at 3 weeks. At 3 weeks, the porous polymer coating was infiltrated by immature and mature collagen. At 15 months, bone was found to have penetrated the coating. No signs of inflammation were noted. After 16 months, the rotational strength of the interface was 6 kg/cm^2. Shear occurred through the Proplast coating as half of the porous coating remained attached to the femoral bone while half adhered to the prosthesis.

There are currently several prosthetic designs clinically available which employ a porous surface for fixation by bone ingrowth. There are several practical problems associated with this mode of fixation [32]. There is the possibility of long-term corrosion; the surface area of a porous implant is approximately 18 times the surface area of a solid implant of the same size. Intimate contact between bone and the implant must be attained at the time of implantation to inhibit fibrous encapsulation of the prosthetic stem. Also, motion at the prosthesis-bone must be temporarily restricted to allow bone ingrowth. Finally, the mechanical interlocking between bone and the porous implant may be so complete that to remove the prosthesis would be surgically impossible; the prosthesis must be failure-free.

PRESENT RESEARCH

In 1975 the NASA's Lewis Research Center initiated a program to utilize benefits resulting from ion thruster technology [33]. Ion beam bombardment of a material alters the surface characteristics chemically and morphologically.

One such application is the sputter texturing of dental implants [34]; the target's surface is micro roughened by ion beam bombardment using a screen for selective texturing.

A textured surface can also be created by an acid etching technique. The surface of the metal is coated with light sensitive chemicals which is then photochemically altered through a patterned screen. Those areas not photochemically treated are more susceptible to acid attack.

The present study is being undertaken to elucidate the feasibility and possibility of firm fixation of the grommet stems in the intramedullary cavity by direct apposition of bone on the textured outer surfaces. The initial study is being conducted to test the fixation strength and mechanisms of bone apposition in the intramedullary cavities of goose ulna by using Co-Cr-Mo and Ti6Al4V alloy, with and without textured surfaces contacting bone. Only the Co-Cr-Mo alloy preliminary results will be presented in this report.

Materials and Methods

Implants Fabrications

Co-Cr-Mo alloy was cast in a cylindrical form (6.08 I.D. × 6.32 O.D. × 12.7 mm long) by Davis Laboratory, Grand Rapids, MI. Half of the twenty-two samples were further textured outside surface by ion thruster technique by Dr. A. J. Weigand of Lewis Research Center, National Aeronautics and Space Administration, Cleveland, OH.

The Ti-6Al-4V cylinders (6.3 I.D. × 6.45 O.D. × 12.7 mm long) were pressed from smooth and chemically textured (Tech-Etch, Plymouth, MA) sheets of the alloy. Figures 1 and 2 show the sample dimensions and SEM pictures of the surfaces from Co-Cr-Mo and Ti-6Al-4V alloy.

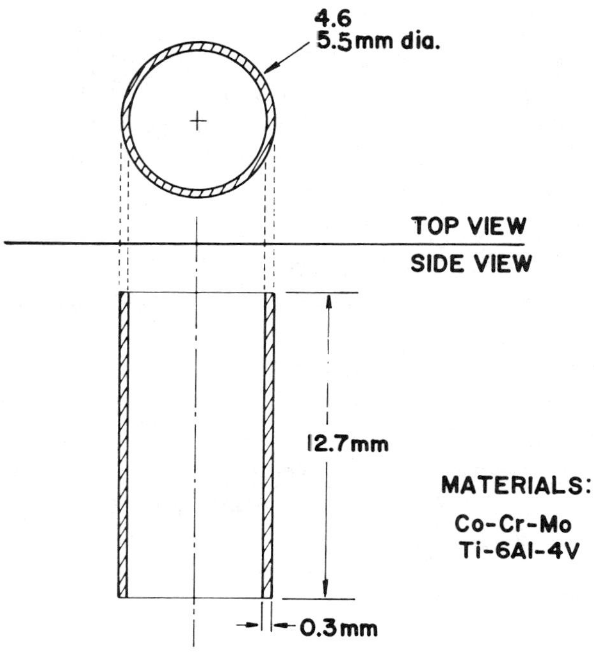

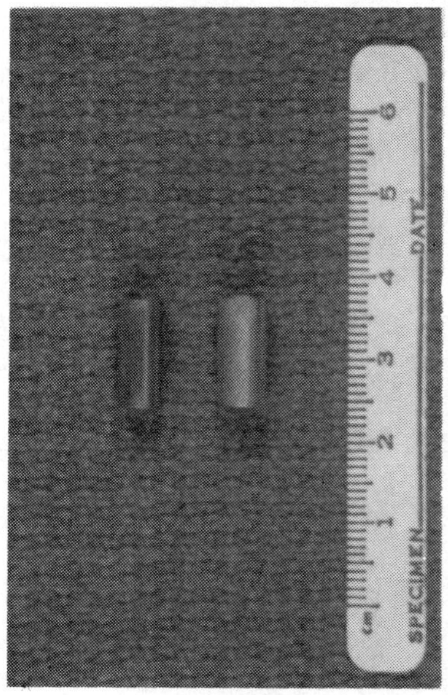

Figure 1. Dimensions and actual photographs of smooth and textured implants (only Ti alloy photograph is shown).

Implantation

Mature male geese (*anser anser)* were used as the host animal since their ulnae are similar to the finger joints biomechanically and have round intramedullary canals up to 2 to 3 cm from distal ends (Figure 3). After two weeks of clinical observations in an outdoor pen the animal was anesthesized by 3 ml of 4 volume % thiamylal sodium; 0.01 mg/kg atropine sulfate was also injected intravenously to reduce salvation. The goose was intubated with a 4 mm O.D. tracheal tube and anesthesia was maintained with methoxy fluorane with oxygen as the carrier gas. Manual respiration is generally required, 20 breaths/minute, with a maximum inspiratory pressure of 4 cm H_2O.

The feathers were removed from both wings and the bird was placed in a body stocking

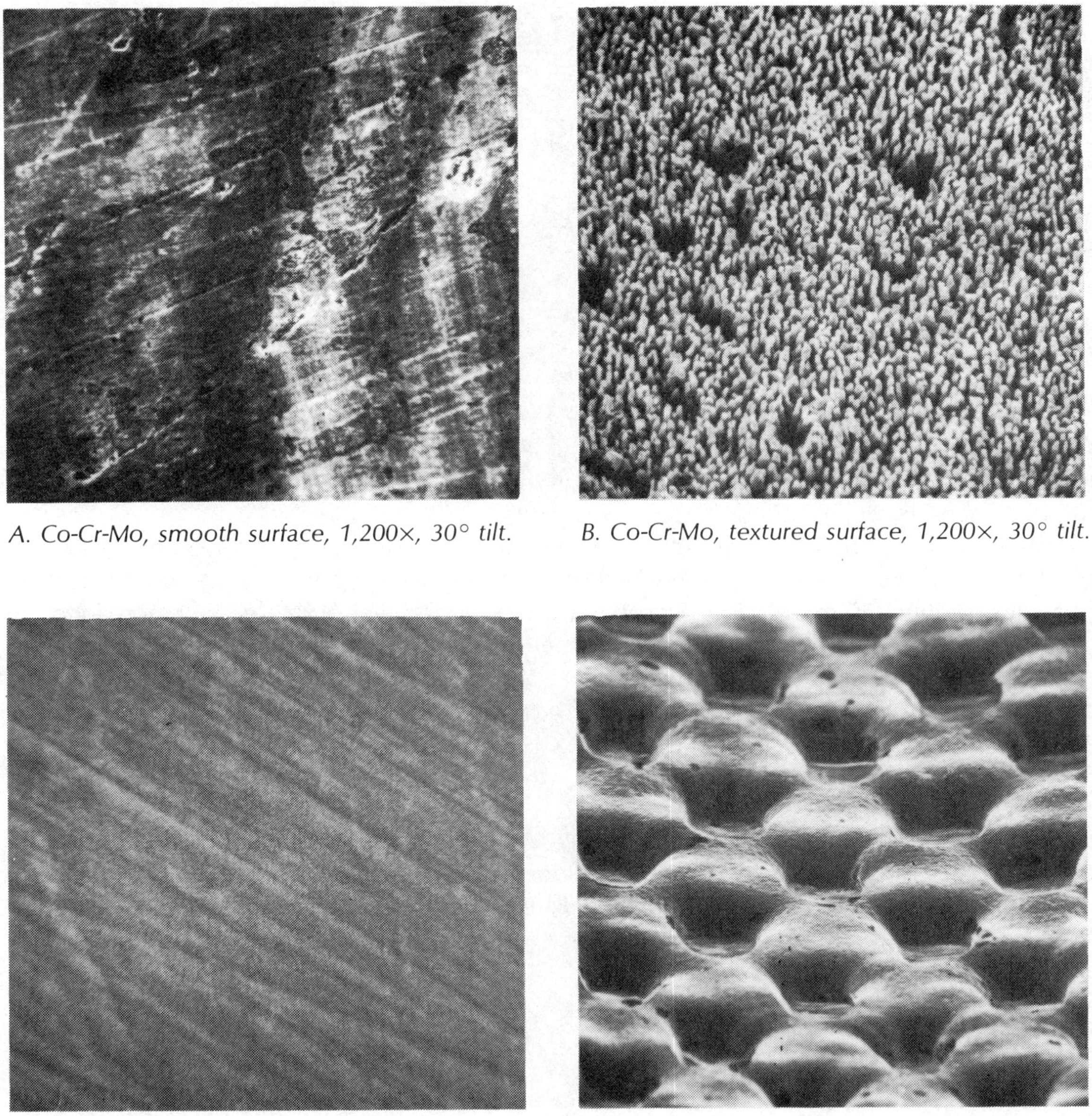

A. Co-Cr-Mo, smooth surface, 1,200×, 30° tilt. B. Co-Cr-Mo, textured surface, 1,200×, 30° tilt.

C. Ti-6Al-4V, smooth surface, 1,500×, 30° tilt. D. Ti-6Al-4V, textured surface, 120×, 70° tilt.

Figure 2. SEM pictures of smooth and textured surfaces of Co-Cr-Mo and Ti-6Al-4V implants.

with the goose in dorsal recumbency, both wings were scrubbed three times alternately with betadine and 70% ethanol solution. The wings were placed within sterile stockenettes and draped. Sterile surgical technique was enforced throughout the surgery.

After the surgical site was exposed the wing was amputated at the radio-ulna-carpal (antebrachio-carpal) joint. The soft tissue was retraced approximately 6 cm. Both the radius and ulna were transected approximately 3 cm above the distal condyles with a Hall II air drill and side cutting burr. The intramedullary canal was prepared with a round cutting burr and

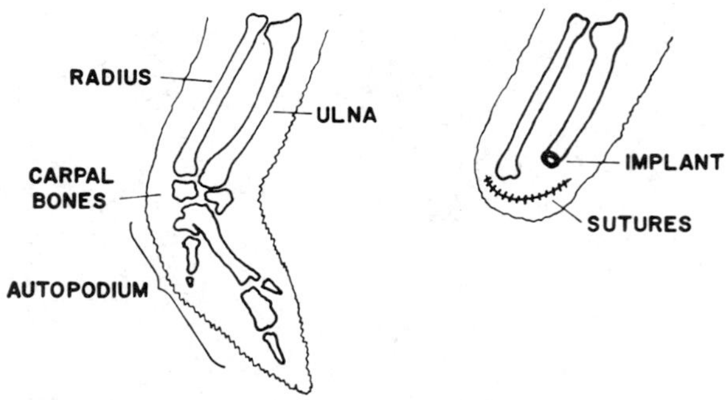

Figure 3. Schematic drawing of the wing of the goose before and after surgery.

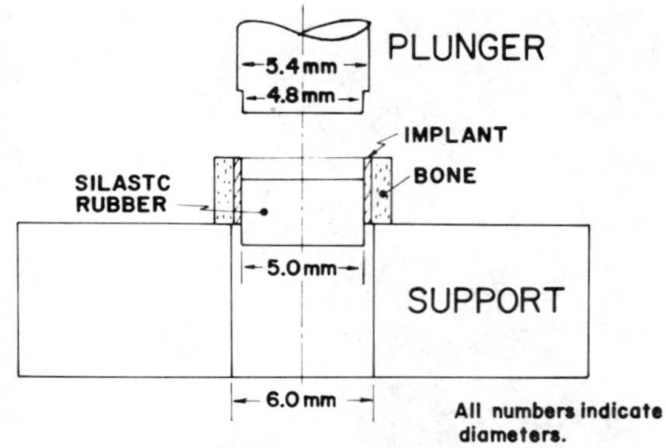

Figure 4. Push-out test arrangement.

the implant was inserted by hand although the last few millimeters generally required impaction. A "snug" fit of the implant was achieved in this manner. The soft tissue was sutured about the implantation site and the incision was closed.

The same procedure was peformed on the contralateral wing. At completion of the implantation procedure, radiographs were taken from each wing, both in a bilateral and an anteposterior position (50 mA, 40 KV, 0.1 seconds). The wound was protected by a non-adhesive gauze pad. Nitrofurazone antibacterial ointment was applied topically to the wound. The goose was maintained in a recovery cage over 5 days for observation. Food and water were provided *ad libitum*. This surgical procedure has been well tolerated by the goose.

Mechanical Sample Preparation

The geese were sacrificed at 4 or 8 weeks following implantation and radiographs were taken. The ulnae were dissected free and the bone with the implant intact was sectioned with a diamond saw while tap water was running. Five sections of approximately 2.5 mm were obtained. The distal, middle and proximal sections were used for histological purposes, the other two for mechanical testing.

Mechanical Testing

A push-out test was performed for each sample by using an Instron Hydraulic Tension/Compression machine. The sample was placed on a support and an appropriate plunger was used to push out the metal implant at a constant strain rate of 0.254 mm/minute which corresponds 0.1 mm/minute for our sample dimension as shown in Figure 4. Maximum shear stress between bone and implant was calculated by knowing the shearing area ($\pi \times$ outer diameter of implant $\times$ thickness) and the maximum force recorded on a chart as shown in Figure 5.

Results and Discussion

The maximum interfacial shear stresses of bone and implants are summarized in Table 1 and plotted in Figure 6. As can be seen, the interfacial strength is greater in the proximal

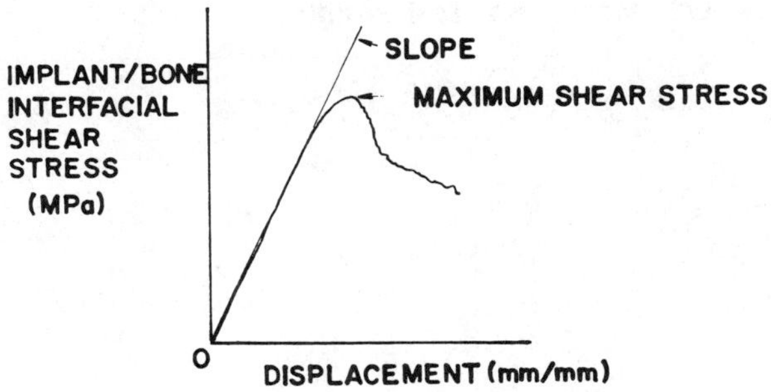

Figure 5. Force (changed to shear stress) versus displacement tracing of push-out tests.

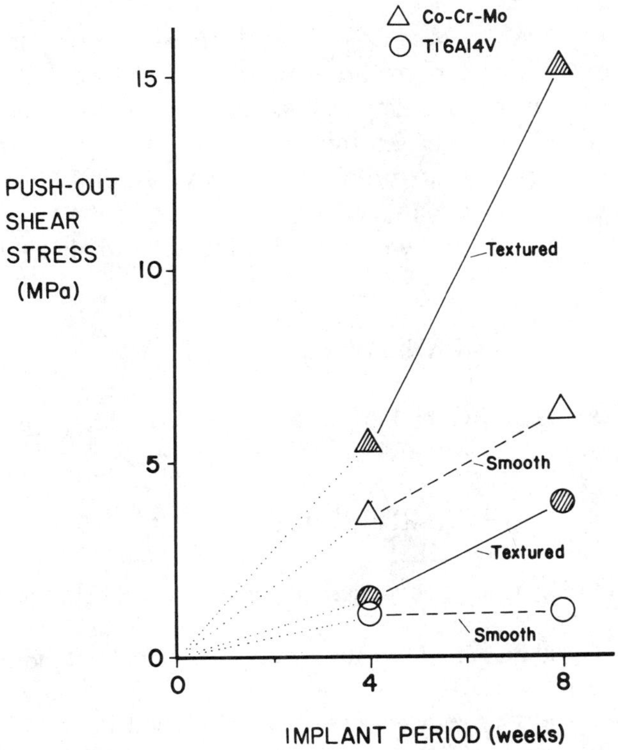

Figure 6. Push-out interfacial shear stress versus implant period.

portion than the distal portion for the textured Co-Cr-Mo implants. This is mainly due to the lesser movement of implant in the proximal region than the distal. It is generally believed that the initial phase of the bone fracture or wound healing is faster with a firmer fixation. Some even apply compressive forces in fracture healing; dynamic compression plate, DCP [35].

It is also true that the interfacial shear strength is greater for the textured implant than the smooth although it is not statistically significant due to the very limited number of samples. Similar results were obtained by Gibbons [36] who implanted four 0.25 inch diameter and

Table 1. Summary of Push-Out Mechanical Test Results

Implant Type	Implant Period (wks)	MAX. PUSH-OUT SHEAR STRESS (MPa)					
		SMOOTH			TEXTURED		
		Distal	Proximal	Overall	Distal	Proximal	Overall
Ti6Al4V	4	0.65±0.56(5)*	1.72±2.68(5)	1.18±1.91)10)	1.68±1.44(5)	1.26±1.24(4)	1.49±1.28(10)
	8	0.99±0.91(6)	1.30±0.68(7)	1.17±0.78(13)	3.60±2.80(5)	5.80±5.70(6)	4.81±4.54(11)
Co-Cr-Mo	4	5.45±2.47(4)	3.19±3.48(4)	4.04±3.17(8)	1.02±0.75(4)	9.78±13.5(4)	5.40±10.01(8)
	8	5.64±3.18(4)	7.05±5.07(4)	6.34±3.99(8)	8.44±1.50(4)	18.50±13.78(5)	15.24±9.80(9)

*Mean ± One Standard Deviation (No. of Samples).

0.375 inch long Co-Cr-Mo and MP 35N samples in each canine femur. After 8 weeks, push-out tests were conducted, and the maximum forces were used to calculate the shear strengths. According to the recalculation by us using values taken from the chart and assuming the thickness of cortical bone to be about 2.5 mm, the shear strength of the control (smooth) samples was about 1.3 MPa and the textured samples was about 2.1 MPa. These values are smaller than the porous Co-Cr-Mo implants which reached up to 8.4 MPa after about 7 weeks in dog femurs [37]. Many other studies with porous metallic implants showed similar results [38-42].

ACKNOWLEDGEMENT

The help of Drs. D. Powers and G. H. Kenner and A. F. Von Recum is acknowledged. This research was supported in part by a NASA grant, NAG 3116.

REFERENCES

1. Brannon, Col. E. W. and Klein, G.: Experiences with Finger Joint Prosthesis, *J. Bone Joint Surg., 41 A*:87-102, 1959.
2. Flatt, A. E.: Restoration of Rheumatoid Finger-Joint Function: Interim Report on Trial of Prosthetic Replacement, *J. Bone Joint Surg., 43 A*:753-774, 1961.
3. Flatt, A. E.: Follow-up Notes on Articles Previously Published in *The Journal:* Restoration of Rheumatoid Finger-joint Function, *J. Bone Joint Surg., 45 A*:1101-1103, 1969.
4. Girzadas, D., and Clayton, M. L.: Limitations of the Use of Metallic Prosthesis in the Rheumatoid Hand, *Clin. Orthop. Rel. Res., 67*:127-132, 1969.
5. Flatt, A. E., and Fisher, G. W.: "Biomechanical Factors in the Replacement of Rheumatoid Finger Joints, *Ann. Rheum. Dis., 67*:127-132, 1969.
6. Swanson, A. B.: A Flexible Implant for Replacement of Arthritic or Destroyed Joints in the Hand, *N.Y. University Inter-Clin. Inform. Bull., 6*:16-19, 1966.
7. Niebauer, J. J., Shaw, J. L., and Doren, W. W.: The Silicon-Dacron Hinge Prosthesis: Design, Evaluation and Application, *J. Bone Joint Surg., 50 A*:639-641, 1968.
8. Calnan, J. S., and Reis, N. D.: The Development and Use of an Artificial Finger Joint for Rheumatoid Arthritis, *J. Biomed. Mater. Res., 3*:314-319, 1968.

9. Swanson, A. B. *Flexible Implant Resection Arthroplasty in the Hand and Extremities.* The C. V. Mosvy Company, St. Louis, 1973.
10. Beckenbaugh, R. D., Dobhns, J. H., Linscheild and Bryan, R. S.: Review and Analysis of Silicone Rubber Metacarpophalangeal Implants, *J. Bone Joint Surg., 58-A:*483-487, 1976.
11. Gschwend, N.: Comparison of Results Obtained by Excisional Arthroplasty and Silicone Rubber Prostheses, *Ann. Rheum. Dis. Suppl. 28:*104-106, 1969.
12. Hirayama, T., and Ikuta, Y.: Experiences with Silicone Rubber Implants for Replacement of Proximal Interphalangeal Joints Destroyed by Trauma, *Hiroshima J. Med. Sci., 20:*47-54, 1971.
13. Swanson, A. B.: Finger Joint Replacement by Silicone Rubber Implants and the Concept of Implant Fixation by Encapsulation, *Ann. Rheum. Dis. 28:*47-55, 1969.
14. Hagert, C. G.: Metacarpophalangeal Joint Implants, *Scand. J. Plast. Reconstr. Surg., 9:*158-164, 1975.
15. Gillispie, T. E., Flatt, A. E., Youm, Y., and Sprague, B. L.: Biomedical Evaluation of Metacarpophalangeal Joint Prosthesis Designs, *J. Hand Surg., 4:*508-521, 1979.
16. Moore, A. T.: A Metal Hip Joint, a New Self-locking Vitallium Prosthesis, *Southern Med. J. 45:*1015-1017, 1952.
17. Adell, R., Hansson, B. O., Brainemark, P. I., and Breine, U.: Intraosseous anchorage of dental prosthesis, II, Scand. *Plast. Reconstr. Surg., 4:*19-22, 1970.
18. Sarmiento, A.: Austin Moore Prostheses in the Painful Hip; Experiences with 224 Patients, *Clin. Orthop., 82:*14, 1972.
19. Homsy, C. A., Cain, T. E., Kessler, F. B., Anderson, M. S., and King, J. N.: Porous Implant Systems for Prosthesis Stabilization, *Clin. Orthop., 89:*220-35, 1972.
20. Cohen, J.: Tissue Reaction to Metals – The Effect of Surface Finish, *J. Bone Joint Surg., 43 A:*687-99, 1961.
21. Struthers, A. M.: An Experimental Study of Polyvinyl Sponge As A Substitute for Bone, *Plastic Reconstr. Surg., 15(4):*274-89, 1966.
22. Henefer, E. P., McFall, T. A., and Hauschild, D. C.: Acrylate-Amide Sponge for Repair of Alveolar Bone Defects, *J. Oral Surg., 26:*577-81, 1968.
23. Smith, L.: Ceramic-Plastic Material as a Bone Substitute, *Arch. Surg., 87:*653-61, 1963.
24. Welsh, R. P., and MacNab, I.: Ceramics in Surgery, *J. Biomed. Mater. Res. Symp., 5:*231-49, 1971.
25. Hirschhorn, J. S., McBeath, A. A., and Dustoor, M. R.: Porous Titanium Surgical Implant Materials, *J. Biomed. Mater. Res. Symp., 5:*49-67, 1971.
26. Lueck, R. A., Galante, J., Rostoker and Ray, R. D.: Development of an Open Pore Implant to Permit Attachment of Bone, *Surg. Forum, 20:*456-7, 1969.
27. Klawitter, J. J., and Hulbert, S. F.: Application of Porous Ceramics for the Attachment of Load Bearing Internal Orthopaedic Applications, *J. Biomed. Mater. Res. Symp., 5:*161-229, 1971.
28. Galante, J., Rostoker, W., Lueck, R., and Ray, R. D.: Sintered Fiber Metal Composites as a Basis for Attachment to Bone, *J. Bone Joint Surg., 53 A:*101-14, 1971.
29. Sedlin, E. D.: A Rheological Model for Cortical Bone: A Study of the Physical Properties of Human Femoral Samples, *Acta Orthop. Scand. Suppl., 83:*1-77, 1969.
30. Evans, F. G.: Region Differences on Some Physical Properties of Human Spongy Bone, *In Biomechanical Studies of the Musculo-Skeletal System,* ed. by F. G. Evans, Springfield, Illinois, Charles C. Thomas, 1961.
31. Ducheyne, P., De Meester, P., and Aernoult, E.: Influence of a Functional Dynamic Loading on Bone Ingrowth Into Surface Pores of Orthopedic Implants, *J. Biomed. Mater. Res., 11:*811-38, 1977.
32. Pilliar, R. M., Cameron, H. U., and MacNab, I.: Porous Surface Layered Prosthetic Devices, *J. Biomed. Mater. Res., 10:*126-31, 1975.
33. Banks, B. A.: Ion Beam Applications Research – a 1981 Summary of Lewis Research Center Programs, for: Fifteenth International Electrical Propulsion Conference, Las Vegas, Nevada, April 21-23, 1981.

34. Weinstein, A. M., Cook, S. D., Klawitter, J. J., and Zide, M.: Ion Beam Texturing for Dental Implant Retention, p. 71, Trans. 7th Ann. Soc. Biomaterials Meeting, R.P.I., Troy, N.Y. 1981.
35. Allgower, M., Matter, P., Perren, S. M., and Ruedi, T.: *The Dynamic Compression Plate, DCP,* N.Y., Berlin, Springer-Verlag, p. 18, 1973.
36. Gibbons, D. F.: Push out test of untextured and ion textured MP35N and Co-Cr-Mo bone implants, Report to NASA Lewis Research Center, NASA/164530/Y057265, 1980.
37. Salman, N. N., and Park, J. B.: The Effect of Direct Electrical Current Stimulation on the Bone Porous Metallic Implant Interface, *Biomaterials, 1:*209-13, 1980.
38. Karagianes, M. T., Westerman, R. E., Rasmussan, J. J., and Ludmell, A. M., Development and Evaluation of Porous Dental Implants in Miniature Swine, *J. Dent. Res., 55:*85-93, 1976.
39. Hahn, H., and Palich, W.: Preliminary Evaluation of Porous Metal Surfaced Titanium for Orthopedic Implants, *J. Biomed. Mater. Res., 4:*571-7, 1970.
40. Nilles, J. L., and Lapitsky, M.: Biomechanical Investigations of Bone Porous Carbon and Porous Metal Interfaces, *J. Biomed. Mater. Res., 7:*63-84, 1973.
41. Cameron, H. U., Pilliar, R. M., and MacNab, I.: The Effect of Movement on the Bonding of Porous Metal to Bone, *J. Biomed. Mater. Res., 7:*301-11, 1973.
42. Cameron, H. U., Pilliar, R. M., and MacNab, I.: Porous Vitallium in Implant Surgery, *J. Biomed. Mater. Res., 8:*283-9, 1974.

Chapter 29

The Role of Fibronectin in the Bioreactivity of Material Surfaces

Frederick Grinnell
Department of Cell Biology
The University of Texas Health Science Center at Dallas
Dallas, Texas 75235

ABSTRACT

The roles of fibronectin in wound healing, thrombosis, and fibroblast adhesion are discussed. Evidence is reviewed indicating that fibronectin adsorbs to wettable and non-wettable material surfaces in different conformations, which results in differences in the biological activity and antibody reactivity of the adsorbed fibronectin.

I. INTRODUCTION

The development of suitable materials of appropriate blood and tissue reactivities for use in surgical implants and extracorporeal organ assist devices remains a major problem in biomaterials research. Surface properties such as charge, texture and wettability are clearly important in determining material reactivity [1], but the relative significance of these parameters and the biochemical basis for their effects are unknown.

Three general approaches to understanding biomaterial reactivity have developed based upon a consideration of initial protein interactions with the material surfaces, which occurs immediately upon their exposure to blood [2,3]. The views are similar except in their emphasis. The first is that surface reactivity is promoted by adsorption of certain proteins in appropriate conformations [2-5]; the second is that surface reactivity is prevented if there is preferential adsorption of serum albumin relative to other proteins [6]; and the third is that surface reactivity is least pronounced if protein adsorption on the surfaces is minimized [7].

The influence of several different plasma proteins on material surface reactivity has been described [see ref. 1-7]. Recently, however, considerable interest has developed in understanding the possible role of plasma fibronectin in blood-material and tissue-material interactions. Fibronectins are a group of glycoproteins found in plasma and other body fluids and secreted by a variety of cells of epithelial and mesenchymal origin. The plasma form of fibronectin has also been called cold insoluble globulin and alpha-2-opsonic protein. It is present in plasma at a concentration of about 30 mg% and circulates as a disulfide-cross-linked dimer with a molecular weight of 440,000 [8,9].

Our investigations on fibronectin function developed in the context of studies on fibroblast adhesion. Subsequently, it became clear that fibronectin is important in wound healing and in thrombosis. As a first step to determining whether fibronectin adsorption on material surfaces is a major factor in their reactivity towards blood and tissues, we have carried out studies on the adsorption properties of fibronectin on material surfaces. In this review, some aspects of the work on the role of fibronectin in wound healing and thrombosis are presented in Part II. Also, in Part II, there is a brief description of the role of fibronectin in fibroblast adhesion. Then, in Part III, the results of our studies on fibronectin adsorption to material surfaces are described.

II. ROLE OF FIBRONECTIN IN WOUND HEALING, PLATELET ADHESION, AND FIBROBLAST ADHESION

A. Fibronectin and Wound Healing

The role of fibronectin in wound healing has been studied by making full thickness wounds on the backs of guinea pigs and then analyzing the distribution of fibronectin by indirect immunofluorescence during subsequent formation of the granulation tissue [10]. Figure 1 shows the organization of fibronectin in normal skin. It is absent from the epidermis but prominent in the basement membrane region (Figure 1A,B). Fibronectin is also associated with some of the collagen fibrils at the papillary level of the dermis (Figure 1A,B) and to a lesser extent with collagen in the reticular dermis (Figure 1C,D). Fibroblasts in the dermis are found in a fibronectin meshwork (Figure 1C,D), which is probably important in the sessile nature of these cells [11]. Other basement membranes in skin such as hair follicle epithelium and vascular endothelim

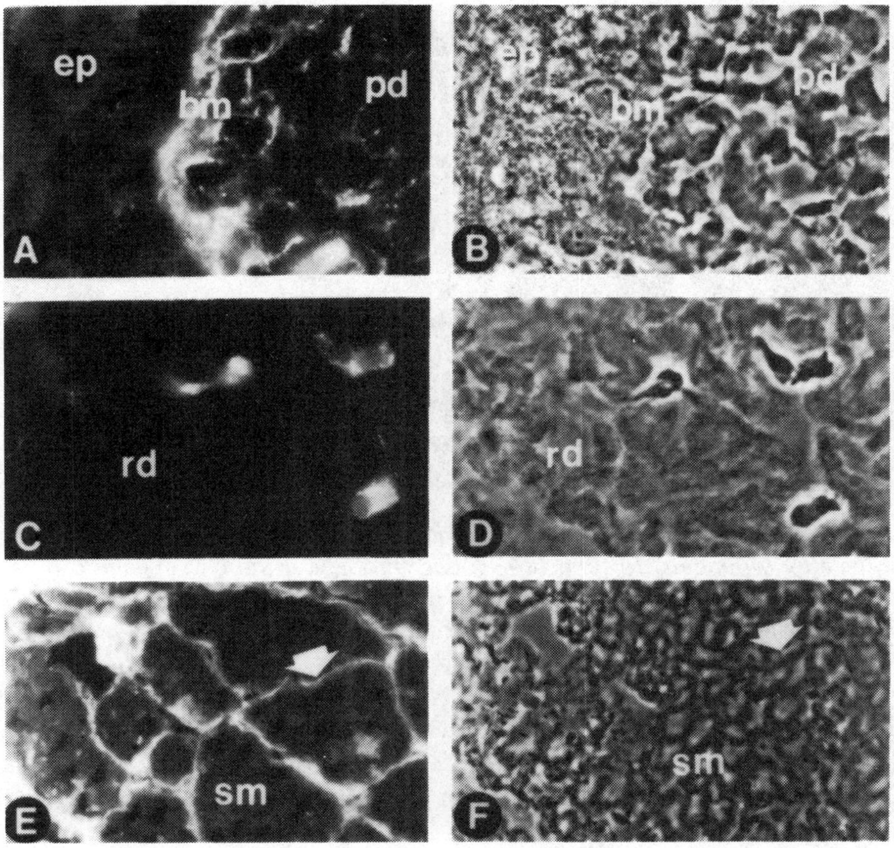

Figure 1. Fibronectin distribution in normal guinea pig skin. The samples were taken at the time of wounding. A,B: Fibronectin is found in the basement membrane (bm) underlying the epidermis (ep) and to a lessor extent in the papillary dermis (pd). C,D: Little fibronectin is found in the reticular dermis (rd) except in association with fibroblast surfaces. E,F: Fibronectin is also found in other basement membranes such as the endomysium (arrow) of skeletal muscle (sm). A,C,E: fluorescence; B,D,F: phase contrast, × 750. See ref. 10.

are also fibronectin positive, as is the basement membrane of skeletal muscle underlying the hypodermis (Figure 1E,F). (See also refs. 12 and 13).

Following wounding, fibronectin is found localized in the clot in association with individual strands of fibrin (Figure 2). The primary source of the fibronectin is probably the plasma. In biochemical studies, it has been shown that fibronectin can bind both covalently and non-covalently to fibrinogen and fibrin. The covalent interaction is mediated by plasma transglutaminase (Factor XIII) [8,9].

The fibronectin in the clot constitutes a highly localized center since there is little fibronectin in the adjacent reticular dermis (Figure 2A,B). This provides a specialized fibronectin-coated substratum for the ingrowth of fibroblasts and endothelial cells. Also, some evidence suggests that fibronectin is chemotactic for fibroblasts and endothelial cells [14,15]. The significance of the fibronectin-coated substratum is further demonstrated by *in vitro* studies in which fibroblasts were found to require fibronectin in order to attach to fibrin [16]. Moreover,

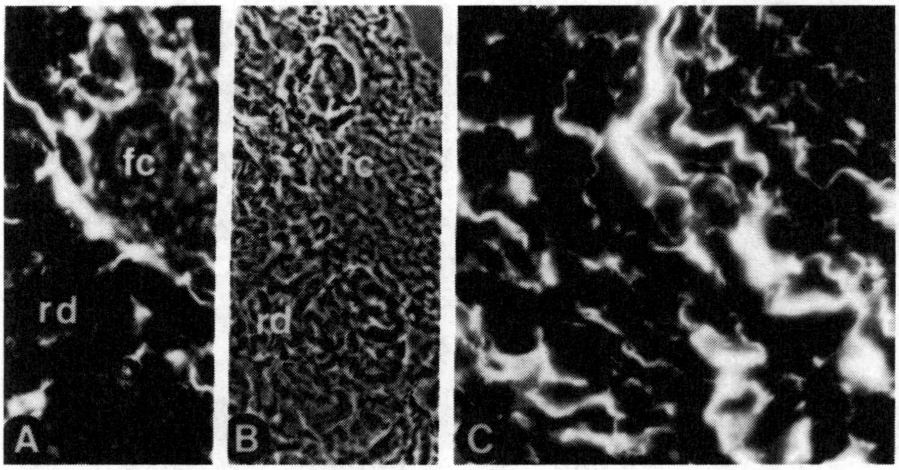

Figure 2. Fibronectin distribution in the initial clot. The samples were taken 5 hours after wounding. Fibronectin is found throughout the clot (fc) and can be seen to coat individual fibrin strands (C). Little increase in fibronectin staining of the reticular dermis is seen. A,C: fluorescence; B: phase contrast. A,B: × 600; C: × 950. See ref. 10.

optimal fibroblast attachment activity required covalent crosslinking of fibronectin to fibrin by Factor XIII. Taken together these observations suggest a possible molecular explanation for the wound healing problems encountered with some individuals who are deficient in Factor XIII [8].

During the early stages of formation of granulation tissue there is vigorous migration of fibroblasts from the hypodermis into the region of the wound. The substratum for migration is fibronectin-coated fibrin and denatured collagen [10]. In regions where the epidermis migrates back over the granulation tissue, basement membrane region fibronectin reappears (Figure 3A,B) (see also ref. 17). Although fibronectin is not one of the basal lamina components synthesized by epidermis, recent *in vitro* experiments indicate that the presence of fibronectin is required for the organization of the secreted epidermal components into a formed structure [18]. Also, there is extensive deposition of fibronectin in association with newly secreted Type III collagen fibrils in the granulation tissue (Figures 3C,D), which is thought to be important in the organization of the dermal matrix [19]. As the wound matures and Type I collagen becomes the predominant component of the matrix, the fibronectin levels diminish markedly [20].

It also should be pointed out that in the granulation tissue fibronectin is found on surfaces of mononuclear cells, which are probably macrophages [10]. Fibronectin binds to a variety of materials such as denatured collagen [21] and certain bacteria [22] as well as fibrin. It also promotes the phagocytosis of particulate material by monocytes [23], macrophages [24,25] and fibroblasts [26]. Thus, fibronectin is probably very important in the clearance of debris from the wound and in tissue remodeling. Related to this, fibronectin has been proposed to be a general opsinin in the systemic function of the reticuloendothelial system [27].

In summary, it appears likely that fibronectin plays a role in several phases of wound healing. First, it forms part of the plasma clot and provides a localized center for fibroblast migra-

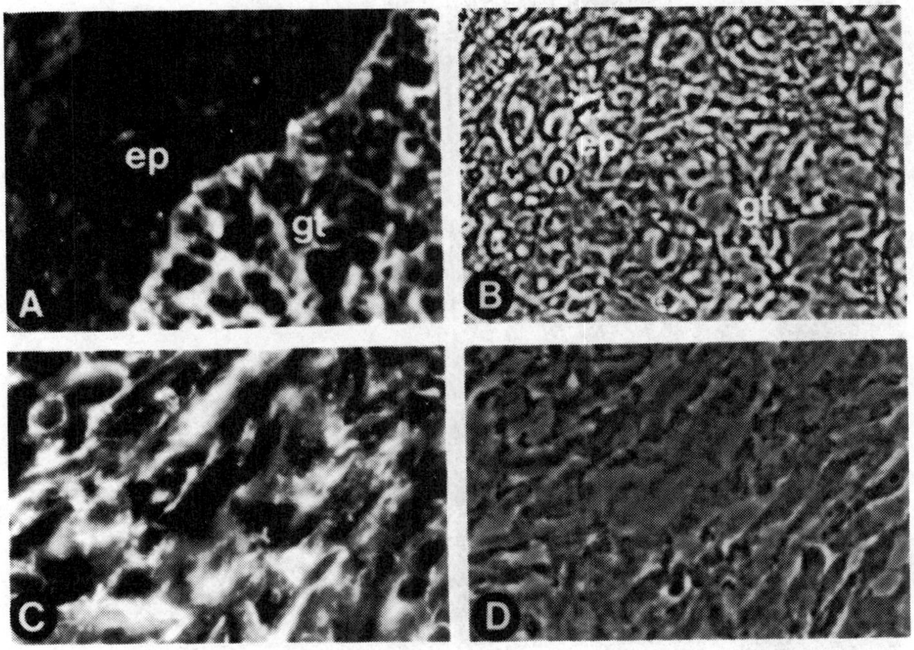

Figure 3. Fibronectin distribution in organized granulation tissue. The samples were taken at Day 9. A,B: Fibronectin is found in the basement membrane where the epidermis (ep) has migrated back over the granulation tissue (gt). C,D: Throughout the granulation tissue, fibronectin is found coating newly deposited collagen fibrils, which were also determined to be positive for reticulin staining. A,C: fluorescence; B,D: phase contrast. × 950. See ref. 10.

tion during formation of the granulation tissue. Second, it both opsinized particulate material for phagocytosis by macrophages and fibroblasts and promotes the phagocytosis of particulate material (coated with other opsinins) by monocytes. Third, it is involved in reformation of the epithelial basement membrane region that is necessary for epidermal cell migration over the granulation tissue. Fourth, it is involved in the organization of the newly synthesized connective tissue matrix.

B. Fibronectin and Thombosis

Fibronectin has been found within platelets and is released following stimulation [28,29] at which time specific, saturable receptors for fibronectin appear on the platelet surface [30]. In *ex vivo* shunts, the presence of fibronectin has been found to promote thrombus formation [31].

Indirect immunofluorescence analysis has been used to study the distribution of fibronectin in freshly formed blood clots [32] (Figure 4). Fibronectin is found distributed along fibrin strands (Figure 4A,B, arrows), which is consistent with the *in vivo* wound healing studies (above), as well as the biochemical studies [8,9]. The possibility should be considered that fibrin strands formed *in vivo* are actually a fibrin-fibronectin copolymer.

Platelets were observed to be the only peripheral blood cells coated with fibronectin in

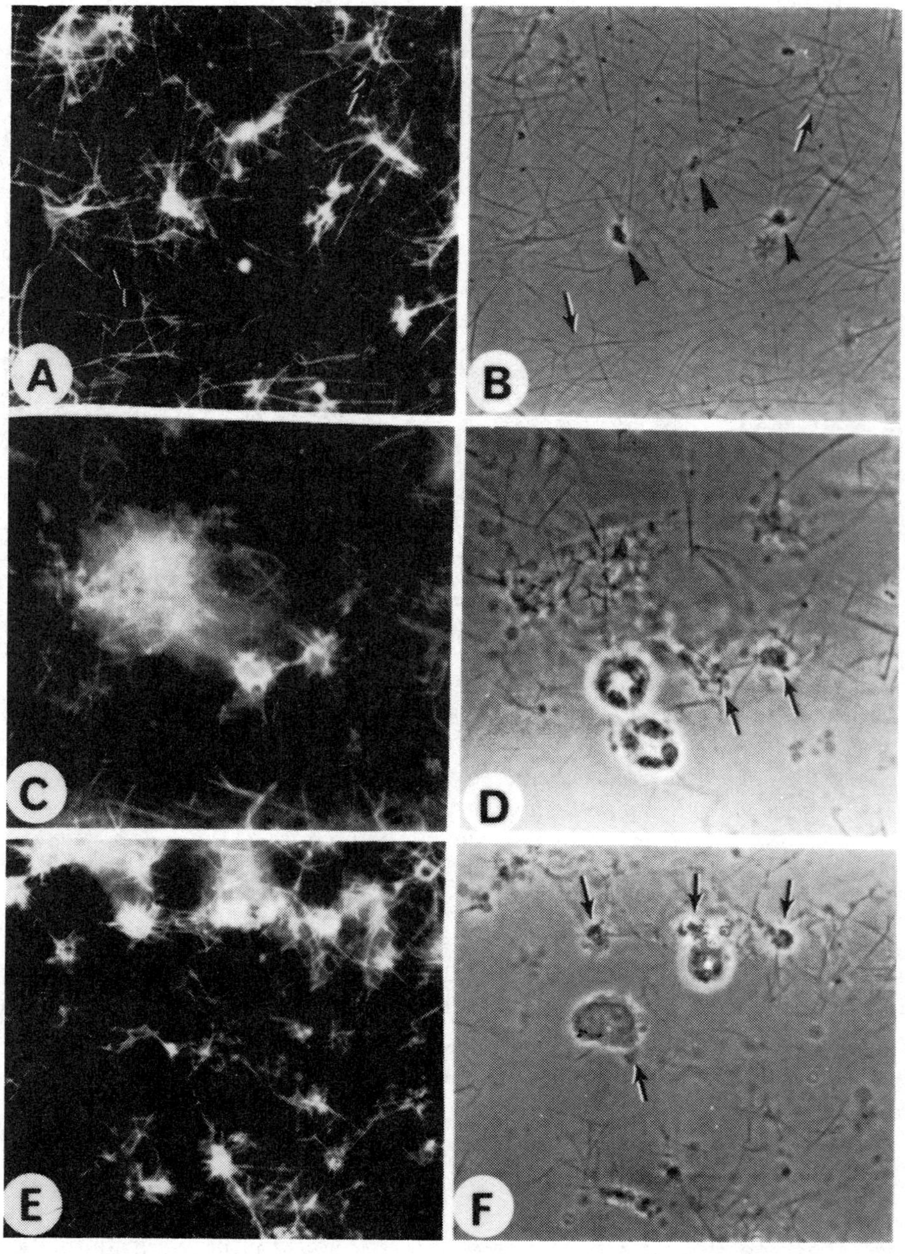

Figure 4. Fibronectin distribution in blood clots. Fibronectin is observed to coat fibrin strands (A,B, arrows) and platelets (A,B, arrowheads). Fibronectin was absent from the surfaces of neutrophils (C,D) and monocytes (E,F). In C-F, arrows point to platelets that are useful for orientation purposes. A,C,E: fluorescence; B,D,F: phase contrast × 750. See ref. 32.

blood clots (Figure 4). Platelets enhance fibronogen polymerization and also interact better with polymerizing fibrin than with fibrinogen or fibrin molecules formed *in vitro* [33]. This may reflect the release of fibronectin from platelets by thrombin stimulation [28,29], the binding of fibronectin to fibrin, and the subsequent binding of platelets to the copolymer. Moreover, the presence of a continuous layer of fibronectin in association with platelets and fibrin probably provides substantial mechanical stability that might be necessary for clot retraction.

Fibronectin has also been demonstrated on platelets following platelet adhesion to collagen [34]. Although no direct role of fibronectin in platelet-collagen adhesion has been found [35], the presence of fibronectin may be important in platelet shape change [36]. Platelets can assume a series of morphologies when interacting with material surfaces as illustrated in Figure 5. Following formation of filipodia (Figure 5C), platelets can either spread (Figure 5D,5F) or lyse (Figure 5E). As shown in Table 1, for both collagen-coated and fibrinogen-coated surfaces, the presence of fibronectin did not affect the extent of platelet attachment to the surfaces but did have a marked effect on the transition of the filipodial form to the spread or lysed forms.

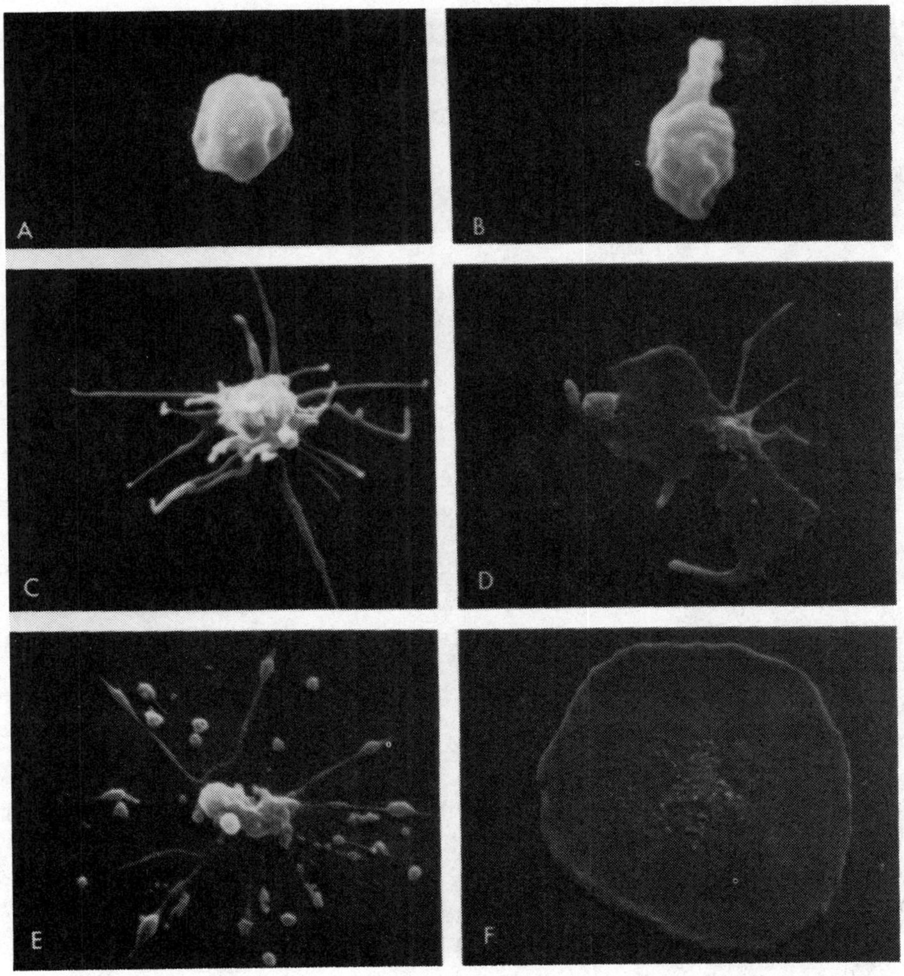

Figure 5. Appearance of platelets interacting with tissue culture dishes as observed by SEM. The incubations contained washed platelets in Tyrode's solution and were carried out at 37° for various times periods up to 20 min. A: round; B+C: filipodial extension; D+F: spreading; E: lysis. × 4500. See refs. 36 and 57.

Table 1. Attachment and Morphological Changes of Platelets on Collagen and Fibrinogen Substrata in the Presence and Absence of Fibronectin[a]

Substratum / Incubation Time	% Attachment		% Attached Platelets in Spread or Lysed Morphologies	
	- pFN	+ pFN	- pFN	+ pFN
Collagen				
2 Min	28 ± 6	16 ± 1	0	6 ± 1
5 min	29 ± 5	18 ± 2	10 ± 5	49 ± 5
20 Min	34 ± 6	21 ± 1	30 ± 6	74 ± 8
Fibrinogen				
2 Min	12 ± 2	12 ± 4	0	10 ± 1
5 Min	14 ± 1	15 ± 6	2 ± 1	29 ± 7
20 Min	18 ± 2	23 ± 1	8 ± 3	68 ± 3

[a]Incubations were carried out for the time periods designated with 30 μg/ml pFN added as shown. Immediately prior to addition of platelets, substrata were coated for 10 min at 22° with rat tail collagen (ca. 2 mg/ml in 0.1% HAc) or fibrinogen (Pentex, plasminogen free, 5 mg/ml in phosphate buffered saline). Data are the average and deviation of 2 experiments. See ref. 36.

The results on fibronectin and platelet function are suggestive although inconclusive. It seems likely that the interaction of platelets with fibrin – both attachment and spreading may involve fibronectin. In platelet-collagen interactions, however, fibronectin seems to be involved only in spreading.

C. Fibronectin and Fibroblast Adhesion

The studies on fibronectin function in wound healing and thrombosis are of relatively recent origin. The area in which fibronectin function has been most thoroughly characterized is that of fibroblast attachment and spreading. In order to clearly discuss the role of fibronectin in fibroblast adhesion, some preliminary comments would be useful.

Under routine tissue culture conditions, fibroblasts placed on material surfaces undergo morphological changes somewhat similar to those demonstrated for platelets. This is shown in Figure 6 in which initially attached, round fibroblasts (Figure 6A) are observed to extend filipodia (Figure 6B) and subsequently spread (Figure 6C) [37]. A closer analysis of the cell-surface interface (Figure 7) has revealed the presence of extracellular material deposited from serum in a thin layer on the surface (Figure 7A). With fully spread cells, many areas can be observed where there is close apposition (<10 nm) between components of the cell glycocalyx and the serum layer (Figure 7B, arrows).

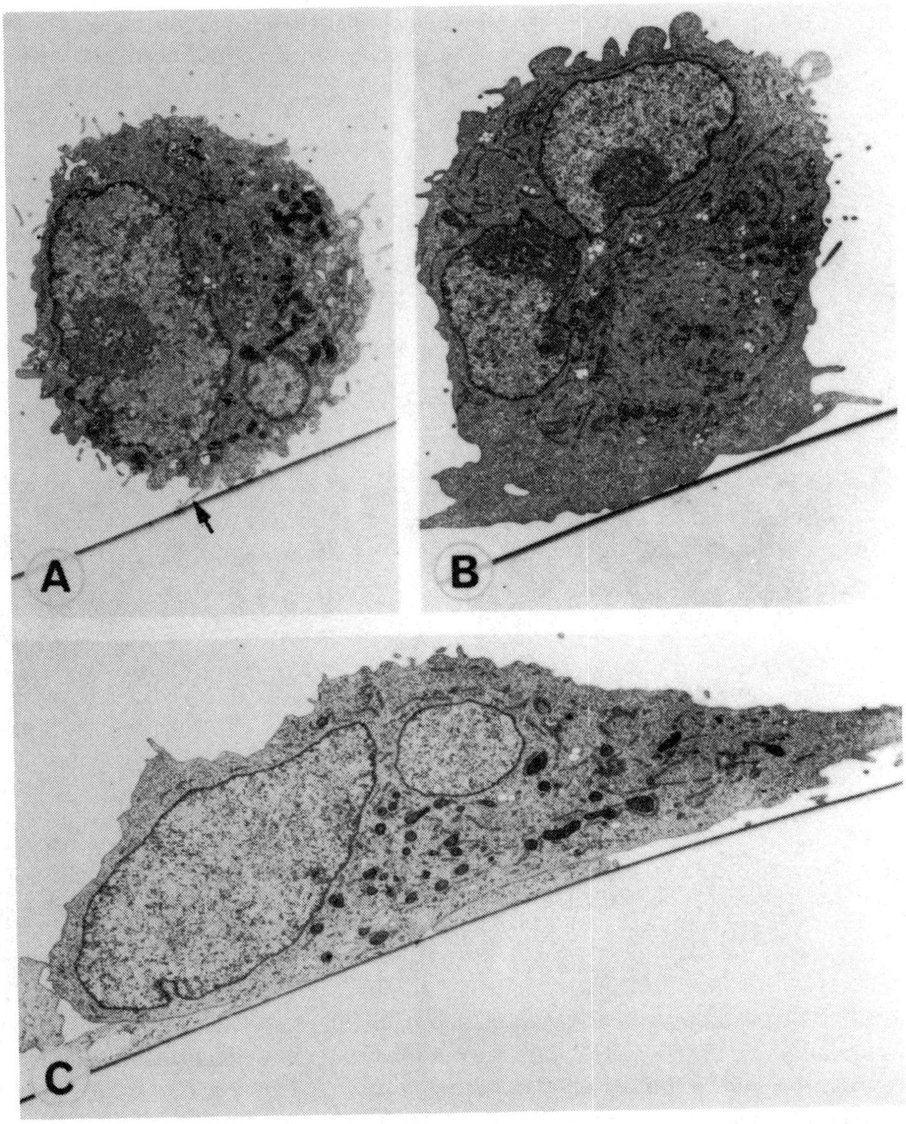

Figure 6. Appearance of baby hamster kidney (BHK) cells interacting with tissue culture dishes as observed by TEM. The incubations contained BHK cells in modified Dulbecco's PBS and 5% fetal calf serum and were carried out at 37° for various time periods. A: After 15 min the cells are rounded; many microvilli are apparent and microvilli probably mediate initial cell-surface interactions (arrow). B: After 30 min cell flattening has begun by filipodial extension. C: After 1 hour cell flattening is essentially complete. × 5000. See ref. 37.

A variety of studies have shown that fibronectin is a major serum component that can promote cell attachment and spreading [38,39]. In general, however, a variety of cell surface ligands have been shown to have a similar effect when they are adsorbed onto surfaces [40]. Included among these are lectins, polycationic materials, and antibodies directed against the cell surface. Cell spreading on the polycationic protein, polycationic ferritin, is shown in Figure 8. At the cell-surface interface it is possible to observe a monolayer of ferritin molecules (de-

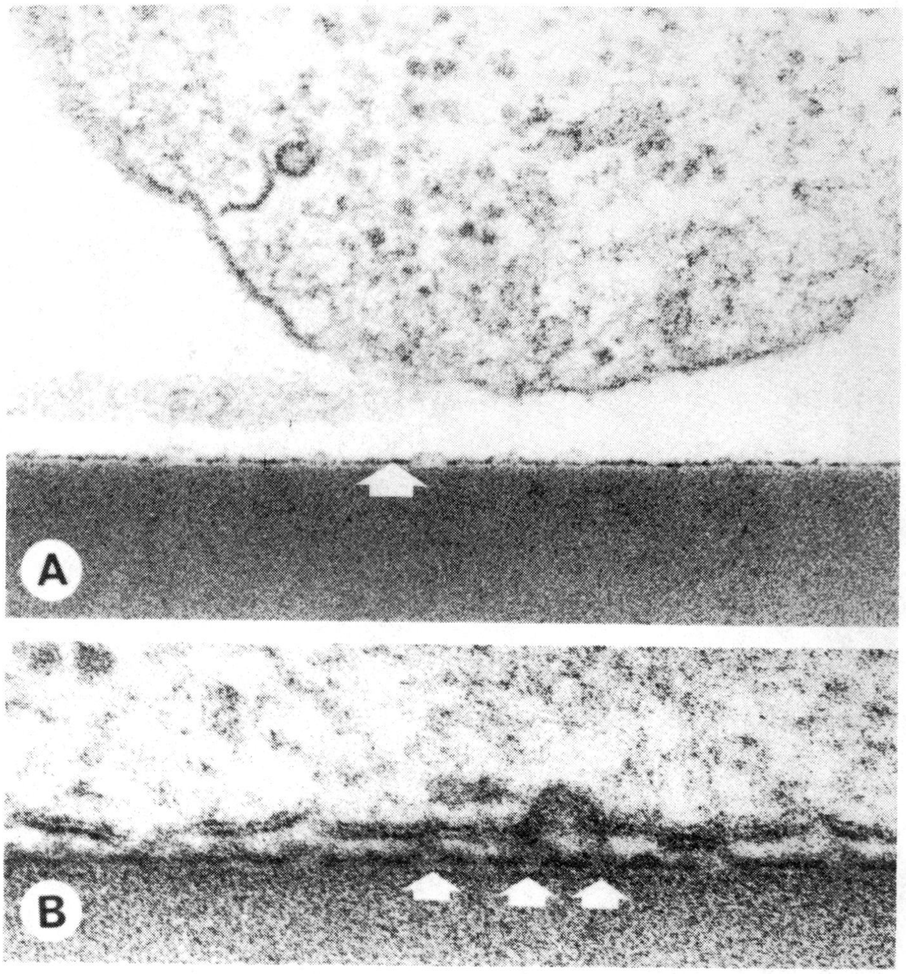

Figure 7. Appearance of cell-substratum surface interface of attached BHK cells. A: Detail of cell in Figure 6A showing microvillus approaching the cell surface; the serum layer on the surface is apparent (arrow). B: Detail of underside of cell attached for 60 min showing close interactions between the cell glycocalyx and the serum layer (arrows). Visualization of the glycocalyx in "B" was enhanced by tannic acid fixation. × 132,000. See ref. 37.

tected in the electron microscope by their iron cores) to which the cells are attached (Figure 8B). As a result of these and similar studies, a general ligand-receptor model for cell-surface interactions has been developed as shown in Figure 9. This model is analagous to the more generalized vesion of ligand-receptor interactions in the control of cell adhesion and recognition, which was proposed more than 30 years ago [41,42].

The observation that first brought to our attention the possible importance of the chemistry of material surfaces in cell-surface interactions is shown in Figure 10. On a series of different surfaces there was a general correlation between hepatoma cell attachment and surface energy [43]. Subsequent studies using several different lines of baby hamster kidney fibroblasts confirmed these findings and demonstrated a relationship between cell attachment

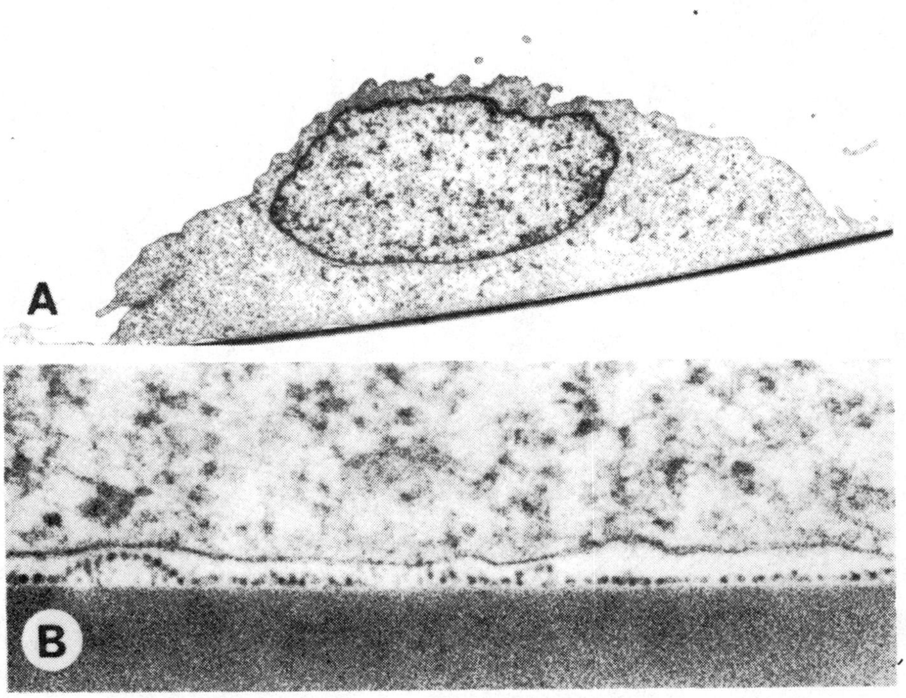

Figure 8. Appearance of BHK cells interacting with polycationic ferritin coated substratum. A: The morphology of cells spread on polycationic ferritin-coated surfaces is similar to that found with cells on a serum layer except that there is continuous apposition of the cells to the surface. B: Detail of the cell-substratum surface interface showing a monolayer of bound polycationic ferritin molecules and close interactions between the cells and the polycationic ferritin. A: × 5000; B: × 200,000. See refs. 37 and 40.

and surface wettability in which surfaces with air-water contact angles below 60° were able to support cell attachment much better than surfaces that had air-water contact angles above 60° [44]. In light of the more recent studies, which have demonstrated a role for particular surface-adsorbed serum components in fibroblast adhesion, the following question became relevant. Did the differences in the adhesion of fibroblasts to the various surfaces depend upon the amount of adsorption or conformation of fibronectin or other serum components on the surfaces? This question is analogous to that posed for protein-surface interactions and thrombogenicity, which was discussed in the Introduction. It was in the context of these considerations, then, that a systematic investigation of fibronectin adsorption on materials surfaces was undertaken.

III. FIBRONECTIN ADSORPTION ON MATERIAL SURFACES

Several different kinds of measurements have been used in our studies on fibronectin adsorption. First, the amount of fibronectin adsorbed has been determined directly by using radiolabeled fibronectin and recovering the adsorbed material from the surfaces being studied [45]. Second, the quantitative interaction of anti-pFN antibodies with adsorbed fibronectin has

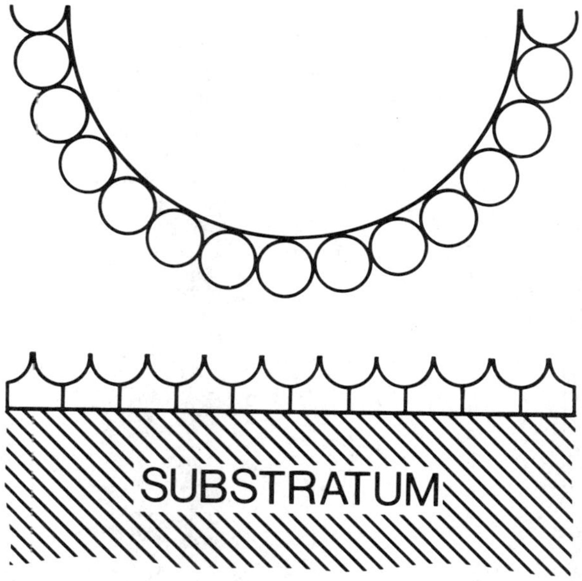

Figure 9. Ligand receptor model for cell adhesion. Receptors on the cell surface interact with ligands adsorbed to the substratum surface. See refs. 38 and 40.

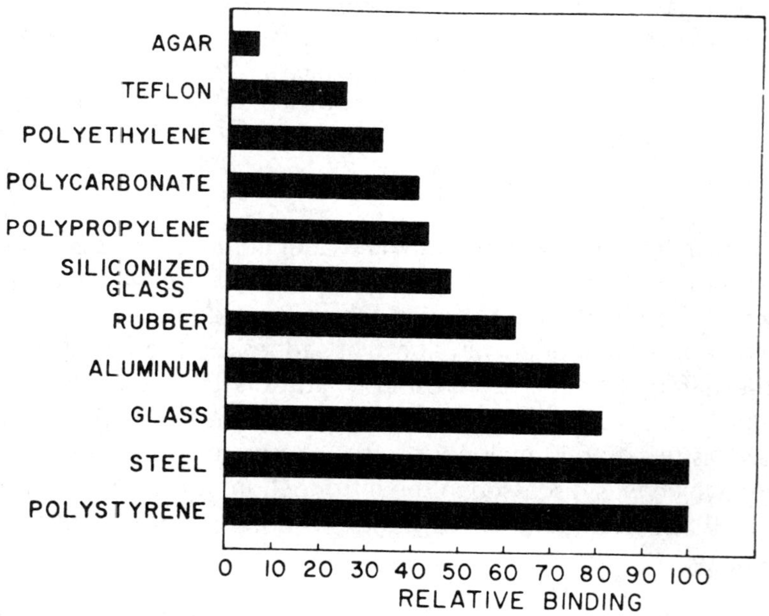

Figure 10. Attachment of rat hepatoma (HTC) cells to various surfaces. The incubations were carried out at 37° for 60 min with cells in modified Dulbecco's PBS supplemented with 5% bovine serum. Tissue culture polystyrene (glow discharge treated) is denoted polystyrene. Other details can be found in ref. 44.

been measured using an indirect assay with radiolabeled anti-immunoglobulin [46]. Finally, the biological activity of adsorbed fibronectin has been measured using assays for fibroblast attachment and spreading [45,46]. The choice of these latter assays was made for several reasons. The roles of fibronectin in fibroblast adhesion to material surfaces [38] and biological surfaces such as fibrin [16] and collagen [39] have already been discussed. Fibroblast adhesion assays are relatively rapid and easy to carry out. Also, it has been suggested that fibroblast adhesion assays might be useful for assessing blood-material interactions [47]. Moreover, fibroblast adhesion is directly relevant to questions of tissue-material interactions where fibroblast interactions are of considerable importance.

The material surfaces studied in our experiments were wettable tissue culture dishes (TC) and non-wettable bacteriological dishes (BACT) (Falcon Plastics). The dishes are made from polystyrene and are exactly the same size and shape. They differ essentially in that the BACT dishes are hydrophobic, whereas the TC dishes have been glow discharge treated, which oxidizes the polymer chain resulting in increased surface wettability [38,48]. The underwater contact angles for the BACT and TC dishes are 88° and 31°, respectively [48]. The use of these material surfaces was made for several reasons. From a technical point of view, the dishes are readily available, inexpensive, and packaged in sterile condition. More substantively, as mentioned above, fibroblasts attach and spread better on wettable surfaces than on non-wettable surfaces. Therefore, it was worthwhile to determine any differences in fibronectin adsorption on these particular surfaces.

A. Fibronectin Adsorption in Relationship to Biological Activity

The first series of experiments were carried out to measure fibronectin adsorption isotherms on the dishes and at the same time to determine the ability of cells to spread on the surfaces that had different amounts of adsorbed fibronectin [45]. With low concentrations of fibronectin in the incubation media more adsorption occurred to BACT dishes than to TC dishes (Figure 11A). The ability of adsorbed fibronectin to promote cell spreading, however, was markedly greater on TC dishes than on BACT dishes. Complete cell spreading on TC dishes required about 14.6 ng/cm^2 of fibronectin, 2×10^{10} molecules/cm^2 based upon a molecular weight of 440,000. On the other hand, complete cell spreading on BACT dishes required 99 ng/cm^2 or 1.4×10^{11} molecules/cm^2. At higher concentrations of fibronectin (Figure 11B), saturation of the surfaces occurred at about the same level, i.e., 320 ng/cm^2 or 4.5×10^{11} molecules/cm^2. This value is slightly lower than that reported for saturation of Nunclon tissue culture dishes by fibronectin, i.e., 698 ng/cm^2 [49].

The data in Figure 11A were obtained with radiolabeled fibronectin. In Figure 11B the radiolabeled material was diluted with increasing amounts of nonradiolabeled fibronectin. No obvious differences in the binding of radiolabled and nonradiolabled fibronectin to the surfaces were apparent.

The results of the preceding experiments suggested that fibronectin could adsorb onto TC and BACT dishes by different mechanisms leading to different conformational states of the adsorbed protein. On TC dishes, the adsorbed protein appeared to be more biologically active than on BACT dishes.

To test the possibility of different chemical interactions of fibronectin on the different surfaces, the ability of various chemical treatments to remove fibronectin from TC and BACT dishes was measured. Adsorbed fibronectin appeared to be much more firmly bound to BACT

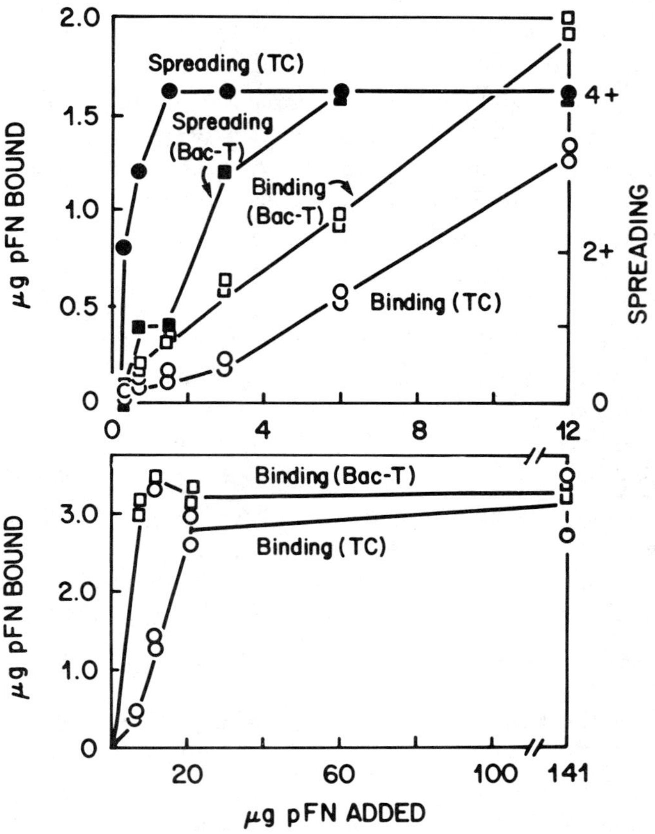

Figure 11. Adsorption isotherms at 22°C for radiolabeled pFN binding to BACT and TC dishes. A: Dishes were incubated for 10 min at 22°C with 1 ml of Tris saline containing the amounts of radiolabeled pFN indicated. B: To obtain the higher concentrations (i.e., above 12 μg), radiolabeled pFN was diluted with increasing concentrations of unlabeled pFN and the specific activities used to calculate binding were adjusted accordingly. At the end of the incubations, the dishes were rinsed and used to determine the amount of bound pFN or cell spreading. See ref. 45.

dishes than to TC dishes as judged by resistance to removal by NaOH, SDS, urea, or guanidine HCl [45]. It has been previously suggested that resistance of adsorbed proteins to removal by NaOH can be taken as an indication of hydrophobic bonding interactions, whereas the more easily removed protein is bound to the material surface by ionic bonds [50]. According to this interpretation, fibronectin adsorbed on BACT dishes would be bound by a more hydrophobic mechanism than fibronectin adsorbed on TC dishes, which is consistent with known differences in hydrophobicity of the surfaces.

It has also been reported that hydrophobic bonding interactions between proteins and surfaces are less susceptible to pH changes than ionic interactions [50]. When the pH dependence of fibronectin adsorption was determined, it was found that adsorption to BACT dishes was relatively insensitive to pH changes, whereas the TC dishes there was a marked decrease in the extent of fibronectin adsorption and biological activity as the pH was increased from 3 to 11 (Figure 12). It should be mentioned that concentations of fibronectin used in these experiments were chosen to give complete cell spreading at pH 7.

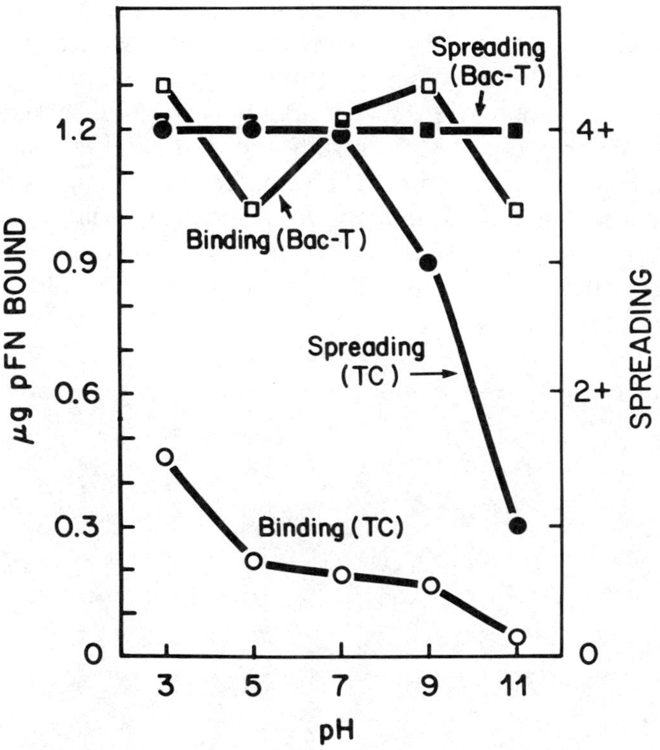

Figure 12. Adsorption of pFN to BACT and TC dishes at different pH's. Dishes were incubated for 10 min with 1 ml of 2.5 mM borate, 2.5 mM citrate, or 2.5 mM phosphate buffer adjusted to the indicated pH's containing 1.8 μg of radiolabeled pFN (TC dishes) or 7.2 μg of radiolabeled pFN (BACT) dishes. At the end of the incubations, the dishes were rinsed and used to determine amount of bound pFN or cell spreading. See ref. 45.

The major ionizable groups on the TC dish surface are probably carboxyl groups [38,48] which would be maximally charged at high pH. Similarly, fibronectin would have its maximal negative charge at high pH. The resulting electrostatic repulsion might account for the decreased adsorption of fibronectin. On the other hand, there probably would be no pH-sensitive ionic groups important in hydrophobic interactions. It also should be pointed out, however, that fibronectin changes shape and is in a more "open" conformation at pH 11 compared to pH 7 as determined by hydrodynamic studies [51].

B. Effect of Bovine Serum Albumin on Fibronectin Adsorption

One explanation for the differences in adsorption and biological activity of fibronectin on TC and BACT dishes was that fibronectin changed to an inactive conformation when it is adsorbed on the BACT dishes at low concentrations. At high fibronectin concentrations, however, packing requirements of the fibronectin molecules on the dish surface may not permit this change to occur. Changes in the molecular conformation of the adsorbed species has been described for some proteins [52-54]. To test the possibility that packing might influence fibronectin conformation, adsorption of fibronectin was measured in the presence of low concentrations of bovine serum albumin (BSA). As evident in Figure 13, simultaneous treatment of the BACT dishes with fibronectin and BSA resulted in a marked increased in cell spreading (Figure 13C) compared to dishes treated with fibronectin alone (Figure 13A). No cell spreading occurred if the dishes were treated sequentially with fibronectin followed by BSA (Figure 13D) or with BSA followed by fibronectin (Figure 13B). Therefore, in order for the biological activity of fibronectin to be enhanced by addition of BSA, both proteins had to interact with the dish surfaces at the same time.

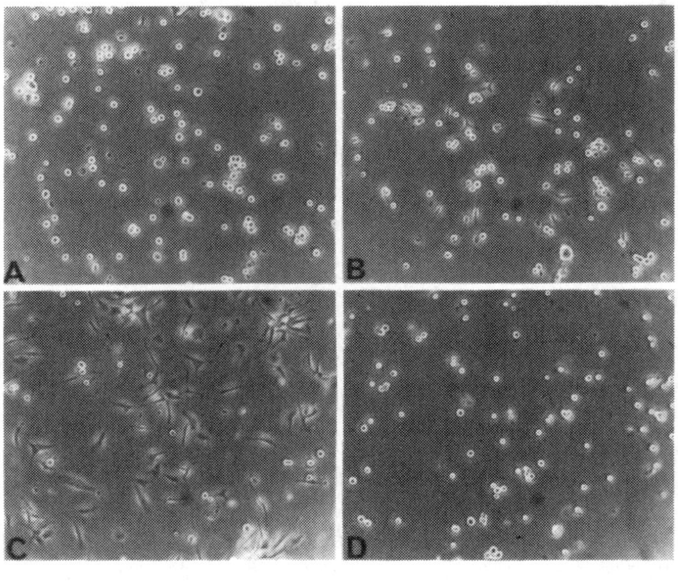

Figure 13. Morphology of BHK cells spread on BACT dishes with pFN in the presence and absence of BSA. The experiment was carried out using 2.9 μg of radiolabeled pFN and 50 μg/ml BSA. (A) pFN alone, (B) BSA then pFN, (C) pFN plus BSA, (D) pFN then BSA. Cells are well spread when pFN and BSA are added simultaneously, but not otherwise. × 80. See ref. 45.

The time course of fibronectin adsorption was measured in the presence or absence of BSA (Figure 14). Under either condition, with BACT or TC dishes, binding to the surfaces was essentially maximal by 10 min. Different concentrations of fibronectin were used on the BACT and TC dishes to maximize the BSA effect. Nevertheless, it can be appreciated that in the absence of BSA the biological activity on BACT dishes was much lower than on TC dishes at all times

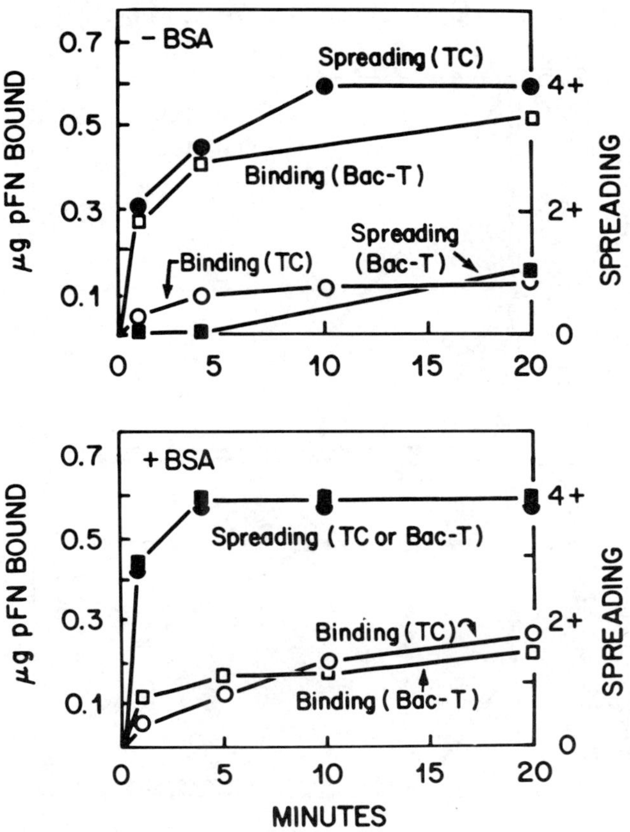

Figure 14. Time dependence of pFN adsorption in the presence and absence of BSA. TC or BACT dishes were incubated at 22°C for the time periods shown with 1 ml of Tris saline containing 0.9 or 3.6 µg of radiolabeled pFN, respectively. At the end of the incubations, the dishes were rinsed and used to determine amount of bound pFN or cell spreading. See ref. 45.

tested, even though more fibronectin was adsorbed. On BACT dishes, when BSA was added there was a marked increase in biological activity that was accompanied by *reduced fibronectin adsorption.* On TC dishes, on the other hand, increased adsorption of fibronectin was observed when BSA was added!

C. Competition Between Fibronectin and Other Proteins for Surface Adsorption Sites

It was of interest to compare the adsorption characteristics of fibronectin with some other plasma proteins. Fibrinogen was selected because it has been characterized as a major component rapidly adsorbed out of plasma onto material surfaces [3]. Albumin was studied because of its ability to passivate surface thrombogenicity [55,56]. Heat denatured albumin was also tested because it passivates surfaces with respect to fibroblast adhesion better than albumin [57].

The competition experiments between fibronectin and the other proteins were carried out

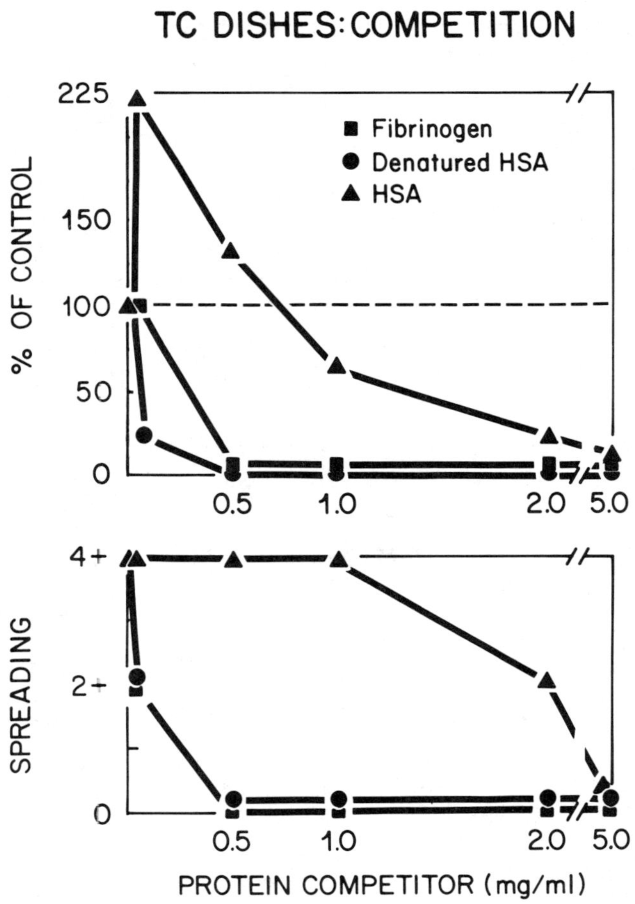

Figure 15. Competition between pFN and other proteins for TC dishes. Dishes were incubated for 10 min at 22°C with 1 ml of Tris saline containing 1.8 μg of radiolabeled pFN in the presence of the proteins at the concentrations indicated. At the end of the incubations the dishes were rinsed and used to determine the amounts of bound pFN or cell spreading. See ref. 45.

with TC dishes (Figure 15) and BACT dishes (Figure 16). At low concentrations of human serum albumin (HSA) (i.e., 50 μg/ml, the same concentration that resulted in cooperative effects with BSA), the amount of fibronectin adsorbed on TC dishes was increased (Figure 15) and on BACT dishes was decreased (Figure 16). With TC dishes, in order to completely suppress the adsorption that occurred with 1.8 μg/ml of fibronectin in the incubations, it was necessary to add 5 mg/ml of HSA; 1 mg/ml of HSA reduced the amount of fibronectin adsorption only slightly and had no effect on the biological activity (Figure 15). With BACT dishes, the adsorption of fibronectin was somewhat more sensitive to albumin (Figure 16): with 7.2 μg/ml of pFN in the incubations, the addition of 1 mg/ml of albumin inhibited binding by more than 90% and partially suppressed biological activity. The results with fibrinogen indicated that on TC dishes, the addition of 50 μg/ml fibrinogen with 1.8 μg/ml of fibronectin partially suppressed both adsorption and biological activity. At 500 μg/ml of fibrinogen, suppression was complete.

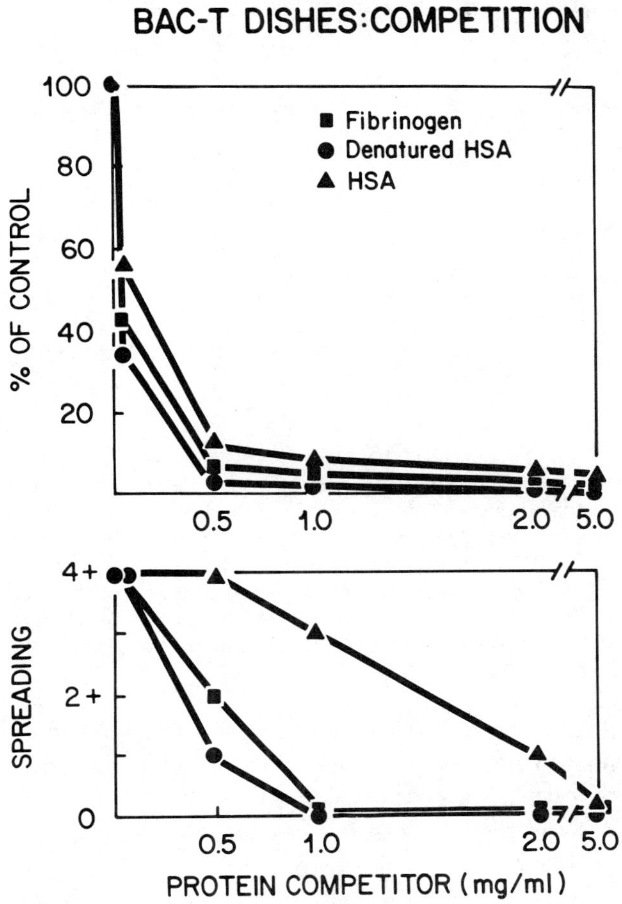

Figure 16. Competition between pFN and other proteins for BACT dishes. Dishes were incubated for 10 min at 22°C with 1 ml of Tris saline containing 7.2 μg of radiolabeled pFN in the presence of the proteins at the concentrations indicated. At the end of incubations the dishes were rinsed and used to determine the amounts of bound pFN or cell spreading. See ref. 45.

The most surprising results were with HSA denatured by brief heating at 80°C, which causes aggregation [58]. The heat denatured HSA was about as effective as fibrinogen in competing with fibronectin, which indicates that its affinity for the dish surfaces was increased at least 10-fold compared to native HSA.

Another approach to studying reciprocal interactions between fibronectin and other proteins on the surface was to pretreat the surfaces with the various proteins and then determine how well fibronectin could bind. In these experiments, the protein concentrations used (5 mg/ml) were able to completely prevent fibronectin adsorption if added simultaneously with fibronectin (see above). Following pretreatment of TC dishes with 5 mg/ml of HSA, incubation with fibronectin still resulted in 67% of the amount of binding obtained with untreated dishes after a 60-min incubation (Table 2). Much lower amounts of fibronectin adsorbed, however, when the dishes were pretreated with heat denatured HSA. After fibrinogen pretreatment of

Table 2. Binding of pFN to Protein Treated Surfaces[a]

Pretreatment of Surface	% PFN Bound After 1 hr Compared to Control	
	TC Dish	BACT Dish
HSA (5 mg/ml)	66.8	15.2
Denatured HSA (5 mg/ml)	5.5	4.9
Fibrinogen (5 mg/ml)	20.2	18.4
Plasma	68.2	9.5
Plasma = 2mM $CaCl_2$	25.9	8.4

[a]Dishes were incubated for 10 min at 22°C with 1 ml of Tris saline containing proteins, dialyzed plasma, or recalcified dialyzed plasma as indicated. They were then incubated with 2 μg of radiolabeled pFN (TC dishes) or 8 μg of radiolabeled pFN (BACT dishes) in 1 ml of Tris saline for 60 min at 37°C. The amount of radioactivity bound to the dishes at the end of the incubations was determined and compared to control experiments in which dishes were treated with Tris saline alone i.e., in the absence of any proteins, and then with pFN. See ref. 45.

the dishes, binding of fibronectin was reduced but not as much as with denatured HSA (Table 2). Experiments were also carried out in which plasma (under clotting or nonclotting conditions) was used to pretreat the dishes. It was found that fibronectin could bind to dishes about 68% as well as controls if the dishes were pretreated with plasma under nonclotting conditions. If the dishes were pretreated with plasma under clotting conditions, less binding of fibronectin occurred. Because of the complexity of the protein components in plasma and the possibility that fibronectin binds to fibrin under these conditions, interpretations of these results is at present ambiguous. Similar experiments carried out on BACT dishes indicated that of the three proteins, HSA, fibrinogen, and denatured HSA, pFN adsorbed better to dishes pretreated with HSA and fibrinogen than denatured HSA.

D. Fibronectin Adsorption in Relationship to Antigenicity

The foregoing experiments suggested that fibronectin adsorbed on BACT and TC dish surfaces in different conformations with the more biologically active form on the TC dishes. In order to obtain additional information about possible conformational differences in fibronectin on the surfaces, experiments were carried out to determine the interaction of anti-pFN antibodies with adsorbed fibronectin [46].

Since in these experiments it was necessary to measure fibronectin adsorption on dishes subsequently incubated with antibodies, control experiments were carried out to analyze whether anti-pFN treatment would cause desorption of adsorbed fibronectin. It was determined that up to 10% of the adsorbed fibronectin on the dishes could be desorbed by sequential incubations with anti-pFN followed by anti-immunoglobulin. It was found, however, that fixation of adsorbed fibronectin almost completely prevented subsequent desorption. Fixation was accomplished by treatment of the adsorbed protein with formaldehyde.

Aside from preventing desorption, fixation of adsorbed fibronectin appeared to have little effect on its biological activity. For instance, Figure 17 shows adsorption isotherms and biological activity for fibronectin that had been subjected to fixation. The results are very similar to those presented in Figure 11. It should be pointed out that the binding data are shown as CPM bound (Figure 17) rather than as μg of pFN bound (Figure 11). The data can be converted by taking into consideration the radioactivity of the pFN preparation used (about 5000 cpm/μg).

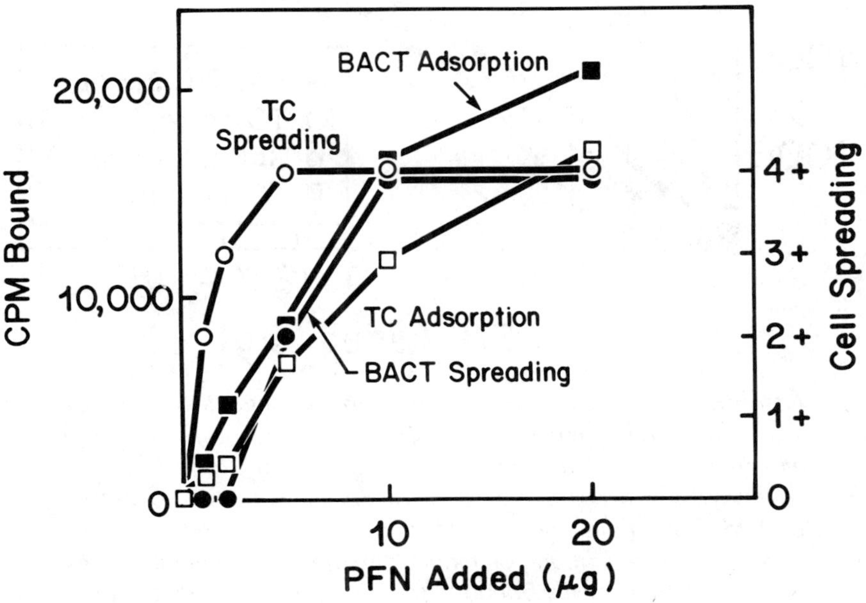

Figure 17. Adsorption of fibronectin in relationship to cell spreading activity. Pairs of TC and BACT dishes were treated with radiolabled pFN at the concentrations indicated in PS buffer for 10 minutes at 22°. At the end of the incubations, the dishes were rinsed and fixed. Subsequently, one dish from each of the pairs was used to determine the amount of pFN adsorption and the other dish was used to determine cell spreading activity. See ref. 46.

Figure 18 shows an isotherm for fibronectin adsorption measured by the direct method using radiolabeled fibronectin compared to the amount of adsorbed fibronectin determined indirectly by anti-pFN binding. The isotherms determined by the direct assay are similar to those already presented. With the antibody assay, however, it can be seen that much less of the adsorbed fibronectin could be detected on the BACT dishes. It should be pointed out that essentially identical results for the antibody assay were observed in experiments using unlabeled fibronectin. Therefore, the anti-pFN antibody appeared to react less well with fibronectin adsorbed on BACT dishes than with fibronectin adsorbed on TC dishes and this difference was particularly pronounced at low concentrations of fibronectin. These results are analogous to those found by the biological activity measurements and are further evidence supporting the idea that fibronectin is adsorbed on the TC and BACT dishes in different conformations.

The effect of increasing concentrations of albumin on cell spreading and on the binding of anti-pFN to adsorbed fibronectin is shown in Figure 19. All of the incubations contained 2 μg/ml

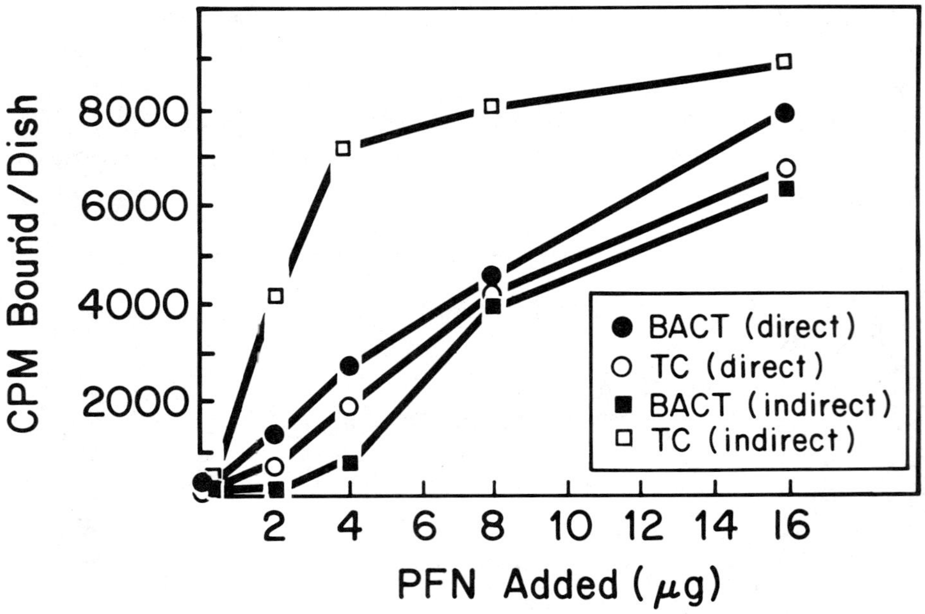

Figure 18. Adsorption of fibronectin in relationship to antigenicity. Pairs of TC and BACT dishes were treated with radiolabeled pFN at the concentrations indicated in PS buffer for 10 minutes at 22°. At the end of the incubations, the dishes were rinsed and fixed. Subsequently, one dish from each of the pairs was used to determine the amount of pFN adsorption directly. The other dish was processed with anti-pFN and radiolabeled anti-IgG. The amount of binding in the indirect antibody assay was calculated as the total radioactivity bound to the dishes less the radioactivity bound in the direct assay. See ref. 46.

of fibronectin. In the absence of albumin there was complete cell spreading on TC dishes but only 1+ cell spreading on BACT dishes. Concentrations of albumin as low as 2 μg/ml stimulated spreading on BACT dishes and at 5 μg/ml there was complete cell spreading. The effect of albumin on the antibody assay was also marked. Compared to the results in the absence of albumin, there was a 10 fold increase in the amount of fibronectin detected by the antibody assay on BACT dishes when 10 μg/ml of albumin was present. Control experiments indicated that these results were not due to the presence of fibronectin in the crystalline albumin preparations or in cross-reactivity of the anti-pFN or anti-immunoglobulin antisera with albumin. Also, as described previously, the albumin had to be added with the fibronectin; there was no effect if the surfaces were treated with the proteins sequentially (Figure 13). An increase in antibody binding to adsorbed fibronectin on TC dishes and a decrease in antibody binding to fibronectin on BACT dishes were observed at higher albumin concentrations. This is consistent with the previous findings using the direct assay in which albumin was observed to cause an increase in the absolute amount of fibronectin bound to the TC dishes but a decrease in the absolute amount of fibronectin bound to the BACT dishes (Figure 14-16). Low concentrations of albumin, therefore, are able to cause a change in the conformation of fibronectin adsorbed on BACT dishes permitting increased binding by the antibody, as well as full biological activity.

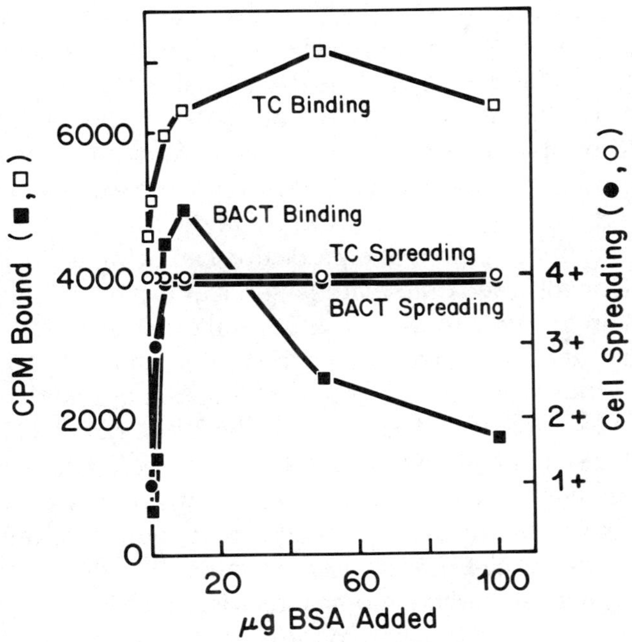

Figure 19. Effect of serum albumin on fibronectin adsorption and spreading activity. Pairs of TC and BACT dishes were treated with 2 μg/ml of unlabeled pFN in the presence of bovine serum albumin in the incubations indicated in PBS buffer for 10 min at 22°. At the end of the incubations, the dishes were rinsed and fixed. Subsequently, one dish from each of the pairs was used to determine the amount of antibody binding to pFN in the indirect assay and the other was used to determine cell spreading activity. See ref. 46.

E. Implications and Future Studies

The results of these studies permit several important conclusions with regard to the adsorption properties of plasma fibronectin. Perhaps the most interesting finding is that the biological activity of adsorbed fibronectin is not directly related to the amount of adsorbed fibronectin when comparing the results on wettable (TC dishes) and nonwettable (BACT dishes) surfaces. It seems that on the BACT dishes, at low concentrations, fibronectin is able to adsorb in a manner that does not permit full expression of cell spreading activity. Similarly, anti-pFN reacted poorly with fibronectin adsorbed on BACT surfaces compared to fibronectin adsorbed on the TC surfaces. These findings indicate that fibronectin is adsorbed on the surfaces in two different conformations with the more biologically active and antigenic conformation on the wettable surfaces.

Direct evidence for different conformations of adsorbed fibronectin on surfaces of high and low wettability has recently been obtained by physical studies [59]. Following saturation of silanized quartz surfaces with fibronectin, the receding contact angle of H_2O on the surfaces went from 60° to 10°; on plain quartz surfaces, the receding contact angle went from 0° to 31°. This suggests that adsorption of fibronectin on the more hydrophilic surface was accompanied by the exposure of more hydrophobic side chains and/or domains of the protein than were exposed following adsorption of fibronectin on the hydrophobic surface.

The studies with albumin further support the differential conformation hypothesis since addition of small amounts of albumin was able to modify fibronectin adsorption on the surfaces in a fashion such that both the active cell spreading conformation and the antigen reactive conformation were exposed on the hydrophobic surfaces. The explanation for how albumin is altering the way in which fibronectin interacts with the hydrophobic surface is still not clear.

Based upon the results of our studies, the prediction can be made that fibronectin will be a major protein component adsorbed onto material surfaces exposed to blood. Considering the high affinity of fibronectin for surfaces relative to several other major plasma proteins studied (fibronogen and albumin), it is likely to be among the proteins that are directly adsorbed. If this is the case, then the effect of the surfaces on the conformation of adsorbed fibronectin may be an important clue to understanding surface reactivity with blood. In addition, fibronectin may associate with the surfaces indirectly by binding to adsorbed fibrinogen/fibrin. What is now necessary is to analyze the adsorption of fibronectin on surfaces exposed to plasma and whole blood, and to determine bioreactivity of adsorbed fibronectin using assays more relevant to thrombosis such as platelet adhesion or activation.

The final important point established in our studies is the ability of mild heat denaturation to dramatically increase the affinity of albumin for surfaces. Albumin has been demonstrated to passivate surfaces *in vitro* [55,56] and is sometimes used clinically to decrease the thrombogenicity of extracorporeal circuits such as in membrane oxigenators [60] and detoxification devices [61]. The drawback with this technique is the ability of albumin to rapidly exchange off the surface [62]. Because of its much higher affinity and decreased exchange on surfaces, heat-denatured albumin may be more valuable as a passivating agent. The interactions of heat-denatured albumin-coated surfaces with blood, however, have yet to be determined.

ACKNOWLEDGEMENTS

The author's research has been carried out by grants from N.I.H., CA14609 and HL24221. Dr. William Snell, Nancy Oppenheimer-Marks, and Doug McAbee provided helpful comments about the manuscript.

REFERENCES

1. Olsen, D. A. and Kletschka, H. D. (1973). Biophysical interactions of blood proteins with polymeric and artificial surfaces. Progress in Surface and Membrane Science *6:* 331-364.
2. Baier, R. E., Loeb, G. I. and Wallace, G. T. (1971). Role of an artificial boundary in modifying blood proteins. Fed. Proc. *30:* 1523-1538.
3. Vroman, L., Adams, A. L. and Klings, M. (1971). Interactions among human blood proteins of interfaces. Fed. Proc. *30:* 1494-1502.
4. Nyilas, E., Morton, W. A., Lederman, D. M., Chiu, T-H. and Cumming, R. D. (1975). Interdependence of hemocynamic and surface properties in thrombosis. Trans. Amer. Soc. Art. Int. Organs *21:* 55-69.
5. Ratner, B. D., Horbett, T., Hoffman, A. S. and Hauschka, S. D. (1975). Cell adhesion to polymeric materials: Implications with respect to biocompatibility. J. Biomed. Mat. Res. 9: 407-422.
6. Lyman, D. J., Metcalf, L. C., Albo, D., Jr., Richards, K. F. and Lamb, J. (1974). The effect of chemical structure and surface properties of synthetic polymers on the coagulation of blood. III. In vivo

adsorption of proteins on polymer surfaces. Trans. Amer. Soc. Artif. Int. Organs. *20:* 474-479.
7. Andrade, J. D., Lee, H. B., Jhon, M. S., Kim, S. W. and Hibbs, J. B. Jr. (1973). Water as a biomaterial. Trans. Amer. Soc. Artif. Int. Organs. *19:* 1-7.
8. Mosher, D. F. 1980. Fibronectin. Prog. Hemostasis & Thrombosis *5:* 111-151.
9. Mosesson, M. W. and Amrani, D. L. (1980). The structure and biological activities of fibronectin. Blood *56:* 145-158.
10. Grinnell, F., Billingham, R. E. and Burgess, L. (1981). Fibronectin during wound healing *in vivo.* J. Invest. Dermatol. *76:* 181-189.
11. Grinnell, F. (1981). Fibronectin and wound healing. Am. J. Dermatopathology. In Press.
12. Stenman, S. and Vaheri, A. (1978). Distribution of a major connective tissue protein, fibronectin, in normal human tissues. J. Exp. Med. *147*: 1054-1064.
13. Linder, E., Stenman, S., Lehto, V-P and Vaheri, A. (1978). Distribution of fibronectin in human tissues and relationship to other connective tissue components. Ann. NY Acad. Sci. *312:* 151-159.
14. Bowersox, J. C. and Sorgente, N. (1980). Chemotactic response of vascular endothelial cells to fibronectin. J. Cell Biol. *87:* 64a.
15. Gauss-Muller, V., Kleinman, H. K., Martin, G. R. and Schiffman, E. (1980). Role of attachment factors and attractants in fibroblast chemotaxis. J. Lab. Clin. Med. *96:* 1071-1080.
16. Grinnell, F., Feld, M. and Minter, D. (1980). Cell adhesion to fibrinogen and fibrin substrata; role of cold insoluble globulin (plasma fibronectin). Cell *19:* 517-525.
17. Fujikawa, L. S., Foster, C. S., Harrist, T. J., Lanigan, J. M. and Colvin, R. B. (1981). Fibronectin in healing rabbit corneal wounds. Lab. Invest. In Press.
18. Brownell, A. G., Bessem, C. C. and Slavkin, H. C. (1981). Possible functions of mesenchyme cell-derived fibronectin during formation of basal lamina. Proc. Natl. Acad. Sci. *78:* 3711-3715.
19. Wartiovaara, J. and Vaheri, A. (1980). Fibronectin and early mammalian development. Development in Mammals *4:* 233-266.
20. Kurkinen, M., Vaheri, A., Roberts, P. J. and Stenman, S. (1980). Sequential appearance of fibronectin and collagen in experimental granulation tissue. Lab. Invest. *43:* 47-51.
21. Ruoslahti, E., Engvall, E. and Hayman, E. G. 1981. Fibronectin: Current concepts of its structure and function. Coll. Res. *1:* 95-128.
22. Kuusela, P. (1978). Fibronectin binds to *Staphylococcus* aurerus. Nature *276:* 718-720.
23. Bevilacgua, M. P., Amrani, D., Mosesson, M. W. and Bianco, C. (1981). Receptors for cold-insoluble globulin (Plasma fibronectin) on human monocytes. J. Exp. Med. *153*: 42-60.
24. Gudewicz, P. W., Molnar, J., Lai, M. Z., Beczhold, D. W., Siefring, G. E. Jr., Credo, R. B. and Lorand, L. (1980). Fibronectin mediated uptake of gelatin-coated latex particles by peritoneal macrophages. J. Cell Biol. *87:* 427-433.
25. Van de Water, L. III, Schroeder, S., Crenshaw, E. B. III and Hynes, R. O. (1981). Phagocytosis of gelatin-latex particles by a murine macrophage line is dependent on fibronectin and heparin. J. Cell Biol. *90:* 32-39.
26. Grinnell, F. 1980. The fibroblast receptor for cell-substratum adhesions: studies on the interaction of baby hamster kidney cells with latex beads coated by cold insoluble globulin (plasma fibronectin). J. Cell Biol. *86:* 104-112.
27. Saba, T. M. and Jaffe, E. 1980. Plasma fibronectin (opsonin glycoprotein): Its synthesis by vascular endothelial cells and role in cardiopulmonary integrity after trauma as related to reticuloendothelial function. Am. J. Med. *68:* 577-594.
28. Ginsberg, M. H., Painter, R. G., Birdwell, C., Plow, E. F. and Forsyth, J. (1979). The detection, immunofluorescent localization, and thrombin induced release of human platelet-associated fibronectin antigen. J. Supra. Struct. *11:* 167-174.
29. Zucker, M. B., Mossesson, M. W., Brockman, M. J. and Kaplan, K. L. (1979). Release of platelet fibronectin (cold-insoluble globulin) from alpha granules induced by thrombin or collagen; lack of requirement for plasma fibronectin in ADP-induced platelet aggregation. Blood *54:* 8-12.

30. Plow, E. F. and Ginsberg, M. H. (1981). Specific and saturable binding of plasma fibronectin to thrombin-stimulated platelets. J. Biol. Chem. In Press.
31. Ihlenfeld, J. V., Mathis, T. R., Barber, T. A., Mosher, D. F., Riddle, L. M., Hart, A. P., Updike, S. J. and Cooper, S. L. (1978). Transient In Vivo thrombus deposition onto polymeric biomaterials: Role of plasma fibronectin. Trans. Am. Soc. Artif. Intern. Organs *24:* 727-735.
32. Grinnell, F. and Feld, M. (1982). Distribution of fibronectin on peripheral blood cells in freshly clotted blood. Thromb. Res. In Press.
33. Niewiarowski, S., Regoeczi, R., Stewart, G. J., Senyi, A. F. and Mustard, J. F. (1972). Platelet interaction with polymerizing fibrin. J. Clin. Invest. *51:* 685-700.
34. Hynes, R. O., Ali, I. U., Destree, A. T., Mautner, V., Perkins, M. E., Senger, D. R., Wagner, D. D. and Smitt, K. K. (1978). A large glycoprotein lost from the surfaces of transformed cells. Ann. NY Acad. Sci. *312:* 317-342.
35. Santoro, S. A. and Cunningham, L. W. (1979). Fibronectin and the multiple interaction model for platelet collagen adhesion. Proc. Nat. Acad. Sci. *76:* 2644-2648.
36. Grinnell, F., Feld, M. and Snell, W. 1979. The influence of cold insoluble globulin on platelet morphological response to substrata. Cell Biology Inter. Reports *3:* 585-592.
37. Grinnell, F., Tobleman, M. Q. and Hackenbrock, C. R. (1976). Initial attachment of baby hamster kidney cells to a substrata. Ultrastructural analysis. J. Cell Biol. *70:* 707.
38. Grinnell, F. (1978). Cellular Adhesiveness and extracellular substrata. Inter. Rev. Cytol. *53:* 65-144.
39. Kleinman, H. K., Klebe, R. J. and Martin, G. R. (1981). Role of collagenous matrices in the adhesion and growth of cells. J. Cell Biol. *88:* 473-485.
40. Grinnell, F. and Hays, D. G. (1978). Induction of cell spreading by substratum adsorbed ligands directed against the cell surface. Exp. Cell Res. *116:* 275-284.
41. Tyler, A. (1946). An antigenantibody concept of cell structure in growth. Growth *10.* Suppl. 6th Symp. pp. 7-19.
42. Weiss, P. (1946). The problem of specificity in growth and development. Yale J. Biol. Med. *19:* 235-278.
43. Grinnell, F., Milam, M. and Srere, P. A. (1972). Studies on Cell Adhesion II. Adhesion of cells to surfaces of diverse chemical composition and inhibition of adhesion by sulfhydryl binding reagents. Arch. Biochem. Biophys. *153:* 193-198.
44. Grinnell, F., Milam, N. and Srere, P. A. (1973). Attachment of normal and transformed hamster kidney cells to substrata varying in chemical composition. Biochem. Med. *7:* 87-90.
45. Grinnell, F. and Feld, M. K. (1981). Adsorption characteristics of plasma fibronectin in relationship to biological activity. J. Biomed. Mat. Res. *15:* 363-381.
46. Grinnell, F. and Feld, M. 1982. Fibronectin adsorption on hydrophobic and hydrophilic surfaces in relationship to biological activity, antigenicity, and cell adhension in serum-containing medium. J. Biol. Chem. Submitted.
47. Ratner, B. D., Horbett, T., Hoffman, A. S. and Hauschka, S. D. (1975). Cell adhesion to polymeric materials: Implications with respect to biocompatability. J. Biomed. Mat. Res. *9:* 407-422.
48. Smith, L. W. (1979). Cell adhesion as influenced by substrate surface properties. Ph.D. Thesis, University of Utah.
49. Hughes, R. C., Pena, S. D. J., Clark, J. and Dourmashkin, R. R. (1979). Molecular requirements for the adhesion and spreading of hamster fibroblasts. Exp. Cell Res. *121:* 307-314.
50. Dillman, W. J., Jr. and Miller, J. F. (1973). On the adsorption of serum proteins on polymer membrane surfaces. J. Coll. Int. Sci. *44:* 221-241.
51. Alexander, S. S., Colonna, G. and Edelhoch, H. (1979). Structure and stability of human plasma cold insoluble globulin.J. Biol. Chem. *254:* 1501-1505.
52. Kochwa, S., Litwak, R. S., Rosenfield, R. E. and Leonard, E. F. (1977). Blood elements at foreign surfaces: A biochemcial approach to the study of the adsorption of plasma proteins. Ann. NY Acad. Sci. *283:* 37-49.

53. Morrissey, B. W. (1977). The adsorption and conformation of plasma proteins: A physical approach. Ann. NY Acad. Sci. *283:* 50-64.
54. Soderquist, M. E. and Walton, A. G. (1980). Structural changes in proteins adsorbed on polymer surfaces. J. Coll. Sci. *75:* 386-397.
55. Packham, M. A., Evans, G., Glynn, M. F. and Mustard, J. F. (1969). The effect of plasma proteins on the interaction of platelets with glass surfaces. J. Lab. Clin. Med. *73:* 686-697.
56. Lyman, D. J., Klein, K. G., Brash, J. J., Fritzinger, B. K., Andrade, J. D. and Bonomo, F. S. (1971). Platelet interaction with protein-coated surfaces: an approach to thromboresistant surfaces. Thromb. Diath. Hemorrhag. Suppl. *42:* 109-114.
57. Grinnell, F. and Feld, M. (1979). Initial adhesion of human fibroblasts in serum-free medium. Possible role of secreted fibronectin. Cell *17:* 117-129.
58. Lin, V. J. C. and Koenig, J. L. (1976). Raman studies of bovine serum albumin. Biopolymers *15:* 203-218.
59. Stoker, R. L. (1981). Adsorption of plasma fibronectin on quartz and glass substrates. M.S. Thesis, Department of Bioengineering, University of Utah.
60. Lande, A. J. (1972). Assisted circulation with membrane oxygenators. In: "Artificial organs and cardiopulmonary support systems" (ed. F. T. Rapaport and J. P. Merrill) Grune and Stratton, New York, pp. 85-88.

Chapter 30

Adhesion of Fibroblasts to Artificial Substrata

Lloyd A. Culp
Department of Microbiology
Case Western Reserve University
School of Medicine
Cleveland, OH 44106

ABSTRACT

The molecular mechanism(s) by which fibroblasts adhere to a model extracellular matrix, tissue culture glass or plastic substrata, has been explored. The complexity of the serum proteins which bind to the substratum and mediate adhesion is determined by the chemical nature of the substratum, primarily via the nature of disulfide-crosslinked complexes formed among some commonly-bound proteins. Plasma fibronectin, in complexed form, is critical to the physiologically-compatible adhesion of cells. On the other hand, evidence is accumulating that one or more substratum-bound serum proteins other than fibronectin is also important in adhesion.

Detachment of cells from the substratum leaves tight, focal, footpad, adhesion sites as substratum-attached material (SAM). SAM is a specialized region of the cell surface enriched in cellular fibronectin, proteoglycans, the glycosaminoglycan hyaluronic acid, the subunit protein of the 10nm filaments of these cells, and several proteins associated with microfilaments. A variety of approaches have been used to probe the molecular organization of these so-called "cell surface adhesion complexes". These studies have led to molecular models of the adhesion and eventual detachment of cells based on the coordinate interaction of both forms of fibronectin, proteoglycans, and cytoskeletal elements.

I. INTRODUCTION

Understanding and utilization of the mechanism(s) by which animal cells adhere to various extracellular matrices have become increasingly important in a wide range of biological systems and applications. Solid tumor cells, in order to undergo metastasis in the animal, must dissociate from the primary tumor site, circulate, and then reimplant in distant tissues by interacting with various basal lamina in those tissues and particularly with the extracellular matrix (ECM) underlying the endothelial cell lining of blood vessels of those tissues [1]. Embryonic cell populations organize into tissues by depositing ECM that directs specific cellular interactions [2]. Wound healing requires the re-formation of basal laminae which give structure to newly-formed tissues. Finally, implantation of artificial substances into the body, including plastics, metals, and ceramics, has become increasingly important to provide tissue function after longterm failure or accidental abuse (see other chapters in this text for complete descriptions of these uses). For a better understanding of these and other biological phenomena, it is important to acquire an understanding of the molecular biology of animal cell adhesion and detachment from ECM.

Unfortunately, it has been extremely difficult to obtain natural ECM in sufficient quantities to perform the necessary biochemical and structural analyses, although some progress has been recently reported [3,4]. To circumvent this problem, many laboratories have resorted to the study of this interaction with a model ECM, tissue culture plastic or glass surfaces, that can be obtained in large quantities and can be readily manipulated to obtain sufficient quantities of adhesive material to do structure-function analyses. This review will focus attention on the molecular mechanism(s) by which one prominent cell type in the animal, fibroblasts, adheres to physiologically-compatible tissue culture substrata, with some later comments on other differentiated cell types. These studies provide insight on two major issues: (a) how cells may interact with "natural" ECM in the animal and (b) how to chemically and structurally provide artificial implant materials which are more compatible with the biological system.

II. SERUM PROTEINS REQUIRED FOR CELL ADHESION TO ARTIFICIAL SUBSTRATA

Early studies on the requirements for survival and growth of many aneuploid cell lines grown in tissue culture determined that serum protein binding to glass or plastic is required for their attachment [5,6,7]. On the other hand, attachment to naked glass or plastic surfaces was found to be nonphysiological and resulted eventually in cell death. Subsequently, it has been found that the only exceptions to this rule are cell lines or cell strains which secrete large amounts of collagen, fibronectin, or other adhesion-promoting proteins which coat the glass or plastic surface and to which the cells can successfully "crawl" onto [8]. The serum proteins which bind to artificial substrata are not passively engaged in the adhesion process but are enriched in proteins which bind to cell surface receptors with a specificity reminiscent of antigen-antibody or enzyme-substrate binding. It is also important to differentiate attachment and cell spreading processes of cells [11] – attachment will occur transiently on substrata coated with virtually any protein (including the inactive component serum albumin) but spreading requires appropriate adhesion-promoting factors in the serum layer.

A. Studies on Proteins Which Bind to Various Substrata

Culp and his collaborators [9,10] first extracted the serum proteins which bind to tissue

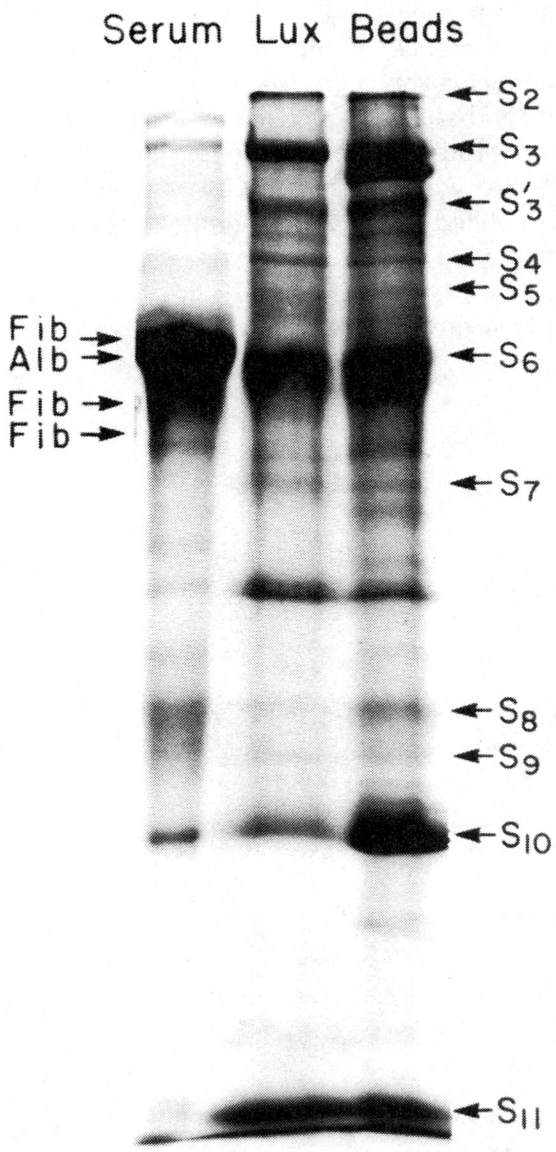

Figure 1. Substratum-attached serum proteins from glass microbeads and tissue culture plastic. Bovine fetal calf serum (Serum) was adsorbed to glass microbeads (Beads) or tissue culture plastic dishes (Lux) as described previously [14]. The beads and plastic dishes were rinsed well and treated with 0.2% SDS in water to solubilize a major portion (but not all) of the tightly bound serum protein. The samples were concentrated and electrophoresed in an SDS-PAGE gel under thiol-reducing conditions. The gel was stained with Coomassie blue and the migration positions of the three chains of fibrinogen (Fib) and albumin (Alb) are denoted. The sizes of major adsorbed serum proteins are provided in Table 1. (Taken from reference 14).

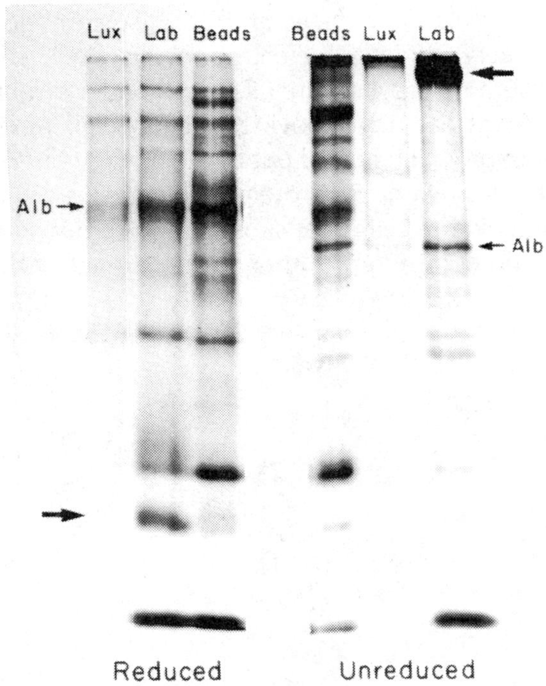

Figure 2. Substratum-attached serum proteins from three chemically different substrata after electrophoresis under thiol reduced *or unreduced conditions. Bovine fetal calf serum proteins adsorbed to tissue culture plastic (Lux), bacteriological plastic (Lab), or glass microbeads (Beads) were solubilized with SDS and analyzed by SDS-PAGE as described in reference 14 under thiol-reduced or -unreduced conditions with Coomassie blue staining. Marker bovine albumin (Alb) is denoted with the thin arrow. The thick arrows at the left and right denote major protein components unique to bacteriological plastic surfaces. (Taken from reference 14).*

culture plastic surfaces and showed an enrichment for twelve major proteins separable by polyacrylamide gel electrophoresis (PAGE) in the presence of the denaturing detergent sodium dodecyl sulfate (SDS) and under disulfide-reducing conditions (see Figure 1 and Table 1). Many batches of bovine sera (fetal calf, newborn, and calf) generated the same spectrum of proteins which bound out of the literally hundreds of proteins which are found in animal sera. The prominent S_6 protein is bovine serum albumin, which fails to catalyze cytoplasmic spreading of cells over substrata when bound in its purified form [12,13] and therefore cannot be the adhesion promoting receptor activity in this layer.

Table 1. Substratum-bound Serum Proteins on Tissue Culture Plastic[1]

Serum Protein	Molecular Weight
S_1 and S_2	very large (>500,000)
S_3	175,000
S_3'	140,000
S_4	85,000
S_5	73,000
S_6 (albumin)	65,000
S_7	49,000
S_8	29,000
S_9	27,000
S_{10}	23,000
S_{11}	11,000

[1] These are the approximate molecular weights determined by SDS-PAGE under reducing conditions using bovine serum albumin, actin, myoglobin, myosin, and E. coli β-galactosidase as markers. These proteins are extractable from tissue culture plastic made by several different manufacturers using 0.2% SDS in H_2O for 30 minutes at 37°C.

Haas and Culp [14] then characterized the serum proteins which bind to three different substrata – bacteriological plastic which is not compatible for attachment and growth, tissue culture plastic, and glass microbeads which were treated in such a manner as to make them compatible for cell attachment, cytoplasmic spreading, and growth. When the serum proteins adsorbed to these three substrata are solubilized with SDS and fractionated by SDS-PAGE under reducing conditions (Figure 1 and Figure 2), the banding patterns are remarkably similar except for two prominent proteins at the top of the gel which bind to glass beads but not to plastic surfaces and for a small protein (arrow at bottom lefthand side of Figure 2) which binds to tissue culture plastic and glass beads *but not to bacteriological plastic.* When these preparations are electrophoresed as unreduced samples (righthand side of Figure 2), the profiles are very different. These results indicate that the chemical nature of the substratum determines the spectrum of serum proteins which bind; the considerable differences in the disulfide-cross-linked complexes indicates that either substrata bind out specific preformed complexes from the serum (but whose subunit composition may be similar, as reflected in the similarity of reduced SDS-PAGE profiles) or substrata bind similar proteins but in a topographically different way that permits different disulfide-crosslinked complexes to form on the substratum surface. The mechanism of formation of these complexes has not been resolved and it is becoming increasingly clear that single proteins do not catalyze adhesion; several different proteins in high molecular weight and multivalent complexes may be the true adhesion-promoting activities.

An independent approach has also established the importance of disulfide-crosslinked complexes for mediating fibroblast adhesion to tissue culture substrata. Grinnell [13] fractionated fetal calf serum on a DEAE-cellulose column and obtained a high molecular weight fraction which catalyzed cytoplasmic spreading of cells when adsorbed to the substratum, thereby termed "spreading factor" (SF). SF is obtained from a wide variety of animal sera [13]. When SF is analyzed by SDS-PAGE under reducing conditions [12], it generates eight Coomassie-stainable protein bands, the major component of which was identified as cold-insoluble globulin (or, as it is more commonly referred to, plasma fibronectin). This approach, as well as several other approaches, led many laboratories to investigate the role of plasma fibronectin in mediating adhesion of cells as a component of the adsorbed serum layer.

B. Role of Plasma Fibronectin

Several laboratories independently discovered that plasma fibronectin (pFbn), when purified from animal sera or plasma by affinity chromatography on gelatin-Sepharose columns

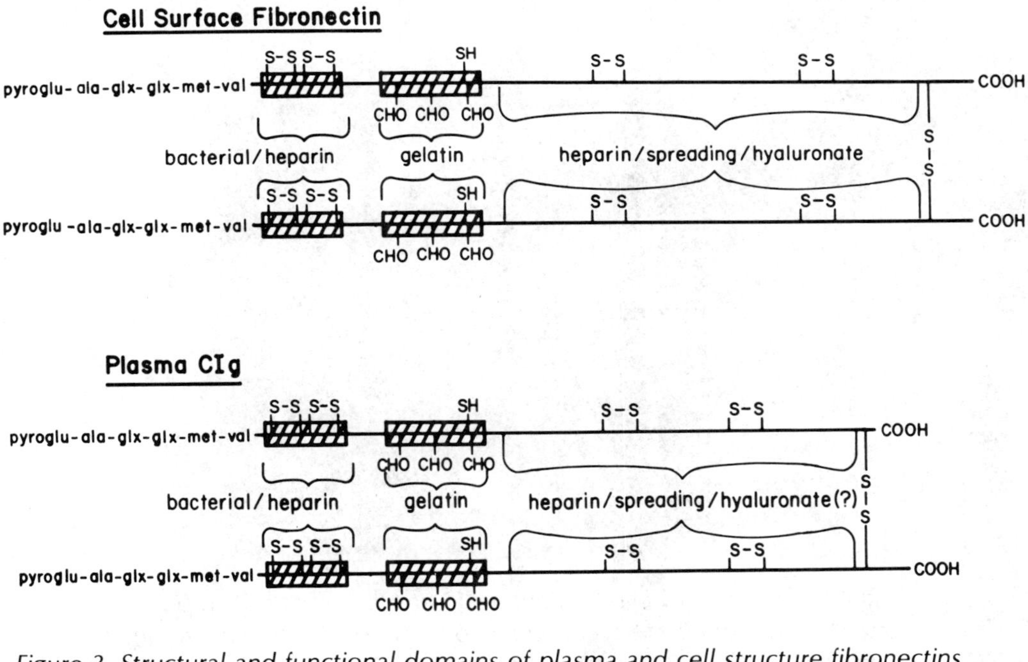

Figure 3. Structural and functional domains of plasma and cell structure fibronectins. Both molecules occur most commonly as a dimer of disulfide-crosslinked chains. However, plasma fibronectin (cold-insoluble globulin of CIg) contains two shorter polypeptides than cFbn with differing C-termini. Both forms share common structural and functional binding sites at the N-terminal ends but differ significantly at internal sequences. CIg apparently does not have a hyaluronate binding site whereas cFbn does [17b]. Whether the internal cell spreading site is identical or different from the heparin binding site has not been established. CHO represents the oligosaccharide side-chains on the molecule.

and subsequently bound to the tissue culture dish, catalyzed physiologically-compatible adhesion and cytoplasmic spreading of a wide variety (but not all) cell types, including fibroblasts (reviewed in 15). pFbn contains two polypeptide chains of approximate molecular weight 220,000 which are disulfied-crosslinked to each other and which are of slightly differing lengths as a result of one of the two chains having a shortened C-terminal sequence (Figure 3). The cell surface form of fibronectin (cFbn) contains two identical chains disulfide-crosslinked, both chains of which are slightly longer than the chains from pFbn (Figure 3). There is increasing evidence that pFbn and cFbn are structurally and functionally different (probably products of separate genes). Atherton and Hynes [16] have identified internal amino acid sequences using monoclonal antibodies which are unique to pFbn or cFbn. Laterra and Culp [17b] have established that pFbn lacks a binding site for hyaluronic acid which is "expressed" on cFbn when the protein aggregates into high molecular weight multimers (see section III D for a discussion of the significance of this finding). However, both pFbn and cFbn have binding sites in distinguishable molecular domains for heparin or heparan sulfate, fibrin, the α_1 chains of collagen, and certain bacterial polysaccharides [18] (Figure 3).

The mechanism by which pFbn binds to tissue culture plastic or glass has unfortunately not been thoroughly investigated. Saturation levels are probably one-two molecules thick [19] and some of the substratum-bound pFbn exists as multimers which are covalently crosslinked by bonds other than disulfide linkages [20]. When serum proteins are extracted off the substratum with SDS alone and then analyzed by SDS-PAGE under reducing conditions [14], there is no detectable pFbn band in the gels (Figure 4); however, when a reducing agent is

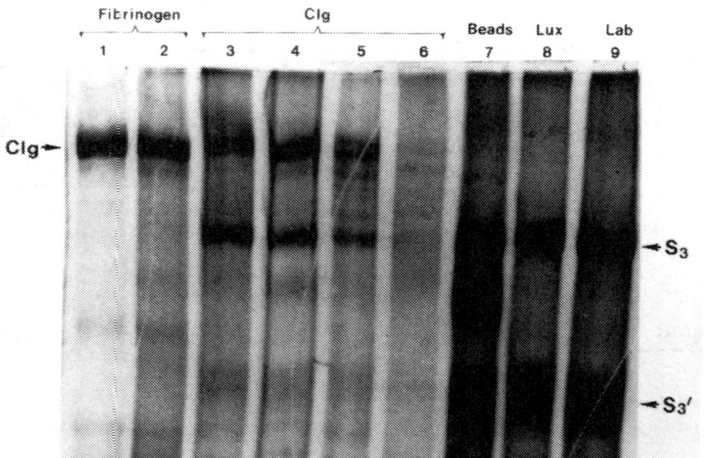

Figure 4. Absence of plasma fibronectin in substratum-bound protein extracts without thiol extracting conditions. Substratum-bound serum proteins (wells 7-9) from glass microbeads (well #7), tissue culture plastic (well #8), or bacteriological plastic (well #9) were electrophoresed on low-crosslinked SDS-PAGE gels under thiol-reduced conditions and Coomassie stained. Bovine fibrinogen was also electrophoresed in wells 1 and 2 (note the prominent contamination of plasma (Clg) and human plasma fibronectin in wells 3-6 (Clg) at various concentrations. Note the absence of a plasma fibronectin band in the adsorbed serum preparations (wells 7-9), even though it can be readily detected by immunofluorescent methods in the adsorbed serum layer (see Figure 6). (Taken from reference 14).

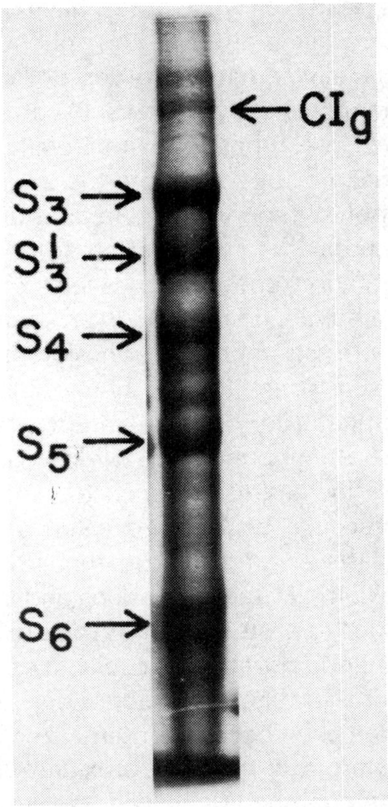

Figure 5. Plasma fibronectin in substratum-bound protein extracts using thiol extractants. The serum proteins bound to tissue culture plastic were solubilized with 0.2% SDS in H_2O and 0.1% mercaptoethanol. In contrast to Figure 4 where no plasma fibronectin band can be detected, there is plenty of plasma fibronectin (CIg) in this preparation as detected by Coomassie blue staining.

included with SDS during the extraction step, sizable amounts of pFbn are observed in gels (Figure 5) (Haas and Culp, unpublished data). This suggests that pFbn is bound in the substratum-bound serum layer to itself or to some other protein by disulfide linkage and this unknown "anchoring" component is not extracted off the substratum with SDS. The possible significance of this "anchoring" component will be discussed in Section II C.

This leads into a discussion as to why negatively-charged tissue culture polystyrene is so proficient for adhesion and spreading of fibroblasts whereas bacterial polystyrene is so unsatisfactory. It is becoming increasingly clear that tissue culture plastic binds quantitatively more pFbn (relative to the concentrations of other serum proteins) than bacteriological plastic as determined by immunoaccessability of pFbn in the serum layer to antibody to Fbn [19] and as determined on SDS-PAGE gels of SDS-mercaptoethanol-extracted material (Haas and Culp, unpublished data). When various ratios of bovine serum albumin and pFbn (mixed previously in solution) are bound to substrata and cells tested for cytoplasmic spreading capacity, the critical concentration is approximately 0.1-0.2 mg of pFbn per 10 mg of BSA (Laterra and Culp, unpublished data). Below this concentration, cells attach but do not spread and at this concentration some cells have spread well while others have not spread at all. This latter finding suggests that cytoplasmic spreading is an all-or-none phenomenon requiring some critical concentration of pFbn in the extracellular matrix in order to "trigger" the cell's signal to spread. These data indicate that the chemical nature of the substratum determines whether a sufficient concentration of pFbn binds in competition with literally hundreds of other serum proteins. Another possibility that has not been explored is a differing conformational change upon pFbn binding to charged polystyrene which generates a higher association constant of binding to the cell surface receptor. It is clear that some proteins, such as fibrinogen and γ-globulin, change their conformation considerably when they bind to artificial substrata whereas other proteins, such as albumin, do not [21]. In any case, it will be imperative to study the physical chemistry of binding of this important adhesion-promoting factor in extracellular matrices to artificial substrata used for implants in humans; the nature of this binding may reflect the compatibility or incompatibility of tissue and/or blood components.

Cellular interaction with substratum-bound pFbn will be discussed more fully in molecular terms below. However, there is increasing evidence that cells "metabolize" pFbn off the substratum. Early immunofluorescence analyses revealed a halo of "cleared" fibronectin around the periphery of fibroblasts and to some extent under fibroblasts [19] (Figure 6). However, these experiments are complicated by masking and inaccessibility of both pFbn and cFbn at the cell substratum interface to proteins such as trypsin, lactoperoxidase, and antibody [20]. Avnur and Geiger [22] have demonstrated that cells "clear" rhodamine-conjugated pFbn off the substratum directly under their tight focal adhesion sites but not at the periphery of these sites. Some of this rhodamine-pFbn becomes internalized into cells. Similar evidence has been demonstrated by our laboratory using lactoperoxidase-radioiodinated pFbn bound to the substratum (Haas and Culp, unpublished data); cells catalyze the evolution of a small portion of the radioiodinated material into the culture medium and to a more limited extent into the cell itself. Some of this "metabolized" pFbn is conserved as a 220,000 MW species while some of it is proteolyzed into smaller fragments. These experiments indicate two very important considerations – (a) cells may have at least two mechanisms for adhering at their tight focal contacts, one of which is an Fbn-independent mechanism; and (b) Fbn bound to the extracellular matrix is not metabolically-inert but is constantly turning-over in response to cell surface contact-mediated processes.

C. Involvement of Serum Proteins Other Than Plasma Fibronectin

There are several independent lines of investigation which demonstrate that fibronectin is not the only adhesion-promoting factor in the substratum-bound serum layer. As we reviewed in the paragraph above, rhodamine-conjugated pFbn is cleared off the substratum under tight focal adhesion sites which indicates that a secondary non-Fbn-dependent adhesion process is taking over [22]. Rees and his collaborators [23] using interference reflection microscopy have shown that rat fibroblasts adhering to pFbn-coated dishes do not make focal tight (10nm distance) contacts characteristic of cells adhering to serum-coated substrata. These data suggest an important function for one or more of the other substratum-bound serum proteins [14] in forming tight focal adhesion sites. Murray et al. [19] compared the biochemical composition of cellular substratum-attached material left bound to pFbn-coated serum-coated tissue culture plastic after EGTA-mediated detachment of cells; pFbn-attaching cells deposited much more hyaluronate and chondroitin proteoglycan than serum-attaching cells, providing further

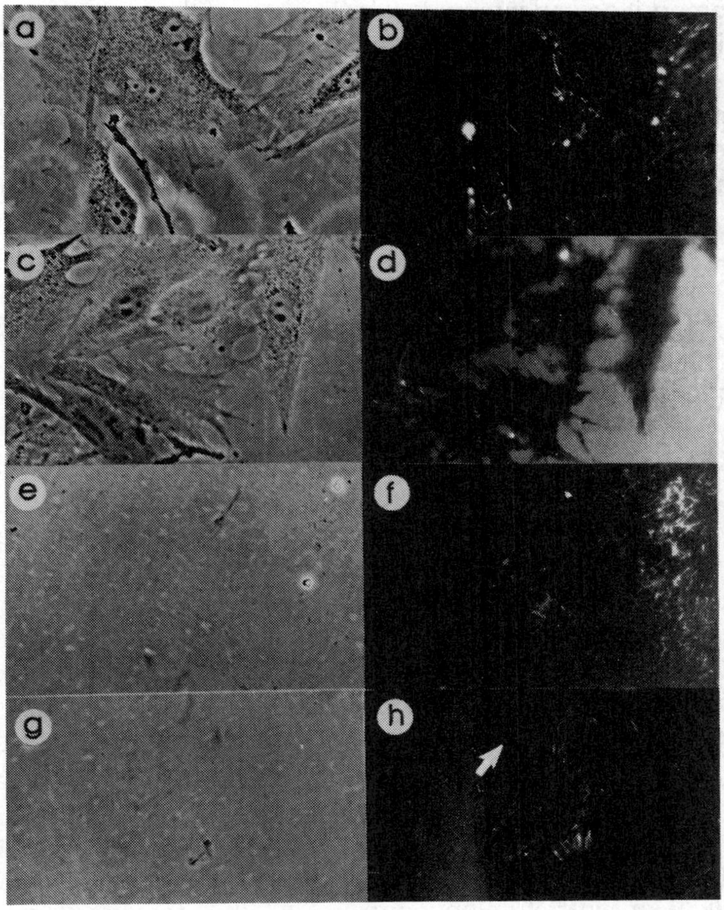

Figure 6. Immunofluorescent localization of plasma or cell surface fibronectins using antibody specific to each fibronectin. Balb/c 3T3 cells and SAM were prepared for immunofluorescence microscopy 24 hours after seeding onto plastic tissue culture dishes precoated with medium containing 10% calf serum (a,b,e,f) or with 30 μg/ml human plasma fibronectin (pFbn) in PBS (c,d,g,h). Cultures were stained with rabbit antibody to human plasma fibronectin and visualized with FITC-conjugated goat anti-rabbit Ig as described [19,20]. (a) 3T3 cells on serum-coated substratum, phase contrast photomicrograph; (b) same field stained with anti-pFbn preadsorbed such that it specifically stains cell surface fibronectin (note the focal, fibrillar staining); (c) 3T3 cells on pFbn-coated substratum, phase contrast; (d) same field stained with anti-pFbn showing an even layer of fluorescence around cells but most of the undersides of cells fail to stain because of masking of fibronectin in adhesion sites [20] and "metabolism" of some of the pFbn off the substratum; (e) 3T3 SAM on serum-coated substratum, phase contrast; (f) same field stained with anti-pFbn specific for cell surface fibronectin and showing concentrated fibrillar staining; (g) 3T3 SAM on pFbn-coated substratum, phase contrast; (h) same field stained with anti-pFbn (note the "sole plate" left bound to the substratum at the arrow; also, the contrast of this photomicrograph was modified to reduce the background fluorescence of the pFbn on the dish and to amplify the fibrillar fluorescence of cellular fibronectin in the adhesion sites in the original print). (Taken from reference 19).

support that the composition and intermolecular bonding of the serum layer are as important as Fbn alone in adhesive interaction. Knox and Griffiths [24] have fractionated animal sera and have identified a second protein of MW 70,000 which is not realted to Fbn and which may be critical for the proper adhesion of fibroblasts to tissue culture dishes. Interestingly, this activity promoted a slower initial adhesion of a variety of cell lines to dishes but a more stable longterm spreading of the cells. Perhaps, this is the factor which assumes a secondary adhesion-promoting role under the tight focal sites as suggested by the evidence of Avnur and Geiger [22].

III. CELLULAR COMPONENTS OF TIGHTLY-APPOSED FOCAL ADHESION SITES

A. General Considerations from the Cell's Perspective

On the serum-coated tissue culture substratum, fibroblasts appear to make two different types of adhesions as distinguished by interference reflection microscopy [25] – (a) small focal adhesions spaced approximately 10nm from the substratum and concentrated around the periphery of the cell and (b) broader contact regions of 30nm spacing under the leading lamellae of moving cells. The tight focal adhesion plaques appear to form as specialized regions of the broader contact regions of the cell. The tight focal adhesions also develop by an independent mechanism after trypsin- or chelation-mediated detachment of cells [27] – extension of 0.1 μm-diameter filopodia across the substratum, branching into finger-like structures, and membrane extension between the fingers to form footpad-like structures (Figure 7A).

When cells are detached by chelation or trypsinization, they undergo readherence to a substratum coated with pFbn in a tissue culture medium that contains very high concentrations of pFbn. Why doesn't the medium-contained pFbn bind to cell surface receptors and inhibit binding to substratum-bound pFbn? There may be two reasons why medium pFbn cannot compete successfully with substratum-bound pFbn [26,28]. In the first place, pFbn binding in solution to cells is extremely weak and dimeric pFbn is constantly shuffling on and off receptors. On the other hand, substratum-bound pFbn provides an array of "fixed" pFbn binding sites which recruit many cell surface molecules into an adhesion site. [The nature of these cell surface receptors will be discussed in section III D.] Weak monomeric binding is overcome by a high concentration of bound molecules which develop into a very tight-binding adhesion site. This recruitment is probably the major obstacle that the cell must overcome after trypsinization or chelation by resynthesizing new surface molecules and mobilizing them into patching networks. A second alternative explanation is conformational change of pFbn when it binds to the substratum providing much stronger binding to the surface receptor than displayed by Fbn in solution. Using low molecular weight heparin binding to pFbn or cFbn in solution or to Fbn bound to various inert matrices as a model system, we have been unable to detect any stronger binding of this glycosaminoglycan to matrix-bound Fbn [17]. Therefore, the cooperativity provided by many pFbn molecules "fixed" on the artificial substratum may be the major contributing factor in tight adhesion with cells bathed by high concentrations of adhesive molecules.

B. Composition under Various Physiological Conditions

Chelating agents, such as the more Ca^{++}-specific agent EGTA, were used to detach cells

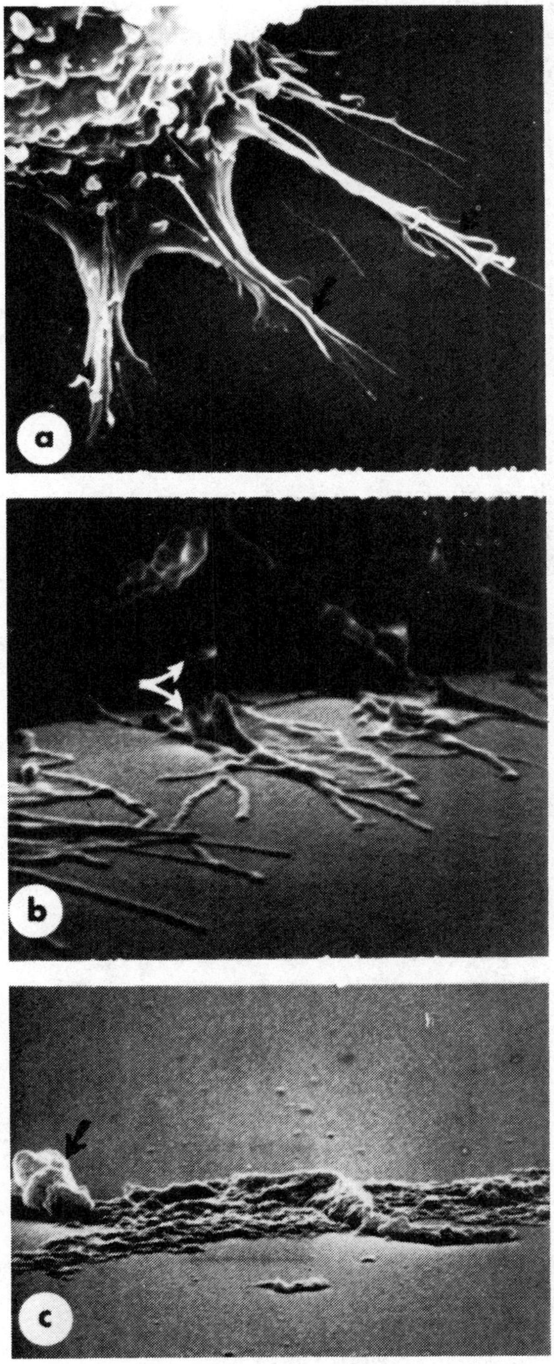

Figure 7. Scanning electron microscopic visualization of fibroblast adhesion sites. Swiss 3T3 cells growing in tissue culture dishes were detached by EGTA treatment and permitted to reattach for one hour to fresh dishes (a). Typical footpad-like adhesion sites are depicted by the arrows in "a". Detachment of cells by EGTA is depicted in (b) where the fragile elastic retraction fibers connecting the cell body and footpad adhesion sites are breaking (at the split arrows). A pool of one footpad adhesion site as SAM is depicted in (c) with a nub of membrane at the arrow where the retraction fiber has broken away. a: 30° tilt, 2500X; b: 80° tilt, 12,500X; c: 80° tilt, 22,000X. (Taken from reference 26).

and offered several advantages for biochemical characterization of cellular adhesive material [29]. (a) EGTA is a potent inhibitor of Ca^{++}-requiring proteases in cells. (b) It avoids destruction of cell surface proteins which occurs during protease-mediated detachment of cells. (c) Detachment occurs, not by dissociation of cell surface molecules in the adhesion site as a result of Ca^{++} chelation, but by collapse of the membrane-bound cytoskeleton of cells [27,29]. (d) Adhesive material is left as SAM while the rest of the cell is liberated into suspension (Figure 7B and C). SAM is essentially a one hundred-fold purification of cellular adhesive material containing protein and polysaccharide with virtually no RNA or DNA (Figure 7C).

An important artifactual source of SAM would be secretion of components from the cell and their rebinding to the serum-coated substratum. These proteins could rebind after secretion during the long periods of growth of these cells or after secretion during the EGTA treatment. Such an occurrence would seriously interfere with various biochemical analyses. The former process is unlikely because of the massive amounts of serum protein in the tissue culture medium which greatly dilutes the specific radioactivity of components made and secreted by the cell and which would bind cellular materials, thereby preventing any binding to the substratum.

Several experimental approaches were used to determine that SAM resulted from cell contact-mediated deposition and not artifactual rebinding. Adding *non-radiolabeled* components identified in SAM during growth of cells or during the EGTA treatment failed to diminish the amounts of *radiolabeled* SAM components [10,12,26]. The relative proportions of SAM components distinguished on SDS-PAGE gels were invariant and therefore inconsistent with a rebinding process that would fluctuate from experiment-to-experiment [10]. High resolution autoradiography experiments demonstrated that the radiolabeled cellular proteins and polysaccharides occurred on the substratum only where cells had grown and not on areas unoccupied or in very close proximity to cells [10,12]. These radiolabeled components were concentrated in small focal pools similar in density to the morphologically-identified tight focal footpad adhesion sites [25,27]. A careful scanning electron microscopy (SEM) study during the EGTA treatment (see Figure 7 and 8) provided evidence of cell body rounding and

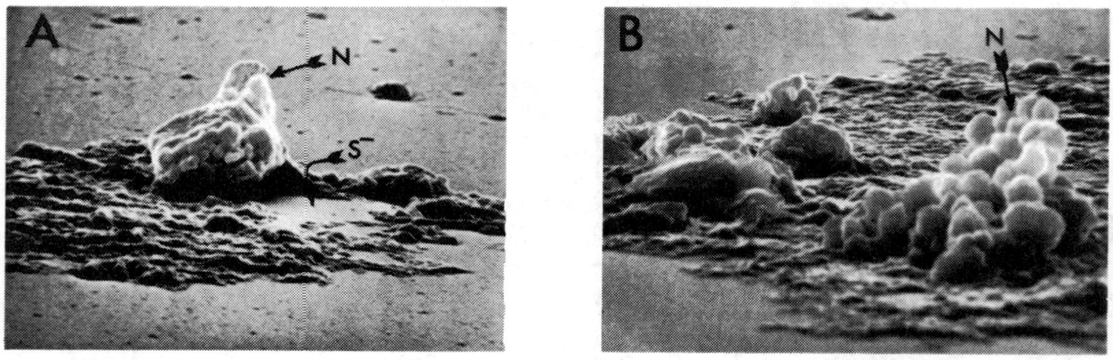

Figure 8. Morphology of SAM from attaching or well-spread cells. Swiss 3T3 cells were EGTA-detached and permitted to reattach to serum-coated glass coverslips for one (A) or 24 (B) hours, the latter cells being highly flattened on the substratum [27]. Cells from the two cultures were EGTA-detached, the substratum rinsed with PBS, and SAM prepared for scanning electron microscopy. A nub (N) of membrane is identifiable on both types of SAM where the retraction fiber has presumably broken away from the footpad. Attaching-cell SAM (A) frequently contains internal regions where membranous material is missing (S^-), presumably because adhesive functions have not matured over this short a timespan. SAM from well-spread cells (B) appears to be virtually intact footpads. (Original magnification X26,000; 80° tilt.)

pulling away from the footpad adhesion sites; culture agitation breaks the elastic retraction fiber stretched between the cell body and the footpad, leaving footpad adhesion sites as SAM (Figure 7C). SAM from newly-formed adhesion sites contains components which are labile to the EGTA treatment in the center of the footpad (Figure 8A); long-term generated SAM contains components which are stably bound across the entire footpad (Figure 8B). This is further evidence for two different adhesive mechanisms under the footpad site. All of this evidence indicates that SAM of the cell lines used in our studies are tight focal footpad adhesion sites and virtually no other cellular material in a non-contact-mediated fashion. However, it should be reiterated that these studies have focussed on cell lines* growing in serum-containing medium and that cells growing in chemically-defined serum-free media may very well secrete components that rebind to the substratum and may affect in one way or another cell growth and social behavior.

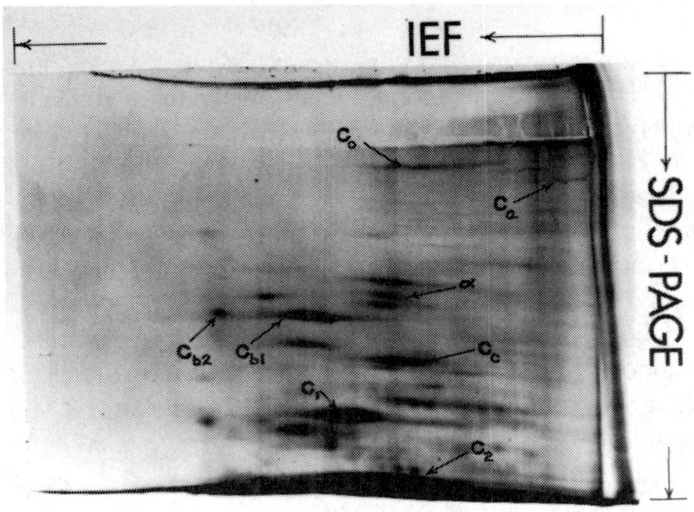

Figure 9. Two-dimensional electrophoresis of fibroblast SAM proteins. Balb/c SVT2 murine fibroblasts were grown for 72 hours in medium containing ^{14}C-leucine in tissue culture plastic dishes. Cells were rinsed and detached by treatment with 0.5mM EGTA in PBS. SAM was solubilized with SDS, concentrated, and loaded onto a disc gel for isoelectric focussing (IEF) between pH 3 and 10 as described previously [26]. After separation based on the isoelectric points of individual proteins under disulfide-reducing conditions, the IEF gel was loaded onto the top of a slab gel for electrophoresis into the slab in the presence of SDS and a thiol. The two-dimensional gel was dried and exposed to autoradiography film for several weeks to detect the cell-synthesized ^{14}C-radiolabeled proteins in SAM. The autoradiogram is shown in this figure. The following proteins have been characterized in SAM: C_o, cell surface fibronectin; C_a, myosin; α, α-actinin; C_{b1}, C_{b2}, and C_c, three prominent cytoskeletal proteins enriched in SAM; C_1, the subunit protein of the 10nm filaments of these cells; and C_2, actin. (Taken from reference 26).

*Cell strains, such as human diploid fibroblasts, have been shown to deposit some extracellular matrix components such as collagen as a continuous layer bound to the substratum rather than small focal pools [30]. It is not clear that fibroblasts adhering to a collagenous matrix make footpad-like adhesion sites.

Several complementary biochemical and immunochemical approaches were used to identify some of the major proteins and polysaccharides in fibroblast adhesion sites from several species [26,28,31]. Because of the appreciable size of footpad sites and their noted resistance to chemical dissociation from the substratum (requiring SDS for quantitative removal), it is likely that the prominent proteins and polysaccharides in SAM are the choicest candidates for mediating adhesive bonding. A two-dimensional gel of SAM proteins is depicted in Figure 9 after longterm-radiolabeling of cells. Protein C_2 splits into two components identified as the β and γ forms of actin, whose relative proportions in SAM are identical to that in the rest of the cell. Protein C_1 is the subunit protein of the 10nm filaments of fibroblasts (termed vimentin) and this protein interestingly contains no tryptophan [10,26]. There is also a prominent protein between C_1 and C_2 of approximate molecular weight 49,000 which shares some metabolic properties with fibronectin (see below). C_a has been identified as myosin. The most prominent glycoprotein in SAM is cell surface fibronectin (C_o), although there are two minor glycoprotein components of MW 140,000 and 175,000. When the composition of SAM is compared with that of whole surface membranes, SAM is enriched in fibronectin and some cytoskeletal components (some of which remain to be identified), although some cytoskeletal proteins such as tubulin and α-actinin (Figure 9) are depleted in SAM making it unlikely that they play a role in binding the cytoskeleton to the interior of the surface membrane. Therefore, the footpad adhesion sites of cells are biochemically-specialized regions of the surface membrane of the cells. The *coordinate deposition* of fibronectin and these cytoskeletal proteins into SAM under all attachment conditions suggested that they form a cell surface complex designed specifically for adhesive functions [31].

Polysaccharide analyses have also confirmed the specialized nature of SAM, which is enriched in glycosaminoglycan (GAG) and depleted of glycoprotein-derived glycopeptide [28]. The distribution of hyaluronic acid (HA), the chondroitin sulfates (C-4-S, C-6-S, C-0-S), dermatan sulfate (DS), and heparan sulfate (HS) are very different in SAM and surface membrane preparations. Furthermore, EGTA-detached and reattaching cells deposit principally HS in their newly-formed footpad adhesion sites, even though there are sizable pools of all GAG's on the cell surface conserved during EGTA-mediated detachment. This and other data discussed below suggest that HS proteoglycans play a direct role in mediating adhesion of cells to the substratum (at least in terms of an initial adhesive mechanism). In contrast, as cells initiate movement across the substratum, HA and CS accumulate in SAM. This evidence, coupled with data showing very high concentrations of HA in easily-detached cells [28], suggests that these components play some role in detachment of cells.

To a limited extent, the metabolism of some of the components in SAM has been explored [33,31,26]. When cells are pulsed with radioactive leucine for only two hours during exponential growth, SDS-PAGE analyses of pulse-labeled SAM reveal all of the proteins identified in longterm-labeling experiments such as that depicted in Figure 9, with the exception of two proteins that are very heavily radiolabeled in the autoradiograms (see Figure 3 of reference 31). Fibronectin is heavily labeled, as well as an unidentified protein C_d of MW 48-49,000. When these pulse-radiolabeled cells are chased with medium containing *nonradioactive* leucine for 24 hours and then their SAM analyzed by SDS-PAGE [31], most but not all of the heavily radiolabeled fibronectin and C_d protein have disappeared from SAM; the remaining radioactive C_o and C_d are metabolically stable. In contrast, the radiolabeling of the cytoskeletal proteins is conserved.

These experiments establish several important properties of adhesive material. (a) The conservation of radiolabeled cytoskeletal protein in SAM after the chase period, during which cells have moved considerable distances from their original location, provides biochemical evidence that cells leave "footprints" of their adhesive material during natural cell movement in a fashion similar to the effects of EGTA treatment – that is, cells leave their adhesive anchors behind and no doubt effect movement by rearranging their intracellular cytoskeletal networks rather than by breaking their extracellular adhesive contacts. (b) The failure to dilute the radioactivity in cytoskeletal proteins during the chase period indicates minimal exchange of actin and the 10nm-filament subunit protein with microfilaments and filaments anchored to the surface membrane. In other words, once formed, the membrane-associated cytoskeletal elements in adhesive footpads are relatively stable. (c) The similarity in synthesis, incorporation into SAM, and subsequent turnover of cell surface fibronectin (C_o) and the C_d protein suggests that they are complexed on the cell surface and play a coordinated functional role. Perhaps the C_d protein is the membrane anchorage protein for cell surface fibronectin. Several experimental approaches will be required to address this important issue.

C. Approaches for Studying Topography and Intermolecular Interactions in These Sites

When gross compositional studies of SAM were relatively complete, we began probing the supramolecular organization of SAM using several complementary experimental approaches. These included selective extraction with various reagents, susceptibility to digestion with specific enzymes, and availability to binding proteins such as antibodies.

Extraction of SAM was tested using various detergents and chaotropic agents [32]. Nonionic detergents were very ineffective at extracting protein from SAM but was able to extract some of the polysaccharide. Sodium deoxycholate extracted a limited amount of protein and polysaccharide. Urea, on the other hand, extracted increasingly greater amounts of either component with longer extraction periods. A mixture of ATP and KCl readily solubilized approximately one-half of the actin from SAM while the remainder was highly resistant to extraction.

Several distinguishable pools of cell surface fibronectin have now been identified in SAM (Table 2). Treatment of SAM with lactoperoxidase and radioactive iodine does not identify a pool of fibronectin which is easily accessible to the enzyme, in contrast to Fbn on other regions of the cell surface which is readily iodinated [32]. The longterm-radiolabeled Fbn in SAM is also resistant to trypsin, whereas the pulse-radiolabeled and metabolically-labile Fbn discussed above is very labile to this protease [33]. Similarly, the longterm-radiolabeled Fbn cannot be solubilized from SAM with testicular hyaluronidase treatment, whereas the pulse-radiolabeled form can be quantitatively solubilized, suggesting that the latter species is somehow associated with hyaluronate- and/or chondroitin sulfate-containing species. Using antibody to Fbn, most of the immunofluorescent detectable Fbn in SAM can be removed by a very gentle trypsin treatment which leaves eighty percent of the Fbn unaffected [20]. Testicular hyaluronidase has no adverse effect on detectability of Fbn with antibody. Although the SAM from confluent cells contains the expected concentration of Fbn as determined on SDS-PAGE gels, it cannot be detected on the substratum using antibody. These experiments all confirm that most of the fibronectin in substratum adhesion sites is inaccessible to protein reagents, even after various fixation protocols. Small amounts of Fbn are accessible to hyaluronidase and protease under the appropriate metabolic conditions.

The distribution of Fbn in SAM after various treatments was compared to the distribution

Table 2. Different Subsets of Cell Surface Fibronectin in Substratum Adhesion Sites[1].

Amount of Particular Subset	Metabolically Labile	Susceptible to Trypsin	Solubilized by Hyaluronidase	Detectable by Immuno-fluorescence
80 - 85%	-	-	-	-
10 - 15%	-	+	-	+
2 - 5%	+	+	+	+

[1] Cellular fibronectin in fibroblast adhesion sites was tested for several properties after EGTA-mediated detachment of cells and the amounts quantitated in each class by differential SDS-PAGE analyses as described in references 20,28, 32, and 33. Properties described are: metabolic lability (whether it turns over with a rapid half-life after a 2-hour pulse metabolic radiolabeling of SAM followed by a chase period); susceptibility to trypsin (whether the particular pool rapidly disappears upon gentle treatment of SAM with the protease trypsin); solubilization by hyaluronidase (whether it can be solubilized off the substratum by gentle digestion with testicular hyaluronidase); detectable by immunofluorescence (whether it is lost as determined by anti-fibronectin binding and indirect immunofluorescent detection).

of GAG's after identical treatment [33]. Although trypsin could remove most of the HA and CS from SAM, heparan sulfate resisted solubilization, along with Fbn and cytoskeletal protein [33]. Similar results were obtained for testicular hyaluronidase treatment, which removed virtually all of the HA and CS. These data suggested that (a) HA and CS are not integral components in the adhesion sites of these cells, (b) HS is not bound in SAM by HA- or CS-dependent structures, and (c) HS may be complexed with cFbn in the adhesion site.

These results led us into a direct analysis of pFbn's ability to bind to various GAG's [17]. When pFbn was linked covalently to a Sepharose column and challenged with polysaccharide preparations from cells or SAM, only highly N-sulfated HS bound to the column [17a]. Similar results were observed for cFbn linked to a column [17b], in contrast to the results of Yamada et al [34] showing that cFbn aggregated in solution binds HA as well. Further analyses demonstrated that pFbn as a dimer or as an aggregate in solution was unable to bind HA [17b]. This provides the molecular explanation as to why HA does not mediate adhesion of fibroblasts to tissue culture substrata [33]. cFbn, on the other hand, does not bind HA as a dimer but acquires the ability to bind HA when it aggregates into multimers [17b]. Some evidence indicates that the aggregated protein changes its conformation in such a way to generate a new HA binding site but this question must be examined more carefully.

Most of the CS and HS in SAM is proteoglycan and not free GAG chains. The potential of these proteoglycans to aggregate was explored using methodologies found successful in analyzing cartilage proteoglycan aggregates [35]. Approximately sixty percent of the GAG can be extracted from SAM with the dissociative reagent 4M guanidine hydrochloride (GuHCl) (the GuHCl-resistant material is highly enriched in HS) [28]. When [GuHCl] is reduced to allow reassociation of components in this extract and then analyzed by Sepharose gel filtration chromatography, much of the GAG appears in supramolecular aggregates. There appear to be two distinguishable classes of aggregate – one which is dissociable with 4M GuHCl and a second which requires a detergent for complete dissociation. Because of the central role played by HA and the proteoglycans in adhesion of cells (see below), it will be imperative to better characterize these intermolecular associations.

D. A Prospective Molecular Model of One Type of Adhesion Process in Focal Sites.

The evidence described above has led us to propose molecular models for adhesion and detachment of cells with specific functions assigned to plasma and cell surface fibronectins and the glycosaminoglycans [26,28]. Since focal adhesion sites are relatively large "organelles" of specialized cell surface function and are very tightly bound to the substratum, it appears likely that their binding is mediated by major components identified in SAM and not by minor components. Collagen has not been found in the adhesive material of many aneuploid cell lines grown on tissue culture substrata [36], and therefore our attention has been drawn to fibronectin and proteoglycans as the major interactive components on the outer cell surface. It should also be stated that these models do not exclude other adhesive mechanisms, such as the rearrangement of molecules within the adhesion site leading to a different molecular mechanism. This latter possibility is suggested by at least two independent lines of evidence – (a) the importance of plasma proteins other than CIg which bind to artificial substrata and mediate adhesion and (b) the scanning electron micrographs of Figure 8 which show poor molecular organization at the interior of newly-formed footpads and "strengthening" of this interior with time. In any case, evidence is becoming overwhelming for the central role of fibronectin and proteoglycans in adhesion (Figure 10).

In Figure 10A is presented a model of initial footpad formation. Multivalent heparan proteoglycans aggregate into patching networks on the cell surface. These proteoglycans bind to literally hundreds of CIg molecules in the substratum-bound serum layer. Although there is weak unimolecular binding between CIg and heparan sulfate, the coordinate binding of hundreds of molecules generates a tightly bound matrix. The heparan proteoglycans, in turn, would be linked to the cell surface by two possible mechanisms, only one of which is shown here. They probably bind to cell surface fibronectin molecules which are, in turn, linked across the plasma membrane by some unidentified protein to the actin-containing microfilaments of the cell. Alternatively, some of the heparan proteoglycan may have hydrophobic protein cores which are embedded directly in the phospholipid bilayer.

The ramifications of the model in Figure 10A are multiple. In the first place, the chemical nature of the artificial substratum determines the topography and amounts of plasma fibronectin bound, thereby effecting the distribution and size of cellular footpad adhesion sites. Insufficient amounts or arrangements of plasma fibronectin on the substratum would lead to poor development of footpad sites, such as found on bacteriological plastic, and to improper reconstruction of the cell's cytoskeleton which is critically important for growth and movement. This mechanism also provides a transmembrane control which works in both directions – elements on the outer surface of the cell must be arranged properly to allow proper cytoskeletal organization within the cell and vice versa. Therefore, the cell can control its own adhesiveness from within by manipulating membrane-associated microfilament organization. By this process, cells leave "footprints" by disorganization of their microfilaments at posterior regions of the cell surface and retraction of the elastic plasma membrane away from the footpad site.

One possible mechanism for detachment of cells is presented in Figure 10B. Considerable evidence discussed above suggests that hyaluronic acid plays a central role in the detachment of cells. The data of Laterra and Culp [17b] suggests the molecular basis for this phenomenon. Hyaluronate cannot bind to plasma fibronectin and therefore does not mediate adhesion of cells to artifical substrata. On the other hand, HA binds to the aggregated form of cell surface

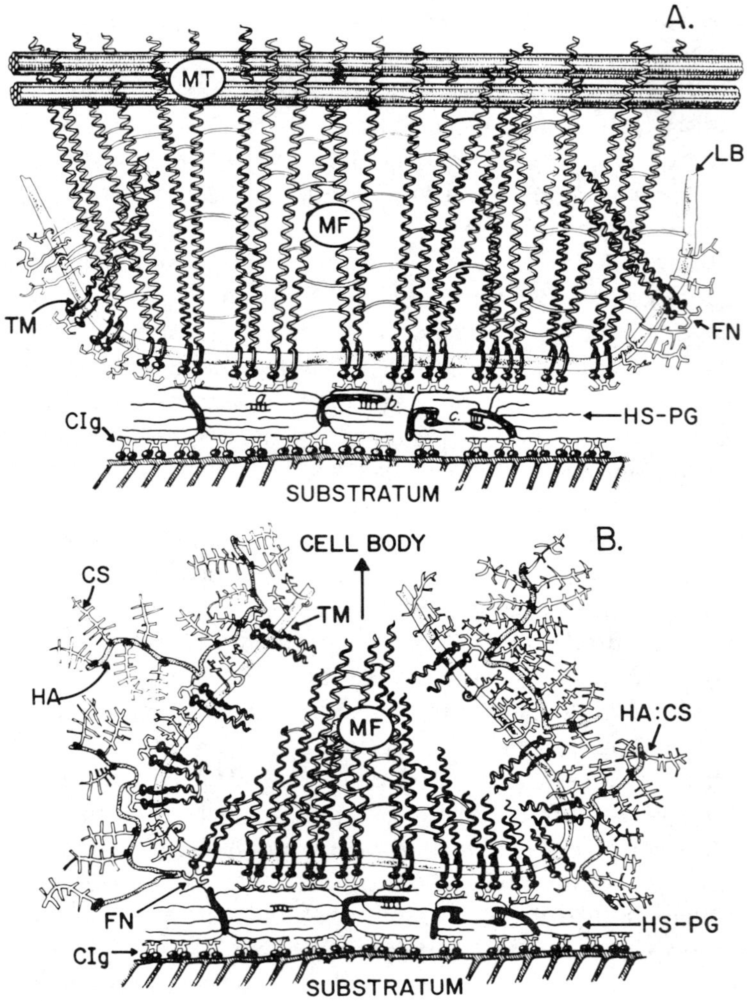

Figure 10. Prospective models for the initial adhesion and eventual detachment of cells. The initial events in formation of an adhesive bond between the cell surface and the serum-coated substratum are depicted in A. Dimeric plasma fibronectin (CIg) molecules on the substratum probably bind to aggregated heparan sulfate proteoglycans (HS-PG) on the cell surface; HS-PG aggregation may occur by unknown mechanisms involving polysaccharide chain:chain interaction (a), core protein:GAG chain binding (b), and/or the involvement of a "link" protein which crosslinks GAG chains (c). HS-PG would then bind to cell surface fibronectin (FN) forming an ordered array of these latter molecules. FN would bind to some unidentified transmembrane protein (TM) which also binds to microfilaments on the interior of the lipid bilayer (LB). Microfilaments (MF) would be crosslinked into bundled arrays and may interact with the microtubules (MT) of the cell. Such a mechanism provides a cascade of molecule ordering processes from the distant outer cell surface into the interior of the cell. Detachment is depicted in B. Complexes composed of hyaluronic acid (HA) and chondroitin sulfate proteoglycans (CS) accumulate at the periphery of the adhesion site. HA binds specifically to cell surface fibronectin, a process which competes with HS-PG binding and which causes disordering of FN at the adhesion site periphery. Disordering of FN leads to disorder in the microfilaments. With disorder in the cytoskeleton, there is retraction of the elastic plasma membrane leading to pinching off the adhesion site, leaving a "footprint" on the substratum. (Taken from reference 28).

fibronectin. HA may accumulate in mature footpad adhesion sites at localized regions and bind to cell surface fibronectin in such a way that fibronectin matrices become disorganized; this subsequently results in disorganization of intracellular microfilaments because of transmembrane linkage. HA may also compete with heparan proteoglycans for binding cell surface fibronectin freshly incorporated into the adhesion site. Another possibility is that HA; fibronectin complexes are labile on the cell surface to proteolysis, a process which perturbs footpad and cytoskeletal organization.

Although these models in Figure 10 are still speculative, they provide frameworks on a molecular basis for testing various aspects of the adhesive properties of cells. Various GAG components must be localized in footpad sites by sophisticated ultrastructural techniques. Interactions between plasma or cell surface fibronectin and various GAG's in the test tube must now be examined directly in the adhesion site itself. Much more must be learned about association of proteoglycans with themselves and other components on the cell surface. In any case, we are getting closer to an accurate understanding of the molecular events in cell adhesion to tissue culture substrata and this model system will provide insight as to how cells adhere to natural collagenous matrices, a process which also requires binding of fibronectin to the "inert" collagen matrix.

E. Comparison of Fibroblast Adhesion with Adhesion Processes of Other Differentiated Cells

By far the easiest cells to grow *in vitro* have been fibroblasts, which has been the principal reason more is known about fibroblast adhesion to extracellular matrices than adhesion of other differentiated cell types. Studies are now being initiated into the molecular mechanism of adhesion of muscle cells, macrophages, neutrophils, T lymphocytes, endothelial, and epithelial cells. Letourneau [37,38] initiated studies into neuronal cell adhesion to tissue culture substrata by chemically modifying the substratum and by demonstrating selectivity of both cell bodies and neurites for adherence to specific coated surfaces. Neuronal cells attach, spread well, and extend neurites on substrata coated with pFbn [39].

Culp et al. [39] detached neuroblastoma and glioma cells from tissue culture plastic using EGTA and examined the composition of their SAM's. Several similarities to fibroblast SAM content were observed. The highly motile glioma cells deposited large quantities of hyaluronate in their SAM, whereas the relatively immobile neuroblastoma cells deposited only small quantities. The SAM of both cell types contained considerable heparan sulfate and actin-containing microfilament proteins. The neuroblastoma SAM was enriched for a 220,000 MW glycoprotein which was immunologically related to fibroblast fibronectin but which only shared some cross-reactivity. This molecule may be a neuron-specific analog of fibroblast fibronectin and may function in the specific adhesiveness of these cells.

The SAM of the neurite-containing cells was compared with that of nonneurite-containing neuroblastoma cells to provide some indication of different mechanisms by which growth cones adhere to the tissue culture substratum as compared to the cell bodies of neuronal cells [39]. Neurite SAM contained an unknown and uncharacterized high molecular weight polysaccharide (I_o) never before observed in fibroblast, glioma, or nonneurite neuroblastoma SAM's. The distribution of 10nm filament proteins changed considerably in neurite SAM. Scanning electron microscopic evidence indicates that the ultrastructures of adhesion sites under neurites or cell bodies are significantly different [40]. Cells are attached under their central cell bodies by small, periodic contacts no more than 0.2–0.5 microns in diameter; footpad adhesion sites commonly observed in fibroblasts are not observed under the cell bodies of these neuroblastoma cells. However, growth cones at the tips of neurites adhere to the substratum over broader and tighter regions of the undersurface somewhat characteristic of fibroblast adhesion sites [40]. From these preliminary experiments, there is suggestion that neuronal cells may adhere to the tissue culture substratum by a mechanism similar to that of fibroblasts, but differentiated function, as displayed by neurite extension over the substratum, requires cell type-specific adhesion properties. Whether other differentiated cells have unique mechanisms for adhering remains to be seen.

REFERENCES

1. Poste, G. and Fidler, I.J. (1980) The pathogenesis of cancer metastasis. Nature *283,* 139-145.
2. Letourneau, P.C., Ray, P.N. and Bernfield, M.R. (1980) In *Biological Regulation and Control,* ed. R. Goldberger, Plenum Press. pp. 339-376.
3. Rojkind, M., Gatmaitan, Z., Mackensen, S., Giambrone, M.-A., Reid, L.M. Ponce, P. (1980) Connective tissue biomatrix: its isolation and utilization for long-term cultures of normal rat hepatocytes. J. Cell Biol. *87,* 255-263.
4. Gospodarowicz, D., Delgado, D. and Vlodavsky, I. (1980) Control of cell proliferation *in vitro* by extracellular matrix. Proc. Natl. Acad. Sci. U.S.A. *77,* 4094-4098.
5. Taylor, A.C. (1961) Attachment and spreading of cells in culture. Exp. Cell Res., Suppl. *8,* 154-173.
6. Weiss, L. (1959) Studies on cellular adhesion in tissue culture. I. The effect of serum. Exp. Cell Res. *17,* 499-507.
7. Lieberman, I. and Ove, P. (1959) Growth factors for mammalian cells in culture. J. Biol. Chem. *234,* 2754-2758.
8. Grinnell, F. and Feld, M.K. (1979) Initial adhesion of human fibroblasts in serum-free medium: possible role of secreted fibronectin. Cell *17,* 117-129.
9. Culp, L.A. and Buniel, J.F. (1976) Substrate-attached serum and cell proteins in adhesion of mouse fibroblasts. J. Cell. Physiol. *88,* 89-106.
10. Culp, L.A. (1976) Electrophoretic analysis of substrate-attached proteins from normal and virus-transformed cells. Biochemistry *15,* 4094-4104.
11. Grinnell, F., Hays, D.G. and Minter, D. (1977) Cell adhesion and spreading factor. Exp. Cell Res. *110,* 175-190.
12. Culp, L.A. (1978) "Biochemical determinants of cell adhesion" in *Current Topics in Membranes and Transport,* Vol. 11, pp. 327-396.
13. Grinnell, F. (1978) Cellular adhesiveness and extracellular substrata. Int. Rev. Cyt. *53,* 65-144.
14. Haas, R. and Culp, L.A. (1979) Adhesion of murine cells to glass microbeads: substrate-adsorbed serum proteins. J. Cell. Physiol. *101,* 279-292.
15. Yamada, K.M. and Olden, L. (1978) Fibronectin: adhesive glycoproteins of cell surfaces and blood. Nature *275,* 179-184.
16. Atherton, B.L. and Hynes, R.O. (1981) A difference between plasma and cellular fibronectins located with monoclonal antibodies. Cell *25,* 133-142.

17a. Laterra, J., Ansbacher, R. and Culp, L.A. (1980) Glycosaminoglycans that bind cold-insoluble globulin in cell-substratum adhesion sites of murine fibroblasts. Proc. Natl. Acad. Sci. U.S.A. *77,* 6662-6666.

17b. Laterra, J. and Culp, L.A. (1982) Differences in hyaluronate binding to plasma and cell surface fibronectins: requirement for aggregation. J. Biol. Chem. *257,* 719-726.

18. Mosher, D.F. (1980) "Fibronectin" in *Progress in Hemostasis and Thrombosis,* Vol. 5, ed. T.H. Spaet, Corune and Stratton, Inc. pp. 111-151.
19. Murray, B.A., Ansbacher, R., Culp, L.A. (1980) Adhesion sites of fibroblasts on CIg-adsorbed substrata. J. Cellular Physiol. *104,* 335-348.

20. Murray, B.A. and Culp, L.A. (1981) Multiple and masked pools of fibronectin in murine fibroblast cell-substratum adhesion sites. Exp. Cell Res. *131*, 237-249.
21. Morrissey, B.W. (1977) The adsorption and conformation of plasma proteins: a physical approach. Ann. N.Y. Acad. Sci. *283*, 50-64.
22. Avnur, Z. and Geiger, B. (1981) The removal of extracellular fibronectin from areas of cell-substrate contact. Cell *25*, 121-132.
23. Thom, D., Powell, A.J. and Rees, D.A. (1979) Mechanisms of cellular adhesion IV. Role of serum glycoproteins in fibroblast spreading on glass. J. Cell Sci. *35*, 281-305.
24. Knox, P. and Griffiths, S. (1980) The distribution of cell-spreading activities in sera: a quantitative approach. J. Cell Sci. *46*, 97-112.
25. Izzard, C.S. and Lochner, L.R. (1976) Cell-to-substrate contacts in living fibroblasts: an interference-reflexion study with an evaluation of the technique. J. Cell. Sci. *21*, 129-159.
26. Culp, L.A., Murray, B.A. and Rollins, B.J. (1979) Fibronectin and Proteoglycans as determinants of cell-substratum adhesion. J. Supramol. Str. *11*, 401-427.
27. Rosen, J.J. and Culp, L.A. (1977) Morphology and cellular origins of substrate-attached material from mouse fibroblasts. Exp. Cell Res. *107*, 139-149.
28. Rollins, B.J., Cathcart, M.K., and Culp, L.A. (1981) "Fibronectin:Proteoglycan binding as the molecular basis for fibroblast adhesion to extracellular matrices" in *The Glycoconjugates,* Vol. III, ed. M.I. Horowitz, Academic Press, Inc., N.Y. pp. 289-329.
29. Culp, L.A. and Black, P.H. (1972) Release of macromolecules from Balb/c mouse cell lines treated with chelating agent. Biochem. *11*, 2161-2171.
30. Lembach, K.J., Branson, R.E., Hewgley, P.B. and Cunningham, L.W. (1977) The synthesis of macromolecular 3-hydroxyproline by attaching and confluent cultures of human fibroblasts. Eur. J. Biochem. *72*, 379-383.
31. Culp, L.A. (1976) Molecular composition and origin of substrate-attached material from normal and virus transformed cells. J. Supramol. Str. *5*, 239-255.
32. Cathcart, M.K. and Culp, L.A. (1979) Initial studies of the molecular organization of the cell-substrate adhesion site. Biochim. Biophys. Acta *556*, 331-343.
33. Culp, L.A. (1978) Two functionally distinct pools of glycosaminoglycan in the substrate adhesion site of murine cells. J. Cell Biol. *79*, 788-801.
34. Yamada, K.M., Kennedy, D.W., Kimata, K. and Pratt, R.M. (1980) Characterization of fibronectin interactions with glycosaminoglycans and identification of active proteolytic fragments. J. Biol. Chem. *255*, 6055-6063.
35. Hascall, V.C. (1977) Interaction of cartilage proteoglycans with hyaluronic acid. J. Supramol. Str. *7*, 101-120.
36. Culp, L.A. and Bensusan, H.B. (1978) Search for collagen in the substrate adhesion site of two murine cell lines. Nature *273*, 680-682.
37. Letourneau, P.C. (1975) Cell-to-substratum adhesion and guidance of axonal elongation. Dev. Biol. *44*, 92-101.
38. Letourneau, P.C. (1979) Cell-substratum adhesion of neurite growth cones, and its role in neurite elongation. Exp. Cell Res. *124*, 127-138.
39. Culp, L.A., Ansbacher, R.A. and Domen, C. (1980) Adhesion sites of neural tumor cells: biochemical composition. Biochem. *19*, 5899-5907.
40. Domen, C. and Culp, L.A. (1981) Adhesion sites of neural tumor cells: morphogenesis of substratum-attached material. Exp. Cell Res. *134*, 329-338.

ACKNOWLEDGEMENTS

The author acknowledges support for these studies from American Cancer Society research grant BC217; National Institutes of Health research grants CA31513, CA27755, AM25646, and NS17139; and a Career Development Award from the NIH (KO4-CA70709).

IV

Emerging Technologies

Chapter 31

Synthesis, Characterization and Fabrication of High-Purity Biomedical Grade Silicone Rubbers

Henry M. Gajewski
Travenol Laboratories, Inc.
Corporate Materials Development
Route 120 & Wilson Road
P.O. Box 490
Round Lake, Illinois 60073

ABSTRACT

A historical perspective of silicone gum synthesis is explored to serve as a background in showing how silicone gums, high purity silica fillers and crosslinking agents are blended to prepare biomedical grade silicone rubber. Rubber fabrication techniques are presented appropriate for manufacturing medical devices from silicone rubber. Properties and applications of biomedical grade silicone rubber are examined.

SYNTHESIS

The evolution of silicone technology has its basis in the classical studies of F.S. Kipping in organosilicon chemistry [1]. During the period from 1899 to 1944, Kipping investigated the preparation and properties or organosilicon compounds and coined the word "silicone" to describe monomeric structures analogous to the ketones of organocarbon chemistry. Presently, "silicone" is the designation for polymeric siloxane products which include fluids, resins, and gums. These materials have in common a molecular structure consisting of alternate atoms of silicon and oxygen making up the "back-bone" of the polymers.

Silica is the basic raw material for the synthesis of silicones. It is reduced to the element silicon in an electric furnace in the presence of carbon.

$$SiO_2 + 2C \rightarrow Si + 2\,CO$$

The elemental silicon is then converted to chlorosilanes, the monomeric intermediates that are building blocks for the silicone polymers.

Various routes are commercially effectual for the manufacture of chlorosilanes. Three processes that had gained commercial importance are the "direct process," the "Gringard process," and the "olefin addition method" [2].

The "direct process" was discovered by Dr. E. G. Rochow of the General Electric Company [3]. In this process chlorosilanes are produced in a single stage by the reaction of silicon with an alkyl or aryl halide in the presence of a suitable catalyst. The primary aim of the direct process is to produce difunctional chlorosilanes which are required in the production of silicone polymers. Methyl chlorosilanes are produced in a "direct process" reaction by reacting silicon with methyl chloride in a reactor in the presence of a copper catalyst. The reaction is controlled within the temperature range 260°C-300°C and within the pressure range of 1-3 Kg/cm^2

$$2\,CH_3\,Cl + Si \xrightarrow[CAT]{*Cu} (CH_3)_2\,Si\,Cl_2$$

The "Gringard process" developed to full commercial scale by the Dow-Corning Corporation [4] is no longer used for the production of methyl chlorosilanes. Its main purpose is in the manufacture of chlorosilanes for which the direct process is not suitable.

The "olefin addition method" for producing chlorosilanes was used on a manufacturing scale in conjunction with the direct process by Union Carbide Corporation [5]. The method is limited to reactions where the olefin compounds are readily available and inexpensive.

The production of silicone gum is the basis for preparing silicone rubber. Silicone gums are produced by base-catalyzed (anionic) polymerization. When dimethyl dichlorosilane is hydrolyzed, a mixture of linear and cyclic siloxanes of relatively low molecular weight are formed. Upon separation, the cyclic siloxanes are polymerized to high molecular weight polymers by the catalytic action of potassium, sodium or triethylammonium silanolates.

$$(CH_3)_2\,Si\,Cl_2 + 2\,H_2O \rightarrow (CH_3)_2\,Si\,(OH)_2 + 2\,HCl$$

$$HO - \overset{CH_3}{\underset{CH_3}{\overset{|}{\underset{|}{Si}}}} - OH + HO - \overset{CH_3}{\underset{CH_3}{\overset{|}{\underset{|}{Si}}}} - OH + HO - \overset{CH_3}{\underset{CH_3}{\overset{|}{\underset{|}{Si}}}} - OH \rightarrow$$

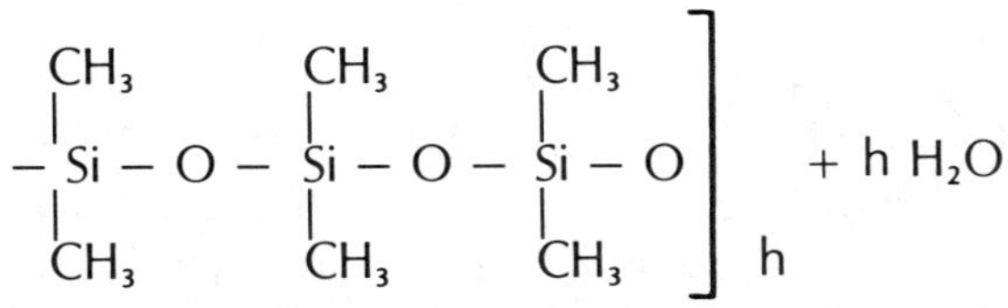

Polymerization is terminated by the addition of end block, mono functional trimethyl units.

To enhance vulcanization characteristics a small amount (less than one half of one percent) of the methyl groups ($-CH_3$) can be replaced by vinyl groups ($-CH = CH_2$).

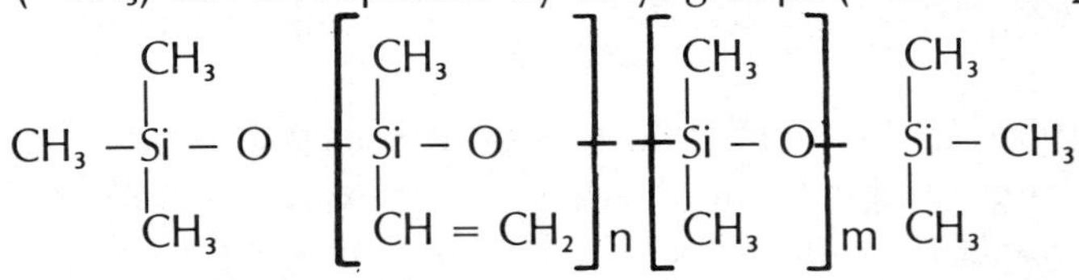

This results in a more efficient use of the vulcanization agents producing a cured rubber with better overall properties. Vinyl modified gums are available commercially and have become standard.

The excellent low temperature properties of the silicone rubbers can be further improved by the substitution of phenyl ($-C_6H_5$) groups for some of the methyl groups attached to the polymers chain.

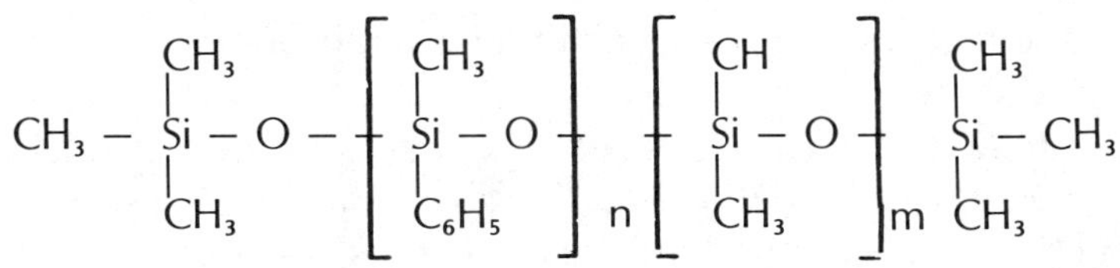

If 5 to 10% of the methyl groups are replaced it will lower the crystallization temperature flexibility to below −90°C.

To improve the solvent resistance of the silicone rubber, a more polar group such as trifluoropropyl ($-CH_2\,CH_2\,CF_3$) is substituted for one of the two methyl groups attached to the silicon atom.

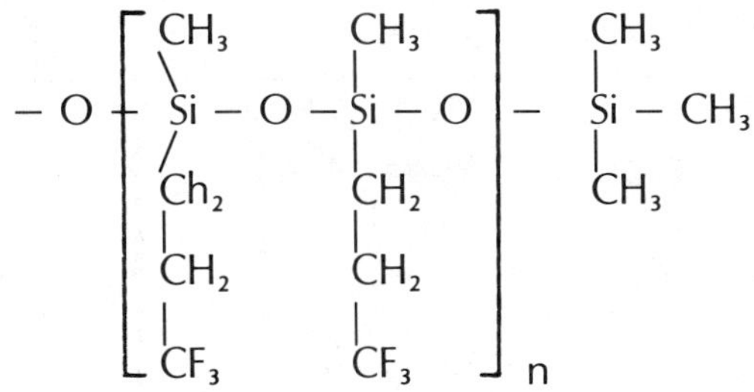

This class of silicones are known commercially as the fluorosilicones and are produced by Dow-Corning.

CHARACTERIZATION

Mechanical Properties

The term "silicone rubber" covers a range of materials with an equally broad range of properties. They are elastic thermosets which remain elastic over a temperature range of −75°C to 240°C. Physical properties are retained even after repeated steam auto-claving.

Hardness of rubber materials are measured by using an instrument that measures the resistance of the rubber to indentation of a ball-point. This instrument, the Shore durometer [6], gives a relative hardness reading on a scale of 0-100. Soft rubber materials are measured on the Shore A gauge. Silicone rubber can be compounded to have a hardness range of 25 Shore A (soft) to 90 Shore A (hard). Variations of hardness are obtained by increases in the amount of filler to silicone gum in the compound. No plasticizers or softeners are used.

Ultimate tensile strength is a measure of the stress required to cause the rubber to rupture in tension [7]. Silicone rubbers are compounded to have ultimate tensile strength in the range of 15-20 Kg/cm² to a high of 100-110 Kg/cm². In comparison to organic rubber the silicone rubber is generally of lower tensile strength, however their strength is retained over a wider temperature range.

Ultimate elongation is the percent stretch of the silicone rubber before it ruptures in tension. Elongation is measured in conjunction with tensile strength using a standard method for tension testing of vulcanized rubber. It is calculated by the equation:

$$\text{Elongation, percent} = \frac{S_B - S_o}{S_o} \times 100$$

where S_B = observed distance between bench marks of the stretched specimen at rupture, and S_o = the original distance between bench marks. Elongations of over a 700% can be obtained with silicone rubber.

One of the outstanding mechanical properties of silicone rubber is its resistance to *compression set.* Compression set is defined as the ability of a test specimen of the rubber to return to its original thickness after undergoing a compressive stress for a prescribed period of time. Under the specifications of the test, values of 7% to 10% for silicone rubber can be obtained.

A summary of physical properties at room temperature is shown in Table 1.

Table 1. Summary of Physical Properties of Silicone Rubber at Room Temperature

DUROMETER HARDNESS, SHORE A	25-90
TENSILE STRENGTH, Kg/CM^2	UP TO 110
ELONGATION, %	UP TO 700
TEAR RESISTANCE, Kg/CM	UP TO 45
COMPRESSION SET, %	DOWN TO 5

(Published couresty of General Electric Company, Silicone Product Division, Waterford, New York).

Thermal Properties

Silicone rubber can be compounded to operate at exceptional temperature extremes. Under normal operating conditions silicone rubber can retain useful physical properties at temperatures as high as 260°C and as low as −100°C. In comparing useful life at 200°C of silicone rubber to organic rubber, (Figure 1) it is readily apparent that silicone rubber far outperforms the organic rubber in spite of the fact that the organic rubber had superior tensile strength before aging.

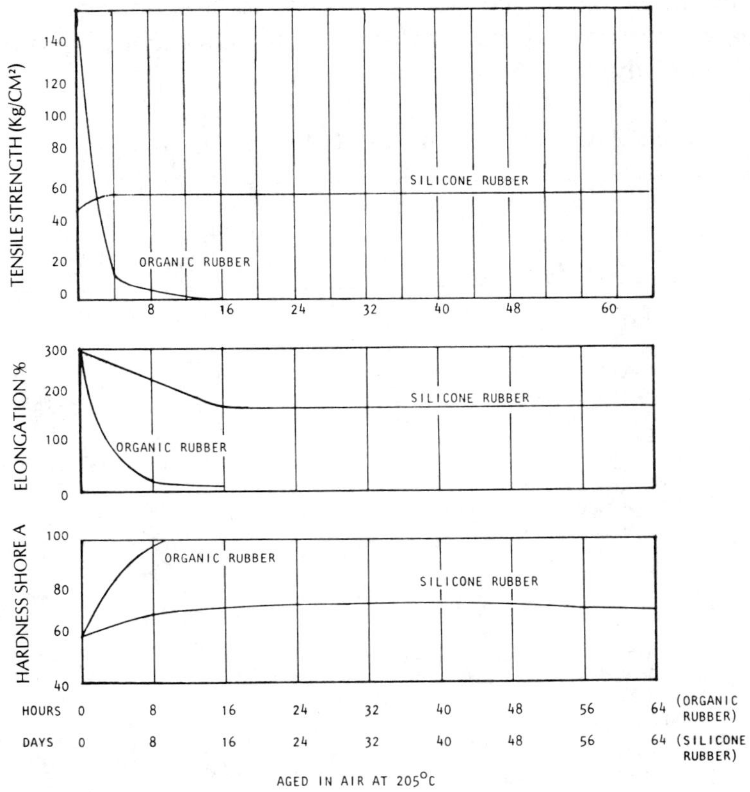

Figure 1. Effects of heat aging on a "heat resistant" organic rubber & a silicone rubber of identical initial hardness. (Published courtesy of General Electric Company, Silicone Products Division, Waterford, New York. Use of General Electric Company data in this article is for illustrative purposes only and does not constitute a recommendation to use General Electric Company silicone products.)

Flexibility at low temperatures can be enhanced by using silicone gums containing phenyl groups. Serviceability at temperatures of −85°C to −90°C with brittle points below −100°C silicone rubber greatly outperforms commonly used "low temperature" organic rubbers.

The thermal expansion coefficient of silicone is high:

$$\text{Volumetric expansion} = 6\text{-}8 \times 10^{-4}/°\text{C}$$

$$\text{Linear expansion} = 2\text{-}3 \times 10^{-4}/°\text{C}$$

The thermal conductivity of silicone rubber increases with filler loading and ranges from 0.3 to 0.5×10^{-3} gr-cal/sec/cm²/cm/°C.

Specific heat of silicone rubber varies from about 0.3 to 0.35 cal/gr./°C and goes down with filler loading.

Chemical Properties

The chemical resistance of silicone rubber is excellent for acqueous systems, i.e. acids, bases and salts with the possible exception of concentrated sulfuric acid and nitric acid. Data on weight change, volume change and hardness change (durometer) is shown in Table 2 after one week immersion of the test specimen at 25°C.

Table 2. Chemical Resistance of Methyl-Vinyl Silicone

Material	Weight Change %	Volume Change %	Durometer Change Points
ACIDS			
Nitric conc.	+10	+10	-30
Nitric 7%	< 1	< 1	-2
Sulfuric conc.		DISINTEGRATES	
Sulfuric 10%	< 1	< 1	-2
Acetic conc.	+2	+3	-4
Acetic 5%	+4	+4	-8
Hydrochloric conc.	+1	+1	-6
Hydrochloric 10%	+2	+4	-4
Hydrochloric 3%	< 1	+1	-2
BASES			
Sodium Hydroxide 20%	< 1	< 1	-2
Sodium Hydroxide 1%	< 1	< 1	-4
Ammonium Hydroxide conc.	+2	+2	-4
Ammonium Hydroxide 10%	+3	+2	-6
SALTS			
Sodium Chloride 10%	< 1	< 1	-2
Sodium Carbonate 2%	< 1	< 1	0
SOLVENTS			
Ethyl Alcohol	+5	+6	-10
Acetone	+5	+15	-15
Toluene	+75	+120	-30
Gasoline, Regular	+65	+130	-25
Gasoline, Aviation	+60	+110	-30
Mineral Spirits	+65	+110	-30
Carbon Tetrachloride	+130	+110	-25
OILS			
Caster Oil	< 1	< 1	-4
Lard Oil	< 1	< 1	-4
Linseed Oil	< 1	< 1	-2
Mineral Oil	+5	+6	-6
ASTM #1 Oil[2]	+3	+5	-6
ASTM #3 Oil[2]	+20	+31	-20
Silicone Oil SF96 (100)[2]	+25	-35	-25
Silicone Oil 42,000 cstk.[2]	+9	+10	-12
OTHER			
Water	< 1	< 1	< 1
Hydrogen Peroxide 3%	< 1	< 1	< 1
Pyranol 1476	+4	+4	-8

[2]70 hrs @ 150°C. (Courtesy of General Electric Co. Silicone Prod. Div.)

Silicone rubber has a high permeability to organic solvents. As a result the rubber absorbs solvents with a corresponding weight change and volume swell. If the solvent is allowed to evaporate, the silicone rubber retains its original shape with no apparent change in physical properties. This property of the silicones can be put to good use. Molded parts and extruded shapes of silicone rubber prepared for medical applications can be effectively cleaned prior to final packaging in a ultrasonic solvent bath. The swelling of the rubber in combination with the ultrasonic action helps sweep out residual catalyst and other contaminants that may have worked themselves into the bulk of the rubber during processing. It is important to note that silicone devices that have been bonded to a substrate or to itself cannot be cleaned in a solvent bath because the swell of the rubber will destroy the bond.

Gas sterilization with ethylene oxide has been successfully carried out on devices made from silicone rubber even those that have an adhesive bond.

Water and steam has very little effect on silicone. Autoclaving of silicone rubber medical devices is also a good means of sterilization.

Radiation Resistance

The radiation resistance of silicone rubber at normal temperatures is similar to that of many of the organic rubbers. Silicone rubber based on a methyl-vinyl retains usable physical properties when exposed to radiation in the range of 50 to 100 megarads. Silicone rubber based on gums containing phenyl groups can tolerate higher radiation (Table 3). The usual doses of radiation used in sterilization of medical devices 1-3 megarads, has little effect on the silicone rubber.

Table 3. Radiation Resistance-Silicone Rubber

	Methyl-Vinyl		Methyl-Phenyl-Vinyl	
Dosage (Rads)	Elongation (%)	Tensile Strength (Kg/cm^2)	Elongation (%)	Tensile Strength (Kg/cm^2)
None	200	84	600	84
5×10^6	130	70	450	77
5×10^7	50	63	225	63
1×10^8	20	42	75	60

(Courtesy of General Electric Co. Silicone Prod. Div.)

Permeability

At room temperature silicone rubber has a high permeability to gases (Table 4). This high permeability is applied in the design of membrane oxygenators and other gas separation devices.

Table 4. Permeability Rate for Silicone Rubber[1]

GAS	RATE	GAS	RATE
Carbon Dioxide	290	Carbon Disulfide	7500
Oxygen	55	Methane	80
Nitrogen	25	Ethane	210
Hydrogen	55	Ethylene	115
Helium	30	Propane	340
Carbon Monoxide	30	Butane	750
Hydrogen Sulfide	840	Formaldehyde	925
Nitrogen Dixoide	635	Carbon Tetra-chloride	5835
Sulfur Dioxide	1250	Air	26

[1] 10^{-9} CM^3 of gas (STP) that would permeate through 1 CM^2 of membrane 1 CM thick in 1 second at a pressure gradient across the membrane of 1 CM of Hg.
(Courtesy of General Electric Silicone Products Division, Waterford, N.Y.)

FABRICATION

Compounding

A biomedical grade silicone rubber compound is manufactured by blending a *silicone gum*, a *reinforcing filler*, a *processing aid* with a *peroxide curing agent*. Additives and color pigments are sometimes used for special purposes; generally the biomedical grade silicone vulcanizates are clear.

The *silicone gum* is a highly viscous material with a molecular weight of around 500,000. Before it is used in a medical grade formulation the silicone gum is subjected to a series of quality and safety tests, such as

1. **Infra-Red Scan** — The gum, as received from the vendor, is analyzed by infra-red spectroscopy in order to ascertain its identity. The infra-red scan must match that of a standard I.R. scan previously run for this gum.
2. **Heavy Metals Test** — A sample of the gum is chemically analyzed for "heavy metal" content and must pass a "less than -" specification.
3. **Contamination Test** — A sample of the gum is dissolved in an appropriate solvent filtered thru a 1.2 micron filter and observed for contaminants.
4. **Vacuum Volatiles** — The amount of volatile matter of a sample of the gum is measured after it is placed in a vacuum oven for 4 hrs. at 200°C. The percent volatiles must not exceed a specified amount.
5. **Biological Testing** — Depending on the intended application of the silicone several biological tests may be prescribed, however the bulk of the biological tests are carried out on the fully compounded vulcanizate.
6. **Average Molecular Weight** — The silicone gum must meet prescribed limits on specified, average molecular weight.

A silicone gum that meets the requirements of these tests is released for use in the blending process. It is important that good records be kept and traceability be established for not only the gum but all the ingredients of a formulation.

Fillers are used in silicone rubber to reinforce the silicone gum so that a vulcanizate with useful physical properties results. The fumed process silicas of extremely fine particle size (10-15 millimicrons) and high specific surface are very efficient reinforcing fillers for silicone gums. They have features which enhance their use in medical grade silicone rubber compounds. They are chemical inert toward the other rubber components, they are of high purity and are stable to the environmental conditions which the silicone rubber will encounter.

As with the silicone gum the filler is checked for quality prior to use in a medical grade silicone. Contamination, pH, bulk density and moisture content are some of the quality tests that are employed.

To improve the processing characteristics and to decrease the moisture absorption of the fumed silicas, they can be treated with a reactive silane. The silane replaces the hydrophilic hydroxyl groups on the silica with a hydrophobic methyl group. Particle size and specific surface area remains essentially unchanged. These treated silicas are commercially available and provide a viable alternative to the silicone rubber compounder.

When using highly reinforcing fillers in silicone rubber compounds it is desirable to use a *process aid.* A process aid has a softening effect on the unvulcanized compound and tends to retard its "structuring" or "crepe aging." This "crepe aging" is a phenomenon that occurs in unvulcanized silicone compounds due to the high reactivity of the silica filler with the silicone gum. The more common process aids are proprietary silicone fluids mixed with a silicone gum and/or silica filler.

The organic *peroxides* are the most commonly used *crosslinking or curing agents* used for silicone rubber. They are free-radical producing materials that at elevated temperatures initiate a chemical crosslinking of the rubber, resulting in a permanent elasticity. Table 5 describes some of the commercially available peroxides that are used in silicone rubber compounds. The primary consideration in the selection of a peroxide for a biomedical grade silicone rubber is active concentration, decomposition products and the volatility of the

Table 5. Commercially Available Peroxides for Vulcanizing Silicone Rubber

PEROXIDE	ACTIVE CONC.	PRIMARY DECOMPOSITION PRODUCTS	VOLATILITY OF DECOMP. PRODUCTS	GENERAL CURE TEMP (°C)	RECOMMENDED USE
Benzoyl Peroxide	99%	Benzene Benzoic acid Carbon dioxide	Volatile	115 - 137	For molding, solution coating, adhesive bonding
2,4-Dichloro-Benzoyl Peroxide	50%	2,4-Dichloro-Benzoic Acid 2,4-Dichloro Benzene	Fairly Volatile	105 - 121	For molding Cont. Hot Air Vulcan.
Tert-Butyl Perbenzoate	100%	Benzoic Acid Acetone Methane	Volatile	142 - 155	Sponge Rubber Vulcanization
Di-tert-Butyl Peroxide	Masterbatch in Silicone Gum	Acetone Methane	Volatile	170 - 182	For molding thick section, can only be used with vinyl containing gums
Dicumyl Peroxide	99%	α,α-Dimethyl Benzyl Alcohol Acetophenone	Fairly Volatile	160 - 170	For molding thick sections, can only be used with vinyl containing gums
2,5-Bis(tert-Butyl Peroxy) 2,5-Dimethyl Hexane	95%	Acetone, Methane 2,5 - Hexane Dione	Volatile	165 - 177	For molding, can only be used with vinyl containing gums.

decomposition products. The active concentration should be as close to the pure, 100% peroxide as possible to avoid the addition of carrier materials to the compound. If it is necessary to use a peroxide with a carrier, the use of a silicone gum master-batch or a silicone fluid as a carrier should be considered. Decomposition products and their volatility should be ascertained so that a proper post-cure schedule can be established. Solubility of the decomposition products would also help to design an effective solvent cleaning procedure.

The blending of a medical grade silicone requires a piece of equipment whose size and type depend on the quantity of rubber needed for a particular application. Equipment used for blending organic rubbers is also used for silicone rubber. The equipment most often used to blend small to medium quantities of silicone rubber i.e. 0.5 Kg to 25 kg is the two roll mill. The two-roll mill consists of two steel rolls which rotate in a direction opposite to each other. One roll positioned toward the work space rotates at a faster speed than does the other. Roll speed ratios of 1.2 to 1.4 with a speed of about 30M/min for the fast roll are suitable. The blending of the silicone rubber occurs at the space between the rolls (See Figure 2).

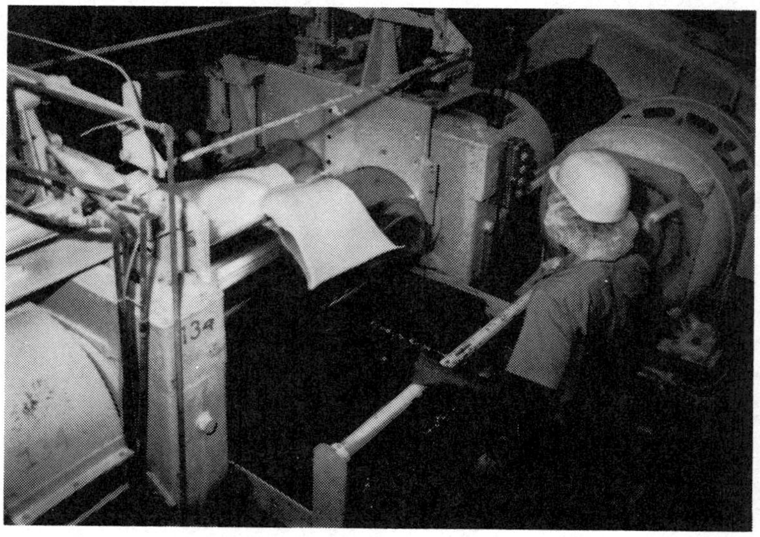

Figure 2. Two roll mill. Blending of silicone rubber on a two roll mill. The dispersion of ingredients takes place at the space between rolls. (Courtesy of Travenol Laboratories, Inc.).

The blending process begins by adding a preweighed amount of silicone gum to the mill and allowing it to spread on the rolls. The process aid is then added to the gum, if one is to be used. Incremental additions of filler are then made, allowing each addition to be thoroughly worked into the mix before the next is added. It is essential that a slow addition be adhered to, when using the reinforcing silica fillers to avoid filler-rich areas in the gum which are difficult to disperse. A scraper blade on the fast roll is essential to facilitate cross blending of the mix. Because of the heat generated during the milling operation, the rubber mix must first be cooled before the peroxide crosslinking agent is added to the mix to avoid partial prevulcanization. Two roll mills for rubber mixing are equipped with water cooled-rolls. The rubber mix temperature can be cooled to below 45°C by allowing cold water to circulate within the rolls. The crosslinking agent is then added across the band of rubber mix. Cross blending is exercised to assure good dispersion of the crosslinking agent.

Throughout the blending operation cleanliness is of utmost importance. Contamination, even by small amounts of organic materials can interfere with the cure of the rubber or effect the toxicity characteristics of the vulcanizate. It is essential that the milling operation for medical product applications be isolated from other plant operations. Mill operators should be garbed in lint-free suits and hair covers. When the catalyzed mix is stripped from the mill, the mix should be formed into a roll and covered tightly with a polyethylene film for storage. Although some compounds can be used immediately after mixing, certain properties of the vulcanizate can be enhanced by bin storage of 48 hours or longer before use.

For blending larger batches of silicone rubber, 25 Kg to seveal hundred Kg, the operation can be carried out in a dough mixer or a Banbury mixer. The addition of compounding ingredients is carried out in the same sequence as in the two roll mill operation. Mixing is very rapid but tends to cause a high heat build up of the rubber. If the mixer is equipped with cooling, crosslinking agent addition can be carried out in the mixer. Otherwise the final incorporation of the crosslinking agent is carried out on the cold rolls of a two roll mill. Each batch of silicone rubber must be clearly identified so that traceability of the raw materials going into the batch can be established. Although maximum quality control of ingredients in a medical grade silicone formulations is obtained by doing "in-house" blending, there may be occasion when control can be relinquished for convenience.

In many non-critical applications a compounder may choose to purchase gums that have been previously reinforced with filler and processing aids by the vendor. These so called R-gums allow for the use of a base material for several compounds of various hardnesses. The compounder would need only to add filler to increase hardness. The R-gums can also be chosen for special purposes such as low compression set, long term high temperature stability, low temperature flexibility or high strength.

Since the R-gum represents a mixture of at least two and usually more ingredients and since they are proprietary formulations held trade secrets by the vendor very little control of what goes into the R-gum is available to the compounder.

A more extreme position in relinquishing control of medical grade silicone is the use of commercially available compounds which come from the vendor ready to use. They are usually compounded by the vendor to a specified set of physical properties (hardness, tensile strength, elongation, etc.) and can be received catalyzed with the proper amount of peroxide catalyst.

The decision as to which route to establish for a particular application (1) complete "in-house" blending, (2) R-gum blending (3) commercial compounds, depends on several factors. The extent of government regulatory control inherent to a particular product, the need for unique properties unavailable in commercial compounds, the criticality of the application, i.e. a silicone gasket or silicone flow valve versus a silicone implant and not least of all the economic impact on the product of the cost of compounding are all considerations which must be analyzed prior to making a decision. Each approach may have its place in manufacturing medical products from silicone rubber.

Prior to use in a production process the silicone rubber compound is evaluated for its rheology properties. This gives one information on the vulcanization rate and completeness of cure of the compound.

There are several instruments on the market that measure the vulcanization rate of the silicone rubber. The oscillating disk rheometer [8] provides a continuous measurement of the

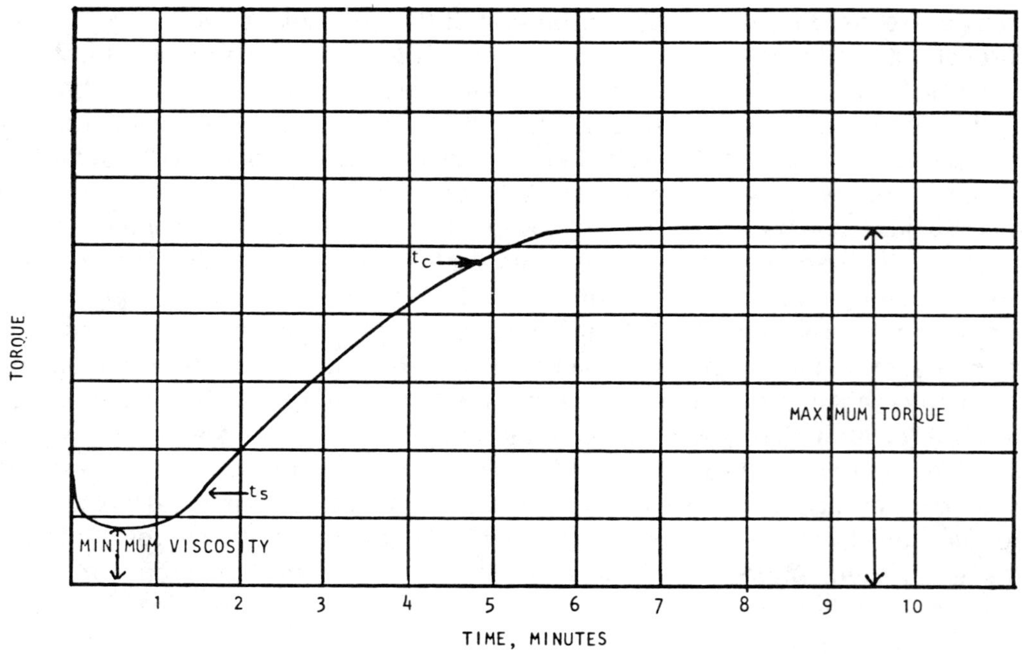

MINIMUM VISCOSITY May be considered a measure of "Mooney Viscosity" i.e. the relative ease at which a rubber will flow in a mold or through an extruder at the test temperature.

t_s - Time to incipient cure, is a measure of processing safety at the test temperature.

t_c - Time to attain 90% of final cure.

MAXIMUM TORQUE - A measure of the shear modulus or stiffness of the fully cure vulcanizate. An increase in Max. torque results in an increase in durometer, modulus and a decrease in elongation.

Figure 3. Typical rheometer curve.

change in torque vs time for a test specimen undergoing a shear force brought about by the oscillation of a disc into which it is inbedded (Figure 3). The torque is directly proportional to the stiffness (shear modulus) of the specimen. Therefore at a particular test temperature as the modulus increases with vulcanization, the curve generated describes the entire curing cycle of the specimen. In this way one can determine batch-to-batch variation, proper catalyst level in the batch, effect of moisture in the filler on cure and make gross prediction of physical properties of the mixed batch.

In addition to its rheology properties the cured silicone rubber is subjected to biological and chemical assays to establish its safety in use. The tests that a particular silicone rubber compound will undergo will depend on the extent to which the rubber comes into human contact during use. Biological assays consist of:

1) Tissue culture assays [9]
2) Systemic injection and intracutaneous reactivity (Extract) [10]
3) Implant assay [10]

In conjunction with the biological assays, chemical assays are designed to indicate the potential extraction profile of both organic and inorganic leachables. The silicone is extraced with water at a fixed surface to volume ratio at elevated temperature. The extract is assayed against a negative control.

MOLDING OF HEAT VULCANIZING SILICONE RUBBER

The standard methods used throughout the rubber industry can be used to mold silicone rubber. The method chosen for a particular application will depend on such factors as: size of the part to be molded, number of parts needed, complexity of the parts, the need for an isolated operation and the economic factors associated with relative tool and machine costs.

Freshening the silicone rubber compound that has been stored, requires a remilling operation prior to molding or other fabrication process. The remilling or "freshening" breaks up a "crepe-aged" compound and softens it to the point where it will flow easily during molding or extrusion. The rubber is placed on a cold two-roll mill and cross blended several times to the desired consistency. The freshened stock may also require a "screening" operation. Here the rubber is extruded through a series of stainless steel screens of various mesh sizes to remove undispersed filler lumps or other contaminants.

Compression moldings is by far the most popular method overall, for molding rubber. In this method the silicone rubber is pre-weighed or preformed to the appropriate size, placed in an open heated mold, the mold is closed and placed in the compression molding press where it is held at a pre-set temperature and time. Upon completion of the cycle the mold is opened, the part is removed, the mold is cleaned of any remaining molding flash, in preparation for the next cycle. The molds are relatively simple two or three part steel molds, preferably chrome plated. Compression molding presses consist of two or more heated platens that are hydraulically actuated to close on the heated mold. In the compression molding process pressures of 56 Kg/cm^2 to 140 Kg/cm^2 and temperatures of 95°C to 190°C are used.

Time and temperature of cure are determined by the choice of peroxide curing agent and the geometry of the part to be molded. Mold release agents should be avoided. If it is absolutely imperative to use a mold release, a dilute water solution (0.5%) of a detergent can be brushed or sprayed on the mold. Parts that have release agent must be washed thoroughly before any post-molding operation.

Transfer molding of a silicone rubber can result in faster cycles than compression molding because generally preparation of the rubber for molding is simpler. Whereas in compression molding when using a multicavity mold, each cavity must be filled individually with a preweighed or preformed "shot," with transfer molding a single preform is all that is required. That is because the transfer mold, in addition to the two or more plates that define the geometry of the part, has a "transfer pot" that is connected by means of a sprue to each individual cavity. The material preform in the pot is transferred to the cavities of the mold through these individual sprues by a piston that can either be part of the mold or part of the press. Presses designed for transfer molding have double rams or pistons, one to clamp the mold in the press, the other to transfer the material into the mold cavities in a two stage operation. Upon curing, the part of the preform not used to fill the mold can be easily stripped from the pot with attached sprues, leaving the parts clean at the gate.

Pressures and temperatures appropriate for transfer molding are similar to those used for compression molding.

When high volume production and complex parts are required, *injection molding* can well be the molding method of choice. Because silicone rubber has good flow characteristic and can be quickly cured at high temperatures, it is a material well suited for the injection molding process. The injection molding press has an injection cylinder with a reciprocating screw or a ram-type piston that injects the silicone material into the mold cavities at very high pressures (500 to 1500 Kg/cm²). Injection times are approximately 5 to 10 seconds and mold temperatures are relatively high at 200-200°C. As a result vulcanization takes place very quickly resulting in mold cycles in the range to 30 to 90 seconds (Figure 4 and 5).

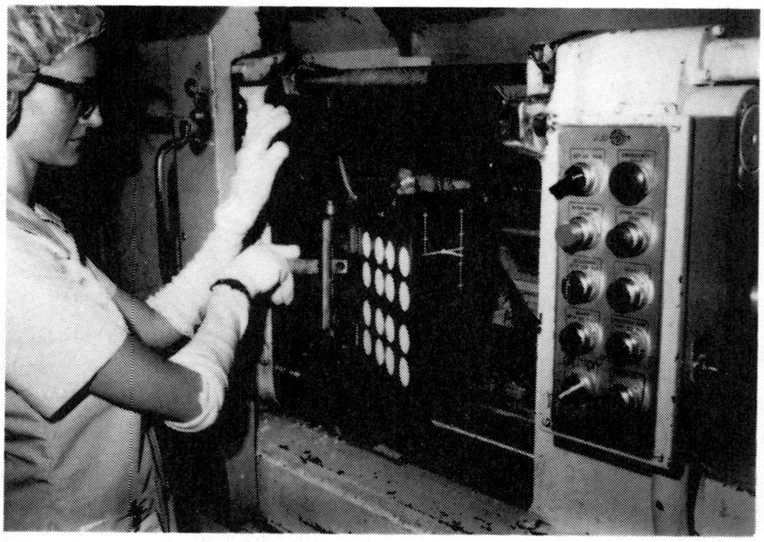

Figure 4. Injection molding of silicone rubber, showing runner system and sixteen cavity mold for molding silicone rubber discs. (Courtesy of Travenol Laboratories, Inc.).

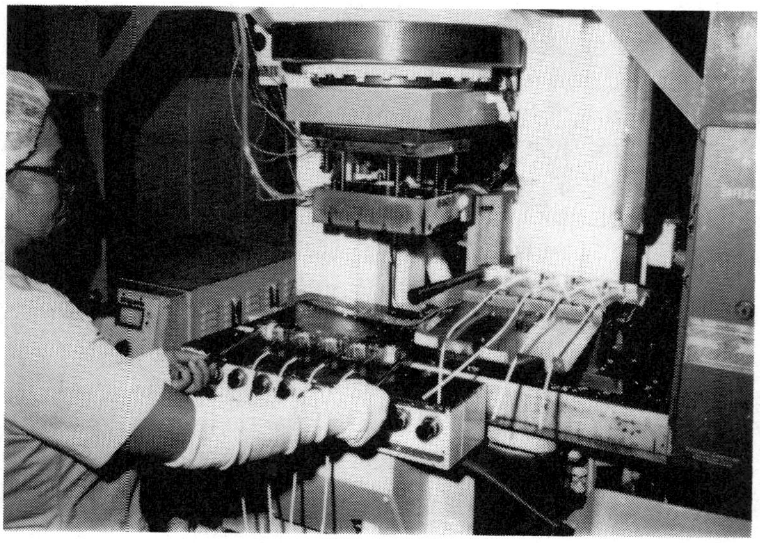

Figure 5. Injection molding silicone rubber catheters on a vertical injection press using a shuttle system to facilitate loading and unloading of cavities. (Courtesy of Travenol Laboratories, Inc.).

In all molding operations special care must be exercised to avoid contamination. Filtered air and positive pressure rooms are required for the molding area. A mold station clean up every shift and two hour quality control checks are common procedures that are followed. Parts that are removed from the mold are kept in covered containers and are transported to and from work stations in this manner.

All molded parts for medical applications benefit from an *oven post-cure*. This involves placing the molded part into a recirculating oven at a temperature and time dependent on the properties needed for the intended application. Oven post curing removes residual peroxide catalyst and other volatile materials from the rubber. What remains is a very pure vulcanized gum reinforced with a high purity silica filler. This fact, in addition to the inertness of the siloxane "backbone" of the polymer is what makes silicone rubber unique as a material for biomedical applications.

Generally silicone rubber in biomedical applications is not required to perform at elevated temperatures. Steam sterilization temperatures are usually the upper limit in thermal requirements. Therefore, the time and temperature of an oven post-cure should be chosen for the purpose of volatilizing the residual catalyst. It can be as short as 1-2 hours at 150°C to as long as 16-24 hours at 200°C, and depends on the type and the amount of catalyst used in the compound. A silicone rubber compounder should be familiar with the kinds of breakdown products associated with the catalysts available for curing the rubber and the difficulty of removing them in an oven post-cure.

Most oven suppliers can supply equipment that can meet the proper rquirements for post-curing silicone rubber.

It must be emphasized that proper post-curing is very important in the manufacture of biomedical grade silicone rubber. In some cases it can mean the difference between success and failure of the silicone rubber in an application. In Table 6 the results of a tissue culture toxicity test indicates that a silicone rubber that is not properly post-cured will elicit a "fail" tissue culture response due to the presence of residual crosslinking peroxide catalyst.

Table 6. The Effect of Post-Cure of Silicone Rubber on Toxicity Response in Tissue Culture

SAMPLE	POST CURE	SOLVENT CLEAN	TISSUE CULTURE RESPONSE
3-20-21-5 LOT RL-12-16-9A1	NONE	NONE	FAIL
3-20-21-5 LOT RL-12-16-9A1	NONE	YES	FAIL
3-20-21-5 LOT RL-12-16-9A1	YES	NO	PASS
5 MO 462 LOT L02A3	YES	YES	PASS

(Courtesy of Travenol Laboratories, unpublished data)

EXTRUSION OF HEAT VULCANIZING SILICONE RUBBER

The extrusion process is a fabricating technique which forms tubing, rod, "U" channels and other profiles. The extruder, by means of a rotating screw forces silicone rubber along the barrel and through a die which forms the uncured rubber into a continuous length of the desired shape.

The extrusion of silicone rubber although carried out on equipment similar to that used for organic rubber has some important differences.

As it leaves the extruder the silicone rubber is still in an uncured state, since the process is carried out at room temperature, i.e. the extruder barrel is not heated as is generally the case when extruding organic rubber. Following extrusion the extrudate is immediately vulcanized by feeding it into a heated tunnel, on a stainless steel endless conveyor belt (Figure 6). The heated air in the tunnel vulcanizes the extrudate as it passes along the tunnel length of roughly 8 meters. This process called hot air vulcanization (HAV) is carried out at temperatures of 400°C to 550°C at speeds of 4-6 meters per minute. Most HAV units are placed tandem to the extruder in a horizontal posture. It was found that a vertical design HAV unit has certain processing advantages. Tubing that requires a close tolerance on wall thickness, or soft stocks that deform by the conveyor belt of the horizontal unit can be more successfully processed on a HAV unit of vertical design. The die can be positioned so that the extrudate leaves the extruder travelling upward into the vertical HAV. The die can be positioned so that the extrudate leaves the extruder travelling upward into the vertical HAV (Figure 7).

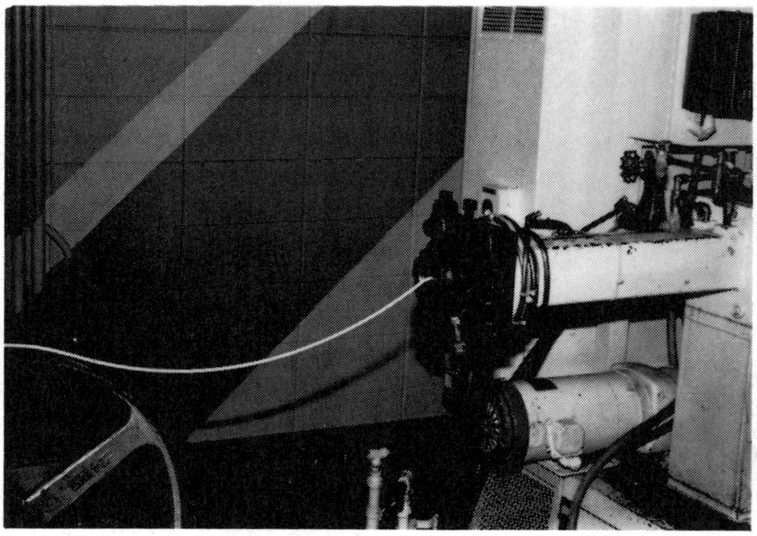

Figure 6. Extrusion of silicone rubber. The silicone rubber extrudate leaves the die of the extruder and is carred to the hot air vulcanizing tunnel on the endless stainless steel belt to be vulcanized. (Courtesy of Travenol Laboratories, Inc.).

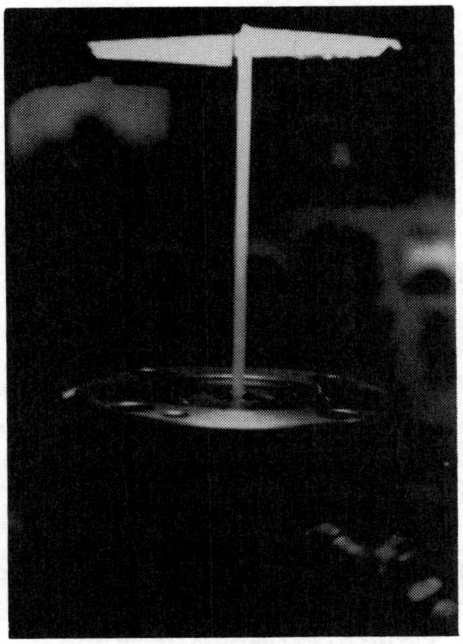

Figure 7. Silicone rubber extrusion into a vertical hot air vulcanizing unit. Using a vertical HAV assures very close tolerances on tubing wall dimensions and tubing concentricity. (Courtesy SIL-MED Corp.).

The only curing agent recommended for hot air vulcanization of silicone rubber is 2,4-dichlorobenzoyl peroxide. The high temperature of the HAV unit causes rapid volatilization of the other peroxide crosslinking agents resulting either in porous or uncured extrudates.

Oven post-curing of extruded silicone rubber is required just as is the case with molded silicone. The continuous length of extrudate is wound on a curing drum, well perforated to allow maximum air access. No more than two or three layers of extrudate are wound on the drum so that complete volatilization of curing agent residual is assured. To prevent staining of the non-post cured silicone rubber, handling of the rubber should be done by workers wearing lint-free cotton gloves and should be kept to a minimum.

Post-cured extruded material that is to be used in subsequent operations is transferred to work stations in covered tote containers correctly identified with batch number, specification number and quality control status.

Cleaning

Silicone rubber parts that have been oven post-cured are subjected to a cleaning procedure. The cleaning procedure is designed with several factors considered; the type of contamination to be removed, the type of device, extent of human contact and whether the device assembly with adhesivie bonds could tolerate a solvent cleaning. If the parts are to be assembled into a device that would make cleaning difficult, the parts are cleaned prior to assembly otherwise the cleaning process is scheduled right before final packaging.

An acqueous cleaning process is very effective in reducing particulate matter that adheres tenaciously to silicone parts. It is used on devices that are adhesive bonded in the assembly process. As an example of such a procedure the following steps are outlined:

1. Load parts into open mesh, nylon laundry bags, ½ full to allow for good agitation.
2.Place in automatic washer using alkali detergent and tap water at 66-77°C.
3. Wash fifteen minutes.
4. Drain and extract (spin) one minute.
5. Rinse with distilled water three minutes.
6. Drain and extract (spin) one minute.
7. Rinse with distilled water three minutes.
8. Drain and extract five minutes. The parts then are placed on cleaned stainless steel trays and dried and cooled under a laminar flow hood. Cleaned and dried parts are placed into clean polyethylene bags and sealed for transfer to the next operation.

Silicone devices that are to be implanted i.e. A.V. shunts, Cannula, catheters are very efficiently cleaned in an ultrasonic solvent cleaning system. Commercial equipment is available that use a series of baths in an ultrasonic environment to clean, rise and dry parts on a continuous basis.

Clean parts and assemblies are placed in the final package as soon as possible after cleaning ready for sterilization.

BONDING OF SILICONE RUBBER

Silicone rubber, molded or extruded into a particular shape assembled into a biomedical device may require the bonding of the silicone rubber to other parts of the device. Silicone rubber can be bonded to itself, to some plastics, to metal, to cloth fabrics and other rubbers.

When bonding vulcanized silicone rubber to a substrate it is essential that the parts to be joined are cleaned prior to bonding. Two methods of bonding may be used:

> (1) A thin layer of unvulcanized silicone can be applied to the substrate. The vulcanized silicone is then placed on the coated substrate and heat and pressure is applied to form the bond. For substrates other than silicone itself, a primer must first be applied to the substrate to assure a good bond. Silicone rubber vendors can supply both information and proprietary primers for bonding silicone to various substrates.
> (2) Bonding can also be accomplished by using a room temperature vulcanizing (RTV) silicone rubber adhesive. To bond cured silicone rubber to itself the use of RTV adhesives is a convenient method to form very strong bonds.

The RTV silicone adhesives are one component solventless pastes that vulcanize by being exposed to atmospheric moisture. The one component silicone adhesive contains a reactive functional group terminating the polymer chain. This end group reacts with moisture as follows:

$$-\overset{|}{\underset{|}{Si}}-O-\overset{O}{\overset{\|}{C}}-CH_3 + H_2O \rightarrow -\overset{|}{\underset{|}{Si}}-OH + HO-\overset{O}{\overset{\|}{C}}-CH_3$$

$$-\overset{|}{\underset{|}{Si}}-OH + CH_3-\overset{O}{\overset{\|}{C}}-O-\overset{|}{\underset{|}{Si}}- \rightarrow -\overset{|}{\underset{|}{Si}}-O-\overset{|}{\underset{|}{Si}} + CH_3-\overset{O}{\overset{\|}{C}}-OH$$

The acyloxy silicone hydrolyzes upon exposure to moisture, giving silanols which may then further polymerize. The carboxylic acid liberated serves as a catalyst. This type of cure is diffusion limited and required a 24 hour cure to develop mechanical strength and a full seven days to develop maximum strength.

An interesting example of the use of RTV silicone adhesives can be found in the assembly procedure used in the manufacture of a silicone Foley Catheter [11] (Figure 8). This involves the RTV bonding of the catheter tip, that is injection molded with a thin-wall section or "skirt" integral to the tip, to an extruded shaft of the catheter. In step one a PVC shrink band is placed

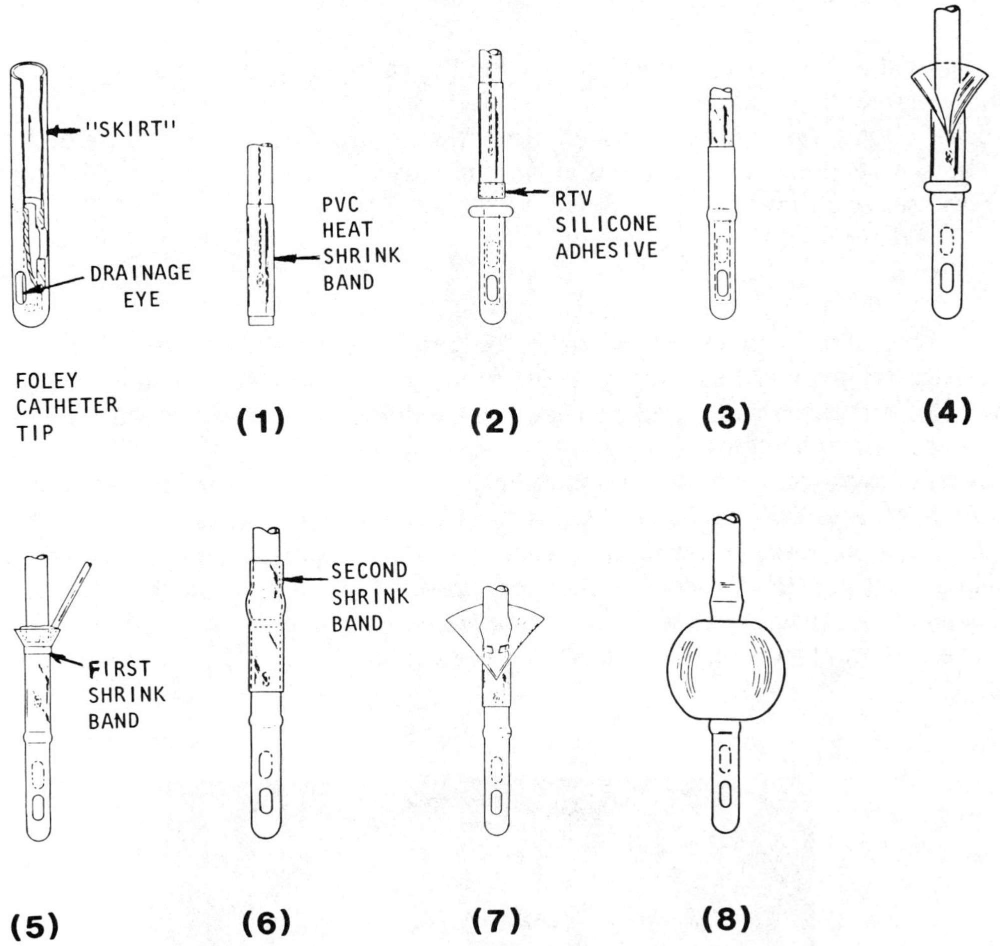

Figure 8. Bonding of Foley Catheter Tip to the shaft. (1) PVC heat shrink band placed on shaft. (2) RTV silicone adhesive applied to shaft. (3) Shaft inserted into tip, "skirt" of tip rolled back. (4) After adhesive is allowed to cure, shrink band removed. (5) Shrink band placed over "skirt," 3mm from end, RTV adhesive applied between "skirt" and shaft. (6) Second shrink band placed over bond and heat shrunk in place to form smooth juncture. (7) After cure of adhesive, shrink bands removed. (8) Adhesive bonded tip inflated.

on the shaft approximately 3 mm from the end to be bonded. The RTV adhesive is applied to the shaft at this end. The "skirt" of the tip is rolled back to prevent the "wet" (i.e. uncured) RTV adhesive to transfer to the "skirt" as the adhesive-laden shaft is inserted into the tip. The "skirt" is rolled back onto the shaft and the bonding junction is allowed to cure overnight. The cure can be accelerated by subjecting the bond to temperatures in the range of 20°C-50°C and relative humidity of 30 to 70%. The PVC shrink band is then stripped off the shaft and a smaller PVC band is applied over the skirt, distal to the first bonding junction and approximately 3 mm from the end. RTV adhesive is then applied around the shaft between the "skirt" of the tip and the shaft. A second heat shrink PVC band is then placed over the junction. Heat is then applied to the area of the junction to shrink the band and form a snug fit around the shaft and a generally smooth gradual taper of the excess adhesive. The adhesive is then allowed to cure.

Upon curing the shrink bands are removed and the catheter is now capable of being inflated to form the retention balloon.

Excellent bonds result from the use of the RTV silicone adhesives. In the case of the silicone Foley, burst tests performed on the bonded balloons shows a rupture of the balloon occurs before the silicone bond breaks.

Applications

Shortly after their introduction as commercial products in the mid-1940's silicones were being investigated for their toxicological properties [12,13]. These studies reported no harmful effects on laboratory animals and signaled the experimental use of silicone rubber in many diverse medical applications.

Extruded tubings is an important commercial medical application of silicone rubber. Clear and non-reactive to body tissue and fluids the silicone rubber tubing is available for clinical and laboratory purposes in size ranging from less than 1 millimeter internal diameter to over 10 millimeters (Figure 9). A silicone rubber compounded for medical applications and properly oven-post-cured is made up essentially of crosslinked silicone gum reinforced with high purity silica. There are no leachable plasticizers and the silicone rubber will not support bacterial or fungal growth.

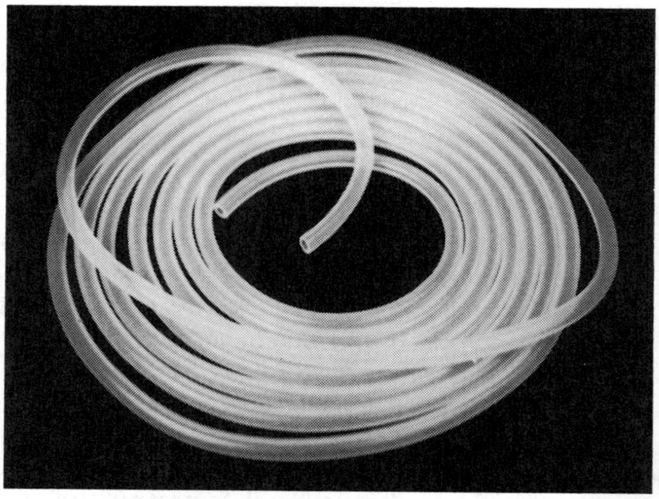

Figure 9. Medical grade silicone rubber tubing properly extruded and post-cured results in a stable inert polymer that exhibits a low order of physiological response and toxicity.

Multi-lumen tubing has found use as the insulating jacket over the wire leads used in the electronic, heart pacemakers (Figure 10). Life saving electronic impulses to make the heart operate are conducted along these leads insulated and protected from the body fluids by the silicone rubber tubing.

Silicone rubber tubing is used as a thoracic drain, abdominal drain and kidney drain. Frequently these tubes are made radiopaque by blending a radiopaque filler such as barium sulfate into the silicone rubber compound (Figure 11).

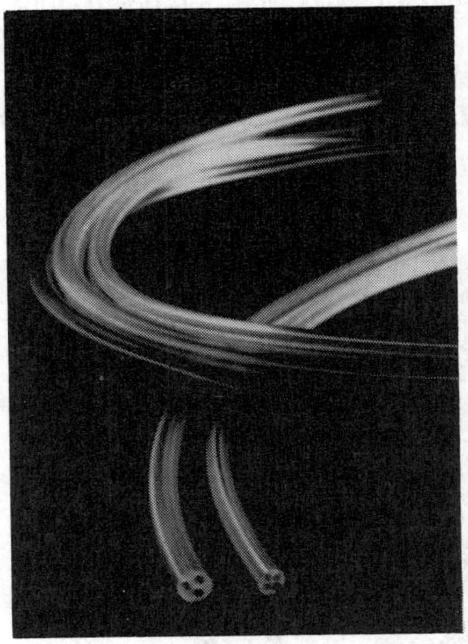

Figure 10. Multi-lumen silicone rubber tubing for pacemaker leads. (Courtesy of SIL-MED Corp., Taunton, Mass.).

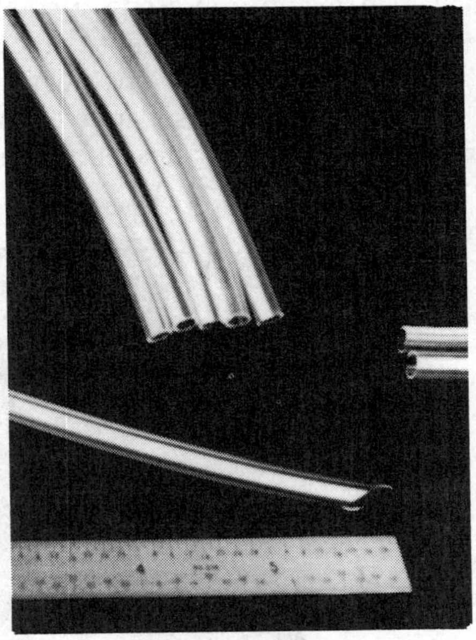

Figure 11. Silicone rubber drain tube with radio-paque stripe formed as an integral part of the tubing wall by a coextrusion process. (Courtesy of SIL-MED Corp.)

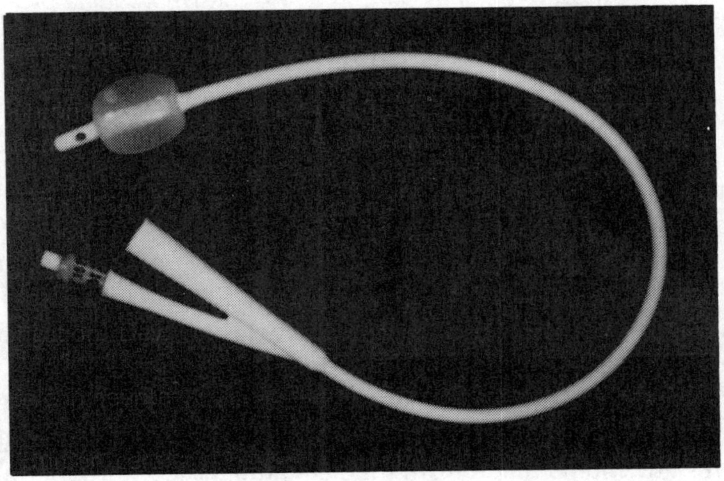

Figure 12. 100% silicone rubber foley catheter used for urinary drainage. (Courtesy of Travenol Laboratories, Inc.).

The silicone Foley catheter (Figure 12) has found increased use as a urinary drain. Clinical studies have shown significantly less tissue reaction, less encrustation of the catheter with insoluble calcification deposits and greater flow rates through the increased size drainage lumen. Silicone Foley catheters are prescribed for long term users of indwelling, urinary retention catheters because they need not be changed as often.

Their manufacture represents a combination of several fabrication methods (Figure 13). The double lumen shaft or drainage tube is formed by the extrusion process. It is then cut to length and used as the insert on to which the "Y" end of the catheter is injection molded. The tip is injection molded in a separate operation and is attached to the shaft by means of an RTV adhesive bonding process described previously (see bonding).

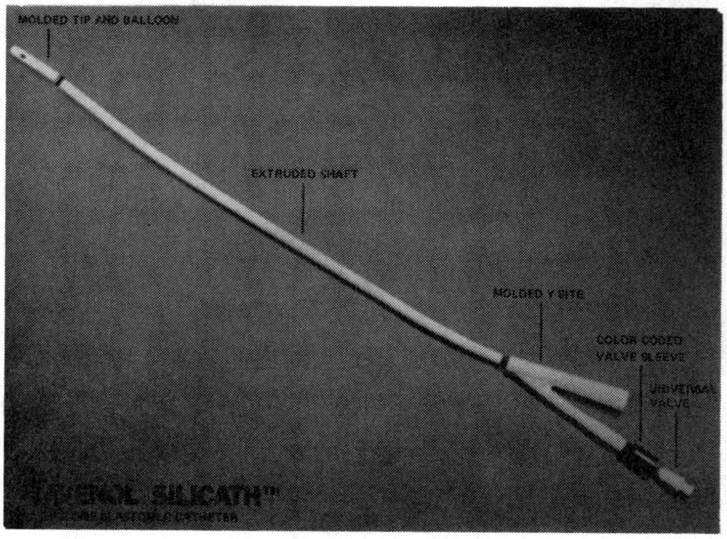

Figure 13. Fabrication of silicone Foley catheter involves an extrusion process to obtain the shaft, an injection molding process to form the tip and "skirt," a RTV adhesive bonding process to adhere the tip to the shaft, an insert injection molding process to mold the "Y" site directly to the shaft. Inflation valve and valve sleeve assembly complete the fabrication. (Courtesy of Travenol Laboratories, Inc.).

Silicone rubber catheters are used for infusion of I.V. solutions required for parenteral nutrition. They allow longer venous tolerance and decrease the incidence of complications such as phlebitis [14]. The reduced thrombogenicity of silicone elastomer suggest that it is preferred to other materials for use as central venous catheters [15]. These catheters, intended for long-term parenteral nutrition are introduced into the subclavian vein and require a radiopaque silicone compound material (Figure 14) to facilitate introduction.

Hemodialysis for patients with chronic kidney failure requires a permanent means of cannulation. Two or three times a week these patients must be connected to the artificial kidney machine. Arterio-venous shunts made from medical grade silicone rubber are implanted into the arm or leg of a patient for quick access to the circulatory system (Figure 15). These shunts are made from extruded tubing compression molded into shape. A polytetrafluroethylene (TFE) tip is bonded to the silicone using a RTV adhesive. To enhance the bond the TFE is first treated (sodium etch) at the surface to be bonded.

The use of A.V. shunts for hemo-dialysis has diminished considerably in recent years because of patency problem associated with thrombus formation. Attempts were made to alleviate these problems with shunt designs which incorporate a non-thrombogenic coating on the I.D. of the shunt tube.

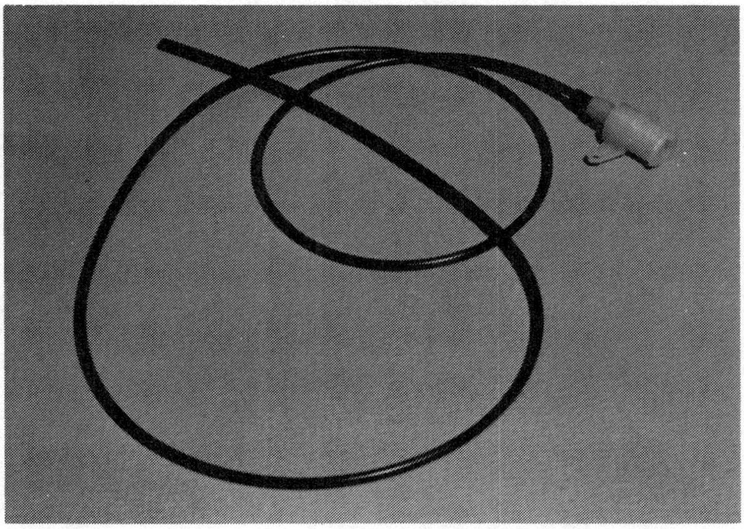

Figure 14. Central venous catheter made from radiopaque silicone rubber. Used for long term parenteral nutrition. (Courtesy Travenol Laboratories, Inc.).

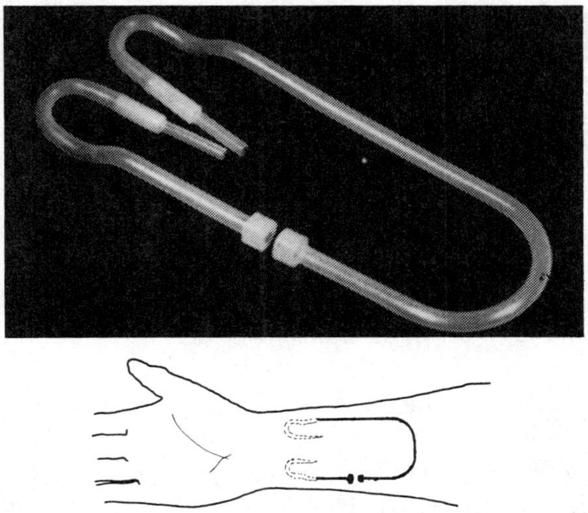

Figure 15. Arterio-venous shunts made from medical grade silicone rubber. Polytetrafluroethylene (TFE) tip is RTV adhesive bonded to the silicone shunt. The A.V. shunt is implanted as shown above to gain access to the circulatory system.

Silicone rubber molded balls and discs are used in heart valves to replace malfunctioning, diseased heart valves (Figure 16). Special care is required to oven post-cure the silicone rubber properly to assure a complete cure of the interior of the ball. It has been demonstrated that if this is not the case absorption of body lipids may occur.

The permeability characteristics of silicone rubber led to the successful use of silicone rubber membranes in blood oxygenators. Membrane oxygenators are used during open heart surgery to supply pulmonary function to the patient.

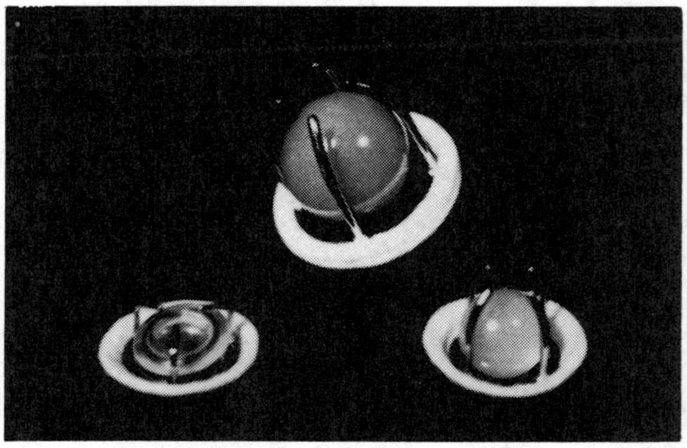

Figure 16. Artificial heart valves. Molded silicone rubber ball used in both large mitral valve and aortic valve. Silicone rubber disc used in alternate aortic valve design.

The oxygenator consists of a series of thin channels through which blood flows on one side of a silicone rubber membrane approximately 1 mm thick. On the other side of the membrane through similar thin channels oxygen or air flows counter current to the blood. Because of the gas concentration gradient across the membrane, the carbon dioxide in the blood diffuses through the membrane into the air flow. The oxygen diffuses through the membrane to oxygenate the blood. Because there is no blood/gas interface, denaturation of blood protein is reduced, platelet function is preserved and there is no increase in particulate microemboli.

Silicone rubber is used with dramatic results in reconstructive surgery. Implants of silicone rubber have been used to augment disfigured facial features. Finger joints made of silicone rubber have restored near normal function to hands disfigured by the crippling effect of arthritis.

For over ten years silicone rubber mammary prosthesis have been used to reconstruct the breast of women who have undergone radical mastectomy due to cancer. There are several designs of mammary implants. One design consists of a thin envelope of silicone rubber filled with a clear silicone gel that is unvulcanized. The filling aperture is then sealed with a silicone adhesive and the gel is then vulcanized by oven heating the implant. The gel upon vulcanization obtains the same general weight and texture as breast tissue.

Uses for silicone rubber in biomedical applications are continually being found. They have attained a reputation as bio-compatible materials through successful use for the past thirty years in a variety of applications. It is estimated that the market for medical silicones will continue to grow at an average annual rate of at least 20%.

REFERENCES

1. Kipping, F. S. Proc. Roy. Soc. (1937) A 159, 139.
2. Fordham, S., Chap. 2, "The Chemistry of Organosilicon Comounds," Silicones New York, Philosophical Library, Inc. 1961.
3. U.S Patent 2,380,995, 1945 (General Electric Co.).
4. McGregor, R. R. "Silicones & Their Uses," New York, McGraw-Hill, 1954.
5. Weaver, D. G. and O'Connors, R. J. Ind. Eng. Chem. (1958) 50, 132.

6. Standard Test Method for Rubber Property – Durometer Hardness. ANSI/ASTM D2240-75. In: 1980 Annual Book of ASTM Standards Part 35. Phildelphia, PA. American Society for Testing and Materials, 1980 pp. 702-705.
7. Standard Test Method for Rubber Properties in Tension. ANSI/ASTM D412-75. in: 1980 Annual Book of ASTM Standards Part 35. Philadelphia, PA. American Society of Testing and Materials, 1980 pp. 148-161.
8. Standard Test Methods for Rubber Property – Vulcanization Characteristics using Oscillating Disk Cure Meter. ASTM D-2084-75. In: 1980 Annual Book of ASTM Standards Part 37, Philadelphia, PA. American Society for Testing and Materials, 1980.
9. Johnson, H., Nortup, S., Seagraves, P., and Thomas, J., "Development of Test Procedures for the Evaluation of Implantable Biomedical Materials *In Vitro,*" U.S. Dept. HEW, Food and Drug Administration, Contract 223-75-5013 (BML), Final Technical Report, Feb. 1978.
10. "Biological tests – plastics" *The United States Pharmacopeia* XX U.S. Pharmacopeial Convention, Rockville, MD, 1980, pp.950-953.
11. U.S. Patent 3,832,253, 1974 (Baxter-Travenol, Inc.).
12. Rowe, V. K., Spencer, H. C. and Bass, S. L. Jour. Ind. Hyg. Tox (1948) 30, 332.
13. Rowe, V. K., Spencer, H. C. and Bass, S. L. Arch. Ind. Hyg. Occ. Med. (1950) 1, 539.
14. Schneider, J. M. "Intravenous Catherization, Traditional Difficulties and a Revolutionary New Technique," Hospital Care, October, 1971.
15. Hoshal, V. L., Dennis, P. R. and Marcus, M. "Experiences with Peripheral and Central Venous Silicone Elastomer Catheters. Scientific Exhibit, American College of Surgeons, 59th Annual Clinical Congress. Chicago, Illinois, October 15, 1973.

Chapter 32

Silicones in Biomedical Applications

Barry Arkles and Peter Redinger
Petrarch Systems, Inc.
2731 Bartram Road
Bristol, PA 19007

ABSTRACT

The chemistry and mechanical properties of silicones including surface treatments, filler-free silicones, low and high consistency silicones and new-generation silicone-thermoplastics is reviewed in the context of medical device applications. Specific medical devices considered are low thrombogenic potential coatings, membranes for oxygenation and dialysis, pressure sensitive adhesives, mammary (soft tissue) prosthesis, cardiovascular devices, microelectrodes and contact lenses. Silicone IPN's silicone-urethanes, silicone-polycarbonates and silicone-methacrylates are emphasized.

Encouraging toxicological data led to the fabrication of the first medical device, a catheter, by 1950 [10]. Silicone polymers now have over thirty years of *in vivo* testing, and are found in an increasingly wide range of medical applications. The silicones that have evolved to meet these requirements have a broad range of properties which are difficult to discuss systematically. This review of silicones will be an overview from the materials perspective illustrated with specific medical device applications.

While applications for biomedical materials may be divided into short-term body contact and long-term implantation, in the case of silicones differences in materials recommendations are associated with manufacturing practice and control. Modifications of mechanical or chemical characteristics of silicones generally play no *a priori* role in determining implantability.

Several basic fabrication techniques are associated with silicones incorporated into medical devices.

Coating	Sealing
Bonding	Casting
Encapsulation	Molding

The selection of a particular silicone is dictated both by its fabrication and performance characteristics. A single silicone material frequently is not limited to a single fabrication technique. Widely different silicones fabricated by different techniques can satisfy the same application requirements.

Silicone materials used in biomedical applications can be classified as follows:

1 Monomers and Low Molecular Weight Resins
- 1.1 Surface treatments and molecular coatings
- 1.2 Monomers for cureable systems and crosslinking

2 Prepolymer Fluids and Unfilled Polymers
- 2.1 Filler-Free Silicone Rubber
- 2.2 Pressure Sensitive Adhesives
- 2.3 Gels

3 Elastomers (including RTV, LTV and HTV systems)

The most general purpose and widely recognized silicones including those used in many soft tissue replacement, catheter, flexing joint, drain, shunt, adhesive and impression applications.
- 3.1 Adhesives and Sealants
- 3.2 Low-Consistency Elastomers
- 3.3 High-Consistency Elastomers

4 Thermoplastics

"New-generation" silicones with greater mechanical properties including copolymers, graft polymers and IPN's used in cardiovascular devices, contact lenses and membranes.
- 4.1 Silicone-Urethanes
- 4.2 Silicone-Polycarbonates
- 4.3 Silicone-Methacrylates

REVIEW OF SILICONE CHEMISTRY

The simplest silicones are the polydimethylsiloxanes. The polymers, when not cross-linked, have found widespread use in the manufacture of cosmetics, food-processing materials, and deflatulant preparations. They are valued for their lubricity, ability to lower surface tension and act as antifoam agents. Polydimethylsiloxanes exhibit the basic structure of the silicones.

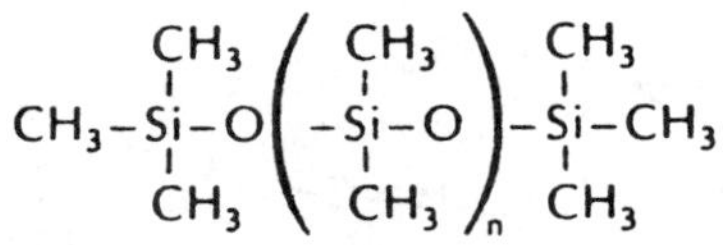

The repeating unit of the polymer

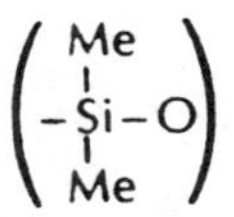

the dimethylsiloxane unit, is referred to as a D unit, while the termination unit (Me_3SiO-), the trimethylsiloxy group, is referred to as an M unit. The structure shown above can thus be described as an M unit. The silicones do not have to remain linear; they can obtain branch points,

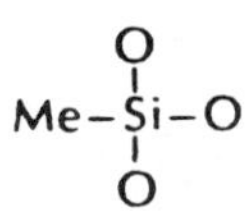

and

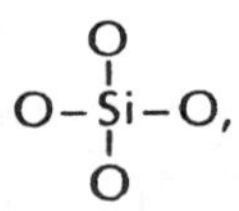

referred to as T groups and Q groups, which introduce rigidity into the structure. This relatively simple chemistry results in fluids at low molecular weights and leads to cross-linkable gums at high molecular weights.

Table 1. Silicone Substitutions.

Structure	Name	Application
CH_3–	methyl	Basic substitution found in virtually all silicones; a cross-linking point with peroxide cures
C_6H_5–	phenyl	Increases modulus, thermal, and UV stability; raises refractive index; decreases reactivity with peroxides
$CF_3CH_2CH_2$–	trifluoropropyl	Increases stability, increases solvent resistance
H–	hydride	Introduces metal-catalyzed and vinyl-addition cross-link sites
HO–	silanol	Cross-linking point for condensation and metal-catalyzed cross-linking
CH_2=CH–	vinyl	Increases peroxide reactivity; introduces cross-link points for vinyl addition

A variety of groups, including phenyl, vinyl, and hydrogen can substitute for the methyl group in a silicone. This is significant inasmuch as the substitution, branching and molecular weight of a silicone polymer will dictate the method by which curing or cross-linking can be accomplished. Fundamentally, there are four processes employed to cure silicones. In high temperature vulcanizing (HTV) systems, polymers containing methyl or vinyl groups are cross-linked with peroxides. In room-temperature vulcanizing (RTV) systems, two cure methods are used. In the older methods silanols are condensed with a moisture

Peroxide

$$\equiv Si-CH_3 + CH_2=CH-Si\equiv \xrightarrow[\text{peroxide}]{} \equiv Si-CH_2CH_2CH_2-Si\equiv$$

Condensation

$$\equiv Si-OH + HO-Si\equiv \xrightarrow[H^+]{} \equiv Si-O-Si\equiv + H_2O$$

Metal salt

$$\equiv Si-H + HO-Si\equiv \xrightarrow[\text{metal salt}]{} \equiv Si-O-Si\equiv + H_2$$

Vinyl addition

$$\equiv Si-H + CH_2=CH-Si\equiv \xrightarrow[Pt]{} \equiv Si-CH_2CH_2-Si\equiv$$

Figure 1. Silicone-curing systems.

sensitive silane cross-linker or a metal salt catalyzed reaction between silicon hydrides and silanols takes place. The latter reaction liberates hydrogen which can be used to produce foamed products. Vinyl addition systems in which a platinum complex catalyzes the addition of silicone hydrides to vinyl substituted silanes was initially used in low temperature vulcanizing (LTV) systems but has been gradually extended to RTV's and HTV's.

The primary monomeric raw materials for silicone polymers are chlorosilanes. These materials are corrosive, flammable and generally difficult to handle. They are used directly or as their alkoxy derivatives only in surface treatment applications. The direct intermediates for polymers are cyclic siloxanes and low molecular weight silanols. It is important to note that biological inertness of polymers derived from these monomers does not imply biological inertness of the monomers themselves. The biological activity of many low molecular weight silanes has been established. The commonly used monomers shown in Figure 2 have been shown to have extremely low levels of toxicity.

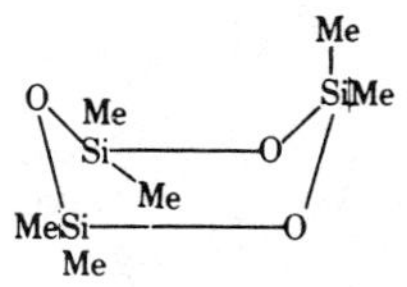

hexamethyl-
cyclotrisiloxane

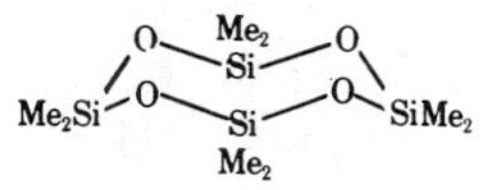

octamethyl-
cyclotetrasiloxane

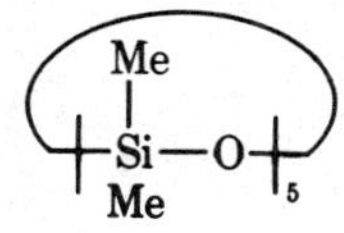

decamethyl-
cyclopentasiloxane

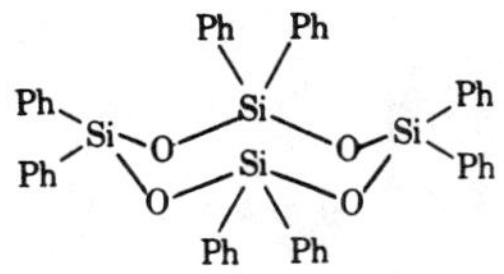

octaphenylcylco-
tetrasiloxane

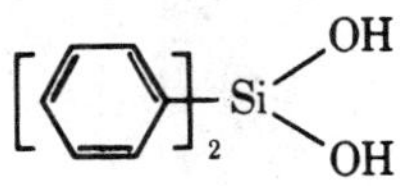

diphenylsilane-
diol

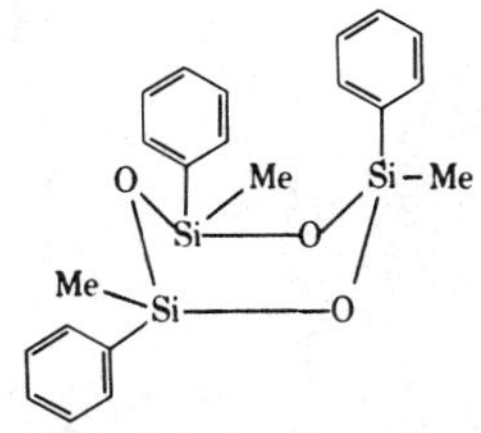

trimethyltriphenyl-
cyclotrisiloxane

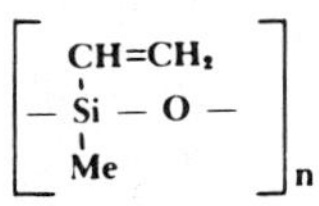

vinylmethyl-
cyclosiloxanes

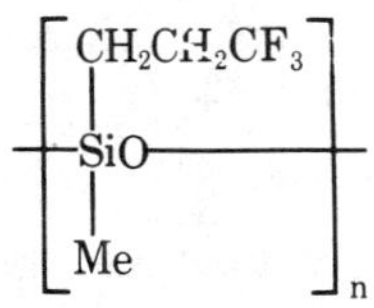

trifluoropropylmethyl-
cyclosiloxanes

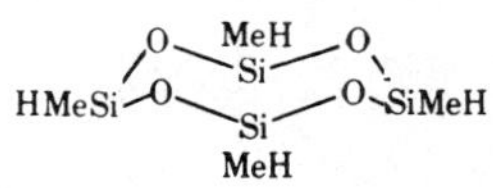

methylhydro-
cyclosiloxane

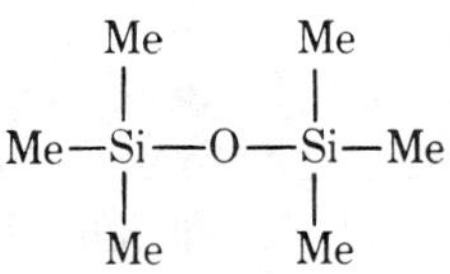

hexamethyl-
disiloxane

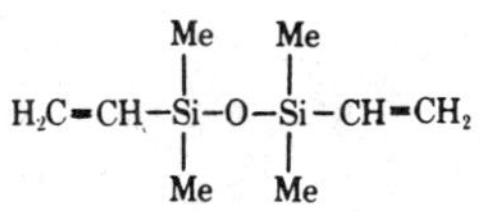

divinyltetra-
methyldisiloxane

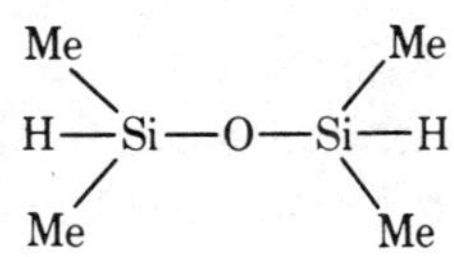

tetramethyl-
disiloxane

Figure 2. Silicone monomers and terminators.

Two general methods are employed to produce silicone polymers. Gums and non-silanol terminated fluids are produced by base catalyzed (anionic) polymerization. Under typical conditions, potassium, sodium, or tetramethylammonium silanolate catalysts are introduced into a mixture of monomers and end-cappers. The mixtures are equilibrated by heating under moderate conditions (60-150°C) [11,12]. Silanol terminated polymers are produced by a variety of techniques including hydrolysis of chlorosilanes with water or indirectly with methanol, metal salt catalyzed telomerization of cyclics in the presence of dimethyl-

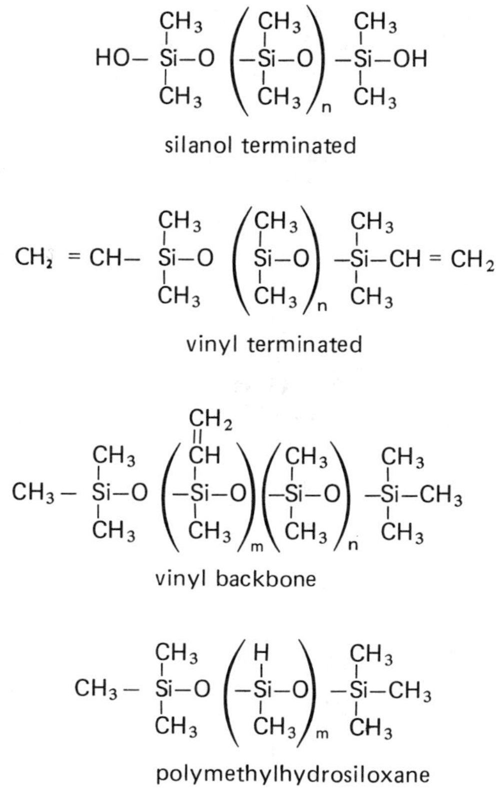

Figure 3. Silicone prepolymers.

dichlorosilane followed by hydrolysis, and equilibration of cyclics with low molecular weight silanol fluids which act as chain terminators [13,14,15]. Typical reactive silicone polymers are shown in Figure 3. They include silanol, vinyl and hydride functional materials of various degrees of polymerization.

Most silicones are filled with particulate silica. Particulate silica has a reinforcing effect on silicone elastomers that results in increased modulus, tensile strength, tear strength and abrasion resistance. The reinforcing effect depends on three properties of the filler: particle size, structure, and surface interaction. The particle size together with the filler loading determines the area available for surface interaction. The structure determines the extent polymer movement is restricted under deformation. The surface interaction determines the effectiveness with which particle size and structure control elastomer properties. Parameters associated with surface interaction include population and type of hydroxyl groups, adsorbed moisture and chemical treatment. It is postulated that the redistribution of stress among polymer chains in reinforced systems is accomplished by two-dimensional mobility of polymer chains that are otherwise bound tightly to the silica surface.

Chemical treatment of silica may greatly change its interaction with silicone polymers. Fumed silica behavior can be altered by inactivating the isolated silanol groups with various silanes. Materials used to modify surface characteristics include hexamethyldisilazane, divinyltetramethyldisilazane and cyclic and short linear siloxanes. Under-treatment of silica results in "crepe hardening," a characteristic condition in which uncured elastomer exhibits crumbling rather than plasticity under applied stress. Over-treatment of filler results in non-responsive or "dead" elastomers. High tear strength elastomers result from filler treatments which introduce vinyl groups.

1 Monomers and Low Molecular Weight Resins

1.1 Surface treatments and molecular coatings

Reactive monomeric and oligomeric silanes are employed to impart specific surface properties to inorganic and silicone substrates. The materials have the general structure: $R_{4-n}SiX_n$ where n = 1 to 3. R is an organic radical in which a carbon is bound to silicon. X is an electronegative moiety such as alkoxy or chlorine. The organic radical is hydrolytically stable and the electronegative moiety is not. The electronegative group is removed by hydrolysis to form an unstable silanol which condenses with the -OH group of substrates. If there are three hydrolyzeable moieties telomerization occurs during the deposition process and coatings 6-8 molecular layers thick usually result. Details of this chemistry have been reviewed [16].

Monomeric and oligomeric silanes are not sold as medical grade materials. They are widely used in industrial products including composites, coatings and adhesives. They are used to form water-repellent surfaces. It is imperative that the user of these materials for medical devices insures that excessive monomer and hydrolysis byproducts are removed after surface treatments.

Silane surface treatments are employed in clinical analytical techniques to reduce interaction of blood with hydrophilic surfaces. Water-soluble derivatives of octadecylsilane are employed in the treatment of glassware to reduce adsorption of erythrocytes. Oligomeric silanes with active chlorine or alkoxy termination not only exhibit the hydrophobicity of octadecyl surface treatments, but have a high degree of oleophobicity as well. They reduce protein adsorption on glass surfaces. Other silanes perform more active roles, enhancing adsorption or bonding of specific proteins such as heparin, bioactive groups such as fungistats, or whole cells and cell organelles. Silanes have been employed to covalently bond enzymes and cofactors to inorganic substrates. A summary of surface treatments is found in Table 2.

Table 2. Surface Treatments and Molecular Coatings

Silane Type	Application	Tradename	ref.
Octadecyl	reduces protein adsorption reduces thrombogenicity	Glassclad® 18 Siliclad	18,19
Chlorinated siloxane telomer	reduces protein adsorption reduces thrombogenicity increases oleophobicity	Glassclad® 6C Dri-Film®	17
Aminopropyl	adsorbs heparin		17
Polyethylenimine	adsorbs proteins	Glassclad® IM	19
Ethyl	adsorbs erythrocytes		19
Octadecyl Quat	fungistatic treatment	D.C.® 5700	20,21
Amine, p-nitrobenzamide, mercapto	immobilization of enzymes		22,23
Heparin	anticoagulant	Glassclad® HP	24

Glassclad® J.M. of Petrarch Systems, Dri-Film J. M. at General Electric D.C. T.M. at Dow Corning

1.2 Monomers for Cureable Systems

The hydrolysis and condensation of alkoxysilanes leads to resinous products which have traditionally been used as coatings and encapsulants. In a manner consistent with this chemistry, slow release anti-tumor devices have been produced by hydrolyzing the silanes in the presence of various drugs [25].

The direct polymerization of monomeric siloxanes such as hexamethylcyclotrisiloxane (D_3) and octamethyl-cyclotetrasiloxane (D_4) is of current interest in the preparation of filler-free silicone rubber (FFSR). On many occasions undesireable biological responses to filled standard silicone rubber (SSR) has been attributed to the filler rather than the silicone itself. Physiological reaction to fillers is especially noteable in devices with large surface areas such as oxygenator and dialysis membranes. FFSR is more often achieved by reaction of prepolymers than polymerization of monomers. The monomeric approach is discussed in this section. The prepolymer approach is discussed in the next section.

Plasma and radiation polymerization of D_3 has been reported by Chawla for the production of filler-free silicone coatings and bulk moldings [26-29]. In this method D_3 is melted and cast or applied to a polymer substrate then subjected to high energy polymerization. The materials have tensile strengths of 2.5 MPa and an elongation of 500%. In work with whole canine blood adsorption of platelets and leukocytes is reduced 30–35% when compared to SSR.

2 Prepolymer Fluids and Unfilled Polymers

2.1 Filler-Free Silicone Rubber

Filler-free silicone rubber can be prepared by cross-linking unfilled silicone gum stocks. Membranes for artificial lungs, are fabricated by a method in which 1-1.5% dichlorobenzoyl peroxide is used to cross-link a polydimethylsiloxane gum. The gum is cured at 100°C, for five minutes, followed by a four hour postcure at 150°C. Another method that lends itself to the preparation of thin films requires that a vinyl-modified dimethylsiloxane gum and peroxide be dissolved in toluene and cast into a film. After the film is dried at 75°C, it is cured in air at 180°C and subjected to ultraviolet radiation from germicidal lamps [30,31].

The importance of silicone membranes in oxygenation and dialysis cannot be overemphasized. The permeability of oxygen through silicones is more than ten times greater than permeable materials like natural rubber and low density polyethylene. It is over 100 times greater than butyl rubber and nylon. The permeability (P) of selected gases through polydimethylsiloxane elastomer has been reported [32]. An incomplete summary follows.

Permeabilities of Gases through Polydimethylsiloxane Elastomer

$$\frac{\text{cc of gas} \cdot (\text{cm})}{\text{sec} \cdot \text{cm}^2 \cdot \text{cmHg}} \times 10^9$$

water	3600	nitrogen	28
carbon dioxide	325	methane	95
oxygen	60	methanol	1390

In order to grasp the significance of the permeation rates, it is useful to make some conversions and approximations of the reported units, simplifying it within 10% to the following:

$$P = \frac{\text{liter, mil thick}}{\text{hour, meter}^2\text{, atmosphere}}$$

This indicates, for example, that oxygen would diffuse at approximately 60 liters per hour through a square meter of silicone one mil thick under a pressure of one atmosphere. Man at rest consumes 18 liters of oxygen per hour.

2.2 Pressure Sensitive Adhesives

Most of the unfilled cured silicone polymers employed in medical devices can be described as pseudointerpenetrating polymer networks. The materials contain two polymer components. One silicone is a matrix material with a linear structure. The second silicone component has a branched or cross-linked structure that extends homogeneously throughout the matrix. The systems behave in a uniform cohesive manner, although unlike true interpenetrating polymer networks only one component is cross-linked.

Pressure sensitive adhesives are generally formulated from a high viscosity silanol terminated fluid and a low molecular weight resinous silicone. The two component system is supplied in a solvent. The materials are used externally for adhering ileostomy and colostomy appliances, attaching electrodes and adhering maxillofacial medical devices. The properties of silicone PSA's are exemplified by Dow Corning® 355.

Silicone Pressure Sensitive Adhesive

solids content, %	18.5
solvent	trichlorotrifluoroethane
adhesive strength Al/Al, oz/in.	100

2.3 Gels

Silicone based pseudointerpenetrating polymer networks which result in clear resilient gels with cohesive properties are useful in orthopedic pads [33]. The gels used for orthopedic pads in breast implants are generally produced by vinyl addition chemistry. The first gels used for these purposes were linear siloxanes with low levels of cross-linking; for example, a 500-700 centistoke dimethylsiloxane fluid with 1.0% vinylmethyl backbone was cross-linked by platinum-catalyzed addition to 4 to 5 ctsk polymethylhydrosiloxane [34]. In most updated formulations, vinyl terminated siloxanes of 1000 ctsk or greater are cross-linked with a methylhydro-dimethylsiloxane copolymer using a complex of neutralized chloroplatinic acid in divinyltetramethyldisiloxane or vinylmethylcyclosiloxanes. However, this cross-linked system constitutes only 10-20% of the gel weight; the matrix material is 350 to 1000 ctsk polydimethylsiloxane. The cross-linked silicone produces an interpenetrating polymer network within the matrix silicone, which creates a responsive gel with good cohesion [35-38]. Another approach to gel formation is to produce a hydrophilic copolymer between a vinylsiloxane with hydrolyzeable groups and vinylpyrrolidone [39,40].

An undesireable property of pseudointerpenetrating silicone networks is for a small portion of the matrix polymer to bleed out. The matrix material can bleed through fully cross-linked polydimethylsiloxane mammary shells. Methods of reducing bleed include coating or preparing shells from phenyl or trifluoropropyl containing siloxanes [41]. The different solubility parameters for these materials allow them to behave as barriers for polydimethylsiloxanes.

3 Elastomers

The most widely recognized silicones are filled or reinforced elastomeric products. The two main classifications of materials are: low-consistency – not requiring simultaneous application of heat and pressure for processing; high-consistency – requiring simultaneous application of heat and pressure. All of the cure systems mentioned earlier are employed in the elastomeric products. The multitude of products allows the selection of only the most representative examples in this section.

3.1 Adhesives and Sealants

Silicone adhesives and sealants are low consistency room temperature vulcanizing liquid rubbers which offer considerable latitude in formulation and properties. The main components of condensation cure RTV's are silanol terminated polydimethylsiloxanes. The viscosity of the polymer can range from 500 to 1,000,000 ctsk. Often a blend of polymers will be used in compounding. This allows variations in cross-link density, cure times and working consistencies.

Most RTV's of this class have moisture sensitive cure systems. They contain a silane cross-linker with moisture sensitive hydrolyzeable groups. The most common systems are listed below:

ACYLOXY	≡Si-OH	+	AcOSi≡	$\longrightarrow$	≡Si-O-Si≡	+	AcOH
AMINE	≡Si-OH	+	$Me_2NSi\equiv$	$\longrightarrow$	≡Si-O-Si≡	+	Me_2NH
OXIME	≡Si-OH	+	$R_2C=N\text{-}OSi\equiv$	$\longrightarrow$	≡Si-O-Si≡	+	$R_2C=NOH$
ALKOXY	≡Si-OH	+	MeOSi≡	$\xrightarrow[\text{Catalyst}]{}$	≡Si-O-Si≡	+	MeOH

The reactions of these systems are often catalyzed with carboxylic acid salts of tin, zinc or iron. A fast catalyst is tin octoate. A slow catalyst is dibutyltin dilaurate. Titanates are also used to catalyze these reactions. In general, amine and oxime materials react the fastest, followed by acyloxy then alkoxy. Excess silane gives slower reacting materials with longer pot-life. Adjusting cure times is best accomplished during compounding.

Choosing a material for a particular application requires consideration of physical properties and processing. One part RTV's tend to be used as adhesives. Two part RTV's tend to be used as sealants and encapsulants. Either type can usually be dispersed in solvents as required for processing.

3.2 Low-Consistency Elastomer – Addition Cure

Addition cure materials tend to have greater strength than condensation cure products. They are thought of as clean systems since there are no by-products or hydrolyzeable leaving group during cure. Cure rate may be adjusted from minutes to hours depending upon the use of inhibitors or level of catalyst.

The viscosity of material may vary from 1000 to 1,000,000 ctsk. Lower molecular weight polymers are used to formulate dental impression materials [42,43], while higher molecular weights are used in liquid injection molding compounds. Higher molecular weight, high consistency products with properties similar to traditional HTV's are available but will not be discussed here.

Addition cure materials are supplied as two part systems. Generally the catalyst, a platinum complex, is in the "A" part and the cross-linker, a hydride, is in the "B" part. Cross-link density may be adjusted by the distribution of hydride along the siloxane chain and length of the chain. Short chains with high hydride give material with a "snappy" character and are used in formulating products with high tensile and tear strengths. Longer chains with lower hydride content give greater elongations. Typical levels of platinum in these formulations range from 5 to 15 ppm. Inhibitors may be used to moderate the rate of cure. They differ from "poisons" in that their interaction with the platinum complex is reversible. Poisons include sulfides and sulfur containing rubbers and certain amines.

Very few of the additional cure systems are sold specifically as medical grade materials. One such material which is used for biomedical encapsulating and moldmaking is Dow Corning® MDX-4-4210. Typical properties are given below.

viscosity, as supplied, ctsk.	80,000
Cured Properties	
Durometer, Shore A	>25
Tensile Strength, MPa	>3.8
Elongation, %	>350
Specific Gravity	1.12

3.3 High Consistency Elastomers

The oldest and most widely used silicones are the peroxide cure high temperature vulcanizing (HTV) systems. They are used for extrusion of catheter tubing, compression molding of shunts and flexing joints and calendering sheeting, both Dacron reinforced and non-reinforced. Uncured forms can be fabricated by manual or "lay-up" techniques. The reader is referred to Lynch [2] for an excellent review of processing and properties of HTV's.

Table 3. Typical Properties of High Consistency Silicone

specific gravity	1.12-1.25
durometer Shore A	25-75
tensile strength, MPa	5.9-8.3
elongation, %	350-700
tear strength, lb-in	70-160
compression set, 24 hours at 175°C	10-40%
dielectric constant	2.8-2.9
dissipation factor	$6.0\text{-}9.0 \times 10^{-4}$

4 Thermoplastic Silicones

Thermoplastic silicones include silicone copolymers, block copolymers and some alloys. A substantial portion of the polymer composition does not contain a siloxane backbone. Generally speaking the materials have radically different properties than conventional silicones. Mechanical strengths are higher, but a variety of other striking property differences are introduced.

4.1 Silicone-Urethanes

The mechanical, fatigue and physiological response characteristics of silicone homopolymers are not comparable to those of silicone-urethanes used in blood pumps, intra-aortic balloons, total heart replacements and related devices [44]. Fatigue strength, toughness, flexibility and low interaction with plasma proteins are bio-engineering criteria applicable to silicone-urethanes. The most widely recognized material in this category is Cardiothane 51 (formerly Avcothane 51) produced by Kontron Cardiovascular, Inc. The material is described as a copolymer of aromatic polyether urethane and polydimethyl-siloxane [45]. The copolymer is proposed to crosslink by the interaction of acetoxy-terminated siloxane blocks with substituted urethane nitrogens [46]. The polymer is not homogeneous and may be described as a mixture of 10% moisture cured polydimethylsiloxane in a urethane matrix, with bulk phase separation prevented by small amounts of silicone-urethane surfactant formed during cure [47]. Cardiothane is primarily a casting resin. Molding and extrusion grades of silicone-polyester urethane IPN's are available from Petrarch Systems.

While not yet available on a commercial basis, several true urethane-siloxane copolymers with promising properties are in development. One approach is to use a carbinol (C-OH) transition between the siloxane and urethane [48,49]. A carbinol terminated silicone can be created by reacting silanol-terminated polymers with ethylene oxide to yield a hydroxyethyl ether ($SiOCH_2CH_2OH$), and by adding allylic alcohols to hydride-terminated polymers to give materials with greater hydrolytic stability ($SiCH_2CH_2CH_2OH$). A second approach is to use a urea transition between the siloxane and urethane which results from an aminoalkyl terminated siloxane [50]. (Table 4).

Table 4. Silicone-Urethane Mechanical Properties

name	Cardiothane 51	PTUE 102
manufacturer	Kontron	Petrarch
processing	dipping, casting	molding, extrusion
silicone %	10	10
specific gravity	.95	1.00
tensile strength, MPa	43.8	41.4
elongation, %	525	450
tear strength lb/in	490	750
water absorption, 24 hr	1.6%	.03%
hardness, Shore	A72	D50

4.2 Silicone-Polycarbonates

The earliest silicone-polycarbonates were produced by condensing preformed silicone blocks with Bisphenol A by phosgenation in the presence of amine [51-54]. Later syntheses of these materials improved reproducibility and properties of these materials by using polycarbonate prepolymers and amine terminated siloxane blocks [55]. The physical characteristics of these materials have been extremely well defined [56,57]. Silicone-polycarbonates have high mechanical and tear strengths, while maintaining a high degree of oxygen and water permeability. Films may be extruded or cast at thicknesses below 1 mil.

Blood oxygenation, dialysis and microelectrode membranes are the usual biomedical applications for silicone-polycarbonates. The simple unmodified materials are used in blood oxygenation [58]. Techniques for preparing thin high temperature membranes for oxygen transport have been described [59-61]. Silicone-polycarbonates have been cast as defect free membranes 0.015 microns thick.

In microelectrode applications simple block copolymers of Bisphenol A polycarbonate have inadequate hydrolytic stability and their dielectric constants are too low to permit ion transport. For this reason, many current microelectrode materials incorporate ion-carrier groups in the siloxane block to allow molecular transport as well as a urethane transition to the polycarbonate to increase hydrolytic stability. The combination of mechanical, dielectric, permeation and film formation properties has allowed the preparation of membranes useful for monitoring physiological changes in concentrations of hydrogen, potassium, sodium and ammonium ions [62-65]. A typical structure is:

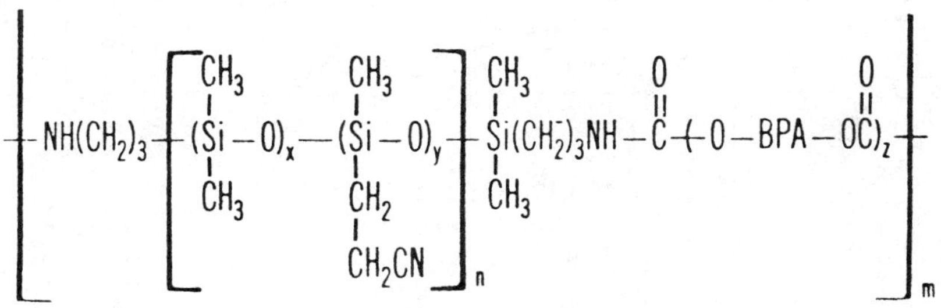

Silicone-polycarbonates can be injection molded and extruded. Perhaps their most unique process characteristic is the abiity to cast films from solutions in methylene chloride or trichloropropane by dropping the solutions onto warm water and allowing the solvent to evaporate. The mechanical properties of these materials are far greater than unfilled silicones.

SILICONE-POLYCARBONATE 50:50 BLOCK COPOLYMERS

specific gravity	1.07–1.08
tensile strength	19.0-22.0 MPa
elongation	270–350%
water vapor transmission	16–20 g/24hr/100m²/mil

4.3 Silicone-Methacrylates – Ophthalmic Materials

Once it was recognized that maximum contact lens comfort was achieved when the eye could "breathe," silicones became likely candidates for lens materials. The primary design parameters which lead to selection of silicone materials are permeability (Dk) and Equivalent Oxygen Percentage (EOP), a finished lens measurement that considers oxygen demand of occular tissue. Other parameters which require modification of basic silicone properties are wettability (contact angle), dimensional stability and refractive index.

A minimum EOP of 5-7% has been proposed for finished lenses [66,67]. This is equivalent to the oxygen available to the eye during sleep (closed eyelid). An EOP below 2 is known to cause corneal edema. Figures 4 and 5 show how the EOP relates to permeability for various lens thicknesses and various lens materials.

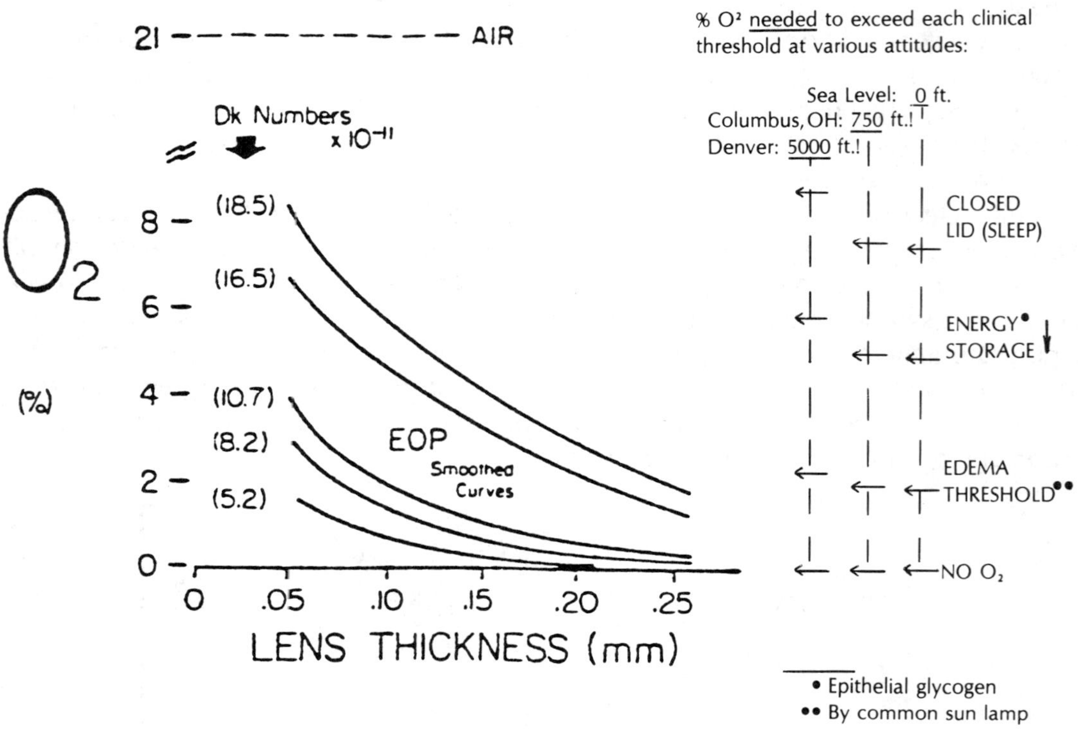

Figure 4.

Trends in the early '70s toward soft lenses bolstered interest in pure siloxane backbone materials which have the highest Dks. A variety of mechanical, optical and wetting problems posed a considerable challenge. No siloxane backbone lenses have achieved commercial acceptance. A recently introduced lens which incorporates siloxane backbone technology is offered by Dow Corning as Silsoft®. A newer approach is to employ siloxane modified methacrylate copolymers. This polymer technology leads primarily to hard lenses and is now an established commercial technology. The most conspicuous example is the Polycon Silofocon® lens offered by Syntex.

The enhancement of oxygen permeability in siloxane lens systems is associated with high relative proportions of silicon – oxygen and silicon-carbon bonds. These long bonds lead to a free volume element which is in the case of polydimethylsiloxane 5-6 times greater than that in polymethacrylates [68]. Both polydimethylsiloxane and polyvinyltrimethylsilane exhibit high oxygen permeability when introduced into copolymer systems. It appears that a maximum disordering of polymer structure – i.e., random copolymers or terpolymers – is desireable. Polymers should be designed to exclude microblock regions that are large enough to phase

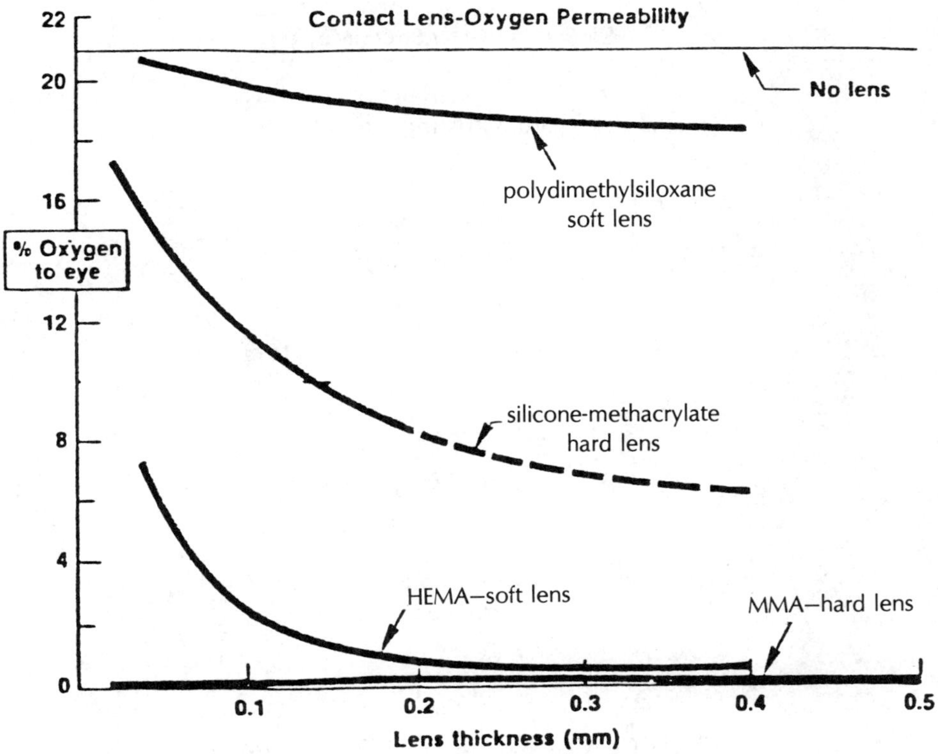

Figure 5.

separate. In order to provide satisfactory dimensional stability the systems are cross-linked.

The earliest lens materials were dimethyl-phenylmethyl-siloxane copolymers containing sufficient phenyl groups (10—15 mole percent) to match the refractive index of the polymer to silica reinforcing fillers. These were peroxide cure elastomer systems [69-71]. Lenses based on this chemistry were extremely hydrophobic, causing discomfort and in many instances damage to the corneal epithelium. While the lenses had high oxygen permeability, the permeability of water was also high. Water permeated through the lenses from the surface of the eye. Since these unmodified siloxanes are extremely hydrophobic, water is unable to return to the tissue under the lens and dehydration of tissues along with adhesion of the lens takes place [72].

Approaches toward improving the hydrophilic properties of siloxane backbone lenses have included both plasma and radiation treatment [73-5]. Siloxane polymers can also be blended or grafted with hydrophilic polymer systems such as vinylpyrrolidone and glycidyl methacrylate [76-79]. Surface siloxane bonds have been hydrolyzed by titanates [80].

Probably the most significant new technology in silicone hard lens materials is that disclosed by Gaylord for the production of siloxane-modified methacrylate copolymers [81,82]. In the simplest example, methacryloxypropyltris(trimethylsiloxy)silane is copolymerized with other methacrylate monomers, by which means the oxygen permeability of siloxanes is combined with the mechanical and optical properties of the methacrylates. This technology is the basis of the Syntex Polycon® lens, which is said to employ a methacryloxypropyltris(pentamethyldisiloxanyl) silane [83]. Several research groups have found other siloxane-modified methacrylates not described in the Gaylord patent [84-6]. Toyo Contact Lens, for example, has

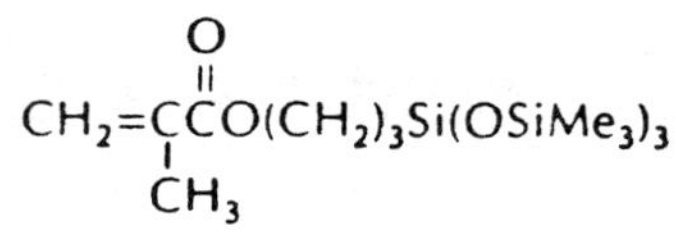

methacryloxypropyltris(trimethylsiloxy)silane

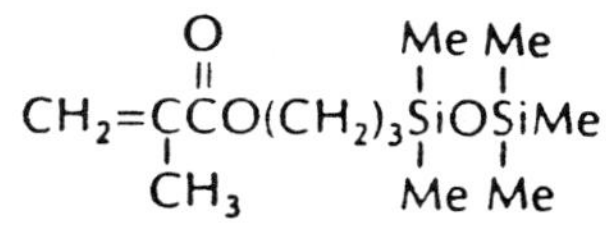

methacryloxypropylpentamethyldisiloxane

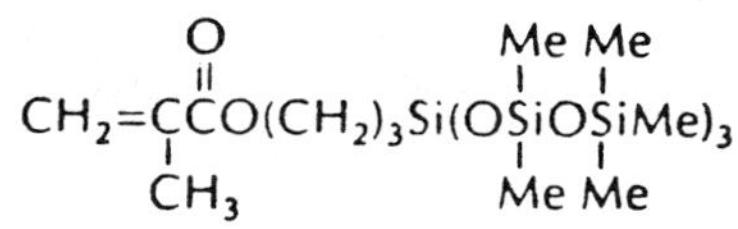

methacryloxypropyltris(pentamethyldisiloxanyl)-
silane

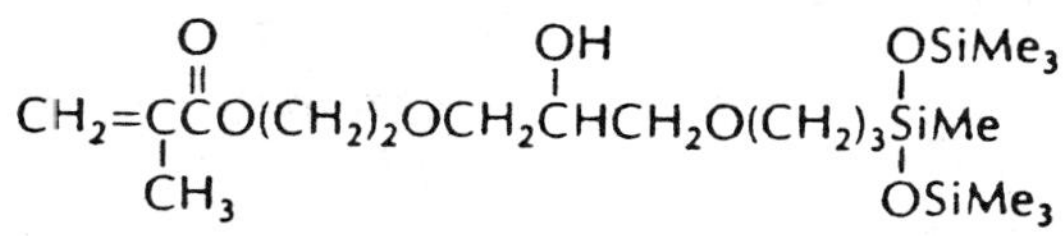

methyldi(trimethylsiloxy)silylpropylglycerol-
methacrylate

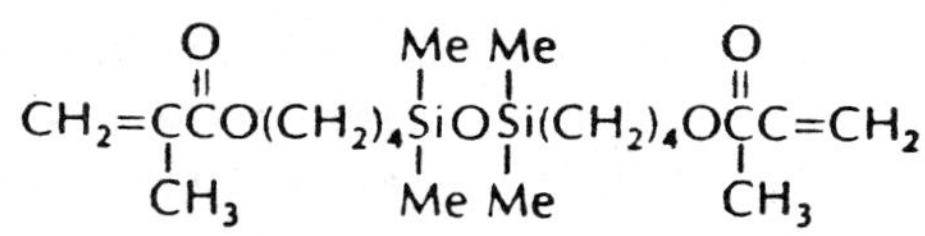

bis(methacryloxybutyl)tetramethyldisiloxane

Figure 6.

prepared siloxane modified hydroxyethylmethacrylate monomers that have pendant hydroxyl groups which suggest improved hydrophilicity [87]. This chemistry has also been translated to soft contact lens systems [88].

Other siloxane-modified methacrylate technology which appears to have considerable obstacles for commercialization is that of Bausch and Lomb, in which a bis(methacryloxybutyl) end-blocking unit is prepared and then polymerized with D_4 [89-92]. This long, oxygen permeable group acts as a difunctional cross-linking unit in the polymerization of a variety of monomers. The result is a soft lens system that is both oxygen permeable as well as hydrophilic. An analogous result with a different technology, reported by Ciba-Geigy, employs a urethane bridge from a polysiloxane to hydroxyethylmethacrylate [49].

While not currently directed toward contact lens formulations, silicone-acrylate copolymers develop properties that suggest future evaluation [93-5]. Hard contact lenses have been produced by application of high pheny content silicone casting resin-technology [96]. It also should not be surprising to see some of the silicone-polycarbonate and other oxygen permeable membrane technologies translated to contact lens materials.

Many other thermoplastic silicones have been reported. Materials which appear promising for biomedical applications include silicone-polyamides IPNs [7], silicone-methylstyrene block copolymers [97], and silicone-polypeptide block copolymers [98]. An important review which discusses silicone rubbers from a biocompatibility and surgical approach has recently been published [98].

REFERENCES

1. W. Noll "Chemistry and Technology of Silicones" Academic Press, New York 1968.
2. W. Lynch "Handbook of Silicone Rubber Fabrication" Van Nostrand-Reinhold, New York, 1978.
3. M. Ranney "Silicones" Noyes Data, Park Ridge, N.J., 1977.
4. G. Bendz, I. Lindqvist "Biochemistry of Silicon and Related Problems" Plenum, New York, 1978.
5. R. Tacke, U. Wannagat, M. Voronkov "Bioactive Organosilicon Compounds: Topics in Current Chemistry" Springer-Verlag, New York, 1979.
6. M. Voronkov, V. Mileshkevich, Yu Yuzhelevski "The Siloxane Bond" Plenum, New York, 1978.
7. B. Arkles, W. Peterson, R. Anderson "Organosilicon Compounds: Register and Review" Petrarch Systems, Bristol, Pa. 1982.
8. E. Warrick, O. Pierce, K. Polmanteer, J. Saam *Developments in Silicone Elastomer Chemistry* Rubber Chem. and Tech. *52(3)*, 438-525, 1979.
9. O. Dolgov, M. Voronkov, M. Grinblat "Organosilicon Liquid Rubbers" Rubber and Plastics Research Associates (RAPRA) Shawbury, England, 1977.
10. R. DeNicola *Permanent Artificial Urethra,* J. of Urol. *63,* 168, 1950.
11. R. Mansfield *Polydimethylsiloxane Gum* Macromolecular Syntheses Col. Vol. 1, 451, 1977.
12. J. McGrath, J. Riffle in reference 7.
13. W. Sorenson, T. Campbell "Preparative Methods of Polymer Chemistry, Wiley, New York 1968, p. 383.
14. R. Lewis, E. Martin *Process for making siloxanediols,* U.S. Pat. 4,066,680, 1978.
15. S. Borisov et al Zh Obsch Khim *38,* 2794, 1968.
16. B. Arkles *Tailoring Surfaces with Silanes,* CHEMTECH, *7,* 713, 1977.
17. R. Merker et al *The heparinization of silicone rubber using aminoorganosilanes* in Proc. Artif. Heart Prog. Confr. U.S. Dept. HEW 1969.
18. E. Sako, O. Kawamura *Polycarbonate container for medical applications* U.S. Pat. 3,746,196 1973.
19. B. Arkles, W. Brinigar, A. Miller *Whole cell and cell organelle immobilization on siliceous surfaces* in "Silylated Surfaces" ed. D. Leyden, W. Collins, Gordon & Breach, New York, 1980.

20a. A. Isquith, E. Abbott, P. Walters *Surface bonded antimicrobial activity* Appl Microbiol *24,* 859, 1972.

20b. E. Abbott, A. Isquith *Method of inhibiting the growth of bacteria using organosilicon amines* U.S. Pat. 3,794,736 1974.

21. W. Fudy *Organosilicon quarternary ammonium antimicrobial compounds* U.S. Pat. 4,282,366 1981.
22. R. Messing, H. Weetall *Chemically coupled enzymes* U.S. Pat. 3,519,538 1970.
23. G. Royer, F. Liberatore *The use of silylated derivatives of porous glass as enzyme supports* in "Silylated Surfaces" ed. D. Leyden, W. Collins, Gordon & Breach New York 1980.
24. A. Nagata, J. Iyoda *Anticoagulant organosilicon polymers* Germ. Off. 2,647,389, 1975.
25. Japan Atomic Energy Institute *Antitumor Device* Jap. Pat. 26,910, 1981.

26. A. Chawla *Pure and filler free silicone rubber biomaterial* J. Bioeng. *1,* 51, 1976 and *2,* 231, 1978.
27. A. Chawla *Preparation of silicone coated biomaterials* Trans Am Soc Artif Organs *25,* 287, 1979.
28. A. Chawla *In vivo interactions between novel filler free silicone rubber and blood* ACS Org Coat Poly Proc *37,* 291, 1977.
29. A. Chawla *Blood interaction of filler free silicone rubber* Biomaterials *2,* 83, 1981.
30. T. Kolobow, F. Hayano, P. Weathersby *Membrane Lung* U.S. Pats. 3,819,772, 1974, and 3,969,290, 1976.
31. T. Kolobow, E. Stool *Ultrathin silicone rubber membranes for use in membrane lung* in "Artif Lungs Acute Resp Failure" ed. W. Zapol Academic Press, New York, 1976.
32. W. Robb *Permeability of Silicone Rubber* Ann. N.Y. Acad. Sci. *146,* 119, 1968.
33. Cronin *Implantable Breast Prosthesis* U.S. Pat. 3,293,663, 1965.
34. M. Nelson *Organosiloxane potting compound* U.S. Pat. 3,020,260, 1962.
35. E. Jeram *Organosiloxane Gels* Germ. Off. 2,616,057, 1976. U.S. Pat 4,072,635 1978.
36. D. Sierawski *Preventing discoloration of platinum containing gels* U.S. Pats. 4,100,627 and 4,122,246 1978.
37. A. Brill *Silicone gels and flexible articles filled with them Germ. Off. 2,* 711, 383, 1977.
38. Dow Corning *Gel filled flexible articles and gels therefore* Brit Pat. 1,582,081, 1980.
39. Institute for Production and Development Science *Biocompatible gels from polyvinyl alcohol and ethyl silicate* Jap. Pat. 06, 385, 1980.
40. K. Polmanteer *Hydrophilic water swellable copolymer gel for prosthesis* U.S. Pat. 4,138,382, 1979.
41. W. Larson *Silicone gel filled silicone rubber aticle possessing reduced surface bleed* Eur. Pat. 30,838, 1981.
42. P. Hittmaier, W. Hechtl, H. Eckhart *Dental Impression Material* U.S. Pat. 3,950,300, 1976.
43. P. Hittmaier, W. Hechtl, H. Eckhart *Dental Impression Material* U.S. Mat. 4,035,453, 1977.
44. T. Honda et al *One 25 day survivor with total artificial heart* J. Thorac Cardiovasc Surg *69,* 92, 1975.
45. E. Nyilas *Development of blood compatible elastomer* 23rd Ann Conf Eng in Med and Bio 1970.
46. E. Nyilas *Polysiloxane polyurethane block copolymers* U.S. Pat. 3,562,352, 1971.
47. R. Ward, E. Nyilas *Production of biomedical polymers* in "Organometallic Polymers" ed. C. Carraher, J. Sheats, C. Pittman Academic Press New York 1978, p. 219.
48. E. Bennet Germ. Off. 2,215,393 1972.
49. K. Mueller, E. Kleiner *Polysiloxane hydrogels* U.S. Pat. 4,136,250 1979.
50. R. Ward, P. Litwack, R. Rodvien *Improved Blood Compatibility of Modified Thermoplastics* Proceedings Society for Biomaterials 1982.
51. E. Goldberg *Copolymer polycarbonate* and *polysiloxane constituents* U.S. Pat. 2,999,845, 1961.
52. H. Vaughn Jr., *Organosiloxane Polycarbonate Block Copolymer* U.S. Pat. 3,189,662 1965.
53. W. Merrit, L. Vestergard *Block Copolymers* U.S. Pat. 3,821,325 1974
54. D. Laurin *Thermoplastic copolymer of polysiloxane polycarbonate and polyester constituents,* U.S. Pat 3,994,988 1976.
55. J. Riffle, R. Freelin, A. Banthia, J. McGrath *Phase-transfer catalyzed synthesis of polycarbonate polysiloxane block copolymers* J. Macromol Sci. Chem. *A15,* 967, 1981.
56. D.G. LeGrand *Mechanical and Optical studies of Poly(dimethylsiloxane) bisphenol A polycarbonate copolymers* J. Polym. Sci. B7, 597, 1969.
57. D.G. LeGrand, J. Magi a *Physical Properties of Block Copolymers of Polydimethylsiloxane and Polycarbonate* Polymer Eng. & Sci. *10* 349, 1970.
58. E. Pierce, N. Dibelius *Membrane Lung: Studies with a New High Permeability Copolymer Membrane* Trans Am. Soc. of Art. Int. Organs *14,* 220, 1968.
59. W. Robb, D. Reinhard *Gas Separation by Differential Permeation* U.S. Pat. 3,335,545 1967.
60. S. Kantnor, P. Juliano *High Temperature Membrane Material* U.S. Pat. 3,781,378 1973.

61. W. Ward, W. Browall, R. Salemme *Ultrathin silicone-polycarbonates for gas separation processes* J. Membr Sci. *1(1)*, 99, 1976.
62. P. Kinson, C. Orland, J. Klebe *Chemical Modification of Siloxane Copolymers for Use as Membranes in pH or K^+ Electrodes* 11th Organosilicon Symp., 1977.
63. J. Brown, G. Slusarczuk, O. LeBlanc *Ion-specific membrane* U.S. Pat 3,743,588 1973 Germ offen. 2,254,524 1973.
64. J. Montalvo *Ammonium ion-specific electrode* U.S. Pat 3,869,354 1975.
65. O. LeBlanc, W. Grubb *Long lived potassium ion selective polymer membrane electrode* Anal Chem. *48(12)* 1658 1976.
66. R.B. Mandell *Corneal Physiology and Permeable Materials* Contact Lens Mfrs. Assoc. paper 10-81-200 1981.
67. R. Hill *The Oxygen Connection* Contact Lens Mfrs Assoc. Paper 10-81-240 1981.
68. K. Ziegel, F. Erich J. Poly. Sci. Part A2 *8* 2015 1970.
69. W. Beker *Corneal contact lens fabricated with silicone,* U.S. Pat. 3,228,741 1966.
70. E. Travnicek *Optically clear filled silicone elastomers for contact lenses and eye implants* U.S. Pat 3,996,187 & 3,996,189 1976; Germ. Offen. 2,616,147 1976; Can. Pat. 1,043,491 1978.
71. M. Takamizawa *Siloxane contact lenses* Jpn Tokyo Kokai 81,363 1979.
72. M. Refojo, F. Leong Water pervaporation through silicone rubber contact lenses Contact Intraocul Lens Med. J. *7(13)* 226 1981.
73. E. Masuhara, N. Tarumi, M. Tsuchiya et al., *Hydrophilic silicone contact lenses* Fr. Dem. 2,407,232 1979.
74. R. Chen *Putting a hydrophilic coating on a hydrophobic lens* U.S. Pat. 4,143,949 1979.
75. B. Deubzer, J. Burkhardt, E. Brunner, K. Sallersbeck *Hydrophilic crosslinked modified organopolysiloxanes* Germ. Offen. 2,917,754 1980.
76. G. Wajs *Grafted silicone polymers and their use for contact lenses* Germ. Offen. 2,813,558 1978.
77. A. Baszkin, G. Wajs, S. Tchaliovska et al., *Silicone grafted with polyvinylpyrrolidone for contact lenses* J. Bioeng *2* 1978 pg. 527.
78. W. Covington *Method of molding an ocular membrane* U.S. Pats 4,169,119 & 4,182,723 1980 & 4,245,069 1981.
79. S. Chang, *Hydrophilic, soft and oxygen-permeable copolymer compositions* U.S. Pat 4,182,822 1980.
80. D. McVannel, J. Mishler, K. Polmanteer U.S. Pat 3,350,216 1976.
81. N. Gaylord *Oxygen permeable contact lens composition* U.S. Pat 3,808,178 1974 Braz. Ped 03,534 1974.
82. N. Gaylord *Oxygen permeable contact lens composition* U.S. Pat 4,120,570 1978.
83. M. Refojo *Contact Lenses* "Kirk-Othmer Encyclopedia of Chemical Technology," Vol. 6 New York Wiley 1979.
84. E. Ellis, J. Salamone *Silicone containing hard contact lens composition* U.S. Pat 4,152,508 1979.
85. N. Novicky Oxygen permeable contact lens compositions U.S. Pats 4,216,303, 4,242,483, 4,248,989, 4,303,772 1980.
86. A. LeBoeuf *Contact lens material* Germ. Offen. 3,023,096 1980, U.S. Pat. 4,246,389 1981.
87. K. Tanaka, K. Takahashi, M. Kanada *Copolymer for contact lenses* U.S. Pat 4,139,692 1979.
88. K. Tanaka, K. Takahashi, M. Kanada *Copolymer for soft contact lenses* U.S. Pat. 4,139,513 1979.
89. W. Deichert, K. Su, M. Van Buren *Polysiloxane composition and contact lens* U.S. Pats. 4,153,641 1979 & 4,189,546 1980; Neth. Appl. 07,333 1979; Fr. Pat. 2,398,782 1979.
90. R. Chromecek, W. Deichert, J. Falcetta, M. VanBuren *Contact lens from a copolymer of polysiloxane, acrylic acid or methacrylic acid* Germ. Offen. 3,034,505 1981.
91. G. Friends, M. VanBuren *Contact lens from polymers of polysiloxane and polycyclic esters of acrylic acid or methacrylic acid* U.S. Pat. 4,254,248 1981.
92. P. Keogh, J. Kunzler, G. Niu *Hydrophilic contact lens* U.S. Pat 4,259,467 1981.
93. E. Martin *Acrylate functional polysiloxane polymers* U.S. Pat. 3,878,263 1975.

94. P. Juliano *Substantially transparent polydimethylsiloxane-polymethylalkylmethacrylate compositions* U.S. Pat. 3,663,650 1972.
95. S. Varshney, C. Beatty *Synthesis and characterization of polymethylmethacrylate and polydimethylsiloxane block copolymers* Polymer Preprints 1981 152.
96. A. Birdsall, J. Fitzgerald, D. Jones, K. Polmanteer *Silicone Resin Optical Device* U.S. Pat 4,198,131, 1980.
97. J. Saam, F. Fearon *Properties of polystyrene-polydimethylsiloxane block copolymers* Ind. Eng. Chem. Prod. Res. *10,* 10, 1971.
98. C. Kania et al. *Preparation of poly(dimethylsiloxane)-polypeptide block copolymers* J. Apply Poly Sci., *27,* 139, 1982.
99. R. von Noort, M. Black Silicone Rubbers for Medical Applications in "Biocompatibility of Clinical Implant Materials", ed D. Williams CRC, Boca Raton, Fla.

Chapter 33

Silicone Elastomers for Implantable Biomedical Devices

T. Deva Devanathan
Product Development Engineer
Hexcel Corporation
P.O. Box 2312
11711 Dublin Boulevard
Dublin, California 94566-0705

ABSTRACT

With the widespread use of silicone elastomer in medical devices, greater attention has been focused on its properties regarding contact with blood and living tissue. The compounding of the polymer and the processing steps have to be monitored carefully to achieve a final elastomer which would be suitable for long term implantation. The thermal crosslinking of a widely used silicone polymer, poly dimethyl siloxane is discussed here.

The effects of catalyst concentration and processing time and temperature on the final properties of the elastomer are discussed. While the catalyst concentration appears to have a significant effect on the mechanical properties, the post curing time and temperature have a profound impact on the hemolytic properties of the silicone elastomer.

INTRODUCTION

Silicone elastomers are a class of polymers that have witnessed a phenomenal growth in commercial applications over the past forty years. A large number of those applications are in the fabrication of medical devices. No other polymer to date has proved to be as versatile as silicones for applications requiring total implantation, chronic or acute, in living human tissue. Some of the medical devices fabricated using silicone elastomers are blood pumps, cardiac pacemaker leads, heart valve poppets, contact lenses, medical adhesives, drug delivery systems, oxygenators, contraceptive devices, finger joints, etc. The properties that tend to make silicone rubber such an excellent candidate for biomedical applications are its soft touch, low toxicity, ability to be modified to fit various biomedical needs and good engineering properties.

Although regarded as the most stable and safest of implant materials, silicone elastomer devices have failed *in vivo*. Carmen and Kahn [1] report on failure of silicone rubber heart valve poppets while failures of replacement finger joints made of silicone rubber are brought to light by Meester and Swanson [2]. The mechanism of degradation of the physical properties of silicone elastomer *in vivo* is not well understood. A possible candidate could be the effect of absorption of lipids into the polymer. But again, Swanson *et al.* could find no correlation between the amount of lipid uptake and the condition of the implant upon removal or the period of implantation [2,3]. Ward and Perry have pursued further work along these lines by studying the effect of immersion in distilled water and in pseudo-extra cellular fluid at 37.5°C for up to four months [4]. Changes in the polymer properties were found to be independent of the sample surface area. Small amounts of moisture uptake were detected but did not cause the observed changes in the mechanical properties.

It appears that the service life of a silicone elastomer device is dictated not only by parameters, such as period of implantation, surface area of the implant exposed to blood or tissue fluids, but also by certain other conditions prior to implantation. The physical composition of the silicone elastomer and its process history while being incorporated into a medical device can play an important role on the behavior of the polymer *in vivo*. Therefore, it is important to understand the basic chemistry, formulations, and processing techniques that are integral to the manufacture of silicone rubber.

Silicone Elastomer Chemistry

The special properties of silicone elastomer result from its unique molecular structure as shown in Figure 1.

While organic polymers have a backbone of carbon-to-carbon atoms, the silicone backbone is composed of Silicon-oxygen linkages. It is this unique backbone structure which gives silicone elastomer its inertness towards the deteriorating effects of ozone, corona weathering, hydrolytic attack, etc. However, organic side chains attached to the silicon atoms incorporate excellent flexibility in the polymer allowing the design of compounds without the use of liquid plasticizers which generally tend to be toxic. Low molecular weight silicone polymers tend to be liquids, while at higher molecular weights we get silicone gums that may be crosslinked to yield silicone elastomer.

The methyl group in the poly di methyl siloxane can be substituted by a variety of groups, including phenyl, vinyl and hydrogen as shown in Table 1 [5]. The substitution, branching and

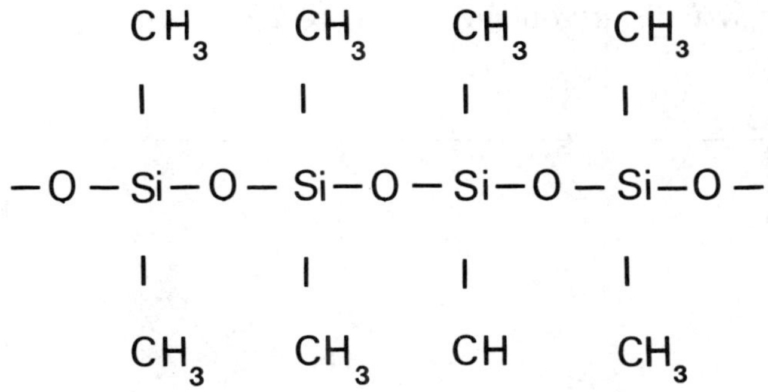

SILICONE POLYMER

Figure 1. Structure of silicone polymer, poly dimethyl siloxane.

Table 1. Silicone Substitutions

Structure	Name	Application
CH_3-	Methyl	Basic substitution found in virtually all silicones; a cross-linking point with peroxide cures
C_6H_5-	Phenyl	Increases modulus, thermal, and UV stability; raises refractive index; decreases reactivity with peroxides
$CF_3CH_2CH_2$-	Trifluoropropyl	Increases stability and decreases reactivity
H-	Hydride	Introduces metal-catalyzed and vinyl-addition cross-link sites
HO-	Silanol	Cross-linking point for condensation and metal-catalyzed cross-linking
CH_2=CH-	Vinyl	Increases peroxide reactivity; introduces cross-link points for vinyl addition

(Courtesy of Petrach Systems, Bristol, PA).

molecular weight of a silicone polymer will dictate the method by which curing or crosslinking should be accomplished. The most common method of curing of silicone polymer in the medical devices applications is the high temperature vulcanization technique. Polymers containing methyl or vinyl grups are crosslinked with peroxides.

In room temperature vulcanizing (RTV) systems, two cure methods are used. In the older method silanols are condensed with a moisture sensitive silane crosslinking agent. In the newer metal salt catalyst method, polymers containing silicon hydrides are reacted with polymers containing silanols. In the low temperature vulcanizing vinyl addition systems, a platinum complex catalyses the addition of silicon hydrides to vinyl substituted silicones.

These silicone curing systems are outlined in Figure 2.

Peroxide

$$\equiv Si - CH_3 + CH_2 = CH - Si \equiv \xrightarrow[\text{peroxide}]{} \equiv Si - CH_2CH_2CH_2 - Si \equiv$$

Condensation

$$\equiv Si - OH + HO - Si \equiv \xrightarrow[H^+]{} \equiv Si - O - Si \equiv + H_2O$$

Metal Salt

$$\equiv Si - H + HO - Si \equiv \xrightarrow[\text{metal salt}]{} \equiv Si - O - Si \equiv + H_2$$

Vinyl addition

$$\equiv Si - H + CH_2 = CH - Si \equiv \xrightarrow[Pt]{} \equiv Si - CH_2CH_2CH_2 - Si \equiv$$

Figure 2. Silicone curing systems.

Processing Techniques and Requirements

The final properties of the silicone elastomer are governed to a great extent by the kinds and amounts of filler used and by the conditions of vulcanization. The amount of catalyst used also plays a definitive role in predicting the final properties of the elastomer. Since the most widely used silicone elastomer for implantable medical devices is of the high temperature vulcanization type, we would restrict our discussions to this type of polymer only. The room temperature vulcanizing silicone elastomer finds extensive application as an adhesive for bonding silicone elastomer to metals and other polymers. The reader is referred to an excellent work by Mayhan *et al.* for further detailed information on RTV silicone elastomers [6].

The most commonly used catalyst in the high temperature vulcanizing system is dichlorobenzoyl peroxide. The unfilled elastomer has very poor tear strength and fumed silica is added as the reinforcing filler. Because of the highly branched structure of the filler, small quantities can increase the polymer viscosity tremendously as shown in Table 2 [7]. Silicone oils are added to afford the plasticizing effect for ease of process blending and also to enhance elastomer flexibility. In special cases where the elastomer has to be radiopaque, Barium sulphate is added as an additional filler. The filler, silicone oil and the silicone polymer are all blended in a roll mill. The catalyst is added as the final step to reduce premature dissociation of the catalyst. The curing or the vulcanization is done at 121°C for 10 minutes followed by a post cure at a higher temperature around 180°C for four hours.

Table 2. Effect of Filler Concentration on the Viscosity of Di-methyl Siloxane

Filler	Vol. %	Viscosity (MPa)
None	-	1.64
TiO_2	5	2.62
TiO_2	10	5.82
SiO_2	2	21.30

Silicone Elastomer Characterization

Infra-red Spectroscopy

The base polymer, polydimethyl siloxane is easily identified by infra-red spectroscopy. A typical I.R. spectrum is shown in Figure 3. Silicone polymers are readily identified by strong bands in the 1200-1000 cm^{-1} region due to the Si-o-Si stretching vibrations. Often several distinct bands appear in this region of the spectrum. Silicones also show CH_3 stretch near 2900 cm^{-1} a sharp band in the 1270-1250 cm^{-1} region (symmetrical CH_3 banding) and sharp band in the 874-740 cm^{-1} region (CH_3 rocking). In Figure 4 we compare the I.R. spectrum of a silicone elastomer containing dimethyl and methyl vinyl groups, before and after crosslinking. The effect of crosslinking on the CH_3 stretch near 2900 cm^{-1} is quite obvious. A modern I.R. spectrophotometer is shown in Figure 5.

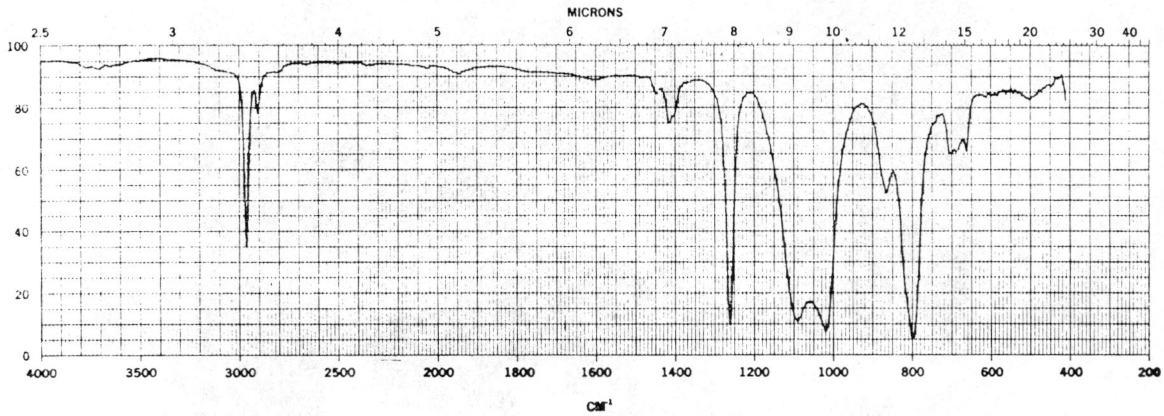

Figure 3. Infra-red spectrum of silicone polymer, polydimethyl siloxane.

Other techniques such as nuclear magnetic resonance and gel permeation chromatography have been attempted to determine the vinyl or active hydrogen content in silicone polymers, but are not very successful when the active groups are in extremely low concentrations. (Less than one reactive group occurring per 100 monomer units) [7].

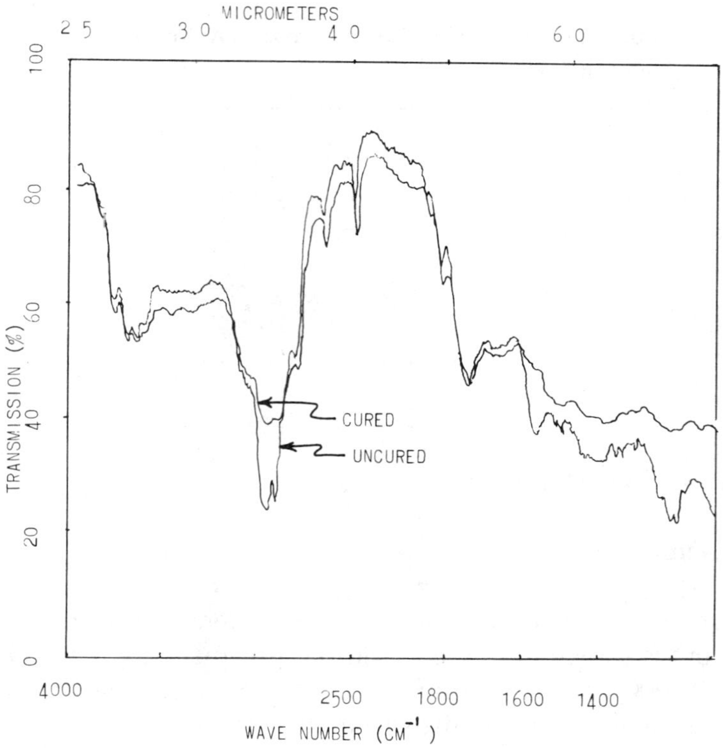

Figure 4. I.R. spectrum of silicone polymer before and after crosslinking.

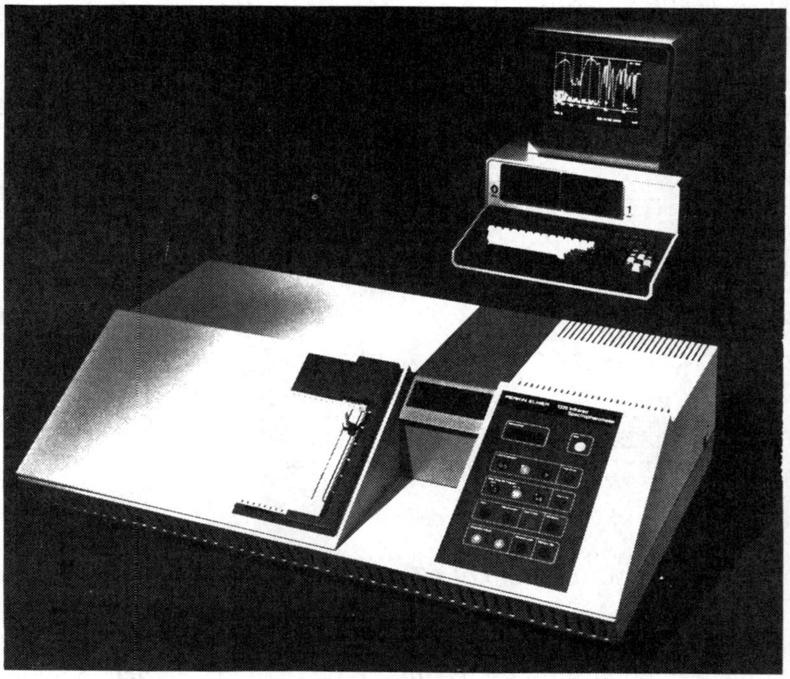

Figure 5. A modern I.R. spectrophotometer. (Courtesy of Perkin Elmer Corp., Norwalk, Conn.).

Differential Scanning Calorimetry (DSC)

As the temperature is elevated, materials undergo physical or chemical transitions which are accompanied by either absorbance or liberation of heat. The DSC measures the enthalpies of these processes by measuring the diffential heat flow required to maintain a sample of the material and an inert reference at the same temperature. For a detailed bibliography of literature on DSC the reader is referred to an excellent compilation by the Perkin Elmer Corporation [8]. A modern DSC is shown in Figure 6.

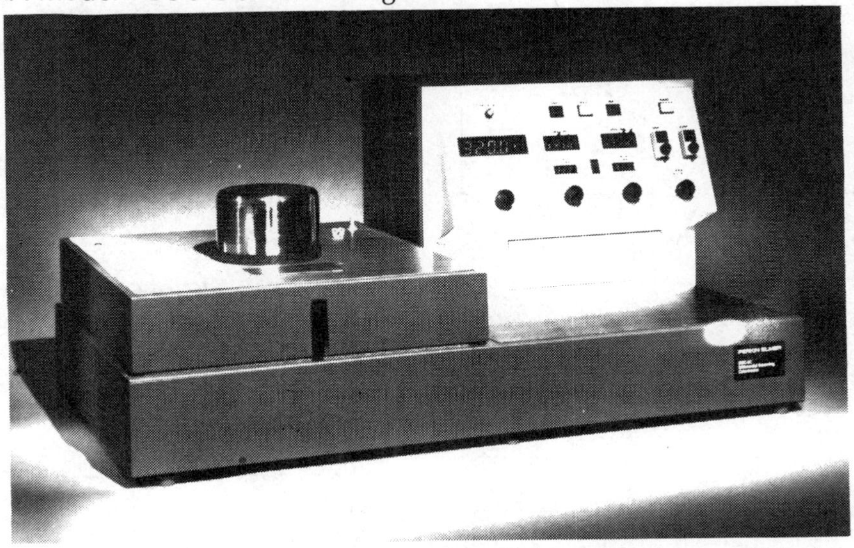

Figure 6. A modern differential scanning calorimeter. (Courtesy of Perkin Elmer Corporation, Norwalk, Conn.).

The crosslinking reaction of silicone elastomers is exothermic. The rate at which the reaction proceeds fastest is detected by the peak exothermic temperature on a typical DSC curve as shown in Figure 7. The effect of catalyst concentration on the peak exothermic temperature is shown in Figure 8. We see that with increasing catalyst concentration there is a gradual drop in the peak exothermic temperature. Using a calibration curve, one could use this technique to predict the amount of catalyst present in a random batch of compounded silicone polymer.

Effect of Catalyst Concentration on the Mechanical Properties of the Elastomer [8].

Durometer Hardness

The silicone elastomer hardness is measured using a type A shore hardness tester. This is a simple device in which one measures the depth of penetration of a pointed probe that is pressed onto a flat elastomer surface. The effect of catalyst concentration on the durometer hardness of the elastomer is shown in Figure 9. With increasing catalyst concentration the degree of crosslinking also increases leading to an overall increase in the elastomer hardness.

Ultimate Tensile Strength

The effect of catalyst concentration on the ultimate tensile strength of the elastomer is

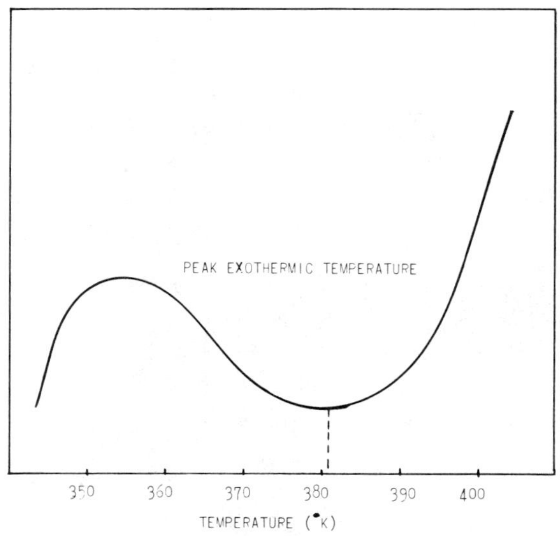

Figure 7. A typical DSC scan of a peroxide cured silicone polymer.

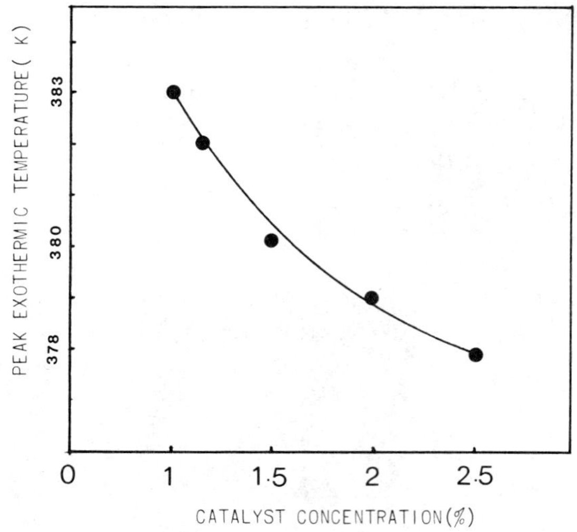

Figure 8. The effect of catalyst concentration on the peak exothermic temperature of silicone elastomer.

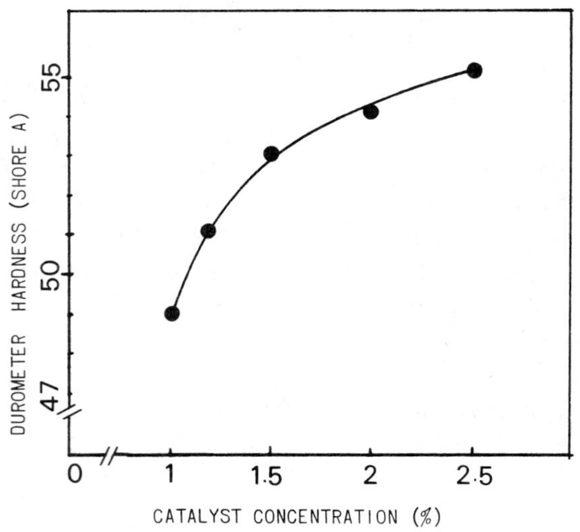

Figure 9. The effect of catalyst concentration on the durometer hardness of silicone elastomer.

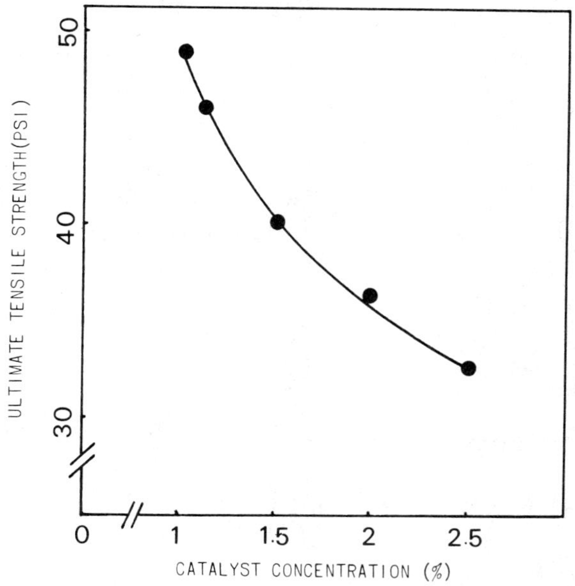

Figure 10. The effect of catalyst concentration on the ultimate tensile strength of silicone elastomer.

shown in Figure 10. At lower catalyst concentration, higher strength is obtained followed by a gradual drop in value as the catalyst concentration is increased. This could be explained by lower linear chain polymerization due to higher crosslinking at greater catalyst concentration. The highest ultimate tensile strength is obtained at a catalyst concentration of about 1%.

Extraction Studies

In the cured silicone elastomer, although the bulk of the polymer is in a stable, well crosslinked, three dimensional matrix, one would expect to find chemical species that are loosely bound or merely physically interlocked. Chief among them could be, residual peroxide catalyst, by-products such as benzoic acid (from benzoyl peroxide), low molecular weight fractions of the polymer, etc. The silicone elastomer can be analyzed for these species by extraction studies in a suitable solvent for the uncured polymer. All extractions were done in reagent grade toluene in which the elastomer swelled to three times its original volume. The extraction was carried out for 24 hours at room temperature in glass test tubes which were agitated at regular time intervals of 2 hours. The agitation serves to break up any concentration gradient being set up in the solvent and provides for fast diffusion rates of the extractables into the solvent. The swelled samples are then dried in a forced draft oven at 60°C to drive off all the solvent. The difference in the weight of the elastomer before and after extraction is the weight of the extractables.

The effect of catalyst concentration on the percent extractables is shown in Figure 11. The lowest value of the total extractables from the elastomer occurs in the vicinity of catalyst concentration of about 1.4%. At low catalyst concentrations we tend to extract more low molecular weight polymer chains due to incomplete crosslinking while at higher catalyst concentrations we create more by-products and residual catalyst.

Effect of Postcuring on Percent Extractables

Figure 12 shows the effect of catalyst concentration on the percent extractables in a silicone elastomer subjected to different post-curing conditions. The 82°C vacuum bake was an attempt to keep the post curing temperature low and achieve total volatilization of all by-

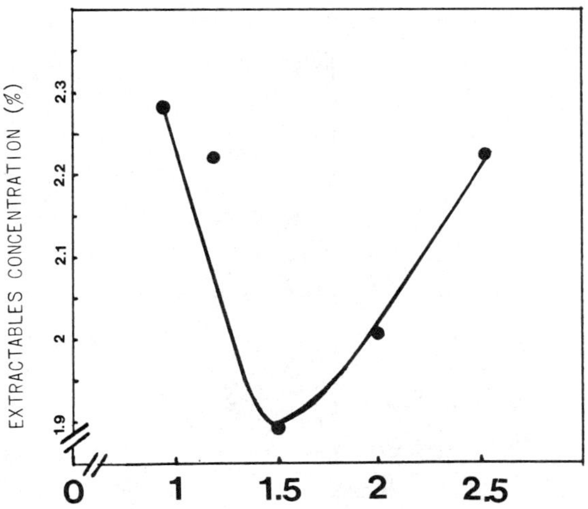

Figure 11. The effect of catalyst concentration on the extractables concentration of silicone elastomer.

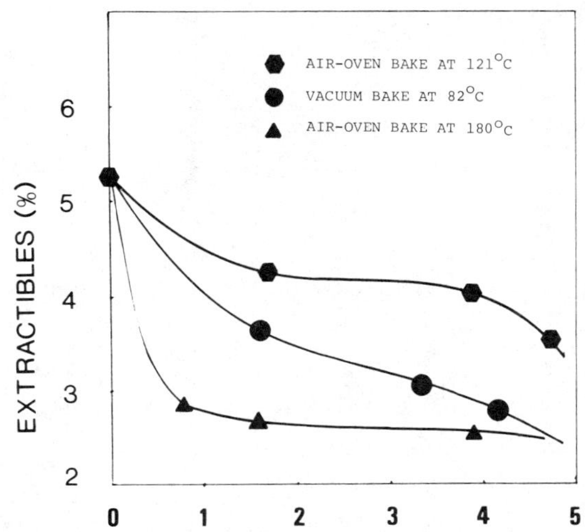

Figure 12. The effect of post curing on the extractables concentration of silicone elastomer.

products. This is significant as there are occasions where a medical device fabricated from silicone elastomer may also contain some other materials of construction that may not withstand higher post curing temperatures. A typical example is a polyurethane cardiac pacemaker lead [9]. The tubular insulation over the electrode coil is made of a tough elastomeric polyurethane while the connector that plugs into the pulse generator is made of silicone elastomer because of its superior compression set properties.

Unless the silicone elastomer is properly post cured, the impurities would leach out into the adjacent tissue fluids on implantation over a period of time. A postcure at 180°C in air appears to be the most efficient method to obtain an elastomer with minimum extractables.

Effect of Postcuring on the Hemocompatibility of Silicone Elastomer

The hemocompatibility of the elastomer was measured by determining the degree of hemolysis of the elastomer surface. The degree of homolysis was determined by making optical density measurements. Five grams of test sample were placed into each of three tubes containing 10 ml of normal Saline. After temperature equilibration to 37°C, 0.2 ml of oxylated, diluted rabbit blood was added to each tube. A control was prepared using water. All tubes were incubated for one hour and centrifuged. The optical density (O.D.) of the supernatent is determined at 545 um. The percent homolysis is calculated from the average optical density value using the following formula:

$$\% \text{ Hemolysis} = \frac{(\text{O.D. test sample}) - (\text{O.D. negative control})}{(\text{O.D. positive control}) - (\text{O.D. negative control})} \times 100$$

The results are illustrated in Figure 12.

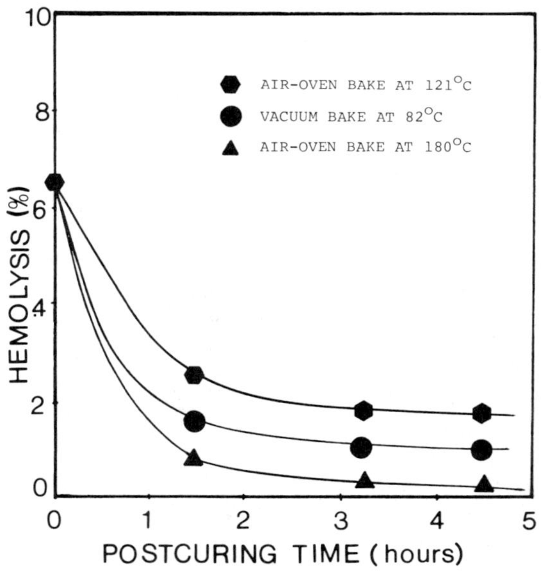

Figure 13. The effect of post curing on the surface hemolysis of silicone elastomer.

The purpose of the postcure is to volatilize any residual peroxides, benzoic acid and contamination such as sweat. It also serves to complete the crosslinking reaction to the maximum. If a cured silicone elastomer is not postcured, it exhibits a phenomenon called "blooming." A white powdery coating appears on the surface, which is in fact the peroxide catalyst and by-products of the crosslinking reaction. The presence of these reactive chemicals on the elastomer surface, causes it to exhibit a high degree of hemolysis. These residual chemicals would eventually diffuse to the surface of the device *in vivo*, causing undesirable tissue and hemolytic reactions. While the postcuring at 180°C appears to be the most efficient, the vacuum bake technique at a reduced temperature appears to be a good second choice.

CONCLUSION

The processing of silicone elastomer for implantable biomedical device applications has to be monitored under stringent conditions to ensure that the final elastomer would be truly biocompatible. The characterization techniques for the physical properties of the elastomer are well established and relatively easy to perform. We hope that the methods outlined here would pave the way for better characterizationof silicone elastomer for long term implantable applications.

REFERENCES

1. Carmen, R. and Kahn, P. "In Vitro Testing of Silicone Rubber Heart Valve Poppets for Lipid Absorption," *J. Biomed. Mat. Res.*, 2, 457-464, (1968).
2. Meester, W. D. and Swanson, A. B., "*In Vivo* Testing of Silicone Rubber Joint Implants for Lipid Absorption," *J. Biomed. Mat. Res.*, 6, 193-199, (1972).
3. Swanson, A. B., Meester, W. D., Swanson, G., Rangaswamy, L., Deg., and Schut, G. E. D., *Ortho. Clin. N. Am.*, 4, 1097, (1973).
4. Ward, T. C. and Perry, T. J., "Dynamic Mechanical Properties of Medical Grade Silicone Elastomer Stored in Simulated Body Fluids," *J. Biomed. Mat. Res.*, 15, 511-525, (1981).
5. Arkels, B. C., "New Generation Silicones for Medical Devices," *Medical Device and Diagnostics Industry*, Vol. 3, No. 4., April, 1981.
6. Mayhan, K. G., Hahn, A. W., Dortch, S. W., Wu, S. H., Peace, B. W., Biolsi, M. E., and Bertrand, G. L., "The Effect of Catalyst Concentration on the Cured Properties of a Medical Grade RTV Silicone Elastomer," Intern. J. Polymeric Materials, 1977, Vol. 5., pp. 231-249.
7. Warrick, E. L., "Silicone Rubber: A Perspective," Rubber Chemistry and Technology, V. 49., (4), pp. 909-936, (1976).
8. James, M. P., Barrall II, E. M., Dawson, B., and Logan, J. A., "Crosslinking of Methyl Silicone Rubbers, Part II. Analysis of Extractables from Samples Crosslinked under Various Conditions." Polymer Characterization by Thermal Methods of Analysis; Editor Jen Chiu, New York, Marcel Dekker, 135-155, 1974.
9. Devanathan, T., and Carr, R., "Silicone Rubber: Some Simple Characterization Techniques," Presented at SPE, ANTEC N.Y.C., May 1, 1980.
10. Devanthan, T., Sluetz, J. E., and Young, K. A., "In Vivo Thrombogenicity of Implantable Cardiac Pacemaker Leads," *Biomat. Med. Dev. Art. Org.*, Vol. 8, No. 4., 1980.

Chapter 34

An Overview of Current Biomedical Considerations Involving Electrodes for Chronic Neural Stimulation

David J. Burke
Biomedical Engineer
Biomedical Systems Division
Thermo Electron
Waltham, MA 02254

ABSTRACT

An overview of current biomedical considerations involving electrodes for chronic neural stimulation is presented. Tables and text summarize the results of recent investigations concerning tissue reactions and electrode degredation as a result of long term neural stimulation.

INTRODUCTION

In recent years considerable research has been directed toward the development of sophisticated neuroprosthetic devices for use in the central nervous system. Before such devices can become a clinical reality, fundamental questions involving the safety and reliability of functional neural stimulation must be answered. It is not the purpose of this discussion to present a comprehensive review. Rather it is to provide a brief overview of the salient materials and electrochemical aspects of chronic neural stimulation with emphasis on current areas of concern.

ELECTRODE MATERIALS

The ideal neural electrode material is one that will perform reliably and predictably for many years under conditions of continuous electrical stimulation. Criteria for the selection of such a material include: (1) good mechanical stability, (2) high resistance to corrosion, (3) minimal toxicity to body tissues, and (4) long term electrical stability. Unfortunately, in practice no presently available material fully satisfies all of these criteria. Material selection often involves compromises based on its particular application.

Of the many potential electrode materials studied, passive corrosion and tissue toxicity have precluded the use of several candidate materials [14,22,28,42,44]. Studies involving copper and silver have consistently shown these materials to be toxic and necrotic to neural tissue [3,14,26]. Similarly, the propensity for corrosion exhibited by stainless steel when pulsed biphasically has limited its use in chronic stimulation [19,28,43,44]. However, there is some evidence that biphasic pulsing employing a small charge imbalance may significantly reduce the amount of corrosion with stainless steel electrodes [30]. Platinum and platinum alloys have been the most extensively investigated electrode materials and consistently display the best overall electrode characteristics. Despite its relative inertness, in vitro studies have shown that platinum is susceptible to severe damage when pulsed for long periods of time at high current densities [22,24]. These studies have also shown that rhodium is only moderately damaged at the same current densities. A recent study by Robblee et al. [36]. indicates that the addition of human serum albumin to their saline test solutions drastically reduced the dissolution of platinum electrodes. Interestingly, the application of current is required to initiate this corrosion resistance but is not necessary to maintain it.

Other electrode materials such as gold, irridium, and tantalum have been subject to considerable study although none have received the general acceptance accorded platinum and its alloys. Table 1 presents results from some of the more recent studies concerning electrode dissolution and electrical instability involving the aforementioned materials.

ELECTROCHEMICAL CONSIDERATIONS

Charge Transfer

As with any electrical circuit the use of bioelectrodes to convey information requires a flow of current through the system. The flow of current within a metallic electrode is due to the movement of electrons. Current flow within a liquid system, biological fluids in this case, requires the migration of ions. It is at the electrode-tissue interface that electron conduction is

Table 1.

MATERIAL	ENVIRONMENT	STIMULATION PARAMETERS	EVALUATION	RESULTS	REF.
Pt	Cat brain	Bi, .5msec, 50Hz, 0.6A/cm^2, 300μC/cm^2/phase, 40 hrs.	Pathology	Significant damage	5
Pt	NaCl sol'n	Bi (AF), 4.0msec, 50Hz, 10.0mA/mm^2, 120 hrs. (max).	Electrode dissolution	Significant dissolution	7
Pt	Monkey brain	Bi, 1.0msec, 10Hz, 0.5μC/phase, 7.4μC/cm^2/phase, 205 hrs.	Pathology	No damage	8
Pt	Monkey brain	Bi, 1.0msec, 10Hz, 22.0μC/phase, 323.4μC/cm^2/phase, 205 hrs.	Pathology	Extensive damage	8
Pt	NaCl sol'n	Bi (CF), 33Hz, 100mA/real cm^2, 200μC/real cm^2, 22 hrs.	Chloride oxidation	Insignificant amounts	9
Pt (platinized)	NaCl sol'n	Bi (CF), 33Hz, 100mA/real cm^2, 300μC/cm^2,	Platinum dissolution	Minimal dissolution	9
Pt	Monkey brain	Mono, 1.0msec, 10Hz, 30.0mA/cm^2, 30μC/cm^2, 2.4μC/phase, 205 hrs.	Pathology	Extensive damage	12
Pt	Human Cochlear	Bi, mono, 0.25msec, 200Hz.	Impedance and Threshold	Stable	15
Pt	Simulated CSF	Bi (CF), 0.5msec, 50Hz, 1.0A/cm^2, 1100 hrs. (max).	Corrosion damage	Severe damage	24
Pt	Simulated CSF	Bi (AF), 0.5msec, 50Hz, 0.1A/cm^2.	Corrosion damage	Moderate damage	24
Pt	NaCl sol'n	Bi (CF), 50.0mA/cm^{-2}, 400μC/cm^{-2}, 12 hrs. (max).	Electrode dissolution	Significant dissolution	29
Pt	NaCl sol'n	Bi (CF), 200 mA/cm^{-2}, 100μC/cm^{-2}, 12 hrs. (max).	Electrode dissolution	Slight dissolution	29
Pt	Cat brain	Bi, 0.25msec, 50Hz, 3.0mA, 0.75μC/phase, 48.7μC/cm^2/phase, 36 hrs.	Pathology	Minimal damage	35
Pt	Cat brain	Bi, 0.5msec, 50Hz, 6.0mA, 3.0μC/phase, 300μC/cm^2/phase, 36 hrs.	Pathology	Significant damage	35
Pt-10%Ir	Stimulated CSF	Bi (CF), 0.5msec, 50Hz, 1.0A/cm^2, 1582 hrs. (max).	Corrosion damage	Severe damage	24
Pt-10%Ir	Simulated CSF	Bi (CF), 0.5msec, 50Hz, 0.1A/cm^2, 1582 hrs. (max).	Corrosion damage	Moderate damage	24
Pt-10%Ir	Cat Cochlear	Bi, 0.1msec, 25Hz, 200μC/real cm^2/phase (max), 1000 hrs. (max).	Pathology	Significant damage	41
Pt-10%Rh	Simulated CSF	Bi (CF), 0.5msec, 50Hz, 1.0A/cm^2, 500 hrs.	Corrosion damage	Severe damage	24
Pt-10%Rh	Cat Cochlear	Bi, mono, 0.1msec, 30 months.	Pathology	No stimulation damage	37
Au	Cat brain	Bi, 0.5msec, 50Hz, 0.6A/cm^2, 300μC/cm^2/phase, 40 hrs.	Pathology	Significant damage	5
Au	Stimulated CSF	Bi (CF), 0.5msec, 50Hz, 1.0A/cm^2, 1582 hrs. (max).	Corrosion damage	Massive damage	24
Au	Simulated CSF	Bi (CF), 0.5msec, 50Hz, 0.1A/cm^2, 1582 hrs.	Corrosion damage	Very light damage	24
Ir	Simulated CSF	Bi (CF), 0.5msec, 50Hz, 1.0A/cm^2, 736 hrs.	Corrosion damage	Severe damage	24
Ir	Simulated CSF	Bi (CF), 0.5msec, 50Hz, 0.1A/cm^2, 736 hrs.	Corrosion damage	Very light damage	24
Rh	Cat brain	Bi, 0.5msec, 50Hz, 0.6A/cm2, 300μC/cm^2/phase, 40 hrs.	Pathology	Severe damage	5
Rh	Simulated CSF	Bi (CF), 0.5msec, 50Hz, 1.0A/cm^2, 2972 hrs. (max).	Corrosion damage	Light damage	24
Rh	Cat brain	Bi, 0.4msec, 50Hz, 3.0ma, 1.2μC/phase, 120μC/cm^2/phase, 36 hrs.	Pathology	Significant damage	35
Ta_2O_5	Cat brain	Mono, 0.25msec, 50Hz, 3.0ma, 93.5μC/cm^2	Pathology	Minimal damage	6
Ta_2O_5	Cat brain	Bi, 01.msec, 500H[illegible] 3.0ma, .3μC/phase, 38μC/c[illegible] /phase, 36 hrs.	Pathology	No damage	35

translated to ionic conduction and the actual charge transfer process occurs. The electrochemical nature of this change transfer process is the primary determinant of the efficacy of a particular electrode systen.

The application of a potential, lower than its galvanic potential, to an electrode initiates a non-faradaic (capacitive) charge transfer process. This is due to the formation of a charge gradient known as the electrical double layer at the electrode tissue interface. Following a very brief surge of current, the electrode surface contains an excess of electrical charges of one polarity. In turn, these charges attract the mobile ions in the surrounding solution to form a layer of opposite charge directly adjacent to the electrode surface. This charged layer is composed of two distinct regions. The first contains the inner Helmholtz portion involving strongly adsorbed ions. In combination with this is the outer Helmholtz portion involving somewhat more loosely adsorbed ions. These two portions are collectively termed the rigid double layer [4]. The second region is more diffuse in nature. Here the predominance of one particular charge decreases as a function of the distance from the electrode. This continues until the ratio of signs equals that of the bulk of the solution. The double layer charging mechanism continues until the applied potential (overvoltage) exceeds the specific polarization potential of the electrode material. At this point the electrode is polarized and current flow is due to the predominance of faradic reactions. Within limits, the corresponding oxidation-reduction reactions proceed in proportion to the applied potential.

Polarization

Electrochemical polarization is an integral, albeit undesirable component of the faradic process. At low current densities an electrode behaves as a fairly linear resistance that approximately follows Ohm's law [18]. However, at current densities commonly used for neural stimulation there is a sharp departure from linearity manifested as a decrease in resistance and an increase of capacitance at the electrode [13,32,38]. The practical consequences of this process result in a significant waste of applied energy as well as potential electrode degradation [27,18].

The polarization effects that must be overcome to maintain a continuous current flow may be divided into three general groups: 1) ohmic, 2) concentration, and 3) kinetic [27,39]. The ohmic potential is simply a measure of the electrical potential necessary to overcome the ionic resistance to movement toward the electrode. The required potential is proportional to the current flow and follows Ohm's law. Certain localized effects such as concentration variations and deposit formation may cause variations from predicted values [4]. Concentration polarization occurs when the rate of ionic migration from the bulk of the solution to the electrode is insufficient to maintain a current flow commensurate with the ohmic potential. The rate of mass transfer and hence the degree of polarization is determined by diffusion, electrostatic forces, and agitation or convective solution movement. The final polarization effect is that of kinetic polarization. This process has an exponential relationship to current density and is dependent upon the rate at which the electrochemical reactions proceed at the electrode. Unlike concentration polarization, the current flow is controlled by the rate of electron transfer rather than by the rate of mass transfer [39]. The primary contributors to this process are electrode material, current density, and the presence of gaseous reaction products.

Greatbatch, et al. [17,18] have described the polarization effects for several distinct classes of electrode materials based on the chemistry of their coupling reactions. The noble metals, specifically platinum, exhibit very similar polarization voltages under both anodic and cathodic conditions. In addition, at low currents platinum requires low driving voltages. Silver metals are interesting in that they are cathodically polarizable but not polarizable when driven as an anode. However, the apparent toxicity of silver [3,14] generally precludes its use in chronic situations. Finally, the non-noble metals, such as stainless steel, exhibit high polarization voltages for low currents and are susceptible to corrosion under anodic conditions.

Charge Injection

The effectiveness of any chronic stimulation scheme is ultimately bound to successful modulation of the electrochemistry of the charge transfer process. Quite often practical stimulation requires potentials that result in a faradaic charge transfer process [10,13]. An important consideration is the reversibility of the resulting oxidation and reduction reactions. A reversible reaction effectively confines the reaction products to the surface of the electrodes. A much less desirable situation occurs in the presence of irreversible reactions where possibly harmful reaction products may migrate from the electrodes to the surrounding tissue [13].

Brummer and Turner [10] have described several potentially toxic reactions possible with platinum electrodes. The anodic reactions involve the electrolysis of water, oxidation of saline, oxidation of platinum, and the oxidation of organic compounds. The evolution of hydrogen is possible as a cathodic reaction. All of these reactions present the possibility of tissue damage under conditions of long term stimulation. They have also proposed three electrochemically attractive charge injection processes. The first, double layer charging is reversible and non-faradaic. The second is surface oxidation which involves readily reversible oxidation and reduction reactions. The final process is hydrogen atom plating which occurs at low potentials and again is readily reversible. Greatbatch [17] has proposed that the primary charge transfer mechanism with platinum electrodes involves a reversible catalytic adsorption and deadsorption of oxygen on the electrode surface. This process is particularly interesting when considering the very large capacitance [32] often found with platinum electrodes.

There are many factors that determine the class, and consequently the reversibility of the reactions occurring at the electrode surface. Although the geometry of the stimulus waveform and its corresponding charge density appear to be the most influential parameters affecting this process for a particular electrode material [9,10,11,34]. Concern with the possible deliterious effects of the faradaic process has led to the general employment of biphasic stimulus waveforms similar to those proposed by Lily, et al. [25]. In a symmetrical biphasic pulsing regimen a pulse of one polarity is followed by another pulse of opposite polarity and equal magnitude. Theoretically, the ongoing chemical reactions are reversed with each change of pulse polarity resulting in zero net charge transfer. However, several investigators [2,10,13] have noted that a symmetrical waveform does not assure a corresponding symmetry in the resulting chemical reactions. The use of charge balanced waveforms that temporarily compensate for the differences in reaction kinetics alleviates much of the chemical asymmetry [13]. Studies have been conducted [5,9,34] to evaluate dissolution and/or tissue response using smooth and roughened platinum electrodes. The results have indicated that the roughened electrodes caused less tissue damage and have lower dissolution rates than those with smooth surfaces. The correspondingly lower charge density found on roughened electrodes seems to imply that charge density is the major parameter affecting tissue damage and electrode dissolution. There are very definite limits to the amount of charge that can be reversibly delivered using a biphasic pulsing regimen. Brummer and Turner [11] have reported that the maximum theoretica non-gassing limit for platinum electrodes, in simulated CSF, is 350 ± 50 uC/real cm² over a current density range of ±50 to ±450 mA/cm².

TISSUE REACTIONS

The overriding concern of this discussion as well as much of the current neuroprosthetic research [21] involves the long term delivery of safe neural stimulation. Encouraging results have been reported for long term stimulation of peripheral nerves [31,33] and particularly with electrophrenic respiration [16]. In contrast, the assessments of neural damage from chronic stimulation of the brain have been mixed (Table 1).

As previously mentioned, hydrolysis and toxic dissolution products are the primary electrochemical causes of tissue damage. The determining variables of these processes appear to be electrode material, stimulus geometry, and charge/current density. Agnew, et al. [1] have used platinum salt injections to investigate the possibility that platinum electrode dissolution is a significant factor in the cause of tissue damage. Their results showed that pronounced tissue changes did occur although the changes were somewhat different from those observed with chronic stimulation. Rhodium has been reported to be toxic even as a passive implant [5], however previous [14] and subsequent [34] studies have not supported this contention.

A promising alternative to faradaic charge injection with conventional electrodes is the development of capacitor electrodes. This process employs modulation of the double layer which eliminates the undesirable effects of oxidation and reduction reactions. Guyton and Hambrecht [20] have described tantalum-tantalum pentoxide electrodes capable of delivery 2.5 μc in each pulse. Furthermore, studies utilizing tantalum and tantalum pentoxide under active and passive conditions have shown these materials to possess a high degree of inertness in neural environment [3,6,23,28].

Table 1 presents results from some of the more recent studies concerning tissue reactions as a result of electrical stimulation.

REFERENCES

1. Agnew, W. F., Yuen, T. G., Pudenz, R. H. and Bullara, L. A.: Neuropathological effects of intracerebral platinum salt injections. J. Neuropathol. Exp. Neurol. 36:633-46, 1977.
2. Bartlett, J. R., Doty, R. W., Lee, B. B., Negrao, N. and Overman, W. H.: Deleterious effects of prolonged electrical excitation of striate cortex in Macagues. Brain Behav. Evol. 14:46-66, 1977.
3. Bates, J. I., Lewey, F. H. and Reiners, C. R.: The reaction of cerebral tissue to silver, tantalum, and zirconium. J. Neurosurg. 5:349-53, 1948.
4. Bauer, H. H.: Electrodics. George Thieme Publishers Stuttgart John Wiley & Sons, New York — Toronto, 1972.
5. Bernstein,J. J., Johnson, P. F., Hench, L. L., Hunter, G. and Dawson, W. W.: Cortical histopathology following stimulation with metallic and carbon electrodes. Brain Behav. Evol. 14:126-157, 1977.
6. Bernstein, J. J., Hench, L. L., Johnson, P. F., Dawson, W. W. and Hunter, G.: Stimulation of the cortex with tantalum pentoxide capacitive electrodes. In Hambrecht and Reswick, Functional Electrical Stimulation: Applications in Neural Prostheses. P. 465-77. Marcel Dekker, New York, 1977.
7. Black, R. C. and Hannaker, P.: Dissolution of smooth platinum electrodes in biological fluids. Appl. Neurolphysiol. 42:366-74, 1980.
8. Brown, W. J., Babb, T. L., Soper, H. V., Lieb, J. P., Ottino, C. A. and Crandall, P. H.: Tissue reactions

to long term electrical stimulation of the cerebellum in monkeys. J. Neurosurg. 47:366-79, 1977.
9. Brummer, S. B., McHardy, J. and Turner, M. J.: Electrical stimulation with pt electrodes: Trace analysis for dissolved platinum and other dissolved electrochemical products. Brain Behav. Evol. 14:10-22, 1977.
10. Brummer, S. B. and Turner, M. J.: Electrochemical considerations for safe electrical stimulation of the nervous system with platinum electrodes. IEE Trans. Biomed. Eng. 24:59-63, 1977.
11. Brummer, S. B. and Turner, M. J.: Electrical stimulation with pt electrodes: II – Estimation of maximum surface redox (theoretical non-gassing) limits. IEE Trans. Biomed. Eng. 24:440-43, 1977.
12. Dauth, G. W., Defendini, R., Gilman, S., Tennyson, V. M. and Kremzner, L.: Long-term surface stimulation of the cerebellum in the monkey. Surg. Neurol. 7:377-84, 1977.
13. Dymond, A. M.: Characteristics of the metal-tissue interface of stimulation electrodes. IEE Trans. Biomed. Eng. 23:274-80, 1976.
14. Dymond, A. M., Kaechele, L. E., Jurist, J. M. and Crandall, P. H.: Brain tissue reaction to some chronically implanted metals. J. Neurosurg. 33:574-80, 1970.
15. Eddington, D. K., Dobelle, W. H., Brackmann, D. E., Mladejovsky, M. G. and Parkin, J. L.: Auditory research with multiple channel intracochlear stimulation in man. Ann. Otol. Rhinol. Laryngol. 87:1-29, 1978.
16. Glenn, W. W. L., Holcomb, W. G., Shaw, R. K., Hogan, J. F. and Holschuh, K. R.: Long term ventilatory support by diaphragm pacing in quadriplegia. Ann. Surg. 183:566-77, 1976.
17. Greatbatch, W.: Electrochemical criteria for selection of chronically implanted stimulating electrodes. In McCutcheon, Chronically Implanted Cardiovascular Instrumentation, p. 175-83. Academic Press, New York, 1973.
18. Greatbatch, W., Piersma, B., Shannon, F. D. and Calhoon, S. W.: Polarization phenomena relating to physiological electrodes. Ann. N.Y. Acad. Sci. 167:722-44, 1969.
19. Greatbatch, W.: Electrochemical polarization of physiological electrodes. Med. Res. Eng. 6:13-17, 1967.
20. Guyton, D. L. and Hambrecht, F. T.: Theory and design of capacitor electrodes for chronic stimulation. Med. Biol. Eng. 12:613-619, 1974.
21. Hambrecht, F. T.: Neural prostheses. Ann. Rev. Biophys. Bioeng. 8:239-67, 1979.
22. Hench, L. L. and Ethridge, E. C.: Biomaterials – The interfacial problem. In Brown and Dickson, Advances in Biomedical Engineering, p. 116-27. Academic Press, New York, 1975.
23. Johnson, P. F., Bernstein, J. J., Hunter, G., Dawson, W. W. and Hench, L. L.: An in vitro and in vivo analysis of anodized tantalum capacitive electrodes: corrosion, response, physiology, and histology. J. Biomed. Mater. Res. 11:637-656, 1977.
24. Johnson, P. F. and Hench, L. L. An in vitro analysis of metals for use in the neural environment. Brain Behav. Eval. 14:23-45, 1977.
25. Lilly, J. C., Hughes, J. R., Alvard, E. C. and Gallein, T. W.: Brief noninjurious electric waveform for stimulation of the brain. Science 121:468-69, 1955.
26. Loucks, R. B., Weinberg, H. and Smith, M.: The erosion of electrodes by small currents. Electroenceph. Clin. Neurophysiol. 11:823-26, 1959.
27. Mansfield, P. B.: Myocardial stimulation: the electrochemistry of electrode-tissue coupling. Am. J. Physiol. 212:1475-488, 1967.
28. McFadden, J. T.: Metallurgical principles in neurosurgery. J. Neurosurg. 31:373-85, 1969.
29. McHardy, J., Robblee, L. S., Marston, J. M. and Brummer, S. B.: Electrical stimulation with pt electrodes. IV. Factors influencing pt dissolution in organic saline. Biomaterials. 1:129-34, 1980.
30. McHardy, J., Geller, D. and Brummer, S. B.: An approach to corrosion control during electrical stimulation. Ann. Biomed. Eng. 5:144-49, 1977.
31. McNeal, D. R., Waters, R. and Reswick, J.: Experience with implanted electrodes at Rancho Los Amigos Hospital. Appl. Neurophysiol. 40:235-239, 1977-78.
32. Pollak, V.: An equivalent diagram for the interface impedance of metal needle electrodes. Med. Biol. Eng. 12:454-59, 1974.

33. Pudenz, R. H., Agnew, W. F., Yuen, T. G. H., Bullara, L. A., Jacques, S. and Shelded, C. H.: Adverse effects of electrical energy applied to the nervous system. Appl Neurophysiol. 40:72-87, 1977-78.
34. Pudenz, R. H., Agnew, W. F. and Bullara, L. A.: Effects of electrical stimulation of brain. Brain Behav. Evol. 14:103-125, 1977.
35. Pudenz, R. H., Agnew, W. F., Yuen, T. G. H. and Bullara, L. A.: Electrical stimulation of brain. In Hambrecht and Reswick, Functional Electrical Stimulation: Applications in Neural Protheses, p. 437-57, Marcel Dekker, New York, 1977.
36. Robblee, L. S., McHardy, J., Marston,J. M. and Brummer, S. B.: Electrical stimulation with pt electrodes. V. The effect of protein on pt dissolution. Biomaterials.: 1:135-139, 1980.
37. Schindler, R. A., Merzenich, M. M., White, M. W. and Bjorkroth, B.: Multielectrode intracochlear implants. Arch. Otolaryngol. 103:691-99, 1977.
38. Schwan, H. P.: Electrode polarization impedance measurements in biological materials. Ann. N.Y. Acad. Sci., 148:191-209, 1968.
39. Skoog, D. A. and West, D. M.: Principles of Instrumental Analysis. Saunders College/Holt, Rinehart and Winston, Philadelphia, 1980.
40. Vaquero, J., Lozano, A. P., Oya, S., Manrique, M. and Bravo, G.: Chronic implanting of electrodes in the cerebellar vermis of the cat. Acta. Neurochir (Wien). 46:259-66, 1979.
41. Walsh, S. M., Leake-Jones, P. A., Vurek, L. S. and Merzenich, M. M.: Chronic electrical stimulation with intracochlear electrodes. Ann. Otol. Rhinol. Laryngol. 90 (Suppl. 82):27-29, 1981.
42. Weisman, S.: Metals for implantation in the human body. Ann. N.Y. Acad. Sci. 146:80-95, 1968.
43. Wetzel, M. C., Howell, L. G. and Bearie, K. J.: Experimental performance of steel and platinum electrodes with chronic menophasic stimulation of the brain. J. Neurosurg. 31:658-69, 1969.
44. White, R. L. and Gross, T. J.: An evaluation of the resistance to electrolysis of metals for use in biostimulation probes. IEE Trans. Biomed. Eng. 21:487-90, 1974.

Chapter 35

Using Polycarbonate in Biomedical Applications

Stuart L. Cohen, Ph.D.
Mobay Chemical Corporation
Plastics and Coatings Division
Pittsburgh, Pennsylvania 15205

ABSTRACT

An overview of polycarbonate medical applications is provided. Emphasis is placed on sterilization techniques and the effects they have on polycarbonate. Brief discussions of structure and chemistry, chemical compatibility, design, processing and secondary operations are included. Some examples are presented.

I. INTRODUCTION

The medical industry is one of the most demanding market areas for plastic materials. It is not uncommon for a medical device to require clarity, strength and toughness along with blood and/or tissue compatibility. In addition to these, the candidate plastic must be sterilizable by one of several methods. Very few materials can meet such exacting requirements. Polycarbonate (specifically bisphenol A polycarbonate) is a thermoplastic that, in many instances, can meet the needs of the medical market.

In addition to meeting physical property and appearance necessities, polycarbonate has performed admirably when subjected to steam, ethylene oxide or radiation sterilization. Polycarbonate is used in such diverse applications as blood oxygenators and animal cages – applications where its clarity and unique combination of properties make it an ideal choice, whether for single-use items or for repetitive service.

II THE POLYCARBONATE MOLECULE

A polycarbonate is a polymeric ester of a diol and caronic acid. Unlike their polyester cousin, poly(ethylene terephthalate), which can be produced directly from the diol – ethylene glycol and the dicarboxylic acid terephthalic acid via 1, direct combination of a diol and carbonic acid per *2* is not possible. Carbonic acid exists only in meager quantities in dilute aqueous solutions of carbon dioxide.

1 $\text{HO-R-OH} + \text{HOOC-R'-COOH} \longrightarrow (\text{R-OOC-R-COO})_x + H_2O$

R = ethylene $(\text{-}CH_2CH_2\text{-})$

R' = p-phenylene 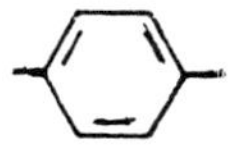

2 $\text{HO-R-OH} + H_2CO_3 \not\longrightarrow (\text{R-OCOO})_x + H_2O$

Like polyesters, however, polycarbonate polymers can be produced by other polycondensation methods, such as those shown in 3 and 4, below. Reaction 4 is usually carried out in the presence of an acid scavenger. An excellent review of polycarbonate history, chemistry and physics is given by Schnell [Ref. 1].

3 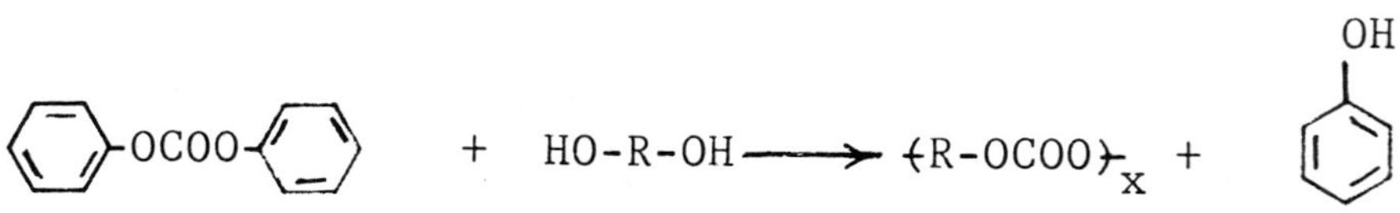

diphenyl carbonate   a diol   a polycarbonate   phenol

4 Cl-CO-Cl + HO-R-OH → $(R\text{-}OCOO)_x$ + HCl

carbonyl dichloride   a diol   a polycarbonate

("phosgene")

For our purposes, polycarbonate will be defined as the condensation polymer of bisphenol A – [2,2-bis(4-hydroxyphenyl)propane] – and phosgene (carbonyl dichloride) according to *5*. Of course, this reaction is generally applicable to any reactive diol and a diacid dichloride.

5 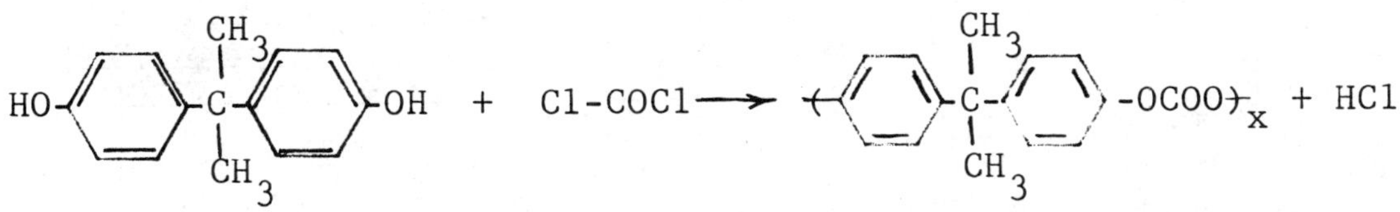

bisphenol A   phosgene   "polycarbonate"

Although a number of polycarbonate and copolycarbonate resins have been prepared (by various methods), the only polymer that has found wide application is the polycarbonate made from bisphenol A. Much of this information is found in the patent literature. Reference 1 may be consulted for a plethora of examples and literature citings.

Polycarbonate is extraordinarily useful as is, but in order to have utility in food contact or biomedical applications, the polymer is freed of extractives down to a maximum of 0.15% by weight of resin in accordance with CFR Title 21, Section 177.1580, p. 216. For a polycarbonate item to be used in blood- or tissue-contact applications, however, the manufacturer of that item also must ensure that it complies with the standards found in USP XX.

III. GENERAL PROPERTIES

Polycarbonate manufacturers commonly supply a variety of grades to meet different molding and performance requirements. The medium molecular weight (M-MW) grade is usually a general-purpose resin which offers good melt flow characteristics for molding parts having relatively thick wall sections. The high molecular weight (H-MW) polymer is well suited to applications requiring the ultimate physical properties of polycarbonate. Lower molecular weight (L-MW) material (than M-MW) is also available; it shuld be used for enhanced flow length in thin sections and when the application does not demand the maximum properties that polycarbonate can offer. In general (as with most thermoplastics), the higher the molecular weight, the better the engineering properties.

Figure 1 shows the different spiral flow lengths obtained from the three molecular weight grades when molded under similar conditions.

IV PHYSICAL PROPERTIES

Table 1 [References 2,3,4] lists the common physical properties of polycarbonate. Among these are:

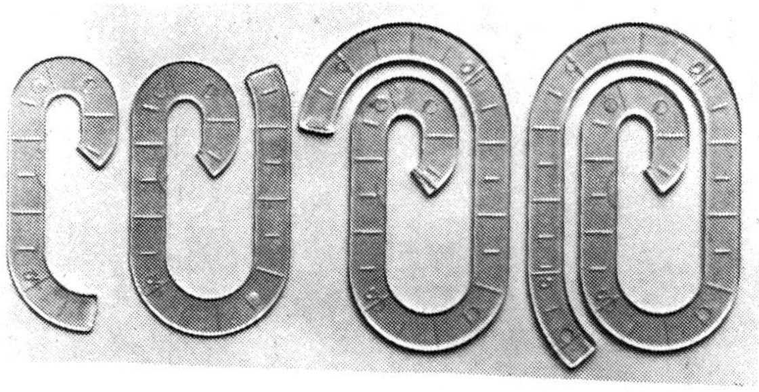

Figure 1. Spiral flow specimens of high, medium and low molecular weight polycarbonate, molded under the same conditions.

Table 1. Physical Properties of Unfilled Polycarbonate Injection Molding Resin

	Units		Properties	
	SI	ENG	SI	ENG
PROCESSING PROPERTIES				
Molding Melt Temp.	°C	°F	271-293	520-560
Linear Mold Shrinkage	mm/mm	in/in	0.005-0.007	
Specific Gravity	-	-	1.20	
Water Abs. (24 hr, Imm.)	%		0.15	
MECHANICAL PROPERTIES				
Tensile Strength @ Yield	MPa	psi	62.0	9000
Tensile Strength @ Break	MPa	psi	65.5	9500
Elongation @ Break	%		110	
Tensile Modulus	MPa	psi	2350	345,000
Flexural Strength	MPa	psi	93	13,500
Flexural Modulus	MPa	psi	2340	340,000
Izod Impact, Notched R.T., 3.2mm (0.125 in)	J/m	ft-lbf/in	745-855	14-16
Hardness Rockwell	M-Scale		62-70	
Hardness, Rockwell	R-Scale		110-120	
THERMAL PROPERTIES				
Coeff. of Lin. Therm. Exp.	1/°C	1/°F	6.8×10^{-5}	3.8×10^{-5}
Heat Deflection Temp.				
@ 0.46 MPa (66 psi)	°C	°F	138	280
@ 1.82 MPa (264 psi)	°C	°F	132	270
OPTICAL PROPERTIES				
Haze	%		1-2	
Transmittance	%		88-91	
Yellowness Index	-		1-4	

Impact Strength: Parts properly fabricated of polycarbonate will sustain an impact force of 300 ft · lb or more without fracturing. In Izod impact tests, using 1/8″ bars, values of 12 to 18 ft · lb per notched inch are attained, placing polycarbonate among the toughest materials in the thermoplastics family.

Transparency: Among plastics, polycarbonate has exceptional optical properties and special grades often are formulated to meet exacting optical requirements. Polycarbonate generally has light transmittance values of 88-91% as compared to 92% for clear plate glass. Distortion is also very low and haze value is only 1-2%.

Dimensional Stability: Polycarbonate has excellent retention of properties in most normal use ranges. Finished part dimensions do not change radically due to environmental conditions such as temperature variations and humidity. This feature qualifies it for very close tolerance requirements.

High Temperature Stability: Polycarbonate has a resistance to heat and moisture at elevated temperatures, which permits sterilization of many properly fabricated parts by low pressure steam methods and autoclaving. It has a heat distortion temperature of 130-140°C (265-285°F) at 1.82 MPa loading and a continuous use temperature of 121°C (250°F) in air. Baby bottles, food containers and steam sterilized medical items often are produced from polycarbonate.

Good Machineability: Parts may readily be shaped, threaded, turned or milled from polycarbonate rod or plate stock using standard metal-working tools and equipment. Parts machined from these materials will possess the approximate properties of injection molded or extruded parts. Rod and plate stock of substantial dimensions are available from commercial suppliers.

V. THERMAL PROPERTIES

Polycarbonate is a linear polymer, which may attain an orderly molecular chain structure in the micro range (i.e., crystallites). These crystallites are smaller, even, than the wavelengths of visible light (400-700 nm), which accounts for its transparency. However, the crystalline melting point of 263°C (505°F) is sufficiently low to permit processing well within practical limits.

Although the principal glass transition of 149°C (300°F) is among the higher thermoplastics materials, there are minor transition points at lower temperatures. It may be due to these that polycarbonate resists embrittlement down to −101°C (−150°F).

The important practical result of these thermal properties is the wide temperature range through which the physical properties of polycarbonate remain essentially uniform.

The melt viscosity – as expected – decreases as temperature increases. The outstanding heat stability of polycarbonate is graphically illustrated in Figure 2. Even after two hours at 300°C (572°F), there is little change in the melt viscosity.

VI. CHEMICAL COMPATIBILITY

Polycarbonate is now being used successfully in a number of different environments. As would be expected, a few environments have been proven hostile to some degree. Certain, more common areas of use are presented; a comprehensive discussion is precluded by space limitations. Data on specific environments and natures of exposure can be obtained from the manufacturer.

Generally, polycarbonate has good room temperature resistance to water, dilute organic and inorganic acids, oxidizing and reducing agents, neutral and acid salts; mineral, animal and vegetable oils and fats; and aliphatic and alicyclic hydrocarbons.

Polycarbonate is attacked by alkalies, amines, ketones, esters and aromatic hydrocarbons such as benzene. Good solvents are methylene chloride, ethylene dichloride, cresol and dioxane.

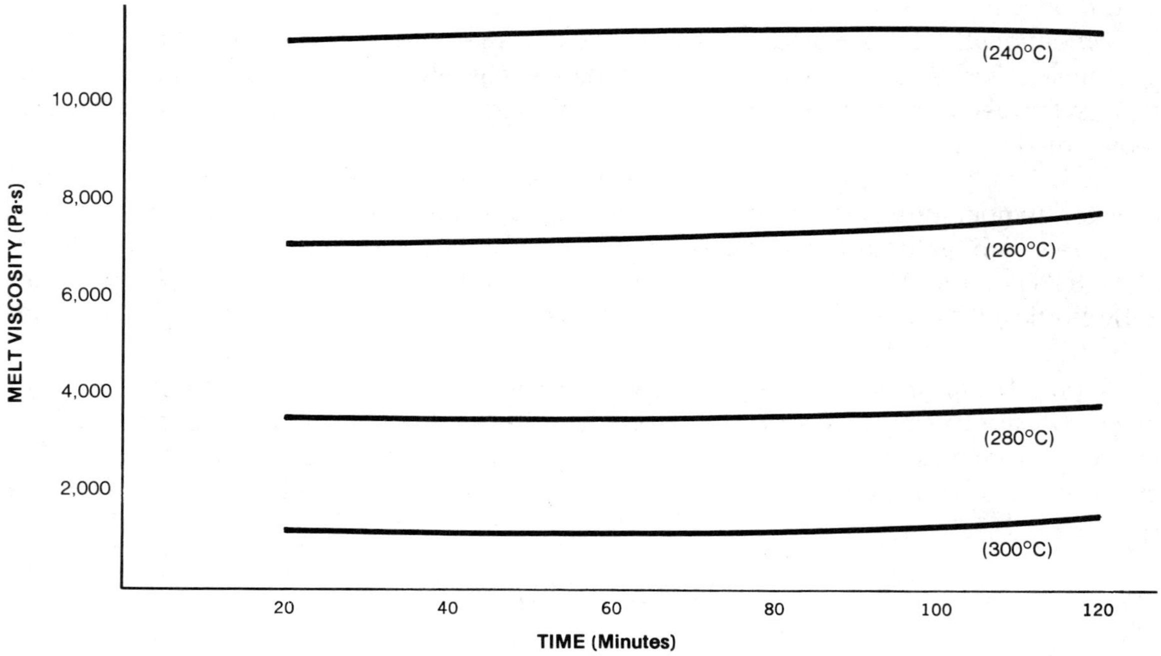

Figure 2. Stability of the melt viscosity of polycarbonate at different temperatures.

The chemical and solvent resistance data found in Tables 2 and 3, which by no means are exhaustive, will assist the designer in determining whether polycarbonate is suitable for a particular environment.

Each application has its own special considerations. In order to determine, quantitatively, the compatibility of stressed plastics with various environments, a test method has been developed by Bayer AG of W. Germany [Ref. 5].

The procedure is to clamp specimens, made from a particular plastic, to fixtures with a known radius of curvature, thus generating a defined outer fiber strain [Ref. 6]. The test environment is then brought into contact with the plastic. After the desired contact period, at a specified temperature, the piece is removed from the fixture and broken on a tensile testing machine. The elongations at break are plotted against the tensile strains applied by the fixtures. Typical results are shown in Figure 3. The critical (applied) strain, in this case 0.8%, is clearly shown as a break in the curve.

VIII. EFFECTS OF ENVIRONMENTAL CONDITIONS

One of the more important features of polycarbonate is its ability to remain dimensionally stable in many kinds of environments. Contributing to the excellent dimensional stability is its low water absorption. As shown in Table 4, this is only 0.35% after room temperature immersion. The dimensional change effects of water absorption are shown in Tables 4 and 5. Figure 4 gives the *percent* water absorption versus time of immersion. Note the rate at which equilibrium is reached.

Table 2. Polycarbonate is Resistant at Room Temperature to:

Chemicals	
Acetic acid (20%)	Nitric acid (10%)
Aluminum chloride	Nitric acid (20%)
Aluminum sulfate	Oleic acid
Ammonium chloride	Oxalic acid
Ammonium nitrate	Pentane
Ammonium sulfate	Petroleum ether
Antimony trichloride	Phosphoric acid, conc.
Arsenic acid (20%)	Propyl alcohol
Butyl alcohol	Potassium aluminum alum
Calcium chloride	Potassium dichromate
Calcium nitrate	Potassium bromate
Chlorinated lime paste	Potassium bromide
Chlorinated lime solution (2%)	Potassium chloride
Chrome alum	Potassium nitrate
Chromic acid (20%)	Potassium perchlorate
Citric acid (40%)	Potassium permanganate
Copper chloride	Potassium persulfate
Copper sulfate	Potassium sulfate
Cuprous chloride	Propargyl alcohol
Cyclohexane	Propionic acid (20%)
Decahydronaphthalene	Silicone oil
Ethyl alcohol (96%)	Silver nitrate
Formic acid (10%)	Sodium bicarbonate
Formalin (30%)	Sodium bisulfate
Glycerine	Sodium bisulfite
Glycol	Sodium carbonate
Hydrochloric acid (10%)	Sodium chlorate
Hydrochloric acid (20%)	Sodium chloride
Hydrogen peroxide (30%)	Sodium hypochlorite
Hydrofluoric acid (20%)	Sodium sulfate
Iron chloride	Stannous chloride
Iron sulfate	Sulfur
Isoamyl alcohol	Sulfuric acid (10%)
Lactic acid (20%)	Sulfuric acid (50%)
Magnesium chloride	Tartaric acid (30%)
Magnesium sulfate	Trichloroacetic acid (20%)
Manganese sulfate	Zinc chloride
Mercuric chloride	Zinc sulfate
Nickel sulfate	

Table 2. Polycarbonate is Resistant at Room Temperature to: (Continued)

Common Household Materials	
Beer	Mineral heating oil
Borax	Mineral water
Cocoa	Mustard
Castor oil	Olive oil
Cement	Onions
Chocolate	Orange juice
Cinnamon	Orange peel
Cod liver oil	Paraffin oil
Cognac	Pepper
Coffee	Rapeseed oil
Detergents (nonionic and anionic)	Rum
Fish oil	Salad oil
Floor polish	Salt solution (10%)
Fruit syrup	Soap (soft and hard)
Glaziers' putty	Table vinegar
Grapefruit juice	Tincture of iodine (5%)
Grapefruit peel	Tomato concentrate
Gypsum	Tomato juice
Ink	Turpentine
Insulating tape	Vodka
Linseed oil	Washing soap
Linseed oil, standard varnish	Water
Milk	Wine
Industrial Petroleum Products	
Axle oil	Petrol
Brake fluid (room temperature)	Refined oil
Compressor oil	Spindle oil
Diesel oil	Transformer oil
Gasoline (low aromatic)	Vacuum pump oil
Polycarbonate has limited resistance to:	
Cyclohexanol	Milk of lime [$Ca(OH)_2$]
Gasoline (high aromatic)	Nitric acid (conc.)
Hydrochloric acid (conc.)	Sulfuric acid (conc.)

(Concluded)

Table 3. Polycarbonate Is Not Resistant to:

Acetaldehyde	Dimethyl formamide
Acetic acid (conc.)	Ethylamine
Acetone	Ethyl ether
Acrylonitrile	Ethylene chlorohydrin
Ammonium fluoride	Formic acid (conc.)
Ammonium sulfide	Freon* (refrigerant & propellant)
Benzene	Nitrobenzene
Benzoic acid	Nitrocellulose lacquer
Benzyl alcohol	Phenol
Bromobenzene	Phosphorous hydroxychloride
Butyric acid	Phosphorous trichloride
Carbon tetrachloride	Propionic acid
Carbon disulfide	Sodium sulfide
Carbolic acid	Styrene
Caustic potash solution (5%)	Sulfuryl chloride
Caustic soda solution (5%)	Tetrachloroethane
Chlorobenzene	Tetrahydronaphthalene
Cyclohexanone	Thiophene
Cyclohexene	Toluene
	Xylene
Polycarbonate is dissolved by:	
Chloroform	Ethylene dichloride
Cresol	Methylene chloride
Dioxane	Pyridine

*DuPont trademark; Freon 113, may be used on unstressed polycarbonate at room temperature.

Table 4. Dimensional Change vs. Percent Water Absorption

Water Absorption %	Dimension Change mm/mm	Conditions
0.0	0.0	50% R.H.
0.15	0.0003	
0.35	0.0008	Room Temperature
0.58	0.0013	Boiling Water

Table 5. Polycarbonate Samples Aged in Hot Water for Six Months (100°C)

Original Dimension (mm)	Dimension after 6 months immersion (mm)
33.97	33.99
33.97	34.01
21.27	22.20

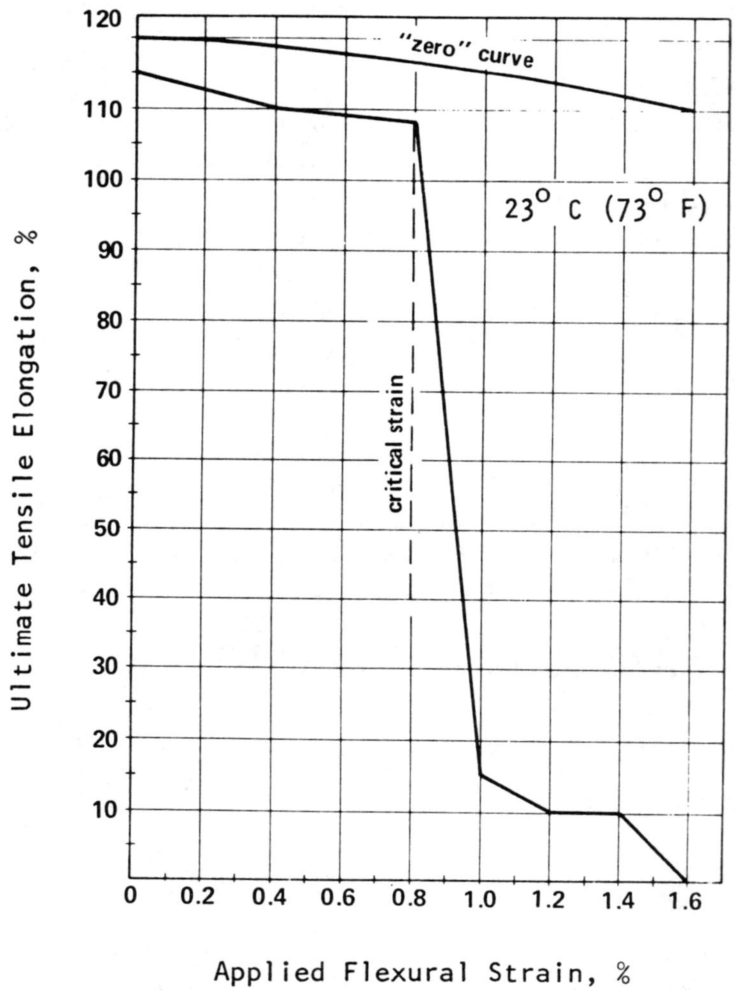

Figure 3. Ultimate elongation of polycarbonate after exposure to test environment at different levels of applied strain.

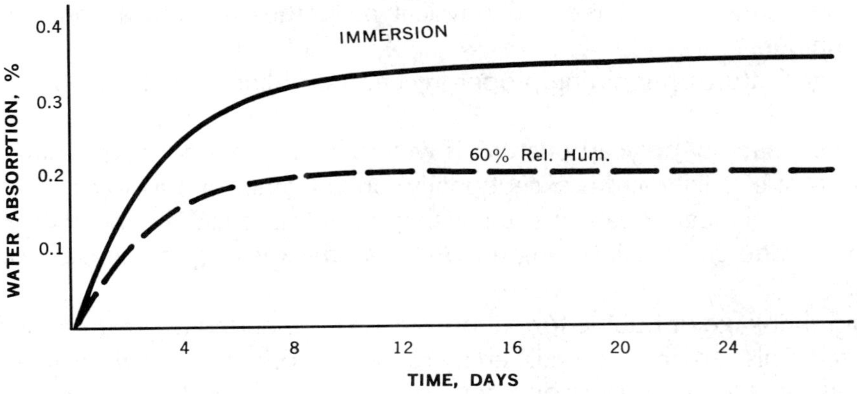

Figure 4. Water absorption of polycarbonate vs. time (per ASTM-D570).

For most practical purposes, polycarbonate has sufficient resistance to water up to approximately 60°C (140°F). Above this temperature, the effect of moisture is time-temperature related. For example, the high temperature resistance of polycarbonate permits the molded part to be autoclaved without deformation, but surface clouding or milky opaqueness may occur after a number of autoclave cycles. In addition, there is a noticeable loss in ductility and impact strength.

Some chemical compounds or their vapors, under certain conditions, will cause stress cracking or crazing of a molded polycarbonate article if the area in contact is under strain. These stresses in a molded piece are generally a direct function of the processing technique and, to some degree, mold design. They can usually be minimized by following proper design and fabricating practices. For example, areas of high stress may be caused by uneven cooling or occur near gates and runner openings where restrictions are put upon the flowing, molten thermoplastic. Ordinarily, compressive stresses present no problem in this respect.

Effort should be made to process polycarbonate so as to avoid extraordinarily high residual stresses. Good standard practices in injection molding, extrusion and other fabricating techniques will usually produce parts in which the residual stresses are minimized. In some cases, it has been found that chemical resistance may be improved slightly by annealing the part, although this may reduce some mechanical properties.

VIII. NOTES ON DESIGN OF POLYCARBONATE PARTS

The performance of any polycarbonate part does not depend only on the quality of the material itself. Appropriate design is, at least, equally important. The design has to be in accordance with the characteristics of polycarbonate and meet the technical requirements of the final article. Since most parts are produced by injection molding, the design must likewise consider the feasibility of this processing technique. No part will perform satisfactorily in service if it cannot be properly molded due to imperfect design. Thus, design considerations have to deal with the following:

1. Structural design resulting from physical and technological properties of polycarbonate.
2. Design parameters based on physical properties as well as on injection molding technique.
3. Design features permitting proper injection molding.

In designing parts of polycarbonate, it is well to keep in mind that the material possesses a high modulus of elasticity and is exceptionally tough. Standard principles normally employed in the design of engineered parts are applicable to this material. This includes the use of fillets, avoidance of undercuts, maintaining uniform wall thicknesses and similar good design considerations.

To avoid shrinkage or bubble formation, it is recommended that extremely heavy sections be eliminated. This can be accomplished by running a core pin through the center of such sections. A draft or taper of at least one degree is recommended to assist in removing the part from the mold or withdrawing the core pins.

Because of the high setting temperature and high viscosity of polycarbonate, it is difficult to mold sections that are less than .038 mm (0.015 in.) thick. In such thin sections, ribs can be used to act both as internal runners and to increase the rigidity of the finished part.

Polycarbonate tends to duplicate the mold surface very accurately. Because of this, it is necessary to have a highly polished mold if a high gloss part is required. A matte finish can be obtained by using a vapor-honed die.

What follows, now, is an abbreviated discussion of polycarbonate design considerations taken from Reference 7. Manufacturers of polycarbonate materials offer design assistance services and design bulletins to aid engineers charged with the responsibility of designing new and often intricate parts for the biomedical industry. *SINCE MANY OF THESE PARTS PROVIDE LIFE SUPPORT FUNCTIONS, PROPER DESIGN IS CRITICAL.*

Most plastic articles which are met in everyday life are not designed to withstand high (static or dynamic) loads. The selected material has to meet specifications for properties such as rigidity, impact strength, heat distortion temperature, optical characteristics, etc., depending on the intended use of the manufactured article. These common data, for polycarbonate, are provided in Table 1.

If vital functions are expected from polycarbonate parts under long-lasting (static or dynamic) loads, the long-term characteristics have to be considered. They differ widely from the data of short-term testing and show that the "apparent" strength decreases with the passage of time, with increased stress and elevated temperatures. The changes result from the creep of polycarbonate, no matter how small the amount actually is. Variations in the apparent modulus of elasticity (initial tensile modulus) are illustrated in Table 6.

Consequently, a constant stress of 13.8 MPa (2000 psi) at room temperature and 10.3 MPa (1500 psi) at elevated temperatures up to about 55°C (130°F) should not be exceeded if the load is applied for months or years. For more detailed information, refer to the polycarbonate manufcturer.

Closely related to the creep properties of polycarbonate is its stress relaxation. The stress resulting from a constant strain decreases slowly from its initial value. Assuming that a part is put together in such a way that the strain is 1%, the initial stress will drop to 14.5 MPa (2100 psi) after 6 minutes and to 11.0 MPa (1600 psi) after 10,000 hours. Taking this fact into account, deformation of a degree that cannot be tolerated under constant load may become permissible.

Table 6. Changes in Modulus Due to Time, Stress and Temperature

Time	Tensile Stress		Temperature		Modulus	
(hr)	MPa	psi	°C	°F	MPa	psi
100	10.3	1500	23	73	2070	300,000
10,000	10.3	1500	23	73	1790	260,000
10,000	20.7	3000	23	73	1380	200,000
100	20.7	3000	60	140	1030	150,000
10,000	20.7	3000	60	140	760	110,000
100	10.3	1500	80	176	1030	150,000
100	20.7	3000	80	176	690	100,000
10,000	10.3	1500	80	176	790	115,000

Those reported data are valid only in air as the environment. Any other environment may change the characteristics considerably. This is especially true if organic solvents or their vapors are involved. In every case, when it is felt that polycarbonate is utilized close to its ultimate strength, testing of machined or molded prototypes would be a wise course of action.

There are specific design parameters which must be taken into account if the part is to be injection molded.

Wall Thickness: It is evident that excessively increased wall thickness does not necessarily provide more strength. If heavier sections appear to be needed for easier grasping or as a spacer, the thick section should be thinned by blind holes, ribbing or the like to maintain a leaner, uniform wall.

On the other hand, the thinnest wall section possible can be correlated to the flow length of the material in the cavity. Figure 5 represents the minimum section thickness for a given flow length of the various molecular weight grades of bisphenol A polycarbonate. Sometimes the flow length can be reduced by using a fan gate or be improved by applying one or more ribs in the appropriate direction – acting like an internal runner.

Ribs: In addition to the ribs acting as "internal" runners, they can also contribute to the stiffness of a wall. Their thickness, however, should not exceed one-half the thickness of the adjacent wall, otherwise a sink mark will appear opposite the rib. Incorrectly placed ribs can also increase the flow of material in a way that can trap air, causing incomplete filling, silver streaking or burned areas.

Radii: Sharp corners should be avoided to improve, among other properties, the impact resistance, since polycarbonate, in spite of its toughness, is a rigid material exhibiting a certain notch sensitivity. Either well-rounded corners or radii at least one-fourth of the wall thickness should be applied. In order not to increase the wall thickness, the internal radius calls for a corresponding external one, as well.

Acute angled transitions tend to cause flow disturbances which become visible flow marks on the surface. Radii can prevent this phenomenon.

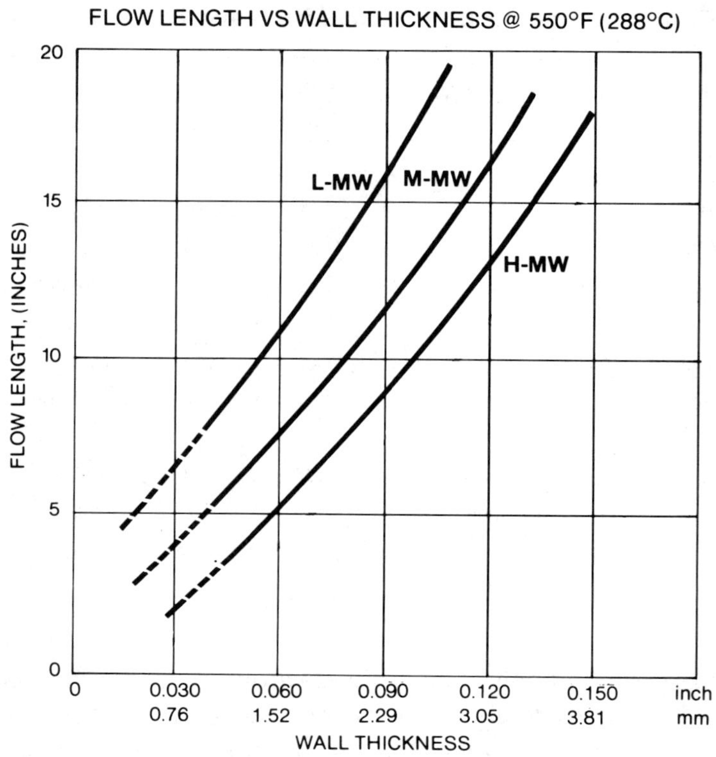

Figure 5. Polycarbonate flow length vs. wall thickness as a function of molecular weight.

Holes: Holes are formed by cores. The length of a pin held at one end only, should not exceed five times its diameter. For cores secured at both ends, a diameter to length ratio 1:10 is the maximum. Longer core pins can be deflected by the pressure of the entering material. These figures are approximate values. Cores may be longer if the section thickness around the core is reasonably above the minimum and if uniform filling can be expected.

Undercuts: Because polycarbonate is a rather rigid material, undercuts cannot be released easily. They generally require sliding side cores or – if internal undercuts are considered – a collapsible core.

Taper and Draft: In order to facilitate the release of a molding, sufficient draft should be applied to all walls in the direction of ejection. A 1° draft is highly recommended; the more the better. With less than 0.5°, ejection may become difficult and special care must be taken not to overpack during filling; otherwise, the mold simply will not open.

Manufacturers often carry grades of polycarbonate containing a mold release agent to facilitate part ejection.

Elements of Assembly: As a general rule, the designer should prefer any assembly design which converts tensile into compressive loads.

Rivets can be used for permanent joining. To better distribute the compressive load, washers are recommended. The travel of the setting tool must be limited to prevent excessive force.

Injection molded threads can be combined with metal or plastic screws permitting indefinitely detachable assembly. Unified and American Standard threads forming pronounced notches reduce impact strength and ultimate elongation; trapezoidal and knuckle threads are slightly better. The used thread length must be more than 1.5 times the diameter; tightening should be limited.

One of the best ways to insert metal components into polycarbonate parts is by using ultrasonic power. If done properly, an almost stress-free bond is introduced.

If metal inserts are to be molded in, choosing the insert must be done carefully and the molding must be done correctly. Knurled inserts with a sharp-edged surface exercise an unfavorable notch effect upon impact. Inserts heavier than 1.5 grams or larger than 6.4 mm (0.250 inch) diameter must be preheated to 175-200°C (350-400°F) before placing them into the mold. The minimum diameter of the boss containing the insert must be 2.2 times the diameter of the insert.

The insert should be at least flush with the surrounding plastic material or, even better, protrude a little to assure a force locking connection between insert and the part to be assembled to it.

Self-tapping screws in accordance with ASA B 18.6.4-1958 or any corresponding type are successfully used for assembly if they are detached only a limited number of times. Type 25 with a more coarse thread is preferred. Using the same screw size without cutting flute after the first detachment will help keep the thread in the plastic undamaged.

Again, the O.D. of the boss should be 2.2 times the I.D. and force locking connection between boss and assembled part must be achieved. If not, failure is likely to occur by fracture of the boss' base.

Snap fits for fast and easy assembly take full advantage of the mechanical properties of polycarbonate. Any deformation during joining, however, should not exceed the 1.5% strain limit and the design must be such that the stress is released completely after assembly.

IX. INJECTION MOLDING POLYCARBONATE

Experience has shown that, although polycarbonate resin has been run successfully using all common types and sizes of injection molding machines, in-line screw injection machines contribute to easier molding. When a choice is available, manufacturers recommend the screw injection machine. If a plunger injection machine must be used, a single stage is usually preferred, since its greater simplicity results in fewer hold-up areas where flushing is difficult. The maximum plunger size should be 20 mm (ca. 0.75-0.80 in.).

In-line screw machines of the reciprocating screw type are satisfactory for molding polycarbonate. The screw preplasticating types have also been used successfully, but they have additional hold-up areas, which are not desirable for polycarbonate processing.

In selecting a screw machine for molding polycarbonate resin, the following features have been found to be important considerations:

- The cylinder should have an Xaloy liner [Ref. 8].
- The screw length should be at least fifteen diameters.
- The screw design normally used is a constant taper transition with a 2:1 to 3:1 compression ratio. Although many types of screws may be employed, the use of rapid-transition (nylon-type) screws is discouraged because of the high power input required and the high temperature rise in a short space.

- Chrome-plated screws are preferred.
- Rotary or other types of valves at the end of the screw and ahead of the nozzle are not necessary nor desirable, since they result in added hold-up of the melt.
- A three piece sliding check ring on the end of the screw is the preferred type of non-return valve.

Because of the relatively short residence time, the screw machine offers more latitude than the plunger machine in shot weight vs. rated machine capacity. Although 50-75 percent of capacity is considered to be the good operating range, a shot weight smaller than 50 percent can be molded successfully.

Whether a screw or plunger type is used, however, the machine should be scrupulously clean and in good condition before attempting to mold any polycarbonate materials.

When processing polycarbonate, the standard rules of good nozzle seating in the sprue bushing should be followed and a nozzle discharge opening slightly smaller than the sprue bushing inlet should be provided. In addition, there are some specific recommendations and suggestions that apply to polycarbonate processing:

- *Materials of Construction:* Standard steel is being used successfully for molding polycarbonate. However, nozzles of stainless steel (No. 420) appear to offer better protection against production problems – particularly black specks, which sometimes occur in long molding campaigns.
- *Nozzle Types:* Open nozzles are used most frequently. A reverse taper at the nozzle exit is preferred because the melt tears off in the interior of the nozzle. As a result, a portion of the material forming a cold slug for the succeeding shot is removed with the sprue.
- *Nozzle Size:* As is the case with runners and sprues, the nozzle should be as short as possible. Nozzle diameter depends upon the length. With short nozzles – up to 15 cm (ca. 6 inches) in length – 6.35 cm (0.250 inch) is probably satisfactory. Longer nozzles should have a diameter of 9.52 cm to 12.70 mm (0.375 inch to 0.500 inch). The bore should taper only toward the end so that an effective short land is obtained. Restricted-type nozzles should be avoided.
- *Temperature Control:* Nozzles, regardless of length, should be equipped with heater bands to prevent cooling or solidifying of the melt in this machine area. Nozzle temperature control should be separate from the front cylinder zone because ideal operating conditions usually require a 10-15°C (ca. 20-30°F) lower temperature at the nozzle to prevent drooling. The best choice is a PID controller. Even a variac is preferred over a slow-cycling controller. PID controllers also are recommended for temperature control of the barrel.

Molds for polycarbonate processing may require clamp tonnages in excess of those specified for other resins because of the higher injection pressures normally required. Predicting the amount of clamp needed for any given mold is not always straightforward. However, experience has indicated that a force of approximately 5.6 kilonewtons per square centimeter (four tons per square inch) of projected area is needed.

A heat exchanger for the mold is a necessity when processing polycarbonate. Generally, water circulating units are sufficient for the normal mold temperature range of 75-95°C (ca. 170-200°F). Separate controllers for each half of the mold are usually desirable desirable because of the frequent necessity of operating the core at a slightly lower temperature to insure retention of the part in that half of the mold.

Material Considerations

For reliable production of good quality parts from polycarbonate resin, it is absolutely essential that all moisture be excluded from the melt. The presence of moisture may cause silver streaking (splay) and bubbles in the molded part; the most damaging effect is a loss in material toughness. For these reasons, *the importance of the following recommended resin handling procedures cannot be overemphasized.*

Polycarbonate, characterized by relatively high melt viscosity, a reasonably broad melting range and higher-than-normal second order transition temperature, requires molding melt temperatures in the range of 275-320°C (ca. 530-610°F). A mold that is to be run with polycarbonate resin should have a section thickness vs. flow length relationship that falls within the range prescribed in Figure 5.

Bisphenol A polycarbonate resin is a hygroscopic material, picking up enough moisture in only ten (10) minutes to cause processing difficulties and a subsequent loss of toughness in the molded part. Figure 6 illustrates the rate of moisture pickup on polycarbonate pellets. The subject pellets were oven-dried at 121°C (250°F), then air-cooled at 50% relative humidity.

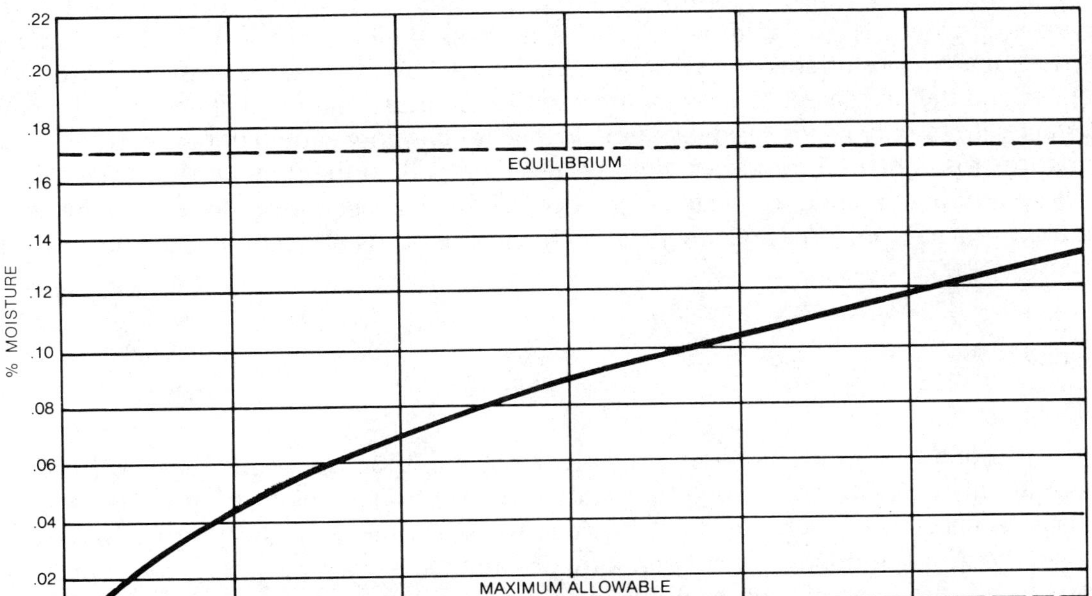

Figure 6. Rate of moisture pickup of dried polycarbonate pellets.

Polycarbonate pellets packaged in polyethylene-lined paper bags (normally 50 lb/22.7 kg) usually will be as dry or as wet as when it was packaged – provided the bag was properly sealed and has remained unbroken. If the resin was dried sufficiently prior to bagging, it should be usable straight from the package. To ensure that the pellets remain dry – 0.01% moisture, *maximum* – a desiccant hopper drier should be used. Manufacturers of polycarbonate materials can supply information about the moisture level of the bagged products they sell.

Polycarbonate sold in bulk, boxes (454 kg/1000 lb) or drums (136 kg/300 lb), normally contains significantly more than 0.01% moisture, the maximum recommended for trouble-free processing.

The preferred method of moisture removal involves the use of a dehumidifying (desiccating) hopper drier capable of delivering air with a dew point of −18°C (0°F) or lower, heated to 120°C (250°F). The drier should be set at 120-130°C (250-260°F) and turned on at least an hour before the polycarbonate is introduced into the hopper or plenum chamber. This procedure allows the air in the system to dry and reach 120°C (250°F). The resin should then be charged to the hopper and exposed to the hot, dry air for a minimum of four hours prior to the start of molding. As the pellets are consumed, additional material should be added, at a rate that will ensure at least four hours drying time.

Circulating air ovens may also be used to dry polycarbonate resin. Material should be transferred from the shipping container onto trays, at a depth not greater than 2.5 cm (one inch). The trays should be placed in an oven that can maintain a temperature of 121-127°C (250-260°F) and left for a minimum of four hours, *but not longer than 24 hours*. The oven must not contain any other types of resin that may contribute to moisture. The polycarbonate resin must be transferred directly from the oven to the hopper, to minimize exposure. If hopper drying equipment is available, it should be used as outlined above in order to maintain dryness. If a hopper drier is not available, strip heaters or a heat lamp must be placed in the hopper and the lid sealed, to prevent ambient temperature and humidity air from coming in contact with the dry resin. Residence time in a heated hopper should not exceed one hour; if the hopper is unheated, residence time should be less than thirty minutes.

Polycarbonate regrind, or virgin polycarbonate that has been exposed to the atmosphere, should be placed in trays and dried in an air-circulating oven according to the procedure discussed above.

Machine Preparation

The cylinder of the molding machine must be thoroughly purged, or (preferably) mechanically cleaned, before polycarbonate resin is introduced into the cylinder. Purging is usually a difficult procedure; the best materials to use for this purpose appear to be reground acrylic sheet or reground polycarbonate, run at a relatively fast rate. Of all the resins, nylon and ABS are the most difficult to purge for molding polycarbonate. The presence of minute amounts of either of these resins in the cylinder at 316°C (600°F) will cause degradation of polycarbonate, evidenced by a deterioration of toughness, dark splotches or streaks in the molded article. In view of this, experience has shown that mechanical cleaning is the more efficient procedure.

During the purge cycle, as the polycarbonate resin is introduced into the machine, the cylinder temperature is raised to slightly above the expected molding level. The polycarbonate is purged by air-shooting as rapidly as possible until the exiting melt is free of contamination.

An examination of the preliminary molded parts will usually reveal the efficiency of the purging step. Quite often, contamination in the part during the early phases of the run originates in the nozzle area. A strong indication of this would be evidence of streaking in the sprue.

With a mold in which polycarbonate has not been run previously, Table 7 shows typical conditions suggested as starting ranges for the screw injection molding machines currently in operation.

Table 7. Suggested Start-up Conditions for Molding Polycarbonate Resin

CONDITION	SCREW INJECTION
Cylinder Temperature, °C (°F)	
Rear	260-280 (500-540)
Middle	270-295 (520-560)
Front	280-305 (540-580)
Nozzle	295-305 (560-580)
Injection Pressure, MPa (psi)	
High	70-140 (10,000-20,000)
Low	40- 85 (6,000-12,000)
Cycle, seconds	
High Injection	3-20
Booster	2- 5
Low Hold	3-10
Clam	5-35
Total	18-80
Hopper Temperature, °C (°F)	120-130 (250-270)
Clamp Pressure	Maximum
Screw Cooling	Neutral
Back Pressure, MPa (psi)	0.70-10.50 (100-1500)
Cushion, mm (in)	nil-3.18 (0-0.125)

From this starting point, changes in machine conditions will have to be made until the mold is filled. Figures 7 and 8 indicate the effect of changes in melt and tool temperatures on flow length in the spiral flow mold. (Also see Figure 1). Of course, the graph is intended to serve only as a rough guide to the temperature changes required.

While the overall cycle depends upon the mold configuration and shot size, in general, the best cycle is one that ensures a relatively fast fill and sufficient holding pressure time only to permit gate setup and curing. For optimum molding conditions, unnecessarily long cycles should be avoided.

Mold temperature should be 75-95°C (150-200°F) before the first shot is made. Initial shots into the mold should be made with less than full injection pressure. To facilitate part removal on initial shots, a generous amount of mold lubricant may be used. Overpacking can also

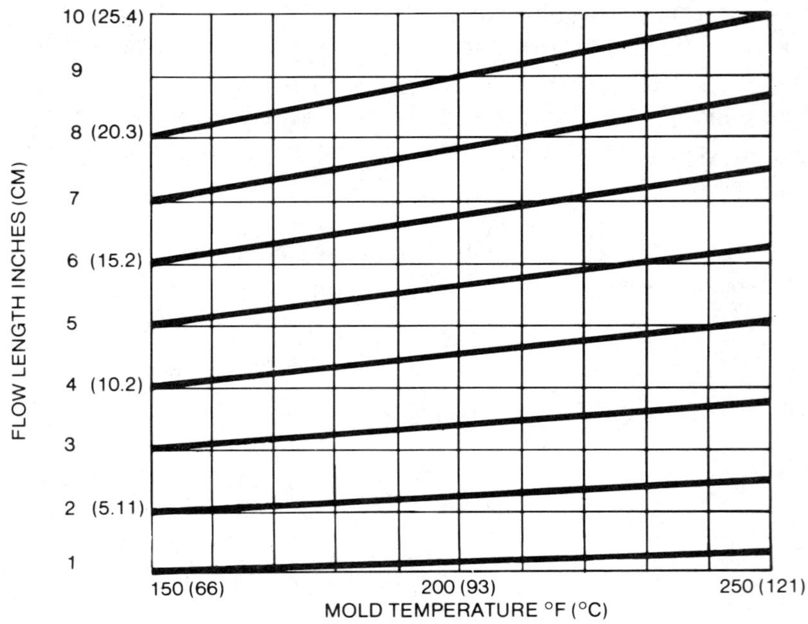

Figure 7. Effect of mold temperature on the flow length on polycarbonate resin.

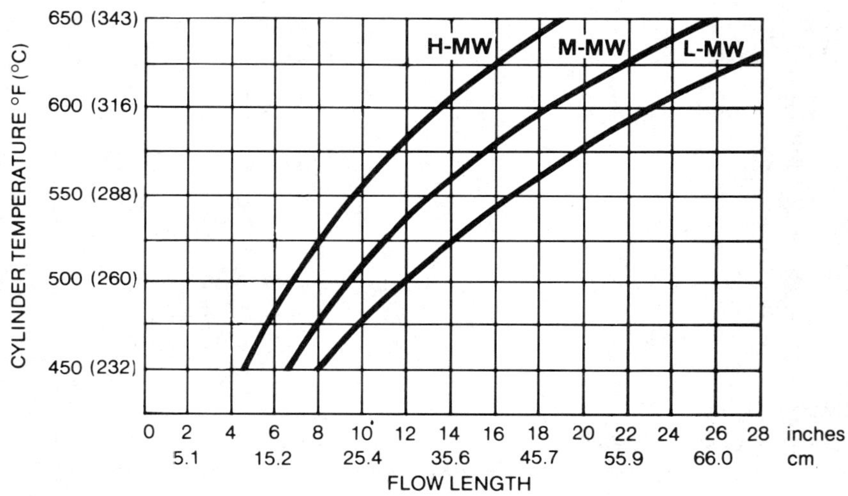

Figure 8. Effect of cylinder temperature on the flow length of the three molecular weight grades of polycarbonate.

occur on initial shots, causing part removal difficulties that are amplified by the natural toughness of polycarbonate resin. The best practice is to start with a short shot – but making sure to reach the ejector pins – then gradually increase feed and pressure until the cavities are properly filled.

General Molding Conditions

Character of the Melt: Polycarbonate resin is characterized by a broad melting range and good thermal stability in the recommended processing temperature range of 270-320°C (530-610°F). Above this range, a darkening of the resin and some loss in toughness can occur due to overheating.

While slow air-shooting the melt from the nozzle, examination should reveal it to be free of bubbles. The presence of bubbles indicates moisture in the pellets, meaning that further drying of the resin is necessary for quality production (See Figure 9).

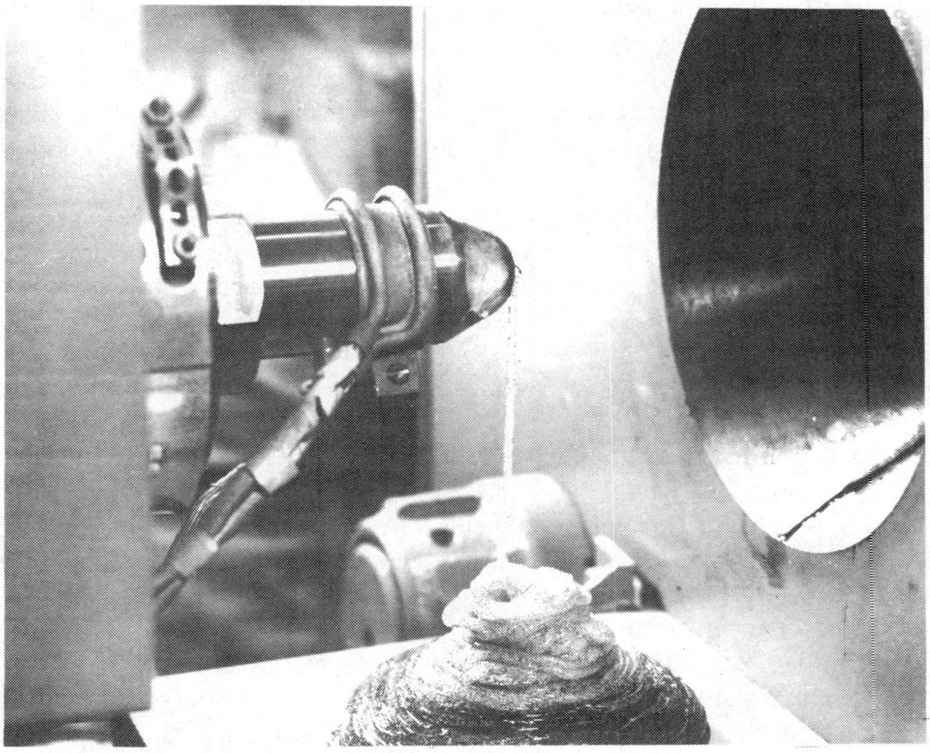

Figure 9. Improperly dried polycarbonate – showing bubbles – as it exits the nozzle of a molding machine.

Injection Pressures: Generally, injection pressures of 15,000-20,000 psi (100-140 MPa) are required in most molds for processing polycarbonate. Second stage or holding pressures are usually in the range of 80-90 percent of injection pressure.

Injection Rates: The rate of injection will, of course, be dependent upon various parameters, such as part geometry and type of machine. In general, the filling should be as rapid as possible to minimize cold flow lines, weld lines and molded-in stresses.

When molding thick sections, 9.5 mm (0.375 in) or more, it may be necessary to employ low injection rates to preclude the formation of internal bubbles. In effect, the slow injection rate allows the molten polycarbonate resin to set up a viscous plastic front as it enters the cavity. The resistance to the incoming melt results in more uniform packing of the cavity.

In some cases, an excessive injection rate can produce a variety of undesirable effects, such as jetting, silver streaking and melt fracture showing as gate blush.

Screw Speed: With screw injection machines, screw speeds of 40-90 rpm have been used. However, the lower levels are normally preferred and will usually provide adequate plastication.

Screw Back Pressure: As a general recommendation, screw back pressure should be kept low. To exclude conveyed air, however, it is occasionally necessary to operate with a back pressure as high as 3.45 MPa (500 psi). Insufficient back pressure will become evident in transparent moldings by the appearance of bubbles which have a partially white, opaque wall due to trapped air.

Resin Feed or Cushion: Best molding results will usually be obtained using little cushion, with either volumetric or weigh feeding. There are two reasons for this: 1) With either screw or plunger, the most effective pressure transmission can be obtained and 2) Excessive shrinks and/or voids due to suck-back of the resin through the runner system will be minimized.

Experience has shown that a 3.2 mm (0.125 in) cushion is the most that is needed to assure reproducible feeding.

Nozzle Temperature: It is important that the nozzle be equipped with heater bands along its entire length to maintain a uniform melt temperature. In most cases, the optimum nozzle temperature is the same as or slightly lower than that of the front cylinder zone.

Drooling is not normally encountered with polycarbonate, but if it should occur, lowering the nozzle temperature 5-10°C (10-20°F) should correct the condition. If drooling should persist, it most likely means moisture is present in the resin; in this case, further drying of the material will be necessary.

It is also important to have the nozzle well seated, since improper seating can cause excessive leakage, resulting in silver streaking from air being pulled into the mold cavity and machine nozzle. Also, the sprue will be diffficult to remove due to the inherent rigidity of the leaked material when it sets up. To prevent these problems, the exit diameter of the nozzle orifice should be slightly smaller than the entry diameter of the sprue bushing.

Mold Temperature and Control: The range of mold temperatures normally used for processing polycarbonate is 75-95°C (170-200°F), as measured on the surface of the cavity or core of the mold. In isolated cases, particularly involving thin sections, it may be advisable to use higher temperatures – up to 120°C (250°F) – to facilitate mold filling. Figure 7 shows the increase in flow length that can be achieved by increasing the mold temperature. It should be noted that greater changes in flow length are usually available by changing cylinder temperatures (See Figure 8).

Generally, both sections of the mold can be operated at the same temperature. In cases of poor part retention on the core when opening the mold, it may be necessary to operate the moving half of the mold at 5-10°C (10-20°F) lower than the stationary half.

Cores and pins may often require special cooling controls through bubblers. Small-diameter core pins are often difficult to cool adequately, and a lower cooling liquid temperature may be required. Inadequate core cooling causes the resin to stick to the pin, resulting in a roughened surface on the part.

Mold Release Agents: In processing polycarbonate resin, it is advisable to keep mold lubrication at a minimum. When part sticking is encountered, it is best to remedy the situation by adjustments in temperature, pressure or cycle. In some cases, further polishing of the mold surface and an increase in knock-out pin area will help. Many mold release agents and lubricants are detrimental to the properties of polycarbonate molded parts, resulting in loss of impact strength, delamination on the part or surface blemish. If a mold release agent is necessary to attain trouble-free production, your supplier's technical representative should be consulted to help work out the best solution to the problem.

Molded-in Inserts: To minimize stresses around metal inserts which are molded-in, it is recommended they be brought to a temperature of approximately 120°C (250°F) at the time of loading into the mold. The purpose of this procedure is to expand the metal insert and help compensate for the greater thermal coefficient of expansion of the plastic.

To this point, we have discussed, albeit in abridged discourses, the chemical structure of bisphenol A polycarbonate, generally applicable physical properties, chemical compatibility and environmental effects. We then pursued, in somewhat more detailed fashion, important part design and injection molding considerations. It is appropriate to reiterate, at this point, that to ensure production of good quality molded parts – such as those we will see in the succeeding sections – the polycarbonate resin must be properly dried and kept dry while in the hopper prior to molding.

X. STERILIZATION OF POLYCARBONATE ARTICLES [Ref. 9]

The three most common methods of biological sterilization of plastics are steam autoclaving, exposure to ethylene oxide (ETO), usually in a mixture with carbon dioxide $(CO)_2$ or Freon 12 [Ref. 10] and gamma irradiation produced by cobalt-60.

Steam Sterilization

Steam autoclaving is the prevalent method of sterilization in use today. Many properly designed and fabricated polycarbonate medical devices are routinely sterilized by this technique, since many of the typical physical properties of polycarbonate are not affected (or only slightly affected) by redundant steam sterilizations. Some properties associated with "toughness," however, are altered; examples are notched Izod impact strength and ultimate tensile elongation. This discussion will review the effects of steam sterilization on the physical properties of polycarbonate, emphasizing those that are affected adversely.

The notched Izod impact strength of all molecular weight grades of polycarbonate decreases with repeated steam autoclave sterilization cycles. The standard cycle is 20-25 minutes at 120°C (250°F).

In order to understand the effect of (even) low pressure steam of polycarbonate's notched Izod impact strength, it first is necessary to understand the phenomenon called critical thickness. Polycarbonate, as well as several other materials, exhibits a dramatic change in notched Izod impact strength when the width (or thickness) of the test specimen or molded part exceeds a specific dimension. This behavior is shown in Figure 10 for three molecular weight grades of polycarbonate; high (H-MW), medium (M-MW) and low (L-MW). Note that in "thin" sections, all grades have high impact strengths (ca. 700–900 J/m; 13–17 ft · lb/in.) and in "thick" sections the impact strengths are low (≤200 J/m; 3.7 ft · lb/in.). The thickness where this abrupt change from high to low occurs is called the critical thickness; it depends upon many factors, including: polymer molecular weight, temperature and notch radius.

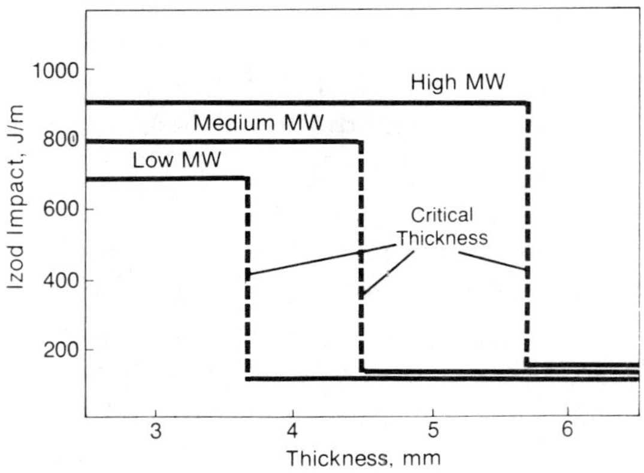

Figure 10. Polycarbonate Izod impact strength versus thickness.

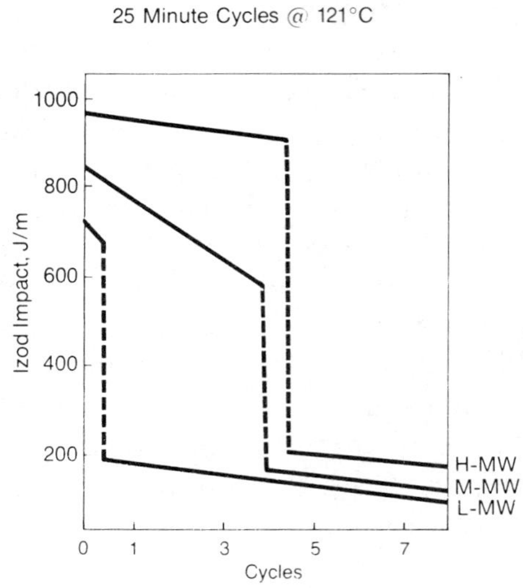

Figure 11. Change in notched Izod impact strength with multiple sterilization cycles.

Figure 11 shows the change in notched Izod impact strength with multiple autoclave cycles for the three molecular weight grades of polycarbonate. The shapes of the curves are similar to those seen in Figure 10. This is due to the decrease in critical thickness due to steam sterilization. For example, since the standard Izod test specimen is 3.2 mm (0.125 in.) thick (wide), the critical thickness of the medium molecular weight grade has been reduced to less than 3.2 mm after about four cycles. Below the critical thickness, the material exhibits only moderate impact strength.

Although the notched Izod impact strength shows discontinuous behavior with increasing steam exposure, the change in critical thickness is continuous, as seen in Figure 12. The critical thickness of M-MW polycarbonate (PC) remains above 3.2 mm after three steam autoclave cycles. After the fourth cycle, however, the critical thickness of M-MW PC will be less than the 3.2 mm thickness of the test specimen and the notched Izod impact strength will be only moderate. This fact notwithstanding, it should be pointed out that even after repeated steam sterilization cycles, Izod impact values for polycarbonate, at 100–200 J/m (1.9–3.7 ft · lb/in.), are still higher than those of many other unsterilized thermoplastic materials (Figure 13).

Summarizing, there is gradual loss of notched Izod impact strength when successive steam autoclaving cycles are carried out. High molecular weight polycarbonate will retain its high impact strength for a greater number of cycles than M-MW or L-MW PC and parts 2.0 to 2.5 mm (0.08-0.10 in.) thick will retain exceptional ductility through many autoclave cycles.

The Gardner impact and dart-drop-impact tests afford other measures of impact performance. Table 8 and Figure 14 illustrate how the "drop impact" behavior of polycarbonate is altered by cyclical steam sterilizations. The table shows, that for all polycarbonate grades, the drop impact values remain high through five cycles; the figure illustrates that even after twenty cycles, M-MW PC retains over half of its original impact strength.

The area under the stress-strain curve is the energy absorbing capacity or toughness of a plastic material. The ultimate tensile strain (elongation at break) is often taken as a measure of

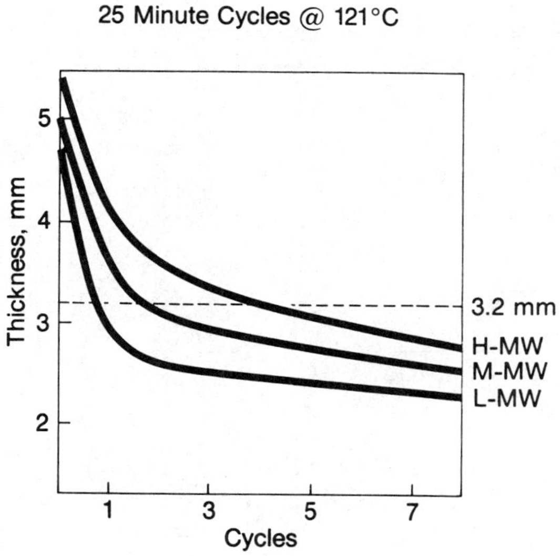

Figure 12. Effect of autoclave cycles on critical thickness.

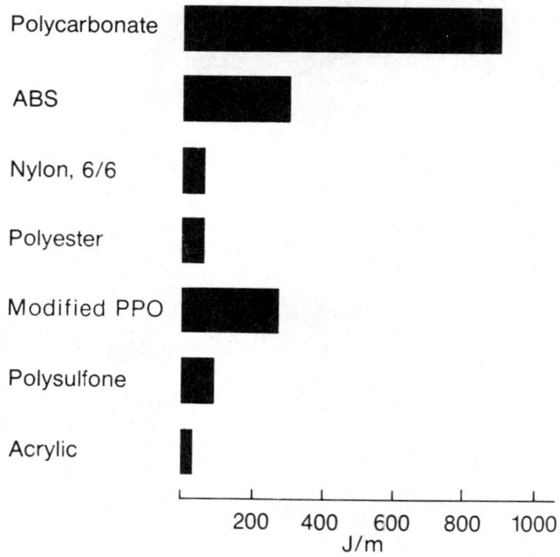

Figure 13. Izod impact strengths of representative thermoplastic materials.

Table 8. Effect of Steam Autoclave Cycles on Drop Impact

	25 Minute Cycles at 121°C Drop Impact Strength, J, 25.4 mm Diameter, 10 Kg Dart		
Grade	Control	1 Cycle	5 Cycles
L-MW PC	197	177	123
M-MW PC	218	216	124
H-MW PC	218	216	171

this property. Table 9 shows the tensile behavior of three grades of polycarbonate after up to five steam sterilization cycles. There is a gradual reduction of the ultimate tensile strain as the number of cycles increases. Also, it is clear from the data that L-MW PC is affected more rapidly than H-MW or M-MW PC.

As stated earlier, many other properties of polycarbonate are not affected significantly by cyclical steam autoclaving. The data in Tables 9 and 10 show that flexural and other tensile properties are relatively unchanged during up to 20 sterilization cycles. Figure 15 illustrates that there is no significant decrease in the ultimate tensile strength of high molecular weight polycarbonate after fifty cycles.

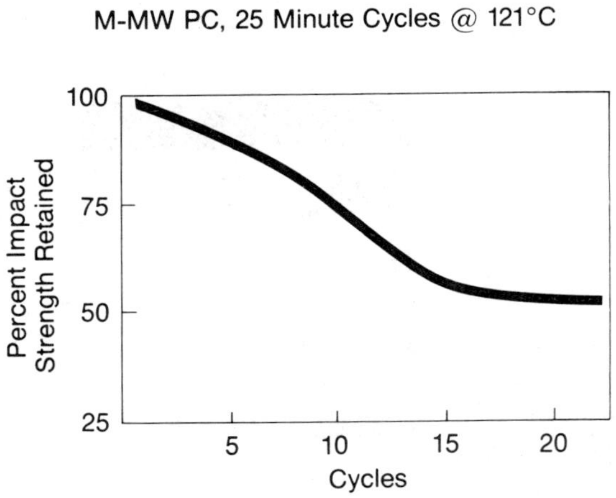

Figure 14. Percent dart drop impact strength retention versus increasing number of sterilization cycles.

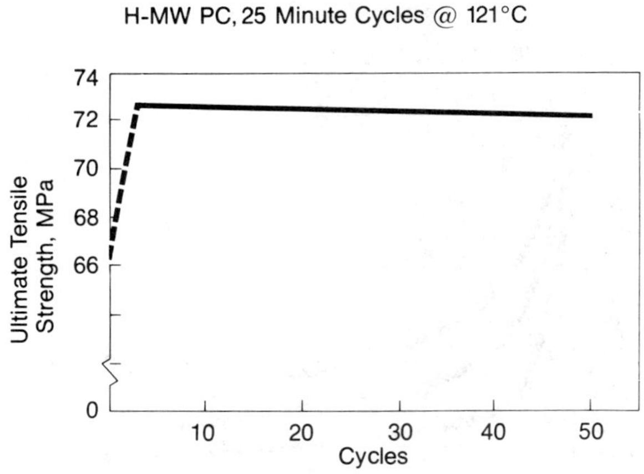

Figure 15. Stability of polycarbonate strength to multiple sterilization cycles.

Table 9. Tensile Properties after Cyclic Steam Sterilization 25 Min. Cycles @ 121 °C

		Tensile Stress, MPa		Tensile Strain, %	
Material	Cycles	Yield	Ultimate	Yield	Ultimate
L-MW PC	0	64	67	5	107
	1	69	69	5	87
	5	--	--	5	42
M-MW PC	0	62	70	5	115
	1	69	69	5	107
	5	69	69	5	67
	20	75	75	5	12
H-MW PC	0	63	72	5	118
	1	68	71	5	112
	5	69	69	5	92

Polycarbonate is an ester and is subject to hydrolysis when exposed to moisture at elevated temperatures. The reaction is shown in 6, below.

6

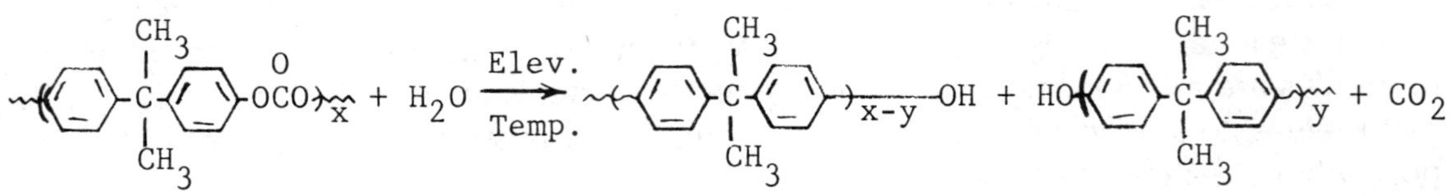

Table 10. Flexural Properties after Cyclic Steam Sterilization 25 Min Cycles @ 121°C

Material	Cycles	Modulus, GPa	Strength @ 5% Strain, MPa	Ultimate Strength, MPa
L-MW PC	0	2.5	88	96
	1	2.3	90	98
	5	2.4	93	103
M-MW PC	0	2.4	88	97
	1	2.3	87	97
	5	2.4	88	99
	20	2.3	94	103
H-MW PC	0	2.4	87	93
	1	2.2	87	97
	5	2.4	90	99

Weight average molecular weight (Mw) and the number average molecular weight (Mn) decrease by approximately 15% after one hundred steam sterilizaton cycles as shown in Table 11 and illustrated in Figures 16A and 16B. The polydispersity of the polymer remains surprisingly constant throughout the one hundred autoclavings. Table 11 also shows the steady decline of other viscosity measurements, such as Mv, Mz and intrinsic viscosity, and the concomitant increase in melt flow rate to nearly two and one-half times the original value (Figure 17). These decreases are caused by hydrolysis of the polymer molecule and is the reason that polycarbonate cannot be steam sterilized indefinitely. These values, however, also illustrate why polycarbonate has found wide acceptance among those who use steam sterilization.

The decrease in molecular weight is very slow; one hundred cycles are required for the polymer to reach 85% of its original MW. Likewise, it takes seventy cycles for the melt flow of M-MW polycarbonate to double its zero-cycles flow rate. This illustrates that even at sterilization conditions, hydrolysis takes place relatively slowly. This also explains why most of the physical properties of polycarbonate are affected only slightly by repeated autoclavings.

Many properly fabricated polycarbonate medical parts are sterilized by the autoclave method, the most common cycle being 20-25 minutes at 121°C (250°F). Very few clear plastics can withstand such temperatures, while maintaining clarity and strength requirements.

Some representative items include an anesthesia canister manufactured by Dryden Corporation, shown in Figure 18. This unit is used to reduce the incidence of post-operative pneumonia, caused by anesthetic gas contamination. The polycarbonate unit replaces a similar unit made of stainless steel. It is re-usable and thus is steam-sterilized repeatedly.

In Europe, animal cages are predominantly polycarbonate and are sterilized repeatedly by steam. The U.S. market is younger and is growing; the method of sterilization is the same.

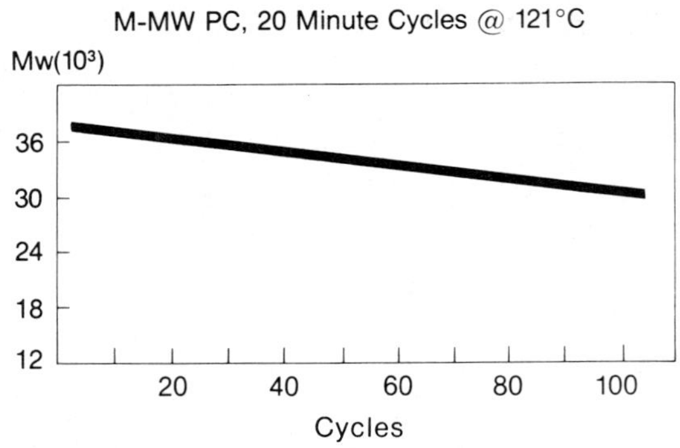

Figure 16A. Effect of steam sterilization on weight-average molecular weight.

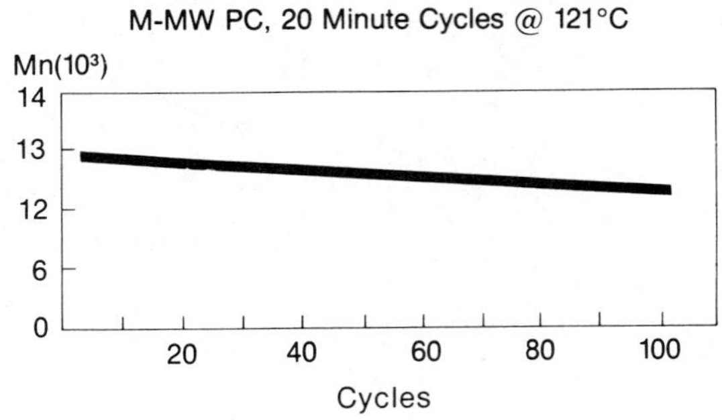

Figure 16B. Effect of steam sterilization on number-average molecular weight.

Table 11. Effect of Cyclic Steam Sterilization on Molecular Properties of M-MW PC

Cycles	$Mw(10^3)$	$Mn(10^3)$	Mw/Mn	$Mv(10^3)$	$Mz(10^3)$	Melt Flow g/10 min	Intrinsic Viscosity
0	38.0	17.8	2.15	35.4	58.4	9.2	0.595
10	36.6	15.6	2.35	33.8	56.8	9.7	0.576
20	35.3	15.6	2.29	32.7	55.1	11.4	0.563
30	34.9	15.4	2.27	32.2	54.5	12.3	0.557
40	35.0	15.6	2.24	32.3	54.3	12.6	0.558
50	33.9	14.5	2.34	31.2	52.6	14.6	0.545
60	33.0	15.4	2.13	30.6	50.9	15.7	0.536
70	32.2	14.6	2.21	29.7	49.7	19.3	0.526
80	31.8	14.6	2.18	29.3	49.5	20.2	0.521
90	30.7	13.5	2.27	28.3	47.6	20.4	0.509
100	30.4	13.9	2.17	30.4	47.3	22.6	0.505

Ethylene Oxide Sterilization

Sterilization by ethylene oxide (ETO, *7*) in the presence of an inert gas is another technique which has been used often in the medical industry. Although some sterilizations are done using undiluted ETO, the ethylene oxide is most often diluted with either Freon 12 (*8*) [Ref. 9] or carbon dioxide (CO_2). ETO sterilizations are performed, commonly, at 49°C (120°F), 45%

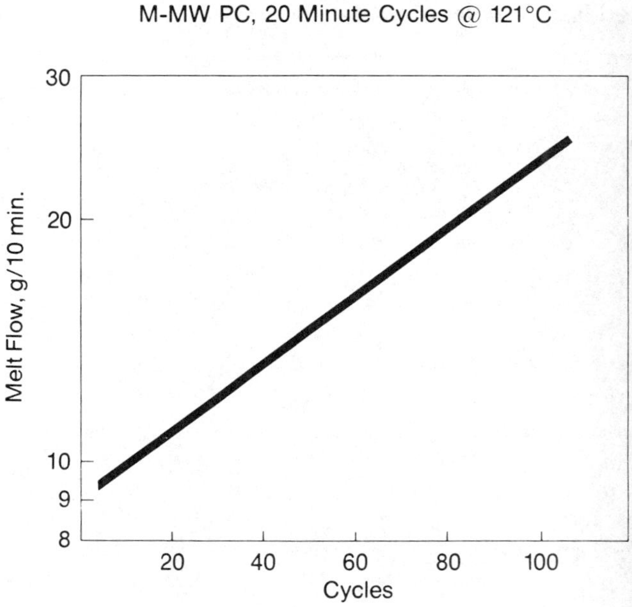

Figure 17. Change in melt flow after cyclic steam sterilizations.

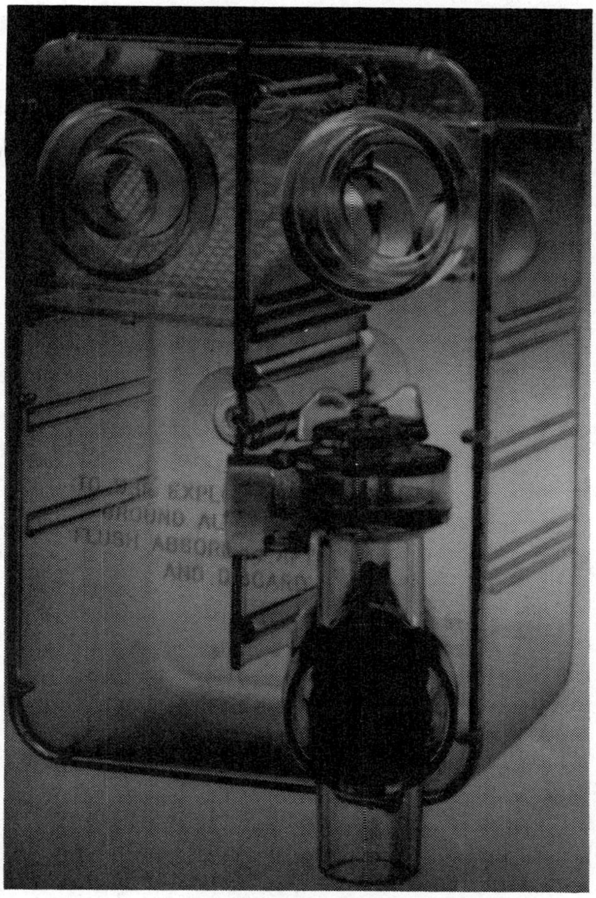

Figure 18. Dryden Corp.'s polycarbonate anesthesia canister.

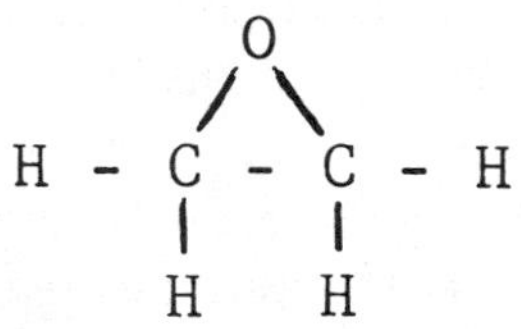

7

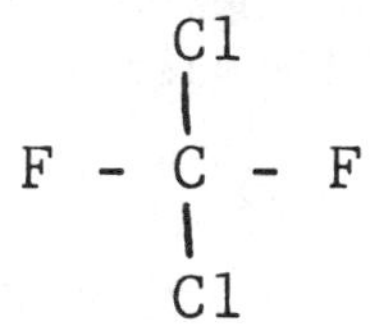

8

Relative Humidity for ten hours under 55 kPa (ca. 8 psig) and 280 kPa (ca. 40 psig) for the Freon 12 and CO_2 systems, respectively. Under these conditions, significant adverse effects upon polycarbonate physical properties have been rare. Retention of residual levels of ETO or its reaction products, ethylene chlorohydrin (ECH, *9*) and ethylene glycol (EG, *10*) have not been a problem in polycarbonate, as shown in Table 12. Both products arise from ring-opening reactions.

Table 12. Ethylene Oxide Residuals in Polycarbonate

Days After Sterilization*	Residual Level (ppm) ETO	ECH	EG
1	119	ND**	ND***
7	19	ND	ND
14	8	ND	ND

*Stored at Room Temperature

**None Detectable at the 1.2 ppm Level

***None Detectable at the 8.7 ppm Level

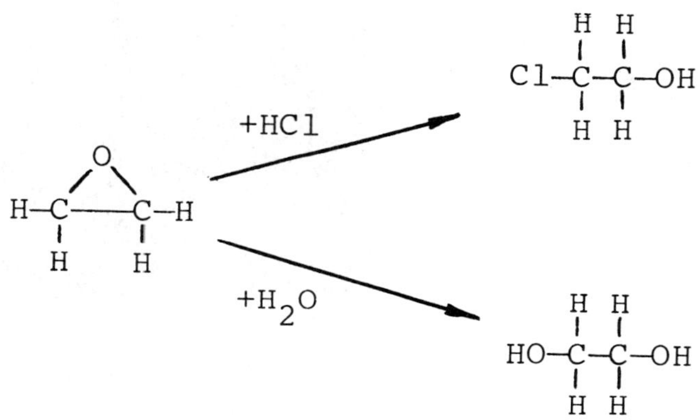

9

10

Because of the origin of these compounds, it is not surprising that no detectable levels of ECH and EG have been reported. Polycarbonate contains no chloride ion or HCl and has a low moisture level.

Table 12 also shows that ETO diffuses out of polycarbonate to very low levels after two weeks when stored at room temperature. Storage at higher temperatures results in more facile diffusion and more rapid achievement of a low residual ETO content. In addition, polycarbonate, when properly manufactured, contains no groups which can react with ETO, so no chemical, physical or FDA status changes can occur.

The effects of repeated ETO/Freon 12 sterilizations on the tensile properties of the three grades of polycarbonate, L-MW PC, M-MW PC and H-MW PC are shown in Table 13. Even after five cycles, there were little changes in tensile srength and elongation for any of the three grades. Similar results are found in Table 14 for the ETO/CO_2 system. Table 15 contains impact and flexural properties of M-MW PC after five ETO/CO_2 sterilization cycles. It also is apparent, from the data shown, that these properties were practically unaffected by the ethylene oxide sterilization technique.

High MW and low MW polycarbonates, when subjected to ETO/Freon 12 sterilization,

Table 13. Tensile Properties of Polycarbonate after ETO/Freon 12[R] Sterilization Cycles

		Tensile Stress, MPa		Tensile Strain, %	
Material	Cycles	Yield	Break	Yield	Break
L-MW PC	0	62	70	5	110
	1	62	70	5	115
	3	65	71	5	125
	5	65	76	5	120
M-MW PC	0	61	68	5	120
	1	61	63	5	100
	3	65	72	5	120
	5	66	68	5	100
H-MW PC	0	62	68	5	110
	1	62	77	5	110
	3	63	72	5	110
	5	63	64	5	90

Table 14. Tensile Properties of Polycarbonate after ETO/CO_2 Sterilization Cycles

		Tensile Stress, MPa		Tensile Strain, %	
Material	Cycles	Yield	Break	Yield	Break
L-MW PC	0	62	70	5	110
	1	63	66	5	105
	5	63	70	5	115
M-MW PC	0	61	68	5	120
	1	65	76	5	125
	5	64	71	5	110
H-MW PC	0	62	68	5	110
	1	66	80	5	115
	5	63	65	5	85

Table 15. Properties of M-MW PC after Five Cycles of ETO/CO_2 Sterilization

Property	Initial Unsterilized	5 Cycles ETO/CO_2
Tensile (DIN)		
Yield, MPa	63	63
Ultimate, MPa	74	73
Ultimate Elong., %	120	97
Flexural		
Strength @ 5% Strain, MPa	87	85
Strength, Ultimate, MPa	92	90
Modulus, GPa	2.3	2.2
Izod Impact		
3.2 mm, J/m	860	907
Critical Thickness, mm	4.6	4.7
Drop Impact, J	218	218

show very slight and moderate decreases, respectively, in *percent* retained ultimate tensile strength at high strain levels. As seen in Figure 19, at 1.6% flexural strain, L-MW PC retains about 70-75% of the initial ultimate strength after five cycles. The H-MW PC, however, retains up to 95% of its strength (Figure 20).

Several polycarbonate parts are sterilized by the 12/88 – ETO/Freon 12^R (12% ETO/88% Freon 12) method. One example is a blood centrifuge bowl (Figure 21). This bowl is manufactured by Haemonetics Corporation to be a component of a hemophoresis system, a continuous flow blood separator/red cell washer.

Haemonetics also manufactures an irrigation bottle spike, which like the bowl (Fig. 18), is a single-use item. This part is about three inches long and is used to regulate the flow of irrigation solutions.

The Avco Medical pulsatile balloon bypass pump (Figure 22) is sterilized using the ETO/CO_2 method. This unit acts as a cardiovascular support system during open-heart surgery. It provides pulsatile flow during bypass operations. Polycarbonate houses the balloons, made of a silicone/urethane copolymer. The connectors to the tubing are polycarbonate and are in contact with blood. The advantages of polycarbonate, here, are its clarity, strength and sterilizability.

Cobalt-60 Sterilization

Over the past few years, there has been a trend toward sterilizing single-use, plastic items

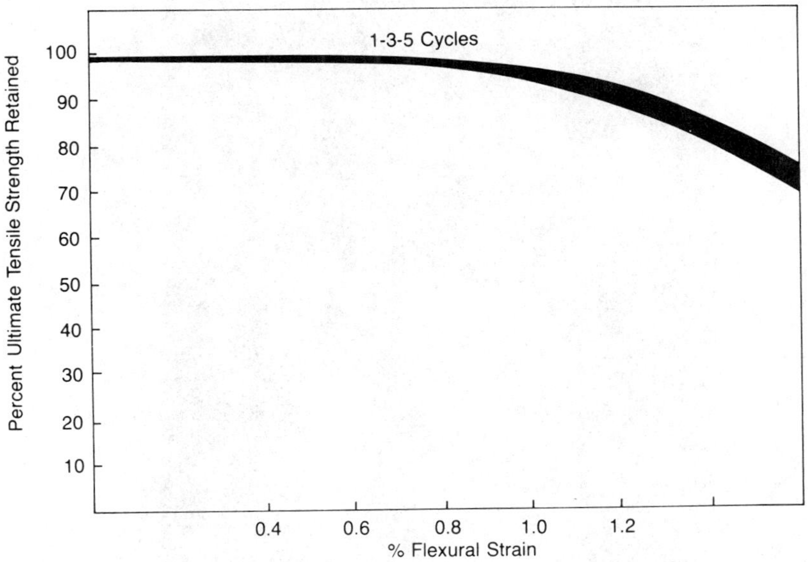

Figure 19. Ultimate tensile strength retention of low molecular weight polycarbonate after ETO/Freon 12® sterilization under induced tensile strain.

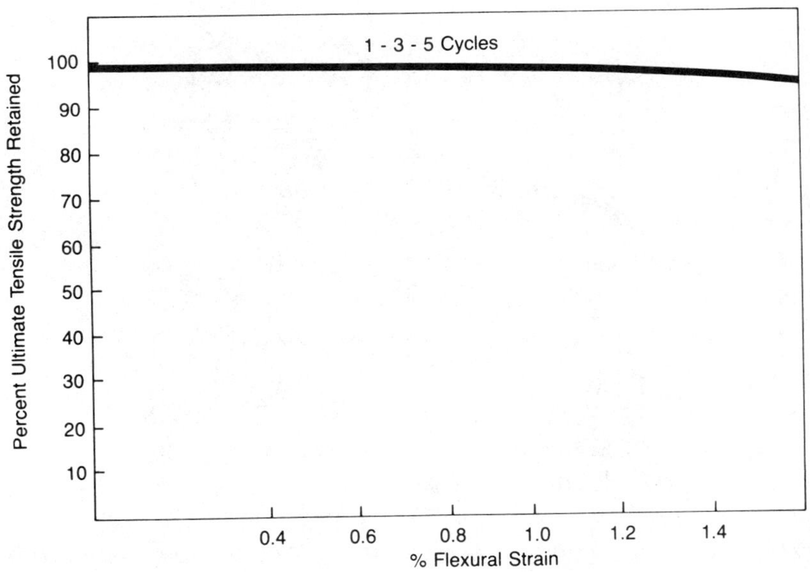

Figure 20. Ultimate tensile strength retention of high molecular weight polycarbonate after ETO/Freon 12® sterilization under induced tensile strain.

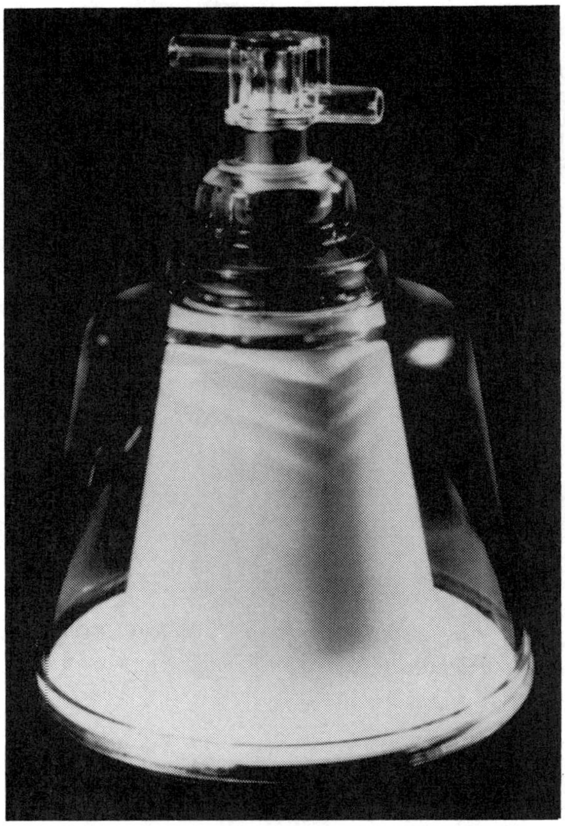

Figure 21. Haemonetics, Inc., polycarbonate blood filter bowl assembly.

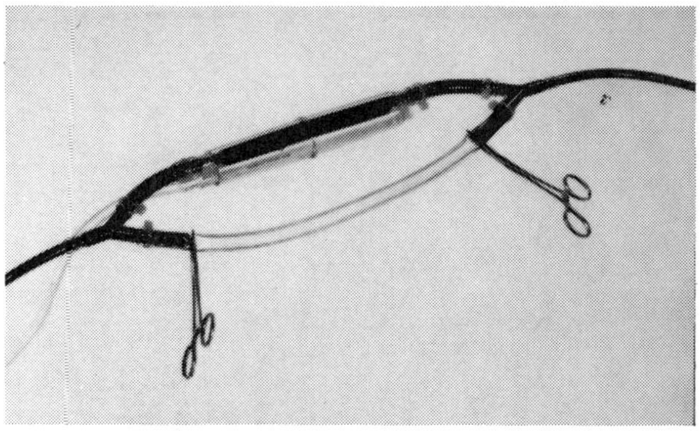

Figure 22. Avco Medical's polycarbonate pulsatile balloon bypass pump.

by high energy radiation. The technique used often is gamma ray bombardment from a Cobalt-60 (Co-60) source. A good basic explanation of this process has been published [Refs. 11,12].

Unlike certain fluorocarbons, acetals and some grades of polypropylene, polycarbonate retains its high strength and toughness even when exposed to signficantly more than the

Table 16. Effect of Radiation Dose on M-MW PC

Gamma Radiation Dosage, Mrads	0	2	4	8
Property				
Izod Impact				
3.2 mm, J/m	859	891	854	843
6.4 mm, J/m	123	128	128	128
Critical Thickness, mm	4.5	4.7	5.0	4.7
Tensile				
Yield, MPa	63	62	61	61
Ultimate, MPa	69	69	68	66
Ultimate Elong., %	115	118	120	112
Flexural				
Strength @ 5%, MPa	88	85	86	87
Ult. Strength, MPa	92	93	92	91
Modulus, GPa	2.3	2.3	2.4	2.4
Dart Drop, Joules	218	--	--	218

"standard dose" (around 2.0 Mrad) of Co-60, gamma radiation. Table 16 shows that impact strength, elongation and both tensile and flexural properties of M-MW PC are essentially unaffected by up to 8.0 Mrad.

In a current study, Izod impact strength of L-MW polycarbonate is being evaluated. Irradiation up to 5.0 Mrad showed no appreciable affect when the exposed Izod impact bars were compared to the non-sterilized controls. Furthermore, Co-60, gamma radiation evoked the same negligible response, whether the bars were notched before or after exposure. These data are in Table 17.

The shelf-life stability of M-MW polycarbonate samples is excellent. As seen in Table 18, both tensile strength and ultimate elongation remain high, one year after exposure to up to 10.0 Mrad. In the present study (Table 19), bars stored for six months (after irradiation) retained the high impact strength for which polycarbonate is noted.

Polycarbonate specimens, of all three grades, were clamped onto the compatibility test jig [Refs. 5 & 6] and irrradiated. Table 20 shows that L-MW PC and H-MW PC are relatively unaffected by 2.0 Mrad and M-MW PC by 8.0 Mrad, even at 1.6% outer fiber strain.

The medical industry has experienced difficulties with certain plastics becoming brittle and losing their strength after being sterilized by gamma radiation. Some grades of aliphatic polymers are known to have poor shelf-life stability, becoming so embrittled after storage at room temperature, they are useless.

This occurs because the energy absorbed from the gamma radiation causes bond breakage, with the concomitant formation of free radicals. These radicals can react with other

Table 17. Effect of Co-60 Gamma Radiation Dose on L-MW PC

Dosage, Mrad	Izod Impact N.B.S.* J/m	Izod Impact N.A.S.* J/m
0	822.2	--
2.5	849.2	791.0
5.0	842.2	775.8

*N.B.S. = notched before sterilization

N.A.S. = notched after sterilization

Table 18. Shelf-Life Stability of Co-60 Gamma Radiation Sterilized M-MW PC

	Ultimate Tensile Strength, MPa		Ultimate Elongation, %	
Mrads	Initial	After 1 Yr.	Initial	After 1 Yr.
0	72	--	130	--
1.2	70	72	130	115
1.7	72	74	115	110
2.8	66	76	120	120
3.9	68	70	125	110
5.7	69	70	125	120
10.0	68	68	130	115

polymer molecules and with oxygen, producing oxidative cleavage of the aliphatic chains. These processes lead to degradation of the physical properties.

Highly aromatic polymers, on the other hand, have low-lying electronic energy states which are responsible for absorption of the effects of radiation, reducing bond breakage and subsequent polymer degradation. Polycarbonate, being largely aromatic (bisphenol A), is fairly stable toward the effects of gamma radiation. The shelf-life stability, discussed earlier, was seen to be excellent.

Table 19. Shelf-Life Stability of L-MW PC Sterilized by Co-60 Gamma Radiation

Dosage*	Izod Impact Strength Initial J/m	Izod Impact Strength After 6 mo. J/m
0, NBS/S	822	818
0, NAS/S	--	753
2.5, NBS/S	849	822
2.5, NAS/S	791	734
5.0, NBS/S	842	828
5.0, NAS/S	776	737

*NBS/S = notched before sterilization and storage
NAS/S = notched after sterilization and storage

Alas, for all of its unique and desirable characteristics, polycarbonate is not perfect. The change that occurs during exposure to Co-60 radiation, is the development of a yellow color, proportional to the dosage. As Table 21 shows, the tensile strength remains reasonably constant, while the Yellowness Index increases nearly fifty-fold. This color development is probably similar to the yellowing of natural polycarbonate when exposed to ultraviolet light. This is believed to occur via a Photofries Rearrangement, which leads to the formation of phenyl salicylates, 2,2′-dihydroxybenzophenones, etc. [Ref. 13]. These products, however, can be formed by reactions within a single polycarbonate molecule, without net bond breakage and reduction in molecular weight. Even reactions leading to polymer bond breakage, result in salicylates and other end groups; yet, the lower molecular weight polymer fragments, thus formed, are non-migratory.

In the case of gamma radiation, the yellow color develops throughout the plastic material and not on the surface alone; still, not enough of the highly colored rearrangement products are formed to significantly affect polycarbonate's physical properties. This is why cutting the Izod notch after sterilization did not give notably different impact strengths than pre-notching the specimens. This color formation, though slight, is objectionable to some medical part manufacturers. Polycarbonate containing standard blue tints tend to become green upon exposure to 2.0 Mrad of Cobalt-60, gamma radiation. The comment heard most often, is that blood "looks sick" when viewed through a yellow or green surface.

There now are polycarbonate grades specially formulated for gamma sterilization. These polymers do not become yellow after a 3.0 Mrad dosage of Co-60 gamma radiation.

Table 20. Ultimate Elongation of Stressed Polycarbonate Bars Sterilized by Co-60 Gamma Radiation

Initial Outer Fiber Strain	Ultimate Elongation				
	L-MW PC	M-MW PC			H-MW PC
	2 Mrad	2 Mrad	4 Mrad	8 Mrad	2 Mrad
(%)	(%)	(%)	(%)	(%)	(%)
0	107	112	100	106	100
0.4	90	105	50	95	110
0.6	100	85	95	95	105
0.8	110	95	100	100	100
1.0	90	90	90	100	110
1.2	100	95	100	100	100
1.4	110	100	100	75	105
1.6	95	90	100	85	85

Table 21. Change in Color of M-MW PC vs. Co-60 Gamma Radiation Dosage

Mrads	Yellowness Index	Tensile Strength, MPa
0	0.9	69
1.2	3.6	69
1.7	6.6	72
2.8	9.2	65
3.9	12.6	68
5.7	20.4	69
10.0	43.0	67

Polycarbonate Film

Polycarbonate film is being used in a growing number of packaging applications, including that of medical items. Even though film is not used in applications requiring multiple sterilizations, it is useful to report results of multiple-sterilization-cycle testing.

The effect of steam sterilization on the properties of PC film, at both 0.025 mm (1.0 mil) and 0.38 mm (15 mil) thicknesses, are shown in Figure 23. Note that after three, standard steam autoclave sterilization cycles, the tear strengths of both the thick and thin polycarbonate films remain high.

Figure 24 shows tensile yeild strengths of polycarbonate film at various thicknesses before and after one sterilization with either ETO/Freon 12 or ETO/CO_2. The data indicate that there are no important deleterious effects from using an ethylene oxide sterilization technique.

The results of radiation sterilization show that polycarbonate film is almost unaffected by dosages up to 8.0 Mrad. Figure 25 graphically illustrates this in the cases of 0.025 mm and 0.38 mm films.

XI. SPECIFIC APPLICATIONS OF POLYCARBONATE IN MEDICAL APPARATUS

Most often, polycarbonate has been used to manufacture medical and surgical articles where clarity was an advantage. Recently, polycarbonate grades also have attracted the attention of design engineers considering materials for opaque parts. Mechanical apparatus, such as surgical staplers are being designed in a number of polycarbonate grades. At this writing, however, most medical applications utilizing polycarbonate call for natural or clear, tinted material. The parts illustrated here all use a clear grade polymer.

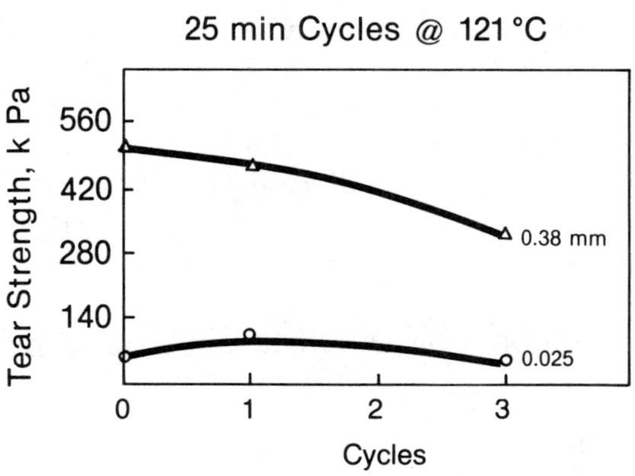

Figure 23. Tear strength of steam sterilized polycarbonate films.

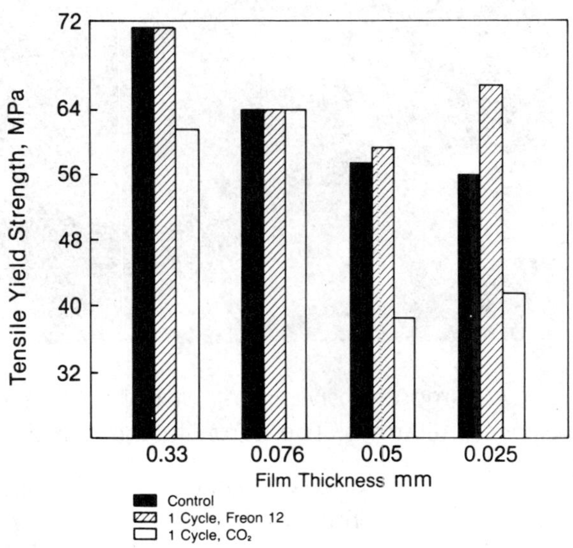

Figure 24. Tensile yield strength of ETO sterilized polycarbonate films.

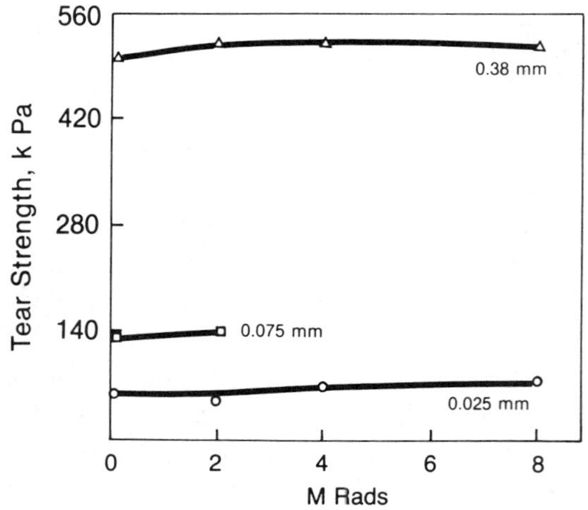

Figure 25. Tear strength of cobalt-60 sterilized polycarbonate films.

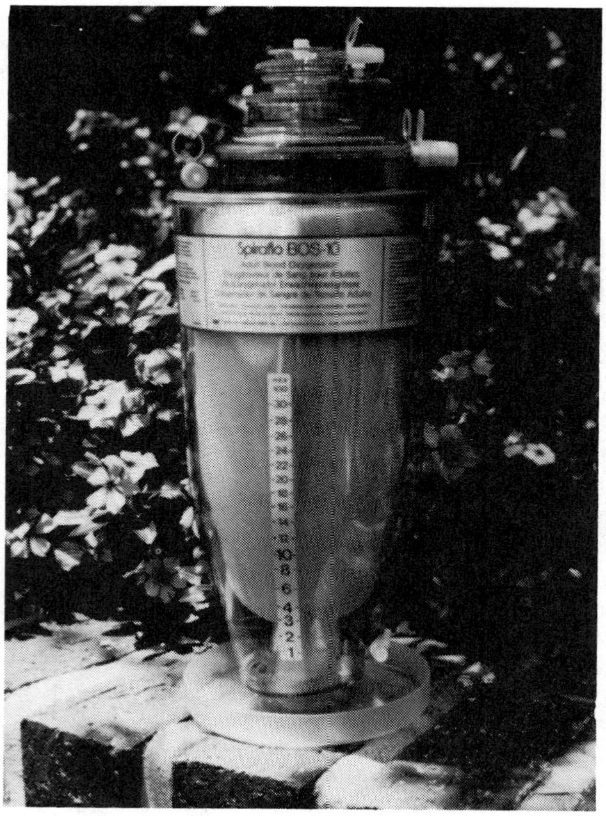

Figure 26. Bentley Laboratories' "Spiroflo BOS-10" Blood Oxygenator. Seven injection molded parts bonded together using the EMABond technique [Ref. 15]. Wall is 8" wide; flowers are 2" across. (Photo courtesy of Mobay Chemical Corporation.)

A comprehensive listing of the medical parts made from polycarbonate is precluded by space limitations. The parts illustrated are:

blood oxygenators	(Figures 26-33)
connector	(Figure 35)
control valve	(Figure 37)
filter bowls	(Figure 34)
transducer domes	(Figure 36)

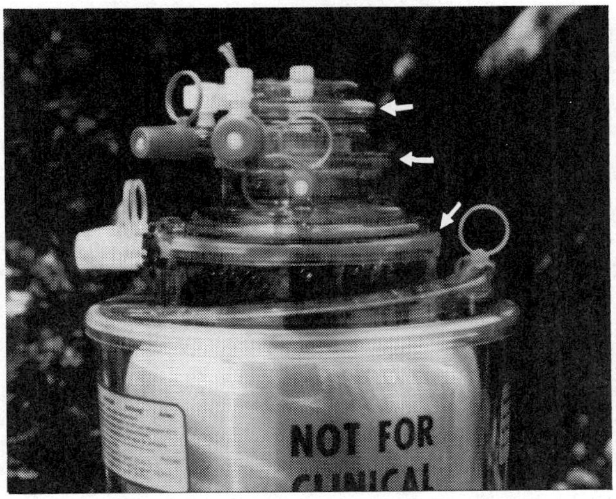

Figure 27. Close-up of top, showing four of five subsections and EMABonds (arrows). (Photo courtesy of Mobay Chemical Corporation.)

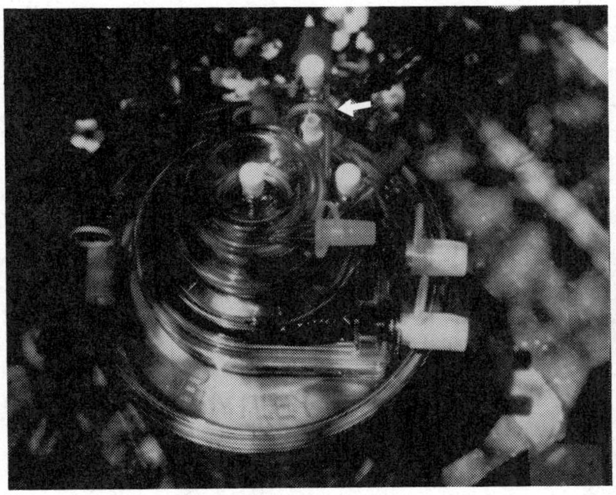

Figure 28. Top view, showing fifth subsection and EMABond (arrow). The various inlets are also clearly indicated: non-oxygenated blood (blue); oxygen port (green); gas vent (yellow); water for temperature control (large white). (Photo courtesy of Mobay Chemical Corporation.)

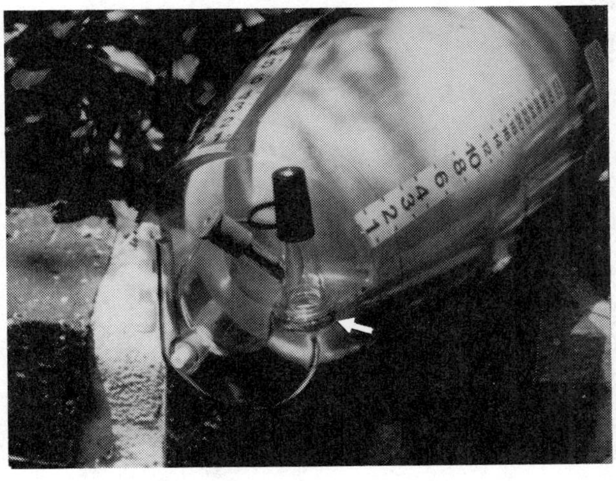

Figure 29. Bottom view, showing oxygenated blood outlet (red) bonded (arrow) to main body section. (Photo courtesy of Mobay Chemical Corporation.)

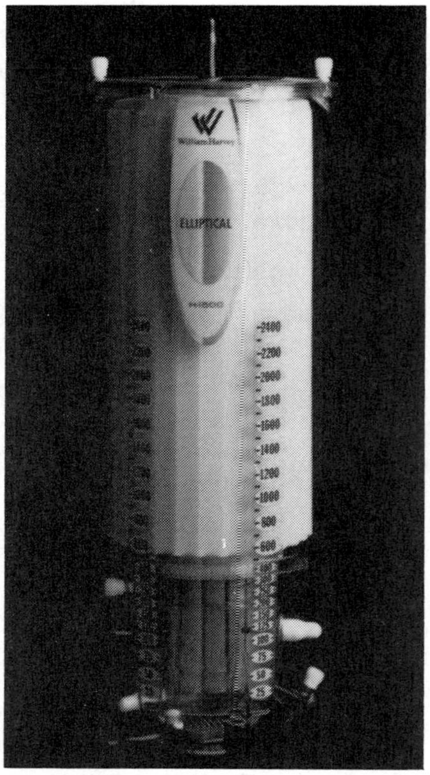

Figure 30. The William Harvey "H-1500" Blood Oxygenator is constructed from injection molded and extruded polycarbonate. Assembly makes use of solvent bonding techniques. The temperature resistance of polycarbonate is especially important in the bottom section, where heater rods are encased in polycarbonate. (Photo courtesy of Harvey Cardiopulmonary Divison, C. W. Bard, Inc.).

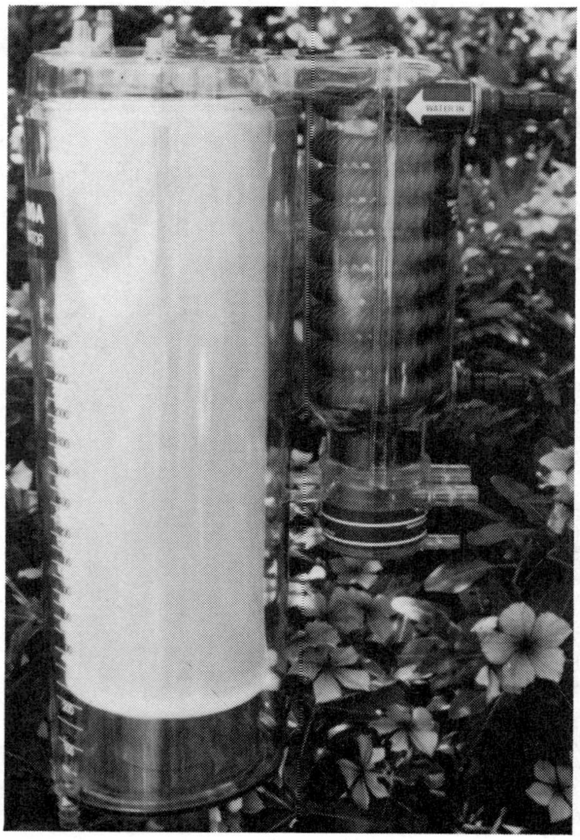

Figure 31. Side view of the complete Shiley 100A Blood Oxygenator. Attached to this side is the blood heater, which warms the vital fluid before introduction to the patient's circulatory system. The warm water enters the heating unit through the top black tube and exits through the lower black tube. (Photo courtesy of Mobay Chemical Corporation).

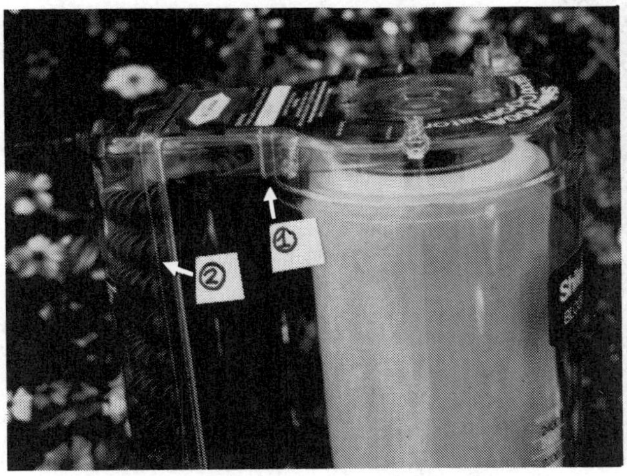

Figure 32. Close-up of top of Shiley oxygenator, where the heater unit is solvent bonded to the main body of the apparatus 1. Note the clarity of the solvent bonds here and at the juncture of the two halves of the heater, 2. Proper solvent bonding of polycarbonate provides strong, durable joints, without loss of clarity. (Photo courtesy of Mobay Chemical Corporation).

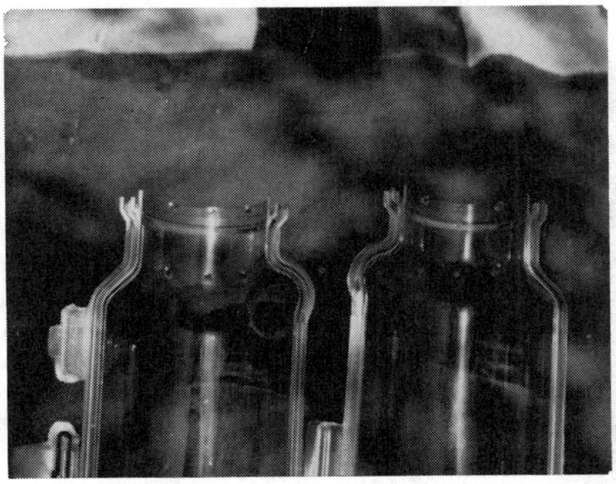

Figure 33. View of the tongue and groove detail of the two halves of the Shiley 100A heater unit.

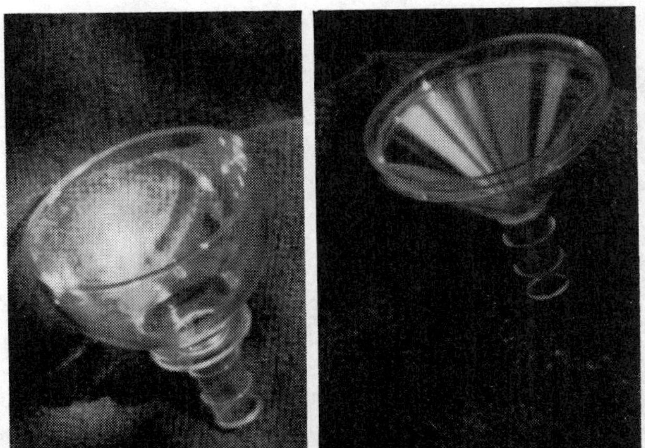

Figure 34. Dome- and Conical-shape filter bowls. A Delta Medical Product molded from low molecular weight polycarbonate. (Photo courtesy Mobay Chemical Corporation).

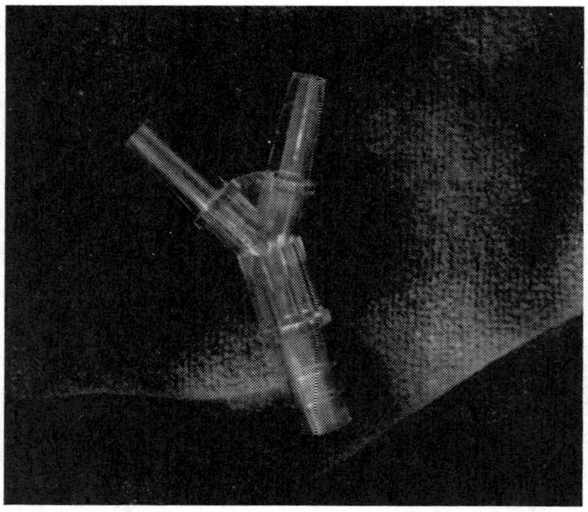

Figure 35. Low molecular polycarbonate was used by Critikon, Inc., to manufacture this connector used in blood contact applications. (Photo courtesy Mobay Chemical Corporation).

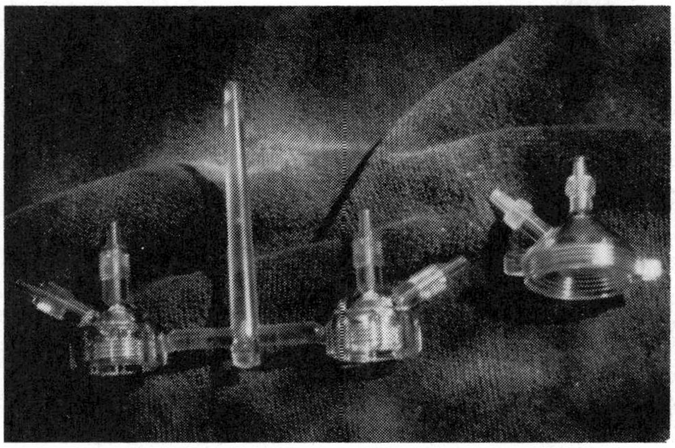

Figure 36. Bentley Laboratories manufactures equipment to sense variations in blood pressure. This transducer dome, molded from polycarbonate, is an important part of this apparatus. (Photo courtesy Mobay Chemical Corporation).

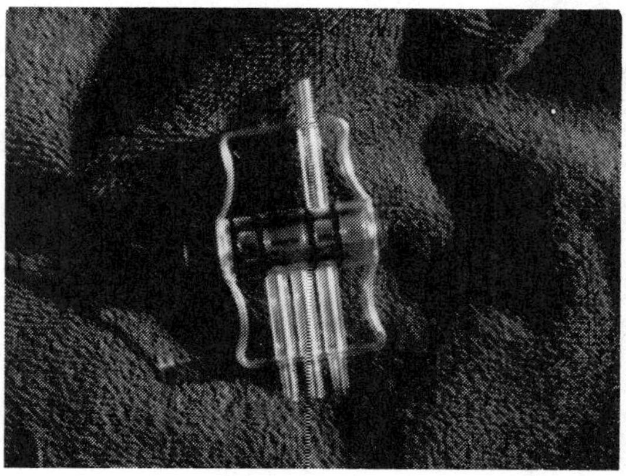

Figure 37. A blood contact application, this piston actuated temperature control valve is molded from medium molecular weight polycarbonate by GICS. (Photo courtesy of Mobay Chemical Corporation).

ACKNOWLEDGEMENT

The author gratefully acknowledges the people whose assistance made it possible to produce this chapter, among whom are: Mrs. Jan Vernillo, who spent many hours at the word processor and was so very patient with me through the seemingly endless minor revisions, uncrossed tees and undotted i's; Ed Kline, who provided most of the photographs; Ken Wobbekind, Rolf Kahl, John Cox, John Bailey, Gene Sokolowski, Steve Drozda, Ms. Chris Schlaegle and Ms. Theresa Lecava, who rendered both technical and syntactical assistance.

REFERENCES

1. Schnell, H., *Chemistry and Physics of Polycarbonate,* Ch. I-III, Polymer Reviews, Vol. 9, H. F. Mark & E. H. Immergut, eds., Wiley-Interscience, NY, 1964.
2. *Guide to Plastics,* p. 17, McGraw-Hill, Inc., NY, 1980.
3. *Merlon Polycarbonate Resin, Basic Grades,* Mobay Chemical Corporation, Plastics Department, Pittsburgh, PA 15205.
4. *Typical Properties of Lexan Resin,* Design Bulletin, General Electric Company, Pittsfield, MA 01201.
5. "Determination of Chemical Resistance of Plastics under Mechanical Stress," Kunststoffe, *65*(3), 155, 1975.
6. A shop drawing for these fixtures and test details are available from Mobay Chemical Corporation, Plastics & Coatings Division, Plastics Department, Penn Lincoln Parkway West, Pittsburgh, PA 15205.
7. "A Processing Guide for Injection Molding," Mobay Chemical Corporation, Plastics Department, Pittsburgh, PA 15205.
8. Registered Trademark of Xaloy, Inc.
9. Masylar, K. D. and Thomas, J. R., "Sterilization of Polycarbonate," presented at the 38th ANTEC, New York City, NY, 1980.
10. Registered Trademark of E. I. du Pont de Nemours and Co., Inc.
11. Chin, Allan, "Gamma Radiation and Single-Use Devices," Medical Device & Diagnostic Industry, Jan. 1980.
12. Chin, Allan, *ibid,* February 1980.
13. Gupa, A., Rembaum, A. and Moacanin, J., "Solid State Chemistry of Polycarbonates," Macromolecules, *11*(b), 1285 (1978).
14. NIOSH, "Ethylene Oxide (EtO): Evidence of Carcinogenicity," NIOSH Current Awareness Bulletin: #35, DHHS (NIOSH) Publication No. 81-130, May 22, 1981.
15. *EMABond* is a registered trademark of EMABond, Inc.

Chapter 36

Case Studies: Synthesis, Characterization and Production of Biomedical Polymers

Barry Ashar
Kontron Cardiovascular, Incorporated
9 Plymouth Street
Everett, MA 02149

ABSTRACT

In this chapter, we have discussed three case studies, undertaken at a biomedical research and development center, on three different biomaterials. This chapter illustrates what goes on behind the synthesis, characterization and production of polymers designed for medical uses. We hope to give a better understanding of biomaterials development to all the professionals in the biomedical field who have come from various disciplines.

The first case deals with the situation where a specific application existed for which a custom made material needed to be designed. The case discusses a methodical approach toward developing a room temperature curing silica-free silicone capable of yielding a microscopically smooth surface. It is presented from a materials design engineer's point of view.

The second case deals with the development of a polycarbonate-silicone co-polymer for which specific uses were not yet defined. The material's usefulness for biomedical applications was defined based on theoretical considerations. This case heavily emphasizes the polymer synthesis and characterization principles. It is presented from a polymer chemist's point of view.

The final case deals with the large scale production of biomaterials. Equally challenging considerations arise when a material moves from a lab set-up to a full scale production, especially when its purity is of extreme importance. This case is presented from a manufacturing engineer's point of view.

INTRODUCTION

As recently as 1960, surgeons who felt uncomfortable with the mechanical aspects of devices, such as rotary pumps and oxygenators, were considered lagging behind in their profession. While some doctors were quite innovative, it became obvious that not all surgeons, at home in the operating room, were efficient at building experimental devices. Engineering help was badly needed. However, a major problem existed; in part because the medical field hesitated to accept non-medical professionals in their circle. Typically, a surgeon could not imagine getting help from an engineer, who knew nothing about blood except that it looked red. Through years of frustration though, this attitude changed, and mechanical and electrical engineers probably became the first non-medical professionals to team up with surgeons and physicians for the purpose of developing improved medical devices.

The current era of a highly interdisciplinary approach to the field of medical science emerged as a result of this sophistication. Biomedical engineering became an offshoot of electronics engineering. Physicists brought the concepts of fluid dynamics to the field. Recently, chemists, especially polymer scientists, have expressed their interest in medical devices. Terms such as "biocompatibility" and "biomedical polymer" are increasingly popular. As an example, a few years ago a cardiac surgeon working with an intra-aortic balloon pump was interested primarily in its ease of insertion and reliable operation. Today, we find many surgical teams working with polymer scientists on the materials research for such devices, and showing interest in their toxicity and biocompatibility characteristics, as well.

Today, both public institutions and private enterprise commit large funds to research work on biomedical polymers. Nearly all of this work is concentrated on in-vitro and in-vivo studies of commercial polymers and their use in medical devices. Institutions, such as NIH and ASTM, have developed extensive guidelines for the characterization of polymers for biomedical applications.

One area significantly lacking in published data involves the synthesis of biomedical polymers. Only a handful of polymers have been specifically designed for medical application and, due to their proprietary nature, hardly any information is available on the various aspects of their synthesis.

The primary goal of this chapter is to address this topic in some detail. First, we present a brief discussion of those concepts of polymer science that relate to the medical applications of polymers. Specific case studies are then undertaken to illustrate the thoughts and considerations of a polymer scientist working to synthesize new biomedical polymers. The interrelationship between the synthesis and characterization of polymers at an early stage of development is described. We illustrate how property requirements of the end user can be translated into measureable characteristics of the raw polymers. The expertise of a polymer engineer, as it applies to the production of biomedical polymers, is shown.

Most professionals working on biomedical polymer synthesis were educated as organic chemists, chemical engineers, surface scientists or biologists. In fact, less than one percent of those working in polymer and plastics related industries have any formal education in polymer science and engineering. We believe that the material presented here will help these professionals to approach their polymer synthesis problems with a better perspective and in a more sophisticated manner. We trust that this chapter also will prove helpful to those who are polymer scientists, by focusing on the application of polymer science to the field of artificial organs and medical devices.

REVIEW

In this chapter, the terms "biocompatibility" and "blood compatibility" are used interchangeably, since most of the materials discussed are for blood contact applications. A blood compatible material, in general, is thought of as one which does not cause thrombosis. In addition, however, experience indicates that blood compatible materials should not lead to the destruction or alteration of blood components; such as, red cells, white cells, platelets, plasma, etc. And, the material should neither deteriorate in the biological environment nor lead to toxicity related issues. Specifics of blood compatability phenomena are defined in detail in the literature [1].

Many authors have reported on the reactions that take place when a material interacts with blood [2,3,4]. However, the factors which initiate or prevent these reactions are still disputed. Various theories have been offered that correlate the blood compatibility of materials with the physico-chemical properties of their surfaces. Electronegatively charged surfaces are believed to behave as vascular walls and thus are expected to show reduced thrombogenicity. Wettability of materials has been related to blood compatibility, and an empirical range of critical surface tension from 20 to 30 dynes/cm has been suggested for good compatibility [5]. In response to these theories, various approaches have been taken toward the development of blood-compatible materials [1]. For example, use of negatively charged groups on polymers, ionically or covalently bonded heparin, hydrogel coatings and glow discharge treatments have been popular.

Nyilas has given a physico-chemical interpretation of the phenomena which occur at the blood/foreign surface interface [6]. On the basis of this interpretation, he has hypothesized that lower heat of adsorption of protein on the surface would favor blood compatibility. The magnitude of heat of adsorption is in turn determined by surface molecular structure. Chemical groups capable of forming hydrogen bonds or those containing highly polarized covalent bonds are undesirable for this application. Instead, groups which are capable of forming only weak bonds, such as van der Waals bonds, are preferred.

Polar groups in polymeric chains can be chemically blocked or be made physically inaccessible through stearic hindrance. Copolymerization is one of the most effective ways to achieve such results. It makes it possible to access the mechanical properties of the polymers containing polar groups, and at the same time have an essentially non-polar surface.

Based on these concepts, a few specific cases are presented to demonstrate how we feel biocompatibility might be achieved through the manipulation of various chemical structures on synthetic polymers. We discuss the chemistry of polymerization, the physico-chemical characterization of polymers, and their relationship to the blood compatibility behavior of polymers. Our approach is highly practical, in the sense that these case studies are actual projects undertaken by a biomedical research and development group. Theory is emphasized only as far as its application is concerned. Approaches taken at the early stages of development, as well as those taken during large-scale production of biomedical polymers, are discussed in detail.

CASE STUDY I

Silica-Free Silicone

Lederman, et al., recognized the importance of having a microscopically smooth blood-contact surface while developing a Left Ventricular Assist Device (LVAD) [7]. The fabrication process involved the dip-coating of a polyethylene glycol mandrel with Cardiothane-51, a polyurethane-silicone copolymer solution. Through numerous manipulations, they were able to obtain an extremely smooth surface on the air-facing side of the film. However, as shown in Figure 1, the surface roughness on the mandrel-facing side of the film was clinically unacceptable. An attempt to solve the problem by precoating the mandrel with a commercial silicone did not succeed. We believed that the basic approach was right, but that the type of silicone available was not suitable for the purpose. At this point, we decided to develop a new silicone system capable of generating an extremely smooth surface for further coating.

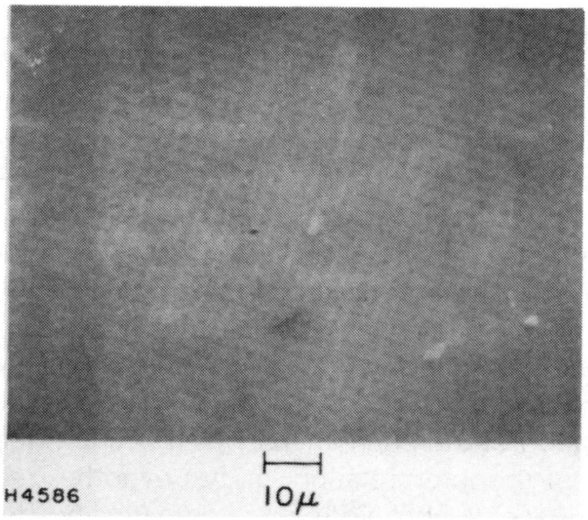

Figure 1a. Air side cured Cardiothane-51 (control for comparison of required degree of smoothness).

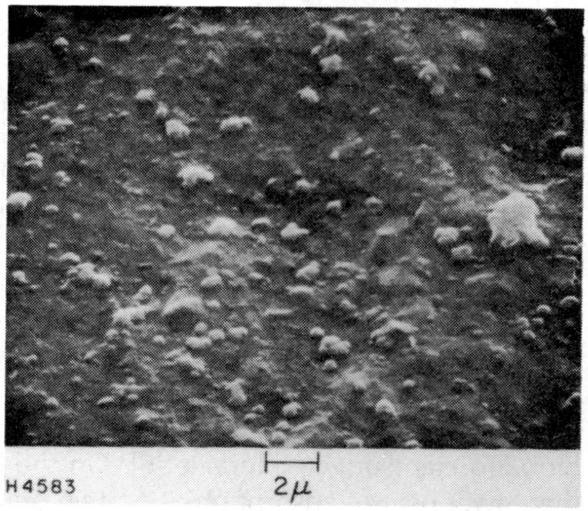

Figure 1b. Mandrel side cured Cardiothane-51, cast on polyethylene glycol.

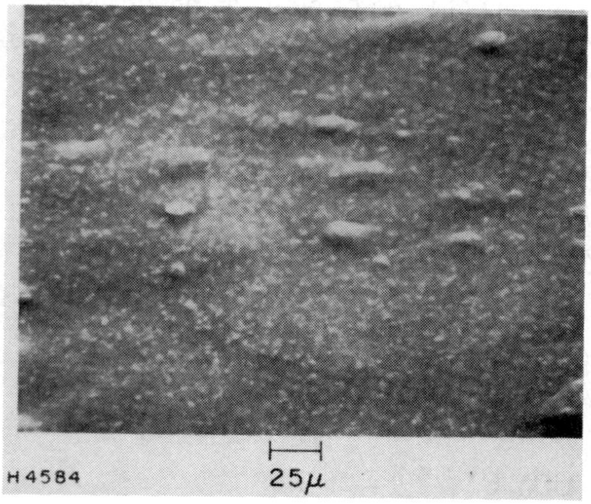

Figure 1c. Mandrel side cured Dardiothane-51, cast on silica-filled silicone coated mandrel.

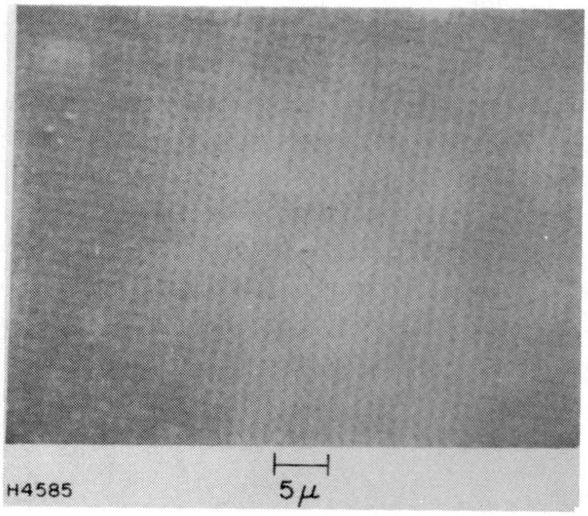

Figure 1d. Mandrel side cured Cardiothane-51, cast on silica-free silicone coated-mandrel.

Figure 1. Scanning electron microscope pictures of blood-contact surfaces. (Note 2).

Based on the already proven fabrication process and other relevant considerations, we established that the silicone materials should:

(a) Contain no fillers
(b) Not adhere to Cardiothane-51
(c) Form a smooth surface
(d) Cure at room temperature
(e) Have viscosity suitable for dip-coating
(f) Be of extremely high purity
(g) Be minimally leachable

As shown in Figure 2, it was clear that the fillers were responsible for the surface roughness of the coatings. Thus we decided to eliminate the fillers. Although this would decrease the mechanical properties of the coating, it would not be detrimental to the fabrication process. Non-adherence to Cardiothane-51 was required so that when the bladder was fabricated, the silicone film could be easily peeled off. Room temperature curing was necessary because of the low melting point of the polyethylene glycol mandrel. Working at room temperature would also give more flexibility to the process. Viscosity requirements were mainly to eliminate the flow-related irregularities of the coating.

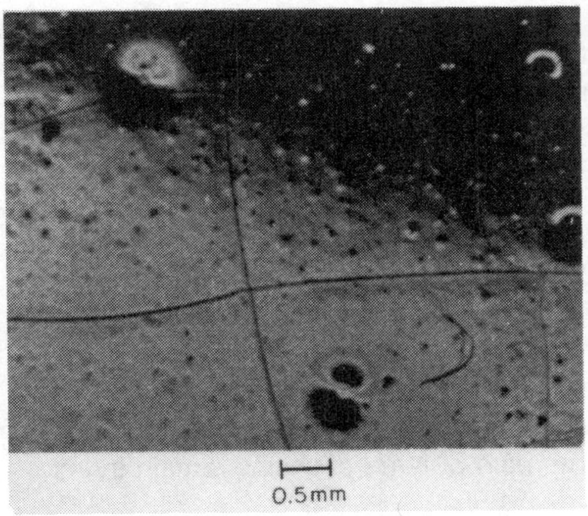

Figure 2a. Surface of a filler-filled silicone.

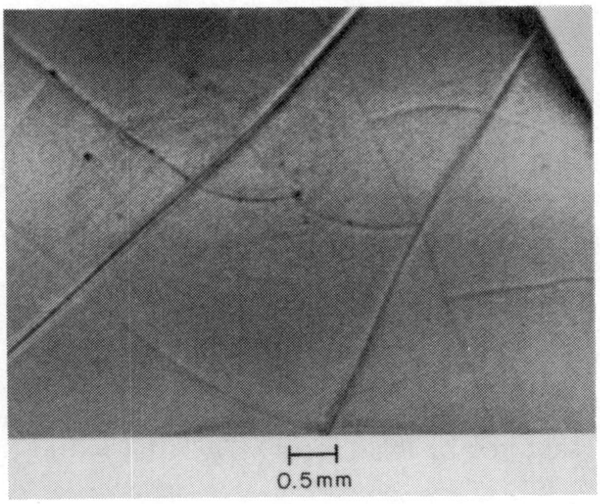

Figure 2b. Surface of a filler-free silicone.

Figure 2. Effect of fillers on the surface smoothness of silicones.

Chemistry

Based on a literature search and previous experience with silicones, we decided that a polydimethyl siloxane polymer terminated in acetoxy end groups would be suitable for the purpose. In addition to room temperature curing, this polymer offers the advantage of being a stable one-component system that cures only when exposed to atmospheric moisture. The principal reactions involved follow.

I.

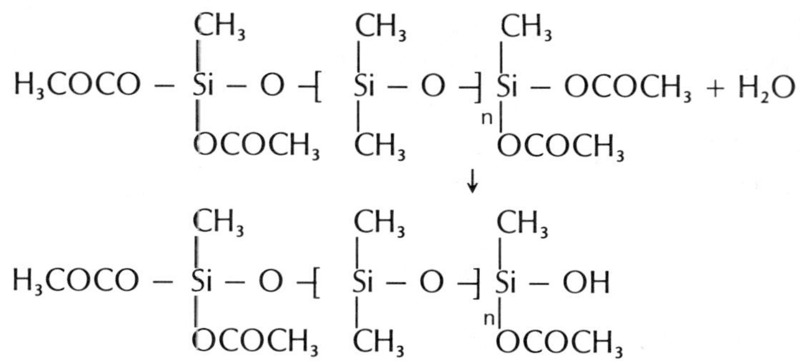

II.

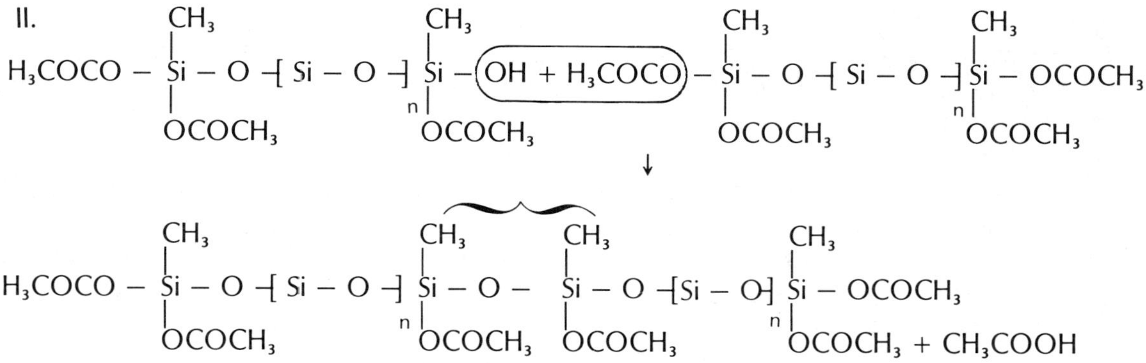

When exposed to moisture, some of the acetate groups in the system undergo hydrolysis. The newly formed hydroxyl (–OH) groups then undergo condensation reactions with the remaining acetate (–OAc) groups, leading to a cross-linked network. This reaction is quite rapid and does not need any additional acceleration. Eventually, however, when only hydroxyl (–OH) groups are left in the system, further condensation is an extremely slow reaction, usually requiring a catalyst. Dibutyl tin dilaurate is probably the most common catalyst used for this reaction.

It was obvious that as the degree of cross-linking was increased, the leachables from the system would decrease. Therefore, we decided to develop polymeric chains with a functionality of at least four. A slight excess of methyl triacetoxy silane (MTAS) over the stoichiometric amount was added so that any incoming moisture during storage would be captured by this excess MTAS. This ensures that the main polymeric chains remain intact.

Physico-chemical Considerations

Extent and rate of curing were the two key parameters to be studied in detail. These would have a direct bearing on the leachables from the system and they would also give an indication of the curing time required before further handling. As shown on the next page thermoset polymers give rise to a cross-linked network on curing.

The cross-linked network is essentially insoluble in solvents. However, some solvents manage to penetrate the network and swell it. Measurements of the extent of swelling lead to a parameter called "molecular weight between cross-links" (M_x) which is a measure of the extent of curing. The greater the curing, the greater the number of cross-link sites in the network, and the lower the molecular weight between consecutive cross-links. Table 1 summarizes the experimental measurements and the equations used in calculating the M_x.

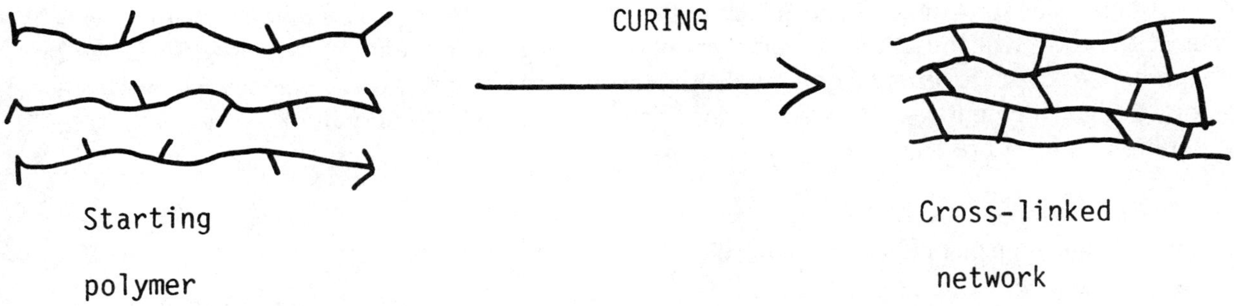

Table 1. Molecular Weight between Cross-Links (M_x)

W_1 = Weight of cured sample

W_2 = Weight of swollen sample

= Weight of cured sample
+ Weight of penetrated solvent
- Weight of extractables from the sample.

W_3 = Weight of dried sample

$(W_1 - W_3)$ = Weight of extractables

W_4 = Weight of penetrated solvent

$= (W_2 - W_3)$

Molecular Weight between Cross-links

$$M_x = \frac{V_1 \rho_2 (C^{1/3} - C/2)}{\ln(1-C) + C + \chi C^2}$$

where ρ_1 = density of solvent

ρ_2 = density of polymer

V_1 = molar volume of solvent

V_s = swollen volume of polymer

$$= \frac{W_3}{\rho_2} + \frac{W_4}{\rho_1}$$

C = Relative concentration

$$= \frac{W_3}{\rho_2} \times V_s$$

χ = Flory-Huggins constant

The values of χ for a given polymer-solvent system are available in literature. For a silicone-toluene system at 20°C, these values are as follows:

	C=0	C=0.2	C=0.4	C=0.6	C=0.8
χ	0.445	0.504	0.59	0.64	0.72

First, we investigated the effect of the following parameters on the extent of curing.

(a) Percent catalyst
(b) Curing time
(c) Curing temperature
(d) Molecular weight of starting silicone
(e) Moisture content of the system

A statistical screening design (Plackett-Burman design; Note 1, see end of chapter) was used to study which of these parameters had any "significant" affect on curing [8]. Table 2 summarizes the experimental conditions, the results and the statistical inferences derived from this design. Percentage catalyst, curing time and curing temperature were the three parameters found to significantly affect the extent of curing.

Table 2. 20-Run Plackett-Burman Design

Variable	Lower Limit (-)	Upper Limit (+)
Percent Catalyst (x_1)	0.005	0.05
Curing Time (x_2), min.	30	240
Temperature (x_3), °C	25	80
Molecular Weight (x_4)	73,000	108,000
Percent Water (x_5)	0	0.05

Run Number	Percent Catalyst (x_1)	Curing Time,min (x_2)	Tempera-ture,°C (x_3)	Molecular Weight (x_4)	Percent Water (x_5)	Response M_x (Y)
1	0.05	30	80	73,000	0	4,531
2	0.05	240	25	73,000	0.05	4,024
3	0.05	240	25	108,000	0	4,887
4	0.05	30	80	108,000	0	65,705
5	0.005	240	25	108,000	0	65,705
6	0.05	30	25	108,000	0.05	22,022
7	0.005	240	80	73,000	0.05	6,392
8	0.005	30	25	108,000	0.05	271,427
9	0.05	30	80	73,000	0	4,907
10	0.05	240	80	73,000	0.05	4,300
11	0.005	30	80	108,000	0	6,854
12	0.005	240	80	73,000	0	4,423
13	0.005	240	80	108,000	0.05	5,480
14	0.05	30	25	73,000	0.05	54,402
15	0.005	240	25	73,000	0.05	33,802
16	0.05	240	25	108,000	0	4,733
17	0.05	240	80	108,000	0	5,782
18	0.005	30	80	108,000	0.05	5,853
19	0.005	30	25	73,000	0	415,541
20	0.005	30	25	73,000	0	254,333
Effect:	-95475	-90581	-107688	-33844	-35852	

Minimum effect for significance: $|E_{min}|$ = 82306
Therefore, x_1, x_2 and x_3 have significant effect

Next, the Box-Behnken statistical design (Note 1, see end of chapter) was used to study the affect of the "significant" parameters in detail. Table 3 summarizes the experimental runs and Figure 3 shows the results in a three-dimensional plot.

Table 3. Three-Variable Box-Behnken Design

Variable	Low (-)	Middle (0)	High (+)
Percent Catalyst(x_1)	$5x10^{-3}$	$5x10^{-2.5}$	$5x10^{-2}$
Curing time(x_2), min.	30	135	240
Curing temp.(x_3),°C	25	52	80

Run Number	Percent Catalyst (x_1)	Curing time,min. (x_2)	Curing temp.°C (x_3)	Response M_x (Y)
1	0.05	240	52	5,179
2	0.005	135	25	158,963
3	0.016	240	25	6,432
4	0.016	30	25	128,842
5	0.016	240	80	4,643
6	0.016	135	52	4,905
7	0.05	30	52	4,229
8	0.05	135	25	4,120
9	0.005	240	52	4,566
10	0.05	135	80	3,811
11	0.016	135	52	5,083
12	0.016	30	80	6,042
13	0.005	135	80	9,000
14	0.005	30	52	19,426
15	0.016	135	52	5,085

At the upper limit of these variables, i.e., when a silicone containing 0.05% catalyst is cured at 80°C for 240 minutes, maximum extent of curing is achieved. However, quite similar results were obtained even at lower values of these parameters. For example, for satisfactory curing at room temperature, 0.05% catalyst is needed if the curing period is restricted to 30 min.; but for a 240-min. curing period, similar results are obtained with only about 0.015% catalyst. In short, when one of the three variables is at its upper limit, acceptable curing is obtained, regardless of what values the other two parameters have taken.

In practical terms, this means that if the process requires frequent handling and a room-temperature operation, then the silicone system used should contain a large amount (0.05%) of catalyst. Otherwise, the amount of catalyst can be reduced almost ten times. This is important for medical polymers where any potential leachables should be kept to a minimum.

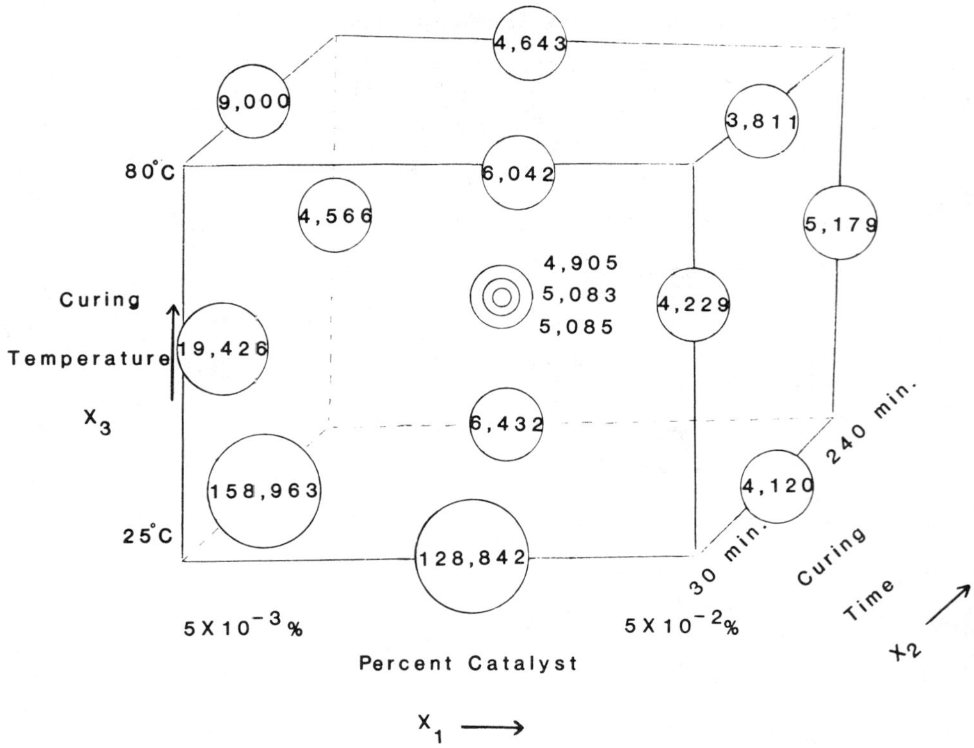

Figure 3. Effect of "significant" parameters on the extent of curing.

Studies on the rate of curing were carried out for practical purposes. For example, one might have to wait until 99.9% curing takes place before further coating the device. However, it might be possible to "handle" the device earlier, say after 80% curing. Some data on the rate of curing would help arrive at numbers, such as the time before further handling and the time before further coating.

A microscope slide was coated with the silicone material containing 0.01% catalyst. A time-driven infrared spectrum was then run on it (at 25°C and 40% R.H.), monitoring the Si—OAc peak at 1740 cm^{-1} as a function of time [9]. Change in concentration of Si—OAc is related to the progress of the curing reaction, since during curing Si—OAc is hydrolyzed to Si—OH, which on further condensation gives Si—O—Si cross-links. Figures 4 and 5 show the results of this experiment.

We concluded that for room-temperature operations, a 24-hour (99.9% curing) waiting time is ideal. However, if the nature of the process requires earlier handling, then a 2-hour (99.0% curing) waiting period might be sufficient.

Because of the metal based catalyst in the system, we decided to study the metal concentration on the surface of the coatings. This is important, especially when the coated device is directly implanted into the blood stream. Neutron activation analysis was used to detect the metal [9]. In essence, this involves irradiating the sample, and then measuring the induced radioactivity of the metal. The amount of catalyst required for suitable curing showed approximately 17 ppm of the metal on the surface. This compared very favorably with the 56 ppm of the metal we detected on the surface of a commercial medical silicone.

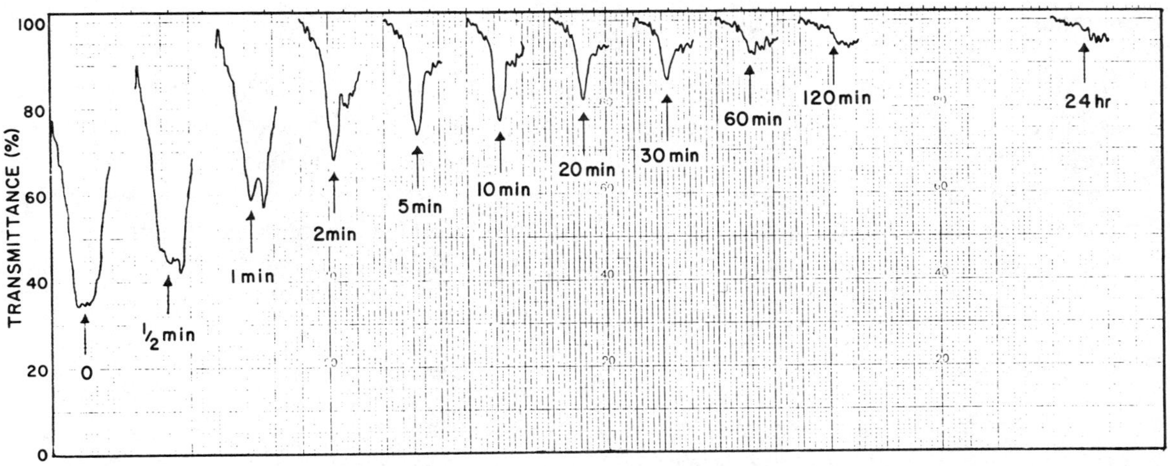

Figure 4. IR transmittance of Si–OAc at different time intervals.

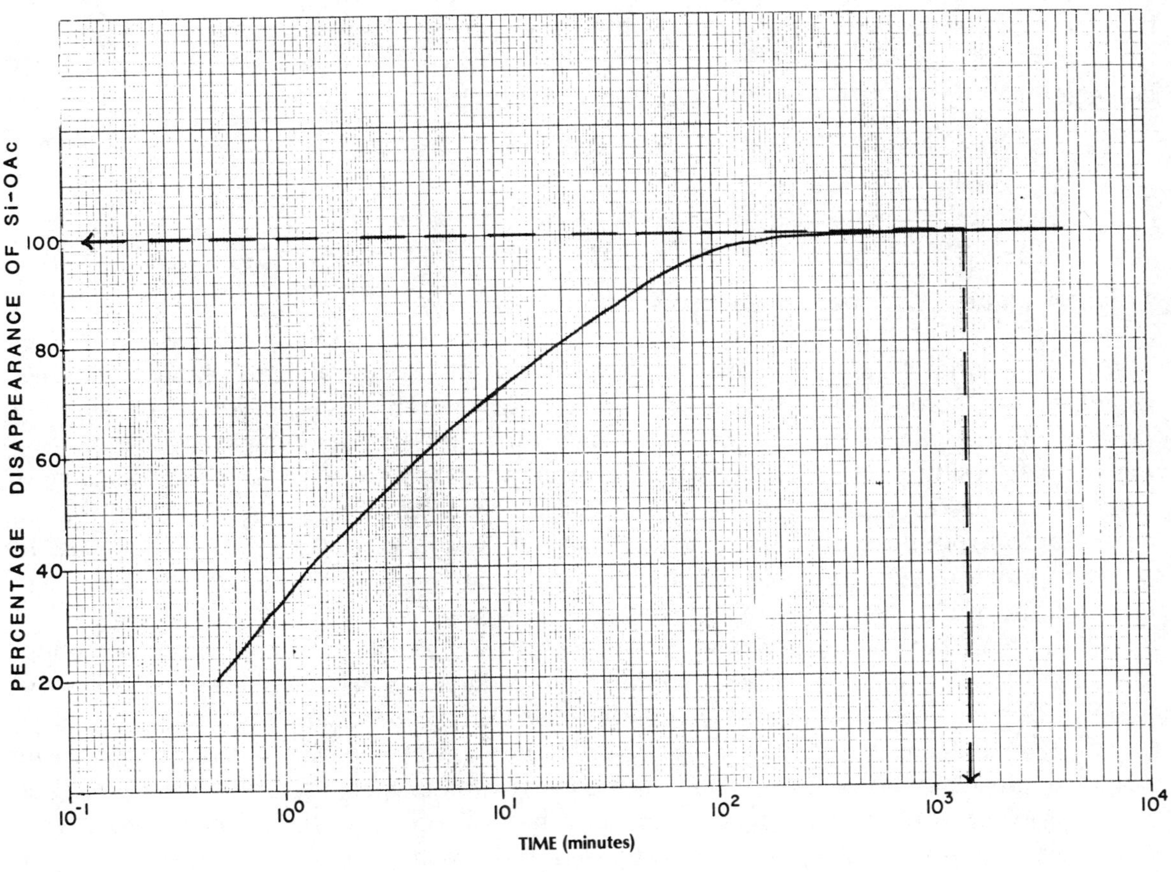

Figure 5. Progress of Si–OAc hydrolysis.

The evaporation rate of solvents and the viscosity of the system influences the flow behavior of the material, and thus the smoothness of the surface. We determined that a 50% solution of the polymer in a 2:1 by volume mixture of tetrahydrofuran and p-dioxane gave a very satisfactory surface [9].

Manufacturing

Large-scale production of medical grade polymers requires special treatment, and is discussed in detail under Case Study III of this chapter. Extreme purity is one of the most important requirements of a medical polymer. To achieve it, we glass distilled and filtered spectrograde solvents. The polymer was filtered through a 0.2-micron size filter before use. For long term use, the material was packaged in thoroughly cleaned and dried glass bottles, blanketed with dry nitrogen gas and sealed using Teflon tape.

Application

As shown in Figure 1, Lederman, et al., noticed a great improvement in surface smoothness, when replacing the previously used silica-filled commercial silicone with this newly developed silica-free silicone.

We also recognized that the material had potential usefulness for various other applications. It was tried and successfully used in the development of seamless tri-leaflet valves [10]. As of today, it has been used in numerous other devices, such as blood-contact silicone gaskets, silicone tubings and conduits, and insulin pumps.

CASE STUDY II

Polycarbonate - Silicone Copolymers

Silicone is one of the most widely used polymers in the medical field, because of its well established biocompatibility. It's uses range from dental and plastic surgery applications to catheters, heart valves and oxygenators. Polycarbonate is gaining increasing popularity in medical devices mainly for its superior mechanical properties. No major studies of its biocompatibility have been reported in the literature. However, the polar groups in polycarbonate are likely to make this polymer reactive to body fluids and tissues. Typical medical uses for polycarbonates range from general purpose housings and connectors to valve occluders and cranioplasty [11].

Recognizing that in many existing and some proposed applications, the combined properties of polycarbonate and silicone would be highly advantageous, we decided to investigate copolymerization technology in this area. We felt that an essentially silicone-type polymer would have enhanced mechanical properties when reinforced with polycarbonate. One potential application for such a polymer is the membrane oxygenator. This technology could also provide a polycarbonate-type material with a siliconized surface. Such a copolymer would enhance the blood and tissue contact performance of devices now made with polycarbonates.

Chemistry

The synthesis, characterization and processing of some polycarbonate-silicone copolymers is described in the literature [12,13]. Basic reactions involve the following:

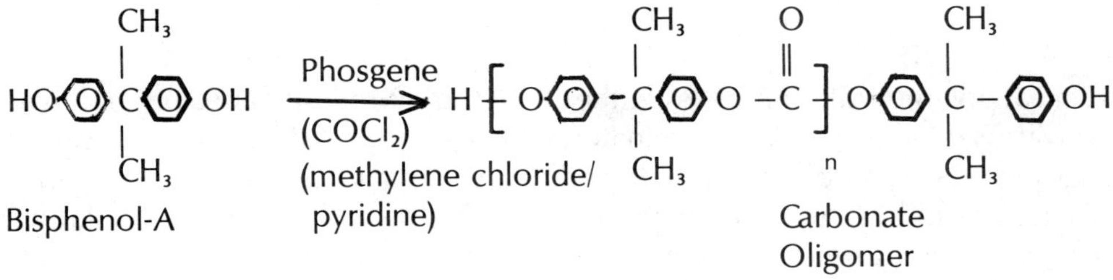

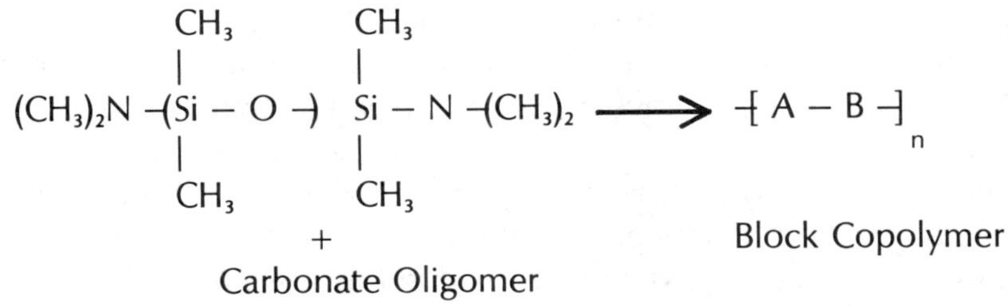

Carbonate oligomers are first prepared by phosgenating high purity Bisphenol A (or many other bisphenols) in a methylene chloride/pyridine mixture to a desired molecular weight, generally in the range of 1,000 to 20,000. Block copolymers are then obtained by the silylamine-hydroxyl reaction carried out in a dehydrated solvent, such as methylene chloride, chloroform or chlorobenzene. This procedure produces alternating block copolymers with very well defined block lengths.

Alternatively, copolymers can be obtained by phosgenating a mixture of Bisphenol A and Bisphenol A-capped siloxane oligomers. Condensation reactions between Bisphenol A molecules themselves and between polycarbonate and siloxane would take place simultaneously, resulting in a random block structure.

Many other approaches have been taken, where different monomers, catalysts, solvents, etc., have been used to obtain copolymers with different properties [14]. In most cases, however, the link between the silicone and polycarbonate blocks has been of the Si–O–C type. This structure has good thermal stability, but relatively poor hydrolytic stability [15].

For biomedical applications, hydrolytic stablity is extremely important. As a result, we decided to develop copolymers with Si–C, rather than Si–O–C, links. Since typical biomedical materials are used at body temperature, the inferior thermal stability of Si–C links would not be detrimental in this application. For the silicone oligomer, we chose bis (hydroxy propyl) terminated polydimethyl siloxane:

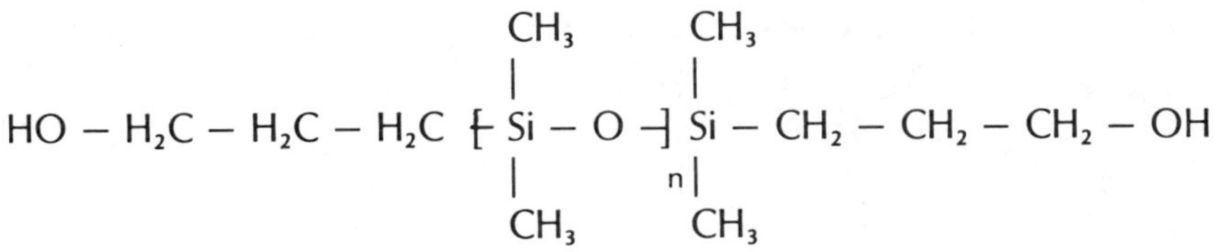

This would react with Bisphenol A and phosgene to give the following structure:

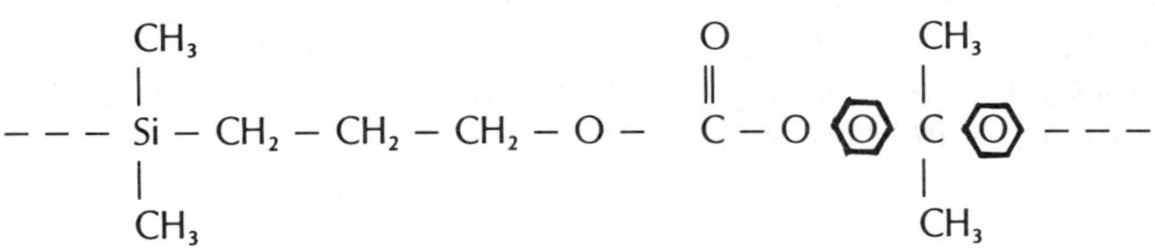

Synthesis

The interfacial polymerization process, rather than the more popular solution polymerization method was used, allowing us to eliminate pyridine, a potentially toxic chemical. Also, in the interfacial process, the polymer is obtained in the organic phase, while the unreacted monomers, catalyst and many other impurities are left behind in aqueous solution. This facilitates the purification process, yielding a polymer of extremely high purity.

The process basically involves dissolving Bisphenol A and sodium hydroxide in water, and dissolving the silicone oligomer in methylene chloride. After vigorously stirring a mixture of these, a phase transfer catalyst is added. We chose tetraethyl ammonium chloride (TEAC). Some of the other popular catalysts give a higher rate of reaction, however, TEAC is water soluble and remains with the impurities in the aqueous solution, leaving a pure polymer in the organic phase. Highly pure phosgene gas is bubbled through the catalyzed mixture. When the reaction is complete, the two phases are separated. The organic phase is then repeatedly washed with water, and finally, excess alcohol is added to precipitate the polymer.

Time, temperature and pH of the reaction have a significant effect on output. Formation of the chloroformate from Bisphenol A and phosgene is a spontaneous reaction:

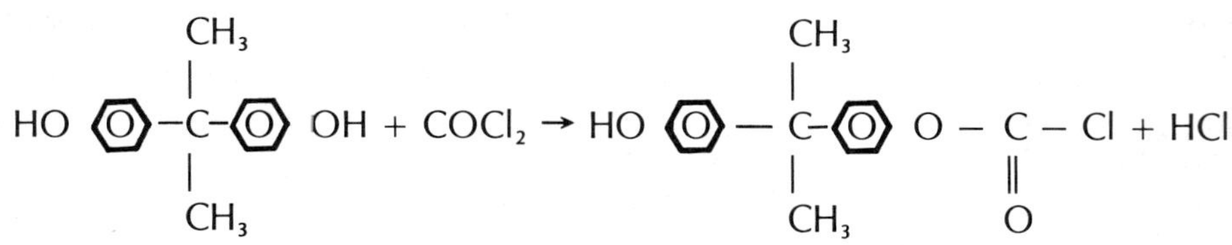

Further condensation of these chloroformates with Bisphenol A to form polycarbonate chains is favored at higher pH (pH > 10). However, silicone oligomers are quite unstable in alkaline conditions. Thus, indiscriminately carrying out the reaction at a high pH would tend to form homopolymers of carbonates with very little silicone incorporated into them.

As the reaction temperature is increased, the reaction rate increases. However, beyond a certain point (T > 35°C), instead of undergoing polymerization, the chloroformates preferably undergo hydrolysis, giving back Bisphenol A. Preference for hydrolysis is especially strong in the case of aliphatic chloroformates formed by the silicone oligomers:

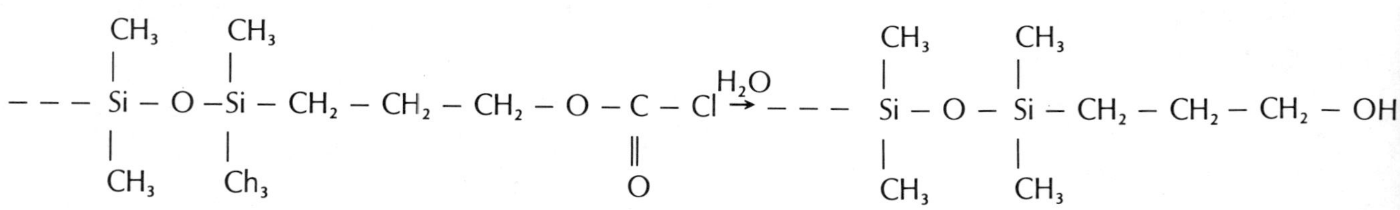

Thus, increasing the temperature to increase the reaction rate may result in the silicone oligomer not being incorporated into the polymer. On the other hand, if the temperature is held low, the rate would be too slow to build up the molecular weight to a useful level.

It was clear that our greatest problem was to achieve copolymerization. One solution was to end-cap the silicone with Bisphenol A to obtain:

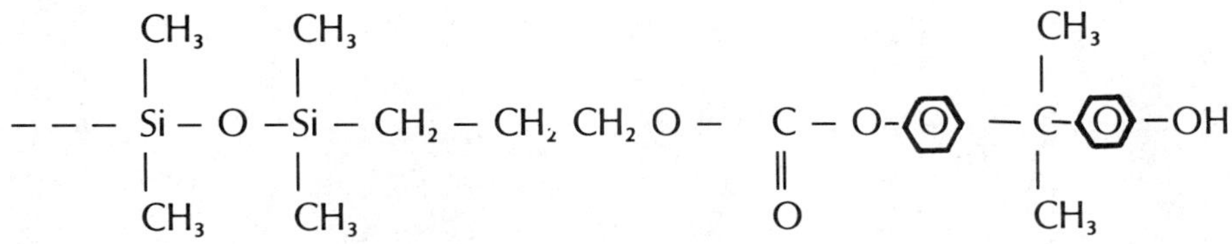

This was then phosgenated along with Bisphenol A. Now the system had essentially all phenolic –OH groups, and hence the reaction was more homogeneous. As a result, we were able to incorporate up to 50% silicone in the copolymer. Another approach, presently under investigation, is to synthesize silicone oligomers with phenolic –OH instead of aliphatic –OH groups on its molecule. One example is:

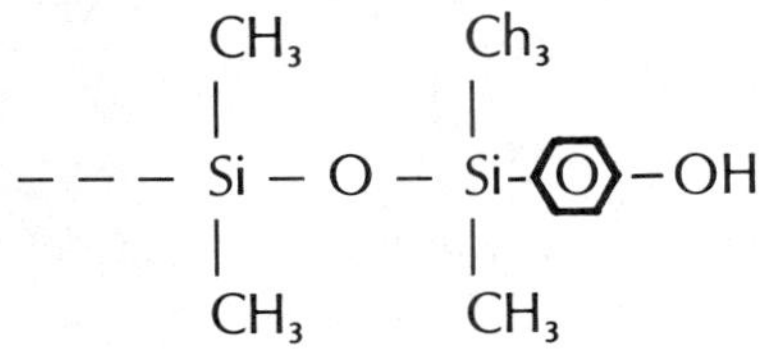

We believe that this method will permit us to have complete control of the copolymer composition.

Characterization

Numerous experiments were carried out under various reaction conditions. Their effect on the end product was studied through the following characterization techniques:

1. Gel permeation chromatography – (GCP)
   Molecular weight and molecular weight distribution
2. Infrared spectrometry (IR)
   Chemical composition
3. Thermogravimetric analysis (TGA)
   Thermal stability
4. Critical Surface Tension (γ_c) and ESCA measurements
   Surface structure

Molecular weight of the polymer gave an indication of the extent of polymerization. In Figure 6, plots A, B and C correspond to the reaction temperatures of 12°, 30° and 41°C. The lower molecular weight at low temperature is due to the slow rate of reaction, whereas that at high temperature is probably due to the preferential hydrolysis of the chloroformates mentioned earlier. We found that it was critical to control the reaction temperature in the range of 26° to 33°C.

Molecular weight distribution gave us an interesting insight into the copolymerization reaction. In the beginning, when we were unable to incorporate any silicone into the product, the GPC plot, as shown in Curve A, Figure 7, was essentially unimodal. Under certain reaction conditions where copolymerization was achieved, we still had a problem. Curve B, Figure 7 shows that the GPC plots obtained on these copolymers were distinctly bimodal. When the

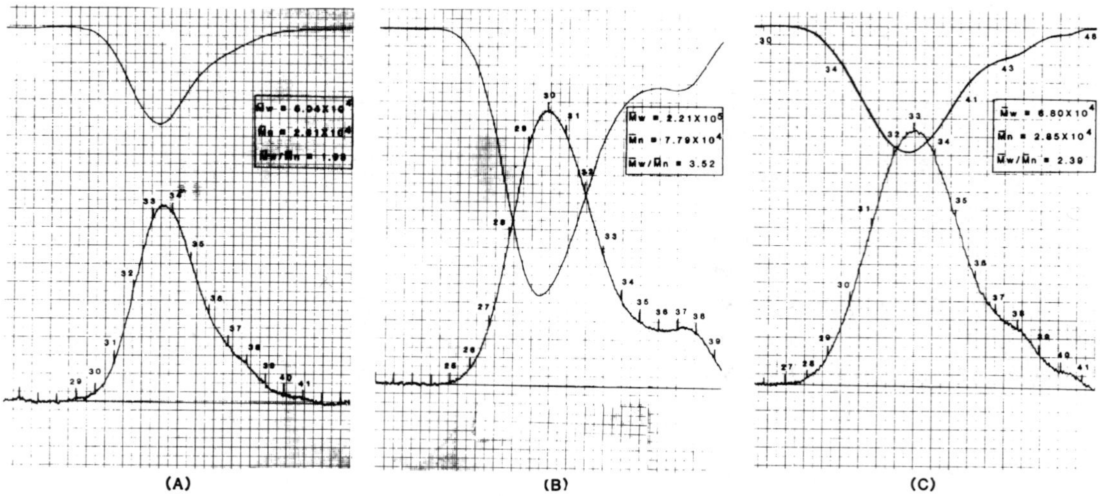

Figure 6. Molecular weight distribution of polymers obtained at different reaction temperatures. (a) 12°C; (b) 30°C; (c) 41°C.

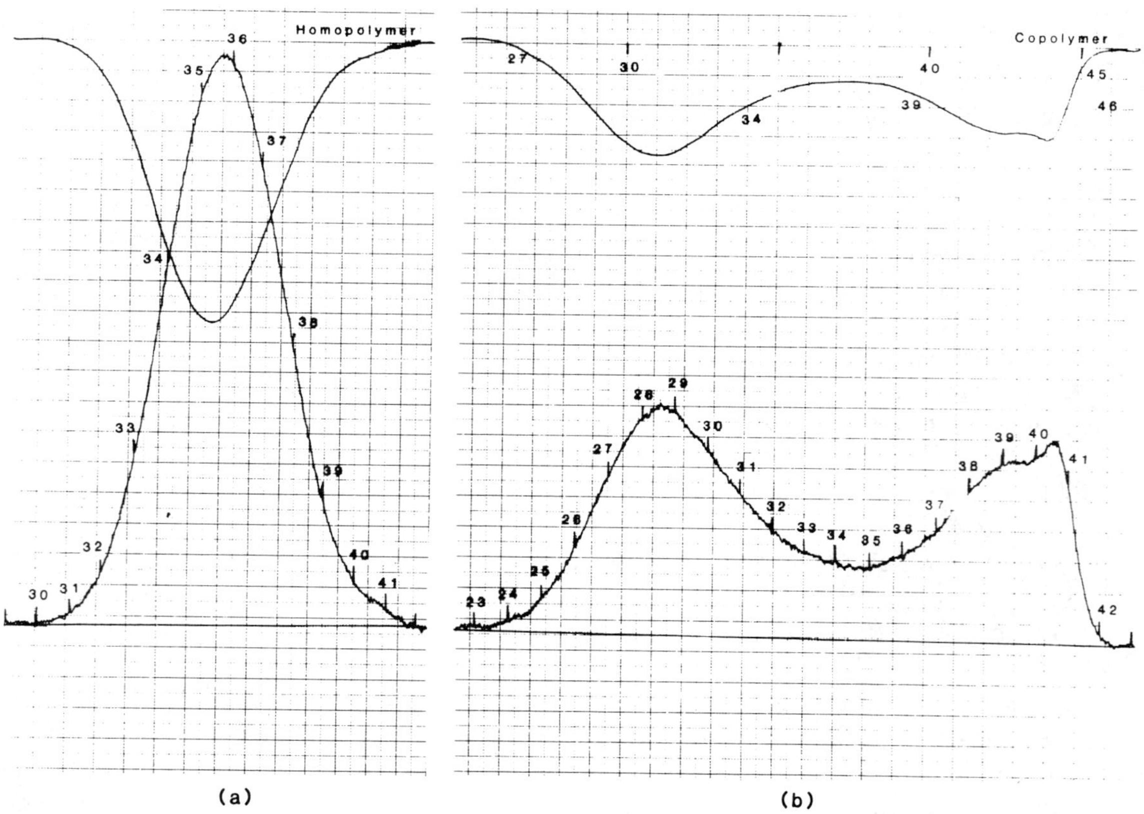

Figure 7. Molecular weight distribution of a homopolymer and a copolymer.

two peaks were separated and analyzed, we found that the higher molecular weight peak corresponded to the homopolycarbonate, while the lower molecule weight peak contained the polymers of polycarbonate and silicone. It was clear that we were not getting a homogeneous reaction. We hypothesized that this was due to the difference in the reaction rates of aliphatic –OH on silicone and phenolic –OH on Bisphenol A. When the silicone oligomers were completely end-capped with Bisphenol A before phosgenating, we obtained copolymers showing unimodal distributions.

Preliminary IR analysis was done by running transmission spectra on thin films of the polymer deposited on NaCl crystals. Presence of strong absorbance peaks at 800 and 1050 cm^{-1} would indicate the presence of silicone in the polymer. A procedure for quantitative analysis was developed. It involved preparing a 5% solution of the sample in CH_2Cl_2, and measuring the CO absorbance band at 1770 cm^{-1}. A calibration curve, shown in Figure 8, was established by measuring this absorbance band for reference samples of known silicone content. Figure 9 shows the 1770 cm^{-1} absorbance band for two samples, A and B. They represent the products obtained under reaction conditions favorable to homopolymerization and copolymerization, respectively. Clearly, this is confirmed by our quantitative analysis.

TGA runs gave us useful information on the thermal stability of the copolymers. Samples were heated from 40° to 900°C at a rate of 20°C/min. in a N_2 gas environment. Weight loss was monitored as a function of time. Figure 10 shows TGA plots for a pure polycarbonate, a bimodal copolymer and a unimodal copolymer. The bimodal copolymer recorded a much

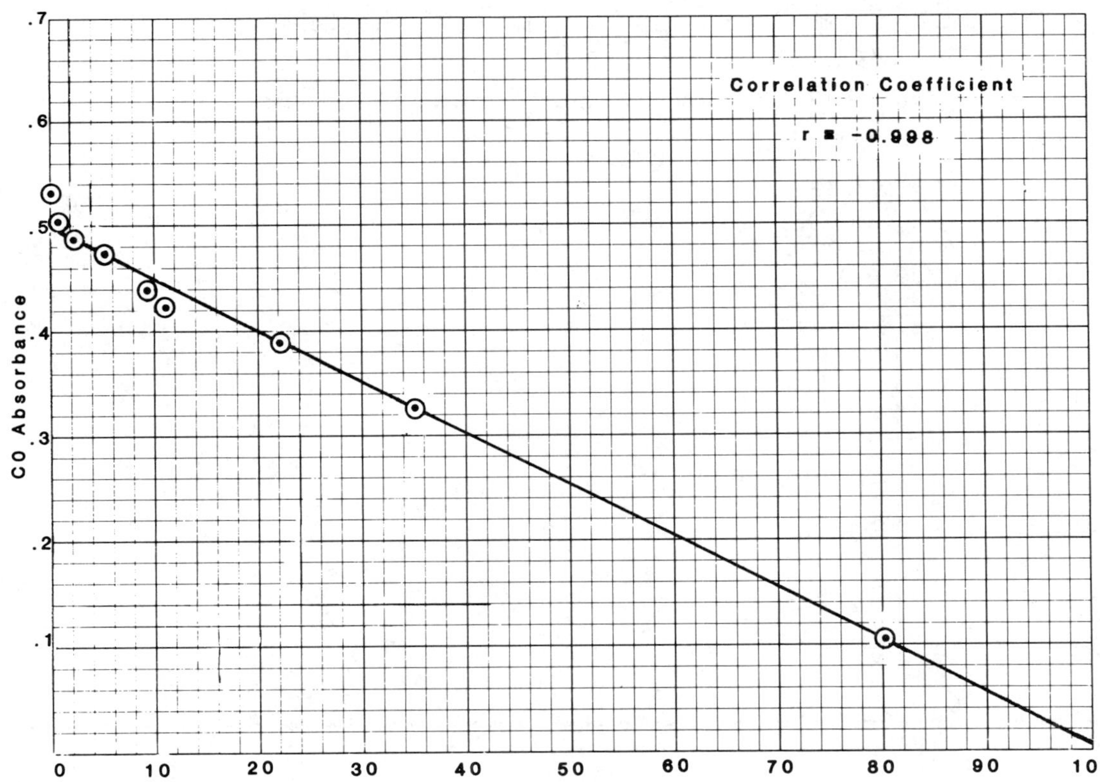

Figure 8. IR calibration curve for percent silicone in the copolymer.

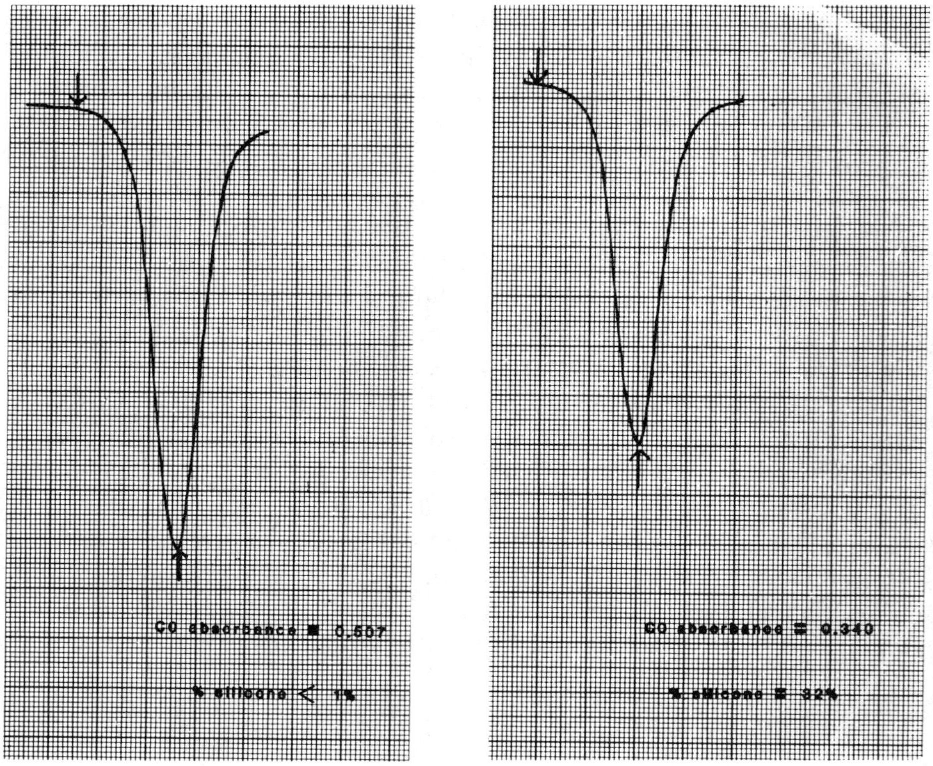

(a) (b)

Figure 9. CO absorbance of a homopolymer and a copolymer.

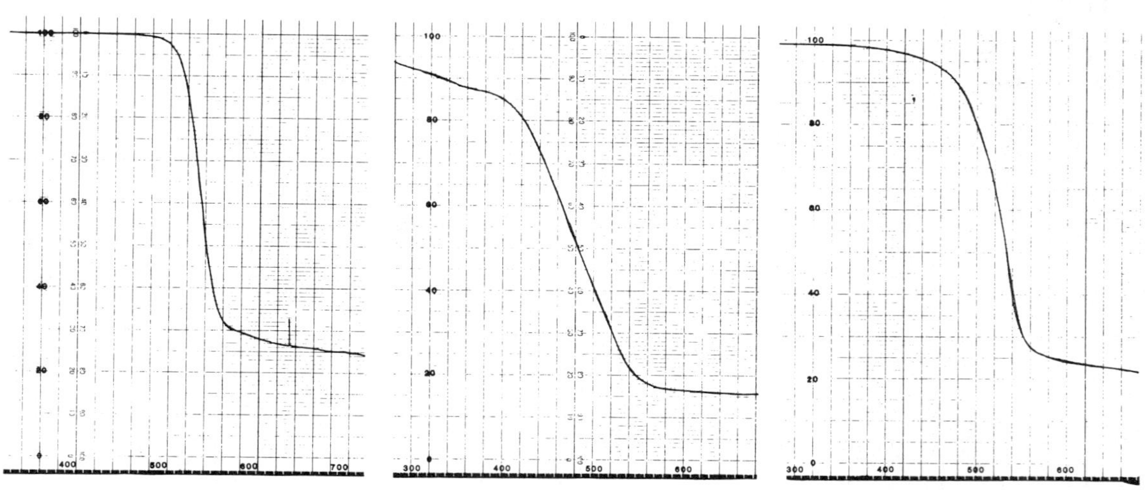

(a) (b) (c)

Fig. 10. Thermogravimetric analysis on (a) homopolymer; (b) bimodal copolymer; (c) unimodal copolymer.

earlier onset of degradation when compared with the unimodal copolymer. A pure polycarbonate run was used as a general reference. It was evident that for the polymer to be melt-processable, a unimodal distribution was needed.

Through critical surface tension measurements, we obtained information on the surface distribution of the two components. Figure 11 shows that films cast from copolymers containing 5% silicone in the bulk, showed a γ_c of 25.5 dynes/cm compared with a γ_c of 30.8 dynes/cm for pure polycarbonate film. However, after the copolymer film was annealed at 120°C for 15 hours, the γ_c value dropped to 22.5 dynes/cm, indicating the migration of silicone toward the surface.

Further surface studies were done by ESCA and, as shown in Figure 12, the relationship between the bulk and surface concentration of silicone was established [13]. A very high surface concentration of silicone at its relatively low bulk concentration makes it possible to have copolymers with the mechanical properties of polycarbonate and the surface properties of silicone.

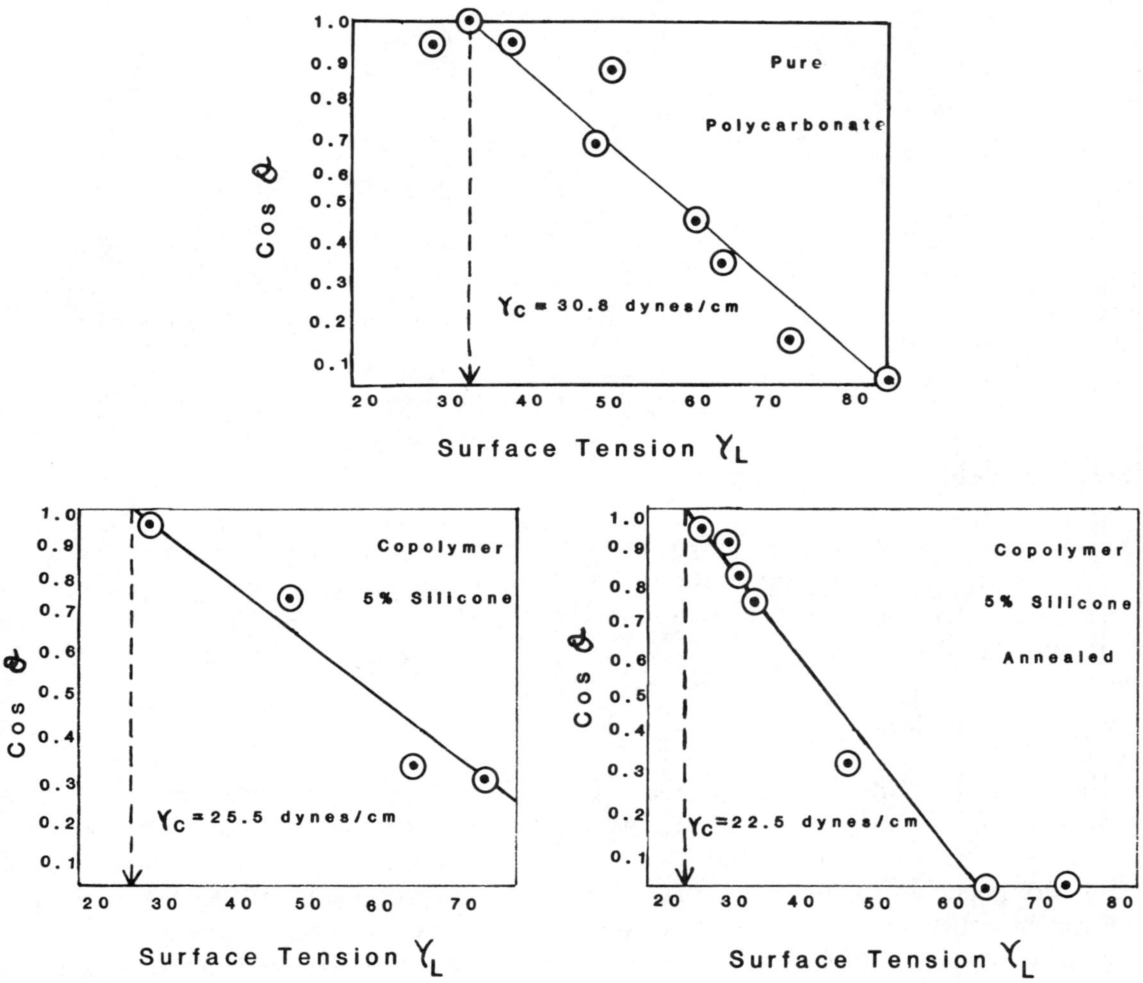

Figure 11. Critical surface tension of a homopolymer and a copolymer; effect of annealing.

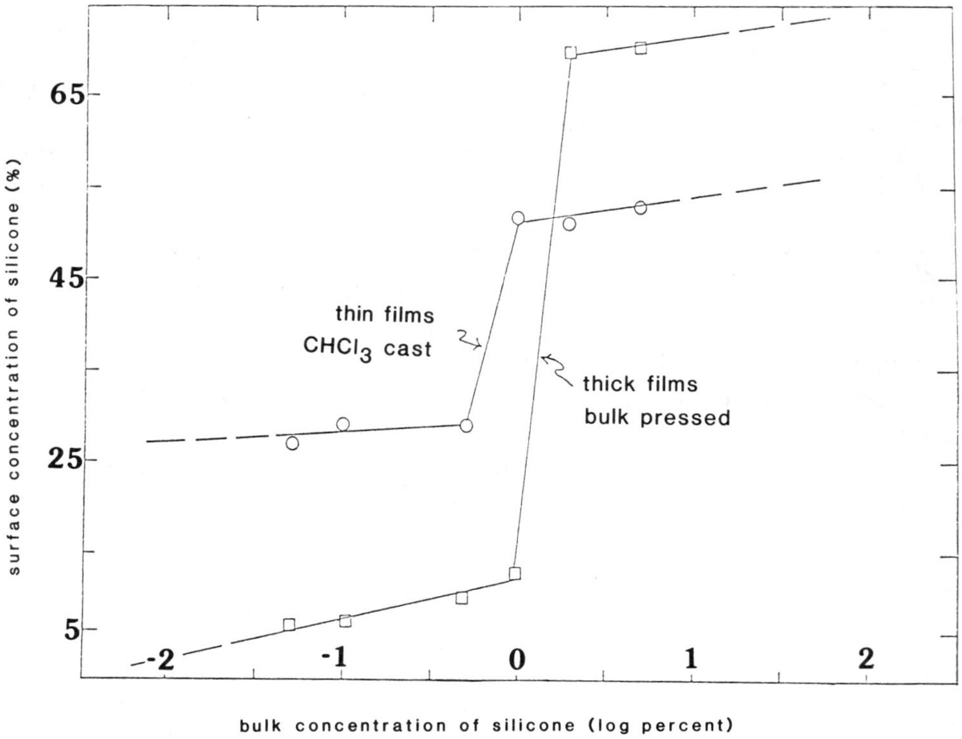

Figure 12. ESCA studies on the copolymers. (Note 4).

In summary, this case study brings into focus the extensive information loop necessary to link the synthesis and characterization of polymers at developmental stages. We have shown how this "feedback" approach was effectively used in developing biomedical polymers with tailor-made properties.

CASE STUDY III

Polyurethane-Silicone Copolymer

Cardiothane-51 copolymer, a polyurethane-silicone system, used for more than 10 years in medical devices for human applications, has an excellent reputation for its blood-contact characteristics. Its biocompatibility is attributed to a unique surface structure and morphology as described in the literature [6,16,17]. Extensive characterization of the material through IR spectrometry, Auger electron microscopy, ESCA and critical surface tension measurements, provides useful guidelines for the surface requirements for good biocompatibility [17,18,19,20].

The single most important application of Cardiothane-51 is the intra-aortic balloon, a temporary cardiac assist device for patients undergoing open heart surgery. In recent years, production of these balloons increased 50 fold, and as a result, the synthesis of Cardiothane-51 moved from bench-scale (~1 gal) to pilot plant (~5 gal) to production (~50 gal). This brought with it numerous technical problems not encountered during the development stage.

It took as much time, effort and money to solve these problems as it did to invent and develop the material. This case study demonstrates that even a well designed and highly developed biomaterial must be properly produced and handled on a large scale in order to obtain satisfactory devices. We show how various quality control standards are established to assure a consistent product, and how the technical expertise of polymer engineers is needed to solve real-life problems in production. We discuss the increased sophistication of process control systems required for large-scale production.

Discussion

A brief discussion of some of the chemical and physicochemical aspects of Cardiothane-51 will help the reader to comprehend the problems discussed. Cardiothane-51 is a mixture of polyurethane, silicone and a copolymer of the two. Its chemical structure is described in detail in the literature [21]. Basically, it contains a segmented polyurethane having a soft segment of polyether structure and a hard segment of aromatic urethane structure. Polydimethyl siloxane is the principal backbone structure in the silicone. The copolymer link is from the reaction between the isocyanate (–NCO, –NHCO) or hydroxyl (–OH) groups from polyurethane and the acetoxy ($-OCOCH_3$) or hydroxyl groups from silicone. This copolymer acts as a "surfactant" and keeps the two homopolymers in one phase. Most of the silicone is acetoxy ($-OCOCH_3$) terminated, and undergoes curing when Cardiothane-51 is exposed to atmosphere in the form of a thin film.

Synthesis and processing conditions have a significant effect on the surface structure of Cardiothane-51 films. Since surface structure is related to the biocompatibility of the material, it is very important to monitor and control the synthesis and processing conditions. In the following paragraphs, we present some of the problems encountered during manufacture and discuss various techniques that were developed to solve them.

Synthesis

When a polymer is to be used for implantables, removal of low molecular weight components is important in order to minimize the leachables. During the development and pilot-plant stages, raw polyurethane was purified by a precipitation method. The polymer was dissolved in a solvent and then precipitated by addition of an alcohol. Low molecular weight impurities were left behind in the solution. This batch mode purification process proved cumbersome and expensive in large-scale production. Leaching of the polymer with a solvent/non-solvent mixture was investigated. Ward presented very interesting results of this study [22]. Figures 13 a and b show the GPC scans on the purified polymer and impurities removed by precipitation and leaching, respectively. By selecting a proper mixture of solvent/non-solvent for leaching, it is possible to purify the polymer to the same level as with precipitation.

The extent of polymerization and copolymerization significantly affects the surface characteristics of a film. As shown in Figure 14, when Cardiothane-51 contains extremely high molecular weight fractions, the resulting surface is relatively rough. This is probably due to the effect of molecular weight on the material's flow behavior and on the mobility of various chemical structures. It is, therefore, very important to control the degree of copolymerization. This is effectively achieved by controlling two retardants to the copolymerization reaction – the moisture and alcohol content of the system. When water or alcohol is present in excess of a few hundred parts per million concentration, the reaction is completely inhibited. At a concentration of less than 50 ppm, a runaway viscosity rise is observed. Delicate control of moisture and alcohol content within a narrow range at such low levels is achieved through sophisticated instruments, such as the Karl-Fisher Titrator

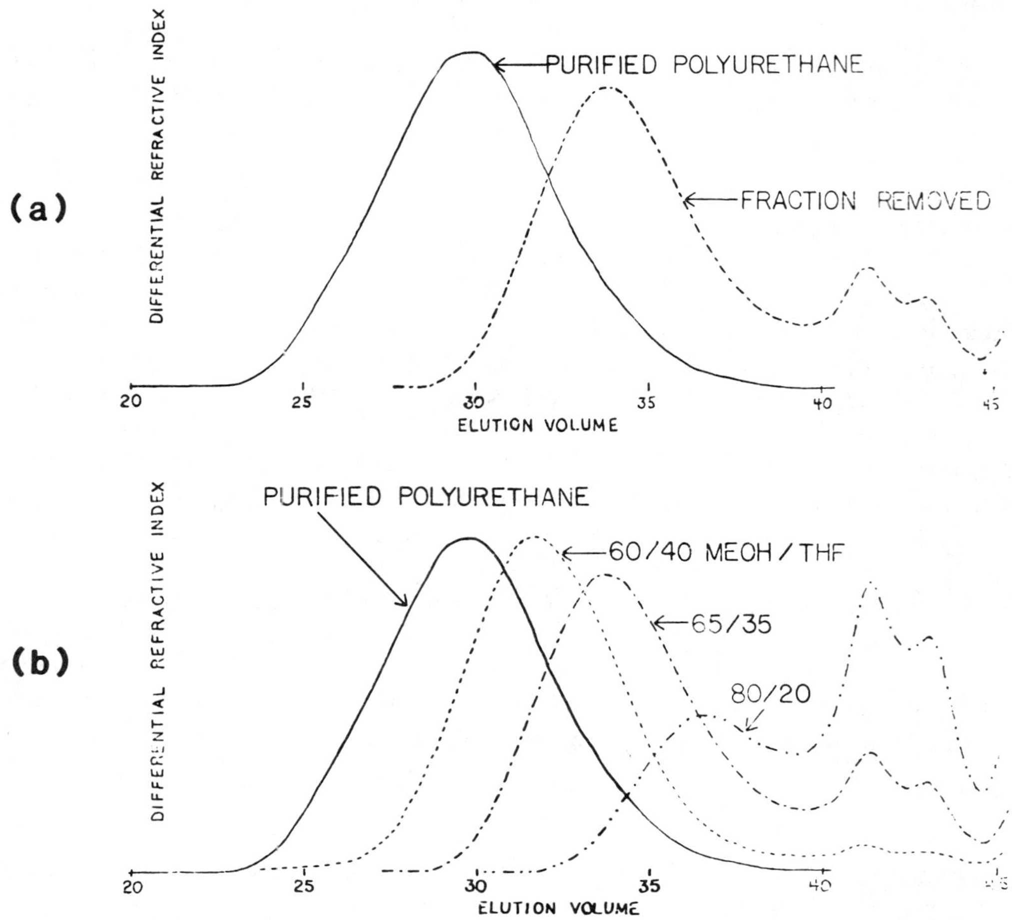

Figure 13. GPC scans on purified polymer and impurities removed by (a) precipitation; (b) leaching. (Note 5).

and Thermogravimetric Analyzer. Solvents are repetitively distilled and dried over a bed of molecular sieves until the desired moisture level is obtained. Polyurethane is vacuum dried at 70°C to achieve the desired water/alcohol content.

Processing

Cardiothane-51 solution is used primarily for dip coating, where a mandrel is dipped into the material, and the film is then allowed to cure at room temperature. Many processing variables such as humidity, moisture content and viscosity of Cardiothane-51, and speed of dipping have a significant affect on the film surface. Typically, the material viscosity is adjusted to about 600 centipoise for the best flow behavior.

If the material is allowed to absorb a lot of moisture during storage or use, its shelf life deteriorates, as evidenced by separation into two layers. This is mainly because the "reactive"

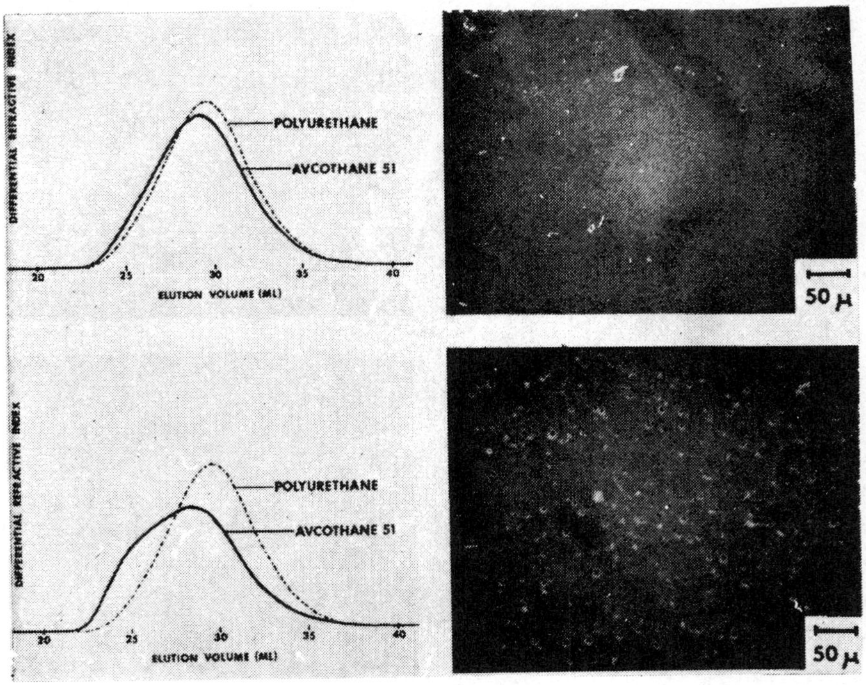

Figure 14. Extent of reaction and resultant surfaces. (Note 5).

silicone in the system, on reaction with water, becomes incompatible with the system. Also, this silicone is now "unreactive," and ends up in a cast film as dispersed oily droplets instead of a cured silicone matrix within a polyurethane matrix.

It is, therefore, extremely important to monitor and control the moisture content of Cardiothane-51. Typically, the material is always handled in enclosed systems equipped with moisture absorbing media. Its only exposure to air is at the final use stage. Its moisture content is monitored frequently using an automatic Karl-Fisher Titrator.

It is also important to control the environmental humidity and temperature where a film is being cured. At high humidity, the silicone cures extremely rapidly, leading to the formation of bubbles and other irregularities on the surface. Also, this leads to silicone entrapment within the bulk of the film, and hence, less than a desirable amount of silicone on the surface. On the other hand, if the humidity is too low, a large amount of silicone ends up on the surface, giving a tacky film. Also, at low humidity, a high static charge is built up, leading to excessive particulate inclusions in the dip-coated films. Proper humidity control and filtered air were effectively utilized in this respect.

Nyilas has related the hemocompatibility of a Cardiothane-51 film to the amount of silicone on its surface [17]. As shown in Figure 15, the amount of silicone on the surface is in turn related to an IRATR index obtained from the Fourier Multiple Internal Reflection (FMIR) infrared spectrscopy. Thus, the IRATR index can be routinely used as a quality control procedure to assure consistency in the surface structure.

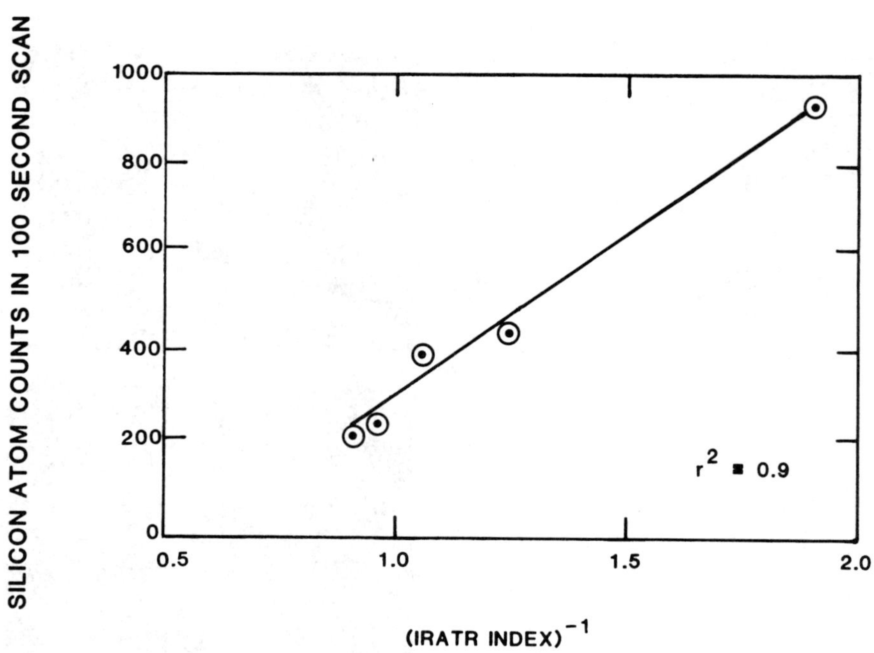

Figure 15. Fourier multiple internal reflection studies for surface silicone concentration. (Note 6).

CONCLUSION

The three case studies discussed here bring into focus the various areas of polymer science as applied in a biomedical materials field. They emphasize the special treatment of synthesis, characterization, and processing of polymers for medical uses. They describe some typical approaches to the research and development, and the production and uses of biomedical polymers.

ACKNOWLEDGEMENT

I thank Linda Turcotte and Lisa Naturman, without whose consistent efforts in our laboratories, results reported here would not have been possible. I am grateful to Marjorie Frith for teaching me effective communication and for offering excellent editorial guidance. I am also thankful to Karen DelVecchio for her beautiful artwork which reflects in the illustrations used in this chapter.

REFERENCES

1. Bruck, S. D., "Polymeric Materials: Current Status of Biocompatibility," Biomat. Med. Dev. Art. Org., 1(1), 79-98, 1973.
2. Petschek, H. E. and Madras, P. N., "Thrombus Formation on Artificial Surfaces," in Proceedings of the Artificial Heart Program Conference, R. Johnson Hegyeli editor, U.S. Government Printing Office, Washington, D.C., 271-290, 1969.

3. Vroman, L., and Leonard, E. F., editors, "The Behavior of Blood and Its Components at Interfaces," Annual N.Y. Acad. Sci., 283, 1977.
4. Halbert, S. P., Ushakoff, A. E., and Anken, M., "Compatibility of Various Plastics with Human Plasma Proteins," J. Biomed. Mat. Res., 4, 549-569, 1970.
5. Lyman, D. J., Brash, J. L., and Klein, K. G., "The Effect of Chemical Structure and Surface Properties of Synthetic Polymers on the Coagulation of Blood," in Proceedings of the Artificial Heart Program Conference, R. Johnson Hegyeli editor, U.S. Government Printing Office, Washington, D.C., 113, 1969.
6. Nyilas, E., "Development of Blood Compatible Elastomers. I. Theory, Practice and In Vivo Performance," 23rd ACEMB, Washington, D.C., 1970.
7. Lederman, D. M., Russell, F. B., Levine, F. H., Singh, P. I., Cumming, R. D., Morgan, R. A., Harpster, N., and Herzlinger, G., "Development of a Seamless Left Heart Assist Blood Pump," Report No. NIH-NO1-HV-7-2937-1, 1978. Available from National Technical Information Service, Springfield, VA.
8. Strategy of Experimentation, E. I. DuPont De Nemours & Co. (Inc.), 1975.
9. Ashar, B., Ward, R. S., Jr., and Turcotte, L. R., "Development of a Silica-free Silicone System for Medical Applications," J. Biomed. Mat. Res., 15, 663-672, 1981.
10. Russell, F. B., Lederman, D. M., Singh, P. I., Cumming, R. D., Morgan, R. A., Levine, F. H., Austen, W. G., and Buckley, M. J., "Development of Seamless Tri-leaflet Valves," Trans. Am. Soc. Artif. Intern. Org., 26, 66, 1980.
11. Szycher, M., "Advances in Biomedical Polymers," University of Lowell Plastics Seminar, Boston, 1981.
12. Vaughn, H. A., "Polycarbonate-Silicone Block Copolymers," Div. of Orgn. Coat. & Pl. Chem., Am. Chem. Soc. Abstracts, 29 (1), 133, 1969.
13. McGrath, J. E., Riffle, J. S., Davidson, T. F., and Webster, D., "Polycarbonate-Polydimethylsiloxane Block Copolymers," Dept. of Chem., Virginia Polytechnic Institute & State Univ., 1978.
14. Kambour, R. P., Corn, J. E., Klopfer, H. J., Miller, S., Orlando, C. M., and Stang, L. D., "BPF Carbonate-Silicone Block Polymers: Improved Synthesis and Further Studies of Mechanical and Flammability Properties," GE Technical Information Series, No. 77CRD172, Schenectady, N.Y., 1977.
15. Noshay, A., and McGrath, J. E., "Block Copolymers: Overview and Critical Survey," Academic Press, New York, 1977.
16. Nyilas, E., "Development of Blood Compatible Elastomers. IV. Performance of Avcothane Blood Contact Surfaces and Correlation with Theory," Presented at AICHE 70th Biomaterials Symposium, Atlantic City, N.J., 1971.
17. Nyilas, E., and Ward, R. S., Jr., "Development of Blood Compatible Elastomers. V. Surface Structure and Blood Compatibility of Avcothane Elastomers," J. Biomed. Mat. Res., 8, 1977.
18. Sung, C. S. P., Hu, C. B., and Merrill, E. W., "Surface Chemical Analysis of Avcothane and Biomer by Fourier Transform IR Internal Reflection Spectroscopy," J. Biomed. Mat. Res., 12, 791-804, 1978.
19. Sung, C. S. P., Hu, C. B., "Application of Auger Electron Spectroscopy for Surface Chemical Analysis of Avcothane," J. Biomed. Mat. Res., 12, 45-55, 1978.
20. Sung, C. S. P., Hu, C. B., "ESCA Studies of Surface Chemical Composition of Segmented Polyurethanes," J. Biomed. Mat. Res., 13, 161-171, 1979.
21. Nyilas, E., "Polysiloxane-Polyurethane Block Copolymers," U.S. Patent 3,562,352, assigned to Avco Corp., 1971.
22. Ward, R. S., Jr., and duBruil, C., "Production of Biomedical Polymers. III. Instrumental Analysis to Assure Biocompatibility," 23rd Annual ISA Analysis Instrumentation Symposium, 49-55, 1977.

NOTES

Note 1: A screening design is mainly used to screen out a few really important variables from a large number of possible variables with a minimum of testing. Plackett-Burman is a type of screening which uses a specific fraction of the 2^P factorial design. Only a 12-run experiment is required to study as many as 7 variables, or a 20-run experiment for 15 variables, or a 28-run experiment for 23 variables.

The only drawback of this design is that it does not give any information on the interaction between variables. However, once the key variables are screened out using this design, further information on interactions can be obtained using more elaborate designs such as the 2^P factorial design or the Box-Behnken design.

Note 2: Reprinted with permission from Ref. #7 in this chapter.

Note 3: Reprinted with permission from Ref. #9 in this chapter.

Note 4: Reprinted with permission from Ref. #13 in this chapter.

Note 5: Reprinted with permission from Ref. #22 in this chapter.

Note 6: Reprinted with permission from Ref. #17 in this chapter.

Chapter 37

Applications of Advanced Composites in Orthopaedic Implants

Kenneth R. St. John
Biomaterials Engineer
Hexcel Corporation
P.O. Box 2312
11711 Dublin Boulevard
Dublin, California 94566-0705

ABSTRACT

While new to the orthopaedic implant field, carbon fiber reinforced materials have been used in other engineering applications for many years.

The use of metals in the manufacture of internal fracture fixation devices and total hip replacement has become common but these implants still present problems. Current research into lower modulus materials for these applications is reviewed and their potential benefits discussed.

Two new materials, carbon fiber reinforced polylactic acid and carbon fiber reinforced polysulfone are discussed in terms of their potential application in the solution of existing problems.

The use of high strength fibers such as carbon, Kevlar® , and fiberglass in conjunction with polymeric resins to form composites with high strength to weight ratios has become quite common. While material costs can be higher than the comparable strength metallic components, offsetting savings and other advantages due to lower weight can make these composites attractive.

Among the many uses of these composites are as facings on homeycomb core materials for the aerospace industry, hollow fishing rods and pole vault poles, low weight laminated structural materials, and experimental uses as weight saving components in the auto industry.

Other advantages over metallic materials are realized in the opportunities which are available to tailor the properties of the material to its particular application. The orientation and volume ratio of fibers in a composite can be varied to provide a wide range of mechanical properties as well as providing local variance within the material by non-uniform dispersion of the fiber.

Hexcel, as a high technology company involved in the development of engineered materials, is in a position to apply the techniques of composite design to the area of interest of its medical division, orthopaedic medical devices.

THE USE OF CARBON FIBER IN MEDICINE

In recent years, carbon fiber has been recognized as a biocompatible material with many exciting applications in medicine. Several commercial products utilize carbon fiber as a reinforcing material which serves to enhance the mechanical properties of the polymeric resin systems in which it is included. Proplast® (Vitek, Houston, TX) is a porous form of polytetrafluoroethylene/chopped carbon fiber composite which has been used or suggested for use in soft tissue augmentation [1], as a surface coating for attachment of orthopaedic implants [2], and in the repair of tendons and ligaments [3]. Poly Two™ (Zimmer, Warsaw, IN) is a composite of chopped carbon fiber and ultra high molecular weight polyethylene which is seeing use as a bearing surface in total joint replacement devices.

The Kronner External Fixation System (Richards Manufacturing, Memphis, TN) was recently introduced into the orthopaedic market. External fixation devices utilize transcutaneous pins which pass entirely through the limb containing a fracture. The fragments of bone are immobilized during the healing period by the attachment of the pins to an external frame by a series of clamps. Due to the need for rigidity, the resultant structure is often very heavy and therefore uncomfortable to the patient. The Kronner system utilizes several composite clamps in its construction, some of which are carbon/polymer composites.

Carbon fiber has also been shown to be compatible in its use as a tendon and ligament repair material and soft tissue repair material in the United States [4], Great Britain [5,6], West Germany [7,8], and South Africa. These investigators have shown that tissue grows around and on the individual fibers implanted as ligament and tendon replacements with little or no adverse reaction to the carbon. This use of carbon fiber is further discussed by Drs Parsons, Alexander and Weiss elsewhere in this publication. When used in fabric form as a patch, the strength of the carbon fabric prevents herniation while providing a biocompatible scaffold for the ingrowth of soft tissue which can eventually take over the function of the patch.

It was our decision based on the excellent mechanical properties of carbon fiber as well as its growing use as a biocompatible structural medical material that it was the fiber of choice for our application.

INTERNAL FRACTURE FIXATION DEVICES

In the treatment of fracture, the orthopaedic surgeon is often unable to achieve acceptable reduction of the bone fragments through the use of non-invasive techniques such as casts, bandages, and braces. These situations necessitate the use of invasive techniques including the external fixators mentioned earlier, intramedullary nails and rods, and bone plates. Bone plates present a challenging area for the application of composite technology due to the nature of the process of bone formation and resorption.

Currently, bone plates are manufactured from stainless steel, cobalt-chromium alloys, and titanium alloys. Attachment of the plate to the bone fragments is accomplished through the use of multiple screws, extending through both cortices of the bone. Frequently, the plate contains one or more oval holes in which the countersink is an inclined plane so that, on tightening the screw, the fracture line is forced together under compression. Plated fractures are held rigidly in close apposition leading to the generation of very little callus during healing.

The rigidity of a plate and therefore the plated system can be an advantage during the period while healing is progressing but the same rigidity can be a strong disadvantage later. It has become apparent over the years that bone remodels itself to most efficiently perform the load bearing required of it. If a plate is not removed once the fracture has healed, it continues to carry a majority of the load over its span and therefore protects the underlying bone leading to osteoporosis and atrophy. At a later date, if removal of the plate becomes necessary, the remaining bone may not be sufficiently strong to support loads. Repair of the fracture which may result will be complicated by the quality of bone present.

Several experimental studies have been reported concerning the effects of plating on the underlying bone. Uthoff and Dubuc [9] report the results of the immobilization of canine femoral osteotomies with metallic plates. The procedure was performed on both femora with at least two weeks elapsing between surgeries. The animals were sacrificed over periods ranging from two weeks to twenty-four weeks. In two animals, the plates were removed after three months then another three months were allowed to elapse before sacrifice. At sacrifice, it was noted that both cortices of bone under the plate exhibited reduction with the greatest reduction occurring directly under the plate. For those animals in which the plate had been removed, a return to normal anatomy was seen to be occurring.

Stromberg and Dalen [10] applied metal bone plates to both femora of seven healthy dogs. No osteotomy was performed and only one plate was left in the animal before closure. After removal of the other plate, the screws were returned to the bone to subject the bone to the surgical trauma without the mechanical effects of plating. After seven months, the dogs were sacrificed and the properties of the plated femur compared with those of the sham-operated femur. Their results show differences in bone mineral distribution, reduction in maximum torque capacity and reduction in the maximum angle of torsion. All differences were significant ($p < 0.05$). At the ends of the removed plates, a bony ridge was observed which was up to 3 mm thick. The plated femur exhibited an average 18.3% reduction in maximum torque and a 22% reduction in maximum torque angle. The conclusions included the observation that treatment of a plated fracture could not be considered complete until the bone had recovered from the effect of the plate after removal.

Uthoff and coworkers [11] compared the result of the plating of canine femora with stainless steel and titanium alloy plates with and without osteotomy. The osteotomized animals were sacrificed at 4, 8, 12, 16 and 24 weeks. The non-osteotomized animals were sacrificed at 24 weeks. Four additional animals were treated with titanium alloy plates, the plates removed at eight weeks, and the animals sacrificed at 24 weeks. At 24 weeks, the thickness of compact bone under the stainless steel was significantly ($p < 0.01$) lower than the unoperated bone while the bone thickness under the titanium plates was lower but not significantly different from the control. For those bones in which the plate was removed at eight weeks, the thickness was significantly higher than the control. No mechanical testing results were reported.

Tonino and coworkers [12] report the results of a bilateral study in canine femora in which one femur was plated with a stainless steel plate (modulus of elasticity approximately 20X bone) while the other was plated with polytriflouromonochloroethylene (PTFCE) with a modulus of elasticity approximately 10% of bone. Comparison of the mechnical properties of the femora by a paired t-test showed significantly weaker bone ($p < 0.05$) under the stainless steel plates. Since this experiment did not involve osteotomized bone, it serves to demonstrate the effect of plate rigidity but does not prove the efficacy of plastic plates.

The same investigators performed an expanded study [13] in which the PTFCE plates were reinforced with metal tubes and applied to radial and femoral osteotomies in dogs. Mechanical testing of the plated radii at one year showed a significantly greater load to failure in bending than for the controls with metal plates. Mechanical testing was not performed on the femoral specimens but there were two non-unions for the steel plates. The authors then report the use of glass fiber reinforced polycarbonate in seven patients for the repair of six tibial and one radial fractures. The fractures were cast immobilized with weight bearing allowed on crutches at three months. All patients were reported to be progressing well.

Brown and Vandergrift [14] have reported the result of a study in which plastic plates were used to fix osteotomies in canine femora. The authors chose this approach based on the hypothesis that healing by primary callus formation (such as occurs when no plate is present) can be augmented if a low modulus plate is used to stabilize the bone fragments. The use of bone plates is different from conventional plating in which the system is rigid enough that very little callus formation occurs. This experiment utilized UHMWPE, Delrin, and polybutylene terephthalate plates on transverse osteotomies. In all animals, the fracture healed without any additional support from an external cast. The authors conclude that similar low modulus plates might have clinical application. As in all other reported studies, the fracture line was an artifically created transverse fracture. This type of fracture probably could be treated by external means in the clinical situation. The severely reduced mechanical properties of plastic plates might be more of a detriment for an oblique or multiple fragment fracture and might prevent early weight-bearing on the affected limb.

The fact that composite material properties can be varied over a wide range by variation of fiber volume fraction and the type and orientation of fiber has lead several researchers to investigate the bone present under a composite plate of reduced stiffness.

Woo and co-workers [15,16] at the University of California at San Diego, have experimented with a polymethyl-methacrylate (PMMA) system reinforced with graphite fiber at $\pm 35°$ from the long axis. Composite plates were fabricated with similar geometry to corresponding metallic plates and a series of comparative studies carried out in osteotomized canine radii and femora. In the comparison of the composite plates to both stainless steel and cobalt-chromium alloy plates, the authors found no evidence of differences in healing time between the high stiffness and lower stiffness plates.

Mechanical testing of the excised bone showed the mechanical properties of the bone material present to be equivalent regardless of which plate was used and it was also found to be equivalent to control bone. Microscopic evaluation of the bones showed the cortical bone under the metallic plate to be considerably thinner than that under the composite plate and the bending load to failure was significantly greater for the composite plates than for the metal. There was no load to failure reported for normal bone.

McKenna [17] also investigated the use of composite bone plates. His plates were glass/epoxy, graphite/polysulfone, and graphite/polypropylene composites. His composites were prepared using various combinations of 0°, ± 45°, and 90° orientations as a stacking sequence. The thrust of this work, as in the previously referenced work, was to produce a plate which would exhibit a lower modulus in bending and therefore provide less shielding of the bone from stress.

A preliminary study using 4-hole plates was found to have disappointing results primarily due to failure of the screw fixation to the bone so a study was instituted using 6-hole plates in which, out of 18 plates placed over transverse osteotomies of canine femora, there were two non-unions and three failed plates. Dr. McKenna also observed one non-union out of four control animals in which stainless steel plates had been placed. The author speculated that the animals in which composite failure occurred may have slipped and overloaded the plates. He also noted that the failed plates had the lowest strengths of the different combinations tested ranged from 2.74 N-m (24.2 in-lb) to 18.1 N-m (160 in-lb).

McKenna found that even when using his plates which had significantly lower flexural rigidity than conventional plates, the bone opposite the plate had significantly higher strength than that under the plate. This would appear to indicate that some degree of stress protection atrophy still occurs.

In Great Britain [18], there has been work performed to evaluate carbon fiber reinforced epoxy as a bone plate material. The authors report the results of a series of tests performed on tibial osteotomies in sheep in which full bone strength is reported to have returned in 24 weeks with the resultant bone having 60% of the stiffness of normal bone. It is reported that the composite design has been in human clinical trials for 18 months with favorable results.

While the thrust of the referenced work was to develop reduced stiffness plates for fracture fixation to reduce osteoporosis, the aim of the work currently being undertaken at Hexcel in conjunction with the College of Medicine and Dentistry of New Jersey is slightly different. This work is an extension of the CMDNJ work undertaken to date in this area and reported in Dr. Alexander's discussion elsewhere in this publication. The aim is to prepare composite bone plates with as high a flexural stiffness as possible for initial stabilization of the fracture site. The use of a biodegradable polymer (polylactic acid) as a matrix material opens up the opportunity to prepare a device which will gradually transfer the load-bearing responsibilities to the bone as the fracture heals.

While the ideal bone plate would lose its mechanical properties at exactly the same rate as the bone gains in its ability to sustain load, such a situation may only be an ideal for which to shoot. It would seem to be more important that the plate maintain its load bearing properties at least as long as needed than that it exactly follow the properties of the bone. Individual differences in healing rates will also mandate a conservative approach to the optimization of degradation rate. The early rigidity of the plates will maintain the fracture segments in close approximation and possibly under compression to minimize callus formation. So long as the degradation is gradual enough that the bone can remodel to accept its additional load bearing duties as required without excessively long maintenance of plate properties, the goal will be achieved.

The design which has been chosen utilizes carbon fiber in a unidirectional "prepreg" of PLA resin. Under pressure and heat, the plate is compression formed from multiple layers, precut in the shape of the plate and laid up so that the fibers are at +15° and −15° alternatively to the long axis of the plate.

This laminated construction for preparing bone plates of this type has been attempted previously at CMDNJ but discarded because of poor fatigue properties [19]. This design will be superior in mechanical strength and stiffness to any random fiber construction like their final design. The current research involves the improvement of the molding conditions to overcome the problems of fatigue delamination in a fluid environment. Once this change has been instituted, *in vitro* and animal testing to refine the design of the plate will commence.

TOTAL JOINT REPLACEMENT

The need to replace one or both of the articulating surfaces of a joint can result from several different conditions. Among them are the arthritic degradation of articulating surfaces leading to pain and decreased mobility, degenerative conditions as a result of complications from previous surgery and cancerous conditions necessitating removal of bone sections in which the only alternative would be amputation of the limb.

Most of the total joint replacement devices implanted in the United States consist of a metallic surface bearing on an ultra high molecular weight polyethylene (UHMWPE) surface. For hip replacement, there is a metallic femoral component consisting of a highly polished spherical head attached to a smaller neck and then widening to a tapered shaft designed to mimic the contours of the medullary canal. The metal is usually a cobalt-chromium-molybdenum alloy or a titanium alloy with mechanical properties and load bearing ability far in excess of those of bone. The opposite bearing surface in the acetabulum of the pelvis is usually UHMWPE molded or machined to closely match the head of the femoral component. As mentioned earlier, one manufacturer has introduced a carbon fiber filled UHMWPE material to perform the same function. In a vast majority of cases, the two components are attached to the remaining bone by PMMA bone cement which has been forced into the cavity after oversize reaming. The implant components are forced into the curing bone cement and attachment is by mechanical interlocking.

Failure of hip arthroplasties have been found to occur in some patients. While there is still some controversy concerning the mechanism of failure and the proper technique for avoiding it, one theory is that resorption of the bone proximal to the implant can lead to cement failure and failure of the replacement. A loose implant cannot function properly and has failed even if physical failure has not occurred. Analysis of the stress patterns present in the prosthesis-cement-bone system at the University of Southern California [20] has led the authors to suggest that a lower modulus stem material may lead to greater transfer of stress to the bone in the calcar region and prevent or lessen the degree of resorption of bone in this region. Based on this concept of reduced stem modulus, titanium alloy hips have been introduced by several orthopaedic manufacturers recently since it has approximately half the modulus of the cobalt based alloys.

Another finite element modeling experiment at the University of Iowa [21] addressed the effects of the properties of the stem as well as four other design aspects of a total hip replacement. In their analysis of the effect of stem modulus, they noted that decreasing the modulus caused greater load transfer to the cement. Based on their assumption that it was important to reduce stresses in the cement to reduce cement failure, they concluded that the modulus of the stem should be high. Their results also showed that reducing stem modulus increased calcar longitudinal and hoop stresses in the bone. It is possible to conclude from their results that reduced stem modulus could lead to more rapid transfer of load to the bone and reduced bone resorption provided that cement failure did not occur.

Composites have begun to be introduced into hip anthroplasty in an attempt to address failure problems. In Germany, several researchers have reported the use of carbon fiber reinforced polymers and carbon fiber reinforced carbon (CFRC). Wolter and co-workers [22,23] have designed a hip which has a CFRC stem and aluminum oxide head which was cemented into place. In ten foxhounds, sacrificed at six or twelve months, no implant failure was seen and the animals were using the joints normally. Reported also was a design concept for non-cemented fixation of a similar prosthesis. Another group [24] presented mechanical data for various polymers in combinations with carbon or glass fibers for prosthetic use. The use of composites in hip prostheses is, however, in its infancy.

The basic thrust of our research is the development of a composite hip design which will have mechanical properties tailored to the application. Our initial design for animal test purposes (Figure 1) is modeled after a similar cobalt alloy implant which will serve as a control. The hip is a laminated structure machined from a solid block. A cast cobalt-chromium-molybdenum alloy head is attached and bears on an UHMWPE acetabular component. While direct load transfer to the femoral bone appears desirable, initial testing is being performed using cement fixation.

The attractive feature of carbon reinforced polymer for this application is that the orientation and fiber content can be varied in the implant to provide the mechnical property orientation necessary for good function. The carbon fiber can be distributed in matrix material to provide strength in only those locations and directions where it is needed. The implant must be designed in such a way that fatigue failure does not occur and the matrix material is not attacked by the physiological environment.

Table 1. Materials (Polymers Tested).

POLYMER	POLYMER TYPE	COMMERCIAL NAME AND MANUFACTURER
Polysulfone	Thermo-plastic	UDEL MG-11, Union Carbide, Dallas,TX
Poly-Methyl Methacrylate	Thermo-plastic	PMMA I.V. 0.4, Rohm & Haas, Philadelphia, PA
Epoxy (Low Viscosity)	Thermoset	Stycast 1267, Emerson & Cuming, Canton,MA
Epoxy (High Viscosity)	Thermoset	C-8W795 & H.R. 795, Hysol Corp., Los Angeles, CA
Polyurethane	Thermoset	Medithane 3190, Hexel Corp., Chatsworth, CA

Table 2. Typical Mechanical Properties of Polymer – Carbon Composites (3 Point Bending)

POLYMER	ULTIMATE STRENGTH (MPa)	MODULUS (GPa)
PMMA	772	55
Polysulfone	938	76
Epoxy		
Stycast	535	30
Hysol	207	24
Polyurethane	289	18

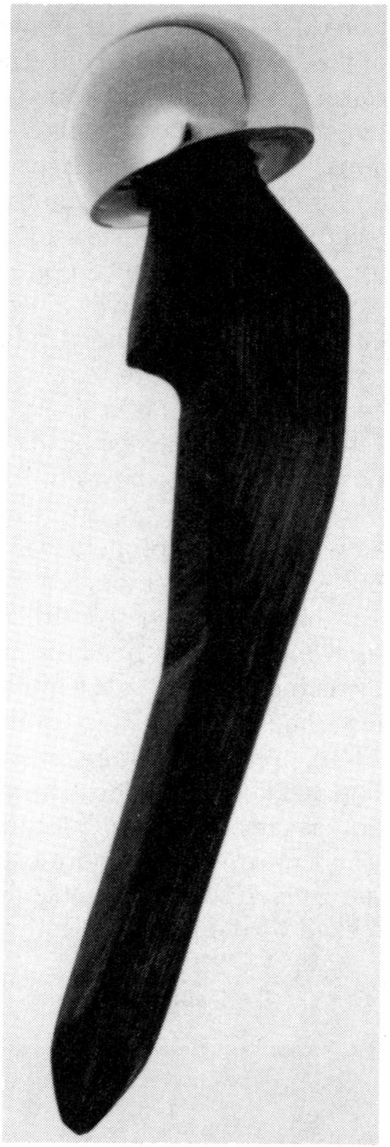

Figure 1. Carbon Fiber/Polysulfone Canine Hip Prosthesis with Co-Cr-Mo Alloy Head.

The matrix materials evaluated are listed in Table 1. These polymers were combined with unsized carbon fiber (Hercules, Inc., Salt Lake City, UT) into ±15° laminated test specimens approximately 2.5 cm × 7.5 cm × 0.3 cm. Testing was performed in three point bending giving the results in Table 2.

These results show that the thermoplastics tested exhibited higher mechanical properties than the thermosets. This diffference was partially due to the problems encountered in achieving high enough fiber loading in the thermosets. The ultimate strength reported for polysulfone composite is equal or higher than that of metals currently used for implants but the modulus is 65% of that of titanium alloy and 30% of that of cast Co-Cr-Mo alloy. These values are typical of those achieved to date. If necessary, lower properties can be achieved by the change of fiber volume or orientation. A composite canine hip prepared from the polysulfone composite had a failure load of 12.46 kN when the load was applied vertically to the ball.

Because a composite hip will be subjected to the physiological environment in use, an accelerated test was performed to evaluate changes in properties. In this test, the samples were immersed in 0.9% saline solution maintained at 90°C for one week. These conditions are extremely severe and can be used to quickly screen out materials with low hydrolytic stability. Bradley and coworkers [18] report similar accelerated test data for epoxy composite in which the bend strength decreased from 84 MPa to 40 Mpa, a drop of 50%. Our results shown in Table 3, show strength losses of 10% for polysulfone, 14% for PMMA, and 40% for epoxy. The apparent superiority of polysulfone in bending strength, hydrolytic stability, and the fact that it

Table 3. Accelerated Test Data.

POLYMER	STRENGTH (MPa)		MODULUS (GPa)	
	Before	After	Before	After
Polysulfone	807	723	77	67
PMA	687	594	76	73
Epoxy (Stycast)	535	323	30	21

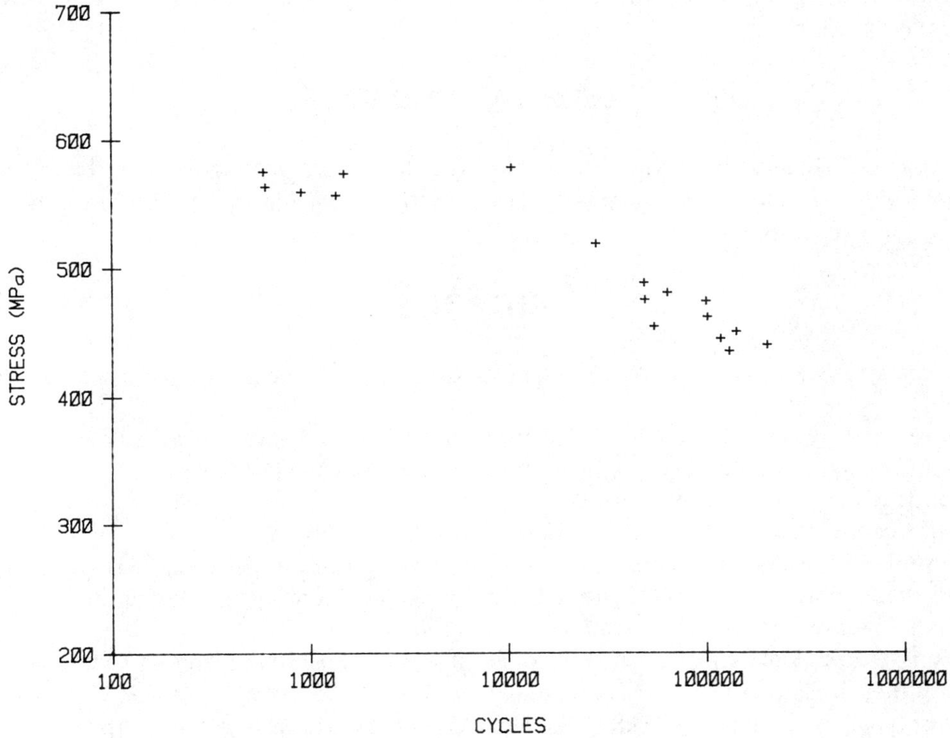

Figure 2. Fatigue Endurance Data for Carbon Fiber/Polysulfone Composite Test Specimens Tested in Air at 3cps.

is commercially available as a medical grade material has led to its choice for further development.

Composites may exhibit fatigue delamination under load because of their layer structures. An experiment is in progress to evaluate the fatigue properties of the polysulfone carbon fiber composite. Specimens approximately 1.3 cm × 7.5 cm × 0.3 cm are subjected to cyclic loading at three cycles per second on a MMED six station fatigue tester (MATCO, La Canada, CA). The stresses used in our tests to date (Figure 2) represent 70-90% of the ultimate stresses for identical implants tested in bending. Even at these loads far in excess of any design limits which would be instituted, the fatigue endurances are high. Further testing is planned at lower stresses and in saline solution to evaluate fatigue under more realistic conditions. Testing of a composite hip under fatigue at 50% of ultimate strength showed no evidence of failure at 10^6 cycles.

Experimentation with the implants *in vivo* as well as further fatigue testing of the implants in a saline environment will yield a total hip replacement which will allow for improved load transfer to the bone of the femur. This work is on-going at the current time.

CONCLUSION

The use of carbon fiber reinforced composites to replace metals in load bearing applications, while new to the orthopaedic implant field, has been used extensively in aerospace and other applications. By the careful application of these techniques to medical applications, engineered materials can be developed whose properties have been tailored to the specific implant application. The two major applications presented here are for a variable stiffness fracture fixation device and a lower modulus total hip replacement device but the results of this work and similar applications of composite technology can lead to a whole new field of materials for implant use.

ACKNOWLEDGEMENTS

The reported studies on composite total hip replacement were performed at Hexcel under the direction of T. Devanathan and S. Lin and their permission to include the results is acknowledged with thanks.

REFERENCES

1. Freeman, B.S.; "Proplast, A Porous Implant for Contour Restoration"; *Br. J. Plast. Surg.;* 29:158-164, 1976.
2. Homsy, C.A., Cain, T.E., Kessler, F.B., Anderson, M.S., King, J.W., "Porous Implant Systems for Prosthesis Stabilization"; *Clin. Orthop. Rel. Res.;* 89:220-235, 1972.
3. Woods, G.W., Homsy, C.A., Prewitt, J.M., Tullos, H.S.; "Proplast Leader for Use in Cruciate Ligament Reconstruction"; *Am. J. Sport Med.;* 7:314-320, 1979.
4. Alexander, H., Aragona, J., Parson, J., Weiss, A., Strauchler, I., Mayott, C.; "A Filamentous Carbon-Absorbable Polymer Medial Collateral Ligament Replacement"; presented at the Thirteenth International Biomaterials Symposium, May 28-31, 1981.
5. Jenkins, D.H.R., McKibbin, B.; "The Role of Flexible Carbon-Fibre Implants as Tendon and Ligament Substitutes in Clinical Practice: A Preliminary Report"; *J. Bone Jt. Surg.;* 62A: 497-499, 1980.
6. Johnson-Nurse, C., Jenkins, D.H.R.; "The Use of Flexible Carbon Fibre in the Repair of Experimental Large Abdominal Incisional Hernias"; *Br. J. Surg.;* 67:135-137, 1980.
7. Neugebauer, R., Burri, C., Claes, L., Helbing, G., Wolter, D.; "The Use of Carbon Fiber Strands for Replacement of Collateral Ligaments at the Knee Joint"; *Langenbecks Arch. Chir.;* 351 (Suppl.): 35-39, 1980.
8. Neugebauer, R., Wolter, D., Claes, L., Bultmann, B.; "Plastic Replacement of the Abdominal Wall by Un-Coated Carbon Cloth"; *Langenbecks Arch. Chir.;* 350: 83-93, 1979.
9. Uthoff, H.K., Dubuc, F.L.; "Bone Structure Changes in the Dog Under Rigid Internal Fixation"; *Clin. Orthop. Rel. Res.;* 81: 165-170, 1971.
10. Stromberg, L., Dalen, N.; "Influence of a Rigid Plate for Internal Fixation on the Maximum Torque Capacity of Long Bones"; *Acta Chir. Scand.;* 142: 115-122, 1976.
11. Uthoff, H.K., Bardos, D.I., Liskova-Kiar, M.; "The Advantages of Titanium Alloy over Stainless Steel Plates for the Internal Fixation of Fractures"; *J. Bone Jt. Surg.;* 63B: 427-434, 1981.

12. Tonino, A.J., Davidson, C.L., Klopper, P.J., Linclau, L.A.; "Protection from Stress in Bone and its Effects"; *J. Bone Jt. Surg.;* 58B: 107-113, 1976.
13. Tonino, A.J., Klopper, P.J.; "The Use of Plastic Plates in the Treatment of Fractures"; *Current Concepts of Internal Fracture Fixation* (H.K. Uthoff, ed.); Springer-Verlag, Heidelberg; p. 342-347, 1980.
14. Brown, S.A., Vandergrift, J.; "Healing of Femoral Osteotomies with Plastic Plate Fixation"; *Biomat. Med. Dev. Art. Org.;* 9: 27-35, 1981.
15. Woo, S.L-Y., Akeson, W.H., Coutts, R.D., Rutherford, L., Doty, D., Jemmott, G.F., Amiel, D.; "A Comparison of Cortical Bone Atrophy Secondary to Fixation with Plates with Large Differences in Bending Stiffness"; *J. Bone Jt. Surg.;* 62A: 68-78, 1980.
16. Woo, S.L-Y., Simon, B.R., Akeson, W.H., McCarty, M.P.; An Interdisciplinary Approach to Evaluate the Effect of Internal Fixation Plate on Long Bone Remodeling"; J. Biomech.; 10: 87-95, 1977.
17. McKenna, G.B.; *The Development of Fiber Reinforced Polymer Composites for Orthopaedic Application;* PhD Dissertation, University of Utah, 1976.
18. Bradley, J.S., Hastings, G.W., Tayton, K.J., Johnson-Nurse, C.; "Carbon Fibre Reinforced Epoxy Resins for Internal Fixation of Bone Fractures"; presented at the Thirteenth International Biomaterials Symposium, May 28-31, 1981.
19. Parson, J., Corcoran, S., Korluk, J., Alexander, H., Mayott, C., Weiss, A.; "In-Vivo Evaluation of Variable Stiffness, Absorbably Bone Plates"; presented at the Thirteenth International Biomaterials Symposium, May 28-31, 1981.
20. Tarr, R.R., Clarke, I.C., Sarmiento, A.; "Loading Behavior of Femoral Stems of Titanium-6A1-4V Compared to Cobalt-Chromium Alloys: A 3-D Finite Element Analysis"; In Press.
21. Crowninshield, R.D., Brand, R.A., Johnston, R.C., Milroy, J.C.; "An Analysis of Femoral Component Stem Design in Total Hip Arthroplasty"; *J. Bone Jt. Surg.;* 62A: 68-78, 1980.
22. Wolter, D., Rose, P.G., Gerstenberger, F.; "In Vivo Studies of Carbon Fibre Reinforced Hip-Joint Endoprosthesis in Fox Hound"; presented at the First World Biomaterials Congress, April 8-12, 1980.
23. Rose, P.G., Gerstenberger, R., Gruber, U., Loos, W., Wolter, D., Neugebauer, R.; "New Aspects of the Design and Application of Carbon Fibre Reinforced Carbon for Prosthetic Devices"; presented at the First World Biomaterials Congress, April 8-12, 1980.
24. Soltesz, U., Richter, H.; "Investigation of Mechanical Behavior of Fibre-Reinforced Materials for Endoprosthetic Devices"; presented at the First World Biomaterials Congress, April 8-12, 1980.

Chapter 38

Absorbable Polymer – Filamentous Carbon Composites: A New Concept in Orthopaedic Biomaterials

J.R. Parsons, Ph.D., Assistant Professor;
H. Alexander, Professor;
and A.B. Weiss, M.D., Professor
Section of Orthopaedic Surgery
College of Medicine and Dentistry of New Jersey
New Jersey Medical School
100 Bergen Street, Newark, New Jersey 07103

ABSTRACT

Composites of filamentous carbon fiber and absorbable polymer form a new and useful class of orthopaedic biomaterials. Ribbon-like composite structures have been utilized in the repair and replacement of tendons and ligaments. When used in this way, the composite acts as a scaffold upon which new collagenous tissue can grow. This technique provides only temporary mechanical integrity until the new tissue can assume the mechanical function.

More rigid structures, plates and rods, have been used to internally fix unstable long bone fractures. Initially, these composite devices have structural rigidities similar to commercially available metallic devices of similar design. With time, however, the composite devices gradually lose rigidity, transferring increasing load to the healing bone. This transference of load permits a more normal healing pattern and avoids detrimental weakening of the bone in the region of the device. Further, the partially absorbable composite devices need not be removed with a second operative procedure as is recommended with metallic devices.

This project has been funded by the generous support of the William Lightfood Schultz Foundation through the Foundation of the College of Medicine and Dentistry of New Jersey and the Hexcel Corporation.

Chapter 38. J.R. Parsons, Ph.D., H. Alexander, Professor; and A.B. Weiss, M.D., Professor

INTRODUCTION

Carbon has been used successfully as an implant material in a number of applications and forms [1-3]. Jenkins et al [4,5], Wolter et al [6], Neugebauer et al [7-9], and Claes et al [10] have shown that tendons and ligaments can be replaced by filamentous carbon implants which act as scaffolds for the development of new fibrous tissue. Carbon succeeds as a scaffolding material for a number of reasons. It provides mechanical strength on implantation, allowing early return of function. The material is extremely compatible, permitting the ingrowth of new aligned fibrous tissue. Finally, the carbon fiber may degrade mechanically as the new tissue matures, allowing for the gradual transfer of load to the regrown tissue structure.

Forster et al [11] and Jenkins et al [4,5], who used spun carbon fiber tows as replacement anterior cruciate ligaments and medial collateral ligaments in sheep, have since proceeded to use this raw, uncoated carbon in humans for various ligament reconstructions [12]. Similarly, Wolter et al [6], Claes et al [10], and Kinzl et al [13] used thick woven tows of carbon to replace medial collateral ligaments in sheep and extra-articular knee and ankle ligaments in humans. In the work of both of these groups, as well as in animal studies conducted by the authors, raw carbon fiber was found to partially fragment during and immediately after the operative procedure and migrate from the implant site before the new fibrous tissue could encapsulate it. Carbon fragments were found in the lymph nodes of the animals and is most likely in the humans into whom the uncoated carbon was implanted. Although not shown to be detrimental in any way, spread of carbon fiber fragments to nearby lymph nodes is clearly undesirable.

This paper reports a program of research in which the authors addressed the problem of the mechanical degradation of the brittle filamentous carbon during its implantation and during the early phases of tissue growth. This premature mechanical degradation, and the resulting migration of carbon fragments from the implant site, was largely eliminated by utilizing a composite of carbon fiber and polylactic acid polymer (PLA). The composite has greatly improved handling characteristics when compared with raw carbon fiber. The PLA-carbon composite, in a ribbon-like configuration, was studied as a patellar tendon replacement and a medial collateral ligament replacement in dogs and as an Achilles tendon replacement in rabbits. In all three studies, the implant material was highly successful as a mechanically degrading scaffold for the development of new soft tissue. The PLA degraded rapidly and completely and the carbon fibers remained benignly within the newly formed tissue. No migration to regional lymph nodes was noted.

During the early phases of the development of this material, it was recognized that composite materials technology could be exploited to design and produce more complex, rigid structures. The natural application in orthopaedics was to produce compatible, partially degradable plates and rods for internally fixing unstable long bone fractures.

Although the metallic bone plates and intermedullary rods currently in use are effective, there are some disadvantages. During early healing, such rigid fixation promotes primary bony union. Unfortunately, as healing progresses, rigid plates and rods can cause bone to undergo a resorptive phase [14-18]. This resorption of bony structure and mass is termed stress protection atrophy and results from the shielding of the bone from normal stresses in the region of the rigid device. The long-term result of stress protection is a mechanically inferior bony structure. As surgical removal of these metallic devices is recommended after healing, refracture of the weakened bone is a very real possibility. Indeed, even without plate or rod removal, refracture sometimes occurs due to the weakened condition of the bone. Protection and limited activity are desirable until the bone can actively remodel and strengthen.

Other investigators [19,21] have proposed the use of intermediately stiff fixation devices. This compromise solution results in some loss of initial rigidity with increased possibility of non-union. However, some reduction in stress protection atrophy is realized.

The possibility of using resorbable fixation devices has also been investigated. In the early 1970's, Cutright and Hunsuck [22,23] and Getter et al [24] used various devices made from polylactic acid polymer to fix orbital fractures in monkeys and mandibular fractures in dogs. These devices were originally designed to eliminate a second operation to remove hardware as with metallic devices. No thought was given the possibility of reducing stress protection atrophy. Unfortunately, the PLA plate and screw system of Getter was not sufficiently strong or rigid enough to fix human long bone fractures. If a sufficiently strong, resorbable plate or rod could be developed, its advantages would be twofold: 1) No secondary operation would be necessary to remove hardware, and (2) such a device would gradually lose rigidity, transferring increasing load to the healing bone, thus preventing stress protection atrophy. It is to this end that composites of carbon fiber- PLA are being applied.

The authors have developed angle-ply and random-oriented laminate bone plates [25-27]. These fixation plates have been mechanically tested in torsion, four-point bending, and in a four-point bending fatigue mode. Subsequent to mechanical testing, these plates were tested in vivo in two experiments in canines.

MATERIALS AND METHODS

Ligament and Tendon Replacement Materials

PLA-filamentous carbon tissue scaffolding ribbons are produced by coating uniaxial filamentous carbon with polylactic acid polymer. The individual carbon fiber tows typically contain 10^4 fibers which are 6 to 10 microns in diameter. The fibers are pyrolized from a polymer fiber precursor. The resulting material is almost pure elemental carbon with mechanical strength and rigidity greater than steel. It has a modulus of over 200 GPa and an ultimate tensile strength of approximately 2.5 GPa. The polylactic acid polymer is produced from L(-) lactide. This cyclic diester, the lactide of lactic acid, polymerizes by an ionic ring opening addition mechanism to a high polymer which can be cast into films, spun into fibers, or extruded into rods similar to the industrial polyesters, such as Dacron® . It is a thermoplastic and can also be dissolved readily in chloroform.

Fabrication of coated fiber tows is accomplished by first preparing a polymer solution in chloroform. Where appropriate, this solution contains polyethylene glycol plasticizer (5-30% polymer by weight). The fibers are coated with the polymer by solution dipping or spraying. For attachment to soft tissues, suture needles are attached to the ends of the fiber tows. The device is then sterilized in ethylene oxide gas or through a dry heating cycle with temperatures below the PLA melt temperature.

The biocompatibility of carbon fiber and polylactic acid have previously been demonstrated. Finely divided carbon particles have been shown to be well tolerated; they do not cause formation of foreign body giant cells in the synovial lining of joints, nor do they produce cytotoxic effects [28]. Studies of tissue tolerance of carbon materials by Christel et al [29]

® Registered trademark Dupont Co., Inc.

have also indicated that carbon materials are well accepted by connective tissues. Filamentous carbon has been used as a component of implants currently in human use, and studies in rabbits and mice indicate good short and long-term biocompatibility of this material. The question of foreign body or physically induced carcinogenicity was addressed in studies conducted by Jenkins [30] and Claes [31] using carbon fiber connective tissue implants. To date, investigators have found no abnormal tumor formation in their studies.

The short and long-term response to polylactic acid has been studied by Cutright et al [32], Brady et al [33], and Kulkarni et al [34]. Polylactic acid has been found to be a biocompatible material that elicits no immunological response, probably due to the absence of peptide linkages. It biodegrades by undergoing hydrolytic de-esterification to lactic acid, a normal metabolic intermediate.

Canine Patellar Tendon

To investigate the response of this tissue scaffold replacement material in a full load-bearing situation, a canine patellar tendon study was conducted in which patellar tendons were removed from fourteen adult beagle dogs [35]. In one series of six dogs, two received patellar tendon prostheses of PLA-coated filamentous carbon tows in one leg and the other leg was unoperated, two received prostheses of uncoated carbon in one leg and the other leg was unoperated, and two received PLA-carbon prostheses in one leg and nylon suture prostheses in the other. These six dogs were sacrified at two months post-implantation. An identical series of six dogs were sacrificed at four months post-implantation. Two dogs with PLA-carbon prostheses in one leg and one leg unoperated were sacrificed at one year post-implantation for a total of fourteen. All of the implants were passed through drill holes in the tibia and through the quadriceps tendon above the patella to form a continuous figure-of-eight repair (Figure 1). The implant was tensioned manually such that the distance between the original tendon insertions was maintained. The ends of implants were tied to each other. Post-operatively, the animals were unprotected and allowed to move freely in their cages. Upon sacrifice, half of the specimens were subjected to mechanical testing in a tensile mode, while the other half were histologically evaluated.

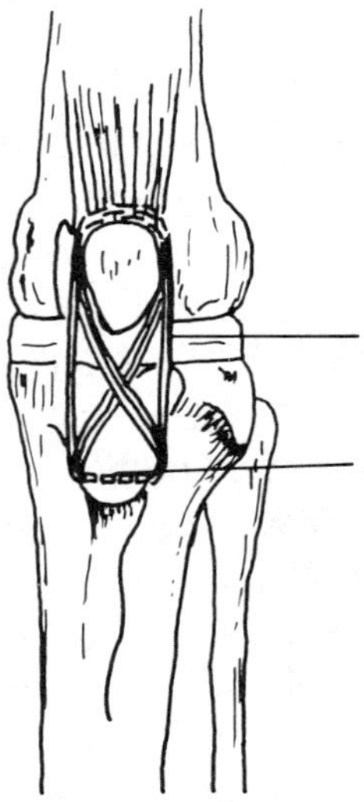

Figure 1. Patellar tendon replacement with PLA-coated filamentous carbon tows.

Rabbit Achilles Tendon

Another factor in the evaluation of the utility of the PLA-carbon composite is its ability to encourage rapid development of secure soft tissue anastomosis. A study was conducted in twenty-three adult male rabbits [36]. In seventeen of the rabbits, the proximal third of the Achilles tendon was removed and replaced by a PLA-carbon composite ribbon. The anastomoses were achieved by use of a new anastomosis technique, the locking weave, which allows the replacement tendon to act as its own suture. This yields a strong juncture between the small diameter composite tendon and the larger diameter muscle or

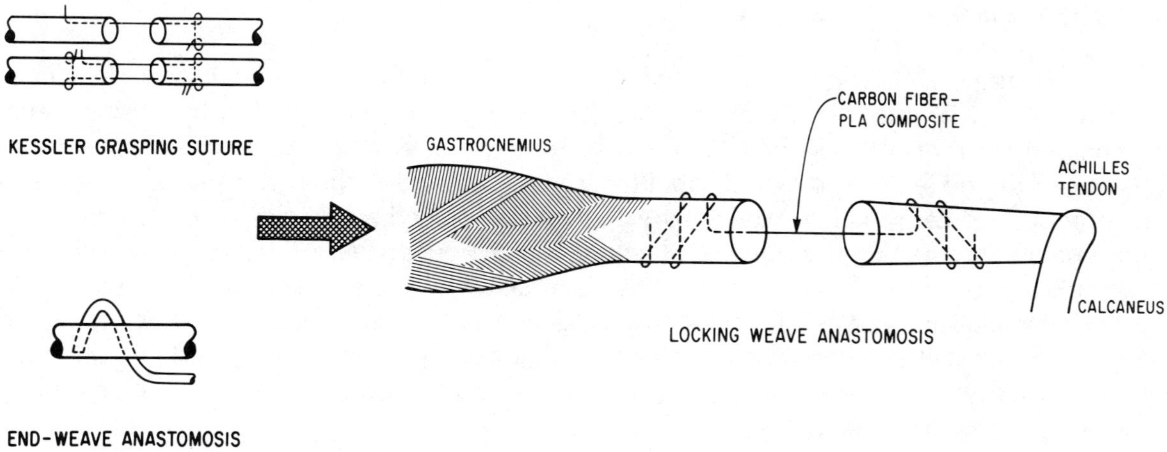

Figure 2. The techniques of the Kessler grasping suture and the end-weave anastomosis are combined to form the locking-weave anastomosis.

tendon remnant (Figure 2). Six rabbits underwent sham procedures in which the proximal third of the Achilles tendon was removed and no replacement was provided. In all animals, the contralateral limb served as a control. No immobilization was applied to the operated limbs, and the animals were free to move about their cages. The animals were sacrificed according to the schedule shown in Table 1.

Table 1. Sacrifice Schedule

	Post-Op	1 Week	2 Week	4 Week	8 Week	12 Week
Carbon-PLA Implants	Mechanical Testing	Mechanical Testing	Mechanical Testing	Mechanical Testing	Mechanical Testing	Mechanical Testing
		2	2	2	2	2
Total = 17	2	Histology	Histology	Histology	Histology	Histology
		1	1	1	1	1
Sham Procedure	Mechanical Testing	Mechanical Testing	Mechanical Testing	Mechanical Testing	Mechanical Testing	Mechanical Testing
	1	1	1	1	1	1
Total = 6						

Canine Medial Collateral Ligament

In this study [37], the medial collateral ligament of adult male beagle dogs was chosen for replacement with the composite material. Under appropriate anesthesia and using sterile technique, the medial aspect of the knee was exposed. The medial collateral was excised from its origins on the femur and tibia. In addition, the medial side of the joint capsule was excised to produce a gross valgus instability. The implant was placed across the joint in an anatomic position and secured using soft tissue attachment techniques (Figure 3) developed in other experiments (see Rabbit Achilles Tendon). The contralateral knee served as a control. A second group of animals served as "shams". These dogs were subjected to identical surgery, only no implant was installed. The surgical wounds were closed in layers in a standard fashion and a bulky "Jones-type" dressing was applied. This dressing provided some immobilization and remained in place for two weeks.

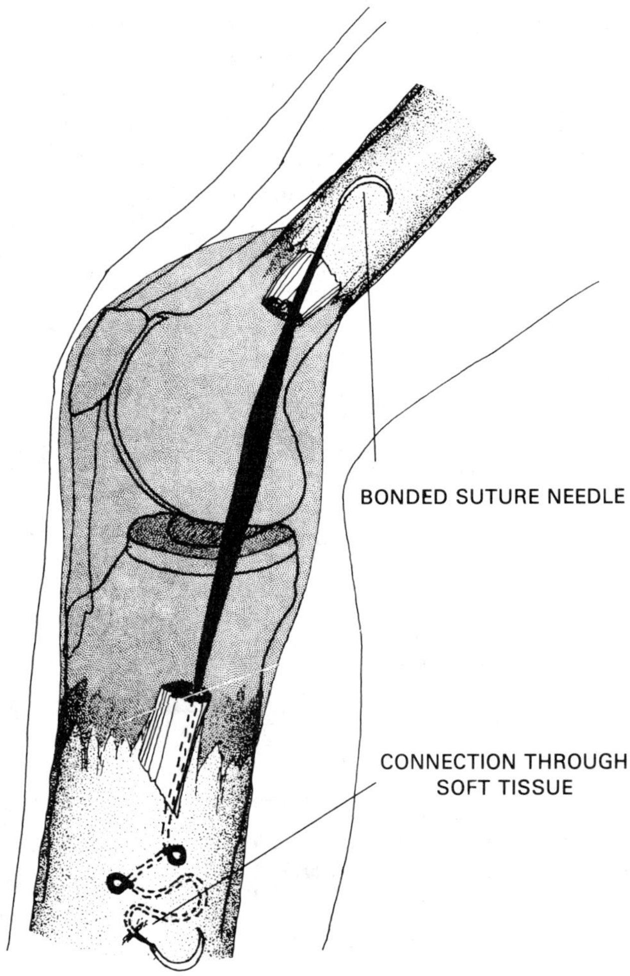

Figure 3. Surgical Technique – The composite ribbon of carbon fiber/PLA is passed through the ligament remnant and woven into the soft tissue and periosteum distally and proximally.

After periods of four weeks, eight weeks, and twelve weeks, the dogs were sacrificed and the regrown medial collateral structures were tested mechanically. All mechanical tests were conducted on a custom MTS servo-hydraulic test machine. The mechanical test procedure included a low force cantilever bending test and a uniaxial tension test to failure. The low force cantilever bending was designed to simulate a clinical valgus stress test for stability. The measure of stability was the opening of the joint at a calculated ligament force of 25 N (Figure 4). The joint was then mounted so a uniaxial tension test could be performed to determine ultimate strengths of the regrown tissue. For this test, all ligamentous and capsular structures were cut, except those in the medial collateral position. The ligaments were tested to failure and the ultimate strengths and slope of the load-elongation curves recorded.

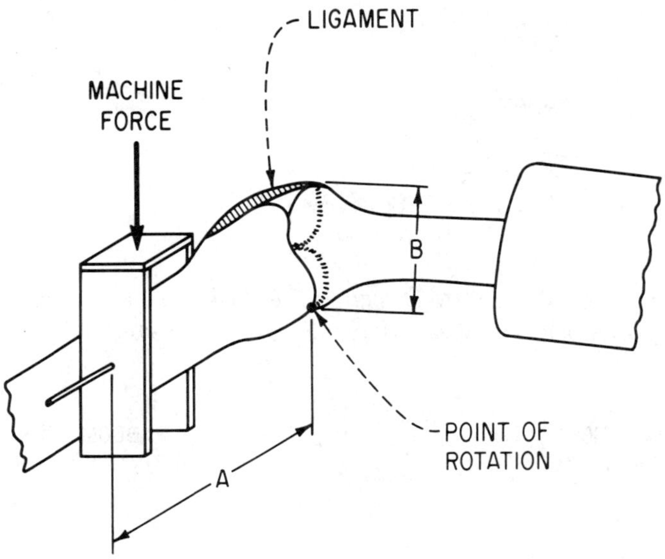

LIGAMENT FORCE = A/B x MACHINE FORCE = 25N

JOINT LAXITY = B/A x MACHINE DISPLACEMENT

Figure 4. Cantilever Bending Test – This low force, nondestructive mechanical test simulates a clinical valgus stress test. Laxity is measured as the opening of the joint in millimeters at a calculated ligament force of 25 N.

Design and Fabrication of Composite Bone Plates

Using an accepted bone plate configuration (Figure 5), angle-ply and random oriented laminated composite bone plates were designed (Figure 6). By varying the matrix polymer properties, the carbon fiber properties, the relative volume fraction of fiber to matrix, and the fiber orientation, composites of widely varying mechanical properties could be anticipated. Based on theoretical predictions [38], plates were produced by molding under heat and pressure above the PLA melt temperature. The nominal materials design parameters are shown in Table 2.

These plates were then mechanically tested to establish their static bending and torsional

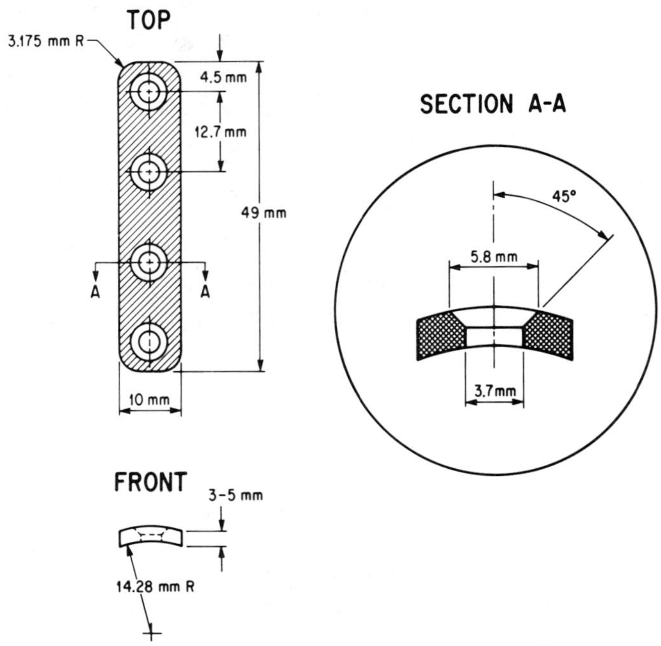

Figure 5. Bone Plate Design – The thickness of the composite plates may vary depending on the desired rigidity.

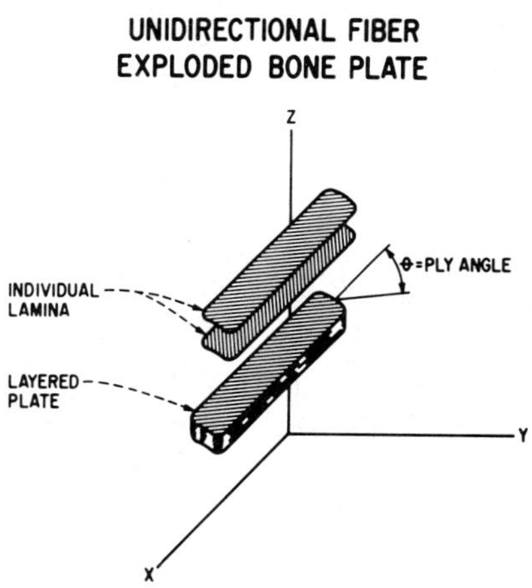

Figure 6a.

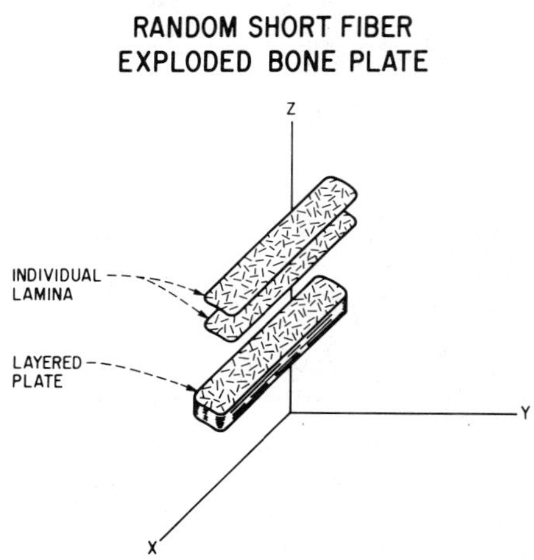

Figure 6b.

Figure 6. Exploded view of composite bone plates. a) Angle-ply laminate. b) Random oriented laminate.

characteristics. Bending tests were of the four point type, conducted at a constant deflection rate. Torsional specimens were fixed with steel screws to transversely osteotomized cadaver canine femurs. This system simulated more closely the actual in-vivo situation. Fatigue tests were conducted in torsion and four-point bending in air, water, and saline environments. Mean stresses of 50% yield ± cyclic stresses of 20% yield were used.

Table 2. Bone Plate Design Parameters

Fiber Type	High Modulus
Fiber Modulus, GPa	330
Fiber Strength, GPa	2.75
Fiber Ultimate Elongation	1.0-1.5%
Polymer Modulus, GPa	6-10
Volume Ratio, V_f/V_{PLA}	40-60%
Ply Angle (Oriented)	15%
Fiber Length (Random)	4-6 mm

Canine Osteotomy Healing Study

To demonstrate the effectiveness of these partially degradable plates in an in-vivo situation, a canine osteotomy healing study was initiated. In this experiment, composite plates were used to fix transversely osteotomized canine long bones [39]. Six German Shepherd dogs were used. In three, a radius was osteotomized and fixed with a composite plate. In the others, a tibia was osteotomized and fixed. In both groups, two dogs were sacrificed after nine weeks and one dog was maintained for long-term study. The healed osteotomies of the dogs sacrificed at nine weeks were examined by x-ray, grossly and microhistologically.

Canine Osteoporosis Study

In order to demonstrate that harmful stress protection atrophy could be avoided with composite, degradable plates, an osteoporosis study was undertaken. Six adult beagle dogs were used. On one intact femur a composite plate was fixed with standard steel bone screws. On the contralateral femur a comparable steel veterinary bone plate was similarly fixed. In this study the intact femur was used to allow determination of osteoporosis independent of possible artifact produced by the healing of an osteotomy. Groups of two animals were sacrificed at six months, nine months, and twelve months. Femurs were excised and examined grossly before and after plate removal. The femurs were fixed and decalcified. Histologic cross-sections were made at regular 1 cm intervals in the region of the plate. Using a light microscope and point counting techniques, the percent porosity of the bone sections was determined.

After removal from the bone, all plates, both steel and composite, were tested to failure in four-point bending. Using the mechanical properties derived from these tests and applying composite beam theory to the bone/bone plate sections, the position of the bone section principal axis and neutral axis were calculated, as were shifts in the neutral axis of plated bone. This analysis allowed determination of the time dependent shift of section neutral axis with plate degradation.

RESULTS

Canine Patellar Tendon Replacement

All of the knees initially regained good function. However, with time, two of the raw carbon fiber prostheses became infected due to migration of the carbon. This unprotected, brittle carbon was found to migrate from its implantation area and in some cases formed sinus tracks through the skin (Figure 7).

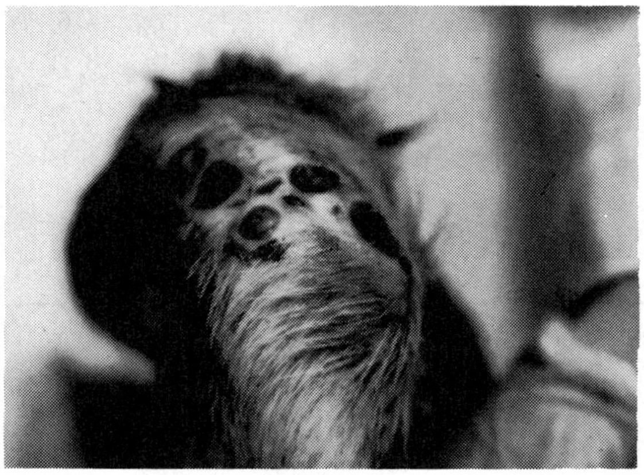

Figure 7. Dog Knee with unprotected carbon fiber fragments from the patellar tendon prosthesis eroded through skin. (4 months post-implantation).

Table 3. Test Results of Study Specimens

DOG	SACRIFICE (mo)	LEG	PROSTHESIS	STIFFNESS (N/mm)	ULTIMATE STRENGTH (N)
1	2	L	None	157	1350
		R	PLA-Carbon	Error in Mech, Test Specimen Destroyed	
2	4	L	None	272	1545
		R	PLA-Carbon	267	1420
5	2	L	None	160	1290
		R	Unprotected Carbon	150	960
6	4	L	None	154	780
		R	Unprotected Carbon	150	780
9	2	L	Nylon Suture	211	1800
		R	PLA-Carbon	167	1380
10	4	L	Nylon Suture	200	1210
		R	PLA-Carbon	208	1560
13	12	L	None	267	1825
		R	PLA-Carbon	367	1940

The dogs with nylon prosthesis ultimately developed limps and passive range of motion was restricted in flexion.

The PLA-carbon prostheses appeared to provide a more consistent return of function than did the other two types. Passive range of motion was normal. In particular, the dogs retained for twelve months both walked with no discernable limp.

The results of mechanical tests are presented in Table 3. The mechanical tests appeared to be valid in that no slippage was detected and the specimens all failed within the central tendon region, away from the grips or tibial attachment.

The PLA-carbon regrown tendons were found to have mechanical properties similar to the contralateral unoperated patella tendons. For both the four month and twelve month data, shown in Figure 8, the slopes of the force-extension curves of the regrown and the natural patella tendons are quite similar. The regrown tendons both have slightly higher ultimate strengths due presumably to some still intact carbon fibers. It appears that the soft tissue remodeling process has resulted in a regrown structure almost mechanically identical to the original patellar tendon.

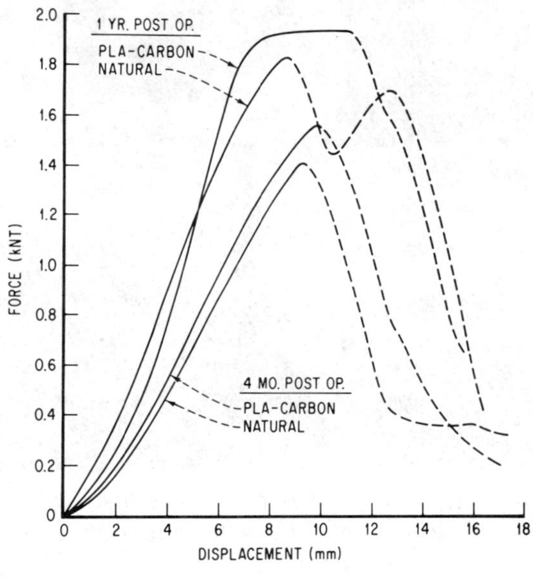

Figure 8. Load-extension response comparison for regrown and contralateral natural patellar tendons at 4 and 12 months.

Absolute values of strength and stiffness for the raw carbon fiber replacements were somewhat lower than for the composite replacements. However, on a paired basis they appeared to be similar to their contralateral normal controls.

The nylon suture prosthesis was successful in that scar tissue growth in combination with the intact suture resulted in acceptable levels of strength. However, mechanical testing suggested most of the load was being carried by the nylon suture. Failure was always preceeded by a loud "snap". The broken suture, which was not biologically attached to the tissue, would slide out of the tissue as the much weaker tissue gradually failed (Figure 9).

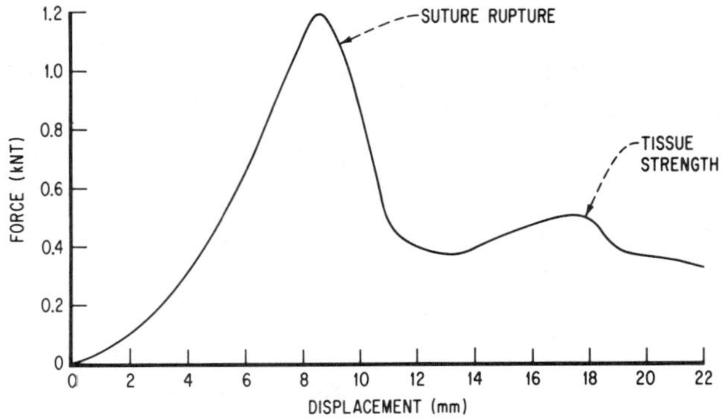

Figure 9. Load-extension reponse for nylon suture regrown patellar tendon at 4 months post-implantation.

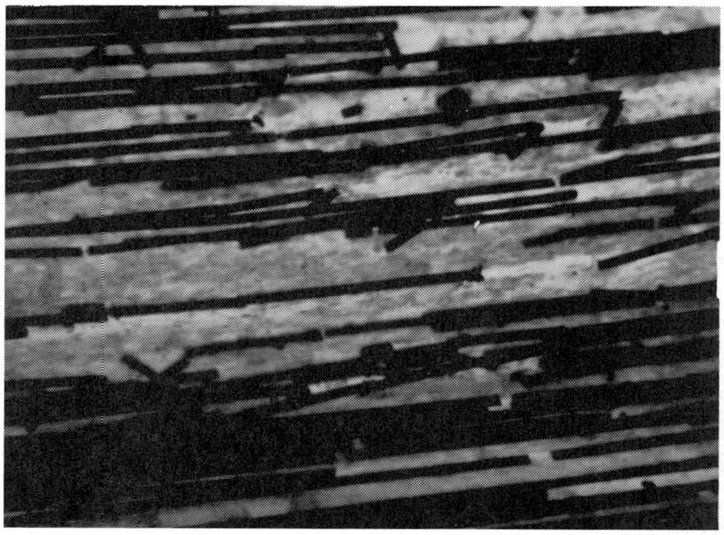

Figure 10. Longitudinal view of connective tissue growth about the PLA-carbon prosthesis after 4 months. (300×).

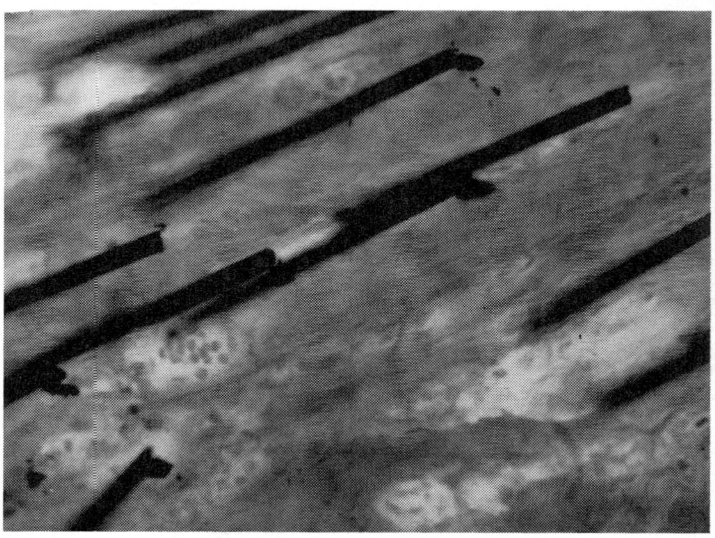

Figure 11. Longitudinal view of connective tissue growth about the PLA-carbon prosthesis after 12 months. (1000×).

Upon sacrifice, gross histological evaluation indicated that the PLA-carbon fiber tendon replacements were freely moveable with no adhesions to adjacent tissue. The carbon was well contained within the regrown tissue. The tissue appeared grossly normal. By contrast, two of the four unprotected carbon prostheses were clearly infected and showed a serious discharge. Carbon fiber had spread to the adjacent subcutaneous tissue. The multi-stranded nylon suture prosthesis elicited an intense fibrous tissue reaction with the development of bulky, space-filling granulation tissue. This tissue reaction most probably led to the unsatisfactory functional results of these replacements.

Microhistology of the carbon-PLA replacements at two months and four months revealed that developing fibrous tissue has well infiltrated the implant, aligning along the axis of the fibers (Figure 10). This infiltration of tissue has spread the fibers and greatly increased the cross-sectional area of the original carbon fiber tow. The implant was well tolerated. No inflammatory or giant cell reaction was evident. At twelve months (Figure 11), the new tissue was similar in appearance to natural aligned patellar tendon collagen with the exception of the embedded carbon fibers. The fibers appear somewhat fragmented, but completely contained. It is unclear whether the fibers had fractured in vivo or if the fractured appearance is a sectioning artifact. The microhistology of the raw carbon replacements which did not become infected was similar to that of the composite replacements. In contrast, microhistology of the nylon implants demonstrated at both two months and four months a disorganized, space-filling granulation tissue.

Scanning electron micrographs of the central tendon region of the patellar tendons regrown about the carbon-PLA scaffold demonstrated extensive ingrowth. A collagen fiber network similar to that of the corresponding region of a normal patellar tendon was found (Figure 12). The developing collagenous network appeared to grow about the carbon fibers as it would about a naturally occurring collagen fiber bundle. The normal collagen fiber bundles of the patellar tendon of the dog were similar in size to the individual carbon fibers. A cross-sectional view (Figure 13) illustrates the extent of collagenous ingrowth.

Bone attachment is a serious concern in all ligament and tendon replacement attempts. At two months, the drill holes in all the tibias were found to have enlarged. However, at four months and twelve months, no additional enlargement was found. At twelve months, microhistological evaluation of tissue within the drill hole revealed calcifying tissue growing in and around the carbon fibers in both the uncoated and polymer coatged replacements (Figure 14). This finding is simlar to that reported by Minns and Flynn [40].

By contrast, the tissue regrown in the bony cavity around the multi-stranded nylon suture material was unorganized granulation tissue. There was no bony growth about the nylon suture and a complete lack of attachment was apparent.

Rabbit Achilles Tendon

Prior to testing it was noted that no composite tendons pulled out of their anastomoses and none had ruptured. There were no infections. The rabbits actively used their limbs with full motion by the fourth post-operative day. Sham procedures resulted in a slower, less predictable return of function with considerable muscle atrophy.

The unoperated gastrocnemius mechanisms of the eighteen control limbs failed in tension by rupture through the belly of the gastrocnemius muscle. The average force to failure was 399 N (Figure 15).

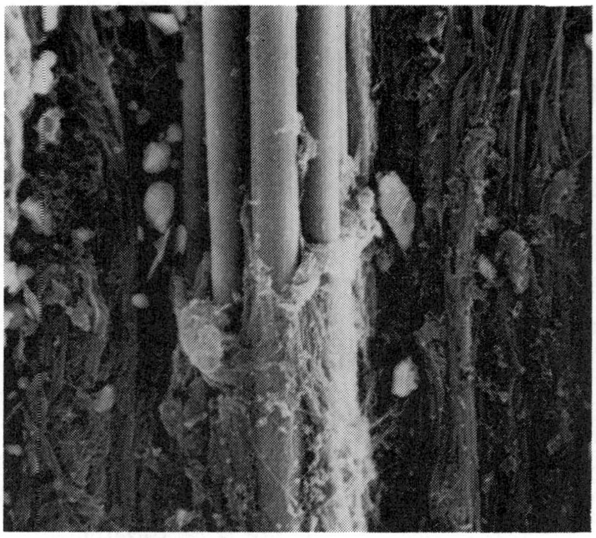

Figure 12a.

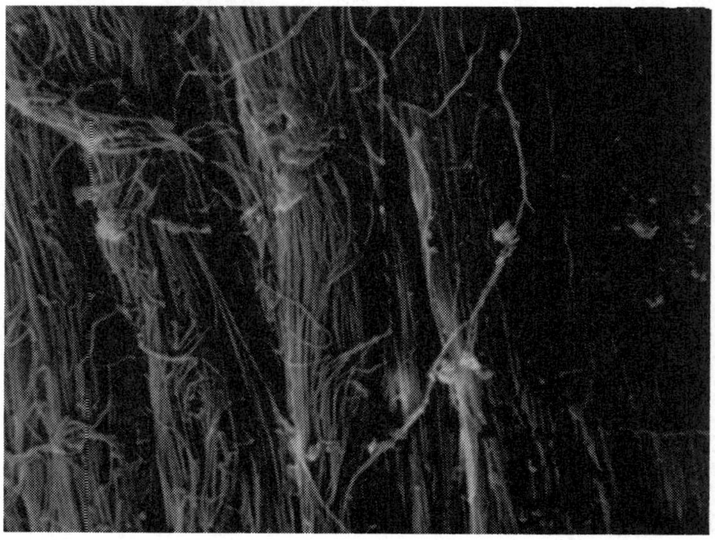

Figure 12b.

Figure 12. SEM comparison of natural and regrown tendons 12 months post-implantation. a) A regrown tendon. Tissue has been stripped away to expose carbon fibers. b) Natural.

During the early post-operative period up to two weeks, the gastrocnemius mechanisms with implants failed by pullout of the carbon-PLA composite from the proximal soft tissue anastomosis. This occurred at average values of 53 N at day 0, 118 N at one week, and 126 N at two weeks (Figure 15).

The shams failed by rupture of the paratendinous soft tissue in the region of resected tendon. This occurred at average values of 20 N at day 0, 50 N at one week, and 100 N at two weeks (Figure 15).

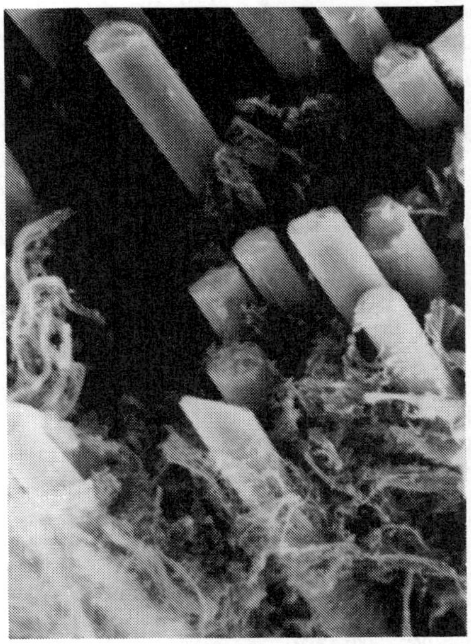

Figure 13. Cross-sectional view of regrown tendon 12 months post-implantation. Collagenous ingrowth is extensive.

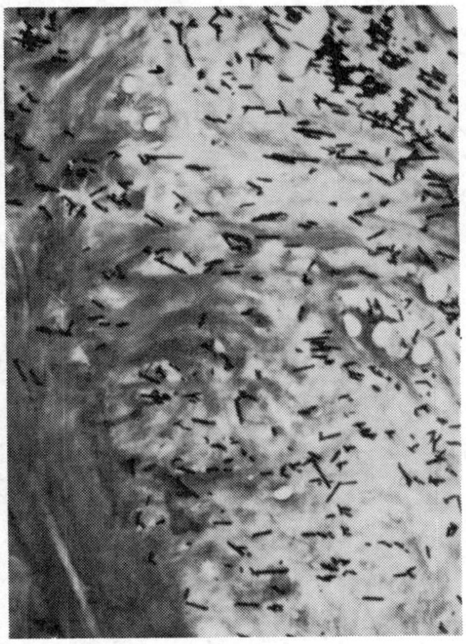

Figure 14. Cross-sectional view of calcifying tissue around PLA-carbon prosthesis in tibial drill hole at 12 months post-implantation. (200×).

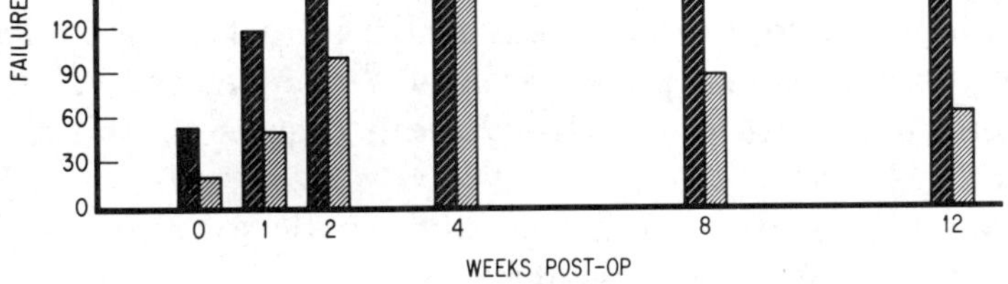

Figure 15. Mean failure strengths and mode of failure for experimental gastrocnemius systems with implants and those with sham procedures.

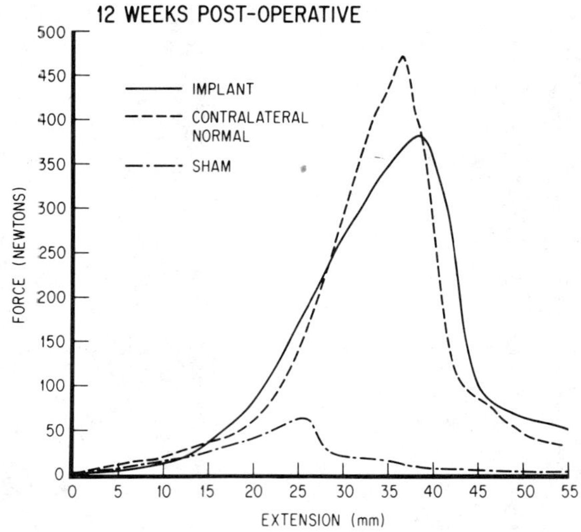

Figure 16. Force-extension curves at the twelfth post-operative week. Unoperated, normal gastrocnemius systems and those with implants show similar mechanical response. Systems having undergone sham procedures are substantially weaker.

During the later post-operative period up to twelve weeks, the gastrocnemius mechanisms with implants now failed by rupture through the belly of the gastrocnemius muscle. This occurred proximal to the level of anastomosis. Average values of force to failure were 329 N at four weeks, 230 N at eight weeks, and 310 N at twelve weeks (Figure 15). The shams continued to fail by rupture of the paratendinous soft tissue in the region of resected tendon. Mean strengths to failure were 220 N at four weeks, 88 N at eight weeks, and 63 N at twelve weeks (Figure 15). In Figure 16, the force-extension curves at twelve weeks of an implant, its contralateral unoperated control, and a sham system are compared.

Examined grossly, the carbon fiber-PLA composites were rapidly incorporated into the proximal and distal soft tissue anastomoses. At one week post-operatively in the area of resected tendon, a large volume of space-filling soft tissue had formed about the implant. In the regions of anastomosis, the implant had likewise been covered with tissue. At one week, the appearance of the sham procedure specimen was similar to that of the implant specimens.

Implant specimens at two weeks post-operatively had increased volumes of enveloping soft tissue. This tissue appeared to be slightly more organized. The sham specimen appearance was similar.

For the implant group and the sham group, surrounding soft tissue appeared to reach a maximum volume at four weeks post-operatively.

Eight weeks post-operatively, remodeling of the soft tissues about the implant had begun to occur. The volume of soft tissue in the area of resected tendon had been reduced. This was true of both the implant specimens and the sham specimens. The tissue about the implant was firm and organized; whereas, the tissue of the sham specimen was thin and attenuated. In both cases, some muscle atrophy was evident but this was not quantitated.

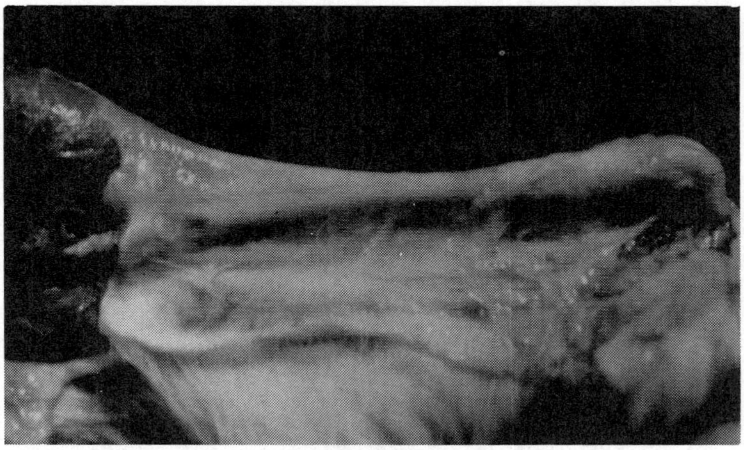

Figure 17a.

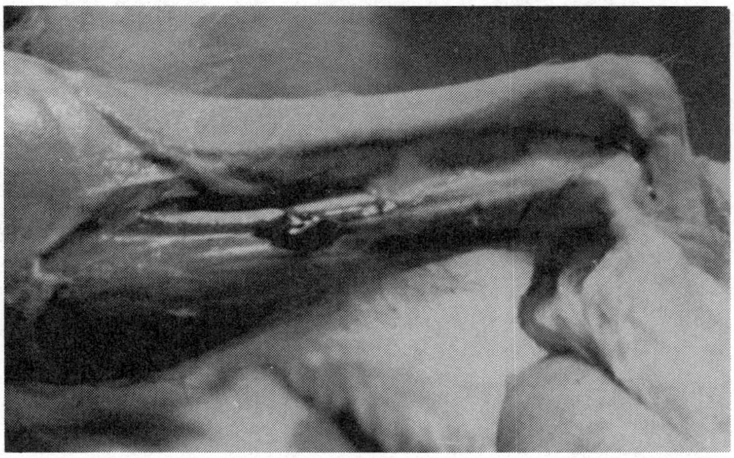

Figure 17b.

Figure 17. Gastrocnemius systems in situ. a) A normal rabbit gastrocnemius system. b) A rabbit gastrocnemius system twelve weeks following implantation of the carbon-PLA composite.

Soft tissue remodeling progressed rapidly. At twelve weeks post-operatively, the gastrocnemius systems with implants closely resembled their unoperated contralateral controls (Figure 17). The tissue in the region of anastomosis appeared normal. Sham specimens had only a filmy, attenuated tissue in the region of resected tendon.

At one week post-operatively, microscopic studies revealed a disorganized space-filling tissue forming about the area of the implant. Implant specimens demonstrated little ingrowth into the composite material at this time (Figure 18a).

At two weeks, the surrounding tissue appeared more organized. Some tissue ingrowth was noted about the periphery of the carbon fiber-PLA implants. Minimal foreign body response was apparent at this time.

At four weeks, infiltration of tissue in the implants was significant in the anastomosis region as well as in the area of resected tendon. This tissue ingrowth caused separation of the carbon

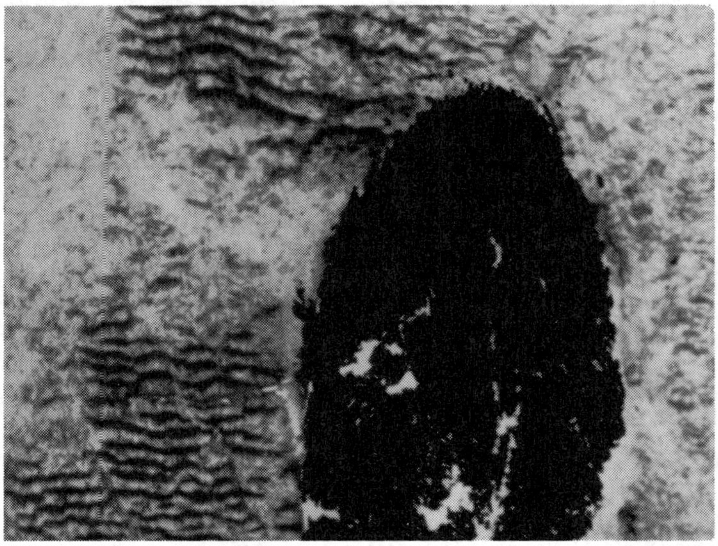

Figure 18a.

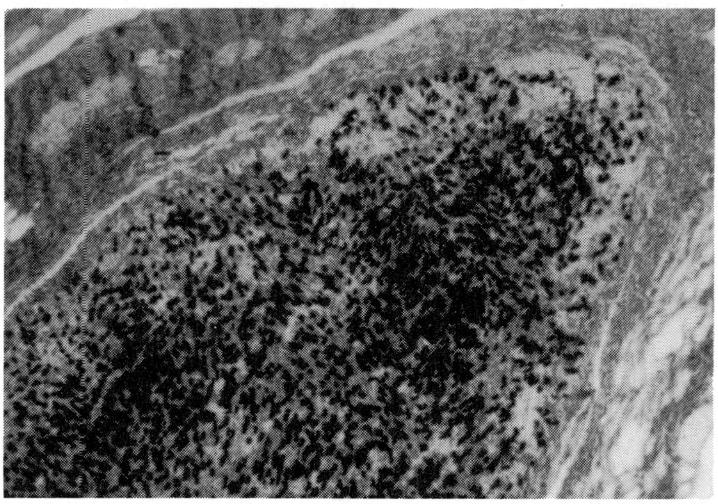

Figure 18b.

Figure 18. Microhistology of the carbon-PLA Achilles tendon implants. a) Cross-section of the implant at the level of the myotendinous anastomosis at one week. There is little tissue ingrowth. The carbon remains in intimate contact with the surrounding soft tissue. There is minimal inflammatory response (200×). b) Cross-section of the implant at the level of the myotendinous anastomosis at 12 weeks. There is significant tissue ingrowth spreading the individual carbon fibers of the implant. The ingrown tissue is highly cellular. There is minimal foreign body or inflammatory response present. This tissue ingrowth provides a secure physiological bond between the carbon-fiber scaffold and surrounding soft tissue.

fibers and hence a volumetric expansion of the composite implant. Around most of the carbon filaments, there were bundles of connective tissue fibers oriented parallel to the carbon filaments and interspaced with fibroblasts. The majority of cells within the confines of the implants were predominantly in parallel alignment.

Tissue remodeling after eight weeks was extensive. The implants were fully infiltrated with oriented collagenous tissue. The volume of soft tissue in the region of resected tendon was reduced. Fibroblasts about the implants appeared mature and well aligned.

Tissue remodeling after twelve weeks of implantation was even more pronounced. The volume of collagenous tissue making up the regrown tendon section appeared normal. The tissue was highly organized with fibroblasts and collagen oriented longitudinally. The carbon fiber composite was completely infiltrated (Figure 18b).

Canine Medial Collateral Ligament

All knees with implants healed uneventfully with no infections. All joints appeared to have a full range of motion and no lameness was detected. Gross inspection of the implants after four weeks in vivo revealed an implant infiltrated with, and covered by, collagenous tissue. There was no obvious spread of carbon fiber beyond the initial site of implantation. The implants examined after eight weeks, twelve weeks, and twenty-six weeks were similar in appearance. There were, however, increasing amounts of collagenous tissue about the implants with increasing time in vivo. No adverse reactions were noted.

Similarly, animals having had sham procedures healed uneventfully. Gross inspection of the site of ligament and capsule resection revealed healing with a space-filling scar tissue.

After twenty-six weeks in vivo, infiltration of tissue into the implant was significant. This tissue ingrowth caused separation of the carbon fibers and, hence, a volumetric expansion of the composite. Histologic appearance was similar to that of the rabbit Achilles tendon at twelve weeks. Viewing under polarized light revealed no trace of residual polymer. The tissue reaction to the implant was remarkably benign in terms of foreign body inflammatory response.

For each time period the sham and implant groups contained four animals. It is difficult to determine with asurity the statistical significance of alterations in mechanical behavior based on samples this small. For this reason, the mechanical data are presented strictly as mean values. The contralateral control joints of these animals, on the other hand, represent a large group (N=32). Thus, for comparison, mean values and 95% confidence intervals are presented for this group.

The stability of all joints was evaluated quantitatively in a low force cantilever bending test that simulates a clinical valgus stress test. The measure of stability was the laxity, or "opening", of the joint in millimeters at a calculated ligament force of 25 N. The results of this nondestructive mechanical test are shown in Figure 19. At all time periods, the knees with implants were more stable than were the sham knees*. In fact, the mean laxity of the joints with implants fell very near or within the 95% confidence interval of the mean for all contralateral normal joints.

---

*The behavior of the implant group in terms of joint stability was so different from that of the sham ($p<0.01$, Student's t-test) that assignment of statistical significance seems justified despite the small number (N=4) of experimental animals per group.

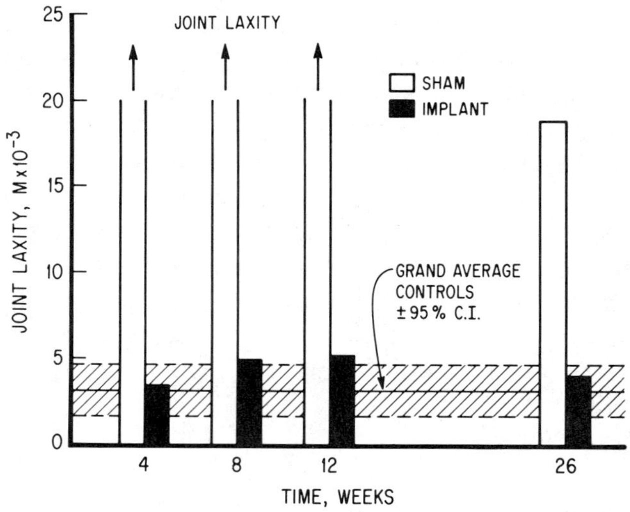

Figure 19. Medial Collateral Joint Laxity – These measurements were made using a low force, non-destructive cantilever bending test which simulates a clinical valgus stress test. Laxity was defined as the opening of the joint in millimeters at a calculated ligament force of 25 N.

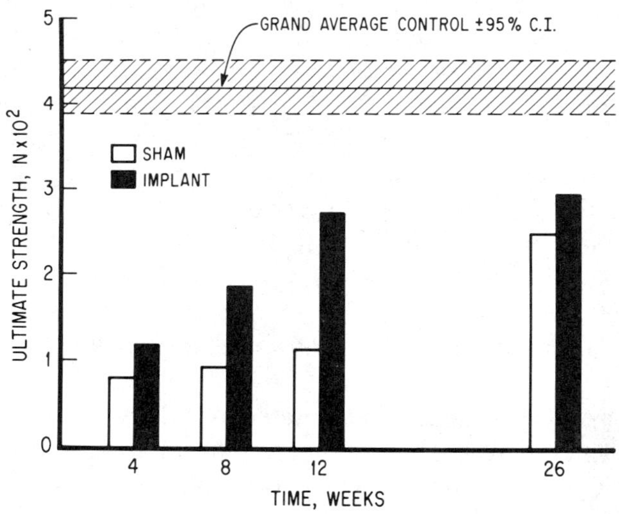

Figure 20. Medical Collateral Ultimate Strength – Ultimate strength of the regrown structures was determined in a uniaxial tensile test. All ligament and capsular structures were cut except a 1 cm band in the medial collateral position.

Following the non-destructive cantilever bending tests, the joints were positioned so a uniaxial tension test could be performed. All ligamentous and capsular structures were cut, except for a 1 cm band regrown in the medial collateral position. In this configuration the

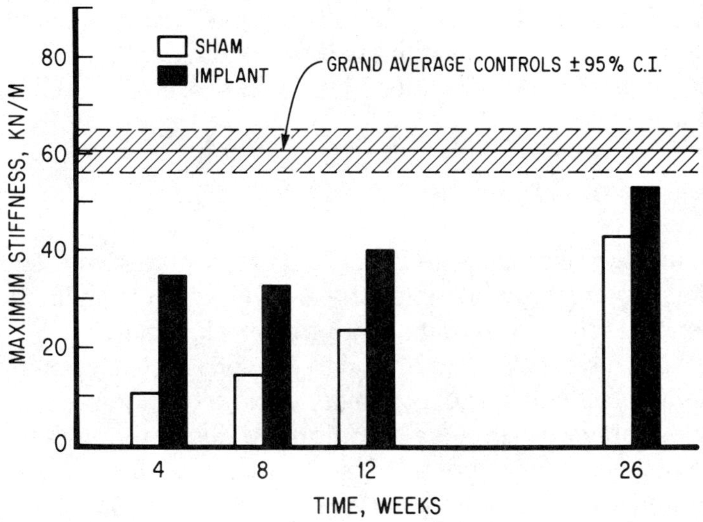

Figure 21. Medial Collateral Maximum Stiffness – The maximum stiffness of the regrown structures is the maximum slope of the force-elongation curve generated in the uniaxial tensile test.

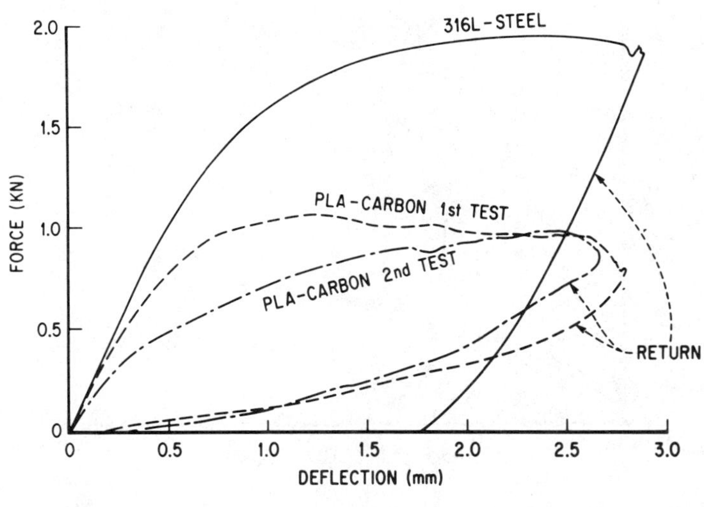

Figure 22. Force-deflection curves for a 4-hole composite plate and a comparable steel plate.

regrown structures were tested to failure and the ultimate strengths and slope of the load-elongation curves recorded. Figure 20 compares the ultimate strengths of medial collateral ligaments regrown about the composite implants and scar regrown in the sham procedure. At all times, the mean ultimate strengths of implant groups were higher than those of the sham group. The mean strengths of the implant groups rose monotomically over the entire period of implantation. A strength three-quarters that of normal was present at twenty-six weeks. This strength is well beyond the "working" range of the normal canine MCL. The tissue regrown following the sham procedure remained weaker, never achieving strengths equivalent to the implants.

Stiffness of the implant system also increased with time (Figure 21). After twenty-six weeks in vivo the implant group had a mean stiffness 90% that of normal. The sham groups for all time periods displayed mean stiffness values less than those of the corresponding implant groups.

Design and Fabrication of Composite Bone Plates

Theoretical calculations had suggested that laminated plates with sufficiently high axial modulus and bending rigidity were possible. The actual mechanical parameters, as determined by four-point bending, agreed favorably with these calculations.

The composite plates have yield strengths up to 70% of a corresponding steel plate, depending on the plate parameters chosen i.e. ply angle, volume fraction of carbon, etc. (Figure 22).

Although the steel plates were irreversibly deformed during the tests to failure, the carbon plates proved more resilient. This is indicated by the return curves (Figure 22). Torsional tests with the plates mounted on osteotomized cadaver dog bone simulate the most severe in vivo case. Results (Figure 23) show that in vivo the weakest link in the bone plate/screw system is the screw fixation to bone. In all tests of this type, the bone fractured through the screw holes. It would thus appear that the composite plate is sufficiently strong in torsion.

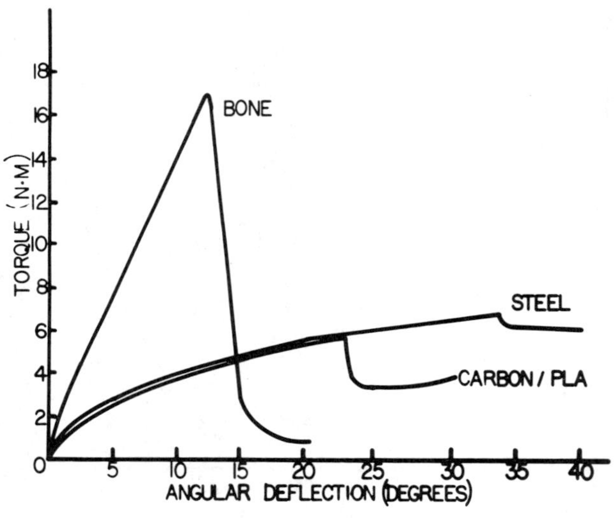

Figure 23. Torsional tests of a 4-hole composite plate and a comparable steel plate mounted to an osteotomized cadver dog bone. A torque-angular deflection curve for an intact unplated femur is shown for comparison.

The fatigue properties of the plates were tested in four-point bending in air, water, and saline (Figure 24). Both angle-ply and random oriented laminated plates performed well in air, surviving over a million cycles at a mean stress of 50% of yield ± 20% yield stress. In water and saline, however, angle-ply laminates, as produced in our laboratory, demonstrated poor fatigue characteristics. Fortunately, the random oriented laminate plates continued to display excellent fatigue properties in these aqueous environments. The random oriented plates were subsequently chosen for use in the animal experiments.

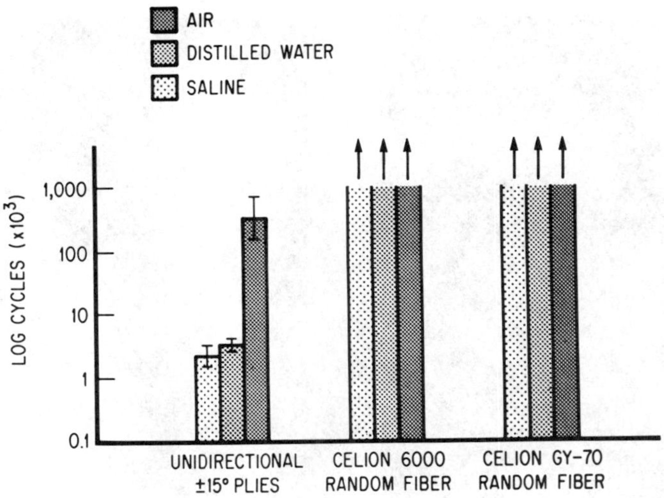

Figure 24. The fatigue properties of composite bone plates of the random and angle-ply varieties in air, water, and saline environments. Four-point bending was utilized with a mean stress 50% of yield ± 20% yield, mean to peak oscillating stress. Designations cellion 6000 and GY-70 (Trademark, Cellanese Corporation, Inc.) refer to high elongation fibers and high modulus fibers, respectively, used in the construction of the plates.

Canine Osteotomy Healing Study

Of the three plated radii, three healed successfully and none failed. Of the three plated tibias, two healed successfully and one failed. This plate, on the tibia of a 40 kg dog, failed soon after plating. The dog was larger than the others in the series and overloaded the plate. None of the dogs were provided with any cast or splint protection.

X-ray evaluation of these osteotomized bones resulted in courses typical of that shown in Figure 25. After nine weeks, the healed fracture is almost identical to the result expected under a steel bone plate. Upon gross examination, the plates were found to be intact at the time of sacrifice. They were firmly encapsulated in soft periosteal tissue and bone (Figure 26). Upon microhistological examination, new bone was seen forming through and across the saw cut, providing the primary osseous union noted in steel bone plating of fractures.

If the composite plate could be removed without being severely damaged, it was then mechanically tested in four-point bending. Before implantation, these plates were found to have a bending rigidity of 10.9 N-m^2 and a maximum bending moment of 10.7 N-m. After eight weeks of implantation, the plates degraded to 28% of their original rigidity and were found to sustain 58% of their original maximum bending moment capability.

Canine Osteoporosis Study

Animals were sacrificed after six months, nine months, and twelve months. All composite plates were carefully removed and tested mechanically in four-point bending. Histology sections were prepared for point counting to determine porosity.

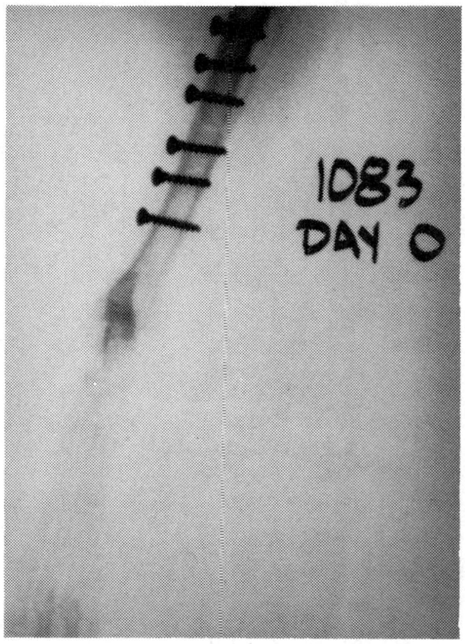

(a)

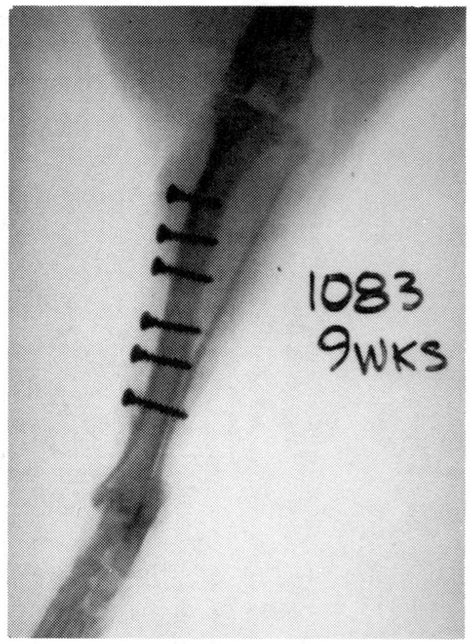

(b)

Figure 25. X-ray evaluation of osteotomized canine tibia with composite plate. a) Post-operative appearance. b) Nine weeks post-operatively, the transverse osteotomy has healed. Note the composite plates are radiolucent aiding greatly in visualizing the bone in the healing region.

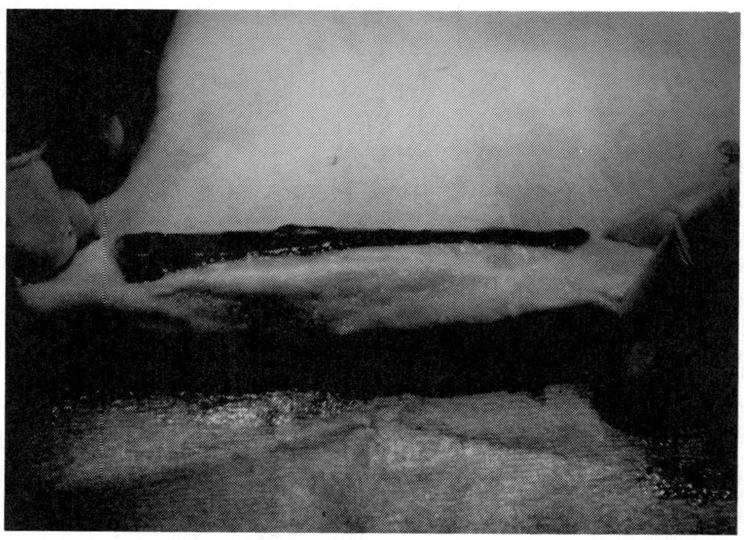

Figure 26. Gross specimen nine weeks post-operatively. The fracture is healed and the tissue reaction to the composite material is excellent.

At six months, there was no significant difference in the amount of cortical porosity in the region of the steel bone plate vs. the contralateral composite plate. Similarly, there was no statistically significant difference in the cortical cross-sectional area. However, after nine

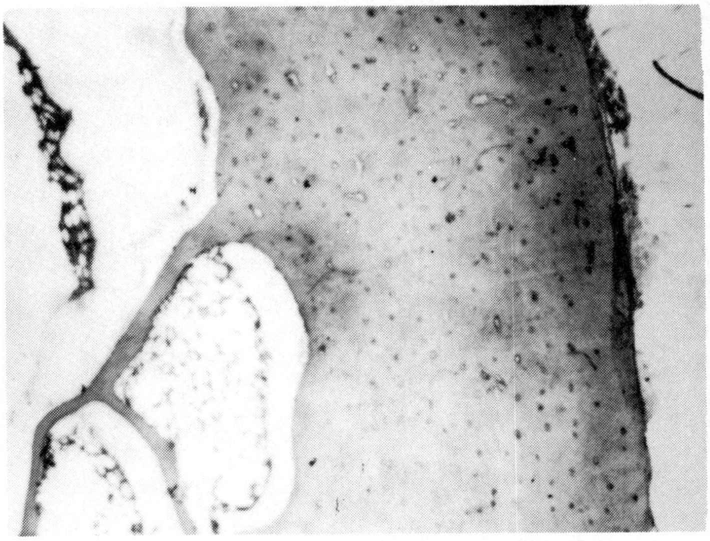

Figure 27a.

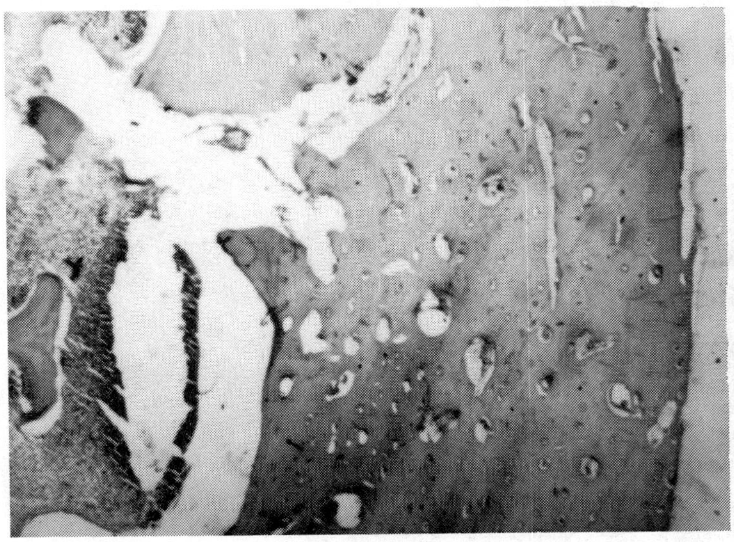

Figure 27b.

Figure 27. Cross-sections of canine femurs plated with carbon fiber composite plates and steel plates after 9 months implantation. Increased osteoporosis is demonstrated with the steel plate. a) Composite plate. b) Steel plate.

months of implantation, the cortex in the region of the steel plate displayed a 56% increase in porosity when compared to the contralateral carbon fiber composite (Figure 27). Further, the cortical cross-sectional area had been reduced by 15%. Although still under evaluation, at one year it appears that the increase in porosity and reduction in cross-sectional area with rigid steel plates is even more severe.

Utilizing typical cross-sections previously prepared for point counting, an analysis of the structural properties of the sections was undertaken. Based on a loading distribution of the

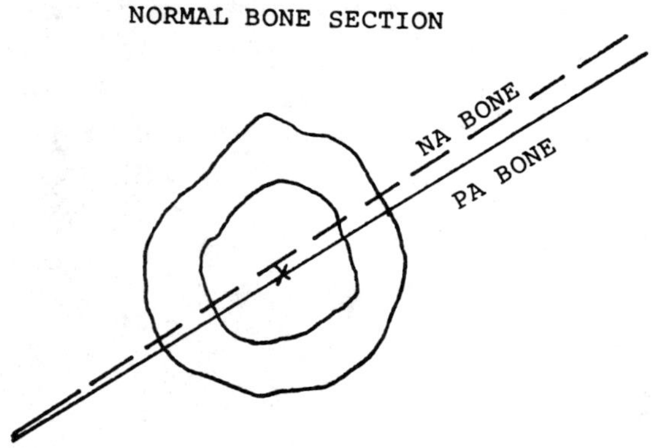

Figure 28a.

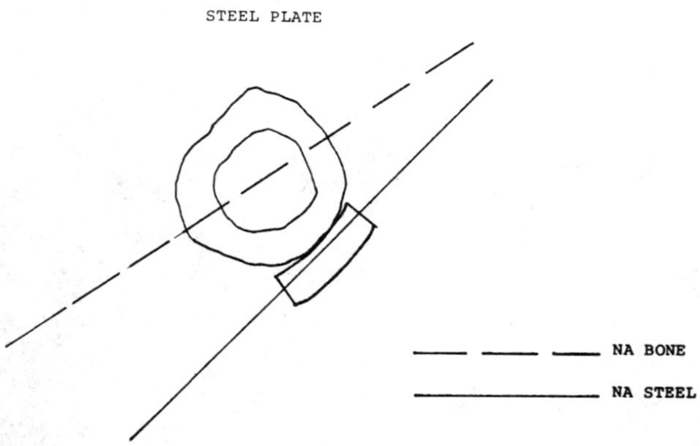

Figure 28b.

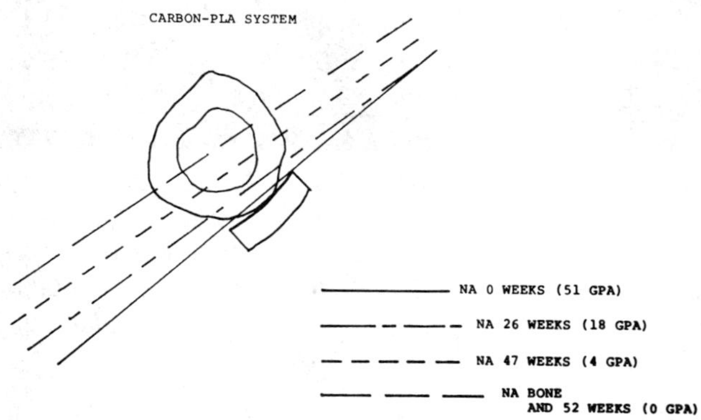

Figure 28c.

Figure 28. The sectional properties of plated bones. a) The neutral axis and principal axis of a normal bone section are nearly coincident. b) Application of a steel bone plate results in a major shift of the neutral axis. The stress distribution within the section is severely altered. c) Application of a composite plate also shifts the neutral axis. However, with time the plate loses rigidity and the neutral axis returns to a normal position. A more natural stress distribution is restored, promoting a beneficial remodeling (strengthening).

canine femur [41], the principal and neutral axis of the bone section alone were determined (Figure 28a). Using composite beam theory, the shift in the neutral axis was predicted for addition of the steel bone plate (Figure 28b). As the properties of the steel plate are static (barring breakage), this shift in neutral axis is effectively permanent. In a similar fashion, the shift in the neutral axis was predicted for application of the composite plate. However, as the composite plate gradually loses rigidity with time, the neutral axis returns to its original position restoring the natural distribution of stress (Figure 28c).

DISCUSSION

Canine Patellar Tendon

Replacement of the canine patellar tendon proved to be a complex experimental system with many variables. However, the success of the carbon fiber-PLA composite in such an elementary design serves to demonstrate the usefulness of this new material.

The carbon fiber PLA scaffold replacements monotonically increased in stiffness and ultimate strength over the twelve month post-operative period. Stiffness increased from 1.57 $\times$ 10N/M^2 at two months to 3.67 $\times$ 10 N/M^2 at one year. Ultimate strength increased from 1.38 KN at two months to 1.94 KN at one year. We believe this increase in strength and stiffness with time is indicative of the regrowth and organization of collagenous tissue on the scaffold replacement. A permanent prosthetic replacement will only become weaker with time. The scaffold approach to replacement permits strengthening with time to some optimal level and maintenance thereafter. On a paired or absolute basis, the mechanical properties of these regrown patellar tendons appear to be indistinguishable from normal.

The ultimate strengths of these replacements are lower than the projected immediate post-operative strength. We must assume some fiber fracture has occurred. It is this gradual mechanical failure of the carbon fiber which transfers load to the developing tissue. We believe this gradual transference of load is critical in the proper development of a well-organized, remodeled structure. The rate of mechanical degradation and transference of load is not known in either the unprotected or polymer-protected replacements. As there were no catastrophic failures of the implants, it seems that the degradation rate is sufficiently slow as to allow adequate regrowth.

Scanning electron micrographs of regrown and natural patellar tendons indicate that the carbon fibers are approximately the same diameter as the naturally occurring collagen fiber bundles. The developing collagen fibers seem to grow around the carbon fibers as they would about a naturally occurring fiber bundle. The result is a structure mechanically and histologically very similar to the natural structure.

Certainly, protection of the carbon fiber with a resorbable polymer is desirable to improve handling characteristics and to prevent the spread of carbon fiber into adjacent tissue. This PLA carbon fiber structure provides mechanal strength upon implantation, allows ingrowth of new tissue, and is thought to mechanically degrade as the new tissue matures. It has been demonstrated, even in this "elemental design" form, to be an acceptable patellar tendon replacement in dogs. The dogs retained for twelve months regained and maintained normal function as a result of this surgery.

Rabbit Achilles Tendon

In the initial two week post-operative period, the mode of failure in tension of the systems with implants was pull-out of the composite from its proximal soft tissue anastomosis. Since no implant separated from its anastomosis prior to testing, it would appear that the "locking-weave" technique of anastomosis provided adequate initial strength (average 53 N) to maintain the anastomosis while tissue ingrowth progressed. At two weeks, the peak force to failure had increased to 216 N. This value represented 66% of the average ultimate strength of the unoperated limbs (339 N).

This progressive increase in strength would seem to correspond with early tissue ingrowth as determined histologically. In addition, there is the formation of a loose, disorganized scar in the region of resected tendon which contributes significantly to these early strengths.

During this same period, the sham procedures failed by separation through the area of resected tendon. This sham procedure produced a regrown structure significantly weaker than systems with implanted composites. As with the implant group, a loose, disorganized scar formed about the area of resected tendon. This volume of scar accounts for the early strength of the shams.

During the four to twelve week post-operative period, an important change occurred in mode of failure. The implants no longer failed by pull-out of the composite from the soft tissue anastomosis. Failure now occurred by rupture through the belly of the gastrocnemius system. This rupture occurred proximal to the anastomosis site. This mode of failure was identical to the failure mode of the unoperated limbs. That is, the ultimate strength of the gastrocnemius muscle is the limiting factor in the gastrocnemius system. The anastomosis between implant and soft tissue was no longer the region of failure. Tensile tests at four and twelve weeks indicate that the strength of the systems with implants were equivalent to the strengths of the unoperated systems. At eight weeks some degree of gastrocnemius atrophy resulted in a decrease of ultimate strength. However, at twelve weeks, this atrophy had resolved and gastrocnemius strength was again normal.

The volume of scar about the implant was reduced greatly during this post-operative period. In fact, the gross appearance of the implant tendons was very nearly normal at twelve weeks. The tissue remaining in region of resected tendon was well organized and vascular. Ingrowth at the tendinous, myotendinous, and central region of the implant was significant. The extent of ingrowth and organization of regrown tissue would seem to account for the normal strengths of the implant systems during this later post-operative period.

During this four week to twelve week post-op period, the sham procedure continued to fail through the area of resected tendon. No tensile strength value of a sham fell within the 95% confidence interval of the normal group. Scar tissue surrounding the sham resulted in a maximum strength at four weeks. During the eight week to twelve week period, this scar resorbed resulting in a weak attenuated and disorganized tissue corresponding to the area of resected tendon.

Comparison of force-extension curves for implant and unoperated systems at twelve weeks showed a mechanically similar response. This mechanical behavior of the implant systems suggests that due to biological fixation and tissue remodeling along the composite scaffold, a structure similar mechanically to the contralateral normal has been regenerated.

The canine patellar tendon replacement proved successful in a highly loaded situation. However, this replacement was a continuous loop of composite material initially anchored in bone. Therefore, this experiment yielded little information regarding the rapidity and security of soft tissue attachment to the composite. A secure soft tissue attachment may be required for many ligament and tendon repairs. The successful replacement of a major portion of the rabbit Achilles tendon utilizing only soft tissue attachment demonstrates this is possible.

Canine Medial Collateral Ligament

Based on the success of earlier soft tissue repairs in animals, human clinical trials of carbon fiber-PLA composites seemed feasible. A human replacement procedure would likely involve the extra-articular ligaments of the knee. Damage to any of the ligaments of the knee is a serious clinical problem. Instability in this joint is debilitating and often leads to chronic progressive osteoarthritis if left unchecked.

Before a replacement procedure could be considered in the human, it was necessary to demonstrate the usefulness of a similar procedure in an animal model. In this study, the medial collateral ligaments and medial capsular structures of canines were resected and replaced with a carbon fiber-polylactic acid polymer tissue scaffold or allowed simply to "scar in". After four weeks, eight weeks, twelve weeks, and twenty-six weeks in vivo, the stability of the knees was quantitatively evaluated and the mechanical properties of the regrown structures determined. Histologic sections of the regrown structures were examined after twenty-six weeks in vivo.

At all time periods, operative knees receiving implants were quantitatively judged to be considerably more stable than sham knees. Further, the structures regrown about the carbon fiber-PLA scaffolds were consistently stronger and stiffer than tissue resulting from the sham procedure. We believe this increase in strength and stiffness with time is indicative of the regrowth and organization of collagenous tissue on and within the scaffold replacement. This concept is supported by the microhistologic appearance of the implant after twenty-six weeks in vivo. The soft tissue attachment technique utilized appears to form a strong, rapid bond as ingrowth proceeds. No adverse tissue reactions were noted and the function of the joints receiving implants was excellent.

In short, the test results presented suggest that carbon fiber-PLA composite ligament replacements may aid significantly in the stabilization of an accutely damaged joint. The improved mechanical performance of implant groups over sham groups suggests repair with a carbon fiber tissue scaffold is superior to simply allowing the ligament deficit to "scar in".

Design and Fabrication of Composite Bone Plates

Angle-ply and random oriented laminate composite bone plates were successfully fabricated. Depending on the design parameters chosen the plates displayed bending rigidities and strengths up to 70% of a corresponding steel plate. These static properties compared favorably with those of titanium alloy and nonabsorbable fiber composite plates.

In torsion, these plates were sufficiently strong as to cause failure of the screw fixation to bone rather than the plate itself.

Unfortunately, the stronger angle-ply composites, as produced in our laboratory, had unacceptable fatigue life in aqueous environments. Manufacturing techniques were, however, crude. Random oriented laminates were shown to have satisfactory fatigue properties and were subsequently used in animal studies.

Canine Osteotomy Healing Study

In this study, composite plates were used to fix transversely osteotomized canine long bones. Six large German Shepherd dogs were used. In three, a radius was osteotomized and in the others a tibia was osteotomized. This represents a severe in-vivo test. A transverse osteotomy is inherently unstable, particularly in torsion. In practice most long bone fractures, except perhaps severely communited ones, have some stability by virtue of the interdigitation of the irregular bone ends.

Despite the severity of the test mode, all radii healed uneventfully. Two tibias healed successfully and one failed soon after plating due to an obvious overload. In retrospect, this failure could have been anticipated. None of the animals were provided with any cast or splint protection. The plate which failed was on the tibia of an active 40 Kg dog. This animal was larger than the other in the series and simply overloaded the device. In medical practice, a larger plate would have been chosen. At the time of this experiment only one plate size was available.

All other plates were intact at sacrifice and the tissue response was excellent. Microscopic evaluation revealed a primary osseous union similar to healing patterns observed with steel plates.

After nine weeks in vivo, the mechanical properties of the plates, most notably the bending rigidity, was reduced. This gradual transference of load to the bone is thought to eliminate stress protection atrophy and promote an earlier return of strength to the bony structure. Further, it is thought that due to the excellent compatibility of this composite material, coupled with its degradation, that there will be no need to remove the device. That is, no secondary operative procedure will be necessary.

Canine Osteoporosis Study

This study utilized six adult beagle dogs. On each dog one intact femur was plated with a standard veterinary steel bone plate. The contralateral femur was plated with a comparable composite plate. Two animals were sacrificed at six months, two animals at nine months, and two animals at one year. Analysis of all of the bone sections revealed a considerable increase in porosity and decrease in cortical area in the steel plated bones when compared to their contralateral carbon fiber composite plated bones. This detrimental remodeling did not become evident until after six months of implantation. The carbon fiber composite plates steadily decreased in rigidity over the test period, having essentially no rigidity at one year.

An analytical study was performed to demonstrate the shift in neutral bending axis associated with plate fixation. Using loading data previously developed by Vasu et al [41], it was determined that the unplated bone neutral axis is quite close to the principal axis of the bone cross-section. This, of course, suggests that nature has provided an efficient structure through evolution and/or remodeling.

Applying a steel plate shifts the neutral axis considerably "off design". In fact, the neutral axis is actually shifted off the bone, significantly altering the stress distribution in the cortex.

Applying a carbon fiber-PLA plate initially causes a similar shift. However, by the time detrimental remodeling can occur, the plate rigidity has decreased enough to shift the neutral axis, and thus the state of stress to a nearly normal position. This would seem to effectively prevent stress protection atrophy.

Human Clinical Trials

Given the success of carbon fiber-PLA composites in animals, particularly with respect to soft tissue repair and replacement, application was made to the Food and Drug Administration (FDA) for limited clinical trials. This initial application has been approved and human clinical trials are now underway. These trials consist of extra-articular repair of soft tissue deficits. To date over 30 patients have received carbon fiber-PLA composite materials for repair of such structures as:

1. collateral ligaments
2. quadriceps-extensor mechanism
3. patellar tendon
4. Achilles tendon
5. shoulder rotator cuff

At this time the oldest case in nine months postoperative. We can report that there have, to date, been no early complications or failures and all patients appear to be doing well. However, no meaningful evaluation of these procedures can be made at this time.

CONCLUSION

Numerous animal experiments have demonstrated the usefulness of carbon fiber-PLA composites for soft tissues repair and replacement. For this purpose the carbon fibers act as a scaffold for tissue ingrowth while the absorbable PLA polymer protects the fibers upon implantation. The composite provides mechanical strength until the new tissue grows and matures. As the new tissue develops, the PLA absorbs and the carbon fibers degrade mechanically. This allows the proper orientation of the developing fibrous tissue as the load is gradually transferred. The controlled degradation of this material allows it to be mechnically and materially replaced by natural tissue. It encourages normal tissue regeneration; however, it does not permanently replace tissue. The system does not, therefore, depend on the long-term integrity of the implant for its strength. The components of this implant are biocompatible materials having been used before in sutures, implants, or implant components. Their use together as an absorbable tissue scaffold is new. The success of this material when used as a soft tissue scaffold has led to approval by the Food and Drug Administration for limited human clinical trials. These trials are now in progress and initial results are promising.

By varying the carbon fiber properties and orientation and by changing the volume fraction of carbon fiber to PLA, rigid structures (bone plates) for the internal fixation of long-bone fractures have been constructed. Such devices have distinct advantages over their commonly used metallic counterparts. First, these bone plates gradually lose strength and rigidity, transferring load to the healing fracture. This effectively prevents stress protection atrophy. As the rigidity of the plates decreases, the stress distribution within the bone section approaches normal, promoting a more active remodeling and return of strength.

Secondly, the materials from which the plates are constructed are extremely compatible. Since no detrimental long-term effects (mechanical or physiological) are anticipated, the plates need not be surgically removed as metallic plates must be. With further animal tests and pending FDA approval, human clinical trials seem feasible.

REFERENCES

1. Benson, J.: Elemental Carbon as a Biomaterial. J. Biomed. Mater. Res., 5:41-47, 1971.
2. von Fraunhofer, J.A., L'Estrange, P.R. and Mask, A.O.: Materials Science in Dental Implantation and a Promising New Material – Vitreous Carbon. Biomed. Eng., 6:114-118, 1971.
3. Mooney, V., Hartman, D.B., McNeal, D. and Benson, J.: The Use of Pure Carbon for Percutaneous Electrical Connector Systems. Arch. Surg., 108:148-153, 1974.
4. Jenkins, D.H.R.: The Repair of Cruciate Ligaments with Flexible Carbon Fibre. J. Bone Jt. Surg., 60B:520-522, 1978.
5. Jenkins, D.H.R., Forester, I.W., McKibbins, B. and Ralis, Z.A.: Induction of Tendon and Ligament Formation by Carbon Implants. J. Bone Jt. Surg., 59B:53-57, 1977.
6. Wolter, D., Fitzer, E., Helbing, G. and Goldaway, J.: Ligament Replacement in the Knee Joint with Carbon Fibers Coated with Pyrolactic Carbon. Trans. Soc. for Biomat., Vol. 1:126, 1977.
7. Neugebauer, R., Burri, C., Claes, L., Helbing, G. and Wolter, D.: The Replacement of the Abdominal Wall by a Carbon-Cloth in Rabbits. Trans. Soc. for Biomat., Vol. 3:135, 1979.
8. Neugebauer, R., Burri, C., Claes, L., Helbing, G. and Wolter, D.: The Anchorage of Carbon Fibre Strands into Bone; A Biomechanical and Biological Evaluation on Knee Joints. Trans. European Soc. of Biomat., Vol. 2, 1979.
9. Neugebauer, R., Burri, C., Claes, L. and Helbing, G.: The Trap Door; A Possibility of Fixation of Carbon Fibre Strands into Cancellous Bone. Trans. World Biomat. Congress, Vol. 1:4, 7, 5, 1980.
10. Claes, L., Wolter, D., Gistinger, G., Rose, P., Huttner, W. and Fitzer, E.: Physical and Biological Aspects of Carbon Fibres in the Ligament Prosthesis. 3rd Conf. on Mech. Prop. of Biomat., Keele Univ., 1978.
11. Forster, I.W., Ralis, Z.A., McKibbin, B. and Jenkins, D.H.R.: Biological Reaction to Carbon Fibre Implants. Clin. Orthop. Rel. Res., 131:299-307, 1978.
12. Jenkins, D.H.R. and McKibbin, B.: The Role of Flexible Carbon-Fibre Implants as Tendon and Ligament Substitutes in Clinical Practice – A Preliminary Report. J. Bone Jt. Surg., 62B:497-499, 1980.
13. Kinzl, L., Wolter, D. and Claes, L.: Aspects of Coated Carbon Fibres in the Ligament Prostheses. Trans. Soc. for Biomat., Vol. 3:71, 1979.
14. Akeson, W.H., Woo, S.L.Y., Rutherford, L., Coutts, R.D., Gonsalves, M., and Amiel, D.: The Effects of Rigidity of Internal Fixation Plates on Long Bone Remodeling. Acta Orthop. Scand., 47:241-249, 1979.
15. Muller, M.D., Allgower, M. and Willenegger, H.: Manual of Internal Fixation. Berlin, Springer-Verlag, 1970.
16. Slatis, P., Karaharju, E., Holmstrom, T., Ahonen, J., Paavolainen, P.: Structural Changes in Intact Tubular Bone after Application of Rigid Plates With and Without Compression. J. Bone Jt. Surg., 60A:516-522, 1972.
17. Tonino, A.J., Davidson, C.L., Klopper, P.J., Linclav, L.A.: Protection From Stress in Bone and Its Effects. J. Bone Jt. Surg., 58B:No. 1, 1976.
18. Uhtoff, H.K. and Bardos, D.: The Use of Titanium-6 A1-4V Plates in the Treatment of Fractures. Trans. Orthop. Res. Soc., Vol. 2:29, 1978.
19. Akeson, W.H., Woo, S.L-Y., Coutts, R.D., Matthews, J.V., Gonsalves, M. and Amiel, D.: Quantitative Histological Evaluation of Early Fracture Healing of Cortical Bones Immobilized by Stainless Steel and Composite Plates. Calcif. Tiss. Res., 19:27-37, 1975.
20. Woo, S.L.Y., Akeson, W.H., Coutts, R.D., Rutherford, L., Doty, D., Jemmott, G.G. and Amiel, D.: A Comparison of Cortical Bone Atrophy Secondary to Fixation with Large Differences in Bending Stiffness. J. Bone Jt. Surg., 58A:No. 2, 1976.
21. Brown, S.A., Mayor, M.B. and Vandergrift, J.: The Use of Polyester Materials for Fracture Fixation. Trans. Orthop. Res. Soc., Vol. 2:3, 1978.
22. Cutright, D.E. and Hunsuck, E.E.: The Repair of Fractures of the Orbital Floor Using Biodegradable Polylactic Acid. Oral Surg., 33:28-34, 1972.

23. Cutright, D.E., Hunsuck, E.E. and Beasley, J.D.: Fracture Reduction Using a Biodegradable Material, Polylactic Acid. J. Oral Surg., 29:393-397, 1971.
24. Getter, L., Cutright, D.E., Bhaskar, S.N. and Augsburg, J.K.: A Biodegradable Intraosseous Appliance in the Treatment of Mandibular Fractures. J. Oral Surg., 30:344-348, 1972.
25. Parsons, J.R., Alexander, H., Corcoran, S.F. and Weiss, A.B.: Development of a Variable Stiffness, Absorbable Bone Plate. Trans. Orthop. Res. Soc., 4:168, 1979.
26. Parsons, J.R., Aragona, J., Alexander, H. and Weiss, A.B.: Medial Collateral Ligament Replacement with a Partially Absorbable Tissue Scaffold. Proc. 9th Northeast Bioengineering Conf., 29, 1981.
27. Parsons, J.R., Alexander, H., Corcoran, S.F. and Weiss, A.B.: Development of a Variable Stiffness Absorbable Bone Plate. Current Concepts of Internal Fracture Fixation, H.K. Uhtoff, Ed., Springer-Verlag, New York, 1980.
28. Haubold, A.: Carbon in Prosthetics. Ann. New York Acad. Sci., 283:383-395, 1977.
29. Christel, P., Buttazzoni, B., Leray, J.L. and Morin, C.: Tissue Tolerance of Carbon Materials. Trans. World Biomat. Congress, 1:4.7.9, 1980.
30. Jenkins, D.: Private Communication.
31. Claes, L.: Private Communication.
32. Cutright, D.E. and Hunsuck, E.E.: Tissue Reaction to the Biodegradable Polylactic Acid Suture. Oral Surg., 31:134-139, 1971.
33. Brady, J.M., Cutright, D.E., Miller, R.A., Battistone, G.C. and Hunsuck, E.E.: Resorption Rate Route Elimination and Ultrastructure of the Implant Site of Polylactic Acid in the Abdominal Wall of the Rat. J. Biomed. Mat. Res., 7:155-166, 1973.
34. Kulkarni, R.K., Moore, E.G., Hegyeli, A.F. and Leonard, F.: Polylactic Acid for Surgical Implants. Arch. Surg., 93:839-843, 1966.
35. Alexander, H., Parsons, J.R., Strauchler, I.D., Corcoran, S.F., Gona, O. and Mayott, C.W.: Canine Patellar Tendon Replacement with a Polylactic Acid Polymer-Filamentous Carbon Tissue Scaffold. Orthop. Review, Vol. X, No. 1, 41-51, 1981.
36. Aragona, J., Parsons, J.R., Alexander, H. and Weiss, A.B.: Soft Tissue Attachment of a Filamentous Carbon-Absorbable Polymer Tendon and Ligament Replacement. Clin. Orthop. Rel. Res., 160:268-278, 1981.
37. Parsons, J.R., Aragona, J., Alexander, H. and Weiss, A.B.: Medial Collateral Ligament Replacement with a Partially Absorbable Tissue Scaffold. Proc. 9th Northeast Bioengineering Conf., 29, 1981.
38. Jones, R.M.: Mechanics of Composite Materials. Washington, Scripta, McGraw-Hill, 1975.
39. Alexander, H., Corcoran, S.F., Parsons, J.R. and Weiss, A.B.: Internal Fracture Fixation with Partially Degradable Plates. Proc. 9th Northeast Bioengineering Conf., 115, 1981.
40. Minns, R.J. and Flynn, M.: Intra-Articular Implant of Filamentous Carbon Fibre in the Experimental Animal. J. Bioengineering, 2:279-286, 1978.
41. Vasu, R., Carter, D.R., Spengler, D.M. and Dueland, R.T.: Intracortical Bone Stress Fields Calculated From In-Vivo Strain Measurements. Proc. 8th Northeast Bioengineering Conf., 425, 1980.

Chapter 39

Hybrid Artificial Liver

Hugo O. Jauregui, Nancy T. Hayner, Barry A. Solomon and Pierre M. Galletti
*Department of Pathology, Rhode Island Hospital
(H.O.J.), Amicon Corporation (B.A.S.) and the Artificial Organ Laboratory
Division of Biology and Medicine, Brown University
Providence, Rhode Island (N.T.H. and P.M.G.)*

ABSTRACT

Our proposed design of a hybrid artificial liver employs a biological component, the hepatocyte, to metabolize toxic substances and to synthesize important products necessary for the maintenance of body functions. This cell should be in intimate contact with the blood circulation (for a fast interchange of metabolic and anabolic substances) through an artificial membrane which allows passage in both directions. Furthermore, to avoid the possibility of immunological rejection, the blood-cell barrier should have a discriminating capacity of restricting antibodies or immune-competent "killer cells". Our model of such an organ is presented here, after a brief description of the liver functional activities and their failure, as well as other past and present attempts to replace impaired liver functions. The coverage of some of the current efforts of liver support in hepatic failure reflects our biased perspective. This is justified by the fact that, although there are commendable technical improvements in the direction of furnishing a replacement for liver catabolic functions, the synthetic (anabolic) functional activity of this organ has received little attention.

The development of a hybrid artificial liver demands a previous treatment of the parenchymal cells "in vitro" and providing that these cells offer a challenge to present tissue culture methodologies, we have emphasized our efforts in that direction. Future research will move, in our judgement, at a fast pace, as soon as a good number of hepatocytes are able to be adapted to "in vitro" conditions, ready to be grafted to the blood circulation without the necessity of tissue matching between donor and recipient animals.

I. INTRODUCTION

A) The Functional Complexity of the Liver In Vivo

The mammalian liver offers to the physiologist, the anatomist, the biochemist, and, consequently, the bioengineer, one of the most complex organs to evaluate and replace. As the main cellular constituent of the liver, the hepatocyte performs multiple and finely tuned functions which are critical for the homeostasis of the human body. Although pathways for synthesis and breakdown of carbohydrates, lipids, amino acids, proteins, nucleic acids and coenzymes can be identified in partial form in many mammalian cells, only the liver cell subsumes all of these biochemical reactions and is able to combine them simultaneously to accomplish a unique biological task (Table 1).

Table 1. Mammalian Liver Functions

1.	Glyconeogenesis.
2.	Glycogen synthesis and storage, glycogenolysis.
3.	Synthesis of serum proteins including albumin, hemopexin, fibrinogen, ceruloplasmin, coagulation factors, α-1 antitrypsin, α fetoprotein.
4.	Conjugation of bile acids.
5.	Conversion of heme to bilirubin or biliverdin.
6.	Lipoprotein synthesis.
7.	Vitamin storage and metabolism.
8.	Detoxification and drug metabolism.
9.	Cholestrol synthesis.
10.	Regeneration.

SOME IMPORTANT HEPATOCYTE FUNCTIONS

Besides the hepatocyte, other cells within the liver perform a number of vital functions. By virtue of the phagocytic sinusoidal (Kupffer) cells (which represent about 2.1 percent of the total liver cell population in the rat [1], the liver represents a major portion of the reticuloendothelial system (RES). As such it contributes to the disposition of particulate bodies carried by the blood circulation, participates in the normal daily breakdown of old erythrocytes, and fights the myriad microbiological agents responsible for a number of infectious diseases. Other liver functions, such as the synthesis of globulins by hepatocytes and resident lymphocytes, also play an important role in regulating the immunological balance of the whole human body. Evaluation and replacement of liver functions present additional complexities because of the interdependence of the liver with the other organs of the portal venous circulation: the pancreas, spleen and intestine. Important, but still poorly understood, stimuli for cell function and cell replication are received via this circulation. Consequently, to isolate the liver from its unique in vivo environment is, by nature, artifactual. Caution must therefore be exerted in interpreting experimental data deriving from experiments with perfusion of the whole liver separated from other portal organs.

B. Clinical Need for Liver Support and Substitution

Partial or total liver replacement is needed in case of transient or permanent failure of vital liver functions. Even with recent advances in supportive therapy, patients with fulminant hepatic failure still exhibit a mortality rate in excess of 80% [2]. This clinical condition may develop in several forms of toxic or alcoholic hepatitis or hepatitis associated with viral infections.

Fulminant hepatic failure is associated with massive necrosis of hepatocytes and concomitant sudden severe impairment of hepatic metabolism. The clinical picture is usually dominated by symptoms of severe attrition of mental functions – a situation which, in most cases, rapidly advances to stupor or coma. An early onset of jaundice is also a characteristic finding and with increments of abnormal enzyme blood levels, these patients usually die within a week.

Acute liver failure demands immediate application of a supportive hepatic system. Although such patients are the most difficult to sustain, they often have good potential for liver regeneration and ultimate recovery.

In chronic liver disease, temporary liver replacement is also needed. Williams has recognized two categoreis of chronic liver patients who could benefit from artificial liver support. First, those patients with chronic liver disease with a temporary and reversible decompensation (e.g. following hemorrhage from bleeding esophageal varices) apparently have a better chance of survival with temporary liver support. The second category of patients includes end stage cirrhotics waiting for liver transplants [3]. Here, the artificial liver is used much as an artificial kidney for preoperative support until a proper donor becomes available. The number of patients in the latter category is impressive. In 1965, this condition caused 12.8 deaths per 100,000 population in the U.S.A., 44.7 in West Berlin, 34.2 in France, and 22.9 in Italy [3].

Both in acute and chronic hepatic failure, there are clinical situations in which damaged liver cells are unable to detoxify toxic nitrogenous products. These toxins are normally absorbed by intestinal capillaries and carried to the liver by the portal system. In addition to the accumulation of toxic products, alteration in acid-base balance, and diminished cerebral blood flow, there seems to be a number of poorly understood metabolic changes which contribute to the general impairment of mental status known as hepatic encephalopathy [4]. Impaired blood coagulation and subsequent gastrointestinal hemorrhages are common in these patients. Such hemorrhages result in double indemnity to the patient: first, they increase the load of previously discussed intestinal nitrogen by-products; and second, they lead to hypotension, which compromises the cerebral circulation, already severely affected by depression of vasomotor centers in the brain.

This all-too-brief review of liver dysfunctions indicates above all the complex and diverse nature of the organ. By consulting specialized texts [4,5], the reader can greatly extend his knowledge of any of the preceding points. However, it must be appreciated that a complete understanding of liver functions is still lacking. While a relatively advanced knoweldge of renal excretory physiology has played an essential part in the successful application of hemodialysis in acute or chronic renal failure, no comparable and organized foundation is available for liver pathophysiology. We have neither detailed information about metabolism of organic anions by liver cells nor a full grasp of the complex biotransformations of the many toxic substances excreted by the hepatocyte.

II. THE ENGINEERING CHALLENGE OF REPLACING LIVER FUNCTION

The complexity of the functions served by the natural liver, the specialization of its cellular components and the fact that fine tuning of its performance requires a continuous, bidirectional exchange of biochemical information with other organ systems, combine to make liver function replacement particularly demanding.

At one end of the spectrum of possible solutions is the global approach represented by conventional liver transplantation in situ, ex vivo liver perfusion of an isolated animal liver connected to the patient's cardiovascular system [7,8,9] and cross-circulation between a subject in end-stage hepatic failure and a healthy individual [10,11]. Theoretically, all of these approaches are therapeutically sound and effective. However, their application is severely limited by the shortage of donors and the complexities of surgical and immune matching.

At the other end of the spectrum are technologies for liver support which proceed from a focus on selected aspects of liver function, such as: 1) hemoperfusion for adsorption of specific toxins, or chemical processing of a specific biological product [12,13]; 2) hemodialysis and hemofiltration for clearance of natural or abnormal compounds within the limits imposed by the diffusive and/or convective permeability of the exchange membrane [14]; 3) plasmapheresis with separation of plasma (whether by filtration or centrifugation) from the cellular elements of blood and chemical processing by appropriate sorbents or reagents before returning it to the circulatory system of the patient [15].

More interactive methods have been proposed such as parabiotic dialysis in which the blood of the patient and that of a donor are made to circulate on either side of a hemodialysis membrane. In this way, the donor's liver and kidneys can actively substitute for the patient's organs inasmuch as the permselectivity of the system will allow [16]. Alternatively, the modern descendant of parabiotic dialysis, the hybrid artificial liver, provides a technique in which live isolated hepatocytes (or cell clusters, or tissue slices) are either encapsulated in a polymer bag or somehow separated by a semi-permeable membrane prior to exposure to blood from a patient in hepatic failure.

The text below reviews some technical and biological aspects of these techniques, and addresses some of the problems encountered in the development of this new biotechnology.

A. Detoxifying Procedures and/or Devices

After initial optimism about the possibility of removing toxic products responsible for hepatic encephalopathy by exchange transfusions [17], investigators agree that results have, in fact, been quite mixed [18]. Similarly, hemodialysis with conventional cellulosic membrane, which has proven so effective in renal failure, has shown no beneficial effect in hepatic coma.

The procedure of direct polyacrylonitrile membranes with hemodialysis has evolved from experimental studies of cross hemodialysis [16]. Opolon and co-workers have applied this procedure (which allows the passage of compounds up to about 15,000 daltons), and observed the recovery of consciousness in 59% of the patients in hepatic coma, but with survival of only about 22% [19,20]. The original report with charcoal hemoperfusion from Kings College Hospital in London was presented in 1974 [21]. Since then, most work has been directed towards the development of biocompatible coatings to separate the charcoal from the blood and thereby avoid the embolization of charcoal microparticles ("fines") and the adhesion of blood formed elements to the hemoperfusion column. The coating ought to be permeable to the toxins to be removed, yet unattractive to leucocytes or platelets so as to avoid thrombus formation. Charcoal granules have been coated with collodion [22], polyhydroxyethyl methacrylate (polyhema) [23], and cellulose [24]. Improvements in biocompatibility have been documented in terms of thrombogenicity in animal studies, but in clinical trial with polyhema coated charcoal, the results have not been as encouraging [25].

Plasma, rather than whole blood, has been proposed for absorbant hemoperfusion as a way of avoiding platelet and other blood cell damage. Nose has developed a system based on a microporous membrane which separates the plasma which, after perfusion over charcoal, is readmitted into the blood flow [15]. This model has been used successfully with calves [26]. A selective removal of serum bilirubin, which is responsible for damage of cerebral tissues in premature babies (kernicterus), was achieved by hemoperfusion runs through a bed of coated anion exchange resins (Amberlite) [27]. Continuous plasma cross circulation after total hepatectomy in dogs proved to be effective in prolonging the life of the animals [99]. These approaches, however, lack controlled human studies [14]. Indeed the design of hemoperfusion columns is difficult since it is not clear which toxins play a decisive role in hepatic encephalopathy [14]. A somewhat different approach was the removal of bile salts by selective membrane separation of plasma followed by absorption which was successful in controlling pruritis in patients with primary biliary cirrhosis [100].

B. Semi-Biologic Liver Replacement Devices

"In vivo" the liver provides a very complicated system of cell compartments. Within the hepatocyte and separated by a sophisticated plasma membrane, we find a microsomal system with an incredible capacity for the disposal of toxic products and xenobiotics carried in by the portal vein. Specifically, the hepatocyte plasma membrane shows (as do other cells in the body) the capacity of regulating passage of active electrolytes and water. In addition, through special receptors for hormones and many other biological and pharmacological agents, the liver cell plasma membrane allows a selective cell internalization of messengers that regulate both hepatocyte growth and synthesis of important products [28-31]. The complexity of this membrane is such that many of its precise chemical constituents are unknown, and much of its structural composition has defied complete ultrastructural analysis.

Quite a number of detoxifying (catabolic) and active synthetic (anabolic) functions of the liver can theoretically be performed by encapsulating multiple combinations of enzymes and reactive pharmacological agents within artificial membranes that allow some selected passage in both directions.

This approach as a whole is not yet feasible at the present time, although trends in that direction can be found in the field of synthetic biomolecular lipid membranes free of proteins (liposomes) which have been used to incorporate receptor proteins in the lipid bilayers [32] or to study adsorption of organic anions [33]. A polyvinylpyrrolidone of 360,000 MW has also been used as an artificial hydrogel entrapment of liver microsomes which were able to metabolize xenobiotics "in vitro" [34].

C. Use of Liver Tissue Slices in Artificial Hybrid Livers

The design of a supportive system for long-term preservation of liver functions seems to demand the incorporation of active living cells in an artificial device that is in contact with the host circulation. This presents problems shared by other mixed cell/artificial supportive systems. In this context, the utilization of liver slices was first advanced in 1959 and was further developed later [35]. This approach (which is one step below whole liver transplantation) has the potential complication of anoxia whenever cells isolated from their normal vascular connections have to function in an overloaded system with poor oxygen supply. To faciliate critical oxygen delivery, incorporation of oxygen carriers such as fluorocarbons (which have already been tested in liver perfusion studies) has been further adapted to liver slices [36]. It is evident that the utilization of liver tissue in assisting devices would be further enhanced by the use of only active elements – the hepatocytes, supported by artificial (although not necessarily inert) polymeric membranes and separated from the blood circulation by similar or specially designed artificial membranes which would allow selective passage in one direction.

III. "CELLULAR" ARTIFICIAL HYBRID LIVERS

Hybrid artificial organs are man-made structures in which functional tissues are housed in a blood-perfused device attached to the blood stream. Prototypes of a hybrid artificial pancreas have demonstrated that surviving pancreatic beta cells, whole islets from donor rats, or insulin-secreting tissue derived from a human endocrine tumor, can provide insulin secretion and glucose balance for extended periods both in vitro and in vivo [37,39]. Typically, the device is attached to the blood stream between an artery and a vein. A permselective membrane, which is an essential component of this biartificial reactor, provides a mechanical barrier against the immune response. In the artificial pancreas application, this membrane features a molecular height cut-off of about 50,000 daltons. It, therefore, allows transport of glucose and other nutrients as well as insulin generated by the beta cells in response to changes in blood glucose [38].

The design and evaluation of a bio-artificial liver is far more complicated than the development of a hybrid endocrine pancreas, because many more functions must be served. The liver possesses a double circulation (hepatic and portal) and a complicated excretory system that utilizes both blood and bile to dispose of its products. Also, the secretory arrangement of many liver functions is mediated by large macromolecules (some of them synthesized by the liver, e.g.: very low density lipoproteins which measure up to 800 Å in diameter).

There are three major options in designing a hybrid artificial liver which incorporates highly purified liver cell populations. The first approach is to use adult liver cells isolated in sufficient numbers, with the expectation that functional activities can be maintained as similar as possible as prevail in situ. The adult rat hepatocyte – the cell used typically in most studies – is separated from neighboring cells and supportive structures, attached to a substrate (hepatocytes are anchor-dependent cells), and then placed in a milieu conducive to a regulated replication with differentiation. Unfortunately, this latter goal has not yet been achieved with "in vitro" adult rat or other mammalian hepatocytes, and long-term maintenance of hepatocyte cultures is still out of reach in spite of recent advances in the control of the process [40,41]. Nonetheless, reliance on adult liver cells characterizes our present approach for the design of an artificial liver, as discussed in more detail below.

A second option, the maintenance of liver tumor cells (which proliferate indefinitely in tissue culture, and can be grafted in an artificial capillary device) is quite attractive. The bundle of synthetic capillaries provides the anatomical substrate for whatever function the cells accomplish. This approach has been pioneered by Wolf [43] who was able to measure bilirubin conjugation by an artificial hybrid liver comprised of hepatoma (tumor) cells. Hepatoma cell lines, originating from either mammalian liver cells transformed in vitro by hepatocarcinogens or from animal experimental liver tumors, are readily available [44,45]. However, these cells show a highly simplified functional cell activity and lack most of the metabolic pathways of "in vivo" hepatocytes [46,47].

A third choice would be the use of cells with replicating capacity, e.g. those obtained from hepatectomized adult animals [48], from embryonal livers [49, 50] or from neonatal animals [51]. This approach has been used by one of us, and the resulting device, seeded with murine neonatal livers cells (which were not fully purified in terms of the hepatocyte content), was shown to produce albumin, to detoxify pharmacological agents such as Diazepam, to metabolize urea and to deaminate cytidine with the generation of uridine [52]. This option has a promising future if one is able to identify, purify and collect a stem cell population of hepatocytes with an enhanced proliferative capacity.

IV. PROBLEMS OF IN VITRO HEPATOCYTE SURVIVAL

The use of adult liver cells in a hybrid artificial liver requires the development of methodology to: A) separate the hepatocytes from other liver constituents, B) attach them to a biocompatible polymeric substrate, C) facilitate oxygen exchange to maintain their viability, and D) identify hormones and growth factors which are critical for liver cell trophism.

A) Separation and Isolation of Adult Rat Hepatocytes

The perfusion of the isolated liver with a mixture of 0.05% collagenase and 0.1% hyaluronidase in a calcium-free buffer has revolutionized the technical aspects of liver cell separation. Yields were initially very low (about 3-5% of the liver mass), but the cells were morphologically intact [53]. The procedure of Howard has been improved by Berry and Friend who separate cells by a recirculating perfusion system in which the calcium-free medium is oxygenated [54]. The softened liver is removed after 20-30 minutes of perfusion, broken up with a blunt spatula, and the resultant cell suspension incubated for an additional 10-15 minutes in a shaking water bath. Hepatocytes are separated from tissue debris by filtration through a nylon mesh followed by differential centrifugations: a yield of 30-50% of the total mass of hepatocytes can be obtained. Most current methods of isolation are based on the procedure of Berry and Friend. Hyaluronidase has been eliminated from many protocols. Indeed, Wagle has reported that it enhances hepatic glycogen degradation [55]. Seglen has introduced a significant variant by preperfusing the liver with a calcium-free medium for 5-10 minutes [56]. This preperfusion fluid (which is not recirculated) is followed by a medium containing collagenase and 5mM calicum chloride which recirculates through the liver for another 10 minutes. Removal of calcium ions in the medium favors cell dispersal at the desmosome junction, a non-reversible process. A modification of the aforementioned separation procedure is used in our laboratory and has been reported elsewhere [57].

The role of collagenase in liver cell separation deserves further comment. Crude extracts of Clostridium histolyticum contain proteolytic activities in addition to collagenase. Variations in the dispersing efficiency of different lots have been noticed in the literature, and are a common nuisance in our laboratory practice (see Table 2). Seglen claims that cell suspensions prepared with purified collagenase have viabilities at least as high as those prepared with crude enzymes [58]. If this is true (we have no definitive proof to the contrary), collagenase

Table 2. Recovery and Viability of Hepatocytes After Isolation

Variable	Collagenase IV Lot 38C-6800	Collagenase IV Lot 88C-6890
Number of Experiments	10	10
Mean Viability of Isolated Hepatocytes $\pm$ SD	82 $\pm$ 4%	89 $\pm$ 3%'
Mean Yield Viable Hepatocytes/Rat $\pm$ SD	324 $\pm$ 78 X 10^6	384 $\pm$ 193 X 10^6
Mean Yield Viable Hepatocytes/ 100 gm wt Rat $\pm$ SD	139 $\pm$ 38 X 10^6	176 $\pm$ 59 X 10^6
Absolute Recovery* (Based on max. potential yield of 630 X 10^6 hepatocytes/100 gm body wt)	22%	28%
Sigma Enzyme Analysis+		
Collagenase U/mg Dry Weight	150	180
Caseinase " " "	30	431
Trypsin " " "	0.02	0.01

*Laishes, B.A. and Williams, G.M. In Vitro, 12:521, 1976

+Sigma Chemical Co., St. Louis, Missouri

is the agent responsible for enzymatic dispersion of the liver when crude collagenase preparations are used. This does not invalidate data from several research groups, indicating that proteolytic impurities of crude collagenase preparations are responsible for better cell separation [58]. At least one manufacturer (Sigma) recommends one of its collagenase preparations as the one best suited for hepatocyte isolation procedures.

The first step in establishing an "in vitro" system of viable, functioning and morphologically-intact liver cells is to isolate them in adequate yields with minimal damage. The task is not an easy one, because information is still incomplete on how the collagenase treatment affects the hepatocyte plasma membrane and other organelles (disruption of subcellular organelles is a distinct possibility, if we accept the claim that the enzyme penetrates the cell [59]).

The differential centrifugation used to purify the adult hepatocytes is based on the observation that damaged parenchymal and all non-parenchymal cells are lighter than intact hepatocytes. Liver cells from rats have also been isolated by centrifugation on Percoll gradients [60]. There is usually an inverse relationship between the yield and the purity of the hepatocyte fraction. Most of the damaged cells in the first suspension are removed by low speed differential centrifugation (approximately 50g). After 3 to 4 centrifugation procedures, the yield is about 40% of the liver weight. Low centrifugation speeds, low temperature, and flat-bottomed beakers have all been recommended by Seglen to minimize the unavoidable cell damage [61].

The activity of collagenase requires an optimum pH of 7.5 which should be maintained within plus or minus 0.2 pH units. The perfused liver acidifies the perfusion very rapidly and, therefore, requires a strong buffer system. If the medium is recirculated, an infusion of NaOH by a pH-stat (automatic pH meter and titration system) or a combination of organic buffers must be used. Although the liver requires good and continuous oxygenation, periods of anoxia of up to 30 minutes are perfectly tolerable. The perfusate flow directly affects the oxygenation of the organ. Flow rates of 3 ml/gm liver/min. with oxygen-saturated perfusate are necessary for maximal oxygenation of 8-10 gm liver when a recirculating perfusion apparatus is used. Certain authors use a non-recirculating perfusion technique with flow rates as low as 5 ml/min. [62].

The separation of liver cells by collagenase perfusion is now a widespread method. The technique is used by biochemists who simply incubate the isolated hepatocytes in buffer solutions for as long as 4 hours for enzymatic studies. Unfortunately, isolated hepatic parenchymal cells show diminished metabolic activity after three to four hours "in vitro" [63]. Furthermore, it appears that certain enzymes, such as ribonuclease, become activated when single cell suspensions are incubated at 37°C in Krebs-Ringer phosphate buffer. The limited viability of freshly isolated hepatocytes, although not affecting some biochemical studies (e.g. glyconeogenesis and fatty acid metabolism), have impaired other investigations, such as those concerned with plasma protein synthesis [64]. The limitation of fresh cells for biochemical studies has motivated a good number of investigators to turn to tissue culture procedures to provide better metabolic conditions for adult rat hepatocytes.

B) "In Vitro" Attachment of Hepatocytes

In vivo, the hepatocytes are attached to basement membranes, which are difficult to visualize even with the aid of the electron microscope. Histologists usually report that the liver cell has a vascular pole which is not directly in contact with the blood sinusoidal capillary (Figure 1), but separated from the capillary endothelial cell by the space of Disse. In this space there are reticulum fibrils which are argentaffin (i.e. react with silver salts). Their chemical composition is a matter of active research, but it seems that type III collagen can be found in these fibrils [65]. Fluorescent antibodies prepared against liver basement membrane collagens and noncollagenous proteins, such as fibronectin (LETS protein) and some acidic glycoproteins show that other proteins are also localized in the so-called reticulum fibrils. Rojkind [66] has isolated, in crude form, different kinds of noncollagen proteins normally present in the space of Disse of the rat liver, and called them "biomatrix." The normal adult liver cell "in vitro" shares with other cells (e.g. normal human fibroblasts) the need to adhere to a solid support in order to thrive. However, attachment alone is not sufficient, and although adult hepatocytes do not proliferate in vitro, they survive only if cell spreading on the substrate follows attachment [67].

The adhesive behavior of rat hepatocytes to polystyrene surfaces was first studied by Williams et al in a series of experiments. Attachment efficiency was related to the degree of viability, and although insulin enhanced the attachment, it did not prolong survival [68]. Dexamethasone supplementation of the culture medium enhanced spreading and increased survival with almost 30% of cells surviving for 8 days [69]. From these experiments, it was concluded that the "number of spontaneously detached floating cells paralleled the number of attached cells," and, therefore, quantification of spontaneously detached cells was used as a

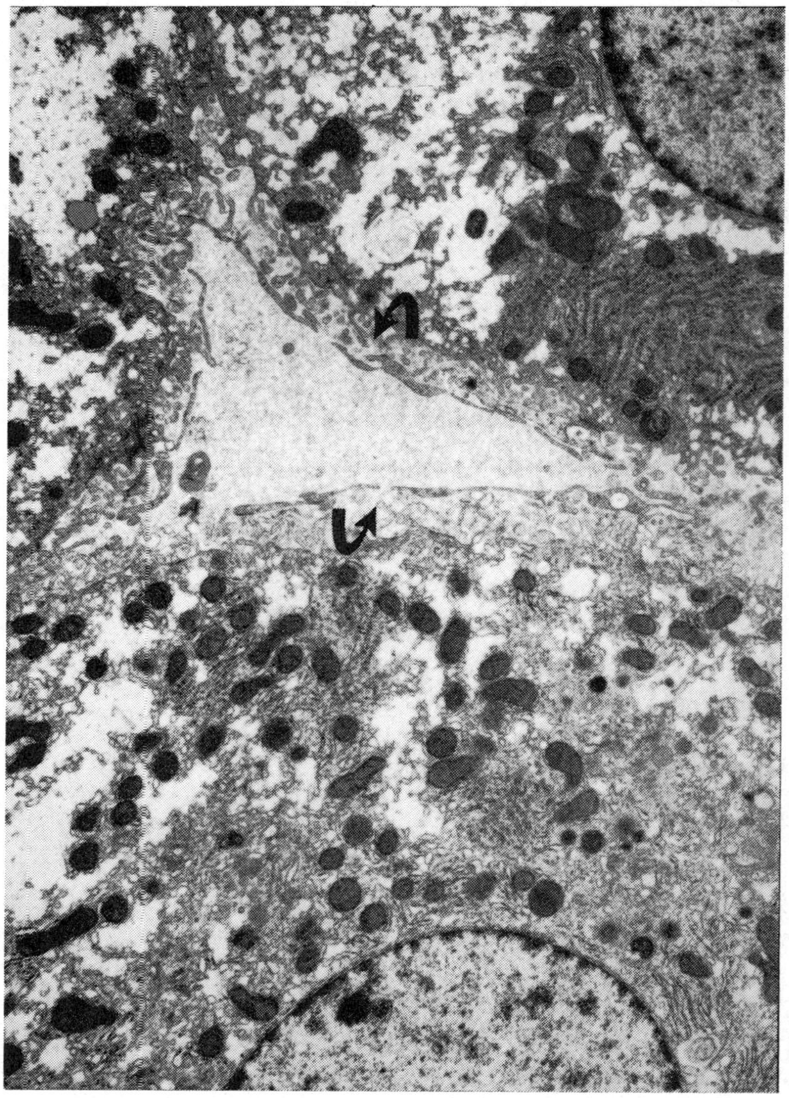

Figure 1. Electron micrograph of a blood capillary at the intersection of 3 rat hepatocytes. Arrows point to the space of Disse. Magnification approximately 12,000.

direct measure of cell loss in the cultures [68].

Our own experience does not confirm this view. The quantification of spontaneously detached cells is not a reliable indicator of cell viability because quite a number of dead cells remain attached, and a small but variable percentage of nonviable cells initially adhere to the polystyrene collagenized surfaces. Pretreatment of polystyrene surfaces with fetal calf serum (FCS) or rat tail collagen promotes attachment equally well, but in addition, the incorporation of 7% FCS in media favored long-term viability [57]. Hepatocyte attachment begins within 30 minutes after the cells are seeded in culture and reaches a maximum after 1½ hours of incubation. A change of culture medium at 4 hours enhances subsequent viability. Although a seeding concentration of 0.5×10^5 hepatocytes/ml furnishes optimal attachment, this concentration is too low for biochemical studies. Furthermore, a higher cell/surface ratio favors survival of the cultures. We suggested that the optimal cell density in seeding hepatocytes in cultures is probably a compromise between the ideal number of cells that will furnish early and optimal cell contacts (known to be necessary for cell survival and function) and an acceptable concentration of oxygen to support the aerobic respiration of a given number of hepatocytes in the first hours of culture.

Hepatocytes attach to a number of substrates made of ligands such as asialoglycoprotein, insulin, epidermal growth factor (EGF), collagen, and fibronectin, but they demand fibronectin or collagen for spreading and, consequently, for subsequent survival [67]. Initial attachment of hepatocytes to collagen depends on the presence of proline and glycine in the collagen chain and proceeds in the absence of fibronectin [70]. Fibronectin is synthesized by hepatocytes in culture. Although this protein is important for hepatocyte spreading on denatured collagen, it seems that it does not affect spreading onto native collagen [67]. Hepatocyte spreading requires a substantial amount of native collagen, and it is probably influenced by the amount of this substrate. Further studies are required to assess the role of native liver-supporting structures such as the liver biomatrix that will enhance both attachment and survival.

In the design of an artificial hybrid liver, we have chosen to incorporate native liver-supporting structures which can be spread on artificial membranes or incorporated into the polymer. We are also turning our attention to the design and testing of bioresorbable polymers that favor attachment. The latter approach probably has the most promise because it will allow the study of chemical groups responsible for the adhesion and survival of cells "in vitro."

C) Oxygen Requirement of Freshly Isolated Hepatocytes

To assess the importance of oxygen supply, a perifusion system was devised in our laboratory in which 37 °C culture medium equilibrated with 5% CO_2 in air was passed through a gas tight chamber containing freshly isolated hepatocytes retained on a nylon mesh screen. The rate of perifusion in this chamber was 0.08 ml/min. and the number of hepatocytes varied between 3×10^5 and 3×10^6 for a total volume of 0.3 ml. At the same perifusion flow rate we also made measurements of O_2 consumption of adult rat pancreatic islets (about 3×10^5 cells). Under these experimental conditions 3×10^5 hepatocytes showed a O_2 depletion of 69 $\pm$ 10 mm Hg. Once equilibrium was reached a larger population of 3×10^6 hepatocytes induced a pO_2 drop of 125 $\pm$ 12 mm Hg. Figure 2 shows oxygen depletion curves of hepatocytes versus pancreatic islets cells demonstrating a dramatic oxygen uptake by hepatocytes and consequently, the need of providing a proper oxygen supply under any tissue culture conditions [71]. This work confirms studies by others [72] showing a high level of respiration in freshly isolated hepatocytes. Furthermore it explains the success of supporting structures, such as collagen membranes [73] or Millipore filters [74] in maintaining liver cell functions at the gas-liquid interphase.

D) Hormones and Growth Factors for Maintenance of Liver Cell Trophism

The composition of media used for monolayer culture of liver cells varies widely. Our choice is Waymouth's medium supplemented with fetal calf serum (1-10%), insulin and glucocorticoids [57]. In adult liver cell cultures in monolayers, insulin and dexamethasone

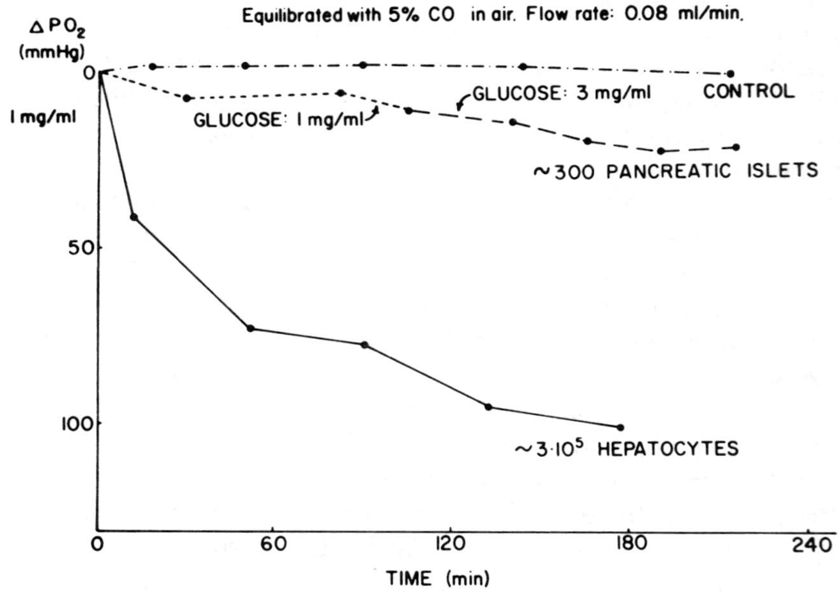

Figure 2. Oxygen depletion of perfused medium by equal number of hepatocytes versus pancreatic B cells.

[68,69,75] have proved to be important in maintaining differentiated functions. Grisham has also proved that insulin plus hydrocortisone promote the highest levels of glycogen metabolism in organ cultures of newborn rat livers [76]. One difficulty in understanding the mechanism of insulin action has been that the hormone exerts many diverse effects on the cell. However, the recent ability to measure directly the specific binding sites at the plasma membrane of hepatocytes has clarified some of these questions [77]. Insulin regulates surface receptors under tissue culture conditions and incubations of hepatocytes with this hormone produce time and temperature-dependent loss of receptors from the cell surface which is reversed by removal of the insulin from the medium [78]. Although the influence of insulin on hepatic metabolism has been well studied in the intact organism and in the isolated perfused liver, the isolation of hepatic cells by the collagenase method has the potential to render the cells insensitive to insulin action. This possible cell surface stripping during the cell separation procedure has not received enough attention in the many laboratories involved in hepatocyte research. In order to assess the potential repair of the cell surface under different culture conditions, we are studying cell surface markers (lectins) that bind to specific sugars [79]. Collagenase action upon all surface receptors is not uniform and certain lots of the enzyme have the potential to alter insulin receptors, whereas others do not [80].

The rate of protein synthesis of freshly isolated hepatocytes is very low but it increases gradually during culture [81]. These cells release branched chain amino acids, particularly valine although they consume other amino acids [82]. Apparently the gradual production of proteinases by hepatocytes in culture is responsible for a negative protein balance and also it seems to be responsible for the degradation of any extracellular matrix into which hepatocytes have been attached [83]. This protein degradation is prevented by the addition of dexamethasone in the culture medium [84]. Moreover, seven amino acids: leucine, asparagine, glutamine, histidine, phenylalamine, tyrosine and tryptophan have been incorporated in excess in a tissue culture medium designed to diminish protein degradation [84].

Accepting the premise that tissue culture in hollow fibers is a prerequisite for successful support of cells and subsequent survival in vivo, one could modify the different tissue culture media to obtain an ideal product that will approach the composition of blood. It seems logical to assume that perfusate such as fresh plasma or serum would be ideal to maintain the performance of hepatocyte function from the very beginning. Unfortunately, there are apparently inhibitors of hepatocyte growth present in the fetal bovine serum which is normally used – a supplement in tissue culture media formulations – to prevent cell attachment and growth in normal epithelial cells. Recent work with fibronectin-depleted fetal bovine serum has shown that its addition improves the survival of neonatal hepatocytes but has no beneficial effect on adult hepatocytes. In fact, when fetal bovine serum was added to tissue culture media of monolayer cultures, it inhibited the enhancement of hepatocyte survival promoted by insulin and dexamethasone [85].

A complete evaluation of hepatocyte function must take into consideration the energy supply of these cells. In this context, fructose and lactate are both oxidized more effectively by hepatocytes than glucose [86]; pyruvate stimulates protein synthesis as well as lactate [84]. Hepatocytes in culture demonstrate a gradual increase of glucose consumption [87], but they have the capacity of surviving in a glucose-free medium [88]. Glycogen is probably the main endogenous energy source in cultured hepatocytes and protein synthesis remains constant for as long as these cells show good glycogen content [89]. In spite of improvements in tissue culture media formulations, we have not yet found the ideal culture conditions to maintain the metabolic pathways of the adult hepatocyte in vivo. In fact, except for one isolated report [90], not confirmed by other laboratories, there is yet no evidence for a net proliferation of adult liver cells in vitro.

V. HOLLOW FIBER MEMBRANES AS THE BASE FOR BOTH TRIDIMENSIONAL TISSUE CULTURE SYSTEMS AND ARTIFICIAL ORGANS

The techniques for three-dimensional cell culture on semipermeable, artificial capillaries was introduced by Knazek et al. in 1972 with the goal of approximating tissue-like cell densities "in vitro" under conditions where cells are separated from their nutrient medium by a synthetic membrane [42]. Thin-walled fibers, i.e., capillaries of about 200 μm internal diameter (ID) and less than 100 μm wall thickness, were used because their lumen provided a ready-made channel for circulating the tissue culture medium and the wall dimensions combined minimal resistance to mass transfer with maximum outer surface for cell implantation. The hollow-fiber membranes were arranged in parallel bundles of a few hundred, their ends sealed off, then potted in a thermosetting resin (silicone, urethane or epoxy), and cut at each extremity to provide a multiperforated "face sheet." Each face was fitted with a funnel-shaped header which allowed for the perfusion of the tissue culture medium from a single tube into all parallel capillaries, and back to a single tube. The bundle of hollow fibers was encased in a cylindrical, transparent, plastic jacket featuring side ports for cell seeding (Figure 3).

The artificial capillaries used by Knazek were provided by the Amicon Corporation and demonstrated a further application of the anisotropic membranes developed by Michaels [91], characterized by a very thin, molecularly discriminating "skin" supported by an open-cell, porous substrate. Anisotropic, tubular membranes with higher hydraulic permeability (water

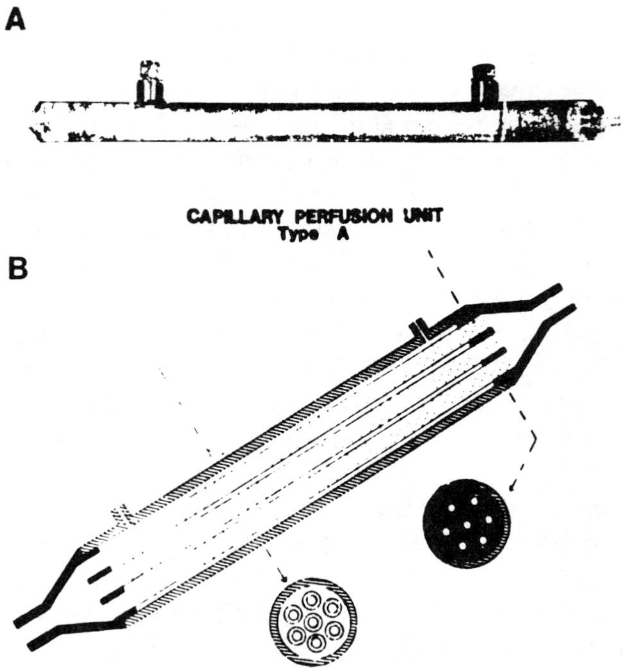

Figure 3a. Photograph of a capillary perfusion unit – length is about 24 cm., diameter is about 2 cm.
Figure 3b. Diagram of the unit.

flux is typically on the order of 2.0 to 20 ml/min-M^2-mm Hg) and higher molecular weight cutoff characteristics than standard cellulosic membrane materials are typically made of either acrylic copolymers or polysulfones. Techniques have been described in the patent literature for casting flat-sheet membranes and spinning hollow-fiber membranes [92,93]. The fabrication of the latter involves specially designed spinnerettes which extrude two concentric fluid streams, the inner (cylindrical) one delivering a precipitating solution and the outer (annular) one providing the polymer casting solution. The control of the transport properties of the thin, semipermeable skin is achieved primarily by: 1) controlling the composition of the polymer solids and solvent system in a casting solution and 2) varying the composition of the precipitating solution to modulate the rate of precipitation of the polymer.

Commercially available hollow-fiber capillary membranes offer molecular weight cutoff values ranging from 2,000 to 100,000 daltons with an ID of 200 ± 20 μm and a wall thickness of 70 ± 5 μm. The research Division of Amicon has fabricated capillary membranes with wall thickness as low as 45 μm and as high as 180 μm for several of our projects.

The molecular weight cutoff of these semipermeable membranes has generally been determined by measuring the fractional filtration of a known molecular weight solute under a standard set of operating conditions, including solute concentration, perfusion rate through the fibers, and average transmembrane pressure. As the transmembrane pressure and consequently the filtration rate decreases, the rejection of a partially permeable solute tends to decrease. Thus, the reported nominal molecular weight cutoffs of different membrane types should be used for comparative purposes as the actual rejection characteristics under cell culture conditions may vary.

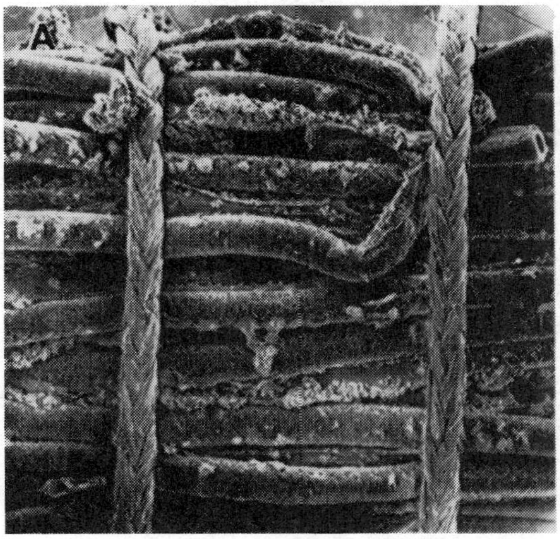

Figure 4a. Scanning electron micrograph of a bundle of Amicon artificial capillaries taken from a 72 hour culture of adult rat hepatocytes.

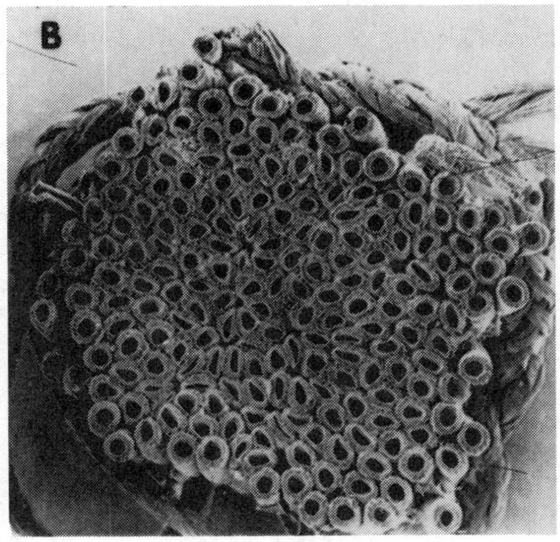

Figure 4b. Scanning electron micrograph presenting a cross section view of the capillary bundle shown in Figure 4a.

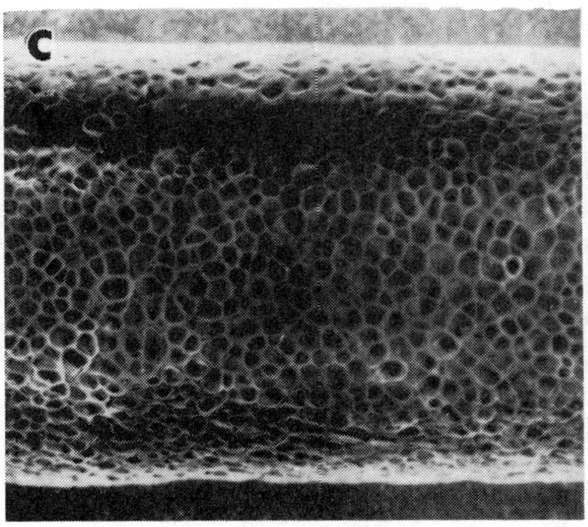

Figure 4c. Scanning electron micrograph of Amicon artificial capillary "21D."

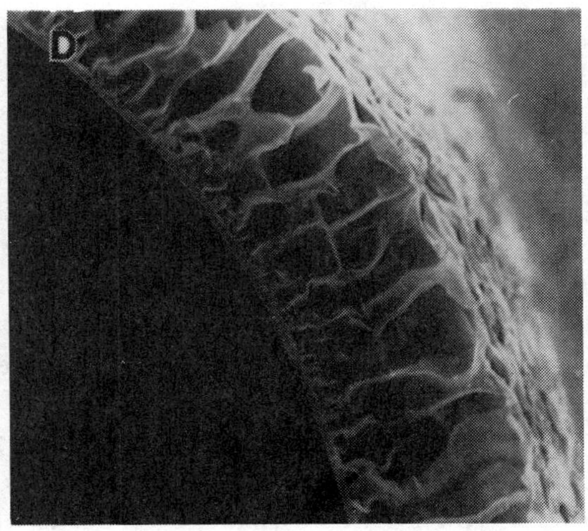

Figure 4d. Scanning electron micrograph of Amicon artificial capillary "23" showing inner skin and convoluted nature of capillary wall.

The outer surface of an anisotropic hollow-fiber or tubular membrane typically presents a reticulated aspect with thin traveculae and polygonal voids on the order of several microns (see Figure 4). The voids in the outer spongy part of the tube wall are typically oriented in a radial fashion, communicate with one another through lateral passages, and extend to within 1 μm of the internal skin. Comparable structures can be prepared by dispersing reinforcing fillers in an organic solvent blended with a bipolar surfactant and mixing the filler solution with an aliquot of the resin in the same solvent. Composite structures in a flat-sheet form have also been prepared by taping a scrim to a flat glass plate, overcoating the scrim with the casting solution, and precipitating the composite in a bath of water.

Quality control of each batch of membranes involves four main steps: 1) measurement of hydraulic permeability to ascertain the rate of ultrafiltration under the transmembrane pressure conditions anticipated in a culture system; 2) measurement of the rejection characteristics of the membranes by calculating the fractional filtration of several solutes of varying molecular weight; 3) scanning electron microscopy to ascertain the surface structure of the material and its bulk architecture; and 4) measurement of a diffusive permeability for a small molecule (typically sodium chloride) and a larger one (typically inulin).

With these membranes, the diffusional supply of nutrients to tumor cells and the clearance of toxic wastes seem to be adequate for cell survival in perfusion capillary chambers. Nonetheless, it is possible to increase the convection of the tissue culture perfusate (to meet the increasing demands of proliferating malignant cells) by incorporating two sets of capillary bundles which carry the perfusion fluid at different intra-luminal pressures [94].

The provision of high mass transfer rates of tissue culture nutrients is critical for the survival and proliferation of tumor cells although there is no definitive proof that this is the case with normal (non-transformed) cells and, indeed, the opposite may be true. In fact, successful tissue culture methods to adapt epithelial, non-transformed cells to "in vitro" conditions rely on variable quantities of "conditioned medium" obtained by culturing other cells which may either release critical "growth factors" or neutralize "growth inhibitor factors" (chalones) [95].

Because hepatocyte attachment to artificial capillaries is a prerequisite for long-term cell survival, a program has been initiated by the Research Division of Amicon Corporation to modify semipermeable, hollow-fiber membranes for hepatocyte culture. Whereas pre-exposure of the hollow fibers to a solution containing a passivating agent, such as bovine albumin or lecithin [96], serves to temporarily decrease enzyme denaturation due to surface interactions, recent advances suggest that a covalent attachment of collagen or polylysine more uniformly and permanently modifies the surface for better long-term hepatocyte attachment. Collagen has been credited with the successful attachment of hepatocytes when put into solution prior to the exposure of the hepatocytes to the fiber surface. Polylysine also has proven useful in promoting attachment and prolonging function of hepatocytes when lysine-coated glass was used as a support.

The hollow-fiber membranes are first etched with a warm solution of NaOH exposing free carboxylic acid moieties. Time, temperature, and etching solution strength have been studied to permit the functionalization to occur without significant modification of the membrane's sieving characteristics. A subsequent activation of the membrane surface through a condensation reaction with N-hydroxy-succinimide results in an active ester, highly reactive to primary amino groups, such as the end chain or epsilon amino groups or either arginine or lysine found in most proteins. Immobilization of collagen or polylysine via this method can then be carried out using a modified technique developed by Solomon et al. [97] for antibodies, based on the original enzyme immobilization work by Adalsteinsson et al. [98]. Concentrations of collagen and polylysine, time of exposure, and pH of solution are varied in the immobilization procedure to achieve different surface coverages of these "attachment promoters." Morphological observations, protein determinations and DNA hepatocyte content are now used to determine the most efficient modification protocol.

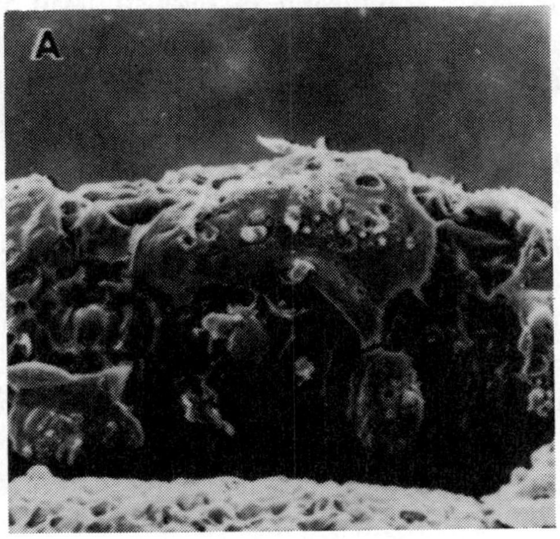

Figure 5a. Scanning electron micrograph of adult rat hepatocytes cultured 48 hours on Amicon artificial capillary bundle.

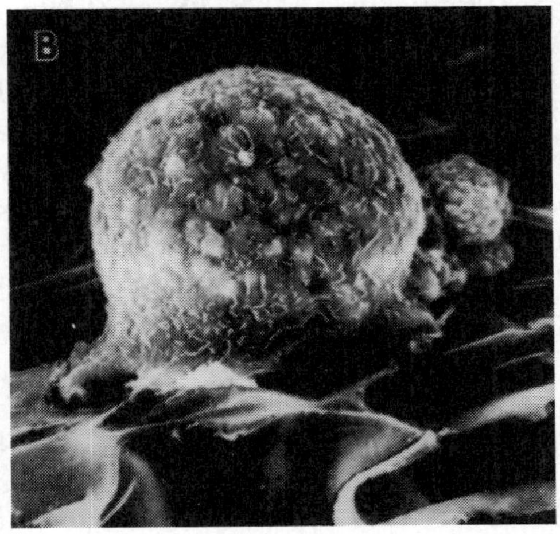

Figure 5b. Scanning electron micrograph of adult rat hepatocyte at 4 hours of culture attached to reticulated surface of Amicon artificial capillary showing numerous microvilli on cell surface.

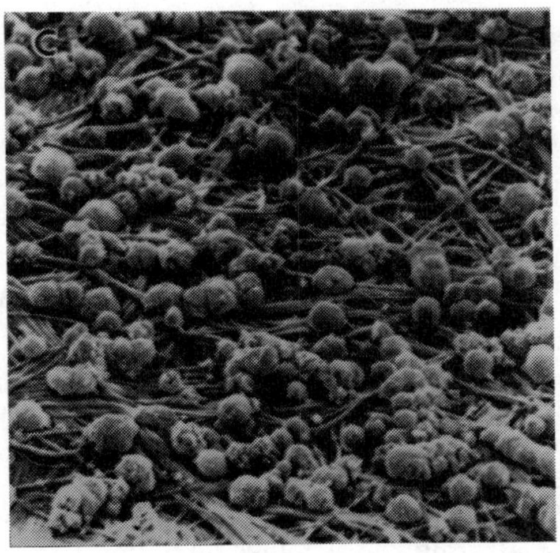

Figure 5c. Scanning electron micrograph of adult rat hepatocytes cultured 24 hours on collagen coated reticulated side of Amicon acrylic copolymer sheets showing strands of "Tyvek" polymer support.

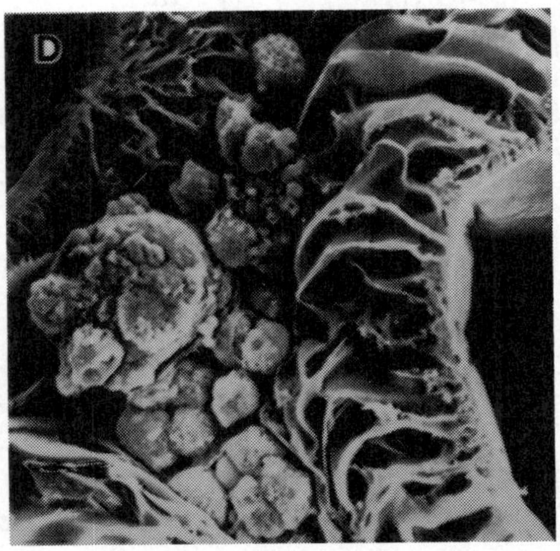

Figure 5d. Scanning electron micrograph of adult rat hepatocytes at 24 hours of culture showing cells growing in the inter-capillary space between three Amicon artificial capillary bundles.

VI. CONCLUSION

The concept of a bioartificial liver is tantalizing, and its ultimate feasibility almost beyond doubt. Yet the production of a therapeutically effective liver substitute faces formidable obstacles. The quantity of liver tissue to be cultured to achieve a "man size" biological reactor is much larger than needed for a hybrid endocrine organ. As a cell type, the hepatocyte is notoriously difficult to maintain in a full functional state for more than a few days. The immune protection of the graft by permselective membranes will be difficult because several key hepatic functions involve the transport of large molecular weight chemical species.

Thus we clearly have a long way to go. A better appreciation of the polymer properties which favor hepatocyte attachment differentiation and growth is still needed, but protocols to address these issues can now be formulated. A better understanding of the biological variables which underlie the functional ability of cultured hepatocytes is a key requirement, but converging information from a wide range of research programs is likely to facilitate progress. In short, the elements of a promising biotechnology have been outlined; the clinical need is acute. Progress is bound to come.

REFERENCES

1. Blouin, A.; Bolender, L. P. and Weisel, E. R. Distribution of organelles and membranes between hepatocytes and non-hepatocytes in the rat liver parenchyme. J. Cell Biol.72:441; 1977.
2. Trey, C.; Davidson, C.S. The management of fulminant hepatic failure. Progress in Liver Diseases, Vol. III:282. Popper, H.; Schafner, F. eds. Grunne & Stratton, New York; 1970.
3. Williams, K. The need for artificial liver support. Proc. of Internatl. Symposium on Artificial Support Systems for Acute Heptatic Failure:3. Williams, R.; Murray-Lyon, J.M. eds. Pitman Med. Pub., Tunbridge Wells, Kent, U.K.; 1975.
4. Zieve, L. Hepatic encephalopathy: Summary of present knowledge with an elaboration on recent developments. Progress in Liver Diseases:327-339. Popper & Schaffner, eds. New York; 1979.
5. Schiff, L. Diseases of the Liver, J. B. Lippincott, Pennsylvania; 1975.
6. Wright, R.; Alberti, K. G. M. M.; Karran, S.; Willward-Sadler, G. H. eds. Liver and Biliary Disease, W. B. Saunders Co., Ltd., Pennsylvania; 1979.
7. Hume, D. M.; Gayle, W. E. Jr.; and Williams, G. M. Cross circulation of patients in hepatic coma with baboon partners having human blood. Surg. Gynecol. Obst. 128:195; 1969.
8. Abouna, G. M. Cross circulation between man and baboon in hepatic coma. Lancet 2:729; 1968.
9. Hollander, D.; Klebanoff, G. and Osteer, R. T. Human-baboon cross circulation for treatment of hepatic coma. JAMA 218:67; 1971.
10. Burnell, J. M.; Dawborn, J. K.; Epstein, R. B.; Gutman, R. A.; Leinbach, G. E.; Rhomas, E. D. and Volwiler, W. Acute hepatic coma treated by cross circulation or exchange transfusion. N. Engl. J. Med. 276:935; 1967.
11. Muller, J. M.; Guignier, M.; Motin, J.; Paliard, P.; and Debru, J. L. Notre experience de la circulation croisee comme method d'assistance hepatique dans les insuffisances hepatiques graves aigues. Ann. Med. Intern. 122:581; 1971.
12. Fennimore, J.; Watson, P.A.; Munro, G. D.; and Kolthammer, J. C. The design and evaluation of a convenient carbon haemoperfusion system. Eur. Soc. Artif. Organs, 1:90; 1975.
13. Rosenbaum, J. L.; Kramer, M. S.; Raja, R. Resin Haemoperfusion for acute drug intoxication. Arch. Text. Med. 136:263; 1976.
14. Silk, D.B.A.; Trewby, P.N.; Chase, R.A. Treatment of fulminant hepatic failure by polyacrylonitrile membrane haemodialysis. Lancet 2:1; 1977.
15. Malchesky, P. S.; Ouchi, K.; Piatkiewicz, W.; and Nose, Y. Membrane Plasma filtration systems with multiple reactors for hepatic support. Artif. Organs 2 (Suppl.):265; 1978.
16. Opolon, P.; Huguet, C.; Granger, A.; Gallot, D.; Bloch, P.; and Bidallier, M. Comparison of single and cross-haemodyalysis with a donor through cuprophan and a new polymer membrane. Proc. of Int. Symp. on Artif. Support System for Acute Hepatic Failure. Page 186. Williams, R.; Murray,

J. M., eds. Pitman Med. Pub., Tunbridge Wells, Kent, U.K.; 1975.

17. Trey C.; Burns, D.; Sanders, S. Treatment of Hepatic coma by exchange blood transfusions. N. Engl. J. Med. 274:473; 1966.
18. Saunders, S. F.; Hickman, R.; Terblanche, T. The treatment of acute liver failure. Progress of Liver Diseases, Vol. IV:333. Popper, H.; Schaffner, F., eds. Grunne & Stratton, New York; 1972.
19. Opolon, P.; Lavallard, M.; Huguet, C.; Bidallier, M.; Granger, A.; Gallot, D.; Bloch, P. Hemodialysis versus cross hemodialysis in experimental hepatic coma. Surgery, Gynecology and Obstetrics, 142:845; 1976.
20. Oplon, P. High permeability membrane hemodialysis in acute hepatic coma; Experimental and clinical results; Proceedings of the Second Int. Symposium for Artif. Organs.
21. Weston, M. J.; Gazzard, B. G.; Buxton, B. H.; Winch, J.; Machado, A.; Flax, H.; Williams, R. Effects of Haemoperfusion through charcoal or XAD-2 resin on an animal model of fulminant hepatic failure. GUT 15:482; 1974.
22. Chang, T. M. S. Removal of endogenous and exogenous toxins by a microencapsulated absorbent. Canadian J. of Phys. and Pharm. 47:1043; 1969.
23. Gazzard, B. G.; Weston, M. J.; Murray-Lyon, I. M.; Flax, H.; Record, C. O., et al. Charcoal haemoperfusion in the treatment of fulminant hepatic failure. Lancet 1:1301; 1974.
24. Courtney, J. M.; Fairweather, I. A.; Gilchrist, T.; Hood, R. G.; Park, C. B.; and Smith, E. M. The design of a polymer coating for activated carbons. Artif. Organs, pp. 133-138. Kenedi, Courtney, Gaylor and Gilchrist, eds. Macmillan, London; 1977.
25. Weston, M. J.; Langley, P. G.; Rubin, M. H.; Hanid, M. A.; Mellon, P. J. and Williams, P. Platelet function in fulminant hepatic failure and effect of charcoal haemoperfusion. Gut 18:897; 1977.
26. Castino, F.; Scheuscher, K.; Malchesky, P. S.; Koshino, I.; Nose, Y. Micro-emboli-free blood detoxification utilizing plasma filtration. Trans. Am. Soc. Artif. Int. Organs, 22:637; 1976.
27. Sideman, S.; Mor, L. and Brandes, J. M. Removal of bilirubin by hemoperfusion with ion exchange resins. Trans. Am. Soc. Artif. Int. Org. 25:497; 1979.
28. Cuatrecasas, P. The insulin receptor. Diabetes 21 (Suppl. 2):396; 1972.
29. Dial, L. D.; Miamoto, S.; Arquilla, E. R. Modulation of 125 I-insulin degradation by receptors in liver plasma membranes. Biochem. Biophys. Res. Communications 74:545; 1977.
30. Leffert, H.; Alexander, N. M.; Faloona, G.; Rubalcava, F.; Unger, R. Specific endocrine and hormonal receptor changes associated with liver regeneration in adult rat. Proc. Nat. Acad. Sci. USA 72:4033; 1975.
31. Accatino, L.; Simon, F. R. Identification and characterization of a bile acid receptor in isolated liver surface membranes. J. Clinic. Invest. 57:496; 1976.
32. Korenbrot, J. T. Ion transport in membranes. Incorporation of biological ion-translocating proteins in model membrane systems. Ann. Rev. Physiol. 39:19; 1977.
33. Beus, R.; Langer, P.; Janko, L. Transport kinetics of hydrophobic ions in lipid bilayer membranes. Charge-pulses relaxation studies. Biochem. Biophys. Act. 455:701; 1976.
34. Denti, E.; Freston, J. W.; Marchisio, M. and Kolff, W. J. Toward a bioartificial drug metabolizing system: gel immobilized liver cell microsomes. Trans. Am. Soc. Artif. Int. Orgn. 22:693; 1976.
35. Mikami, J.; Mito, M.; Nishimura, A.; Sasaki, E.; Nose, Y. and Tedo, I. Surgical treatment of acute liver failure. II. An experimental study of extracorporeal metabolism in the artificial liver using slices of canine liver. Jap. J. Gastroenterol. 56:1022; 1959.
36. Koshino, I.; Sakamoto, H.; Shiada, Y.; Tsuji, Y.; Kawamata, T.; Matsushita, M.; Kon, T. and Kasai, Y. Use of liver slices for an artificial liver. Trans. Am. Soc. Artif. Int. Org. 25:493; 1979.
37. Chick, W.; Like, A. A. and Lauris, V. Beta cell culture on sythetic capillaries: an artificial endocrine pancreas. Science 187:847; 1975.
38. Chick, W. L.; Perna, J. J.; Lauris, V.; Low, D.; Galletti, P. M.; Panol, G.; Whittemore, A. D.; Like, A. A.; Colton, C. K. and Lysaght, M. J. Artificial pancreas using living beta cells: effects on glucose haemostasis in diabetic rats. Science 197:780; 1977.

39. Altman, J. J.; Manoux, A.; Callard, P.; Houlbert, D.; Desplanque, N.; Bruzzo, F.; Galletti, P. Successful pancreatic xenografts using semipermeable membranes. Artif. Organs 5(4):1; 1981.
40. Michalopoulos, G.; Sattler, G. L.; and Pitot, H. C. Hormonal regulation and the effects of glucose on tyrosine aminotransferase activity in adult rat hepatocytes cultured on floating collagen membranes. Lancet Res. 38:1550; 1978.
41. Richman, R. A.; Claus, T. H.; Pilkis, T. T.; and Friedman, D. L. Hormonal stimulation of DNA synthesis in primary cultures of adult rat hepatocytes. Proc. Nat. Acad. Sci. 73:3589; 1976.
42. Knazek, R. A.; Gullino, P. M.; Kohler, P. O.; Dedrick, R. L. Cell culture on artificial capillaries: an approach to tissue growth in vitro. Science 178:65; 1972.
43. Wolf, C. F. W. and Munkelt, B. E. Bilirubin Conjugation by an artificial liver composed of cultured cells and synthetic capillaries. Trans. Am. Soc. Artif. Int. Org. 21:16; 1975.
44. Staedel, C.; Beck, J. P. Resurgency of glycogen synthesis and storage capacity in cultured hepatoma cells. Cell Differentiation 7:61; 1978.
45. Welch, C. L.; Wood, R. Lipids of cultured hepatoma cells: VIII-Utilization of D-(1-14C) glucose for lipid biosynthesis. Lipids 12(3):245; 1977.
46. Weinhouse, S. National Cancer Act of 1971 – an editorial. Cancer Res. 32: i-ii; 1972.
47. Bissell, D. M.; Guzelian, P. S. Microsomal functions and phenotipic change in adult rat hepatocytes in primary monolayer culture. Page 119. Gerchenson, L. E. and Thompson, E. B., eds. Academic Press, New York, 1975.
48. Bissell, D. M.; Hammaker, L.; Meyer, U. A. Parenchymal cells from adult rat liver in nonproliferating monolayer culture. I. Functional studies. J. Cell Biology 59:722; 1973.
49. Nakamura, T.; Kumegawa, M. Induction of key glycolytic enzymes by insulin in mouse fetal liver cultured in a circumfusion system. Biochem. Biophys. Res. Comm. 51:474; 1973.
50. Koch, K.; Leffert, H. L. Growth control of differentiated fetal rat hepatocytes in primary monolayer culture. VI. Studies with conditioned medium and its functional interactions with serum factors. J. Cell Biol. 62:780; 1974.
51. Acosta, D.; Anuforo, D. C.; Smith, R. U. Primary monolayer cultures of postnatal rat liver cells with extended differentiated functions. In Vitro 14:428; 1978.
52. Hager, J. C.; Carman, R.; Stoller, R.; Panol, G.; Leduc, E. H.; Thayer, W. R.; Porter, L. E.; Galletti, P. M.; Calabresi, P. A. A prototype for a hybrid artificial liver. Trans. Am. Soc. Artif. Inter. Organs 24:250; 1978.
53. Howard, R. B.; Christensen, A. K.; Gibbs, F. A.; Pesch, L. A. The enzymatic preparation of isolated intact parenchymal cells from rat liver. J. Cell. Biol. 35:675; 1967.
54. Berry, M. N. and Friend, D. S. High-yield preparation of isolated rat liver parenchymal cells: a biochemical and fine structural study. J. Cell Biol. 43:506; 1969.
55. Wagle, S. R.; Ingebretsen, W. In Methods in Enzymology. Vol. 35 Lipids. Lowestein, J. M., ed. New York Acad. Press, page 579; 1974.
56. Seglen, P. O. Preparation of rat liver cells. II. Effects of ion and chelators on tissue dispersion. Exp. Cell Res. 76:25; 1973.
57. Jauregui, H. O.; Hayner, N.; Laliberte, R.; Lipski, M.; McMillan, P. and Galletti, P. M. Procurement of hepatocytes for a hybrid artificial liver. Trans. Am. Soc. Artif. Intern. Organs 25:487; 1979.
58. Seglen, P. O. Preparation of rat liver cells. III. Enzymatic requirements for tissue dispersion. Exp. Cell Res. 82:391; 1973.
59. Guzelian, P. S.; Diegelman, R. F. Retention of clostridial collagenase by parenchymal cells prepared from adult rat liver. Life Sci. 24:513; 1979.
60. Pertoft, H.; Rubin, K.; Kjellan, L.; Laurent, T. C. and Klingeborn, B. The viability of cells grown or centrifuged in a new density gradient medium, Percoll (TM). Exp. Cell Res. 110:449; 1977.
61. Seglen, P. O. Preparation of isolated rat liver cells. Methods. Cell Biol. 13:29; 1976.
62. Quistorff, B.; Bondensen, S.; Grunnet, N. Preparation and biochemical characterization of parenchymal cells from rat liver. Biochem. Biophys. Act. 320:503; 1973.

63. East, A. G.; Louis, L. N.; Hoffenber, P. Albumin synthesis by isolated rat liver cells. Exp. Cell Res. 76:41; 1973.
64. Jeejeebhoy, K. N.; Phillips, M. J. Isolated mammalian hepatocytes in culture. Gastroenterology 71:1086; 1976.
65. Stern, R. Experimental Aspects of Hepatic Fibrosis. Page 173. Popper, H., Schaffner, F., eds. Progress in liver diseases volume VI. Grunne & Stratton, New York; 1979.
66. Rojkind, M. S.; Gatmaitan, Z.; Mackensen, S.; Giambrone, M.; Ponce, P. and Reid, L. Connective tissue biomatrix: its isolation and utilization for long-term cultures of normal rat hepatocytes. J. Cell Biol. 87:255; 1980.
67. Rubin, K.; Johansson, S.; Hook, M.; Obrink, B. Substrate adhesion of rat hepatoctyes. Exp. Cell Res. 135:127; 1981.
68. Laishes, B. A.; Williams, G. M. Conditions affecting primary cell cultures of functional adult rat hepatocytes. I. The effect of insulin. In Vitro 12:521; 1976.
69. Laishes, B. A.; Williams, G. M. Conditions affecting primary cell cultures of functional adult rat hepatocytes. II. Dexamethasone enhanced longevity and maintenance of morphology. In Vitro 12:821; 1976.
70. Rubin, K.; Johansson, S.; Hook, M. and Obrink, B. Substrate adhesion of rat hepatocytes. Exp. Cell Res. 135:127; 1981.
71. Altman, T. T.; Panol, G.; Hayner, N.; Galletti, P. M. Oxygen requirements of freshly isolated cells for hybrid artificial organs. Proc. Europ. Soc. Artif. Organs 6:282; 1979.
72. Gebhardt, R.; Bellemann, P. and Mecke, D. Metabolic and enzymatic characteristics of adult rat liver parenchymal cells in non-proliferating primary monolayer cultures. Exp. Cell Res. 112:431; 1978.
73. Michalopoulus, G.; Pitot, H. C. Primary culture of parenchymal liver cells on collagen membranes. Exp. Cell Res. 94:70; 1975.
74. Savage, C. R. Jr.; Bonney, R. J. Extended expression of differentiated function in primary cultures of adult liver parenchymal cells maintained on nitrocellulose filters. I. Induction of phosphoenolpyruvate carboxkinase and tryrosine aminotransferase. Exp. Cell Res. 114:307; 1978.
75. Bissell, D. M.; Guzelian, P. S. Phenotypic stability of adult rat hepatocytes in primary monolayer culture – Differentiation and carcinogens in liver cell cultures. Ann. N.Y. Acad. Sci. 349:85; 1980.
76. Reed, G. B.; Grisham, T. W. Insulin and hydrocortisone effects on viability and glycogen stores of postnatal liver organ culture. Lab. Invest. 33:298; 1975.
77. Freychet, P.; Roth, J.; Neville, D. M. Jr. Insulin receptors in the liver: specific binding of (125 I) insulin to the plasma membrane and its relation to insulin bioactivity. Proc. Nat. Acad. Sci. USA 68:1833; 1971.
78. Van Obberglen, E.; DeMeyts, P.; Roth, J. Cell surface receptors for insulin and human growth hormone. Effect of microtubule and microfilament modifiers. J. Biol. Chem. 251:6844; 1976.
79. Jauregui, H. O.; McMillan, P.; Naik, S.; Pajarillo, F.; Lipsky, M. Lectin binding to hepatocyte surfaces – In preparation.
80. Witters, L. A.; Alberico, L.; Avruck, J. Insulin regulation of glycogen synthase in the isolated rat heptocyte. Biochem. Biophys. Res. Comm. 69:997; 1976.
81. Tanaka, K. M.; Sato, M.; Tourita, Y. and Ichihara, A. Biochemical studies on liver functions in primary cultured hepatocytes of adult rats. I. Hormonal effects on cell viability and protein synthesis. J. Biochem. (Tokyo) 84:937; 1978.
82. Tanaka, K. K.; Kishi, K. and Ichihara, A. Biochemical studies on liver functions in primary cultured hepatocytes of adult rats. II. Regulation of protein and amino acid metabolism. J. Biochem. (Tokyo) 86:863; 1979.
83. Williams, G. M.; Bermudez, E.; San, R. H. C.; Goldblatt, P. J.; Laspia, M. F. Rat hepatocyte primary cultures. IV. Maintenance in defined medium and the role of production of plasminogen activator and other proteases. In Vitro 14:824; 1978.

84. Schwarze, P. E.; Solheim, A. E.; Seglen, P. O. Amino acids and energy requirements for rat hepatocytes in primary culture. In Vitro 18:43; 1982.
85. Marcian, N.; Noel, M.; and Deschenes, T. Growth and functional activities of neonatal and adult rat hepatocytes cultured on fibronectin coated substratum in serum-free medium. In Vitro 18:1; 1982.
86. Seglen, P. O. Autoregulation of glycolysis, respiration gluconeogenesis and glycogen synthesis in isolated parenchymal rat liver cells under aerobic and anaerobic conditions. Biochem. Biophys. Acta. 338:317; 1974.
87. Bissell, D. M.; Levine, G. A.; Bissell, M. J. Glucose metabolism by adult hepatocytes in primary culture and by cell lines from rat liver. Am. J. Physiol. 234:C122; 1978.
88. Williams, G. M.; Bermudez, E.; Scaramuzzino, D. Rat hepatocytes primary cell cultures. III. Improved dissociation and attachment techniques and the enhancement of survival by culture medium. In Vitro 13:809; 1977.
89. Wagle, S. R. Interrelationship of insulin and glucagon ratios on carbohydrate metabolism in isolated hepatocytes containing high glycogen. Biochem. Biophys. Res. Comm. 67:1019; 1975.
90. Leffert, H. L.; Moran, T.; Boorstein, R.; Koch, K. S. Procarcinogen activation and hormonal control of cell proliferation in differentiated primary adult rat liver cell cultures. Nature 267:58; 1977.
91. Michaels, A. S. U.S. Patent 3615024, High Flow Membranes, October 26, 1971.
92. Cross, R. W. U. S. Patent 3691068, September 12, 1972.
93. Baker, R. W. U.S. Patent No. 3567810, March 2, 1971.
94. Knazek, R. A.; Gullino, P. M.; Frankel, D. S. Dual circuit woven artificial capillary bundle for cell culture. U.S. Patent H184922, January 22, 1980.
95. Houck, J. C. Chalones: Concepts & Researches. Introduction. p. 1-4. Bullough, W. S. Chalones: Concepts & Current Researches. Chalones: A Review. p. 5-15. Forscher, B. K. and Houck, J. C., eds. Nat'l Cancer Instit. Monograph 38: 1973.
96. Solomon, B. A.; Chen, C. -C. and Colton, C. C. Novel methods for the immobilization of acetate kinase on anisotropic hollow fibers and solid care polymeric beads. Poster paper at 4th International Enzyme Engineering Conference, Bad Neucnahr, W. Germany, September 1971.
97. Pitt, A. M.; Terman, D. S.; Colton, C. K. and Solomon, B. A. Extracorporeal removal of immune complexes: Preparation and characterization of immobilized bovine conglutinin. Int. J. Artif. Org. 3:42; 1981.
98. Adalsteinsson, O.; Lamotte, A.; Baddour, R. F.; Colton, C. K.; Pollak, A. and Whitesides, G. M. Preparation and magnetic filtrationof polyacrylamide gels containing covalently immobilized proteins and a ferro fluid. J. Mol. Catalysis, 6:199; 1979.
99. Takahama, T.; Yamazaki, Z.; Iizuka, I.; Kanai, F.; Wada, T.; Fujimori, Y.; Asano, K.; Inoue, N.; Sonoda, T.; Nogi, T. and Kimura, M. Continuous plasma cross circulation after total hepatectomy in dogs. Int. Symp. on Plasmapheresis, April 1982, to be published. Int. Soc. for Artif. Organs.
100. Carey, W. D. Treatment of chronic liver disease by plasma detoxification. Int. Symp. on Plasmapheresis, April 1982, to be published. Int. Soc. for Artif. Organs.

Sources of Funding:

NIH Grant HL-11945-11
NIH Grant 1-R01-AM26520-01 A1

Chapter 40

Development and In Vivo Testing of an Artificial Endocrine Pancreas

A. M. Sun, Ph.D., G. M. O'Shea, Ph.D., M. F. A. Goosen, Ph.D.
Connaught Research Institute
1755 Steeles Avenue West
Willowdale, Ontario, Canada

ABSTRACT

A bioartificial pancreas has been developed consisting of living pancreatic islets of Langerhans cultured on the outside surface of semi-permeable tubular membranes. When the device was attached as an arterio-venous shunt in unheparinized diabetic animals, such as monkeys, their blood glucose levels dropped to normal for up to 6 days. The biocompatibility of the device was increased by coating the inner surface of the tubular membrane with a blood-compatible heparin-polyvinyl alcohol film.

A second type of bioartificial pancreas, consisting of microencapsulated islets of Langerhans, was also developed. With this sytem, individual viable islets are completely enclosed within a semi-permeable membrane. A single intraperitoneal injection of viable encapsulated islets lowered the blood glucose levels of diabetic rats for up to two months. The encapsulation technique offers the advantage of not requiring surgery for implantation or shunt connection, therefore, reducing the risks of clotting or infection.

Bioartificial pancreas devices have great clinical potential for providing diabetic patients with functional islets which could supply insulin, glucagon, somatostatin, and possibly other unknown chemicals in response to natural physiological demand. In principle, such devices could alleviate all of the disease symptoms of diabetes and constitute a virtual cure.

I. INTRODUCTION

Since the discovery of insulin by Banting and Best six decades ago the lives of millions of diabetics have been prolonged through the injection of exogenous insulin [1]. Insulin therapy, however, often does not prevent the development of chronic complications associated with diabetes, such as retinopathy, neuropathy, nephropathy and premature atherosclerosis. These complications are responsible for the high morbidity and mortality rates in diabetics. It can be postulated that intermittent administration of insulin does not mimic the on-off response to physiologic demand (as is experienced with competent islets of Langerhans) and so results in failure to control the other complications associated with the disease. In addition, islets of Langerhans may have some, as yet undiscovered, functions in regulating the metabolism of vascular and neural tissues.

A promising approach which could effectively cure and prevent the onset of complications is, supplementation of the diabetic's defective endocrine pancreas with a normally functioning transplant. Animal experiments have shown that successful transplantation of synergic islets has a beneficial effect in reversing the kidney and eye damage associated with diabetes [2,3]. However, the problem of immunorejection of the genetically foreign islet cells or organs is a major obstacle.

In this chapter we describe the development and in vivo testing of two types of artificial endocrine pancreas (AEP). With one type, islets are cultured outside a semi-permeable hollow fiber through which small molecules such as glucose and insulin can diffuse freely but large molecules, such as antibodies cannot. The second type of AEP consists of microencapsulated islets wherein individual viable islets are completely enclosed within a semi-permeable membrane. With both such units in which the islets are sequestered from the antibodies responsible for rejection, immunorejection may be overcome.

II. VIABILITY OF ISOLATED ISLETS OF LANGERHANS

To assess the viability and physiologic competence of isolated rat islets and the passage of insulin through the fiber wall, islets were incubated in an AEP unit (capillary fiber bundle unit, see section III for details). The device, containing islets, was perfused with medium CMRL 1969 supplemented with 7.5% fetal calf serum [7]. Samples of the circulating medium from the AEP unit were analyzed for insulin content using a radioimmunoassay method [4]. Islets were isolated from rat pancreata by a conventional collagenase digestion technique and incubated in medium before being transferred to the AEP [5,6].

When islets were cultivated for a prolonged period in the AEP, in the presence of high levels of glucose (300 mg/dl), they remained alive and functional for up to 260 days (Figure 1). The longest survival time for islets cultivated in the presence of low glucose levels (100 mg/dl) was less than 60 days.

Tze and Chen, in a similar study, cultured rat islets in artificial capillary units which were perfused with nutrient medium [8]. In their culture system, the islets remained functioning for at least 97 days. Chick et al. have grown beta cells on the outside surfaces of bundles of hollow fibers [9]. The fibers were perfused with tissue culture medium containing fetal bovine serum and glucose. Their data indicated that the isolated beta cells continued to synthesize, store and release insulin. Although insulin release into the culture medium gradually diminished, measureable quantities of insulin were still being produced after as long as one year.

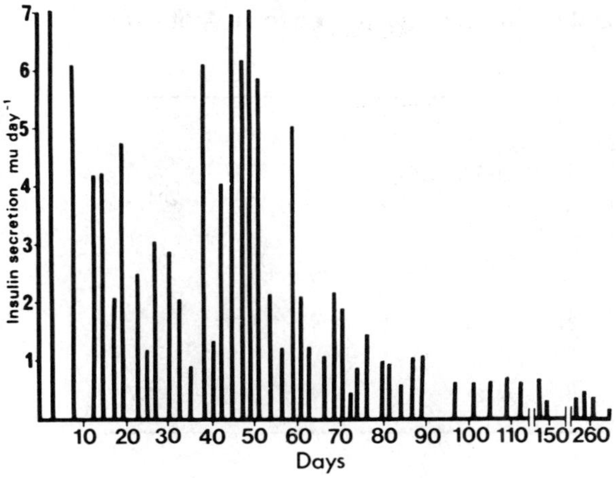

Figure 1. Insulin Release from Islets Cultivated in an Artificial Endocrine Pancreas Unit. One hundred islets were inoculated into the units (see text for the structure of the device), which were perfused with 30 ml of medium CMRL-1969 supplemented with 7.5% fetal calf serum. A high glucose concentration (300 mg/dl) was used after 38 days of cultivation.

In summary, these studies demonstrated that isolated islets and beta cells can be kept alive and functioning in vitro for several months.

III. CAPILLARY FIBER BUNDLE AEP UNIT

The earliest device developed in our laboratory consisted of bundles of capillary hollow fibers (Amicon P-100, 0.50 mm I.D., Amicon Corporation), Figure 2. The fibers are permeable to substances with a molecular weight less than 100,000 daltons. Twenty P-100 fibers were sealed into the ends of an acrylic-plastic jacket with two ports, through which 1,000 to 1,500 islets were injected for rat experiments and 6,000 to 10,000 islets for monkey studies. The seeded islets lodged on the surface of the fibers. Medium was circulated through the interior of the fibers by means of a peristaltic pump (Gilson Millipore II) [10] for two to three days before attachment of the AEPs to the rats and for two to three weeks before attachment to the monkeys.

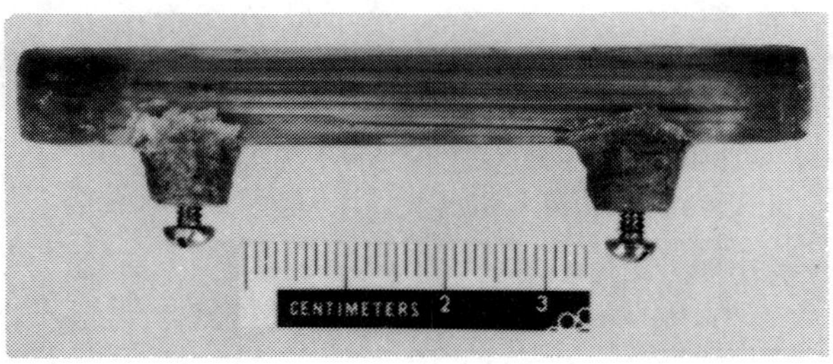

Figure 2. Capillary Fiber Bundle Unit. The AEP unit was fabricated with bundles of capillary hollow fibers and an acrylic-plastic jacket. Islets of Langerhans were inoculated through one of the two ports into the chamber outside the fibers.

When the capillary bundle unit, containing rat islets, was attached as an ex-vivo arteriovenous shunt in streptozotocin-induced diabetic rats, a significant decrease in their blood glucose levels was detected throughout the 48 hour observation period (Table 1, Group A). The blood glucose concentrations in these animals were lowered from an average of 448 mg/dl to 132 mg/dl within the first hour. The levels remained low throughout the remainder of the experimental period. In contrast, when the AEP unit without islets was attached to diabetic rats, Group B, or normal rats, Group C, there was no significant change in the blood glucose levels. With the former group, high blood glucose levels were observed throughout the experiments. All animals received a continuous infusion of heparin while connected to the capillary bundle AEP units.

Table 1. Blood Glucose Levels in Normal and Diabetic Rats Attached to an Artificial Endocrine Pancreas (AEP) Mean ± S.E., n = 6

GROUP	HOURS	0	0.25	0.5	1	2	4	8	18
					Blood glucose - mg/dl				
(A)	Diabetic monkey (AEP with rat islets)	242	185	157	135	112	90	127	204
(B)	Diabetic monkey (control)	157	--	--	280	332	266	353	400
					Blood insulin - μU/ml of serum				
(A)		2	74	93	32	18	15	17	32
(B)		3.1	--	--	4.2	2.5	5.4	6.9	4.7

In monkey experiments, the capillary bundle AEP device was connected to the femoral artery and vein. When the AEP unit containing perfused rat islets was attached to each of these diabetic monkeys, blood glucose levels dropped from 242 mg/dl before attachment of the AEP to 185 mg/dl in 15 minutes and to 90 mg/dl in four hours (Table 2). Serum insulin concentration reached 74 and 93 uU/ml in 15 and 30 minutes, respectively. These early results indicted that insulin released from rat islets in the AEP can modify the hyperglycemic state in both diabetic rats and monkeys. It is also interesting to note that the results of experiments on rats with capillary AEP units, as reported by Tze et al. [11] and Whittemore et al. [12], were in general agreement with those reported by our laboratory [13].

Table 2. Blood Glucose and Insulin Levels in Diabetic Monkeys With and Without Artificial Endocrine Pancreas (AEP) n =3

GROUP	HOURS	0	0.25	0.5	1	4	10	18	24	48
					Blood glucose (mg/dl)					
(A)	Diabetic rats (AEP unit with islets)	448 ±49	--	280 ±40	132 ±28	120 ±19	152 ±21	266 ±32	182 ±27	141 ±18
(B)	Diabetic rats	469 ±58	437 ±65	605 ±40	540 ±38	386 ±32	428 ±41	302 ±40	389 ±51	292 ±29
(C)	Normal Rats	138 ±11	162 ±16	190 ±17	152 ±16	--	--	--	147 ±11	118 ±20

In groups B and C the animals were connected to AEP units without islets.

While blood clotting in the fiber lumen was still a major problem these initial studies indicated that when the AEP device was implanted as an arteriovenous shunt in the vascular system of diabetic rats and monkeys, glucose homeostasis could be restored essentially to normal.

IV. SINGLE FIBER AEP UNIT

With the primary objective of overcoming the problem of thrombosis, more recent devices were fabricated by inserting single lengths of larger diameter fiber (Amicon XM-50, 1.1 mm I.D. and 1.5 mm I.D. nominal molecular weight cut-off of 50,000) into cylindrical plexiglass chambers. The units varied from a long cylinder shown in Figure 3A, to the fairly flat (cylindrically) shaped chamber shown in Figure 3B. In order to make the fiber more blood compatible the lumen was coated with a thin heparin-polyvinyl alcohol (PVA) film using an established procedure [14,15]. The heparin-PVA coating which is also a hydrogel, was found to be irreversibly bound to the fiber surface. The elution rate of heparin from the surface when washed with isotonic saline at pH 7.4 or citrated human plasma was found to be negligible (below the detectable limit of 10^{-4} $\mu g/cm^2/minute$). The heparin-PVA coating does not significantly alter the permeability properties of the fiber with respect to glucose and insulin diffusion.

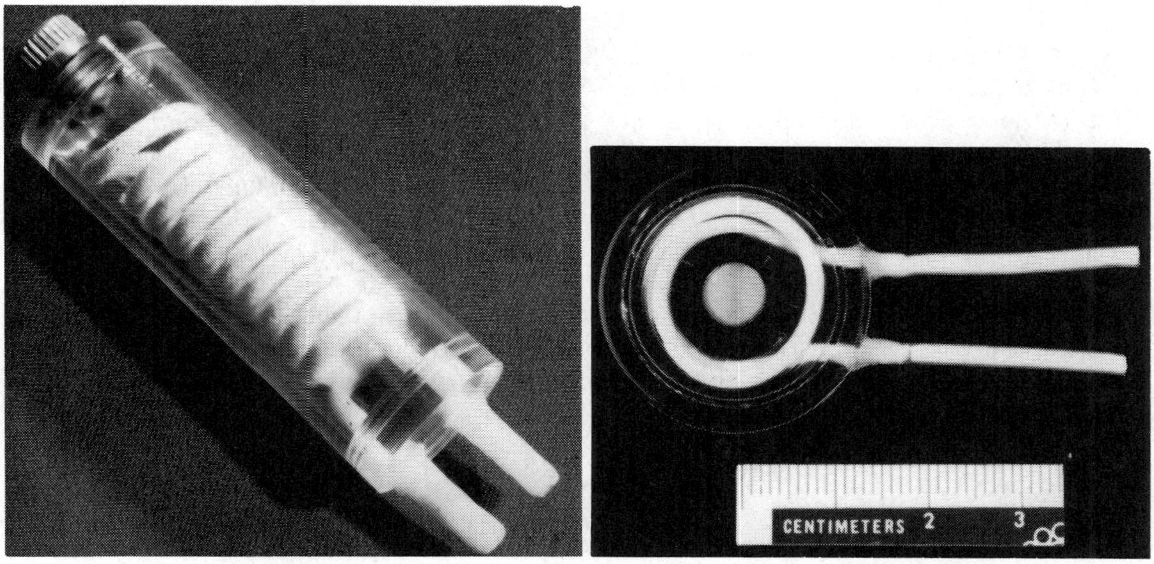

(a) (b)

Figure 3A and 3B. Single Fiber AEP Units. Implantable artificial pancreas units fabricated from single lengths of Amicon hollow fiber. Islets of Langerhans were inoculated through the center ports into the chamber outside the fiber. The units varied from a long cylinder shape, Figure 3A, to the fairly flat shaped chamber shown in Figure 3B.

In animal experiments, the heparin-PVA coated AEP unit (Figure 3B) containing $12 - 15 \times 10^3$ rat islets was attached to each of four unheparinized diabetic monkeys. In all monkeys, hyperglycemia was corrected within two hours. Polyphagia, polydypsia and polyuria were all brought under control, and the monkeys became normally active. In each of three monkeys, the device maintained its functional capacity for two, four and five days, respectively, and in one experiment the unit retained its activity for six days (Figure 4). The blood glucose concentration in this diabetic animal was lowered from 320 mg/dl to 126 mg/dl in two hours. The level remained normal until the sixth day, when it increased to 275 mg/dl. The serum insulin concentration increased from 4 uU/ml before implantation to 42 uU/ml after 4 hours and remained elevated until the unit was removed. Upon removal, the implant was inspected for damage. It was found that a thrombus had formed at the junction of the blood vessel and the fiber thus, presumably, occluding the passage of blood through the device. However, no thrombosis was observed within the fiber itself in any of the four AEPs implanted.

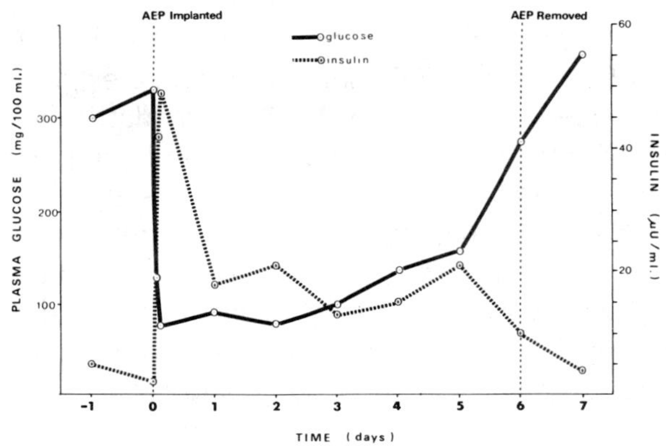

Figure 4. Plasma Glucose and Serum Insulin Levels of a Diabetic Monkey Connected to an AEP Unit. An artificial endocrine pancreas containing 12 × 10³ rat islets was connected to the femoral artery and vein of a depancreatized monkey. The device was removed on Day 6.

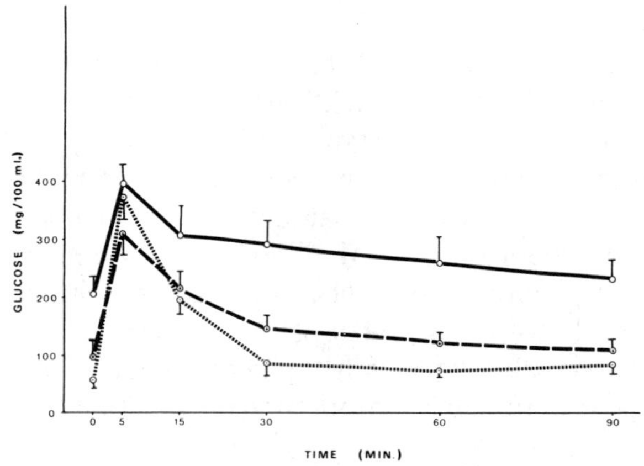

Figure 5. Plasma Glucose Responses in Monkeys Implanted with an AEP. Plasma glucose responses following intravenous glucose (0.5 gm/kg body weight) tolerance tests on four monkeys before (0......0) and after (0–0) pancreatectomy and implantation of an artificial endocrine pancreas containing 12 – 15 × 10³ rat islets (0– – –0) (mean ± S.E.).

Glucose tolerance tests on these animals both pre- and post- pancreatectomy and after implantation with the AEP units showed that improved blood glucose levels (Figure 5) and blood insulin levels (Figure 6) could be achieved in response to a glucose challenge in animals implanted with the AEP.

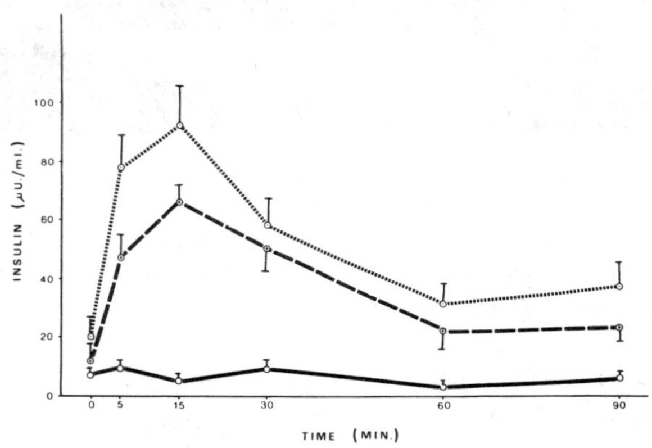

Figure 6. Serum Insulin Responses in Monkeys Implanted with an AEP. Serum insulin responses following intravenous glucose (0.5 gm/kg body weight) tolerance tests in four monkeys before (0.......0) and after (0–0) pancreatectomy and implantation of an artificial endocrine pancreas containing 12 – 15 × 10³ rat islets (0– – –0) (mean ± S.E.).

The AEP device fabricated with a non-heparin-PVA coated fiber remained patent in the monkey for a maximum of a few hours. In experiments with the heparin-PVA coated devices no heparin infusion was employed.

To solve the problem of thrombus formation at the junction of the blood vessel and the AEP, a polyurethane connector was developed and tested in unheparinized dogs. The heparin-PVA coated AEP unit with polyurethane connectors was connected to the femoral artery and vein using microsuture techniques. The results showed that the device remained patent for less than one week with the major problems still occurring at the anastomosis.

Our experiments and studies done by others suggest that silastic arterio-venous (A-V) shunts may provide dependable long-term vascular access for the AEP device [17,18]. Silicone rubber cannulae (2.59 mm I.D. ST-951 and ST-952, Extracorporeal, Markham, Ontario) were implanted as femoral A-V shunts in dogs, and the preliminary results were very promising. Work is presently underway on developing an improved AEP unit by using various semi-permeable tubes with internal diameters greater than 1.5 mm. It is expected that these improvements will significantly increase the patency rate of the single fiber AEP device.

V. MICROENCAPSULATED ISLETS OF LANGERHANS

A second approach to the development of an AEP in this laboratory is the microencapsulation of islets of Langerhans [19,20]. Prolonged survival of islets both in vitro and in vivo has been obtained by using the microencapsulation procedure which comletely encloses viable islets within a semi-permeable membrane. The microcapsular membrane, composed of crosslinked alginate, a nontoxic polysaccharide, polylysine and polyethyleneimine, is permeable to small molecules such as glucose or insulin but totally impermeable to large molecules such as immunoglobulins.

The microencapsulation technique employed can be summarized as follows: Cultured islets were suspended uniformly in a sodium alginate solution in physiological saline. Droplets containing islets were produced by syringe pump extrusion. These islet containing droplets were collected in a calcium chloride solution and coated with polylysine and polyethyleneimine. Finally, they were suspended in isotonic sodium citrate to liquify the alginate gel inside the capsule. The microencapsulated islets were cultured at 37 °C for at least 3 to 4 days before use.

In perifusion experiments, the insulin secretion from the encapsulated islets was comparable with that from the control islets. When the glucose concentration was raised from 50 to 300 mg/dl, for example, there was a biphasic response of insulin release from both groups of islets. However, the encapsulated islets gave a delayed response. This delay could be attributed to the time required for the passage of insulin across the capsular membrane into the medium (Figure 7). The increase in quantity of insulin in the presence of high glucose concentration clearly demonstrated that the viability and function of the cells were retained throughout the process of microencapsulation. It was found that microencapsulated islets remained morphologically and functionally intact for as long as 4 months in culture at 37 °C.

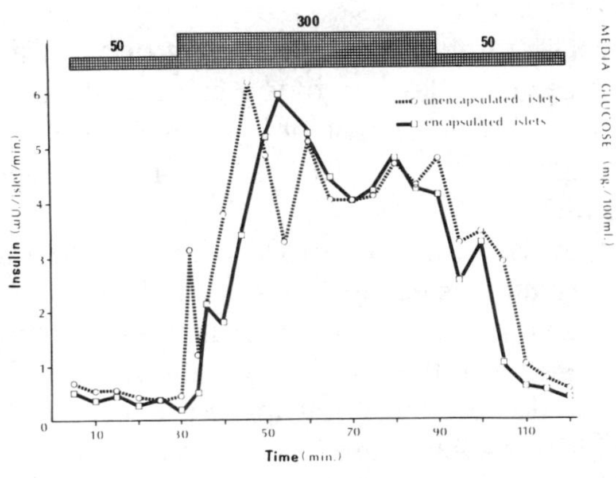

Figure 7. Insulin Release Patterns of Encapsulated and Uncapsulated Islets in Perifusion Study. Both groups showed comparable response to high and low glucose concentrations. Microencapsulated islets appeared to show a slight delay in response initially. The shaded area indicates the level and duration of glucose content (numbers are expressed in milligrams per 100 ml) in the perifusing culture medium.

Experiments were performed to determine whether the encapsulated islets could survive and function in vivo. Wistar Lewis rats were rendered diabetic by an intravenous injection of streptozotocin. The results on intraperitoneal implantation of microencapsulated islets (from Wistar rats) along with suitable controls showed that the unencapsulated islets survived for 6 to 8 days as anticipated. Recipients of microencapsulated islets were normoglycemic for almost 3 weeks (Figure 8); the symptoms of diabetes such as polyuria and polydypsia were markedly reduced.

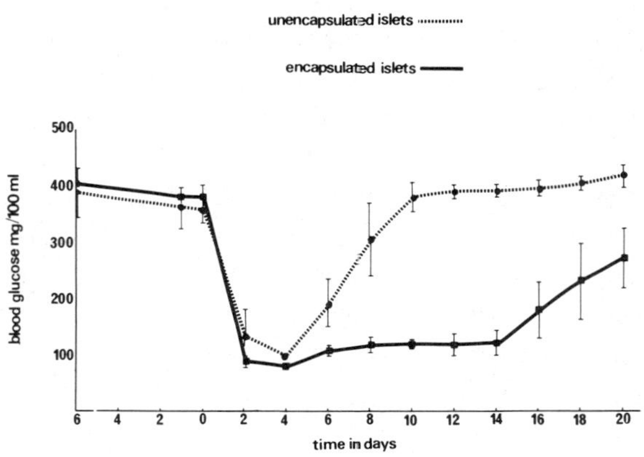

Figure 8. Fasting Blood Glucose Concentrations of Diabetic Rats Before and After Intraperitoneal Transplantation of Unencapsulated and Microencapsulated Islets. A single dose of about 2×10^3 to 3×10^3 microencapsulated islets from Wistar rats was injected into each of five diabetic Wistar Lewis rats 2 weeks after the animals had become diabetic. As controls, five diabetic rats received a transplantation of approximately the same number of unencapsulated islets as the experimental rats. In both situations the blood glucose was returned to normal and remained low for at least 4 days. In the rats that received the unencapsulated islets, the blood glucose increased and by 10 days had risen to the concentration before treatment. In the rats that received the microencapsulated islets, the blood glucose was significantly lower than the controls for 20 days when the experiment was terminated.

Two rats with streptozotocin-induced diabetes received multiple intraperitoneal transplants of approximately 3,000 encapsulated islets. The initial transplants resulted in lowering the blood glucose concentration from > 375 mg/dl to control values (75-150 mg/dl) (Figure 9A). When the animals returned to the diabetic state a second transplant of encapsulated islets was performed and the blood glucose levels were again lowered to within the control range. This pattern was repeated until the animals were sacrificed 90 days after the initial islet transplants. A control group of diabetic rats receiving no transplants or transplants of empty capsules had blood glucose levels higher than 350 mg/dl throughout this study.

The body weight of animals receiving islet transplants increased. In contrast, the body weights of the control diabetic animals did not change significantly over the same period of time.

As is usual in streptozotocin-induced diabetes, the control diabetic animals all developed eye cataracts within 12 weeks of the onset of diabetes. In contrast, the eyes of the two animals receiving multiple islet implants were cataract-free when they were sacrificed at 90 days.

Recently the in vivo viability and function of the encapsulated islets has been extended considerably by modifying the encapsulation procedure. Polyethyleneimine which is not a biocompatible material was omitted, resulting in islets which were coated only with sodium alginate and polylysine. After receiving a single injection of 3,000 encapsulated islets, the blood glucose levels of diabetic rats dropped to normal and remained low for two months as shown in Figure 9B. In contrast, the islets prepared with polyethyleneimine remained viable, in vivo for only two to three weeks (Figure 8 and 9A).

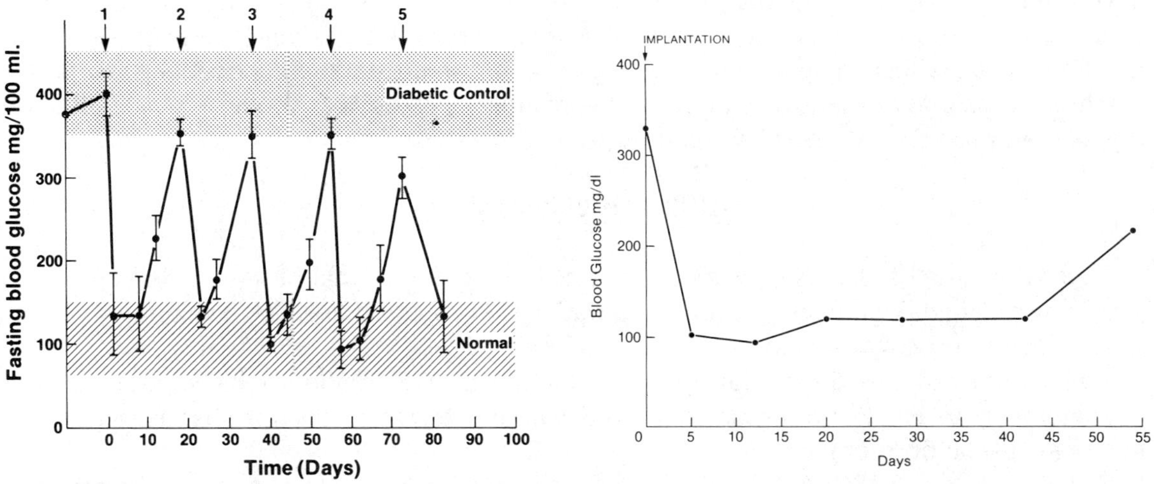

Figure 9A and 9B. Fasting Blood Glucose Levels in Rats Transplanted with Encapsulated Islets. Male Wistar Lewis rats rendered diabetic by i.v. injection of streptozotocin (65 mg/kg) were transplanted with approximately 3,000 encapsulated islets (Wistar donars) on days indicated by arrows. Samples for glucose assay were collected by bleeding through the orbital-sinus complex. The points are mean values from two to four such animals and the bars represent the range. Blood glucose levels in untreated diabetic rats and in normal rats are shown by shaded areas at top and bottom of Figure 9A respectively.

These findings indicate that islet survival and amelioration of the diabetic state can be obtained by intraperitoneal implantation of microencapsulated islets into rats with chemically indiced diabetes. Microencapsulation also provides more options for the method and site of implantation. Unlike the bulky hollow fiber units and diffusion chambers, microcapsules are small enough to pass through a gauge 18 or 19 hypodermic needle.

VI. SUMMARY

Our experiments with rats and monkeys have shown that a hybrid artificial endocrine pancreas (AEP) containing living islets cultured on the outside surface of semi-permeable fibers constitutes an effective means for controlling carbohydrate metabolism in diabetic animals. However, the necessity for continuous heparin injection to prevent blood clotting has made comparable devices inapplicable to human diabetics. In order to devise an implantable AEP which will retain its function for a longer period of time, we have developed a heparin-coated fiber for the AEP. The heparin, although covalently bonded to the lumen of the fiber retains its biological activity and prevents thrombosis.

Thrombosis at the junction of the device and the blood vessel is now the major obstacle which must be overcome before long-term implantation studies can be carried out.

A second approach to the development of an AEP in this laboratory is the microencapsulation of islets of Langerhans. Individual viable islets are completely enclosed within a semi-permeable membrane. In vivo studies with rats have shown that a single intraperitoneal injection of encapsulated islets can lower the blood glucose levels of diabetic rats for up to two months. The process of microencapsulation does not appear to modify the viability or function of the islets. The encapsulation technique offers the advantage of not requiring surgery for implantation or shunt connection, therefore, reducing the risks of clotting or infection.

In conclusion, AEP devices have great clinical potential for providing diabetic patients with functional islets which could supply insulin, glucagon, somatostatin,and possible endorphin in response to natural physiological demand. In principle, such devices should alleviate all of the disease symptoms of diabetes and constitute a virtual cure.

ACKNOWLEDGEMENTS

This work was partially supported by grants from the Industrial Research Assistance Programme of Canada and from Damon Corporation, Massachusetts, U.S.A. We are grateful for their support and encouragement.

We would like to express our appreciation to Dr. D. S. Layne for his support and encouragement, to Dr. P. Vasington for his advice, and to Dr. F. Lim for sharing with us his microencapsulation method.

We wish to thank Mrs. A. Wood, Miss H. van Rooy, Mr. B. Gerrie and Dr. S. Chou for their excellent technical assistance. We also wish to acknowledge the Amicon Corporation for supplying us with the various types of hollow fibers used in this study.

REFERENCES

1. Banting, F. G., Best, C. H., Collip, J. B., MacLeod, J. J. III. The preparation of pancreatic extracts containing insulin. Trans. R. Soc. Can., 16: Sect. V, 27, 1922.
2. Mauer, S. M., Steffes, M. W., Sutherland, D. E. R., Najarian, J. S., Michael, A. F., Brown, D. M. Studies of the rate of regression of the glomerular lesions in diabetic rats treated with pancreatic islet transplantation. Diabetes, 24:280, 1975.
3. Grey, B. N. Prevention of vascular complications of diabetes by pancreatic islet transplantation. Arch. Surg., 111: 254, 1976.
4. Hales, C. N., Randle, P. J. Immunoassay of insulin with insulin-antibody precipitate. Biochem. J., 88: 137, 1963.
5. Lacy, P. E., Kostianovsky, M. Method for the isolation of intact islets of Langerhans from the rat pancreas. Diabetes, 16: 35, 1967.
6. Sun, A. M., Lin, B. J., Haist, R. E. Studies on the conversion of proinsulin to insulin in the isolated islets of Langerhans in the rat. Can. J. Physiol. Pharmacol., 51: 175, 1973.
7. Healy, G. M., Teleki, S., von Seefried, A., Walton, M. J., Macmorine, H. G. Improved chemically defined basal medium (CMRL-1969) for primary monkey kidney and human diploid cells. Appl. Microbiol., 21: 1, 1971.
8. Tze, W. J., Chen, L. M. Long-term survival of adult rat islets of Langerhans in artificial capillary culture units. Diabetes, 26: 185-191, 1977.
9. Chick, W. L., Like, A. A., Lauris, V., Galletti, P. M., Richardson, P. D., Panol, G., Mix, T. W., Colton, C. K. A hybrid artificial pancreas. XXI, T.A.S.A.I.O.: 8-15, 1975.
10. Knazek, R. A., Gullino, P. M., Kohler, P. O., Dedrick, R. L. Cell culture on artificial capillaries: An approach to tissue growth in vitro. Science, 178: 65-67, 1972.
11. Tze, W. J., Wong, F. C., Chen, L. M., O'Young, S. Implantable artificial endocrine pancreas unit used to restore normoglycaemia in the diabetic rat. Nature (Lond), 264: 466-467, 1976.
12. Whittemore, A. D., Chick, W. L., Galletti, P. M., Like, A. A., Colton, C. K., Lysaght, M. J., Richardson, P. D. Effects of the hybrid artificial pancreas in diabetic rats. T.A.S.A.I.O., 23: 336-340, 1977.
13. Sun, A. M., Parisius, W., Healy, G. M., Vacek, I. and Macmorine, H. The use in diabetic rats and monkeys, of artificial capillary units containing cultured islets of Langerhans (artificial endocrine pancreas). Diabetes, 26: 1136-1139, 1977.

14. Goosen, M. F., Sefton, M. V. Heparinized styrene-butadiene-styrene elastomers. J. Biomed. Mater. Res., 13: 347, 1979.
15. Sefton, M. V., Goosen, M. F. A. Irreversible immobilization of heparin for biomaterials. In Chemistry and Biology of Heparin. Lundblad, R. L. (ed.). Symposium at University of North Carolina at Chapel Hill, March 21-22. Dev. in Biochem., 12, Elsevier North Holland, (Publ. 1981): 463-474, 1980.
16. Tze, W. J., Tai, J., Wong, F. C., Davis, H. R. Studies with implantable artificial units containing rat islets on diabetic dogs. Diabetologia, 19: 541-545, 1980.
17. Galletti, P. M., Trudell, L. A., Panol, G., Richardson, P. D., Whittemore, A. Feasibility of small bore A-V shunts for hybrid artificial organs in non-heparinzed beagle dogs. Presented at the XXVII Annual Meeting of the A.S.A.I.O., 1981.
18. Colton, C. K., Solomon, B. A., Galletti, P. M., Richardson, P. D., Takahashi, C., Naber, S. P., Chick, W. L. Development of novel semi-permeable tubular membranes for a hybrid artificial pancreas. In Ultrafiltration Membranes and Applications. Ed. by A. R. Cooper, Plenum Press: 541-555, 1980.
19. Lim, F. and Sun, A. Microencapsulated Islets as Bioartificial Endocrine Pancreas. Science 20: 908-910, 1980.
20. Sun, A. M., Lim, F., Van Rooy, H. and O'Shea, G. Long-term studies of microencapsulated islets of Langerhans: A bioartificial endocrine pancreas. Proceedings of the third meeting of ISAO, Vol. 5, (Suppl.) 784-786, 1982.

Chapter 41

Biomaterials in Maxillo-Facial Surgery

Leonard R. Rubin, M.D., F.A.C.S.
Clinical Professor, Plastic Surgery
Stony Brook School of Medicine
Stony Brook, NY

Director, Plastic and Maxillofacial Surgery and the Burn Center
Nassau County Medical Center
East Meadow, NY

ABSTRACT

Prior to the Second World War, most maxillofacial prostheses were autogenous or homologous bone or cartilate implants. These implants, once vascularized, retained their viability and were incorporated as living tissue into the host. However, these prostheses were limited in availability, moldability and increased patient morbidity.

Since the end of the Second World War, synthetic polymers, such as the acrylics, became available. It was found that on the whole, the human host accepted acrylic prostheses with minor reactions and, if covered with sufficient tissue, repetition was uncommon. More recently, polyethylene, silicones and fluorocarbon polymers have gained popularity with reconstructure surgeons.

INTRODUCTION

This chapter is concerned with the biomaterials used in maxillofacial surgery. Prior to the World War II, most of the implanted solid materials used to repair facial bony defects were autogenous or homologous bone or cartilage grafts. Throughout history, ivory metals, glass and chemicals such as paraffin were used with very limited success, most often being rejected and extruded. As the techniques improved and antibiotics became available, limited successes with homologous bone and cartilage either fresh or preserved were replaced by autogenous fresh bone and cartilage. Such grafts once vascularized, retained their viability and were incorporated as living tissue into the host. However, the disadvantages were limited quantity, limited moldability, and increased patient morbidity. The need for versatile materials which would not elicit rejection by the human host, which could be molded to simulate facial bone contour, which could give underlying bone-like ability and which would be easily fashioned became imperative.

World War II offered this opportunity. There was an experience with certain metal as stainless steel 316L, tantalium and Vitallium in Orthopedic surgery. Solid heat cured acrylics [19] had been used by dentists. It was found that on the whole, the human host accepted these objects with minor reaction and if covered with sufficient tissue, rejection was uncommon. Polyethylene [21] in pure form became available immediately post war, to be followed by silicone rubber (poly-dimethylsiloxane), bone cements such as methylmethacrylate [11], proplast [11] which contained perfluorocarbon polymers, and finally the ceramics.

The advantage of polyethylene and proplast over the silicone and methacrylates was their not needing plasticizers or additives for thermal or chemical stability.

This chapter will omit references to the metals. Except as a cover substitute for skull defects over the brain where vitallium has been molded and as splints for dentistry, their use in the face is limited.

The versatility of molding and altering shapes have made polyethylene, silicone, methylmethacrylate and proplast more popular with reconstructive surgeons. Wire, steel and vitallium mesh used as scaffolds to hold mandibular fragments together when bone grafts are used have gained increased use. The chemical and physical properties of the metals are so varied and complex that special metal studies will have to be made elsewhere.

THE ACRYLICS [19,20]

The acrylics used today are polymerized esters of acrylic acid or esters of methacrylic acid; $CH_2 = CH\ COOH$ – the former; $CH_2 = C(CH_3)COOH$ – the latter. Shortly after World War II, the acrylics used were supplied in solid blocks and carved. The material supplied today comes in a form of previously polymerized polymer granules bonded with newly polymerized monomer. The material is formed by mixing the liquid monome [2] with the powdered polymer. The mixing gives off heat as it cures, resulting in a hard, rigid translucent plastic. It can be ground and then polished; it can be reheated and heat sterilized without any change. The material is not affected by the body fluids nor bacterial degeneration.

Used in maxillofacial surgery the plastic is polymerized outside the body in a mold, removing all possibilities of cytotoxic and cardio-vascular effects of free monomer which might escape polymerization in the body.

TISSUE REACTION TO THE ACRYLICS

Foreign body giant cells appear first to be followed by fibrocytes. These form a layer of fibrous tissue enveloping it. If used as a bone cement, the addition of a catalyst tri-n-butylborane (mng A-TBB system) will provide a chemical as well as a mechanical bond of the cement to the bone with no injury to the adjacent living tissue. New bone may penetrate into the layer.

FORMATION OF THE ACRYLIC IMPLANT

The defect is modeled in wax to the desired form. A negative mold is made of dental Plaster of Paris. The acrylic cement is mixed and placed into the mold and allowed to air cure. After removing from the mold, the implant is polished with fine buffers, making sure the edges are "feathered" to blend into the surrounding bone. Sterilization is accomplished by autoclaving. Fixation to the bone is made with fine #5-0 stainless steel monofilament wires. The implant is made somewhat smaller to allow better blending.

The implant is usually wired to the donor area with 6-0 monofilament stainless steel wire.

POLYETHYLENE [17,18]

Polyethylene was introduced to Plastic Surgery in 1948 by the author of this chapter. First used as tubing for blood transfusions and then as a dural substitute in neurosurgery, the polymer proved to be an excellent filler to replace lost bony tissue in the facial skeleton. The material was found to be non-reactive to human tissue, and as the years passed, this characteristic has been found to be constant. A last survey taken in 1981 showed imbedded implants thirty two years later to be virtually unchanged.

Polyethylene has one of the simplest chemical formulae of all polymers. The polyethylene resins are straight chain aliphatic hydrocarbons.

```
H-H-H-H
| | | |
C-C-C-C
| | | |
H-H-H-H
```

synthesized by the polymerization of ethylene under conditions of high temperature and pressure. The molecular weight controlled by the polymerization procedure, varies from 1000 to 3800.

Polyethylene D.Y.N.H. Bakelite, the material used by this author for 33 years, has a molecular weight of 20 to 21 thousand and has certain definite physical and chemical characteristics:

1. Chemical Inertness
   Resists reaction to concentrated hydrochloric and sulfuric acids as well as concentrated sodium hydroxide;
2. Non-Conductor of heat, cold, and electricity;
3. Insoluble in tissue fluids;

4. No tissue reaction:
5. Physically, the material shaped to the desired contour, resembles a firm cartilage. It is elastic and yet firm.

PREPARATION OF THE POLYETHYLENE IMPLANT

Polyethylene was supplied as white granules of about 2-3 mm. in diameter. A wax model is made of the defect, be it forehead, skull, malar, or mandibular bone. Plaster of Paris or artificial stone two piece mold is made of this wax. The granules are packed into the mold which is now heated to 300°F. The two piece mold is now closed and with hand pressure, the melted granules are fused into the desired shape. The implant can be ground with an emery wheel to the desired shape. Holes of about 4 mm. are made throughout the implant to allow tissue ingrowth which would fasten the implant to the surrounding tissue. The implant cannot be cut easily by a knife; grinding is needed for the final correction.

Sterilization must be performed carefully. The ideal method is to soak it overnight in Betadine Solution. Ethyl chloride may adhere to the surface and must be avoided. Autoclaving would melt the implant.

In the operating room, minor adjustments in size and shape are made using grinding burrs and wheels.

Case #1 – The Use of Polyethylene

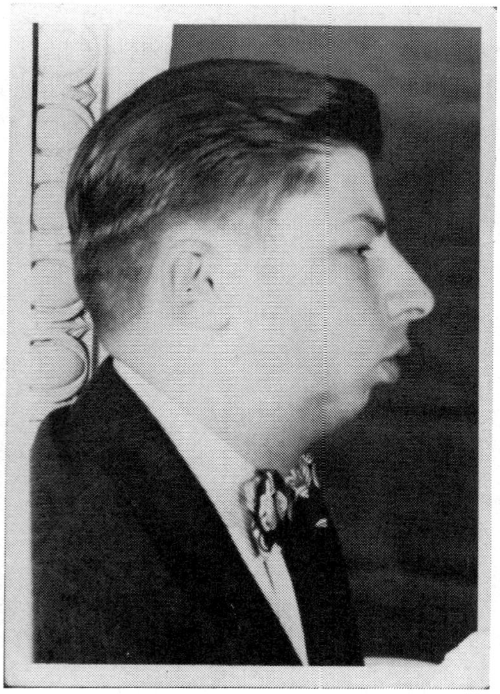

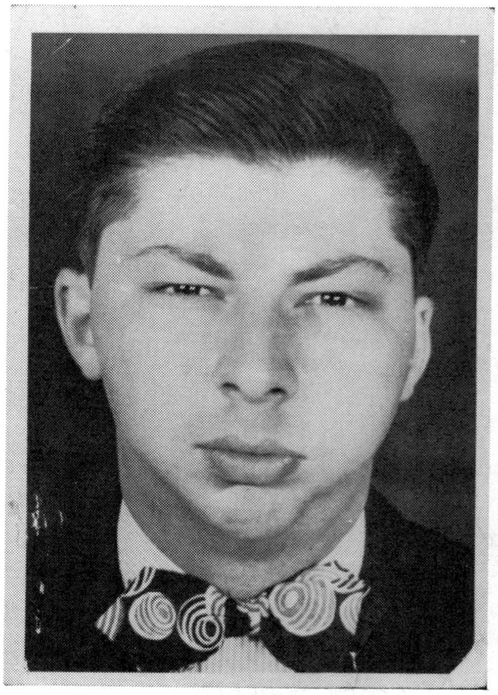

Photo 1 and 2 – Pre-operative views of a 19 year old patient with congenital chin hypoplasia.

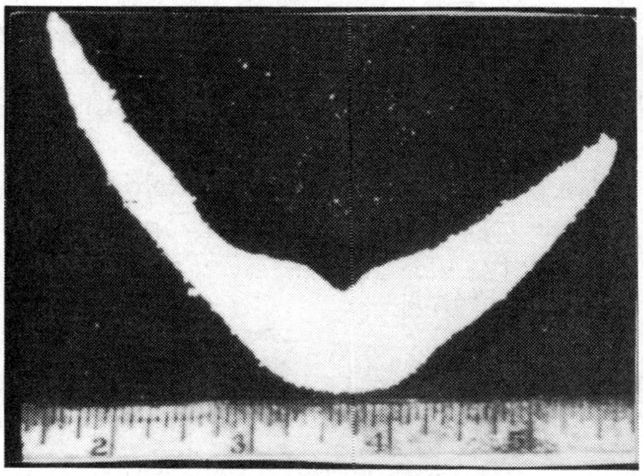

Photo 3. The large chin implant made from polyethylene granules.

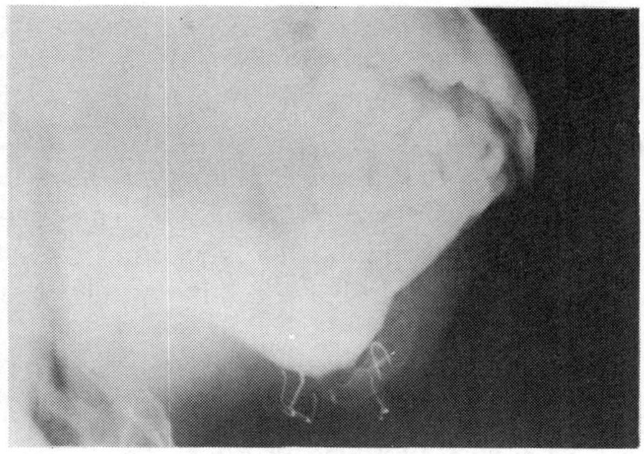

Photo 4. X-Rays showing the chin implant in position 21 years later.

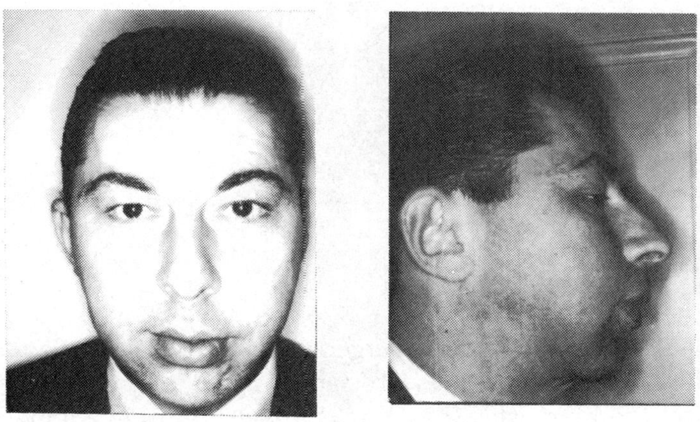

Photo 5 and 6. The patient 21 years later.

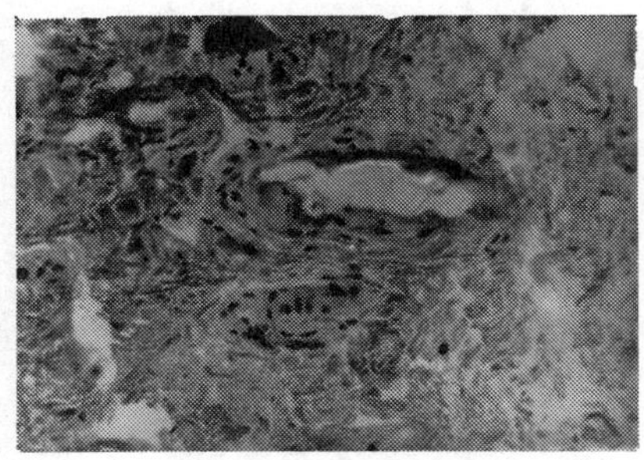

Photo 7. High power field of "capsule surrounding implant 21 years later. Very little reaction is seen.

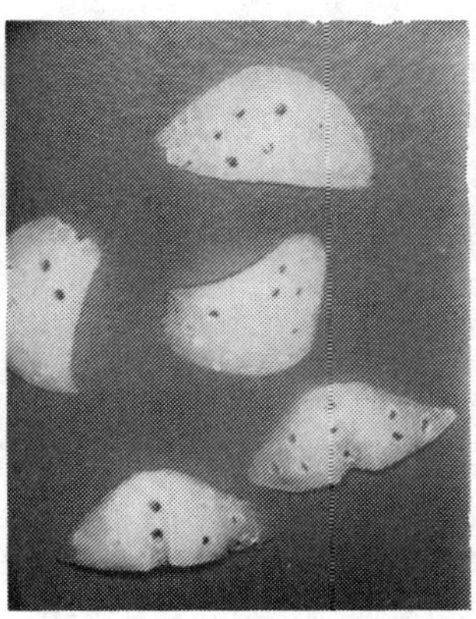

Photograph of different polyethylene implants: Malar, zygomatic, and chin. Holes in the implants allow fibrous tissue ingrowths to ensure firm fixation. Permission granted from author. Reproduced from volume, Biomaterials in Reconstructive Surgery, *Edited by L.R. Rubin, Mosby & Co., St. Louis, In Publication.*

All of the above photos are reproduced from *Biomaterials in Reconstructive Surgery,* Edited by L. R. Rubin, Mosby & Co., St. Louis, In Publication.

The implants have been used as nasal, chin, forehead, malar, and mandibular outlays. After a pocket is made over the soft tissue defect, exposing the deformed bone, the implant is slipped over the defect. A large implant is wired to the underlying bone with #30 stainless steel monofilament wire.

As of this time, about 300 implants have been imbedded by this author. The oldest case was a chin implant over 33 years ago. The observed tissue response to a polyethylene implant is a mild polynorphonuclear reaction, followed by lymphocytes and a few macrophages. These disappear and leave a thin capsule of one to two cell thickness.

CAUTION

A 21 year study of about 200 cases made about 10 years ago showed the necessity of having adequate soft tissue covering the implants. Poor quality skin, tight against an implant, resulted in erosion and extrusion. Implants in the nose and ear were extruded in almost all cases whereas those placed in the forehead, malar, and chin area were rarely lost.

In conclusion, polyethylene, having no plasticizers to leak into the surrounding tissue, has proven to be a most ideal material to reconstruct defects in the facial skeleton.

THE SILICONES [21,22]

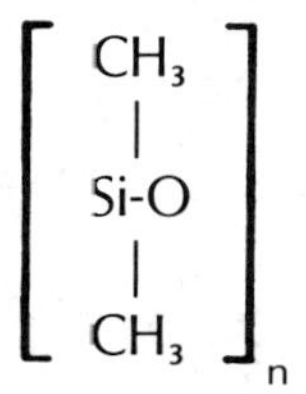

Polydimethylsiloxone

This material has become the workhorse of the restorative surgeon in maxillofacial surgery. It is available as blocks in three different hardness and comes fabricated for use to fill contours in chins, noses, and malar bones. Another form, silastic 382 (Dow Corning) comes in a liquid form and can be placed in a mold and air cure to a solid form.

PHYSICAL CHARACTERISTICS

The material resembles cartilage. It is elastic, and has sufficient body to be hard and yet have the cartilage feel. It can be cut easily with a knife and holes drilled. It can be autoclaved.

All silicone products contain a plasticizer to vary the rubbery consistency. This plasticizer can leak out into surrounding tissue which may alter its physical properties. As an exmaple, sponge soft silicone sheets used as a moderately soft filler for the orbit becomes firm and inelastic after an indeterminable period.

The blocks come in three types of hardness. All can be cut with a knife but cannot be ground because of its rubbery characeristic. Chin implants are often made with an outer envelope of silicone filled with a gel which has the consistency of a heavy oil.

Dow Corning supplies a self-curing elastomer #382. This material can be mixed with a plasticizer and poured into a mold for air curing. When removed, the surface takes on the surface mold characteristics.

As of this time, the silicones can replace hard tissue deformities existing in the forehead, malar, and chin areas.

Case #2 – The Use of Elastomer 218

Patient is a 36 year old female injured in auto accident. (photos courtesy of Vincent DiGregorio, M.D.)

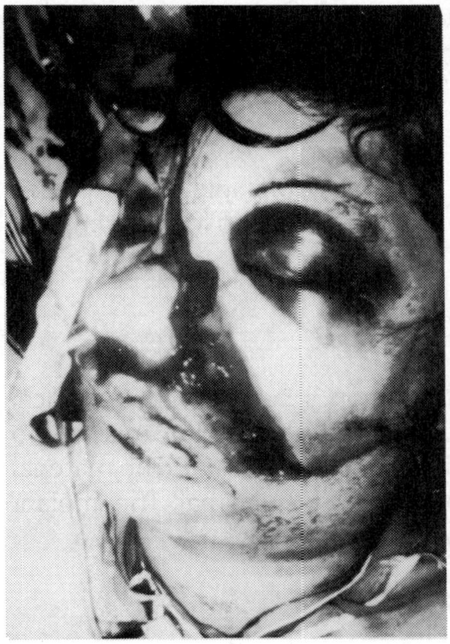

Photo 1. Immediately post-trauma with extensive loss of left malar bone and zygomatic arch.

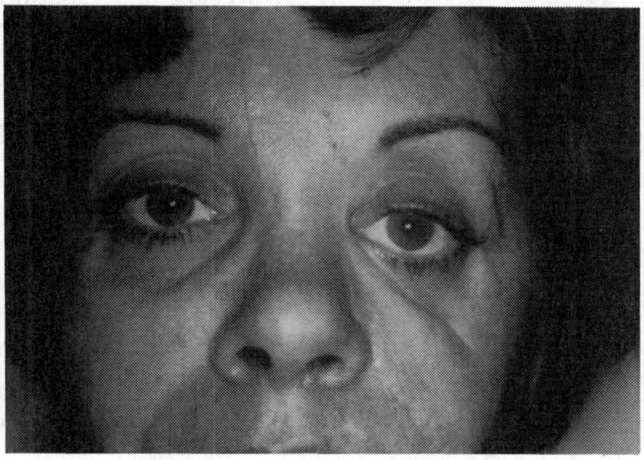

Photo 2. The patient 10 months later. Notice the extensive malar and zygomatic depression.

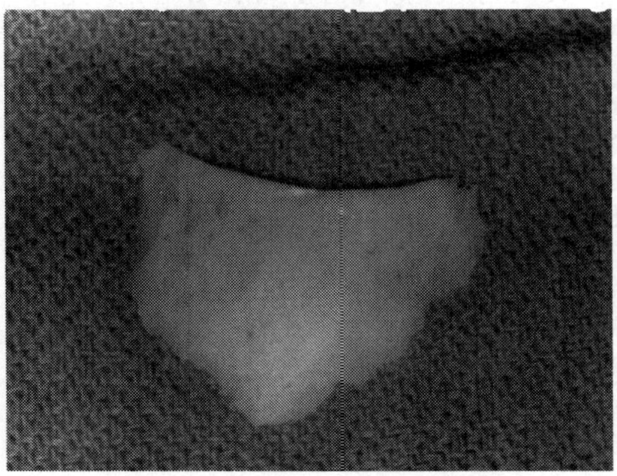

Photo 3. Large malar and zygomatic implant made on the patients plaster cast. The elastomer 218 was placed directly on the cast and the correct shape was sculptured directly like clay. The implant was easily cut by knife and scissors.

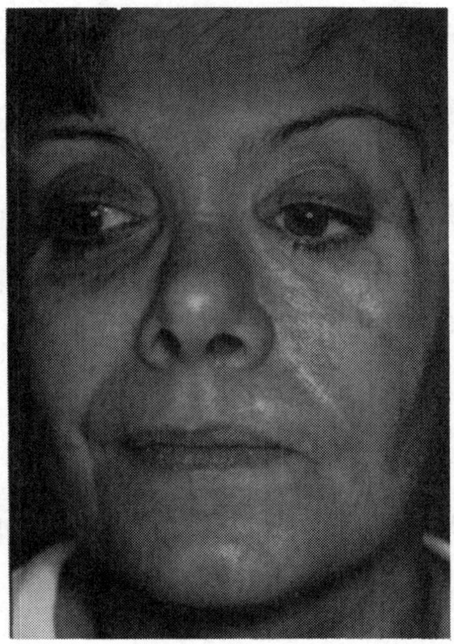

Photo 4. Post-operative photo one year later showing good malar contour.

Nasal implants for profile restoration must be very soft and undercarved where a poor skin cover with scars exists. Underlying pressure will erode through this poor skin cover and extrude. Ear implants are very vulnerable, since the overlying skin is very prone to trauma.

Soft watery gels of silicone have been injected into the dermis and subcutaneous tissue of the face to act as fillers in soft tissue loss (as fatty dysplasia). Unfortunately, the globules of silicones are broken into small particles and transported to the liver and spleen by the reticuloandothelial system.

Soft silicone implants usually are first shaped and then have multiple holes placed throughout the form. This allows fibrous tissue to grow through the holes and lock the implant firmly to the underlying base, preventing movement and displacement.

LIQUID SILICONE SELF-CURING #382 [3]

A liquid self-curing silastic polymer for the do-it-yourself surgeon is the silastic 382 Medical Grade Elastomer, supplied by Dow Corning. The silicone compound is formed by mixing two components resulting in a solid implant which vulcanized by room temperature. The material is non-toxic, non-irritating, and non-sensitizing. Human host reaction is minimal. The implant can be used to fill firm defects in the chin, nose, malar, and forehead region.

PHYSICAL QUALITIES

The implant is soft, resilient, and can be cut with a knife or scissors. The edges can be "feathered" by careful scissor cutting.

FABRICATION

The polymer can be placed directly on the skin over the defect and after mixing the components, it can be shaped roughly to the needed shape. Final shaping is made in the tissue by scissors.

Another method is to make a plaster impression of the defect and fabricating the implant into a two-part mold. It releases very readily from a Plaster of Paris mold.

Sterilization is accomplished by autoclaving. Although Dow Corning states Ethylene Oxide may be used for sterilization, the dangers of absorbed Ethylene Oxide is great and long periods of time may be needed for its removal. This author feels capsule reaction may be a factor by some remaining Ethylene acting as an irritant.

CONCLUSION

Silastic Elastomer Medical Grade #382 is a rapid, accurate implantation material which can be used readily by surgeons with little special skills.

PROPLAST

A new plastic polymer, containing perfluorocarbon polymers have been introduced by Dr. Charles A. Homsey in 1970. These polymers contained carbon, fluorine, and oxygen. The genenic class included:

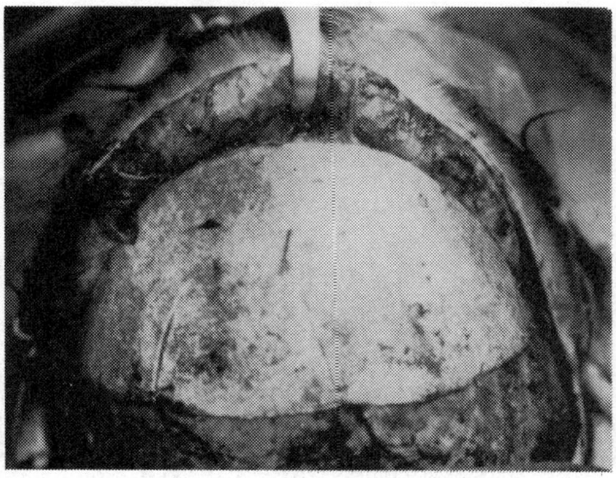

Photo 1. Pre-operative photograph: Shows the deformity of forehead secondary to bilateral frontal sinus crush, exploration and "reconstruction."

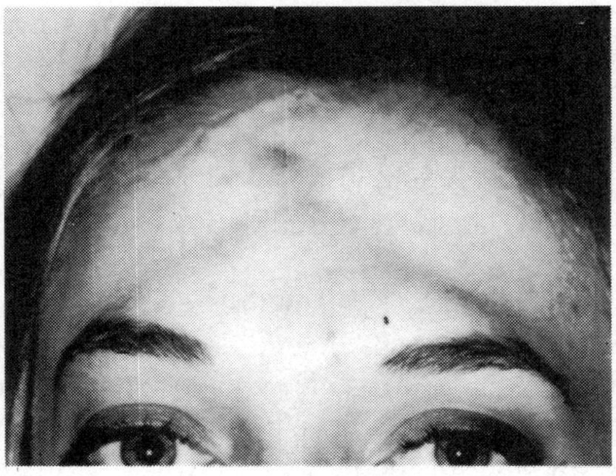

Photo 2. Intra-operative photograph: two millimeter thick proplast sheet, placed directly over peri-cranium has been contoured and tailored to conform with the normal curvature of the frontal bones and avoid neural pressure.

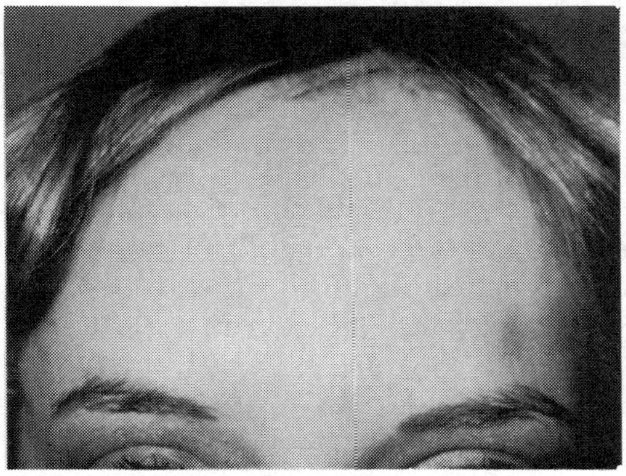

Photo 3. Post-operative photograph: One month after surgery, patient is symptom free and quite happy about her improvement. She will be followed for years.

A) Linear homopolymers of Tetrafluoroethylene (PTFE);
B) LInear regular co-polymers of Tetrafluoroethylene (TFE) and fluorinated ethylene propylene (FEP);
C) Linear regular co-polymers of TFE and perfluoroalkoxyvinyl ether (PFA).

PHYSICAL CHARACTERISTICS

1. Insolubility in all common solvents;
2. No plasticizers;
3. Resistance to chemical reaction (No chemical reaction in the body.);
4. Molecular weight ranges between 300,000 and 500,000 for FEP and PFA, and 6,000,000 to 10,000,000 for PTFE;
5. Extreme inertness;
6. Thermally stable to over 1000°C.
7. PTFE vitreous carbon fiber porous composites (Proplast) has been made specifically for human implantation.

8. Porous composite allows ingrowths of fibrous tissue.
9. Porous composite permits ingrowth of bone cells.
10. Proplast II has the black vitreous carbon of Proplast I replaced with fibers of aluminum oxide, giving it a white color instead of the black of Proplast I.
11. Volume porosity of 75% – Pore size 80 to 400 micra.
12. Elasticity modules approaching soft superficial tissues.

Proplast is supplied in blocks which can be carved to augment defects in the facial skeleton as the skull, maxilla, mandible, and nose. In the mandible it has been used to fill gaps which permitted ingrowths of normal bone from the adjacent edges. Proplast I is sold in blocks of 10 millimeters. Thicker layers can be made by wiring or using adhesives. These carved pieces can be used about the face but because of the bluish tinge seen through the skin, Proplast I has limited use. Proplast II has a normal white color but is firmer and can be used under thin skin as in the orbit, malar prominence, or nose. It doesn't carve well and usually is sold as precarved implants.

The major maxillofacial use has been onlay augmentation of nasal, maxillary, and mandibular defects.

THE CERAMICS [1,5,6,10]

Ceramics have been used by dentists to a great degree as a tooth substitute. The maxillofacial surgeon has looked upon the material primarily as a bone substitute for mandibular bone loss. Ceramic implants composed of aluminum oxide, calcium oxide, and phosphorus pentoxide has shown great promise as a scaffold which would allow ingrowth of normal bone and, as this occurred, a gradual replacement of the ceramic took place.

The problem of facial and bone defects has been solved by inlay or onlay of autogenous bone from the iliae crest or rib; however, limited source, absorption before solid union, difficulty in contouring, and extra surgery (donor area) have led investigators to new areas. Preserved bone by freeze, by allografts, lyophilized bone, heterografts, are all subject to antigen response and cannot be depended upon for the needed results.

At one time, decalcified bone, treated with glutaldehyde to remove the antigenicity was moderately successful as a scaffold to allow new ingrowth of bone. However, limitations of take and absorption before new bone takeover has relegated it to an occasional use.

The use of metals temporarily as a plate fixation material where no bone gap was present presented a good clinical apparatus. However, they could not act as a bridge, and since they eventually caused osteoporosis and bone loss, they had to be removed.

The ceramics seemed to offer a great promise. Resorbable porous ceramics, as described by Bajpai [1], is now being used as a bridging material. A detailed description of the use of ceramics is being described in another chapter in this volume by Dr. Bajpai and to avoid repetition, this author will summarize as follows:

"Aluminum-calcium phosphorus oxide ceramics and phosphorus pentoxide are compatible with the human hosts. They can act as a slowly degradable and absorbing material which is porous and allows ingrowth of bone to bridge a gap. Bone growth is matched by slow absorption of the ceramic bridge.

REFERENCES

1. Bajpai, P. K., et al. "Use of Calcium Aluminate Phosphorus Pentoxide Ceramics as a Bone Substitute." Clin. Res. 24-524A-1976.
2. Bajpai, P. K., "Biogradable Scaffolds in Orthopedic, Oral, and Maxillo-facial Surgery" *Biomaterials in Reconstructive Surgery,* L. R. Rubin – Editor, Mosby & Co., St. Louis, In Publication.
3. Bulletin 51-437 Dow Corning Silastic 382 Medical Grade Elastomer, June, 1979.
4. Burwell, R. G., et al. "Studies in the Transplantation of Bone" *J. Bone and Joint Surgery (Br).* 45-597-1963.
5. Denissen, H. W., Dental Root Implants in Apatite Ceramics. PhD. Dissertation, U. of Amsterdam, Amsterdam, Netherlands, 1979.
6. Ferrow, J. W., "Experimental Evaluation of Ceramic Calcium Phosphate as a Substitute for Bone Grafts," *Plastic and Reconstructive Surgery,* 63-634-1979.
7. Freeman, B. S., "Proplast – A Porous Implant to Contour Restoration," *British J. Plastic Surgery,* Vol. 29, p. 158-64-1976.
8. Freeman, M. J., et al. "Alumino-Calcium Phosphorus Oxide for Rebuilding the Mandible." *Ohio J. of Science,* 80-42-1980.
9. Freeman, B. S., Weiner, D., "Clinical Uses of Proplast-Expectations and Results" *Biomaterials in Reconstructive Surgery,* Edited by L. R. Rubin, Mosby & Co., St. Louis, In Publication.
10. Hassler, C. R., Downes, R. H., McCoy, L. G., Clark, L. C., "Bone Ceramic Interface of Endosseus Alumina Implants," *Biomaterials in Reconstructive Surgery,* Edited by L. R. Rubin, Mosby & Co., St. Louis, In Publication.
11. Homsy, C. H., "Bio-Compatibility in Selection of Materials for Implantation," *J. of Biomed. Mat. Res.,* Vol. 4, p. 341, 1970.
12. Homsy, C. H., "Tissue Reaction to Proplast," *Biomaterials in Reconstructive Surgery,* Edited by L. R. Rubin, Mosby & Co., St. Louis, In Publication.
13. Levander, G. "Study of Bone Regeneration," *Surg. Gynec., Obstet.,* 67-705-1938.
14. Masson, J. K., Payne, W. S., Gonzalez, J. B., "Pectus Excavatim – Use of Preformed Prosthesis for Correction in the Adult," *J. Plastic and Reconstructive Surgery,* 48-599-1970.
15. Roy, D. M., Limehan, J. K., "Hydroxy-Apartite Formed From Coral Skeletal Carbonite by Hydrothermal Exchange" *Nature,* 247-220-1974.
16. Rubin, L. R., et al. "Long Term Human Reaction to Synthetic Plastics," *Surgery Gynecology and Obstetrics,* April 1971, Vol. 132, 603-608.
17. Rubin, L. R., "Polyethylene – A Three-Year Study." *Plastic and Reconstructive Surgery,* 1951-7-131.
18. Rubin, L. R., "Tissue Reaction to Polyethylene – A Thirty-Three-Year Study," *Biomaterials in Reconstructive Surgery,* Edited by L. R. Rubin, Mosby & Co., St. Louis, In Publication.
19. Schultz, R. C., "Acrylics – Reconstruction of Facial Deformities with Alloplastic Materials (Acrylics)" *Facial Injuries,* pps. 434-450, Year Book Medical Publisher, Chicago, 1977.
20. Schultz, R. C., "Restoration of Frontal Contour with Methylmethacrylate," *Annl. Plastic Surgery,* 3(4), 295-303, October, 1979.
21. Speirs, A. C., Blocksma, R., "New Implantable Silicone Rubbers – An Experimental Evaluation of Tissue Response," *Plastic and Reconstructive Surgery,* 31-166-1963.
22. Zaram, H. H., "Silastic Implants in Plastic Surgery," *Surg. Clin. North Amer.,* 48-129-1968.

Chapter 42

Connective Tissue Response To Movement at the Prosthesis/Tissue Interface

Robert L. Whalen
Cleveland Clinic Foundation
Department of Artificial Organs
Cleveland, Ohio
and
Thermo Electron, R&D Center
Biomedical Systems Division
Waltham, Massachusetts

ABSTRACT

A series of experiments designed to evaluate the feasibility of intracorporeal compliance chambers for providing volume compensation to inplantable pulsatile blood pump systems are described. The formation of a dense tissue capsule around the moving implants was initially a serious limitation, but a method for minimizing tissue capsule thickness was developed in which surface morphology of the implant was the important feature. In other applications where tissue capsule formation is undesirable, this method may also be useful.

The sequence of events at the interface between host tissues and an implanted prosthesis is influenced not only by the bulk and surface chemistries of the implant, but also by purley mechanical effects at the interface. While this proposition is generally perceived to be true for orthopedic implants, recent experimental work in our laboratories has demonstrated the importance of mechanical effects on tissue capsule formation for implants in soft tissues.

These investigations were conducted in an effort to resolve one of the most significant problem areas remaining in the development of fully implantable partial and total artificial hearts. For both types of devices, some degree of volume compensation must be provided, as the net volume of the implanted prosthesis must change during normal operation. The problem is more easily appreciated for the partial artificial heart, or left ventricular assist device (LVAD). Figure 1 diagrammatically illustrates the problem for an implanted LVAD. It compares the

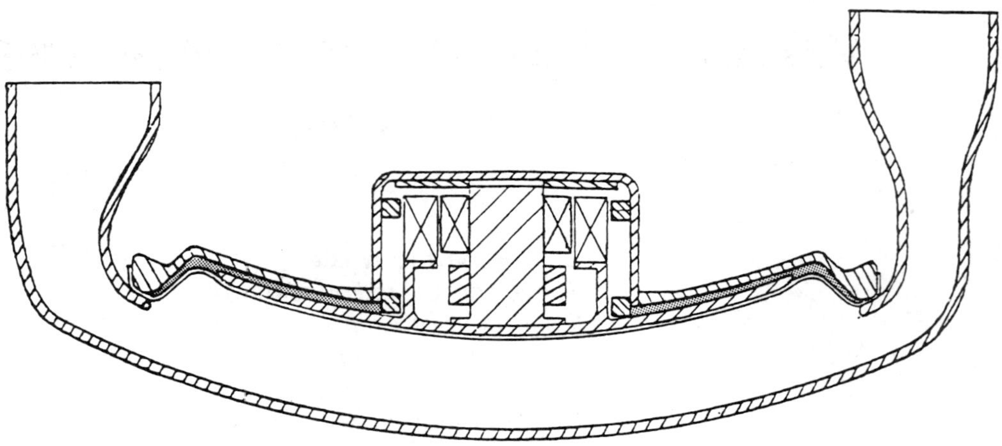

A. With the blood pump full, the compliance volume is the residual space between the housing and the back surfaces of the diaphragm and pusher plate.

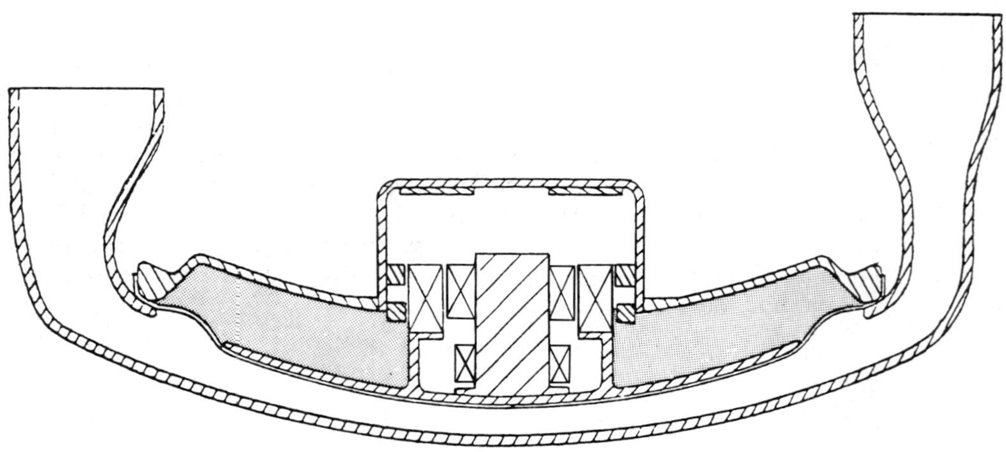

B. At the end of blood pump systole, the compliance volume must be increased by an amount equal to the volume of blood ejected.

Figure 1

residual volume, termed compliance volume, within the device but outside the blood chamber at the end of pump filling versus at the end of ejection. It may be seen that the residual or compliance volume in the pump housing has been expanded at the end of pump ejection by an amount equal to the volume of blood that had been ejected from the pump.

The situation for a total heart replacement device is less severe. It is possible to operate the left and right pumps in a counterpulsation mode, but there is still the need to compensate for differences in right heart versus left heart stroke volumes on a beat by beat basis. It should be remembered that physiologically the left heart output normally exceeds the right heart output by a small percentage (<5 percent) because of the bronchial circulation, or the blood supply to the lung parenchyma which returns to the left artrium, thus constituting a left-to-left shunt. For prosthetic blood pumps, the situation is further complicated by the pressure dependence of valvular regurgitation which can lessen the left heart stroke volume compared to the right heart during periods of increased afterload.

For these reasons, left and right artificial heart outputs are generally "balanced" by either setting their rates independently or by adjusting pumping volumes independently to maintain atrial pressures in the normal range. Pumping output imbalances in the range of 10 to 20 percent are commonly observed experimentally [1]. Thus, while the required volume compensation is less for total heart systems compared to the LVAD, it still appears to be required.

Historically the volume compensation problem did not receive emphasis in the many attempts to develop implantable artificial heart systems because virtually all devices were powered pneumatically by external drive systems. With pneumatic actuation, volume compensation is automatically achieved by the drive gas which is exchanged between the pump and external drive system on each beat. This author first addressed the problem over a decade [2] in connection with the development of nuclear-fueled left heart assist systems, an application in which both the blood pump and its power source are intracorporeal.

When first confronted with the volume compensation problem, it is difficult to intuitively appreciate its significance. One "solution" which comes to mind immediately is to make the blood pump housing sealed and rigid. The pump actuator then must create a partial vacuum in the compliance volume during pump ejection. This may be shown quantitatively, however, to be unfeasible. Figure 2 is a plot of the ratio work required form the pump actuator to produce a partial vacuum in the compliance volume to the work required to pump 90 ml against a mean afterload of 100 mmHg, with respect to the ratio of the compliance volume to the stroke volume. While cumbersome to describe, interpretation of the graph is simple. For example, if the residual volume within the pump at the end of pump filling is equal to the stroke volume, the partial vacuum created in the compliance volume at the end of pump systole would be a significant fraction of an atmosphere, and much more work (approximately a factor of 4) would be needed from the driver to create the partial vacuum than to pump blood at systemic pressures. In practice, since the pump is to be fully implantable, the residual volume in the device is minimized, so the ratio of compliance volume to stroke volume is usually much less than unity. A rigid sealed housing is thus clearly an unacceptable load for any practical pump driver, since the overwhelming fraction of its power output would be wasted doing nonproductive work on the compliance volume. A sealed residual volume in the range of 5 to 10 liters would be required to bring the compliance work within reasonable limits, obviously impractical for a fully implantable device.

Following this line of reasoning, it is apparent that the optimum compliance volume for a sealed system would be infinite such that the compliance work fraction of the driver output

A. With the blood pump full, the compliance volume is the residual space between the housing and the back surfaces of the diaphragm and pusher plate.

B. At the end of blood pump systole, the compliance volume must be increased by an amount equal to the volume of blood ejected.

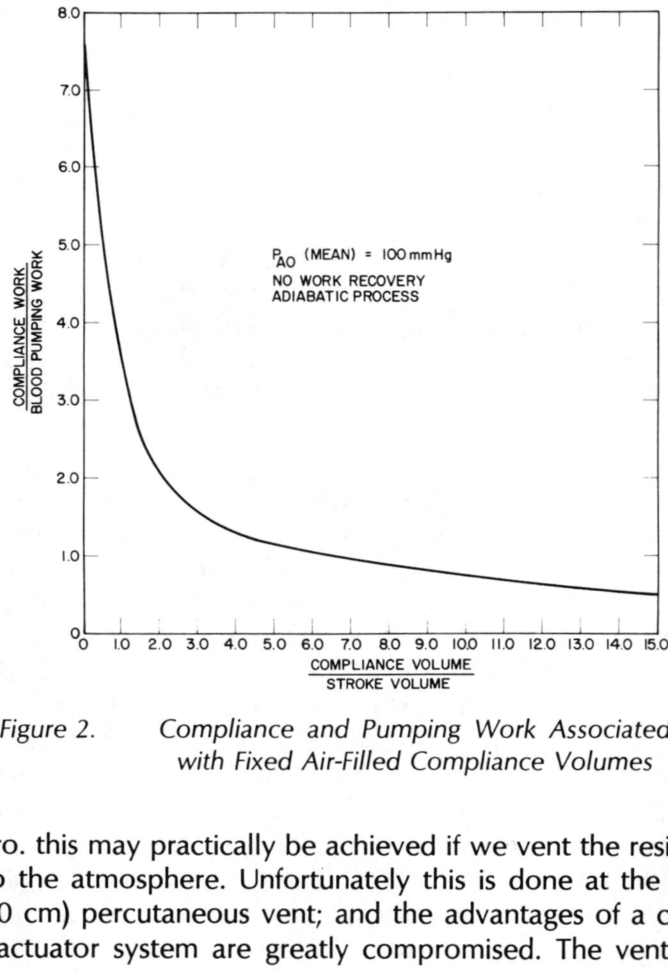

Figure 2. Compliance and Pumping Work Associated with Fixed Air-Filled Compliance Volumes

could approach zero. this may practically be achieved if we vent the residual volume of the implanted pump to the atmosphere. Unfortunately this is done at the expense of a large diameter (0.5 to 1.0 cm) percutaneous vent; and the advantages of a completely intracorporeal pump and actuator system are greatly compromised. The vent is equivalent to a pneumatic driveline, so a logical question is: why not move the pump driver, generally a complex mechanical device possibly prone to failure, to a paracorporeal location? Such systems have, in fact, been proposed. The consensus of investigators working in the field of artificial heart development at the present time, however, is that such systems are undesirable based on quality of life criteria.

If, therefore, the partial or total heart is to be entirely intracorporeal, a volume compensation method is essential. The other obvious option for achieving volume compensation, which avoids percutaneous venting, is to allow the implanted device itself to be flexible; that is, to allow the prosthesis to change its net volume in vivo. This concept at last brings us to the substance of our chapter, for the formation of a fibrous tissue capsule around the implant can seriously limit free movement of the prosthesis and compromise device performance. In our attempts to develop a prosthesis which can freely change its shape so as to function as a volume compensation device for an intracorporeal artificial heart system, the importance of interfacial tissue mechanics as a determinant of tissue capsule morphology was made very apparent.

The design of the implantable compliance chamber to be used in our studies received considerable attention. In order to function well, the chamber must change its volume with minimal change in internal pressure. The reason for this requirement is simple. During pump ejection, the compliance chamber collapses to provide volume to the residual space in the blood pump, and re-expands during blood pump filling. If the chamber geometry is such that it resists shape changes, the chamber will then increase work needed from the pump actuator during ejection or, much more importantly, will serve as a restriction during filling of the blood pump. A lenticular chamber geometry was selected as the best shape to allow for volume and shape changes with minimal expenditure of work in either direction. Basically the chamber changes its volume by having a flexible membrane change from a positive to negative lenticular shape. The bend radii of the material in any position are large, the stress and strain low, and internal pressures required to effect a shape change correspondingly small. The design goal was to provide a chamber with a total capacity of ~50cm³ such that a representative volume change of 90 cm³ could be achieved with a sufficient volume reserve so that small volume losses occurring by diffusion would be insignificant over periods of 2 to 4 days, the interval at which chamber pressure/volume (P/V) characteristics were to be measured during each in vivo study. The P/V data for a segmented polyurethane chamber prior to implantation are given in Figure 3. Over a range of 40 to 130 cm³ internal volume, almost no work is necessary to move the chamber volume in either direction.

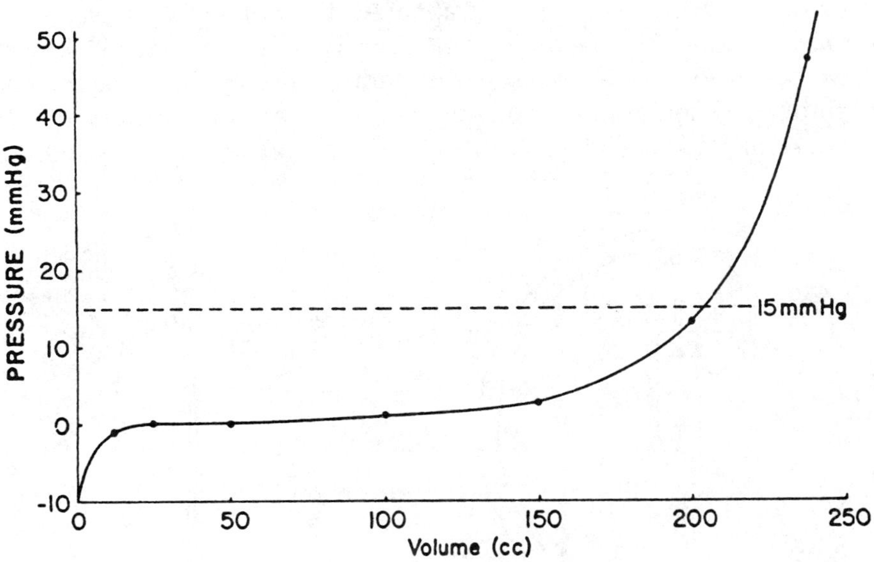

Figure 3. *The pressure required to inflate the chamber represents a filling restriction for the blood pump. Since a design specification for blood pumps is to fill with an inlet pressure of 15 mmHg, this level was assumed as an allowable upper limit for the pressure reuired to inflate the chamber with 100 cc, the approximate stroke volume of the blood pumps. The chamber has a maximum unstressed volume of 150 cc.*

The mechanical design of the implantable compliance chamber is shown in Figure 4. A rigid, curved titanium alloy back plate is used to prevent wrinkling of the chamber membrane following implantation. The curvature of the plate was selected in order for it to rest against the inside surface of the rib cage in 90 kg calves. Rather than couple the chambers to functioning blood pumps and so limit achievable experiment durations, the chambers were independently implanted and driven by an external pneumatic drive source. The pneumatic driveline was positioned so as to exit the thorax in an intercostal space. The driveline was then run subcutaneously for at least a 10-cm distance away from the incision site, brought through the subcutaneous tissues and skin, and secured to a pneumatic stroke volume limit device mounted on a harness positioned on the calf's back. During all experiments the chambers were pulsed at a rate of 80 cycles/min with a collapse-to-expand duration ratio of 0.4.

The P/V data were collected as follows. The chamber was evacuated with a syringe, and air re-introduced in 10 cm^3 increments. At each step, the pressure was measured with a pressure gauge. Increases in the pressure to achieve a given volume provided a measure of the tissue capsule forming around the implant.

The lenticular geometry of the chambers avoids any potential for localized sharp bending during flexing which could provide a focus of irritation to adjacent tissues and thus promote the formation of a thickened tissue capsule. The titanium back plate was fabricated from that metal on the basis of its well demonstrated corrosion resistance and biocompatability. For the chamber membrane itself, initially a segmented polyurethane (Biomer,® Ethicon, Inc.) was selected because of its excellent durability when used as a blood pump diaphragm and also its demonstrated tissue compatability [3,4]. Durability of the chamber membrane is, of course, extremely important, since it is required to flex in the range of 40 million cycles/year.

The efficacy of the chamber design was apparent following in vivo use. An early experiment was terminated after 76 days of implantation when a pneumatic leak was mistakenly thought to have occurred. Figure 5 is a series of photographs of the explanted chamber from that study at autopsy. When examined, the tissue capsule around the implant was thin, comparatively uniform, and basically in accordance with our expectations based on our design analysis.

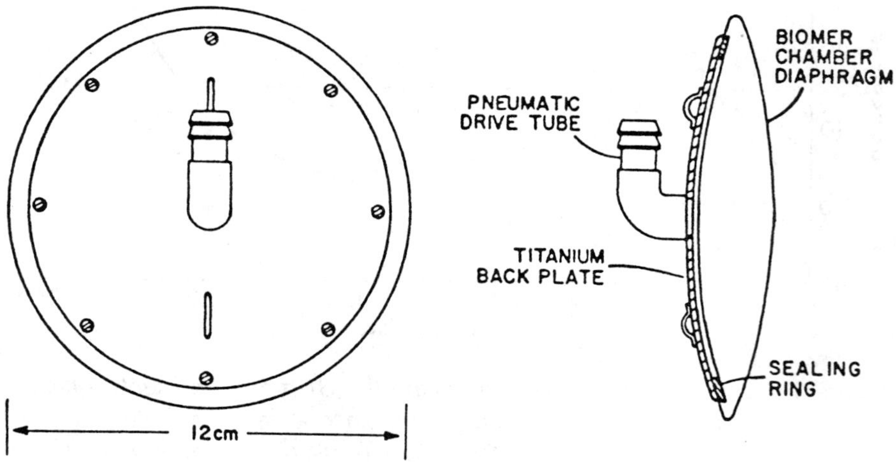

Figure 4. A lenticular shape with the rigid titanium backplate minimizes wrinkling, provides uniform flexing, and has a maximum displacement of about 2.5 cm at the center of the chamber for a volume of 150 cc.

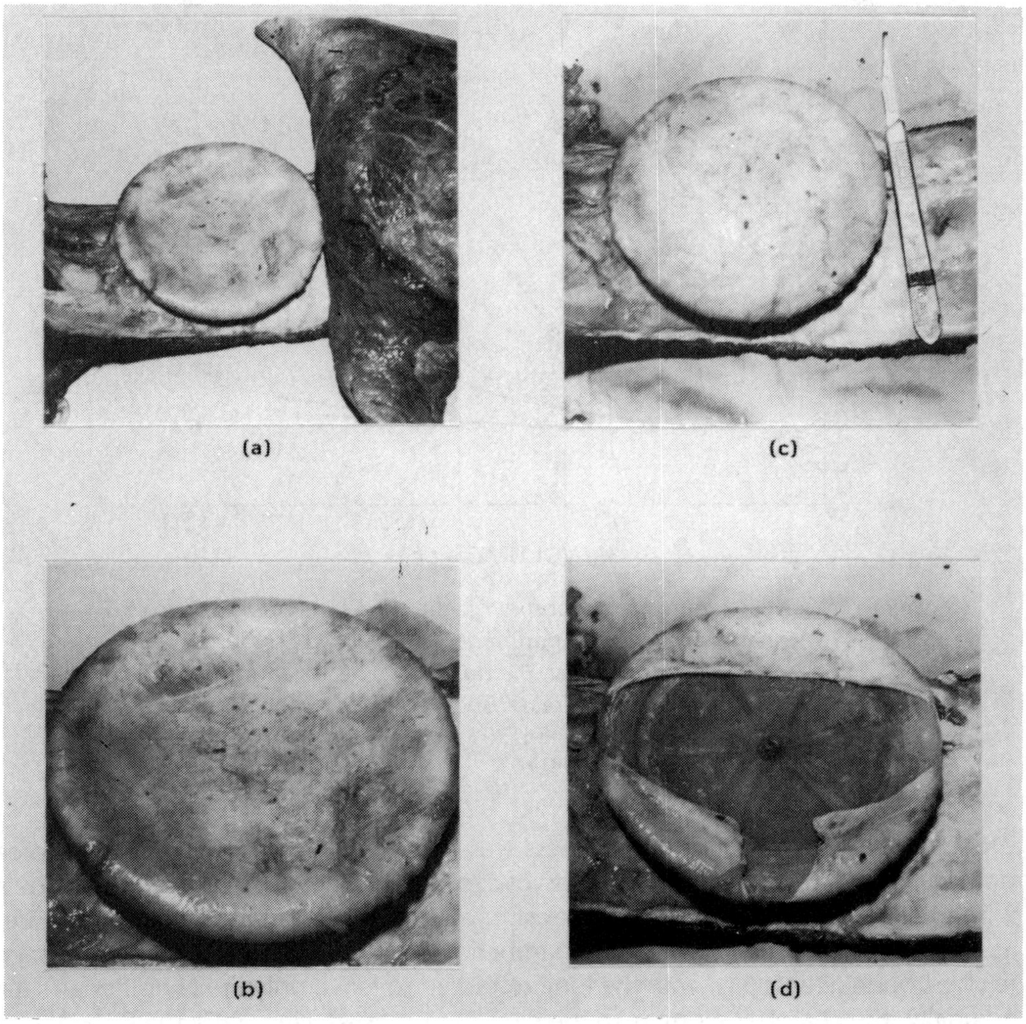

Figure 5. The explanted compliance chamber at autopys. (a) The adjacent lung peeled back, (b) The chamber delfated, (c) The chamber inflated, and (d) The capsule entered to show its thickness.

In the initial series of 6 studies, a single chamber was implanted in each calf. The chambers were positioned in the pleural space with the moving face directly adjacent to the lung. Our plan was to study the tissue capsule around the stationary pneumatic driveline from the chamber as a control.

A disturbing trend in the studies soon became apparent, however, as the experimental durations exceeded the 3 to 4 month range. This trend in the P/V data observed is shown in Figure 6, the record from one of the initial studies. This record is representative of a consistent finding: with increasing implantation duration, drive pressure requirements for the implanted chambers progressively increased such that pressures well in excess of systemic blood pressure were required to change the chamber volume. In other words, the tissue capsules around the chambers were, severely limiting free chamber movement.

The cause for the observed effect was apparent when the longer duration studies were

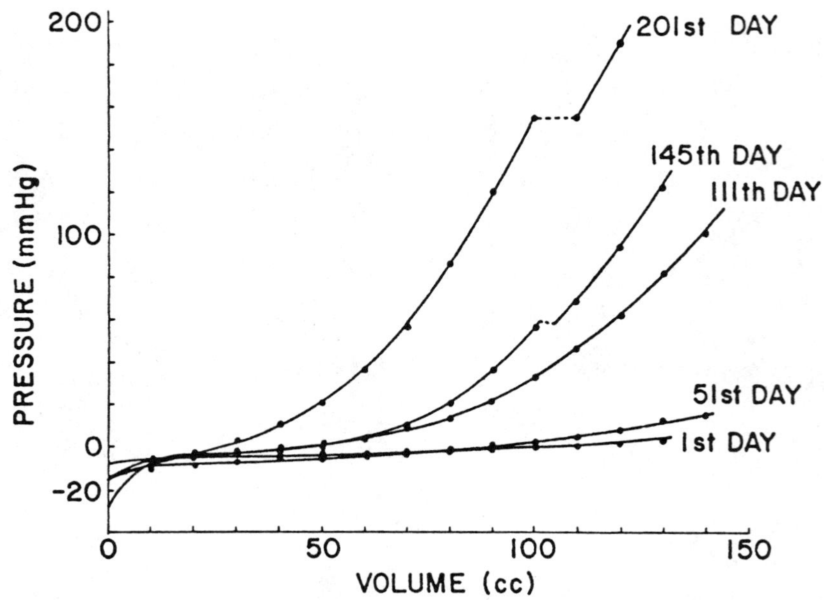

Figure 6. This figure shows some of the pressure-volume curves measured during experiment 78257. Low pressures were measured for the first 2 months, but between the 3rd and 6th month the characteristics changed significantly. The breaks in the curves for 201 and 145 days are due to the measurement technique.

electively terminated. Tissue capsule thickness was in the range of 8 to 10 mm for studies of 6 to 7 month duration. Figure 7 is a compilation of capsule thickness maps from four of the initial studies. There is no doubt that the chamber stiffness resulted from the thickened tissue capsules, as the P/V characteristics for each chamber were measured immediately pre-sacrifice, with the chest open at autopsy, with the lung retracted to leave only the chamber and its capsule, and finally, the chamber alone with the capsule removed. Figure 8 is the P/V data for the prematurely terminated 76-day experiment previously discussed. In this example, the tissue capsule did not have a significant effect on P/V characteristics. Figure 9, in contrast, shows the autopsy data from another study of 189-day duration in which the capsule was the major determinant of chamber P/V characteristics.

None of these initial experiments were compromised by infection. The thickened tissue capsules from the long-term studies all showed a common structure when examined histologically. The capsules were composed of four major tissue layers. From the inner to outermost layers these were: (1) a layer of fibrin; (2) an infiltration of polymorphonuclear and mononuclear cells; (3) a dense connective tissue layer; and (4) a loose connective tissue layer easily separated from the adjacent lung by blunt dissection. This is illustrated in Figure 10. The most disturbing feature of the capsule histology was that even after periods of implantation in excess of 6 months' time, an acute inflammatory process was apparently still in progress at the tissue/prosthesis interface.

The initial series of chambers had been implanted directly in the pleural space. One line of investigation which was followed was to subtly change the implantation site. The pleural space is normally occupied by the pleural fluid only, a proteinaceous liquid thought to provide

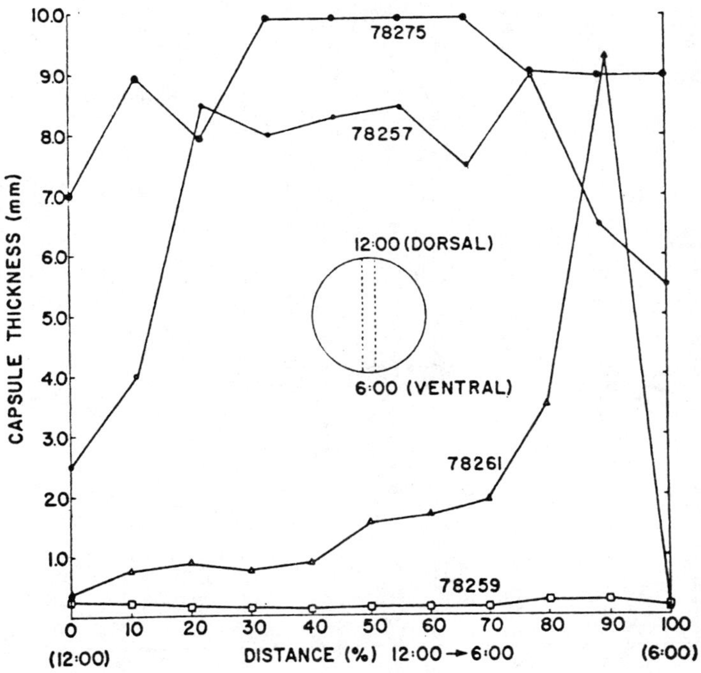

Figure 7. *Compliance capsule thickness mapping for the capsule adjacent to the flexing surface and lung. The thickness varied extensively between experiments. 78259 had pressure volume characteristics well within the limits while 78261 was borderline at the time of sacrifice. 78257 and 78275 were well over the limit.*

a degree of lubrication between the visceral and parietal pleura during lung movement. It is also rich in fibroblasts, a connective tissue cell whose primary function is the synthesis of the structural protein collagen. In order to locate the chambers outside the pleural space but within the thorax, a series of 6 experiments were performed in which the chambers were implanted in a surgically created space between the interior rib surface and the parietal pleura. This implantation site is shown diagrammatically in Figure 11. By isolating the chambers from the pleural space and pleural fluid, it was postulated that tissue capsule formation would be attenuated. Unfortunately, this did not prove to be true, and the extrapleurally positioned chambers performed not significantly different than chambers implanted directly in the pleural space. In addition, the required surgical dissection to create the extrapleural implantation site proved difficult to achieve in practice.

Failing with that approach, we next attempted to change the material of the chamber membrane from segmented polyurethane to test the unlikely hypothesis that the material itself was a problem. In the next series of three studies the chamber membrane material used was silicone rubber, a material with an extensive history of clinical use in reconstructive surgery and excellent demonstrated histocompatibility [5,6]. In this series of studies, an important addition to the experimental design was also included. In each study a nonmoving but identical control chamber was contralaterally implanted in each calf to specifically isolate the effect of chamber movement on tissue capsule morphology. The silicone rubber membrane pulsed and stationary control chambers were implanted in the pleural space.

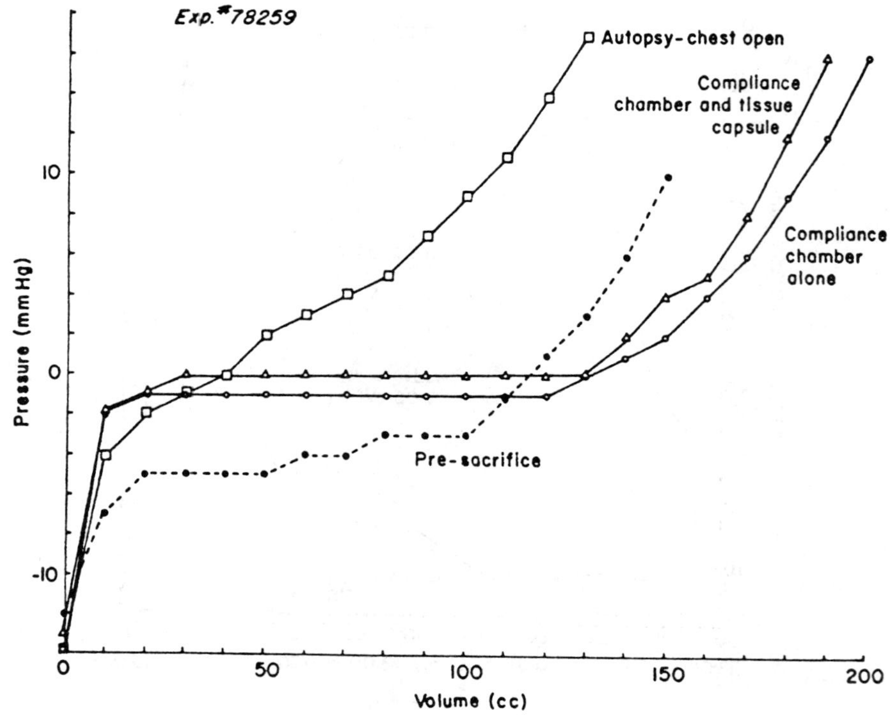

Figure 8. *The pressure-volume curves measured at different stages of the autopsy of experiment 78259. The capsule has very little effect on the pressure-volume characteristics.*

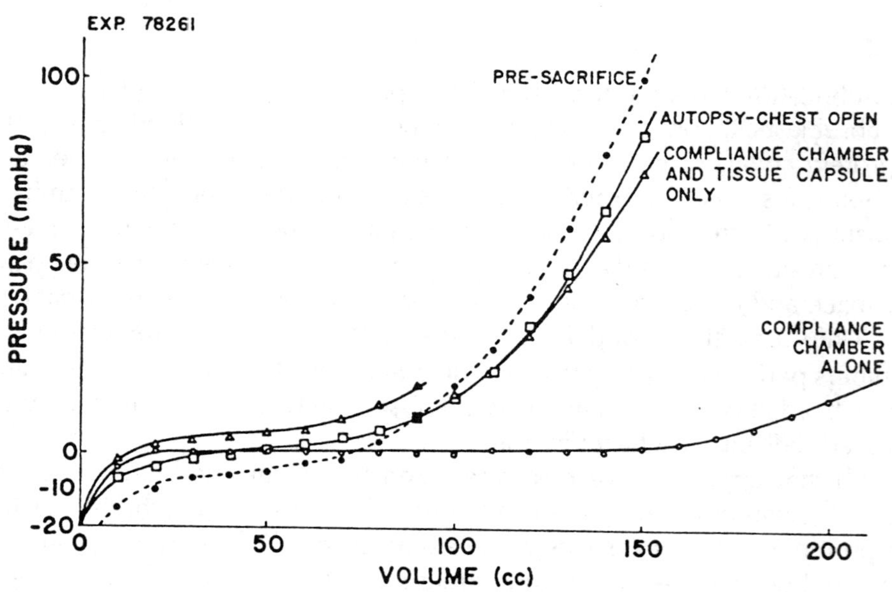

Figure 9. *The pressure-volume curves measured at different stages of autopsy for experiment 78261. Here the tissue capsule has a major effect on the pressure-volume characteristics.*

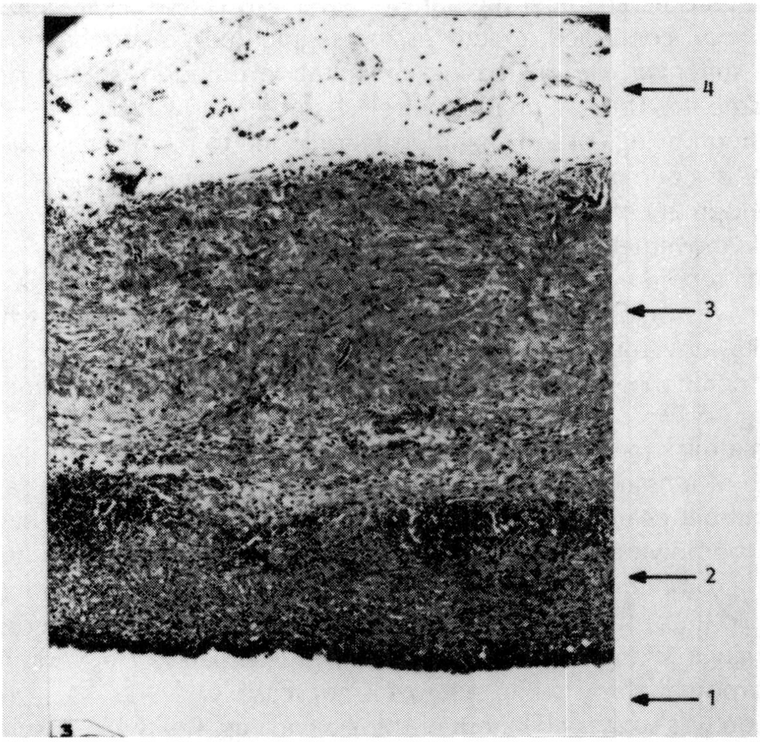

Figure 10. The tissue capsule around a smooth surface chamber is composed of 4 layers: (1) fibrin, (2) inflammatory cells, (3) dense connective tissue, and (4) loose connective tissue, from bottom to top (Exp. 78257, H-E, 40x).

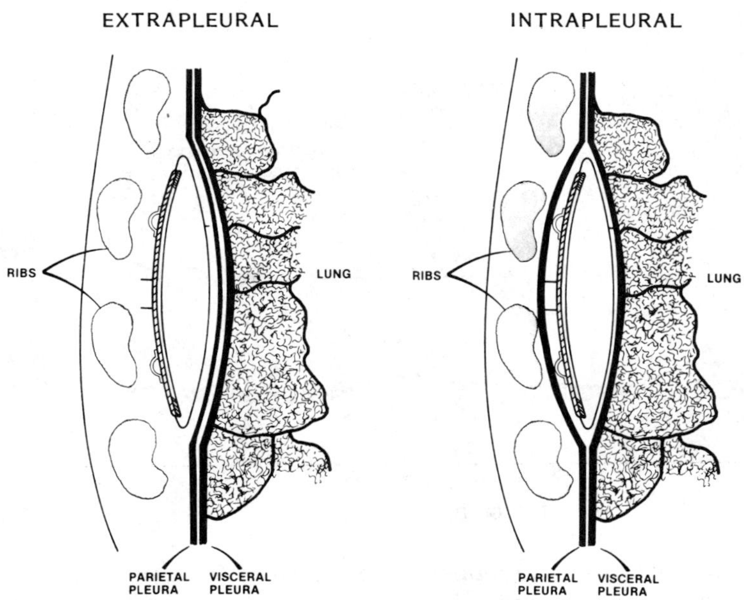

Figure 11. The two possible intrathoracic location for a compliance chamber that are being investigated.

Our expectation that the chamber membrane material was not the stimulus for vigorous encapsulation was soon confirmed. Exactly as the segmented polyurethane chambers had shown progressive stiffening with increasing implantation duration, so too did the pulsed silicone rubber chambers. The stationary control chambers, however, revealed a very different finding. The nonmoving control chambers were found to be minimally or not at all encapsulated when the silicone rubber chamber studies were terminated. The crucial factor that resulted in the development of thick capsule around the implanted chambers had finally been identified. It was the movement of the chamber.

Figure 12 is a data record from one of the silicone rubber experiments. It may be seen that the active chamber was being surrounded by a thickening tissue capsule which was progressively limiting its movement, while the control chamber remained free of movement limitation over the duration of the study. The gross appearance of the chambers from this study is shown in Figure 13, confirming this interpretation. The active chamber, shown on the left, is enveloped in a thick (~0.5 cm) capsule, while the non-moving control chamber on the right is virtually free of a tissue capsule. Histologically, moreover, the tissue capsule around the active silicone rubber chambers revealed the same 4-layer structure that had characterized the capsules of the polyurethane membrane chamber studies previously described.

Having identified chamber movement as the stimulus for thick encapsulation, the question then remained: Could encapsulation of a moving chamber be suppressed in order to permit the chamber to change shape freely? Otherwise, the approach of a flexible compliance chamber for intracorporeal blood pump systems is not feasible.

A possible solution was suggested by our histologic findings. The thick capsules around the active chambers were characterized by acute inflammation at the interface; while any capsule that formed around the stationary controls was free of inflammation. Since movement was apparently the problem, the adjacent lung tissues were examined carefully. The lung tissue adjacent to the central region of the chamber *is* displaced by approximately 2.5 cm in a direction

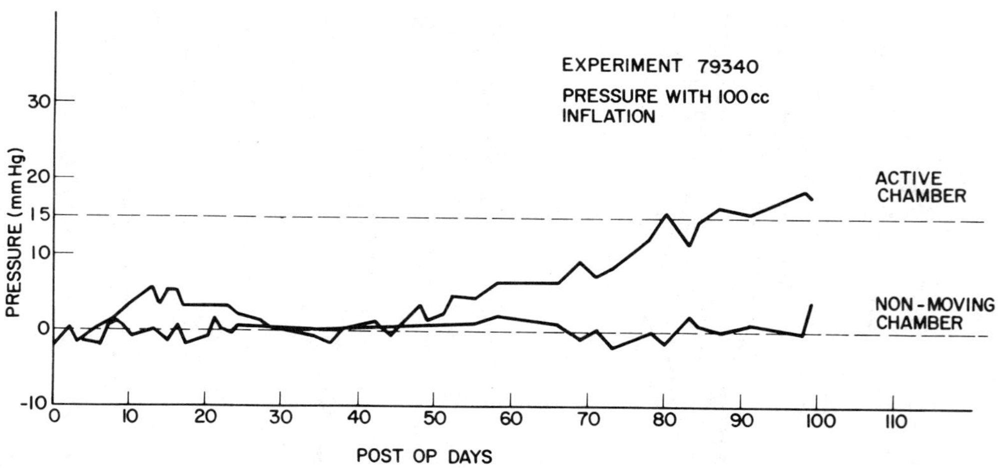

Figure 12. Data from a silicone rubber chamber study. The non-moving control chambers are minimally or not at all encapsulated as evidenced by their stable inflation pressure requirements. The gross appearance of the explanted chambers for this study is shown in Figure 13.

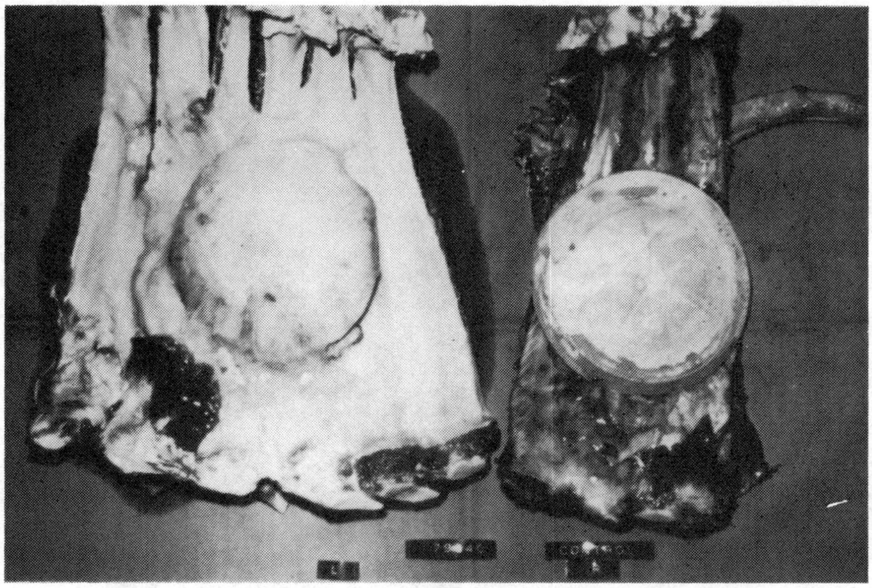

Figure 13. The gross appearance of a smooth surface membrane (silicone rubber) compliance chamber set when explanted. The active chamber is vigorously encapsulated, the control not at all.

normal to the face of the chamber on each inflation/deflation cycle. The lung itself was not signficantly altered by that movement, however. Figure 14 shows the typical histology of the lung adjacent to the moving chambers. The visceral pleura is identifiable and thickened, while the lung parenchyma shows subpleural atelectasis which was relatively superficial. It seemed likely, therefore, that the movement which was damaging was not the displacement of tissue produced by the chamber normal to the surface, but rather was relative to the movement at the interface.

Accordingly, a series of experiments were designed in which relative movement at the tissue/prosthesis interface was prevented. This was accomplished by utilizing a textured surface for the tissue contacting face of the chamber membrane. The textured surface chosen was a polyester velour fabric, a material which has been shown to promote firm tissue ingrowth [7]. Material of this type has been used, for example, as the exterior surface of vascular prostheses, where ingrowth of peri-graft tissues is thought to provide firm anchoring for pseudoneointima at the blood interface [8].

The degree of attachment to this material that is achieved by adjacent tissue is readily understandable on the basis of its structure. Figure 15 is a low-power SEM of the surface as applied to the compliance chamber membranes. The loop structure of the velour permits mechanical interdigitation of the fabric and tissue to occur such that delamination of the tissue is extremely unlikely. The velour was bonded to the polyurethane membranes using the urethane dissolved in dimethlacedamide as a solvent. Since the velour was double sided, delamination of the fabric from the urethane is also unlikely. A photograph of a textured surface compliance chamber so prepared is shown in Figure 16. The fabric was easily molded to the lenticular shape of the chamber membrane with no discontinuities. Because of the lenticular chamber geometry, only comparatively large bend radii are involved in the shape changes of the chamber membrane during flexure. Thus, fatigue failure of the velour fabric

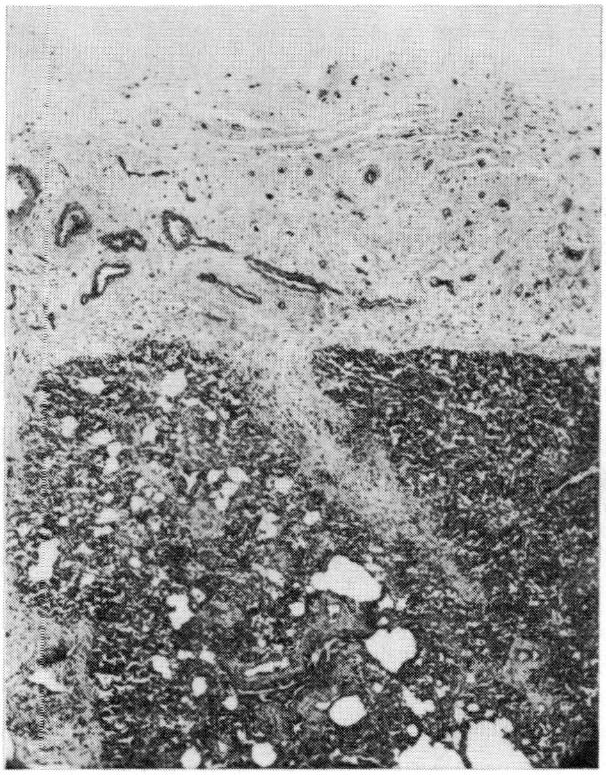

Figure 14. The visceral pleural and lung adjacent to the compliance chamber. The pleura is thickened, and the lung parenchym shows subpleural atelectasis. (H-E, 40x)

was neither expected nor encountered. One effect the velour did have, however, was to give the chamber membrane increased "memory." That is, the membrane had increased the tendency to return to a given shape, since the composite of urethane and fabric had an increased resiliency compared to the urethane alone. For this reason it was found desirable to control the rest position of the chamber by taking advantage of the thermoplastic nature of the urethane. Normally, prior to sterilization, the chambers were run through a residual solvent extraction protocol which consisted of immersion in deionized water at 100°C for a period of two hours. It was observed that even at that temperature (100°C), the urethane would take a set in the position in which it was extracted .While this effect was not significant for urethane membranes, the urethane-fabric composite membranes performed best if heat set in the expanded position of the chamber. Of three pairs of velour-faced chambers prepared, the first pair fabricated was extracted in the empty position. This introduced a fixed offset in the P/V data for that pair, since a positive pressure of 5 to 10 mmHg was needed to expand these chambers in air prior to implantation, while subsequently fabricated chambers heat-set in the full position expanded spontaneously. This difference is apparent in the data to be presented.

The first pair of textured membrane chambers was implanted in a 90-kg calf and followed for a period of 7 months. As just explained, the initial pressure requirements of these

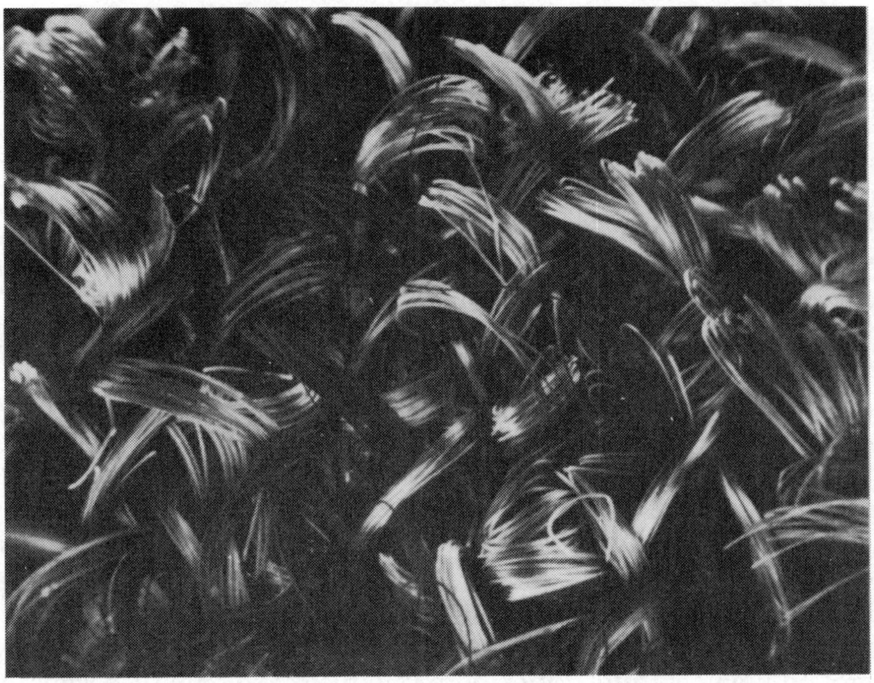

Figure 15. A low-power (40x) SEM of the velour fabric which has been used for the textured surface membranes. The loop structure of the velour is apparent.

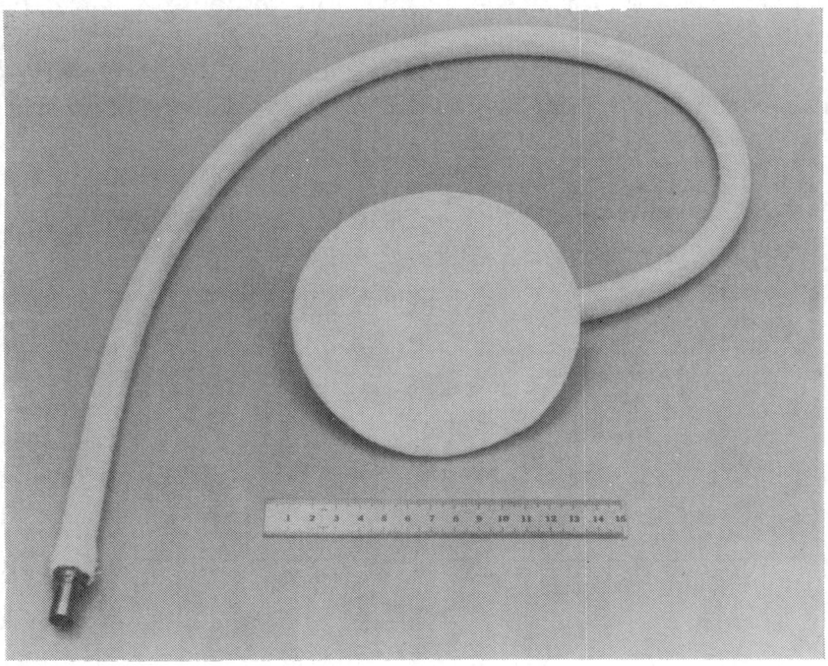

Figure 16. In Vivo Compliance Chamber.

chambers was in the range of 5 to 10 mmHg. Figure 17 is the P/V data from that experiment. At the time of sacrifice, the pressure needed to inflate the chamber was approximately 25 mmHg. However, since the initial requirement at the time of implantation was in the range stated, the total change over the course of the 7-month study was only in the range of 15 to 20 mmHg. This is in marked contrast to the smooth surface membrane chamber studies where, typically, after 6 to 7 months postimplantation, pressures on the order of 200 mmHg or more were needed for inflation. Thus, a full order of magnitude improvement in chamber performance was achieved by utilizing a textured surface membrane. The significance of this change was apparent when the chambers were examined at autopsy.

Referring to the end of the P/V record in Figure 17, it may be seen that the resistance to chamber movement following sacrifice with the lung removed was not significantly different from either the nonmoving control or the initial inflation pressure required when the experiment began. Stated simply, the tissue capsule of the textured surface moving chamber contributed virtually nothing to limiting free chamber movement. In this study, the resistance to chamber movement that was measured can *not* from the tissue capsule of the implant, but from the adjacent lung tissue. The formation of a thick tissue capsule around the moving implant had been suppressed.

This was evident from the gross appearance of the explanted chambers. Figure 18 is a picture of the chamber at the time of removal. Once again, the moving, active chamber is on the left, the control on the right. After 7 months in vivo the shape of the moving chamber in its rest, collapsed state is still apparent. One should compare this to the appearance of a smooth-membrane chamber such as that pictured previously in Figure 13.

Histologically, the comparison between the moving and stationary control chambers is also revealing. Figure 19 compares low power sections from these chambers. There is no significant difference in cell type or distribution between the capsules formed on the moving versus the stationary surface. The active inflammatory response that had been found in association with the moving smooth surface membranes is not in evidence, apparently confirming the hypothesis that relative movement at the interface was the source of the inflammatory response, which in turn was the stimulus for progressive tissue capsule formation.

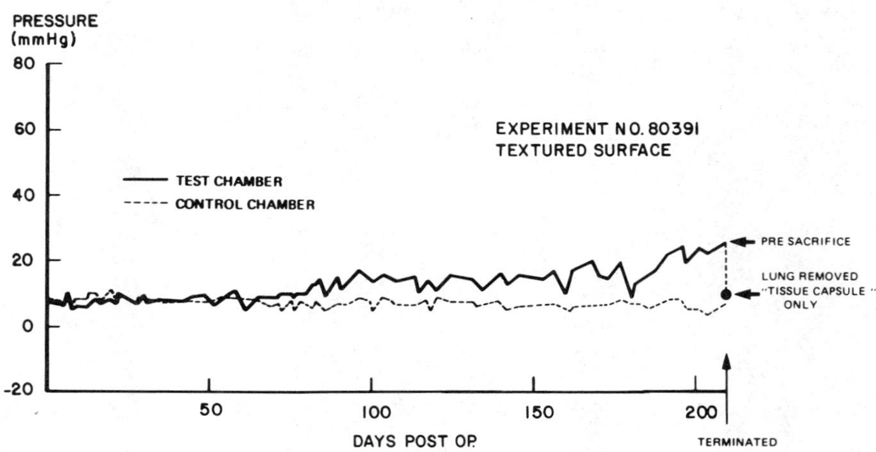

Figure 17. Data from the first textured membrane compliance chamber study which was terminated after 7 months.

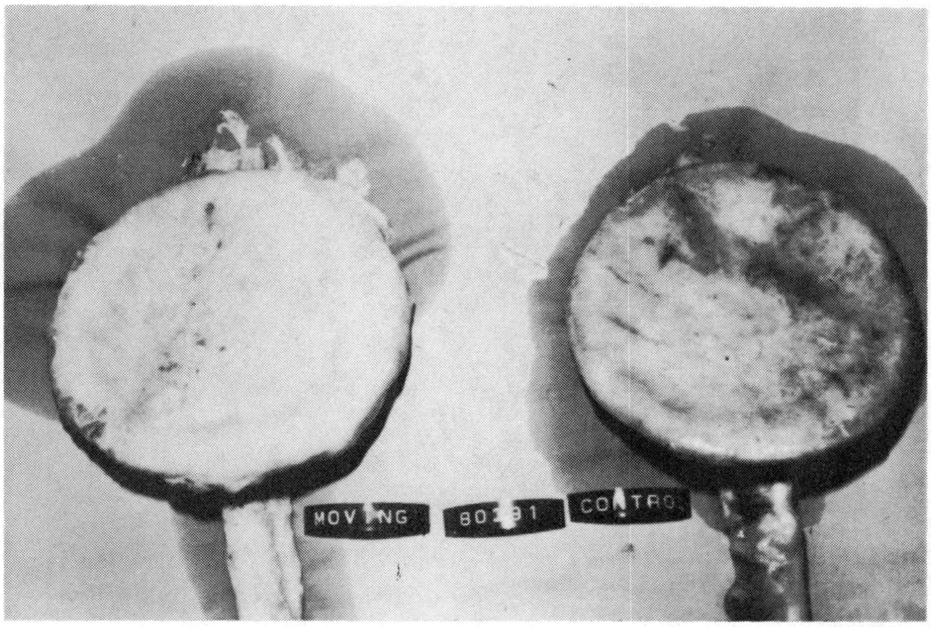

Figure 18. The gross appearance of the first set of textured membrane chambers to be explanted. There was no significant difference in terms of cell type or thickness between the tissue capsules from the active and control chambers.

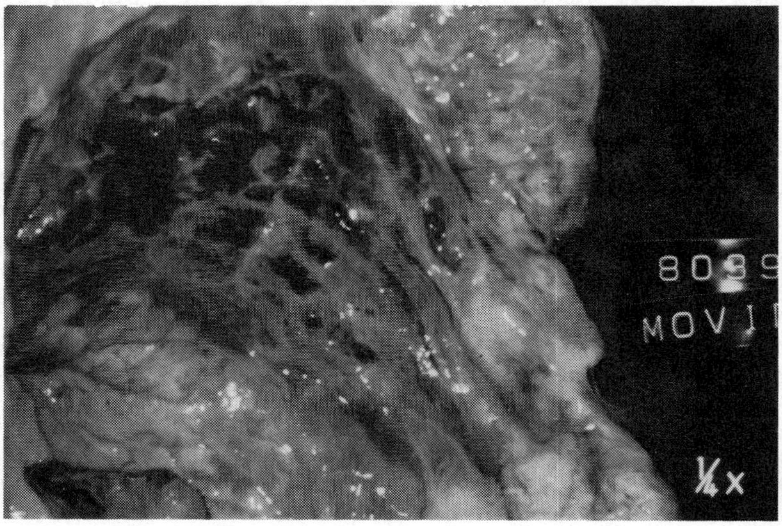

Figure 19A. The lung adjacent to the active chamber in Experiment 80391. There is some superficial subpleural atelectasis.

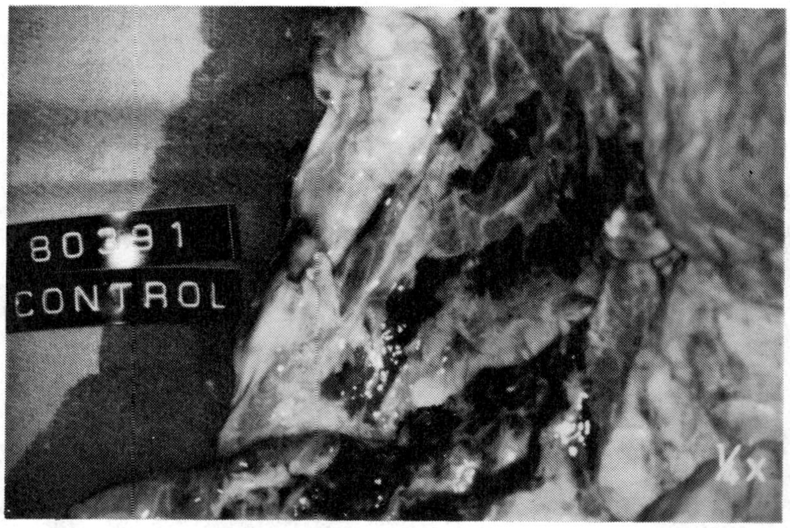

Figure 19B. *The lung adjacent to the control chamber in Experiment 80391. Subpleural atelectasis is also present, and there is little difference compared to the lung adjacent to the moving membrane.*

A question that remains is the potential influence of the textured surface on adjacent tissues. This is especially relevant if resistance to compliance chamber movement now comes almost entirely from adjacent tissues rather than from a tissue capsule around the implant. Figure 19 is the gross appearance of lung tissue adjacent to the textured surface chambers of figure 18. Both the lung adjacent to the moving membrane as well as that adjacent to the stationary control grossly reveal some degree of subpleural atelectasis, but this response is comparable in both. The observed atelectasis thus appears to be chiefly a response of the lung to the presence of a space-occupying foreign body. Mechanically, however, the lung tissue adjacent to the moving chamber was of decreased compliance, since it did, measurably, though not significantly from a functional standpoint, restrict the movement of the active chamber relative to the control.

The remaining two pairs of textured surface chambers were also implanted and carefully followed. These experiments also confirmed the ability of the textured membrane surface to suppress formation of a thick tissue capsule around the moving implant. Figures 20 and 21 are the P/V data for those latter experiments at 8- and 6-month durations, respectively. At this writing, one of those studies was terminated after approximately 1.5 years when infection became a problem, while the last study of our experimental series is approaching 2 years.

Thus, in all cases the textured surface compliance chambers have performed as desired, with tissue capsule formation around the moving implant being adequately suppressed. The compliance chamber concept is thus a possible option for providing volume compensation for pulsatile implantable blood pump systems. More work is clearly indicated, of course, to confirm these results and statistically validate our findings. Currently two other laboratories are, in fact, pursuing this concept for volume compensation of electrically powered fully implantable LVAD systems.

The ultimate significance of this work, however, may well transcend its application in artificial heart development. It would seem that some basic ideas have been elaborated which are at issue with the accepted dogma regarding the interaction of host tissues with an im-

PRESSURE REQUIRED TO INFLATE THE CHAMBER TO 100 cc. VS TIME

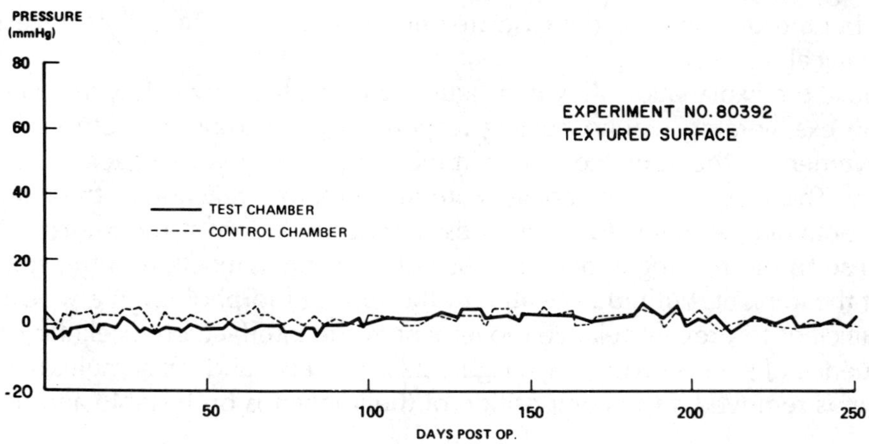

Figure 20. The in vivo data from Experiment 80392, a textured membrane study still in progress at this writing.

planted prosthesis. For example, the notion that a low surface free energy is best for minimizing interaction at the interface is somewhat challenged, for the textutred surface is a high free energy surface if only because its surface area is so much higher than the equivalent smooth surface.

The resolution of this paradox is that in studying the interaction of host tissues with an implant, the macroscopic as well as microscopic effects at the interface must be considered. The

PRESSURE REQUIRED TO INFLATE THE CHAMBER TO 100 cc. VS TIME

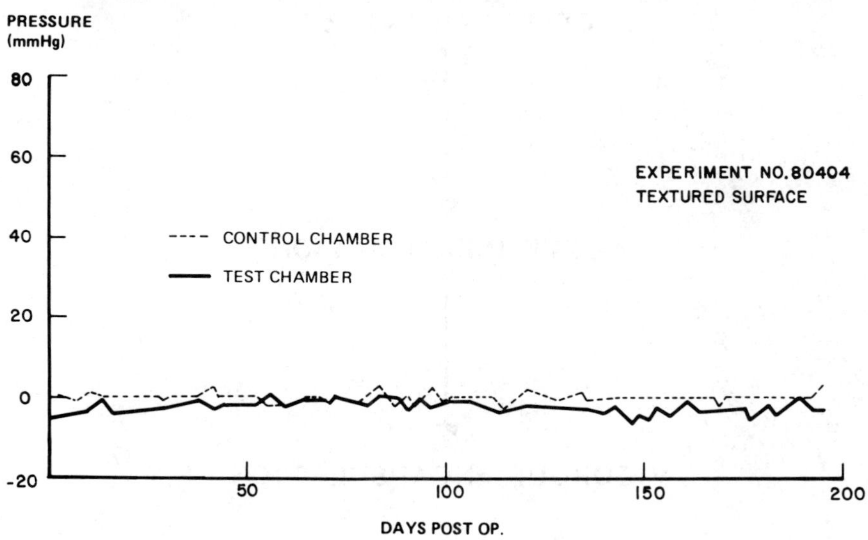

Figure 21. The in vivo data from Experiment 84404, a textured membrane study still in progress at this writing.

high free energy surface does indeed promote enhanced protein deposition and attachment at interface, but the key events in this case are ones that occur on the cellular level in response to the mechanical forces.

We propose the explanation shown in Figure 22 to explain how a low free energy surface produces the exaggerated wound healing response to a moving, smooth surface implant. Relative movement at the interface results in mechanical trauma to adjacent cells producing cellular injury. This results in an ongoing acute inflammatory reaction at the interface which provides a continuing stimulus for fibrous tissue encapsulation of the implant. The overall tissue response to the moving implant is thus not primarily a function of the surface or bulk chemistry of the implant, but rather related to the surface morphology in a specific way. If attachment sufficient to prevent relative movement at the interface on a cellular level is possible, the sequence of events proposed in Figure 22 is blocked, and the stimulus for progressive encapsulation is removed if the composition of the implant is both stable and noncytotoxic.

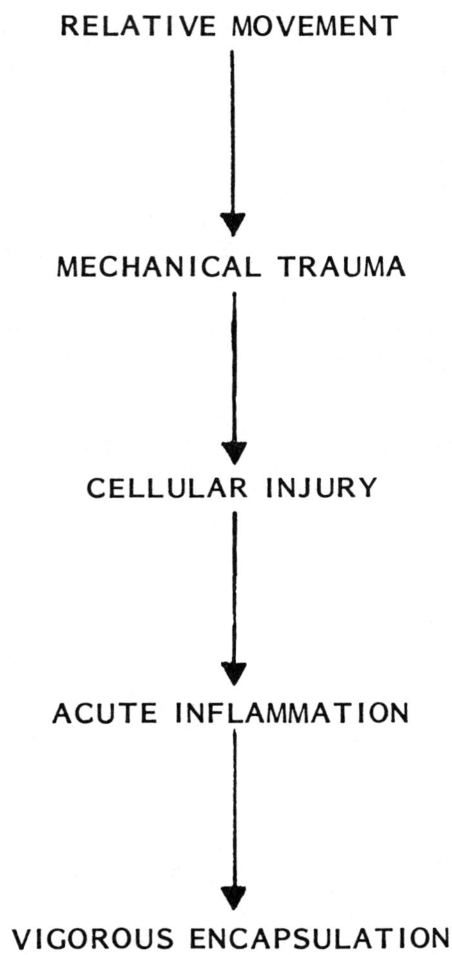

Figure 22. Tissue Encapsulation of a Smooth Surface Moving Implant

While the implantable compliance chambers are an example in which relative movement at the interface is produced by movement of the prosthesis, it is obvious that relative movement can also result from movement of adjacent tissue for implants in soft tissues. Generally speaking, scar tissue formation around prostheses used in breast reconstructive surgery remains a problem which has not been amenable to any known method of prevention. If the problem in that example relates to the events at the interface, it is possible that the choice of implant surface morphology is just as important as the choices to be made among the available tissue compatible elastomers.

Other possible areas of application for the lessons learned from our compliance chamber studies include implantable drug release prostheses, implantable electrode systems, and unipolar type pacemakers, all examples of devices in which tissue capsule buildup can adversely influence device performance. In a manner analogous to that in which hemodynamic conditions affect the course of events at the blood interface in a vascular prosthesis, purely mechanical forces at the interface of a prosthesis in soft tissue can greatly influence the interaction of the host tissues with the implant. For the case of our compliance chambers, the best material to minimize host tissue response was a material (polyester velour) that promotes a definite tissue response rather than the comparatively passive and inert silicone rubber or polyether urethane. The key property in the success of the compliance chamber systems developed was, in fact, the surface morphology, not the surface chemisty.

Inasmuch as this is a book whose emphasis is on the physical and chemical properties of biomaterials, this chapter, which suggests that design of a prothesis on the basis of those properties alone is insufficient, may seem to be at odds with the rest of the text. The reader is urged, however, to take a broad overview of any application of a biomedical material. It is well to remember that the performance of even the best material may be compromised by the final form of the device in which it is used. Ultimately it is the constellation of interactions between the host and the functional device that determine the success of any application using biomedical, synthetic materials.

ACKNOWLEDGMENTS

The author would like to acknowledge the assistance and support of Dr. Yukihiko Nosé, Mr. J. L. Snow, and Dr. H. Harasaki of the Cleveland Clinic Department of Artificial Organs, all of whom participated in the planning and execution of the studies described.

REFERENCES

1. Unger, F., Deutsch, M., Losert, U., Polzer, K., Stellwag, F., Thoma, H., Wolner, E., and Navratil, J., "The Ellipsoid Heart as a Design for Total Artificial Heart Replacement and Left Ventricular Assist Device Driven by an Auotomatic Driving System," Proceedings of the First Meeting of the International Society for Artifical Organs, Artificial Organs, Vol. 2 (Supplement), pp. 200-201 (1978).
2. Whalen, R.L., Harmison, L.T., Molokhia, F.A., Jeffery, D.L., Huffman, F.N., Norman, J.C., "Current Studies with Simulated Nuclear-Powered Left Ventricular Assist Devices," *Transactions of the ASAIO* XVIII: 146-151 (1972).

3. Poirier, V., Szycher, M., and Whalen, R.L., "Comprehensive Real Time Endurance Testing of Cardiac Assist Pump Bladders," ASAIO Proceedings, *XXV:* 319-325 (1979).
4. Boretos, J.W., "Tissue Pathology and Physical Stability of a Polyether Elastomer on Three-Year Implantation," *J. Biomed. Mater. Res.,* 6:473 (1972).
5. Braley, Silas A., "The Chemistry and Properties of the Medical Grade Silicones, J. Macromol. SCI. Chem., *A4*(3), pp. 529-544, May 1970.
6. Braley, Silas A., *Acceptable Plastic Implants,* Chapter 2, Modern Trends in Biomechanics, Butterworths, London, England. 1970.
7. Hall, C.W., Liotta, D., O'Neal, R.M., Adams, J.G., and Debakey, M.E., "Medical Application of Velour Fabrics," Annals of the New York Academy of Sciences, Vol. 146, Article 1, pp. 314-324, Jan. 8, 1968.
8. Sanvage, L.B., Berger, K., Wood, S.L., Nakagawa, Y., and Mansfield, P.B., "An External Velour Surface for Porous Arterial Prostheses," Surgery, Vol. 70, No. 6, pp. 940-953 (Dec. 1971).

V

Processing of Biocompatible Materials

Chapter 43

Sterilization of Medical Devices Based on Polymer Selection and Stabilization Techniques

Harold Landfield
Senior Scientist
Abbott Laboratories,
No. Chicago, Il. 60064

ABSTRACT

Selection of methods of sterilization for medical devices is clarified using two basic parameters:

(a) The effect of polymer structure and
(b) The role of additives for the protection of medical polymers using stabilization techniques.

The most common methods of sterilization, their advantages and disadvantages are discussed relative to medical device manufacture.

Key words:
sterilization, ethylene oxide, gamma radiation, electron beam, antioxadants, stabilizers, plasticizers, megarad

A wide variety of polymer products and devices are used Internationally in the Medical and Pharmaceutical industries.

The use of polymeric materials as components of medical and dental prosthesis has been increasing rapidly and it is interesting to trace some of the past history in these fields. Not too long ago, the only synthetic materials available were cellulosic or phenolic in nature both of which had generally poor physical properties and showed severe degradation on aging.

Some of the illnesses of famous people in the past bring to mind the limited knowledge of polymeric science and sterilization techniques in comparison with today [1]. For example, former President Grover Cleveland's illness was diagnosed in the late 1800's as a malignancy of the jaw. The decision at that time was not to cut away this strange growth because there would be no way to replace the tissue as transplants and plastic surgery were unknown. Lord Byron, who also lived in the 19th century had a poorly formed right foot and continually hid it from sight while he hoped that there would be some way to make it look more natural. Had he been born 100 years later, the art of prosthesis and polymer science would no doubt have come to his aid.

Today, with the need for suitable materials for use in such applications as blood collection, storage and administration assemblies as well as artificial organs, much research is being conducted on existing materials as well as the synthesis of novel candidate materials.

This chapter will cover some of the parameters used in the selection of polymers for medical devices, additives required for polymer stabilization, sterilization techniques and the role packaging plays in producing a satisfactory medical device.

Taking advantage of the relatively non-corrosive and non-deteriorating properties of most plastics, they are increasingly used for both disposables as well as implantation applications in the body.

Table 1 shows some of the important polymers now suggested for use in medical devices [2].

TABLE I

POLYMERS ACCEPTED FOR USE IN MEDICAL APPLICATIONS

Polymer	Application
Acrylics	Hemostatic agents, bone replacement, Corneas, Facial prosthesis
Cellulose Acetate	Nerve regeneration, packaging material
Fluorocarbons	Blood vessels, reconstructive surgery
Polyamides	Syringes, blood transfusion sets, Vascular implants
Polycarbonates	Syringes, containers
Polyetheylene	Tubing, Syringes, heart valves, knee joints
Polypropylene	Syringes, Implants, bones and joints
Polyurethanes	Plastic Surgery, biodegradable sutures, bone adhesive
Polyvinyl Chloride	Surgical tubing, blood collection and administration, blood vessels sets
Silicones	Tubing, catheters, lubricants, tissue substitutes, heart and heart components

A more comprehensive correlation between Device, Function and Biomaterial has been compiled in Table II covering metallic and non-metallic biomaterials [3,4].

TABLE II

Device	Function	Biomaterial
	Sensory and neural systems	
Artificial vitreous humor	Fill the vitreous cavity of the eye	Silicone Teflon sponge: polyglycerylmethacrylate (PGMA)
Corneal prosthesis	Provide an optical pathway to the retina	Polymethylmethacrylate (PMMA); hydrogels
Intraocular lens	Correct problems caused by cataracts	PMMA (lens); nylon, polypropylene, Pt, Ti, Au loops
Artificial tear duct	Correct chronic blockage	PMMA
Artificial eustachian tube	Provide clear ventilation passage	Silicone rubber, Teflon
Nerve tubulation	Align severed nerves	Silicone membrane, porous surgical metals
Middle ear prostheses	Replace diseased bones of the middle ear	PMMA; metallic wire, Proplast (PTFE + carbon fiber); Bioglass
Percutaneous leads	Conduct power to electrical sensory devices	Nylon or Dacron velour, PMMA
Auditory prostheses, visual prostheses	Restoration of hearing & vision	Pt and Pt-Ir wires and electrodes; Ta-Ta_2O_5 electrodes, stainless steel, Elgiloy wires, silicone rubber; PMMA
Electrical analgesia	Eliminate chronic pain	Pt and Pt-Ir wires and electrodes, Ta-Ta_2O_5 electrodes, stainless steel, Elgiloy wires, silicone rubber; PMMA
Electrical control of epileptic seizure	Conduct electrical signals to brain	Same
Electrophrenic stimulation	Control breathing electrically	Same
Bladder Control	Stimulate bladder release	Same

HEART AND CARDIOVASCULAR SYSTEM

Myocardial and endocardial stimulation (heart pacer)	Maintain heart rhythm	Stainless steel, Ti cans; silicone rubber, wax epoxy encapsulant; Pt or Pt-Ir alloy electrode, Elgiloy wire
Chronic shunts and catheters	Assist hemodialysis	Polyethylene, hydrophilic coatings
Cardiac Heart valves	Replace diseased valves	Co-Cr alloys; low-temperature isotropic carbon; porcine grafts; Ti alloy with Silastic or pyrolytic carbon disks or balls
Arterial and vascular prostheses; artificial heart components; heart assist devices	Replace diseased arteries and blood vessels; replace the heart; augment diseased heart	Segmented polyurethanes; silicone rubber or pyrolytic carbon mandrels with Dacron mesh sheaths; heparin + GBH or TGBH coupled coatings on Teflon or silicone rubber; poly-HEMA-coated polymers; Dacron velours, felts, and knits; textured polyolefin (TP) TP with cross-linked gelatin surface: Teflon (PTFE) alone

TABLE II (Continued)

SKELETAL SYSTEM REPAIR AND REPLACEMENT

Artificial total hip, knee, shoulder, elbow, wrist	Reconstruct arthritic or fractured joints	Stems; 316L stainless steel; Co-Cr alloys, Ti and Ti-Al-V alloy; Co-Cr-Mo-Ni alloy cups; high-density, high-molecular weight polyethylene; high density alumina; polyacetal polymer; metal-pyrolytic carbon coating; metal-Bioglass coating; porous polytetrafluoroethylene (PTFE); and PTFE carbon coatings on metal; PMMA-carbon fibers, PMMA-Ceravital powder composite; porous stainless steel; Co-Cr; Ti and Ti alloys
Bone plates, screws, wires	Repair fractures	316L stainless steel; Co-Cr alloys; Ti and Ti alloys; polysulfone-carbon fiber composite; Bioglass-metal fiber composite; polylactic acid polyglycolic acid composite
Intramedullary nails	Align fractures	Same
Harrington rods	Correct chronic spinal curvature	Same
Permanently implanted hip prosthesis	Replace missing extremities	Same plus nylon or Dacron velours on Silastic for soft tissue ingrowth
Vertebrae spacers and extensors	Correct congenital deformity	Al_2O_3
Spinal fusion	Immobilize vertebrae to protect spinal cord	Bioglass
Functional neuromuscular stimulation	Control muscles electrically	Pt, Pt-Ir electrodes; silicone; Teflon insulation

SPACE-FILLING SOFT TISSUE PROSTHESES

Facial contouring and filling prostheses (nose, ear, cheek)	Replace diseased, tumorous, or traumatized tissue	Silicone rubber (Silastic), polyethylene, PTFE, silicone fluid, dissolved collagen fluid, polyrane mesh
Mammary prosthesis	Replace or augment breast	Silicone gel and rubber, Dacron fabric; hydron sponge
Cranial bony defects and maxillofacial reconstruction prostheses	Fill defects	Self-curing acrylic resin; stainless steel, Co-Cr alloy, Ta plates; polyethylene and polyether urethane-coated polyethylene terephthalate coated cloth mesh
Artificial articular cartilage	Replace arthritis deterioration cartilage	Crystallized hydrogel-PVA and polyurethane polymers; PTFE plus graphite fibers (Proplast)

MISCELLANEOUS SOFT TISSUES

Artificial ureter, bladder, intestinal wall	Replace diseased tissue	Teflon, nylon-polyurethane composite; treated bovine pericardium; silicone rubber
Artificial skin	Treat severe burns	Processed collagen; ultrathin silicone membrane, polycaprolactone (PCA) foam-PCA film composite
Hydrocephalus shunt	Provide drainage and reduce pressure	Silicone rubber
Tissue patches	Repair hernias	Stainless steel, Marlex, Silastic, Dacron mesh
Internal shunt	Provide routine access to dialysis units	Modified collagen; Silastic
External shunt	Provide routine access to dialysis	Silastic-Teflon or Dacron
Sutures	Maintain tissue contact to aid healing	Stainless steel, silk, nylon PGA, Dacron, catgut, polypropylene
Drug delivery systems	Release drugs progressively; immobilize enzymes	Silicone rubber, hydrogels, ethylene-vinyl acetate copolymer, PLA/PGA polysaccharides-vinyl polymers
Artificial trachea	Reconstruct trachea	Porous Dacron-polyether urethane mesh, Ta mesh, Ivalon sponge and polypropylene mesh

TABLE II (Continued)

DENTAL

Alveolar bone replacements, mandibular reconstruction	Restore the alveolar ridge to improve denture fit	PTFE carbon composite (Proplast) porous Al_2O_3; Ceravital; hema hydrogel-filled porous apatite tricalcium phosphate; PLA/PGA copolymer; Bioglass
Endosseous tooth replacement implants (blades, anchors, spirals, cylinders natural or modified root form)	Replace diseased, damaged, or loosened teeth	Stainless steel, Co-Cr-Mo alloys Ti and Ti alloys, Al_2O_3 Bioglass, LTI carbon, PMMA, Proplast, porous calcium aluminate $MgAl_2O_4$ spinal, vitreous carbon, dental hydroxyapatite
Subperiosteal tooth replacement implants	Support bridge work or teeth directly on alveolar bone	Stainless steel, Co-Cr-Mo alloy, LTI carbon coatings
Orthodontic anchors	Provide posts for stress application required to change deformities	Bioglass-coated Al_2O_3; Bioglass coated Vitallium

Many of the present medical polymers (Table IIa) would not be available were it not for the rapid progress in the science of stabilization of polymeric materials. The increased use of polymers such as polyvinyl chloride and polypropylene is as the result of the development of additives to protect them from heat and light as well as manufacturing process conditions.

Table IIa. Synthetic Polymers.

Polyvinyl chloride	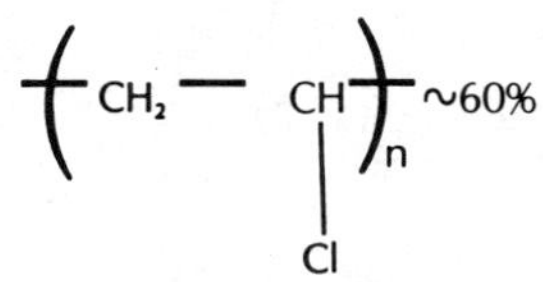 plasticizers ~40%	Blood bags; bubble oxygenators; oxygenator and dialysis tubing; catheters
Polyethylene (high molecular weight)	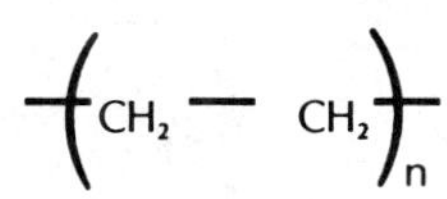	Orthopedic; acetabular cup
Polyethylene terephthalate	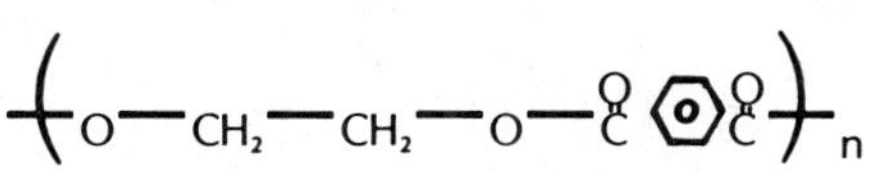	Woven vascular prostheses; heart valve suture rings
Polyacrylonitrile (PAN)	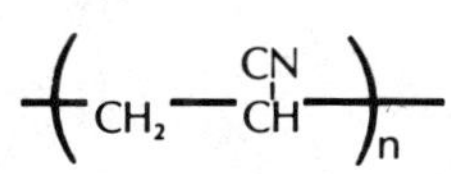	Dialysis membrane
Polytetrafluoroethylene (Teflon TFE[R])	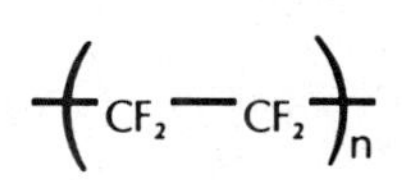	Orthopedic; coating stem prostheses; coating tips; neurosurgery; aneurism clips

Polytetrafluoroethylene-hexafluoropropylene copolymer (Teflon FEP[R])

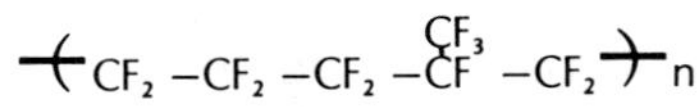

Orthopedics

Polycyanoacrylates

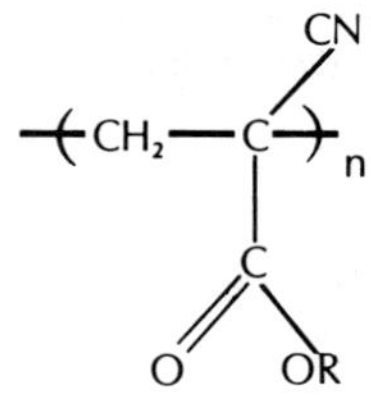

Tissue adhesives

Polymethylmethacrylate

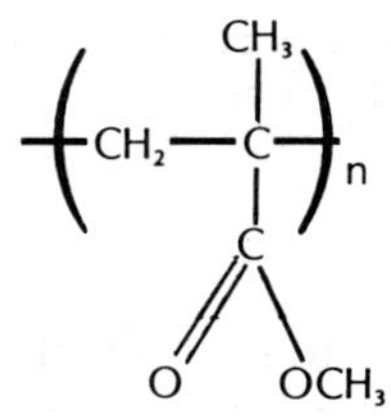

Neurosurgery; cranioplasty; orthopedics; grout for artificial joints; ophthalmology lenses; contact lenses dental

Polyhydroxyethylmethacrylate

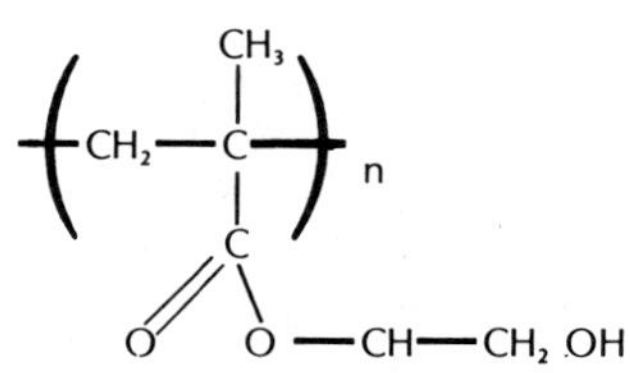

Antithrombogenic surfaces; tubing; plastic surgery; drug release contact lenses

Polydihydroxypropylmethacrylate

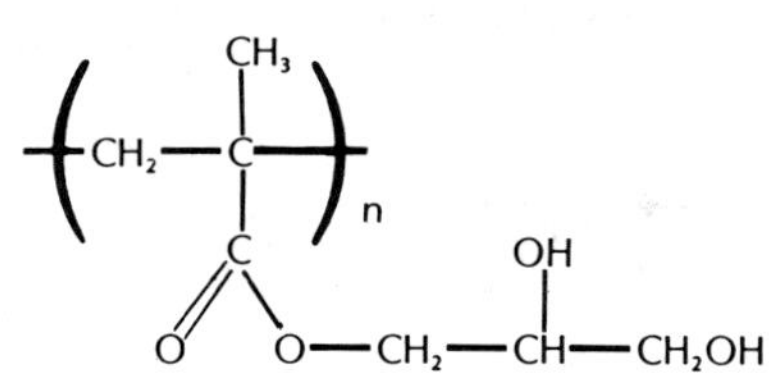

Antithrombogenic surfaces; tubing; plastic surgery; drug release contact lenses

Resin: diglycidyl ether of bisphenol A (DGEBA)

Packaging pacemakers: central restorations

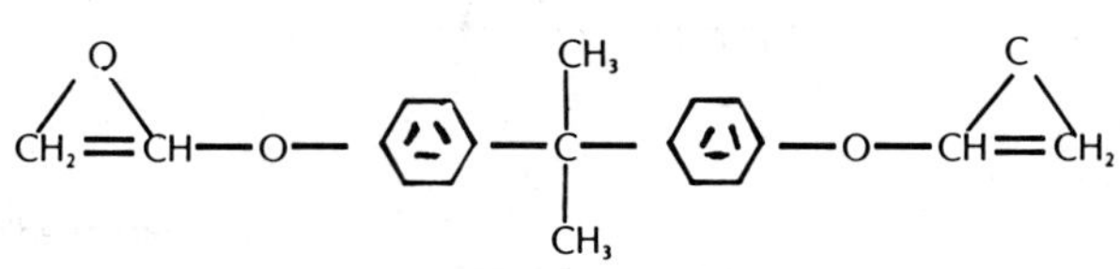

TABLE IIa. (Continued)

	Catalyst: multifunctional amide, e.g., DETA: $NH_2-CH_2-CH_2-NH-CH_2-CH_2-NH_2$, or multifunctional anhydrides	
Polyurethanes (segmented)	Block copolymers of form $[A_x B_y]_n$ where typically x = 10 to 30, y = 1 to 4. A represents the "soft" segment such as polyethers $-[CH(CH_3)CH_2-O]-$ $-[(CH_2)_4-O]-$ or polyester 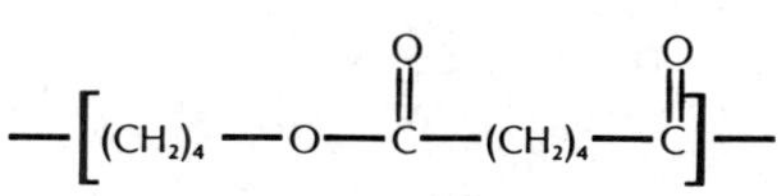 B represents the "hard" segment such as 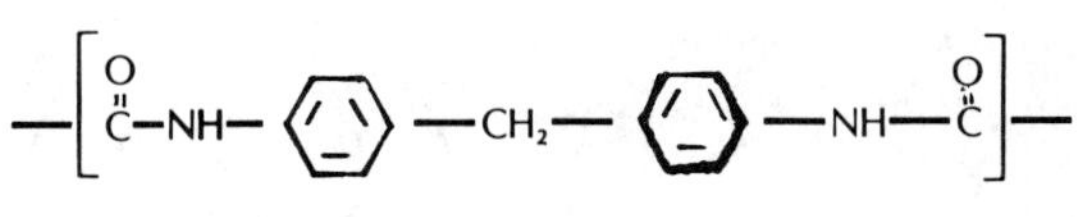	Catheters; tubing; artificial heart ventricles; pumps
Polyglycolic acid	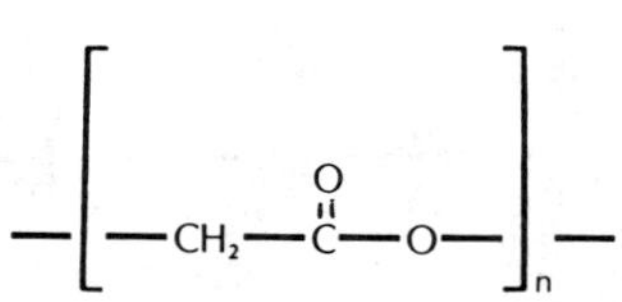	Resorbable sutures
Silicones	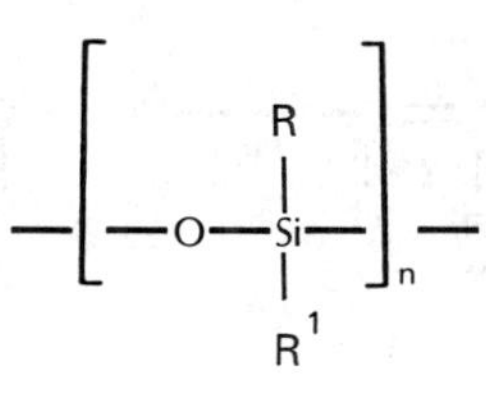	Heart valves; tubing; plastic surgery; oxygenators

TABLE IIa. (Continued)

	where R = CH_3 and R′ = —CH = CH_2, or —  or —CH_3	
Silicone-Polycarbonate copolymer	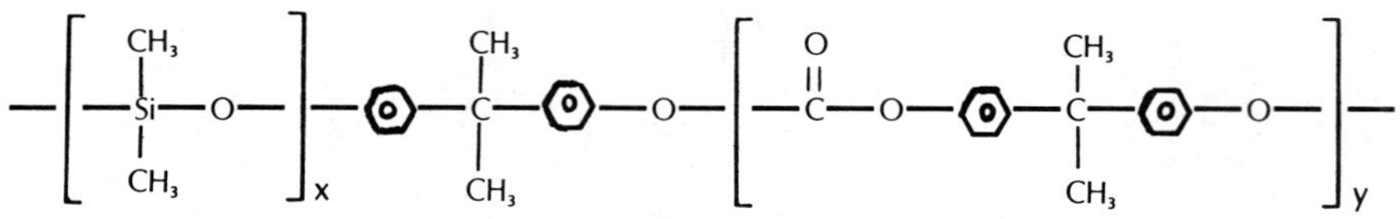 x/y from 1:4 to 1:1	Oxygenator membranes
Copolymer silicone-Polyurethane (Avcothane[R])	$[A_xB_y]_n$ A = polyester or polyetherurethane; B = silicone	**Left ventricular assist devices; intra-aortic balloon pumps**
Polyphenoxy	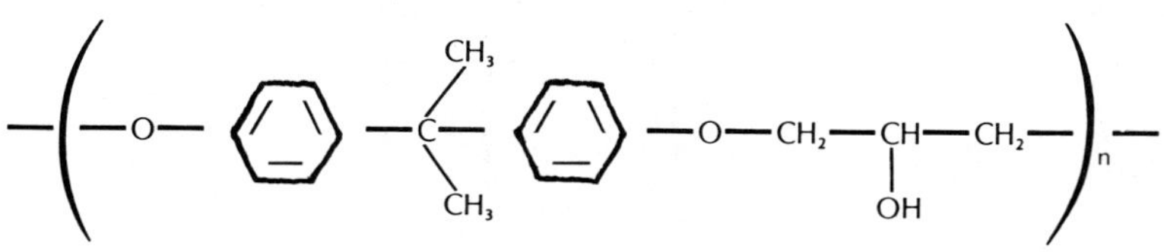	Oxygenator membranes
Polyamide (Nylon 6)	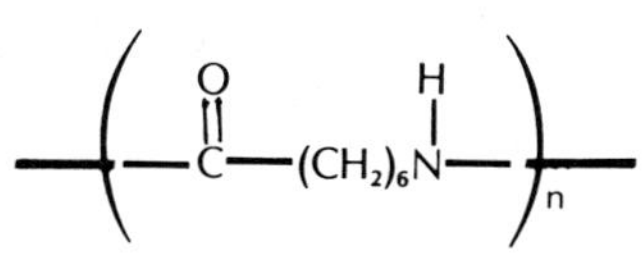	Sutures
Polyformaldehyde (Delrin[R])	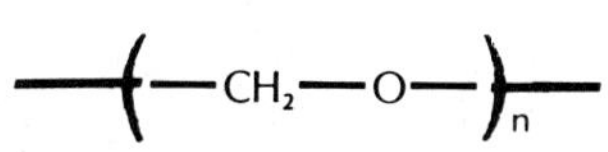	Heart valve occluders general structural polymer
Epichlorohydrin rubber (Hydrin[R])	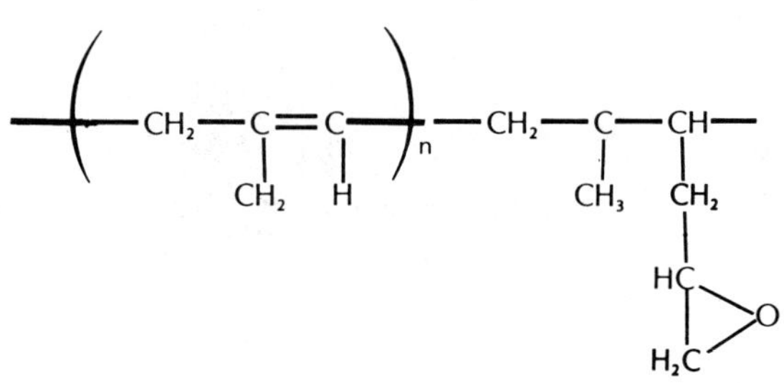	Flexible mold; impression material; dental applications

TABLE IIa. (Continued)

Polycarbonate (Lexan[R])

General use oxygenator valve occluders; cranioplasty

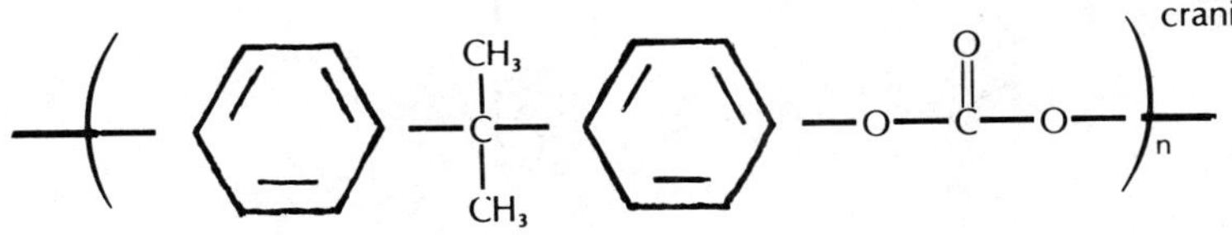

Cellulose

Dialysis membranes

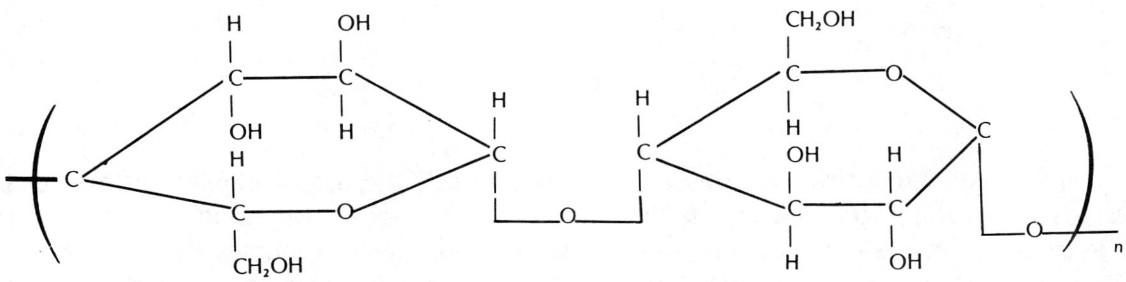

Celluluse acetate

Dialysis membranes

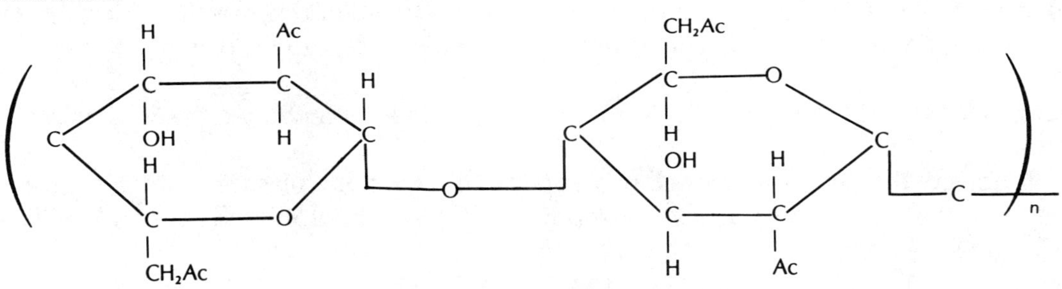

Polyalkylsulphone

Membrane oxygenators

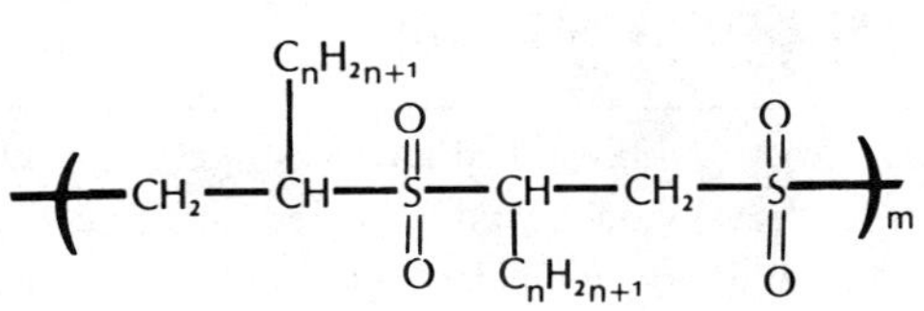

$n \sim 16$

Polypropylene

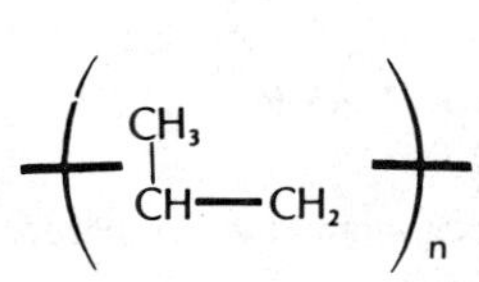

Syringes; catheters; oxygenators; dialysis heart valve occluders sutures

Polyacrylic acid

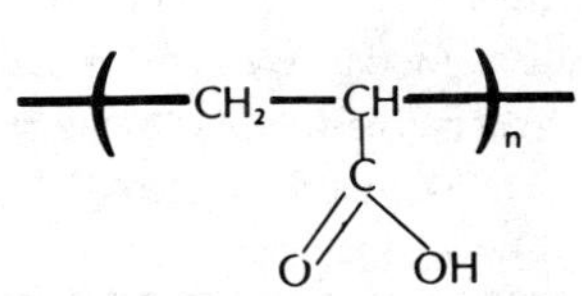

Dental cement

TABLE IIa. (Continued)

Gelatin/resorcinol/ formaldehyde	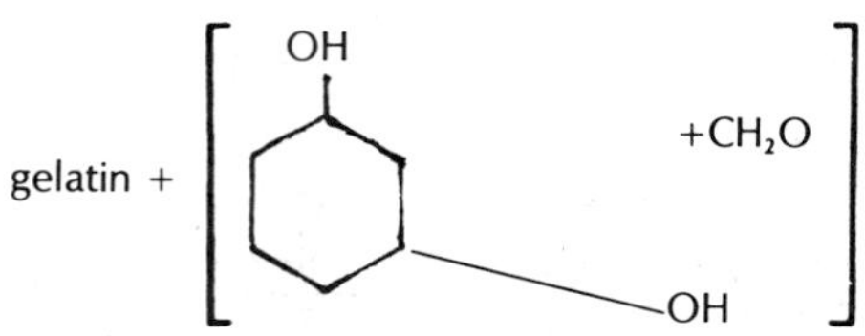	Tissue adhesive
Polysulfide rubber (mercaptan)		Dental impressions

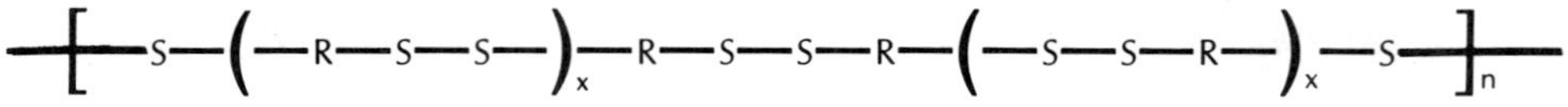

$R = —C_2H_4—O—CH_2—O—C_2H_4—$

$S \approx 23$

As will be seen later, new stabilization techniques enable the use of sterilization methods previously impossible to consider. The most common methods of sterilization of plastics for use in medical devices are heat, gas (ethylene oxide) and radiation sources.

Other sterilization methods are commercially available such as steam, unsaturated chemical vapor, formaldehyde and alkaline Glutaraldehyde but are not generally considered because of the deleterious effect on most medical polymers. The unsaturated chemical vapor sterilization process was developed as a fast and effective method for sterilizing metallic objects, such as cutting instruments and surgical blades, without concern for rusting or corrosion of the metals.

Each of the most common methods of sterilization previously mentioned has its limitations as follows:

Table III depicts the sterilization methods applicable to various plastics materials. Proper stabilization of the polymer again plays an important role in utilization of the various sterilization techniques.

TABLE III
STERILIZATION METHODS FOR VARIOUS PLASTICS MATERIALS

POLYMER	STERLIZATION METHODS
Acrylics	Soften with autoclaving. Radiation may cause chemical degradation but satisfactory with a single radiation sterilization dose. ETO unsatisfactory for molded articles as poor gas penetration results.
Cellulose Acetate	ETO method satisfactory. Radiation may reduce strength.
Fluorocarbons	Heat and gas may be used safely. Radiation unsuitable with PTFE. Fluorinated ethylene/propylene copolymers more radiation resistant.
Polypropylene	May be autoclaved and gas sterilized. Newer types more resistant to radiation.
Silicones	Gaseous methods generally result in slow diffusion of gas out of material. Moderately stable to radiation.
Polyvinyl Chloride	ETO gas satisfactory. ETO may also be used after irradiation if product is properly aerated. Generally discolors and some x-linking with radiation.

HEAT-Generally unsuitable with plastics having low softening points causing distortion and changes in properties.

ETHYLENE OXIDE-Still the most widely used method in the United States as it is relatively harmless to plastic materials. However, surface glazing is possible as well as temporary retention of the gas by plastics.

RADIATION-Very effective with high penetration levels. Until recently, more widely used in Europe but interest in radiation sterilization is now increasing in the United States. Some polymers are attacked causing embrittlement and discoloration while others require special stabilization techniques to protect polymers from degradation. If embrittlement occurs, mechanical failures of medical devices on aging is possible.

As we note that heat is generally unsuitable with polymers having low softening points, i.e. temperature sensitive materials, concentration will now be centered on the two most commercially used sterilization methods for medical devices, ethylene oxide and radiation.

Ethylene Oxide

Historically, this sterilant was investigated by the Army Medical Corps following World War II. In 1949 Phillips and Kaye first established the physical and chemical characteristics of ethylene oxide as a sterilant [5]. The mechanism for the action of ethylene oxide on bacteria, spores and viruses has still not been established with certainty. However, one proposed mechanism is the replacement of the available hydrogen atom in susceptible chemical groups in a protein molecule with its hydroxyethyl radical. Another way of expressing this is that the gas penetrates the micro-organisms and chemically reacts with it's protein. The metabolism and reproduction cycle is disrupted and the cells can no longer survive.

For a successful ethylene oxide sterilization system, four factors must basically be considered; gas concentration, moisture, time and temperature.

Gas Concentration

As pure ethylene oxide is extremely toxic and explosive, it is often but not always mixed with an inert gas to reduce flammability. Typical commercial systems used are:

100% ETO, 12% ETO/88% Freon and 20% ETO/80% CO_2.

Generally the effective concentration may range between 400-1600 mg/liter. In Europe many units operate at the maximum of 1600 mg/liter.

Moisture and Humidity

Moisture is important for improving penetration of the ethylene oxide into the end products and is generally accomplished by preconditioning the medical products in a relative humidity range of 30-60% [6]. Excessive humidity may produce high levels of toxic ethylene glycol which may be difficult to remove from the final product. One trend of thought is that at low temperatures and humidity for longer periods of time, a more uniform penetration results with less chance of significant residuals developing.

Time

This factor depends on the size of the sterilizer, load product, density and composition of product which determines porosity.

Temperature

Typical commercial operating temperatures range from 21.1°C to 65.5°C with higher temperatures allowing more rapid diffusion of the gas into the product in shorter periods of time.

Consideration must be given to toxic by-products which can develop during the ETO sterilization process and how to minimize their formation as well as their removal if necessary from the finished products.

Ethylene glycol formed as the result of the presence of both ethylene oxide and water

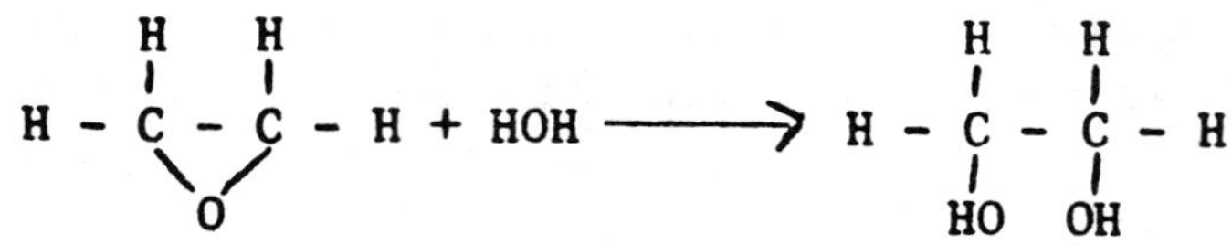

Ethylene chlorohydrin formed by ethylene oxide reacting with chloride atoms

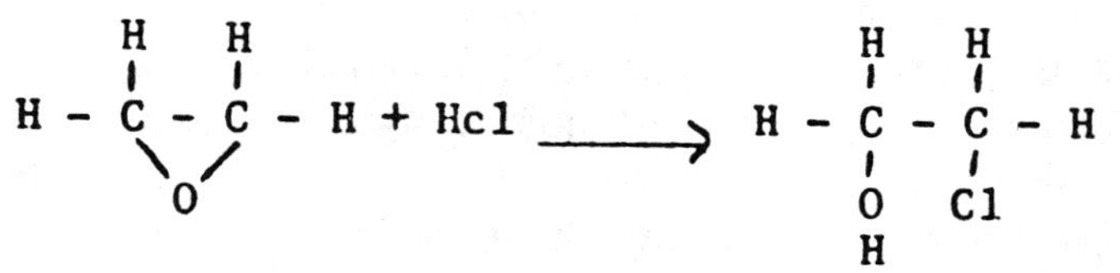

A third but less common by-product is the possibility of diethylene glycol formed by the presence of both ethylene oxide and ethylene glycol under acidic conditions [7].

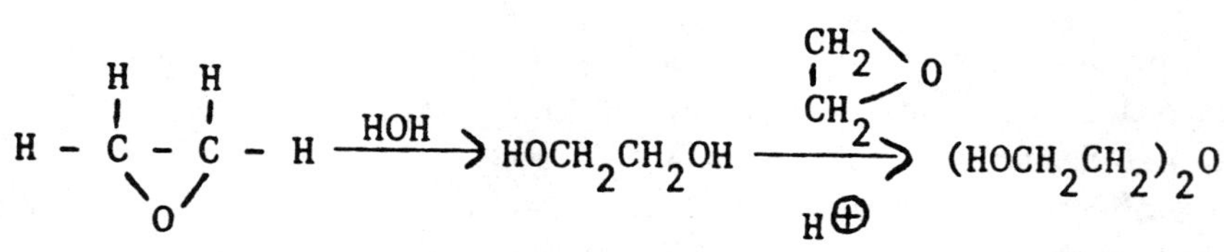

Ethylene glycol — Diethylene glycol

Keeping in mind the consequences resultant from ethylene oxide sterilization residuals remaining

(a) of the gas itself and

(b) it's by-products

commercially gas sterilized medical devices should be carefully monitored for residual levels before marketing. Poorly aerated products can result in skin and mucous membrane irritations or chemical burns, as ETO can react with human protein.

Many factors influence the rate of release of residuals, such as the density and type of polymer. A porous rubber may have high gas absorption levels compared to a rigid polyvinylchloride. Plasticized PVC absorbs and retains a greater amount of ETO versus the unplasticized polymer. Experience has shown that the average medical device containing a plasticized PVC component requires a minimum of two weeks at room temperature for proper aeration. Once high levels of these by-products have been absorbed it is difficult to remove them without using conditions which could affect the performance and properties of the medical device components. To accelerate the removal of residuals, a commercial aerator is suggested containing bacterial filters and operated for 8-15 hours at a minimum of 122°F (50°C.)

Table IV is a comparison which is often made of ethylene oxide parameters versus gamma radiation.

TABLE IV
BASIC COMPARISON OF DIFFERENCES BETWEEN ETHYLENE OXIDE AND GAMMA RADIATION STERILIZATION

Basic Feature	Ethylene Oxide	Gamma Radiation
Physical Parameters	Time, Temperature, RH, Pressure, ETO Concentration	Time
Micro-biological Control	Essential	Not required
Product Mix	Single Product	Mixed Product
Materials of Construction	Most Materials Satisfactory	Most Materials Satisfactory
Packaging	Porous Materials Essential	Hermetic Seal Possible
Radiation System	Batch only	Batch or Continuous

In addition to the above apparent advantages of gamma radiation over ETO, other factors have now become evident accounting for the increasing interest in this method of sterilization.

These are the economics of lower total cost combined with higher process reliability as a method of sterilization for many single-use medical devices. Also enhancing the use of gamma radiation is the Governmental potential tightening of control regulations. This is as the result of reputed mutogenic and carcinogenic effects of continual exposure to ETO and its by-products.

Radiation

There are two methods for radiation sterilization of medical devices: exposing them to intense doses of high-energy electron or gamma radiation.

Basic Principles

In both gamma and electron radiation, the lower energy electrons produce chemical changes in the medium and lead to the destruction of micro-organisms. The degree of sterilization achieved in any device is directly related to the amount of radiation absorbed. The radiation absorbed dose is normally measured in rads. Rad is defined as 100 ergs of absorbed energy per gram of material irradiated. In the case of gamma radiation, sterilization or destruction of live bacteria and other micro-organisms is conveniently carried out by exposing the material to the ionizing radiation emitted from radioactive materials. Sources of radioactive material are gamma rays generated from isotopes such as cobalt 60 or cesium 137. Cesium

137 although having a much longer shelf life requires a greater quantity to obtain the same radiation level. Theoretically, the ionizing gamma radiations absorb energy and the chemical consequences of this energy absorption should kill or inactivate bacteria and micro-organisms. The micro-organisms undergo chain scission of their deoxyribonucleic acid (DNA) and ribonucleic acid (RNA) chains rendering the chains unable to reproduce.

A. Electron Beam

In the past the use of the electron beam as a method for sterilizing medical devices was of little interest in the United States and Europe because of the limited depth of penetration and very uneven absorption. Today with recent advances in accelerator design, many of the previous problems have been overcome including the penetrating power of radiation through the final package. It is now reported that with dose rates as high as 18 million electron volts (MeV) the electrons have a penetrating power for single-pass processing similar to that of the radiation produced by a cobalt 60 gamma source.

Most electron accelerators use a cathode tube to generate electrons. These electrons are then accelerated in a vacuum tube by electrostatic forces or microwaves to increase the energy and penetrability of the electrons. In a typical electron beam processing operation, the parameters to consider are electron current, conveyor speed, electron energy and product area to be irradiated. Today electron beam irradiation is generated by such high voltage machines as the linear accelerator, the Van der Graff accelerator and the Dynamitron. Limitations which still favor the use of gamma radiation over the electron beam are:

1. Heat-sensitive products (product temperature increases)
2. Density factor - higher density products where electron beam still may present poor penetration.

The principal advantage for the electron beam is shorter exposure times resulting in the possibility of less material damage and consequently higher efficiency rates for those materials in which electrons can achieve adequate penetration. It is also a turnkey operation generating radiation as required while with cobalt 60 radiation decay is continuous whether processing or not.

B. Gamma Radiation

As noted from a previous table comparing the ETO sterilization process with gamma radiation, time is the only principle factor involved in gamma radiation. This method because of its many advantages over other sterilization systems is now being adopted by an ever increasing segment of the medical device industry.

In Europe, Alpha, Beta and Gamma type of radiation were studied. Gamma radiation was selected. An important feature of gamma radiation from cobalt 60 (the source commonly used) is that it generates no radioactivity in material exposed to it. It is most useful for radiation sterilization because its high penetration allows material to be treated in bulk. Gamma rays can be regarded as electro-magnetic radiation. Alpha and Beta radiations are relatively poor in penetration and thus restricted in use. Cobalt 60 is preferred for radiation in Europe because it is produced in large quantities in nuclear reactors and has a fairly slow decay rate of 12 1/2%–per annum. The basic sterilization process consists of placing the material to be sterilized near a source of cobalt 60 where it is left until the required Megarad (Mrad) dose has been absorbed.

A typical gamma site is composed of a central gamma cell source around which the product to be sterilized is transported. The product is generally placed in metal totes and exposed to the radiation source in a continuous operation until the required dose level has been obtained. By this procedure both batch and continuous operations are possible. When not in use the radioisotope source, Cobalt 60, is generally immersed 20 ft. below the surface of a pool of water. A blue fluorescent effect develops known as the "Cerenkov effect" which is the consequence of an excited state in the water molecule produced from ionizing radiation.

Disposal of waste or spent cobalt 60 has been a prevalent problem. However, in the U.S. and Europe methods are now being developed to reactivate such material. It is also finding use where low level radiation is required in medical applications.

Dosimetric methods are used to control the radiation process.
Two systems widely used are:
(a) Dyed acrylic-plastic chip and
(b) Radiochromic film dosimeters.
Generally, measurements are made of the optical density changes which take place in proportion to the absorbed dosage. The radiochromic type dosimeters are quite small and can conveniently be placed at almost any point within a carrier in a radiation system. In Europe the general radiation level used is 2.5 Megarads. In the United States, there has recently been much interest in the possibility of using radiation sterilization doses that are lower than 2.5 Mrads, provided that the product bioburden is sufficently low. As a result of this approach, levels of 1.5 Mrads or less are possible for adequately sterilizing medical devices. Some generalizations obtained from recent preliminary field data has shown control of bacteria at 0.3 Mrads, Spores at 1.5 Mrads and most resistant spores at 2.1 Mrads.

There is no residual radiation generated after gamma exposure as gamma rays have no mass. This enables immediate use of products which have been radiation sterilized. This process for microbiological control is a low temperature operation. The complete product and package can be sterilized at under 100ºF with negligible effect on processing time.

There has been much discussion concerning precautions to be taken for PVC medical components which have been gamma irradiated followed by re-sterilization with ETO. Gamma ray sterilization makes chloride atoms readily available for the formation of toxic ethylene chlorohydrin.

The latest data developed indicates that provided recommended aeration times are rigidly adhered to for PVC components following ETO sterilization, previously gamma-irradiated items can be resterilized with ethylene oxide [8].

The radiation resistance of common polymeric materials is shown in Table V. Generally, polystyrene and urethane rubber have the most resistance.

TABLE V
THE RADIATION RESISTANCE OF COMMON POLYMERIC MATERIALS

Material	Stability Effect
Acrylonitrile-Butadiene Styrene (ABS)	Stable for single dose of 2.5 Mrads
Polyamides	Suitable for single doses of 2.5 Mrad level
Polyethylene	Stable under ordinary conditions at 2.5 Mrads
Polypropylene	Embrittles - newer variations more resistant
Poly (vinyl chloride)	Withstands single dose radiation cycle - but discolors - some HCl liberated

TABLE V (Continued)

Polystyrene	Most radiation - stable of common polymers
Poly (tetrafluoroethylene)	Poor resistance to radiation-Copolymers less affected
Polysulfone	Stable under ordinary conditions at 2.5 Mrads (Natural material is yellow)
Polyacetals	Embrittles - discolors
Polyurethane	Stable under ordinary conditions at 2.5 Mrads
Polymethylmethacrylate	Embrittles - discolors
Rubber	
Natural	Stable under ordinary conditions when properly compounded
Butyl	Poor stability at low radiation levels
Silicones	Stable under ordinary conditions at 2.5 Mrads
Urethanes	Excellent radiation resistance

A search of the literature would indicate many areas of disagreement relative to the radiation resistance of basic materials used in the medical field. This is due to the types and purity of polymers available, additive systems and formulations developed for end use application. On this basis as a supplement to Table V the following generalizations can be made:

TABLE VI
The Radiation Stability of Commercial Materials

Material Thermoplastics	Stability	
Acrylonitrile/Butadiene/Styrene (ABS)	Good	
Cellulosics	Fair	Undergoes chain scission, esters more stable
Fluorinated ethylene propylene (FEP)	Fair	Copolymers more resistant than Homopolymer
Polyacetal	Poor	Embrittles
Polyamides		
Aromatic	Excellent	
Aliphatic	Fair	Hardens as levels increased
Polycarbonates	Good	Yellows-mechanical properties unchanged
Polyesters (Aromatic)	Good	
Polyethylene	Good	Lowers melt flow
Polymethylmethacrylate	Poor	Degrades - turns brown
Polyphenylene Sulfide	Good	
Polyproplyene	Fair	Improved stability if properly stabilized
Polysulfone	Excellent	Yellow natural color
Polystyrene	Excellent	
Polytetrafluoroethylene (PTFE)	Poor	Acids evolved
Polyvinylchloride		
Homopolymer	Good	If properly stabilized
Copolymer	Fair	HCl evolved - turns brown
Styrene/Acrylonitrile (SAN)	Good	More resistant than ABS

TABLE VI (Continued)

Material Thermosetting Resins	Stability	
Epoxies	Excellent	Very stable with the use of aromatic curing agents.
Phenol or Urea formaldehyde	Good	
Polyimides	Excellent	
Polyesters	Good	
Polyurethanes	Excellent	
Material Elastomers	**Stability***	
Polyisobutylene (Butyl)	Poor	
Natural	Good	
Urethanes	Excellent	
Nitrile	Good	
Polyacrylic	Poor	
Styrene-butadiene	Good	
EPDM	Good	
Silicones	Good	
Textiles	**Stability**	
Polyesters	Excellent	
Cellulosics	Poor	
Nylon	Fair	

***Additives such as fillers and plasticizers, etc., have a great influence on radiation stability of elastomers. Adhesives made from these polymers show good radiation resistance if the original polymer is satisfactory and with the use of proper additive systems. (Especially those additives containing aromatic group.)**

Manufacturers are learning how to modify and stabilize polymers to enhance radiation sterilization techniques. With the help of additives, this method is being increasingly used throughout the world for medical disposables as shown in Table VII.

TABLE VII
TYPICAL MEDICAL DISPOSABLES USING RADIATION STERILIZATION METHOD

Product	Type of Packaging	Materials	Where Processed
Bandages	paper, plastics	plastic, cotton adhesive non-wovens, polyurethane foam	Europe
Bladder irrigation sets	plastic	PVC	Europe
Catheters	plastic	rubber, plastic, water	Europe
First aid packs	plastic	paraffin, plastic polyurethane foam	Asia
Forceps	paper	polystyrene	Asia

TABLE VII (Continued)

Hypodermic syringes	paper	polypropylene, water filled, SBR rubber, polyethylene, polystyrene	North America
Infusion sets	plastic	plastic, PVC	Europe

Although many polymers may be used by themselves without modification, others require complex formulating. The composition of these formulations may vary from one manufacturer to another due to differences in the additives, methods of blending and processing as well as sterilization selection. Proper selection of polymers and additives is of the utmost importance because of the need for blood and tissue compatibility and mechanically strong materials to suit the end use and device application. Because of the importance of such additives on radiation sterilization stability as well as the general stability of medical polymers, a description of these additives and possible interactions seems appropriate. Additives can be considered as energy absorbers or antirads. As will be seen later, aromatic additives generally help to stabilize polymers exposed to radiation sources.

Radiation commonly used in Europe for the past twenty years in sterilization of medical devices has now become of increasing interest in the U.S. primarily because of recent Government concern on the toxicity levels of Ethylene Oxide.

Moreover, radiation sterilization can result in a high probability of sterility for devices or materials that are not readily sterilized by alternative methods due to sensitivity to temperature, moisture and possibly high ethylene oxide retention.

With the rising costs of Ethylene Oxide, high volume radiation sterilization can result in lower sterilization operating costs especially permitting the use of lower cost packaging materials. These generally are hermetically sealed and prevent penetration of the sterilizing gas.

Depending on the chemical structure of the polymer as well as additives used for stabilization, irradiation may result in crosslinking or degradation of the polymer.

Although many types of additives are available and sometimes necessary for the proper stabilization of medical polymers, it is most advantageous to use the least feasible amount. This minimizes the difficulties which one may encounter due to possible extraction and contact problems which become evident during biological testing of medical devices.

The new polymers available today contain less residuals such as catalysts and monomers which affect the level of additives required. Since not enough is known about interaction between synthetic materials and living tissue, most medical polymers are formulated with some degree of additives to convey specific desirable properties to the polymer. It is especially true in European and other foreign countries where it has been difficult to obtain pure highly characterized polymers completely free of monomer, antioxidants and other additives [9].

Table VIII depicts the many additives to consider in the proper stabilization of medical polymers. Many of these polymers will require some type of heat stabilizer for protection during processing as well as antioxidants to improve aging properties. For flexible products, primary, secondary and specialty plasticizers must be selected for the end use application.

TABLE VIII
ADDITIVES TO CONSIDER IN THE STABILIZATION OF MEDICAL POLYMERS

Heat and light stabilizers
Lubricants
Modifiers (Impact and Processing Aids)
Antioxidants
Plasticizers (Primary, secondary and specialty types)
Pigments
Antistats

The most common primary plasticizer is Dioctyl phthalate used for producing flexible polyvinyl chloride (PVC) components. Specialty plasticizers, such as the epoxidized oils, aid in the stabilization of polymers by a synergistic effect with the primary heat stabilizer. Table IX defines typical available antioxidants of low toxicity levels. The most common primary antioxidants are hindered phenols such as butylated hydroxytoluene (BHT). This antioxidant, while quite fugitive having a low melting point, is necessary during the manufacture of polyethylene resins to prevent deterioration during the manufacturing process. As will be seen later, combinations of low toxicity type antioxidants may be required, depending on the process conditions of the polymer as well as its chemical composition.

TABLE IX
TYPICAL ANTIOXIDANTS OF LOW TOXICITY

1. **Primary antioxidants**
   (usually hindered phenols)

   Butylated Hydroxytoluene (BHT)

2. **Thioester antioxidants**
   (usually derivatives of thiodipropionic acid)

   Dilauryl thiodipropionate (DLTDP)
   Distearyl thiodipropionate (DSTDP)

3. **Phosphite antioxidants**
   (usually derivatives of aromatic phosphites)

   Distearyl pentaerythritol diphosphite
   Tris (nonylphenyl) phosphite

Stabilization problems of typical medical polymers are outlined in Table X. The rubber phase of ABS polymer requires an antioxidant to prevent possible breakdown of unsaturated bonds. Polyesters may discolor under an oxygen atmosphere without the proper antioxidant protection.

TABLE X
STABILIZATION PROBLEMS OF TYPICAL MEDICAL POLYMERS

Polypropylene
Presence of tertiary C-H groups along the polymer chain (susceptible to oxidation)
ABS
Possible breakdown of unsaturated bonds in the rubber phase
Polyethylene
Stabilized during manufacture against oxidation mainly to prevent color development and change in melt viscosity
PVC
Dehydrochlorination results in formation of a conjugated double bond structure (susceptible to oxidation)
Polyester
Discoloration under oxygen atmosphere

Until a proper stabilization system was developed for the polypropylene polymer, it was unsuitable commercially. Polypropylene may show little or no color change but embrittlement may take place initially or on aging especially as a result of trapped free radicals. It has been shown that proper heat treatment of this polymer and processing conditions can sometimes help to release more readily trapped free radicals present. Table XI demonstrates that the tertiary carbon structure must be protected from rapid degradation. This is accomplished by utilizing combinations of alkylated phenols, derivatives of thiodipropionic acid and phosphites. Addition of small amounts of calcium stearate improve the color hold.

TABLE XI
POLYPROPYLENE STABILIZATION

Isotactic PP

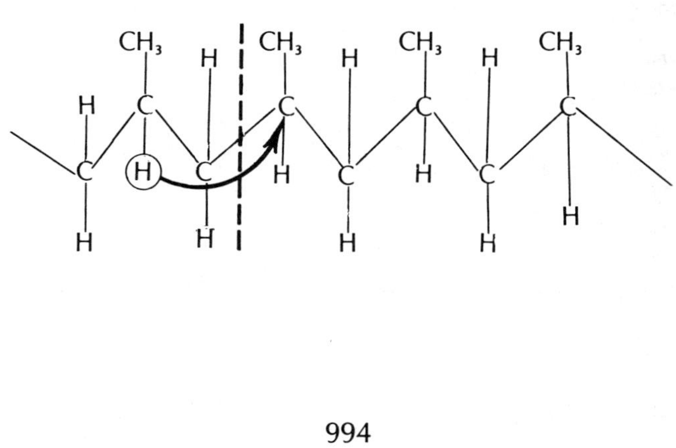

TABLE XI (Continued)

Syndiotactic PP

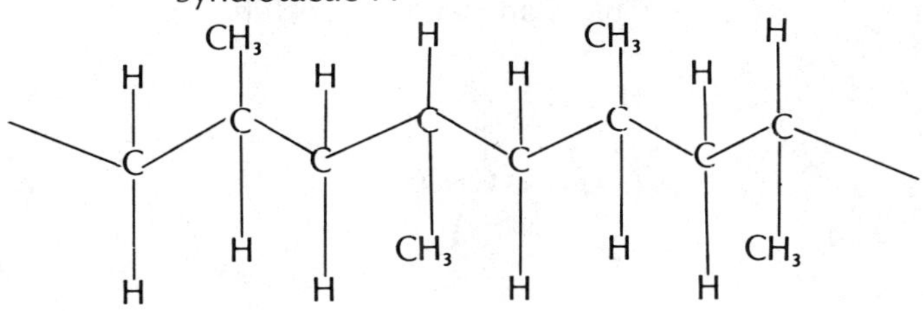

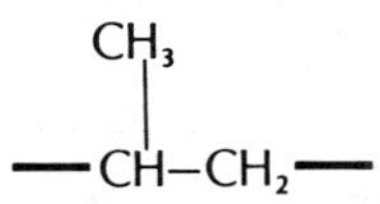

(Tertiary carbon structure)

Stabilization

1. High m.w alkylated phenols-tetrakis (methylene (3,5-ditert-butyl-4-hydroxy-hydrocinnamate)
2. Distearyl thiodipropionate
3. Distearyl pentaerythritol diphosphite
4. Metallic soap ie – calcium stearate (total concentration 0.25 to 1.0%)

The most commonly used polymer for medical applications is still polyvinyl chloride which being more complex requires special and higher amounts of additives. A proposed degradation mechanism for this polymer is shown in Table XII.

A dehydrochlorination by the removal of hydrochloric acid results in a conjugated polyene system which can readily be attacked by oxygen to produce carbonyl groups and free radicals. This product can then result in chain scission as well as cross linking and chromophoric (color producing) groups. To overcome the many possible degradation reactions requires a combination of an acid acceptor, an antioxidant and miscellaneous other materials as defined in Table XIII "Requirements for an Ideal PVC Stabilizer."

TABLE XII
DEGRADATION MECHANISM FOR POLYVINYL CHLORIDE

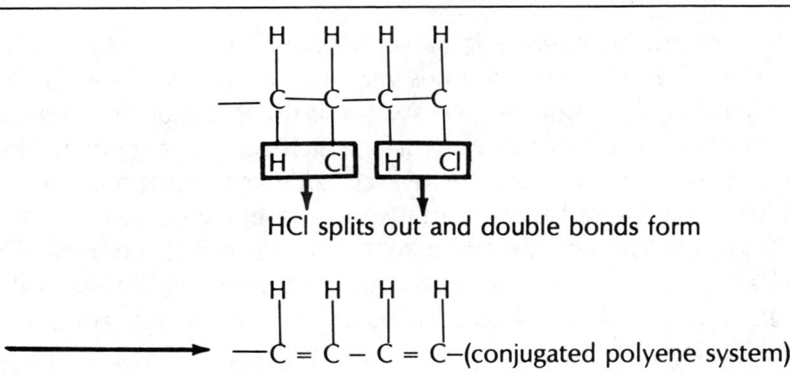

TABLE XII (Continued)

This is attached by oxygen, viz:

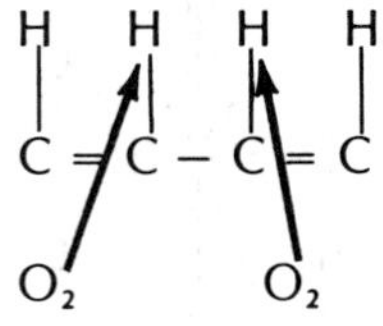

→ C = O (carbonyl groups) and free radicals C –

Ideal stabilizer:
An antioxidant that would be an acid acceptor

TABLE XIII
REQUIREMENTS FOR AN IDEAL PVC STABILIZER

1.	Control release of Hydrogen Chloride evolution from the resin by neutralization and absorption
2.	Displacement of active groups such as the chloride atom attached to a tertiary carbon
3.	Deactivation of stabilizer degradation products such as heavy metal chlorides
4.	Chain reaction disruption e.g. stop progressive unsaturation caused by oxidation and free radical attack
5.	Inactivation of resin impurities, residues, etc.
6.	UV protection

Today with the increasing interest in radiation sterilization, many new problems have developed [11]. Chemical structure becomes very significant in addition to the primary factor of polymer heat stability. For example, polystyrene is notably radiation resistant and superior in this property to the fluorocarbon polymers which have exceptional heat resistance. It therefore becomes necessary to consider overall additives which may possibly sensitize as well as aid in improving the radiation resistance of the many polymers used in the medical field. Some chemical compounds exert apparent radiation resistance by depletion of free oxygen by chemical reaction of oxygen stimulation (metabolic process.) Table XIV reviews typical sensitizers and radiation resistors for consideration should radiation sterilization be used on medical devices.

TABLE XIV
EFFECT OF ADDITIVES ON THE RADIATION STABILIZATION OF MEDICAL POLYMERS

Sensitizers	
1.	Nitrites, nitrates
2.	Quinones
3.	Halides
Radiation Resisters	
1.	Sulfhydryl - containing compounds
2.	Ascorbate
3.	Dimethylsulfoxide
4.	Protein and carbohydrates

Some common plasticizers used in plastic manufacture have been listed in Table XV indicating their general toxicity characteristics. It is evident from frequently released Government bulletins that the most commonly used types such as phthalates and epoxidized soya bean oil are still continually under investigation for toxicity levels. As more sensitive analytical equipment is developed, the regulatory requirements also become more stringent.

TABLE XV
TOXICITY DATA ON SOME COMMON PLASTICIZERS USED IN PLASTIC MANUFACTURE

Plasticizer	Toxicity
Adipates	To date animal experiments indicate possible carcinogenicity
Glycolates	Generally of low toxicity levels. However, studies underway as commercial forms are phthalyl derivatives
Phosphates	Generally cause irritation to skin and mucous membranes
Phthalates	Although commercially used in medical devices, environmental effects and toxicological properties continually under investigation
Epoxidized Soya Bean Oil	Chelating type of plasticizer with low toxicity

The toxicity of commonly used polymer stabilizers and additives are classified in Table XVI. Fatty acid derivatives of calcium, zinc and magnesium provide low toxicity when required for producing PVC medical components. For rigid non-toxic PVC special applications, octyl tin derivatives are available. In France, calcium-zinc metallic soaps have been approved. Both Japan and Germany have limited the use of all tins including the octyl type stabilizer. The U.K.

generally follows very closely the regulatory requirements of the U.S. and, therefore, approves use of similar additives.

TABLE XVI
TOXICITY OF COMMONLY USED POLYMER STABILIZERS AND ADDITIVES

Stabilizer	Toxicity
Fatty acid derivatives of calcium, zinc and magnesium	Low toxicity. Used in non-toxic medical applications
Barium fatty acid compounds	Moderately toxic
Lead & cadmium derivatives	Highly toxic. Not recommended in the U.S. for use in medical applications (cadmium pigments considered of low toxicity in England)
Amines (antioxidants)	Generally toxic, with aromatic amines showing carcinogenic tendencies. Newer types less toxic
Butylated Hydroxytoluene (BHT) (antioxidant)	Considered non-toxic as also used in foods. Recently investigated and found non-carcinogenic
Octyl tin compounds	Only class of tin compounds classified as of low toxicity and used in medical applications e.g. di-(n-octyl) tin maleate polymer

Developers of a suitable medical device must also design a versatile package that will maintain its principle properties following radiation exposure. Table XVII lists some of the most common device packaging materials in use today. Some of the parameters that must be considered in the evaluation of irradiated packaging materials are long term stability, packaging strength retention, seal strength, discoloration of the package and printing ink and durability for shipment [12].

TABLE XVII
MEDICAL DEVICE PACKAGING

Substrate	Properties
Spun bonded polyolefin	Tear and puncture-resistant web. Readily allows the penetration of ETO gas. More costly than most packaging materials.
Plastic film	Semi-rigid (e.g., PVC) Used in kits, sets and trays. Includes coextrusion and copolymer systems. Sterilization methods may vary depending on polymer type and on thickness of material.
Surgical grade	Very economical, but generally poor aesthetically. Protection is sometimes inadequate during shipping and handling of medical devices. More widely used in Europe than in the United States. Readily adaptable to radiation sterilization.

CONCLUSIONS

We have made great strides since the development of the first polymeric materials which had poor physical and aging properties when used in medical devices.

Today with the advances in polymer science, specialty polymers have been developed for specific medical applications. Future technology shows further promise in explaining previously unexplainable phenomena such as rejection of plastic body implants and the control of bacterial infections in these implants.

Ethylene oxide is still the most widely used method in the United States for sterilizing medical devices. However, with the Government's potential tightening of control regulations along with the economics of lower total costs and higher process reliability, gamma radiation is finding its' place in the sterilization of single-use medical devices in the United States.

By utilizing radiation sterilization techniques, a wider range of packaging materials are available in the U.S. and Europe (papers, plastics and laminates.)

The foremost problem in the stabilization of medical polymers is still the difficulty in obtaining pure polymers completely free of monomers, catalyst residues and miscellaneous additives. This is especially true in European and other foreign countries.

Selected additives are needed in minimal amounts to protect medical polymers from external sources of degradation, such as heat and light, as well as to improve aging properties.

Typical commercially approved additives such as antioxidants, plasticizers and stabilizers have been tabulated which satisfy today's medical and regulatory requirements.

Using properly selected and stabilized polymers, the device manufacturer today performs extensive evaluation tests on all materials and components to produce a safe and marketable medical product which can be sterilized by conventional methods used today such as ethylene oxide or radiation.

REFERENCES

1. Stevenson, Robert S. *"Famous Illnesses in History"* London-Eyre and Spottis Woode, 1962
2. Landfield, Harold "Selective Parameters for the use of Plastics in Medical Devices" NATEC 1977 SPE, DENVER, COLORADO, Nov. 8, 1977
3. Gibbons, D.F. Chapter entitled *Biomedical Materials* In the handbook "Engineering in Medicine and Biology," Fleming and Feinberg Editors CRP Press, Cleveland, Ohio 1976
4. Lee, H. Neville, K. Chapter XV in the handbook of *Biomedical Plastics,* Pasadena Technology Press, Pasadena, California 91105
5. Phillips, C.R. and Kaye, S., "The Sterilizing Action of Gaseous Ethylene Oxide," AM. J. Hyg. 50:270-306, 1949
6. Tessler, J. *"Reaction of the Sterilant Ethylene Oxide on Plastics"* App. Microb. 9:256, 1961
7. Roberts, John D. and Caserio, Majorie, C. "Basic Principles of Organic Chemistry" P-410-411 W. A. Benjamin, Inc. New York, N.Y. 1965
8. Roberts, Robert B., M.D. "Respiratory Care" - Mar 1976, Vol 21, No. 3 P-223, 224
9. Private communications with European and U.S. Polymer Producers
10. Nass, E. "Encyclopedia of PVC" Vol I 280 (1976)
11. Landfield, H. "The Effect of Radiation on various materials and the qualification tests required for their use in medical devices." Presented at the Seminar on Radiation Sterilization of Plastics Medical Devices, Cambridge, Mass., Mar 28, and 29, 1979.
12. Landfield, H. " Radiation Effects on device and packaging materials", "Medical Device and Diagnostic Industry" Vol 2, No. 5 May 1980 PP 47-48

Chapter 44

Ionizing Radiation's Effects on Selected Biomedical Polymers

W. E. Skiens
Senior Research Scientist
Battelle Memorial Institute
Pacific Northwest Laboratories
Richland, Washington 99352
and
J. L. Williams
Manager, Materials Research Department
Becton, Dickinson and Company
Research Center
Research Triangle Park, NC 27709

ABSTRACT

Sterilization of plastic medical devices by ionizing radiation has become a well recognized industrial process. Polymeric materials interact with radiation to produce free radicals which in turn react with the polymer chains to cause either crosslinking or chain scission. These reactions may produce a variety of effects in the properties of the irradiated polymer.

The radiation dose necessary to induce significant changes in the properties of polymers varies greatly, ranging from about 10^5 rads with polytetrafluorethylene to nearly 10^{10} rads for polysulfones and polystyrene. The effects of ionizing radiation on a selected group of polymers, thermoplastics, thermosets and elastomers, are detailed with suggestions regarding their applicability to radiation sterilization.

Sterilization of plastic medical devices and supplies by ionizing radiation is increasingly being employed as an alternative to gaseous ethylene oxide sterilization. Ethylene oxide is extremely toxic, is readily absorbed by many polymers, and is not always easily or readily desorbed or eliminated. Many plastic materials cannot be sterilized by techniques which require heat (dry heat or steam), nor is treatment with cold (aqueous) sterilants satisfactory in many instances. Ionizing radiation, therefore, is assuming an increasingly important role in the sterilization of many medical products and, indeed, at this time is becoming a well established industrial process. Although this technique is not limited to the sterilization of polymeric materials, it is probably the most applicable method for many of these materials.

Polymers discussed in this application are organic materials made up of specific molecules-monomers-bonded together in multiple repeat units to form a high molecular weight material (macromolecule). These materials may be either synthetic or natural, although only synthetic or modified natural polymers are commonly used.

The arrangement of molecules in macromolecules may be very regular or completely random, thus providing zones of potentially high crystallinity or those with little or no apparent crystallinity. The degree of crystallinity is highly dependent not only on the molecular makeup, but also upon the processing conditions used to form the material.

In addition to the macromolecules themselves, commercial polymer products frequently contain varying (usually small) amounts of other components to aid in processing, to stabilize the polymer, or to provide particular desirable properties to the product. These additives are generally small molecules which function in the polymer matrix as antioxidants, ultra-violet light stabilizers, plasticizers, inert fillers, processing aids, etc., usually in low concentrations (1% or less), although some additives acting as fillers or reinforcing agents may be used in quantities from 10-70%.

The effects of ionizing radiation's interaction with polymers vary greatly with the basic chemical structure of the polymer. Thus, the dose necessary to produce similar significant effects in two different polymers may vary from values as low as about 4×10^4 rads in polytetrafluorethylene, to 4×10^9 rads or more in styrene or polyimides. These interactions, even at low doses, can significantly effect the mechanical and physical properties of the polymer. For instance, in a typical polyethylene with an average molecular weight of about 100,000, and readily soluble in a solvent such as decalin, only one cross link per 14,000 monomer (ethylene) units can cause gelation (insolubility) (1). Radiation effects on the properties of a polymer are often difficult to predict. Certain additives have very distinct protective action in preventing radiation damage to plastics. These compounds are frequently termed "antirads" and usually are materials which also act as antioxidants. The action of these additives can be either that of a reactant which combines readily with radiation generated free radicals in the polymer, or that of a primary energy absorber preventing radiation's interaction with the polymer itself.

Radition generally interacts with polymers in two basic manners, both resulting from excitation or ionizaton of atoms in the polymer by the high energy source. Alterations in molecular structure of the polymer as a result of these interactions appear as changes in the chemical and physical properties. The two major mechanisms of degradation or change occurring as polymers are irradiated are: 1) chain scission, occurring as a random rupturing of bonds which reduce the molecular weight of the polymer and 2) crosslinking of polymer molecules which results in the formation of large three-dimensional networks. Usually both of these mechanisms occur as polymeric materials are subjected to ionizing radiation, but frequently one mechanism predominates with a specific polymer. As a result of chain scission, very low molecular weight fragments, gas evolution, and unsaturated bonds may appear. Crosslinking generally results in initial increase in tensile strength, while impact strength decreases and the polymer becomes more brittle with increased dose. For polymers with carbon-carbon chains (backbones) it is observed that crosslinking generally will occur if the carbons have one or more hydrogens attached to them, whereas scission occurs at tetra substituted carbons. Polymers containing aromatic molecules generally are much more resistant to radiation degradation than aliphatic polymers. This is true whether or not the aromatic group is directly in the chain backbone or not. Thus, both polystyrene, with a pendant aromatic group and polyimides, with an aromatic group directly in the polymer backbone, are relatively resistant to high doses (10^9- 10^{10} rads). From a product/use viewpoint, the loss of mechanical properties is the most important characteristic affected by irradiation of polymers. These properties include tensile strength, elastic modulus, impact strength, and shear strength as well as elongation. Embrittlement may occur even as irradiated polymers decrease in hardness. Crystallinity and, hence, density characteristics may also change as chain scission continues.

Another consideration resulting from irradiation of polymers is the development of color. This is usually an undesirable development, whether the change results in only yellowing the product or in complete opacity. These changes, which usually occur at widely differing doses in various polymers, are often influenced by the presence of oxygen and may either diminish or develop with storage after irradiation.

A great deal of the information available from government reports, industrial literature, and scientific publications concerning radiation effects on polymers deals with their properties after exposure to extremely high doses and frequently little data is available on biomedical polymers in the exposure range of sterilization.

Radiation dose conditions used for sterilization, although varying significantly from process to process or device to device, generally appear to be in the 1-5 megarad (Mrad) range. It is assumed that the effects of radiation on polymers are cumulative with each subsequent exposure of a device or product.

The polymers described in this chapter are divided into three major types; thermoplastics, thermosets, and elastomers, all of which are used extensively in biomedical applications. Some additional remarks are included concerning fibers, adhesives, coatings, and potting compounds which, although generally polymeric in nature, frequently serve different functions than the usual biomedical plastics.

The conditions of irradiation can significantly affect the properties of the material. The presence of oxygen or air may alter the results of interaction of radiation with polymers. Free radicals produced in polymers by irradiation in air are often rapidly converted into peroxidic radicals (2). The fate of these radicals is dependent both upon the nature of the irradiated polymer, upon the presence of additives, and on other parameters such as temperature, total dose, dose rate, and sample size. Conditions may also change the interaction of radiation with polymer additives resulting in gas evolution and formation of other degradation products from these small molecules, with the possibility of producing irritants or other undesirable products.

THERMOPLASTICS

This large group of polymers constitutes the most widely used type in medical devices, supplies and packaging. These polymers are normally processed by standard polymer melt processing techniques such as injection molding and extrusion or spinning. Many of these materials are briefly described in the following paragraphs.

ABS (Acrylonitrile/Butadiene/Styrene)

Although ABS materials are less radiation resistant than styrene or styrene/acrylonitrile polymers, they are readily processed by standard polymer fabrication techniques and will withstand one or more radiation sterilization procedures of up to 5 Mrads dose with no observable effect on properties (3).

Polyacetals

Homopolymers and copolymers making up the polyacetals are derived from formaldehyde as the primary monomer. Both the copolymers and homopolymers are relatively sensitive to radiation. Radiation doses exceeding 1.0 Mrad appear to cause undesirable changes in these materials and, although they have many desirable properties as structural plastics, they should be used with caution where they may be expected to receive radiation doses in excess of 1 Mrad (3). The radiation damage threshold is estimated at 0.5 Mrad with 25% damage at 1.1 Mrads (4-6).

Polyacrylics

This important group of materials consist of a number of commercially available polymers and copolymers with a wide range of uses and properties. The most commonly used acrylic polymer, polymethyl methacrylate (PMMA), has relatively poor ionizing radiation resistance (7-9). It is certainly capable of withstanding at least one sterilizing radiation procedure in most of its finished product forms without noticeable effect, however, multiple doses in the Mrad range may be expected to affect its mechanical properties significantly. A dose in the 10^7 rads range degrades this polymer to produce an unacceptably brittle product (10-13). Perhaps more importantly, one of PMMA's most desirable properties, optical clarity, is considerably affected. Discoloration may occur at doses as low as 0.5 Mrads and light transmission can decrease by more than 50% after a 5 Mrads exposure. Some recovery of transmission occurs during storage in oil and certain additives help protect the polymer against radiation damage.

Other acrylic polymers such as polyacrylonitrile, polyacrylates, polyhydroxyacrylates and polycyanoacrylates appear to have somewhat better resistance to radiation than PMMA, but none of these materials should be sterilized by radiation many times (11).

Polyamides

These polymers referred to as nylons (in some cases aramids) are among the most commonly used for many applications. The aliphatic polyamides, nylons 6, 66, 6/10, 12, etc., show little difference in their stability to radiation. Nylons of this type generally crosslink under the influence of radiation and initially show increases in tensile strength and hardness, associated with decreasing elongation to break and impact strength (14). Thus, these materials can readily withstand single radiation sterilization; however, the advisability of multiple sterilizations should be questioned, depending upon the use and the particular polymer.

The aromatic family of polyamides called aramids, although most frequently appearing in fiber form, have very excellent radiation (10^9 rads) and thermal stability and can be expected to retain all their properties after multiple sterilizations by radiation or other techniques (15).

Most recently some new transparent (amorphous) polyamides have been made available and may be very useful in some applications, but may be expected to be sensitive to multiple sterilizations.

Cellulosics

The cellulosic polymers considered in biomedical applications are primarily the cellulose esters (including mixed esters) and cellulose ethers, particularly ethly cellulose. They exhibit fair radiation resistance and, although their resistance varies considerably from material to material, an average dose value at which significant (~25%) degradation takes place is, for example, in cellulose acetate about 20 Mrads. Thus, these materials appear to be able to withstand a limited number of sterilizations without significant effect on their properties (16,17).

Fluoropolymers

Fluorinated polymers and particularly polytetrafluoroethylene (PTFE) are renowned for their chemical stability and their high temperature use characteristics. However, some of these materials are extremely sensitive to radiation and are among the poorest known polymers in terms of radiation stability. PTFE, perhaps the best known and most used of the group, shows significant radiation damage at exposures as low as 0.04 Mrads (18) and is, thus, unsuitable for radiation sterilization. PTFE does not crosslink on irradiation, but instead liberates fluorine atoms which in turn react to break carbon-carbon bonds in the polymer, causing severe degradation at low dose.

Other fluoropolymers have somewhat better resistence to radiation. Polychlorotrifluorethylene (PCTFE) reportedly shows threshold radiation damage at about 1 Mrad and 25% damage at 20 Mrads (4). FEP (copolymer of hexafluoropropene and tetrafluorothylene) polymer is considerably more radiation resistant than PTFE and can be sterilized satisfactorily. Other fluoropolymers containing carbons with hydrogen as well as fluorine bonds such as polyvinyl fluoride, polyvinylidene fluoride, and copolymers of ethylene and tetrafluorethylene (PETFE) show much less sensitivity to radiation (100 Mrads), tend to crosslink on exposure, and are capable of multiple sterilizations by radiation (3).

Polycarbonate

The commercial polycarbonate polymers contain aromatic rings in their main chain structure and, as might be predicted, show quite good resistence to radiation (4). Their strength is retained well after exposures up to 800 Mrads. Polycarbonates have excellent impact strength and resist thermal oxidative degradation up to 150°C. They are readily molded, extruded or machined to desired shapes. Severe stress cracking can occur in this polymer under certain preparative and use conditions.

Polyesters (Aromatic)

Aromatic thermoplastic polyesters have been used extensively in structural and biomedical applications in recent years. The most common type of polyester is poly (ethyleneglycolterephthalate) which shows fairly good radiation resistance (25% damage at 90 Mrads) (3). Recently, these materials have appeared in a variety of filled and unfilled as well as transparent (amorphous) products that should find many applications in medical devices and packaging. These materials, of course, can withstand multiple radiation sterilizations without significant degradation.

Polyolefins

These materials are among the most widely used and the most economical thermoplastic materials. They are widely used in biomedical applications and packaging. They are divided into broad groups and one of the most important of the groups, polypropylene, is discussed in detail especially in connection to its response to radiation.

Polyethylene

Polyethylene is produced in differing types known as low density, high density, linear low density and ultrahigh molecular weight varieties by modifying the processes by which the monomer ethylene is polymerized. All forms are reasonably resistant to radiation and can generally withstand (without significant change in properties) doses up to 100 Mrads. Polyethylene reacts primarily with ionizing radiation to crosslink the polymer. Charlesby and Pinner (19) have obtained a value of 0.3 for the ratio of chain scission to crosslinking in irradiated polyethylene, thus indicating that although crosslinking predominates as a mechanism, considerable carbon-carbon bond cleavage also occurs. With irradiation, the average molecular weight increases and the degree of crystallinity decreases (20,21). Some mechanical properties such as tensile strength do show change, with slight increases up to about 10 Mrad followed by a gradual decrease. The modulus of elasticity reacts oppositely, first falling, and then increasing, while the impact strength falls continuously after about 50-80 Mrad.

Polypropylene

Polypropylene is a very important polymeric material used in a wide range of biomedical and medical disposables applications. Both chain scission and crosslinking are observed to occur in irradiated polypropylene at about equal levels (22,23). This might perhaps be predicted since it has a structure intermediate between polyethylene, which primarily crosslinks, and polyisobutylene (quaternary cabon atom), which degrades largely by scission upon irradiation (24). Radiation doses which cause only minor (25% or less) degradation to polyethylene may render polypropylene useless.[(4)] Even a single sterilization of polypropylene may result in problems that may not develop for a period of time after irradiation.

Because of the potential utility and importance of this polymer in medical applications and because it has been thoroughly studied, the following description is given detailing the effects of radiation on polypropylene. This account illustrates problems that may result from the interaction of polymers with radiation, although polypropylene is perhaps an extreme example.

In recent years, radiation sterilization of polypropylene has become increasingly important for industrial purposes due both to economic factors and ease of processability. Polypropylene, which is widely used in numerous biomedical products, degrades very readily with irradiation and suffers more than many other thermoplastic materials. Basically, there are two main degradation problems which arise with irradiated polypropylene. First, polypropylene articles will often discolor during irradiation giving the product an undesirable color tint. The second and more severe problem is the polymer's embrittlement which begins during irradiation. More importantly, the physical properties continue to deteriorate with time following irradiation, often leaving a product highly embrittled after a few months of normal aging. In the current discussion, the effects of irradiation on the mechanical properties of polypropylene syringe barrels has been examined and will be discussed.

Irradiation of polypropylene in air (oxygen containing environment) results in an auto-oxidative reaction as follows:

(1) RM → 2R•
(2) R• + O_2 → RO_2•
(3) RO_2• + RH → ROOH + R•
(4) RO_2• + R• → ROOH

In this scheme R represents the polypropylene chain and R• is the "cleaved" chain which occurs during irradiation. It is important to note in this scheme, that as oxygen is consumed in steps (2) and (3), the free radical (R•) is only consumed in step (4). Therefore, the term auto-oxidative is used to imply that each radical formed will consume numerous molecules of oxygen unless this auto-oxidative reaction is prevented.

Examination of irradiated polypropylene by electron spin resonance spectrometry substantiates the oxidative reaction scheme. As shown in Figure 1 there is a progressive change of the initial polypropylene radical (R•), formed during irradiation in vacuum, to the peroxy radical (RO_2•), formed after the sample has been exposed to the air. When the polypropylene sample is irradiated in air, as would be the case during a sterilization cycle, the oxidative process is initiated at the onset of irradiation.

Discoloration. It has been found that pure polypropylene does not discolor upon irradiation. However, the stabilizers which are added to improve the polymers thermal and irradiation stability can and do often discolor upon irradiation. In general, irradiation imparts a "yellowish" color to the polymer which is essentially permanent, although there is a slight reduction in intensity with time. The discoloration becomes even more pronounced with dose. This coloration problem is best resolved by avoiding the use of any additives which discolor at sterilizing doses of radiation. However, the more severe problem of polymer degradation during irradiation is not as easily resolved.

Physical Properties. Examination of a polypropylene specimen before and after irradiation indicates that the irradiation sterilization cycle embrittles the substrate. When normal molding-grade polypropylene formulations are used to fabricate syringe barrels or related biomedical products several additional practical problems emerge which are related to the fundamental irradiation embrittlement of the polymer:

(1) Flange Breakage
(2) Luer Cracking
(3) Tip Breakage.

All three classes of mechanical failure after irradiation can be characterized physically by stating that the polymer no longer possesses the elongation characteristics needed to accommodate the normal strains encountered in practice. Consequently, items such as syringe barrels, which will be subjected to considerable stress loads in practice, must also fall within product strength specifications after radiation sterilization.

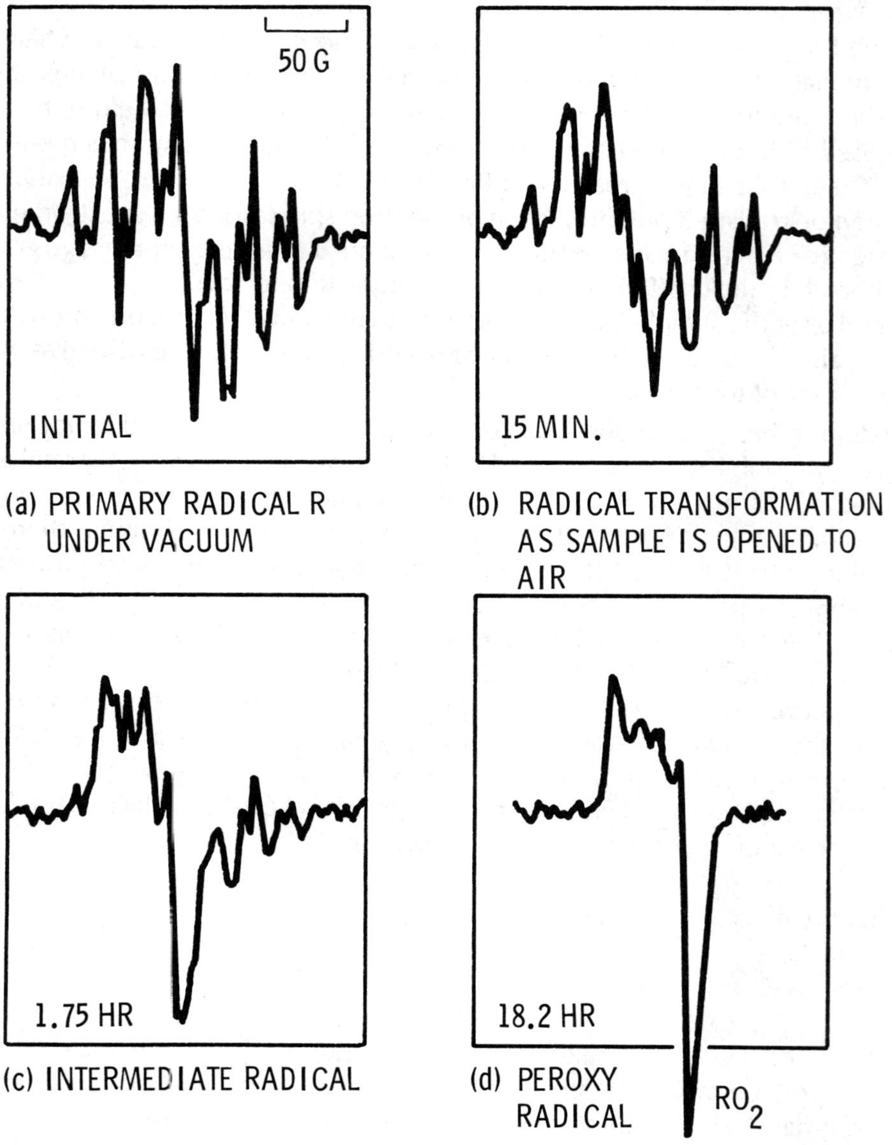

Figure 1. ESR spectra of peroxy radical formation at room temperature (5.0 Mrads).

Considerable effort has been aimed at characterizing (using physical measurements) what happens to a practical property such as flange strength as a function of sterilizing dose. For example, the force required to bend the flange through a given angle is measured and recorded up to the point of breakage. When polypropylene barrels are subjected to various irradiation doses and flange tested there is considerable change in performance as summarized in Figure 2. It is evident that the effect of increasing irradiation dose is to diminish the angle of deflection at which breakage occurs and, consequently, the area under the stress-strain curve. In short, irradiated samples simply cannot undergo the necessary work required in practice. Furthermore, if the irradiated sample is allowed to age, the breaking angle diminishes even further, as shown in Figure 3 for a seven-month aging period. It is obvious that the aged sample has little or no area left under the curve and, consequently, could undergo very little work. This severe embrittlement as a function of time after irradiation is due mainly to post-oxidation which can occur as discussed above. It is for these reasons that products made from a degrading polymer such as polypropylene should be thoroughly checked as a function of aging time.

In summary, the degradation of the polypropylene chain is mainly an auto-oxidative scheme. it is apparent that, if the radical population can be minimized, the possibility of main-chain oxidation occurring can be reduced. There are several variables in polypropylene fabrication which influence the ultimate free-radical population and the net effect of these variables on radical stability can be measured by electron spin resonance. The effects of polymer morphology—especially crystallinity—has a very pronounced influence on the radical population and, consequently, the long-term stability of the polypropylene. Although it is not the intent of the current discussion to resolve the irradiation degradation problem, it is important to recognize that potential embrittlement begins with molding techniques and is further magnified by irradiation conditions.

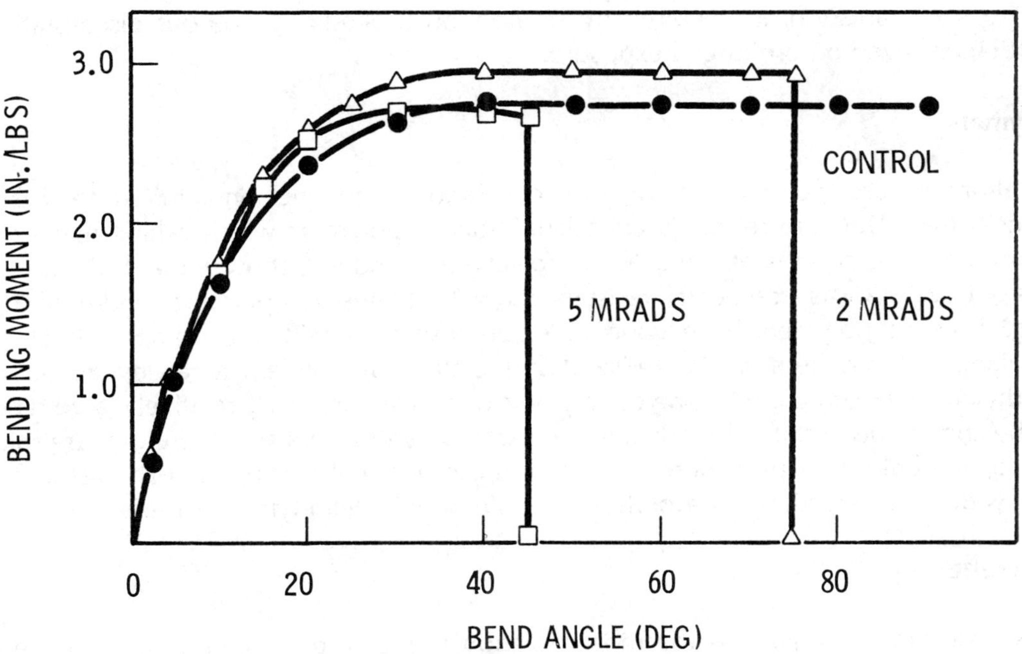

Figure 2. The irradiation effect on the bending angle of polypropylene syringe barrel flange.

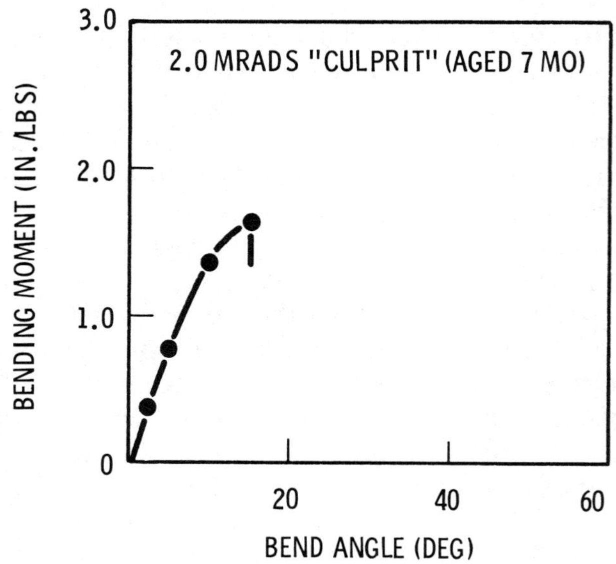

Figure 3. The post-irradiation effect on the bending angle of polypropylene syringe barrel flange.

Polymethylpentene

This transparent polyolefin material has a number of desirable properties and, although not a great deal of information is known concerning its radiation behavior, it is expected to have stability between that of polyethylene and polypropylene. Information from its manufacturer (25) states; "polymer is stable against electron and gamma radiation, and can be subjected to such radiation, as required by sterilization procedures, without discoloration or embrittlement even on prolonged exposure."

Copolymers

Polyallomers are copolymers of ethylene and propylene and in some cases a third monomer. They are relatively crystalline block copolymers which exhibit many of the same properties as polythylene and polypropylene and, indeed, show some of the best properties of both, such as stress-crack resistance, low brittleness temperatures and ease of processing. These copolymers have good radiation resistance with the primary effect being crosslinking and may be multiply sterilized by radiation (3). Poly(ethylene-vinyl acetate) and poly(ethylene-acrylate) are ethylene copolymers normally containing relatively large ratios of ethylene and are quite stable to radiation (similar to polyethylene) and, therefore, are suitable for multiple sterilization procedures. Some of these materials, being almost elastomeric in nature, widen the selection of properties available in polyolefin type polymers.

Polystyrene

This well known polymer is the most radiation stable of the common and inexpensive molding and extrusion materials. Its properties remain unaffected and gas evolution is insignificant to a higher radiation dose than any other plastic in its class. Its stability is believed to be due to the protective action of the pendant aromatic rings (10,26). Crosslinking of styrene occurs almost to the total exclusion of chain scission and a radiation dose of about 4000 Mrads is necessary to cause significant damage (16).

Poly(styrene acrylonitrile) - SAN. Copolymers of styrene, although not exhibiting the same degree of radiation stability as polystyrene itself, nevertheless have reasonably good resistance and may be expected to withstand multiple sterilizations without damage.

Polysulfones

This is a relatively new group of sulfur-containing, aromatic-backbone polymers which, in general, have very promising thermal and radiation resistance properties. There are at least three commercial products available (polysulfone, polyethersulfone, and polyphenylsulfone), all of which reportedly can withstand radiation doses of greater than 1000 Mrads without significant damage (27-29). These polymers also show good chemical resistance, excellent thermal stability and have mechanical properties which make them useful in a range of applications.

Another similar macromolecule of interest, polyphenylene sulfide, although not a sulfone, is a high-performance sulfur containing polymer displaying outstanding radiation stability. Technical representatives of the manufacturer report little change in tensile strength and flexural modulus of this material after exposure to 5000 Mrads.

Polyvinyls

Polyvinyl chloride (PVC) is the most widely used vinyl polymer in medical products and finds application both as a plasticized (flexible) and an unplasticized (rigid) material. PVC is found to crosslink to a considerable extent under irradiation (20,30–32). Its stability to radiation is reported to be very similar to polyethylene—at about 100 Mrads significant damage begins to appear (3). Plasticizers have some effect on PVC's radiation sensitivity and small amounts of HCL are produced as a result of irradiation. PVC is certainly suitable for single and, in most instances, multiple radiation sterilizations. However, radiation may cause undesirable color changes in some PVC products.

Other vinyl polymers. Copolymers of VC as vinyl chloride-vinyl acetate, as well as other vinyls such as polyvinylidene chloride, polyvinylformal and polyvinylbutyral, all appear to be more sensitive to radiation than PVC. Damage with these polymers begins in the range of 1-4 Mrads and 25% damage is observed at about 10-40 Mrads (4). It is therefore probable that these materials can be used in single sterilization, but may not be suitable for multiple materials can be used in single sterilization, but may not be suitable for multiple procedures.

There are many additional thermoplastic polymers which have not been mentioned in this review. An attempt was made to include the major families of thermoplastics and the most commonly used polymers in these groups. There are certainly many other potentially useful materials which might be very applicable for specific purposes. The radiation sensitivity of polymers not mentioned specifically in this review may be roughly forecast based on both the rules set forth earlier in this text and by comparing their structure with that of polymers whose irradiation response is known. However, once a specific material is selected for an application, its radiation sensitivity should be determined on protoypes.

Table 1 summarizes the effects observed as a result of the interaction of radiation with a variety of thermoplastics and estimates their ability to be used in radiation sterilization procedures.

THERMOSETS

Although most thermoset polymers can be sterilized by such techniques as heat or steam sterilization, they will be briefly mentioned here as frequently useful polymeric, biomedical materials that may, in most cases, be multiply radiation sterilized.

Phenol or Urea Formaldehydes

These formaldehyde resins are almost invariably used as filled or reinforced materials. Generally, the addition of mineral fillers increases the radiation stability of these polymers significantly—frequently by as much as 100 fold (3,4). Filled resin of this type usually show good radiation resistance up to 500 Mrads or higher. They can therefore be expected to be suitable for multiple sterilizations by radiation.

Epoxies

Epoxy resins find wide use in many adhesive, potting, coating, and encapsulating applications in medical products. These polymers are above average in radiation resistance, although their stability may vary considerably depending upon the hardner (curing agent) used—products from resins utilizing aromatic curing agents generally are more stable than those using aliphatic hardners. In many formulations these polymers are stable to radiation doses above 1000 Mrads and are capable of surviving many radiation sterilization procedures.

Polyesters (Unsaturated)

Thermoset polyester, which comprise a large group of resins, represented by such systems as styrene or diallylphthalate modified alkyds, have quite good radiation resistance, especially if they contain mineral fillers or glass fibers. Like the phenolic resins, they can be expected to withstand radiation doses of more than 1000 Mrads before evidencing significant damage (4).

Allyl diglycol carbonate, although listed as a polyester, is quite different in structure from most other polyesters and quite distinct in properties and uses. It has good optical qualities and good radiation stability. Exposures to nearly 100 Mrads are required to produce significant damage (25%) to this material (16). Radiation resistance together with its optical properties make it a prime candidate for uses in medical devices requiring lenses or viewing windows.

Polyimides

Polyimides are generally classified as thermosets, although some thermoplastic polyimides are also now available. These materials are well known for their excellent thermal and radiation resistance. They can be expected to withstand radiation doses well above 1000 Mrads.

Poly(Urethanes)

The poly(urethanes) represent a wide variety of polymeric materials with properties dependent upon the monomers and their ratios used in preparation. The most common products are either polyester(urethanes) or polyether(urethanes) and generally show very good resistance to radiation. The urethane's properties vary from those of an elastomer to that of hard, rigid, crosslinked polymer whose mechanical properties showed no reduction after an exposure to 1000 Mrads.

TABLE 1. Effects of Radiation on Selected Thermoplastic Polymers

Polymer	Radiation Stability	Radiation Dose to Produce Significant Damage (Mrads)	Number of Potential Sterilizations*
ABS	Good	100	M
Acetals	Poor	1-2	0
Acrylics		5	
PMMA	Fair	5	1
Others	Fair	10	1-2
Amides			
Alphatic	Fair	50-100	1-2
Aromatic	Excellent	1000	M
Cellulosics	Fair	20	1-2
Fluoroplastics			
PTFE	Poor	1	0
PCTFE	Fair	10-20	1-2
FEP	Fair	20	M
PVF, PVF_2, PETFE, PECTFE	Good	100	M
Polycarbonate	Good	100+	M
Polyesters (aromatic)	Good	100	M
Polyolefins			
Polyethylene	Good	100	M
Polypropylene	Fair	10	1
Polymethylpentene	Good	30-50	M
Copolymers	Good	50	M
Polystyrene	Excellent	1000	M
Copolymer	Good	100-500	M
Polysulfones	Excellent	1000	M
Polyvinyls			
PVC	Good	50-100	M
Copolymers	Fair	10-40	1-2

* Sterilization potential of polymers divided into four categories:
0 - non-sterilizable, 1 - one procedure, 1-2 - somewhat more than one,
M - multiple sterilization possible.

This potential is based primarily on the mechanical properties of the polymers and for other reasons, such as optical clarity or gas evolution, the material may not be suitable for the noted number of sterilizations.

These and other thermoset materials offer a wide variety of properties for a host of applications in the medical area. The polymers listed describe only a few of the most common materials available. A brief summary of the average expected radiation sensitivity of a number of these materials is given in Table 2.

TABLE 2. Radiation Sensitivity of Selected Thermoset Polymers

TABLE 2. Radiation Sensitivity of Selected Thermoset Polymers

Material	Radiation Resistance	Radiation Dose for Significant Damage, Mrads	Suitable for Sterilization*
Epoxies	Excellent	100-10,000	M
Phenol (or Urea) formaldehyde	Good	500	M
Polyesters (unsaturated)	Good	1000	M
Polyimides	Excellent	100-10,000	M
Polyurethanes	Excellent	1000+	M

* This data indicates when the polymer as generally used (formulated) is suitable for: 0-no sterilizations, 1-single sterilizations, or M-multiple sterilizations.

ELASTOMERS

Elastomers (rubbers) represent a large group of polymeric products which have some unique properties quite distinct from those of the thermoplastic and thermoset materials. They have a variety of applications in the area of medical products. Their resistance to radiation varies over a considerable range, although generally not as greatly as with the thermoplastic polymers (6,33). Table 3 lists a selected group of elastomers and compares the average radiation resistance of one of each of these types of rubbers. It suggests radiation doses at which threshold damage occurs (at least one physical property begins to change) and values at which about 25% damage occurs (represented by a 25% change in one property). Although this gives only a brief insight into the radiation stability of these materials, it does permit some selectivity for these materials for use in applications where radiation sterilization may be used.

The figures given in Table 3 are only meant to represent averages and it must be pointed out that fillers, plasticizers, etc., used in the formulation of the elastomers, can have a very substantial influence on radiation stability. For instance, the addition of aromatic plasticizers to neoprene compositions make these rubbers much more stable to radiation (4). The partial substitution of phenyl groups for methyl groups in silicone rubbers increases the radiation stability considerably (34). Most of the elastomers listed, with the possible exception of the first two (polyacrylic and butyl), are certainly capable of being radiation sterilized one or more times.

TABLE 3. Radiation Sensitivity of Selected Elastomers (3,4,34)

TABLE 3. Radiation Sensitivity of Selected Elastomers(3,4,34)

Material (Rubbers)	Radiation Threshold Damage Mrads	Dosage 25% Damage Mrads
Polyacrylic	2-4	10-15
Butyl	2-3	10
Chlorosulfonated polyethylene	--	30
EPDM (ethylene-propylene-diene)	10	100+
Fluoro-	5	50-70
Natural	10	100-200
Nitrile	--	100
Polychloroprene (Neoprene)	6	50
Silicones	--	50-100
Styrene-butadiene	6-8	100+
Urethane	20	600-800

FILMS AND FIBERS

The effects of radiation on thin plastic films and organic synthetic fibers (textiles) may in some cases differ from effects noticed in bulk products manufactured from the same or similar polymers. These variations may be due to differences resulting from processing of these materials. For polymers which may be in the questionable range for the use of radiation sterilization techniques, only testing will determine their applicability.

ADHESIVES, COATINGS AND POTTING COMPOUNDS

These materials generally react to radiation in much the same manner as the plastics or elastomers from which they are derived. Those containing aromatic compounds show good resistance to radiations. Fillers and reinforcing materials usually improve the radiation stability of these products substantially, while also improving other properties.

SUMMARY

Sterilization of plastic medical devices by ionizing radiation is an extremely applicable technique for polymeric materials and its use is rapidly increasing worldwide. Ionizing radiation interacts with polymers in two primary mechanisms: 1) chain scission to reduce molecular weight and 2) crosslinking to generate large polymer networks. Both mechanisms occur in all polymers during irradiation, but one generally dominates. Polymers vary in sensitivity to radiation from polytetrafluoroethylene with damage occurring at doses as low as 0.04 Mrad to polyimides which can tolerate doses as high as 10^4 Mrads without excessive damage. Polymers containing aromatic character have much greater resistance to radiation damage than those with aliphatic structure. Most thermoplastics, essentially all thermosets and most elastomers, can withstand at least one radiation sterilization (~5 Mrads) without significant damage. However, post-irradiation effects can cause severe problems as detailed in the case of polypropylene. Polymeric materials used in adhesives, fibers, films and encapsulants show much the same response to radiation as the bulk polymers, but additives can significantly influence the effects of radiation.

REFERENCES

1. O. Saito, H. Y. Kang and M. Dole, "Theory of Gel-dose Curves for Polymers Undergoing Simultaneous Crosslinking and Scission," *J. Phys. Chem., 46,* 3607-16, 1967.

2. A. Chapiro, "Chemical Nature of the Reactive Species Produced in Polymers by Ionizing Radiation," in *Irradiation of Polymers,* ed. N. A. J. Platzer, Adv. in Chem. Ser., No. 66, pp. 22-30, Amer. Chem. Soc., Washington, D.C., 1967.

3. N. J. Broadway and S. Palinchak, The Effect of Nuclear Radiations on Elastomeric and Plastic Components and Materials, *REIC Report No. 21 (addendum)* AD 454 056, NTIS, August 31, 1964.

4. R. W. King, N. J. Broadway and S. Palinchak, the Effect of Nuclear Radiation on Elastomeric and Plastic Components and Materials, *REIC Report No. 21,* AD 264 890, NTIS, September 1, 1961.

5. Draft Summaries of Properties of Plastics, *FFTF Materials Data Collection Task RM-1,* Battelle-Northwest, Richland, WA, December 1967 (unpublished data).

6. R. Harrington, "Elastomers for Use in Radiation Fields," *Rubber Age, 81,* 971-80, 1957.

7. A. Charlesby, M. Ross, "Breakdown of Methylmethacrylate Polymer by High Energy Radiation," *Nature 171,* 1153, 1953.

8. P. Alexander, A. Charlesby, M. Ross, "Degradation of Solid Polymethylmethacrylate by Ionizing Radiation," *Proc. Roy. Soc. A 223,* 392, 1954.

9. A. R. Shultz, "High Energy Radiation Effects on Polyacrylates and Polymethacrylates," *J. Polym. Sci. 35,* 369-80, 1959.

10. A. R. Shultz, P. I. Roth, G. B. Rathmann, "Light Scattering and Viscosity Study of Electron Irradiated Polystyrene and Polymethacrylates," *J. Polym. Sci. 22,* 495, 1956.

11. A. R. Shultz, F. A. Bovey, "Electron Irradiation of Polyacrylates," *J. Polym. Sci. 22,* 485, 1956.

12. R. W. Kilb, "Effect of Simultaneous Crosslinking and Degradation in the Intrinsic Viscosity of a Polymer," *J. Phys. Chem. 63,* 1838, 1959.

13. A. H. Samuel, J. L. Magee, "Radiation Chemistry: (II) Track Effects in Radiolysis of Water," *J. Chem. Phys. 21,* 1080, 1953.

14. A. Charlesby, "Effect of High Energy Radiation on Long Chain Polymers," *Nature 171,* 167, 1953.

15. H. Lee, D. Stoffey and K. Neville, *New Linear Polymers,* McGraw-Hill Book Co., New York, NY, pg. 154. 1967.

16. J. O. Turner. *Plastics in Nuclear Engineering,* Reinhold Publishing Corp., New York, NY, pg. 131, 1961.

17. D. W. Plester, "The Effects of Radiation Sterilization on Plastics" in *Industrial Sterilization* ed., C.B. Phillips and W. S. Miller, Duke University Press, Durham, NC, pg. 148, 1973.

18. C. G. Collins and V. P. Calkins, Radiation Damage to Elastomers, Organic Liquids and Plastics, *APEX-261, General Electric Co.,* Cincinnati, OH, Atomic Products Div., Aircraft Nuclear Propulsion Dept., pg. 20, September 1956.

19. A. Charlesby, S. H. Pinner, "Analysis of the Solubility Behavior of Irradiated Polyethylene and Other Polymers," *Proc. Roy. Soc. (London),* Ser. A, *249,* 367-386, 1959.

20. E. J. Lawton, A. M. Beuche, J. S. Balwitt, "Properties of Irradiated Polyethylene - Effect of Molecular Weight," *Nature 172,* 76, 1953.

21. M. Dole, *The Radiation Chemistry of Macromolecules,* Vol I, pg. 3, Academic Press, New York, NY, 1972.

22. D. O. Geymer, "The Effects of Ionizing Radiation on the Molecular Weight of Crystalline Polypropylene," *Makromol. Chem. 99,* 152-9, 1966.

23. R. Salovey, F. R. Dammont, "Irradiation of Poly(ethylene oxide) and Polypropylene," *J. Polym. Sci. A1,* 2155-62, 1963.

24. P. Alexander, R. M. Black, A. Charlesby, "Radiation-Induced Changes in the Structure of Polyisobutylene," *proc. Roy. Soc. A 223,* 32, 1955.

25. *TPX, Methylpentene Polymer,* Mitsui Petrochemical Industries, Ltd., Tokyo, Japan, 1975.

26. J.E. Buillet, R.G.W. Norrish, "The Photolysis of Polymethylvinylketone: 1. Reactions and Kinetics II. The Preparation of Graft Polymers," *Proc. Roy. Soc. (London),* Ser. A, *223,* 153-83, 1955.

27. B. D. Gesner, P.G. Kelleher, "Thermal and Photo-oxidation of Polysulfone," *J. Appl. Polym. Sci. 12,* 1199-208, 1968.

28. W. M. Alvino, "Aging Behavior of Poly(arylsulfone) Films," *J. Appl. Polym. Sci. 15,* 2521-37, 1971.

29. L. Kevan, P. L. Hall, E. T. Kaiser, "Sulfur Dioxide Elimination in the Radiolytic Decomposition of Solid Diaryl Sulfones," *J. Phys. Chem. 70,* 853-55, 1966.

30. A. Charlesby, "Effects of High-Energy Radiation in Long-Chain Polymers," *Plastics 18,* 142-5, 1953.

31. A. Chapiro, "The Action of Gamma-Rays on Polymers in the Solid State II Degradation of Polymethylmethacrylate and Cellulose Acetate," *J. Chem. Phys. 53,* 295-305, 1956.

32. S. Stokes, R.B. Fox, "Photolysis of Poly-α-Methylstyrene," J. Polym. Sci. 56, 507, 1962.

33. R. F. Mattia and D. R. Luh, "Radiation Resistance of EPDM, Polychloroprene, and Chlorosulfonated Polyethylene," presented at 1971 Tri-State Regional Mtg. Mass, Conn, and R.I. Rubber Groups, Auburn, MA, May 13, 1971.

34. A. A. Miller, "Radiation Stabilities of Arylmethylsiloxanes," *Ind. Eng. Chem., Prod. Res. Dev., 3,* 252-6, 1964.

35. R. Salovey and D. C. Basset, "Irradiation of Annealed Polyethylene Crystals," *J. Appl. Physics 35,* 3216-21, 1964.

Chapter 45

Polymers, Processes and Properties of Medical Plastics: including Markets and Applications

D. V. Rosato
Program Director
Plastics Seminars
University of Lowell
40 Karen Road
Waban, MA. 02168

ABSTRACT

The prevention, diagnosis & treatment of many health-related problems are facilitated today by an array of devices using medical grade polymers. The important polymers used in these devices are reviewed. Information is presented on their important properties and applications. An up date is provided on the processing techniques used to fabricate these medical devices.

The use of polymers in medical applications and devices continues to increase in significance to our daily activities and to our lives. The prevention, diagnosis and treatment of many health-related problems are facilitated today by an array of new materials, formulations and devices. The different polymers processing techniques used are rather extensive, and they include injection molding, extrusion, compression molding, coating, blow molding, dipping, electrostatic spray, calendering, casting, foaming, encapsulating, thermoforming, reinforced plastics, rotational molding, thermoforming, and others.

Still in the laboratory, and intended to further improve the reliability and utility of present devices, are new generations of technological developments. Included are major developments in the coextruding of different polymers to provide an array of different combinations of properties; such as, sterilization, physical stability, chemical stability, permeability to tissue reactions/gases/moisture/etc., controlled biodegradability, nondegradability, and/or other properties.

Dramatic indeed is the role polymers have played in some of the medical "miracles" of our time. The use of polymers for medical applications constitutes about 4 percent by weight or 6 percent by dollar sales of the total processed plastics/polymers products produced in the United States. This represents an annual 1.8 billion pounds or $3.1 billion sales of plastics processed into end items. [1,2]

The history of biomedical polymers began with the upgrading of natural products such as cellulose or natural rubber. By means of vulcanization, esterification and other chemical reactions, substances were obtained that had new interesting properties but whose molecular structure was at first not accurately known.

The first time a polymer was implanted in the human body was in 1894 when Frankel made use of celluloid to plug gaps in the cranium. Once the fundamental question of their constitution had been clarified and new methods of synthesis had been developed, plastics obtained by entirely synthetic means rapidly gained in significance after about 1930. Today, a large number of high polymers produced solely by syntheses are available on the market; they are tailored to meet the wide variety of demands imposed on them in their applications as engineering materials, raw materials for the production of fibers, auxiliaries, and binders of all descriptions. [3]

Practically all polymers are used in one or more market categories of Intracorporeal, Paracorporeal and Hospital Products, and Rest Homes. The major polymers used are low density polythylene (LDPE) at 22 percent of the total, polyvinyl chloride (PVC) at 20 percent, polystyrene (PS) at 20 percent, high density polyethylene (HDPE) at 12 percent, polypropylene (PP) at 10 percent, thermoset polyesters at 4 percent, polyurethane (PUR) at 2 percent, acrylics at 2 percent, nylon at 2 percent, epoxies at 1 percent, and others at 5 percent (acetals, cellulosics, thermoplastic polyesters, polycarbonates, polysulfones, polyphenyl oxides, silicones, urea formaldehydes, etc.).

Most of the traditional processes are used to produce end items from these polymers. They include extrusion processing 38 percent of the total plastics, injection molding at 32 percent, foam molding at 13 percent, blow molding at 9 percent, reinforced plastics/compression molding at 4 percent, and others at 4 percent (rotational, casting, spray, dip).

The important applications with typical plastics used include:

1. INTRACORPOREAL (Figure 1)
   a. Heart and heart components (polyester, silicone, PVC)
   b. Ear and eye parts (acrylic, PE, silicone, PVC, epoxy)
   l. Esophagus segments (PE,PP,PVC)
   m. Gastrointestional segments (acrylate, silicone, PVC, nylon)

c. Lung, kidney, and liver parts (polyester, polyaldehydes, PVC, SAN)
d. Facial prosthesis (acrylic, PVC, PUR)
e. Soft tissue replacements (PVC, cellulosics)
f. Dentures, cavities (acrylic, UHMWPE, epoxy)
g. Bones and joints (acrylic, nylon, silicone, PUR, PP, UHMWPE)
h. Bone cement (acrylic, propylene vinyl)
i. Repair blood vessels (PVC, polyester)
j. Hydrogel dialysis membranes (acrylate, etc.)
k. Tracheal tubes (acrylic, silicone, nylon, rubber)
n. Laryngeal prosthesis (polyester, acrylate, PP, fluropolymer)
o. Ureter tubings (acrylate, polyester)
p. Face injection, etcs. (silicone)
q. Face implants (fluoropolymer)
r. Surgical dressings (urea formaldehyde)
s. Implant electronic microcircuiting plastic components (PE, acetal, etc.)
t. Membrances (cellulosic, polyvinyl alcohol)
u. Coatings (nylon, acrylic, UHMWPE)
v. Biodegradable sutures (PUR)
w. Others

2. PARACORPOREAL and HOSPITAL PRODUCTS
   a. Catheters (PVC, PE, silicone, polyester, fluoropolymer)
   b. Blood bags (PVC)
   c. Packaging films (PE, PVC, nylon, PUR, PS)
   d. Surgical trays, containers (PS, PE, polyester acrylic)
   e. Bottles (PE, PVC, PS, polyester, PP)
   f. Laboratory analyzer parts/aspirators, optics, etc. (PE, PVC, nylon, etc.)
   g. Medical electronic equipment components (nylon, PP, acetal, etc.)
   h. Heart, lung machine components (polyvinyl pyrilodine)
   i. Medical powder compounds (urea formaldehyde)
   j. Optical and sound wave device parts (acrylic, PC, epoxy, etc.)
   k. Appliances and furnishings (polyester, PE, PP, PVC, PS, acrylic, etc.
   l. Transportation parts/wheelchairs, stretchers, carts, etc. (polyester, PP, etc.)
   m. Food handling equipment (PS, PE, PVC, etc.) Carts, trays, bags, cups, dishes, utensils, microwave oven parts, etc.)
   n. Disposables (PE, PVC, PUR, PS, etc.) Syringes, needles, foam jawlocks, surgical gauze, bandages, identification wrist bands, tracheotomy tube dressings, single use thermometers, surgical gloves, foot guards, air splints, pans, blood bags, pillows, drapes, bedpans, pails, soap dishes, floor mats, moist heat pads, signs, cards, splints, sterilizable pouches, mouth marks, waste can liners, wash cloths, etc.
   o. Medical building products/wall coverings, electrical systems, insulations, etc. (polyester, PVC, PC, ABS, etc.)
   p. Surgical products (PVC, PE, PUR, PS, acrylic, etc.) Sutures, sponges, tubing, forceps, scissors, shoes, gloves, gowns, caps, surgical and nurse masks, etc.

3. REST HOMES, HOMES, DOCTOR's OFFICES, PLANTS (Manufacturing, Industrial, Commercial and Pharmaceutical products)
   Many of the items listed under hospital products are applicable in this category.

Both the commodity type polymers/plastics (such as polyethylenes, polyvinyl chlorides, polystyrenes and polypropylenes) and the engineered or specialty polymers/plastics (such as acetals, acrylics, fluorocarbons, epoxies, and silicones) are used. The commodity plastics are the lower cost materials and used in most medical applications. Engineered plastics are predominately used for intracorporeal applications where significant property performances are required. Table 1 list some of the applications for engineered plastics. [4]

Close to 80 percent of the total sales for plastics parts used in the medical market go into hospital products. About $1.8 billion or 75 percent of hospital products sales are in disposables. In turn this $1.8 billion represents about 60 percent of the total.

Dramatic breakthroughs have been occurring since the mid 1950's in the use of plastics/-medical applications. Many thousands of Americans are living happy, productive lives today, when only a few years ago most of these people would have died or else remained very ill. The use of plastic products in the hospital has made it easier for the patients and employees; also operating cost savings to the hospitals continually exist. With more development now oc-

Figure 1. Intracorporeal
Important Applications for Plastics

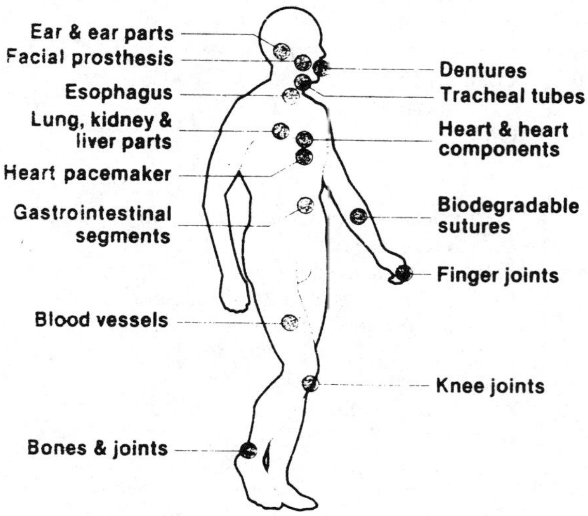

Ear & ear parts: acrylic, polyethylene, silicone, polyvinyl chloride (PVC)
Dentures: acrylic, ultra high molecular weight polyethylene (UHMWPE), epoxy
Facial prosthesis: acrylic, PVC, polyurethane (PUR)
Tracheal tubes: acrylic, silicone, nylon
Heart & heart components: polyester, silicone, PVC
Heart pacemaker: polyethylene, acetal
Lung, kidney & liver parts: polyester, polyaldehyde, PVC
Esophagus segments: polyethylene, polypropylene (PP), PVC
Blood vessels: PVC, polyester
Biodegradable sutures: PUR
Gastrointestinal segments: silicones, PVC, nylon
Finger joints: silicone, UHMWPE
Bones & joints: acrylic, nylon, silicone, PUR, PP, UHMWPE
Knee joints: polyethylene

Table 1

Medical Applications for Engineered Plastics

Location	Device	Etiology	Materials
Eye	Intraocular lens	Cataract removal	Acrylic
2orbital floor	Orbital floor	Orbital blow-out fracture, leading to double vision	Flurocarbon, Silicone Polyethlene, Titanium mesh
	Scleral buckler	Detached retina	Silicone
	Artificial eye	Removal due to trauma or disease	Acrylic
Ear	External ear frame	Congenital or traumatic loss of ear	Silicon, Polyethylene
	Ventilation tube	Middle ear inflecton, occlusion of eustachian tube	Polyethylene, Flurocarbon, Silicone, Stainless Steel
	Stapes prostheses	Stapedectomy	Stainless Steel, Tetrafluorethylene, Gelfoam^R
	Tympanoplasty Prostheses	Reconstruction of the middle ear	Stainless Steel, Fluorocarbon
Nose	Rhinoplasty prostheses	Congenital saddle nose	Silicone
Chin	Chin prostheses	Recessive chin	Silicone
Mouth	Mandibular prostheses	Trauma, ankylosis disease	Proplast$^{T.M.}$
	Dental implants	Trauma, disease	Pyrolitic Carbon
Neck	Trachial stents	Trachial reconstruction	Silicone
	Voice box	Loss of speech due to laryngectomy	Silicone, Acetal, Stainless Steel
Heart & Vascular System	Cardiac pacemaker	Heart block, arrythmia	Epoxy, Silicone, Fluorocarbon, Titanium, Stainless Steel
	Prosthetic valves	Valvular disease	Pyrolytic carbon, Titanium, Fluorocarbon Silicone
	Intra aortic balloon pumps	Patients needing cardiac assist	Urethane-silicone copolymer

TABLE 1 (Continued)

	Blood oxygenators (Heart-lung machine)	Open heart surgery	Polycarbonate, Silicone, Vinyl, Acetal
	Blood storage and delivery systems	Trauma, surgery, disease	Vinyl
	Prosthetic arteries	Atherosclerosis, aneurism, trauma	Convoluted knit Polyester or Flurocarbon
Urinary System	Ureteral stent	Blockage of ureter due to disease	Silicone, Polyethylene
	Urinary sphincter	Urinary incontinence	Silicone
	Wearable artificial kidney	Kidney failure	Nylon, Silicone, Vinyl, Cellophane, Urethane
Sexual	Mammary prostheses	Subcutaneous mastectomy, underdeveloped or asymetrical breasts	Silicone
	Organs		
	Vaginal stent	Reconstruction of vagina due to disease or congenital absence	Silicone, Polyethylene
	Fimbrial implant	Impatent fallopian tube	Silicone
	Penile implant	Erectile impotence	Silicone, Polyethylene
	Testicular implant	Orchidectomy or undescended testicle	Silicone
Skeleton	Skull plate	Trauma	Acrylic, Titanium mesh
	Joints, almost all	Arthritis, trauma	Carbon fibre-Polyethylene composite, Silicone, Steel alloys, Titanium alloys, Acrylic cement
	Artificial tendon	Trauma, tendonitis	Silicone, Polyester
	Passive artificial muscle	Muscle atrophy, trauma, "Dropfoot"	Silicone, Polyester

curring in the use of plastics for implants and hospital products, the growth rate for plastics in this market is expected to be at least 10 percent with potential prospects at 15 percent. Interesting is the fact that plastics are even more firmly entrenched in medical products today than glass and stainless steel were in the 1950's.

When considering medical applications in its broad meaning they include packaging films and plastic bottles for pharmaceuticals, electronic instrument parts, disposable items, diagnostic tools, and devices for prosthetic use outside the body. The problems associated with these applications are far fewer than those for implants because tissue reactions are usually not a concern. Except for the prosthetic devices, many of these are disposable items that find usefulness in hospitals and clinics because of their convenience and/or low cost. At the consumer level, these items represent a very large dollar volume.

WORLD HEALTH CARE

Although developing nations will harbor less than 14 percent of the world's 5.7 billion people, the developed regions will account for over three-quarters of the $1.6 trillion spent on health care in 1995, with per capita expenditures averaging $1,530 (Table 2). They have maintained this ratio of population to health spending since the late 1970's. [5]

The mounting financial burden has led developed regions to turn to cost containment measures. These will include both restructuring health delivery away from in-patient care toward less expensive ambulatory care and stringent price controls on health goods and services. Nevertheless, the efficacy of these measures will be offset by rapid increases in the over sixty-five population segment, a group requiring health care expenditures two to three times the norm. As a result, the developed regions' health expenditures will double by 1995.

Table 2
World Health Care Cost

	1979 ($Billion)	1995 ($Billion)
Developed Nations		
North America	$243.10	$ 440.60
European Community	230.90	436.30
Non-EC, W. Europe	48.90	105.20
Asia/Oceania	81.90	229.00
Total	$604.80	$1,211.10
Developing Nations		
Latin America	$ 22.32	$ 73.35
E. Europe	77.22	151.50
Africa-Mideast	12.16	47.79
Asia/Oceania	22.65	76.72
Total	$134.35	$ 349.36
World Total	$739.15	$1,560.46

Comparatively, the developing regions, which will account for seven-eights of the world's population in 1995, will spend an average of only $70 per capita on health care. The health problems endemic to these regions—poor nutrition, quick transmission of infectious diseases, and inadequate sanitation and hygiene—are the result of rapid population growth.

Although governments have responded by emphasizing family planning and health education pediatric and material nutrition as well as disease control, the lack of infrastructure has impeded implementing these programs.

It is expected that the developing regions will concentrate now on providing services to the rural population through community health centers, paramedics, and low-cost drugs. These efforts will boost expenditures over 6 percent annually to $349 billion in 1995.

The United States alone will account for 26 percent of global health care expenditures in 1995, when spending will reach $404 billion or $1,615 per capita.

MEDICAL DISPOSABLES

It is estimated that the overall market for disposables is about $2½ billion of a total medical market for plastics of about $3.1 billion.

These products have presented significant and steady growth to the plastics industry, well-insulated from the ravages of downswings in the general business economy. But as new, innovative uses of plastics in these devices expand and as the pressure by government and industry for stringent production standards grows, the demands placed on those who choose to serve this market will become even more intense.

Plastics have been important since the first disposable hypodermic syringe was introduced over 30 years ago. The plastic syringe was developed and marketed in the mid-1950's by American Pharmaseal Division of American Hospital Supply Corporation. The first were of injection molded polystryrene and gradually they went to polypropylene.

With this modest beginning there is now a widespread use of plastic materials in health care, in treatment, and in surgical procedures, permitting a standard of hygiene never before available. Examples of a few of the many plastics single-use products are for intubation therapy, IV-connectors, filters, vials, urinary drainage, sanitaryware, and implants.

Plastics have played an important part with the advancement in medical materials performancewise and costwise. The health care industry's first move into plastics was prompted by a growing awareness of cross-contamination between patients due to use of improperly sterilized reusable metal and glass devices. At that time, the cost of sterilization was not as much a factor as it is now.

As labor costs rose in the sterile supply rooms (which reprocessed devices for re-use) costs began to go extremely high. By the mid-1960's, the economics for re-usable vs disposable products crossed, and the major new developments involved more use for plastics.

The doing away of re-usables and the significantly greater use of disposables taught the "medical industry" what other markets had discovered since the coming of age of plastics over a century ago—certain cost advantages exist in developing either small or large production items. [6]

Polymers and Dentistry [7]

Chemists, engineers, and dental professional whose teamwork today produces new dental materials are the current generation in a genealogy that can be traced back 2,500 years or more. Where the first artisans used only metals, today's multidiscipline research teams work with a variety of materials, including an increasing variety of polymers.

The ancient civilization of Babylonia, Assyria, and Egypt (around 4000 B.C) included workers with copper, gold, lead, and silver, and it is possible these materials may have been applied to the relief of dental problems. The Phoenicians (about 500 B.C.) are generally considered to be the first to use gold wire to hold teeth in place. Gold crowns and bridgework were prepared in Etruria and Rome during this period. The teeth in these early devices were generally human teeth or carved from animal teeth.

Following the remarkable achievements of the early civilizations, few advances were made in the area of dental materials for almost two thousand years. Around the 16th century, the science of dentristry began to emerge. During the period of the American Revolution, ivory and gold artificial teeth were one of the products of silversmith (and horseman) Paul Revere. The dental problems and wooden false teeth of George Washington have been widely described. Fused porcelain was first used for teeth during this period. Waxes became widely used, and the first amalgams were introduced for dental use in 1826.

Gutta-percha, as a root canal filling material, and vulcanite, a fulcanized rubber patented for use as a denture base material, were among the earliest macromolecular products to be employed. Until around 1937, when acrylic resins became available, only vulcanite phenolformaldehyde resins, and a few vinyl plastics were widely used for denture base materials. Most of the synthetic polymers only have become available within the last 45 years. Now, a significant number of syntehtic polymers offer at least some of the characteristics desired in a prosthetic or restorative material.

Prior to the last two decades, dentists and others in the medical sciences generally have borrowed from industry a few materials that were designed for other applications, and tried to adapt them to their needs. In a few instances, however, research on dental materials has led to exceptionally developments in polymer science. Included among these efforts were the development of amine-peroxide systems for the curing of acrylics and various epoxy resins.

The recent efforts of multidisciplinary teams of scientists, including biologists, chemists, engineers, and dentists, have allowed great strides to be taken in the development of new and improved polymers for dental applications. Although *the total consumption of polymers in dentistry* is small (about 12½ million pounds per year) when compared to industrial and other consumer applications of plastics and elastomers, the materials are almost always specialty formulation commanding premium rates. Interestingly, the consumption of synthetic polymers in dentistry increased only a few percentage points in the last several years. This is most probably a result of a better public awareness of the advantages of preventive care, and the improved quality and properties of the newer polymers, requiring less-frequent replacement of prosthetic and restorative materials. Equally important are the advances made in the training of dentists who are aware of the material requirements and methods of application.

The availability of several classes of synthetic polymers, and the combined efforts of scientists and clinicians, the processing and performance criteria for an acceptable dental polymer can now be more closely defined. Of course, there requirements vary somewhat depending on the specific application, but in general they include: (1) ease of fabrication, (2) adequate strength and abrasion resistance, (3) dimensional stability, (4) translucence or transparency so that the material can be colored to match tissue, (5) good color stability, (6) resistance to staining, and (7) low toxicity. Unfortunately, at present, only a few materials meet all of these requirements.

Polymers have proven useful as *artificial teeth,* although the amounts used for teeth are low compared to quantities consumed for denture base fabrication. Artificial teeth have been prepared from polyacrylates, polyvinyl esters, polystyrenes, and various combinations of these materials. Plastics teeth are generally softer but tougher than those fabricated from porcelain, the other commonly used material. Neither plastics nor porcelain is an ideal material for artificial teeth, and a material with intermediate properties would probably be more suitable.

The use of acrylic polymers for construction of denture bases is the largest single application of synthetic polymers in dental materials. Acrylics also are widely used in cements, tooth restoration, splints, crown and bridge restorations, and other repair materials. Other polymers that are used less frequently than the acrylics include epoxies, nylons, polycarbonates, polyurethanes, vinyls, and silicones. Compared to the quantities of polymethylmethacrylate consumed annually, the use of these materials is minor. Most of the specialty polymers find applications in tissue conditioners, reliners, sealants, cements, impression materials, maxillofacial prosthetics, and mouth protectors.

The development of unique polymers for dental applications offers a considerable challenge to the material scientist. The development of improved elastomers for use as *resilient denture liners* is a good example. In relining, a thin film of plastic is added to the inside of the denture to obtain an improved fit with the contours of the oral tissues. Of the large number of people who wear dentures, many demonstrate to some degree a senile or presenile atrophy of the denture-supporting tissues. Other denture wearers have chronic soreness that may be caused by an ill-fitting prosthesis that rubs or otherwise irritates the mucosa, or by a surgical procedure, a nutritional disorder, or poor hygiene. The soreness may even result from a denture liner that hardens and cracks on aging and consequently irritates the mucosal surface.

Presently, there are *two categories of soft-liner materials:* the tissue-conditioning materials, which are intended for use over only a short period such as a week; and the so-called permanent soft liner, which, ideally, would serve to eliminate pain or discomfort for the lifetime of the denture base. Natural soft rubber was one of the first materials to be used as a resilient liner. Plasticized polyvinyl chloride, acrylic resins, silicones, and polyvinyl acetate also have been used. Deficiencies shown by these materials include variable bond strenth, poor color, high water absorption, low abrasion resistance, cracking upon aging, and support of fungal growth.

Candidate *reliner materials* representing several classes of synthetic polymers are currently being characterized and evaluated, including unique silicones, polyurethanes, and butadience elastomers. In preliminary studies an aromatic silicone polymer, known as silphenylene has shown promise. This elastomer offers ease of fabrication at moderate temperatures, good adhesion to polymethylmethacrylate, good mechanical properties, and resistance to fungal growth.

Also being studied is a class of solvent-free liquid polymers that recently was introduced commercially. These products, which are terminated with reactive end groups, are formed by the copolymerization of butadiene and acrylonitrile. Copolymers of these two materials have been available for many years, but only recently have the liquid reactive polymers been made available. They add unlimited possibilities for elastomer fabrication.

Polyurethanes have been tried as bone glues, cavity liners, dentures, surgical sponges, and other biomedical products with varying degrees of success. The principal reason for trying them is that they can be cast as liquids and cured rapidly to tough abrasion-resistant rubbers or resilient foams, depending upon the nature of the reactant.

Historically, the magnitude of the research effort in developing a *new dental material* has been dictated by the consumer market for the specific application. Consequently, until recently only token programs have been aimed at developing improved polymers for specialty problems such as external replacement parts for the head and face.

The number of people now afflicted with *facial disfigurement* is not known, but the total number of new patients each year is probably in the range of 500 to 600 and the numbers have been steadily rising. Whatever the origin of the problem, whether injury, birth defect, or disease, lives once lost are now sustained, sometimes by drastic surgery that severely alters facial features. The professional who must eventually assume the burden of restoration, following the earlier efforts of other specialist, is called the maxillofacial prosthodontist.

Of the materials now available for extraoral maxillofacial prostheses, the most commonly used are the vinlys, the silicones, and the polyurethanes. The vinyls offer an acceptable combination of properties but are costly to fabricate because they require metal molds. The silicones are popular for their ease of fabrication but suffer serious property deficiencies. The polyurethanes in general have excellent mechanical properties, but the ones now used for prostheses are weak and give eratic results in fabrication. If the properties of the silicones could be improved substantially without sacrificing their outstanding processibility, an almost ideal material could be provided to the maxillofacial prosthodontists. (Southern Research Institute Bulletin) [7]

Medical and Dental Instruments

The medical and dental instruments market includes X-ray and electromedical equipment ($2.9 billion U.S. shipments in 1980), surgical and medical instruments ($2.6 billion/1980), surgical appliances and supplies ($3.7 billion/1980), and dental equipment and supplies ($1.1 billion/1980). This type of equipment makes extensive use of many different plastics, both commodity and engineered types. [8, 9]

Domestic demand for the products of these industries continues to grow at an average annual rate of about 13 percent, somewhat lower than the 19 percent rate experienced in the mid-1970's. The effects of voluntary hospital cost-containment efforts, regional health planning, and certificate-of-need programs have been felt mostly in capital equipment; the demand growth rates for these industries has been moderate, notwithstanding the added effect of the general economic recession in 1980. Continued growth in export markets for U.S.-produced medical equipment and supplies has helped to offset the softening of the U.S. market.

POLYMERS/PLASTICS

Plastics may be made hard, elastic, rubbery, tough, flexible, crystal clear, opaque, transparent, or practically anything that is wanted depending on the choice of starting materials and the method of manufacture. The physical properties do not alone satisfy all the requirements for these applications. Extracorporal medicine imposes a number of new demands. For example, the materials must be completely inert towards the substances with which they come in contact; they must not be dissolved or swollen by the fluids kept in them; extraction of any one of the ingredients cannot be tolerated, nor can irreversible absorption; and it must be possible to sterilize the plastics.

The conventional method of sterilization, i.e., by heat, cannot be resorted to for many polymers, whose softening point lies below 100°C. They must be made sterile either by immersing them in certain solutions or by exposing them to high-energy radiation or ethylene oxide gas. In the latter case, the gas may not be irreversibly absorbed by the polymer. No method of sterilization is universally applicable. The most suitable method must be selected according to the nature of the plastic, but this is the case for any material in any application, and a compromise must always be made between a number of parameters.

Modern plastics are also used in places where they are not seen: ampules are coated with silicones and thus cannot be wetted by many liquids and can be emptied to the last drop. Hypodermic needles are made smoother by silicone oils. Non-woven fabrics for disposable washing for the sick, diapers, and surgical clothing are held together by plastic binders.

Completely new vistas for application—and more problems—are opened up by the use of plastics parts for temporary or permanent implants within the human body. Fortunately, great progress has been made in the last thirty years in this sector.

Synthetic fibers are largely used for surgical sutures. Examples are polyamide (nylon), polypropylene, and polyester fibers. They are inert, easy to handle, and readily compatible; but this is by no means sufficient reason for surgeons to be fully satisfied with them. Other properties that are difficult to optimize for all requirements are flexibility, texture, and the ability to make strong knots easily. Finally, after they have served their purpose; i.e., holding the wound together until it has healed, the stitches should disappear without leaving a trace of their presence. Today, resorbable suture is available that decomposes almost completely after a few weeks.

An alternative method to stitching for healing wounds is to bond them together. Tissue adhesives allow wounds to be closed sterilely and without suture, i.e., for kidney and liver resections, facial operations, and perhaps soon for eye operations. Encouraging experiments along these lines are in progress. A wound spray contains a solution of a plastic that forms a sterile film after it has been applied.

In ophthalmology, contact lenses made of plastics are widely accepted, and the number of people wearing them in the United States alone is in the millions. However, up to now, about 40 percent have had difficulties in wearing them and have reverted to glasses; the lenses of that time were rigid and comparatively hydrophobic and produced primarily from polymethylmethacrylate. Since then, softer versions have appeared that are manufactured from hydrophilic gels or crystal-clear silicone, but these incur the risk that bacteria may be lodged in the gels with an attendant infection of the eye. Counter measures that were developed were baths of disinfectant in which the lenses could be kept overnight and pharmaceuticals that could be incorporated in the lenses themselves. Vitreous humorous lost from the eyeball can nowadays be replenished by silicones or other synthetic polymers. However, this has led to frequent reports on the appearance of dullness after some weeks or months. There are many problems of long-term compatibility to be solved in this connection. Another method is to inject a collagen gel that acts as a translucent substance and also restores the pressure within the eyeball, with the result that the detached retina is pushed back into position. The compatibility appears to be comparatively good.

Structures of the major commercial thermoplastic polymers are available in the literature. [10] Assuming a chemist of professional qualifications is unfamiliar with a plastics, he would be able from its structure, to indicate the way the polymer was synthesized, the raw materials employed, and to make a reasonable estimate as to the cost of the product in experimental and production quantities. Analysis also would be made to suggest alternate raw materials and synthesis routes to produce species generally similar but with selective modification of properties. [10]

Refinements in depiction of structure would allow to estimate the physical, chemical, and electrical properties and the kinds of processing difficulties which would be encountered in fabrication operations. If required, suggestions could be made in polymer modifications that would result in changing one or more characteristics on a selective basis.

This type of information is routinely applied to the development of new polymers. New polymers are developed either for the purpose of finding a market for an otherwise valueless by-product or for the purpose of exploiting an apparent potential need. The amount of effort that goes into a given plastic from inception to commercial production will involve expenditures of millions of dollars. Under the circumstances, recognize that products designated medical grade plastics in the literature most likely involve no more than special procedures for quality assurance.

There are basically thousands of different plastics available with all combinations of properties; such as, physical, mechanical, fatigue, sterilization, blood compatibility, etc. Figure 2 is an example of mechanical. Recognize that each specific plastics/polymer has its "specific properties" based on type of material, design parameters, and the method of processing. General information follows in regard to typical pıoperties of a few of the plastics that are used in medical applications.[4, 6, 10, 11]

Acetals

Acetals are strong, hard materials with a natural clear white color. They are one of the stronger thermoplastics materials. Abrasion resistance is generally superior to other plastics with the exception of nylon. Another outstanding property is exceptional solvent resistance.

Acetals are unusual among thermoplastics in their resistance to organic solvents. This property gives them excellent stain resistance to tea, catsup, vinegar, margarine, lemon juice, beet juice, and mustard as well as resistance to alcohols, aldehydes, esters, ethers, glycools, hydrocarbons, ketones, and soaps. However, acetals are attached by strong oxidizing agents, mineral acids and bases.

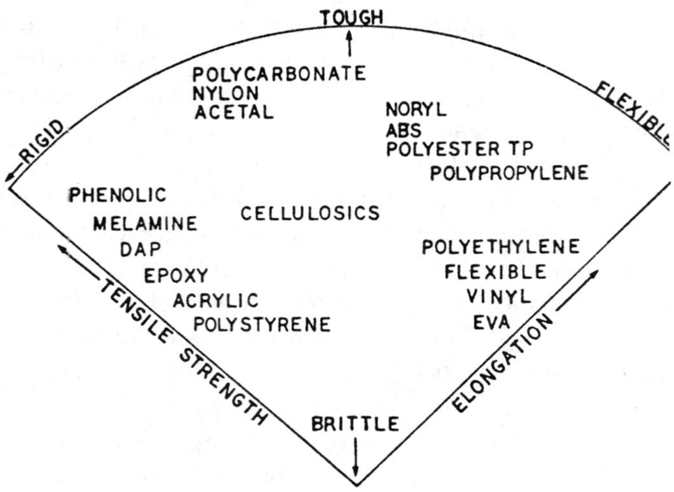

Figure 2.

Acrylonitrile-Butadiene-Stryrenes (ABS)

ABS resins provide a good balance of surface hardness, chemical and heat resistance, rigidity, tensile strength, and impact resistance. Properties that can restrict their use are: lack of transparency, combustibility, and generally limited flexibility. Made with three basic monomers–acrylonitrile, butadiene, and styrene–in varying proportions, ABS materials are almost completely unaffected by water, inorganic salts, alkalies, and many acids.

They are insoluble in most alcohols and hydrocarbon solvents but some of the latter may cause softening and swelling on prolonged contract. Chemicals that may cause cracking include certain alcohols, some vegetable oils and glacial acetic acid. Resistance to staining is characteristic of ABS resins and results in part from low water absorption. Staining that does occur can usually be removed by a shortsoaking in different solutions such as household detergent or bleach.

Acrylics

Acrylic plastics, in generally accepted terminology, are those made, wholly or almost entirely, of methylmethacrylate. Acrylic fibers are polymers made wholly or almost entirely of acrylonitrile. Plastics which use acrylonitrile as ingredients (i.e., ABS and styrene-acrylonitrile copolymers) are not regarded as acrylic plastics since they do not possess the weatherability, tissue tolerance, and clarity of the homopolymers and copolymers made largely of methylmethacrylate. The acrylics encountered in surgical applications are the polymethylmethacrylates, the acrylic hydrogels, $_\alpha$-alkylcyanoacrylates, and the specialized diacrylate dental restoratives.

Polymethylmethacrylate (PMMA) is most widely known. It is encountered in medical practice as post enucleation implants, as contact lenses, as implantable lenses, keratoprostheses, and dentures. It also has been investigated as prosthetic larynx core molds, dental splints, tracheostomy tubes, and buttons. It has been investigated as an implantable drain for the paranasal sinuses and as percutaneous access devices and has been used for experimental tissue windows. In the early surgical practice, PMMA was used extensively for the augmentation of hard and soft facial tissue, in particular for the repair of orbital blow-out fractures, and is still used to some extent in such plastic surgery applications where a hard material is desirable. The precast materials suffer the disadvantage of requiring ionizing radiation or chemical sterilization techniques, since heat procedures are generally unsuited.

PMMA, however, is more widely encountered in surgical practice in the cure-in-place form. It does not provide satisfactory adhesion to bone, but it does serve as a satisfactory substitute or surgical adjunct in a number of operations involving bony tissue. It is used successfully as a fixation agent for intramedullary pins of prosthetic hip joints. PMMA is used for replacing bony defects in the skull attendant on surgical procedures. It has been used for filling space left after mastoidectomy, for replacing ossicular portions in ear operations, and for the fixation of spinal segments. Cure-in-place PMMA formulations also have been used successfully for the reinforcement of cranial artery aneuryms and for filling the aneurysmal sacs of such arteries to stabilize them.

Acrylic hydrogels are produced, essentially, by crosslinking a polymerized acrylic acid copolymer with a polyalcohol. Polymerization and crosslinking occur simultaneously with the amount of water the hydrogel contains being determined by the monomeric materials and by the amount of crosslinks.

The first of the $_{\alpha}$-alkylcyanoacrylates was Eastman 910, based on the methyl species methl-2-cyanoacrylate. When applied as a thin film, where it can pick up sufficient water for catalysis from the atmosphere or the substrate, the material polymerizes rapidly by an anionic rather than free radical mechanism. Higher alkyl species polymerize more rapidly on biological substrates than the lower species and provide less biodegradable polymerized products.

Epoxies

Epoxy resins provide exceptional strength and toughness as well as good resistance to most acids and many solvents. They are fundamentally characterized by deriving at least in part from monomeric compounds containing more than one epoxy group. The epoxy group will react with compounds containing active hydrogens, such as primary and secondary amines and amides, alcohols, organic acids, mercaptans, and phenols. Homopolymerization may be catalized by suitable tertiary amines and some acids. Both thermosets and thermoplastics epoxy formulations are prepared; the usual is thermset.

High molecular weight linear homopolymers are called phenoxy resins, and are available in solution for coatings and as powdered molding compounds. The lower molecular weight monomers are generally liquids and are admired with suitable curing agents to provide cure-in-place formulations. The reaction is moderately exothermic.

Epoxy formulations available commercially nearly always combine a number of ingredients, including fillers, pigments and resinous additives of various kinds, as well as the curing agent. The compounding technology is complex. Formulations have been suggested for use and used with glass cloth for the open reduction and reinforcement of fractures. They have been investigated as bone adhesives, for impregnating aluminum oxide hip joint condyles, for dentures, and direct dental filling resins; they have been used clinically for protecting electronic pacemaker components from body fluids; for tarsorrhaphy; and for reinforcing cranial aneurysms; they also have been used in research for the insulation of electrode brain probes.

Fluorocarbons

Fluorocarbons, also called fluoroplastics, are noted for their resistance to most chemicals and high temperatures. The two most widely used types are polytetrafluoroethylene (TFE) and chlorotrifluoroethylene (CTFE). The chemical inertness of TFE is the highest of any known plastic. Another feature of TFE is its low surface energy. This makes surfaces non-adhesive and slippery.

TFE is more heat resistant (over 500F) than CTFE (390F) and chemical resistance is greater. It is inert to nearly all chemicals. Exceptions: metallic sodium, other alkali metals, certain halogenated chemicals at high temperatures and pressures. Strong inorganic acids and bases, boiling aqua regia, chlorine, bromine, and iodine have no effect on the material.

Although less chemical resistant than TFE, CTFE is inert to most corrosive chemicals and highly resistant to most organic solvents. Usually when a chemical permeates CTFE, only swelling occurs. The material returns to its original state upon evaporation of the solvent. While CTFE is stronger, stiffer, and tougher than TFE, mechanical properties of fluorocarbons are normally low. These properties can be vastly improved when resins are reinforced with fiber glass or inorganic fillers. Both materials are excellent dielectrics, though TFE is better.

Besides TFE and CTFE there are other fluorocarbon plastics. Among these are fluorinated ethylene propylene (FEP) and polyvinylfluoride (PVF).

TFE constructions have been evaluated as prosthetic ureters, bile ducts, tracheas, larynxes, ligaments, and tendons, as artificial blood, prosthetic heart valve leaflets, mandibles, acetabulums, hip joint condyles, and skin. It has been used for the augmentation of soft tissue, for the repair of orbital fractures, and, in mesh form, for bridging tissue defects and for providing tissue fixation through interstitial ingrowth of connective tissue.

TFE foam has been investigated as a replacement for bone, as percutaneous anchoring devices, and as oxygenating membranes for heart and lung machines. It has been used clinically for scleral buckles, as interposition films to prevent adhesions in ear and nose surgery, as esophageal dilators, for heart valve sewing rings, as blood compatible velours, for patching right ventricular outflow tracts, for patching septal defects, as vascular occluders, as sutures, as arterial patches, for wrapping aneurysms, and as endolympatic fluid shunts.

The chief current clinical uses are as arterial prostheses, for coating polyester fiber sutures, as intravascular tips for A-V hemodialysis shunts; in particulate form, for the permanent correction of the nonclosing glottis; and in felt form, for tissue reinforcement in connection with suturing. There are some surgical drains and tubing constructed of TFE.

Polyamides (Nylons) (PA)

Nylon is the generic name of polyamide resins. It is extremely tough, has a high melting point (it can be safely boiled and steam sterilized) and is unaffected by most chemicals, greases, and solvents with the exception of mineral acids. However, it is fairly easily stained by coffee, tea, and colored foods. Nylon has high tensile, impact, and flexural strength. In part, its resistance to hard blows is due to its resiliency, allowing it to give a little when it is hit. Though the glossy surface of nylon is very resistant to abrasion, scouring powders should not be used in cleaning.

Most nylon products are made with nylon 6/6 (hexamethylene diamine adipic acid) or nylon 6 (polycaprolactam). Nylon 6/6 is somewhat harder and more rigid than nylon 6 which generally has more resilience and higher impact strength. A third type, nylon 6/10, resembles nylon 6/6 in many respects. In comparison, it exhibits lower moisture absorption, lower heat resistance and greater flexibility. Unless special grades are used, nylon tends to yellow and become dirty in appearance on aging. Fairly high water absorption may result in swelling which can be a disadvantage—such as when it is used for a close fit with another material.

Typical applications include surgical hand brushes, tubing, nozzles, orthopedic devices, sutures, adaptors, needle hubs in syringes, containers, and film packaging of surgical items, tracheotomy cannula, traction bows, and umbilical cord clamps. Also for prosthetic bile ducts, arteries, tracheas, larynxes, outer ears, bladders, elbow and hip joints, tendons, and artificial skin. They have been used as surgical meshes and as mesh backings for solid constructions to permit tissue fixation; as interpostion films in joints and in the management of extraocular mobility restrictions; as vascular occluders; as microcapsules; and as dialysis membranes. The present clinical use is largely confined to specialized tubing applications, velour for blood contact surfaces, and as sutures. The nylon sutures, the first synthetic sutures introduced, have maintained their popularity over a 35 year span.

Polycarbonates (PC)

Polycarbonate can provide the characteristic of unbreakability for stiff plastics. Other outstanding properties: toughness, impact strength, heat resistance, and transparency.

Polycarbonate has good room temperature resistance to water, dilute acids, oxidizing, and reduction agents, salts, oils, and aliphatic hydrocarbons. It is attacked by alkalies, amines, ketones, esters, and aromatic hydrocarbons. It is dissolved by methylene chloride, ethylene dichloride, cresol and dioxane.

Polycarbonate has good resistance to water up to about 150F but at higher temperatures it slowly crazes and loses toughness. It can be steam sterilized. However, after a hundred or so cycles, its physical properties are reduced significantly.

Speaking comparatively, polycarbonate is not so chemical resistant as nylon or polyolefins (polyethylenes and polypropylenes). Moreover, friction and wear properties do not normally match those of acetals and nylons.

Typical applications include lenses, packaging trays, covers for baby food warmers, baby bottles, blood oxygenators, lighting fixtures, and diffusion panels, glazing (institutional windows). housing, and safety shields.

Polyesters (Thermosets and Thermoplastics)

The term polyester covers a broad group of plastics materials: unsaturated polyesters, saturated types, and alkyds. These compounds are all related since the main polymer backbone is formed by esterification condensation of di- or polyfunctional alcohols and acids. They are produced as high molecular weight linear and branched types from the reaction or organic acids with alcohols in a similar fashion to the polyamide reaction, except that in this case the linkage is an ester group.

Polyesters are generally highly resistant to most solvents, acids, bases, and salt. Water absorption is low. They exhibit fair resistance to aromatics, moderate resistance to dilute alkalies but prove unsatisfactory in the presence of most concentrated acids, strong alkalies, and powerful solvents.

Unsaturated polyesters (thermsets) refer to those that are cured by copolymerizing with vinyl monomer. These are generally used in material reinforced with fiberglass. They are relatively short chain monomers which are subsequently crosslinked by free radical type addition polymerization. Unsaturated polyesters are encountered as cure-in-place systems used for products such as lenses and fabricating light weight glass reinforced prosthetic limbs but are not otherwise often seen in the medical technology.

As for saturated polyesters (thermoplastics) the best known are those employed in fibers and film. Some saturated polyesters are combined with isocyanates to form urethane foams and coatings.

Saturated polyester fiber type meshes have been used in reconstructing the larynx, trachea, ureter, esophagus, and as artificial skin. Surgical uses for the meshes include patching blood vessels and reinforcing aneurysms, ventricular outflow tract repairs, felts for sewing rings for artificial heart valves and suture reinforcement, arterial prostheses, and velours for blood compatible structures, and percutaneous access implants. The filaments are the chief synthetic competitor with nylon as suture materials. Polyester fiber meshes are used for reinforcing silicone rubber and as backings for solid structures to permit tissue fixation. Miscellaneous applications include implants to prevent fistulas and block vein growth after vein stripping.

Polyethylenes (PE)

Polyethylenes are among the most widely used thermoplastics. They are noted for their toughness, low moisture absorption, combined resistance to fats and oil, low water-vapor permeability, high O_2 and CO_2 permeability, overall good chemical resistance, and excellent electrical insulating properties. They fall into various groups, such as, low-density (LDPE), linear low-density (LLDPE), medium-density (MDPE), high-density (HDPE), and ultra-high-molecular weight (UHMWPE). The primary differences between the types are heat resistance, rigidity, and chemical resistance. Broadly speaking, as density increases, hardness, heat distortion point, stiffness, tensile strength, and resistance to permeability increase. As density decreases, impact strength increases.

Original work in the medical applications used LDPE. These did not provide dimensional stability at normal sterilizing temperatures and were replaced in surgical applications by the high density (more crystalline) materials produced with special catalysts at lower temperatures and pressures and introduced commercially in the mid-1950's. By regulating catalyst and reaction condition, a variety of types are produced. The medical literature does not appear to discriminate between them and nothing suggests, in the absence of harmful additives and when suitable sterilization techniques are employed, that tissue response will vary significantly between types.

Typical applications include disposable syringes, tubing, packaging film, cap liners, surgical drapes, disposable examining gloves, denture cups, detergent and bleach bottles, squeeze bottles, sutures, containers such as bottles and other units for administration of drugs and blood and for the collection of body fluids, bottle caps, oxygen tents, pails, repair of incisional hernias and stomach wall support. Surgical uses include prosthetic ureters, bile ducts, tracheas, bladders, acetabulums, hip joint condyles, and tendons. They have been used for tissue augmentation, as sutures, for wrapping aneurysms, for preventing adhesions during healing in vocal cord and middle ear surgery, to fill space after mastoidectomy, and for scleral buckling. Most present clinical use is as drains, catheters, and tubing. Typical of the implanted drains are those used for glaucoma, paranasal sinuses, middle ear vents, tear ducts, and prosthetic vas deferens. The various polyethylenes are gradually being replaced by the more acceptable (from the sterilization standpoint) polypropylene.

Ethylene Copolymers

There are a number of thermoplastic materials that approximate the elastomeric properties of rubber. Among these are chlorinated polyethylenes, internally plasticized vinyls, and ethylene copolymers. The latter are outstanding in such properties as high impact strength, high elongation (they have excellent "snap-back"), and good low temperature flexibility.

Ethylene copolymers include flexible ethylene vinyl acetate (EVA) and ethylene ethyl acrylate (EEA). Both materials resemble polyethylenes in appearance but have properties more like those of vinyl resins.

Food, drug, and medical supply manufacturers now use EVA resins to eliminate possible contamination problems associated with plasticizers used in vinyl compounds or with the additives of rubber products. Typical EVA applications include disposable surgical and enema syringes, squeeze bulbs, dropper for vitamins and drugs, sheeting, baby pants, disposable gloves, food, beverage and medical tubing.

Polypropylenes (PP)

Polypropylenes belong to the same family as the polyethylenes (both are in the family of polyolefins). Their main attributes are high rigidity, resistance to heat and chemicals, and good tensile and impact strength. One property that gives polypropylenes an advantage over other plastics is their great flex life. They are also one of the lightest of plastics materials. Polypropylene is the lowest density of commercial non-foamed plastic formulations, with the exception of polymethyl pentene (TPX).

In general polypropylenes offer good stiffness, yield strength and hardness. Though they are among the harder themoplastics, they are not so hard as polystyrenes, nylon, ABS materials, and acetals. They are essentially unaffected by inorganic salts and their solutions, and higher molecular weight aliphatics. While there is no known solvent at room temperature, lower molecular weight aliphatics, aromatics, and chlorinated hydrocarbons cause them to soften and swell. They are attacked by halogens and other strong oxidizing reagents.

Polypropylenes are generally more resistant than polyethylenes to stress cracking when exposed to polar liquids such as alcohols, soap solutions, and synthetic detergents. They also show very low water absorption. Abrasion resistance is excellent and is normally higher than that of polystyrene and polyethylene but lower than that of acrylic and polyvinyl chloride.

As in the case of polyethylene, FDA-approved antioxidants may be specified when food-contact grades are being produced. Typical applications include disposable syringes, tubing, bottles, bottle caps, jars, cups, pails, basins, sanitary ware, carafes, laboratory ware packaging film and sheeting, sutures, and bedpans.

Polypropylene is used for blood filters and shows promise as prosthetic heart valve leaflets and hip joint condyles. It also has been investigated for prosthetic tracheas, larynxes, and esophaguses—as have many other plastics, pending discovery of clinically satisfactory materials for these applications. Polypropylene velours have been used to obtain blood compatible interfaces and the material has been investigated as sutures.

Polystyrenes (PS)

The name polystyrene designates a family of thermoplastics derived from the basic styrene monomer. Applications depend in many cases on their clarity and rigidity. They also are available as translucent or opaque materials in a variety of colors. Besides general-purpose polystyrenes, there are modified polystyrenes (these contain rubber to improve impact properties), light stable types, chemical resistant types (these are styrene acrylonitrile copolymers—SAN), foams, etc.

Unmodified polystyrenes possess excellent resistance to organic acids, alkalies, salts, lower alcohols, and aqueous solutions of these materials. They are softened or dissolved by many hydrocarbons, ketones, the higher aliphatic esters, and essential oils. Most foods, drinks, and usual household acids, oils, and vinegar have no effect on polystyrenes. This is not true, however, of citrus fruit rind oil, cleaning fluids, gasoline, and turpentine. Typical applications include disposable syringes, suture cutters, thumb forceps, tubing, medicinal nebulizers, medicine cups, wash basins, emesis basins, soap dishes, tumblers, bottle caps, denture cups, and laboratory equipment.

Polysulfone

A high temperature polymer is polysulfone. Among its inherent characteristics are thermal stability, oxidation resistance, and rigidity at elevated temperatures. Heat distortion temperature is 345F, while maximum recommended service temperature in air is 300F.

Polysulfone can be steam sterilized repeatedly without loss of physical properties and will withstand exposure to soap and detergent solutions. The material will also withstand boiling water for long periods, providing low load conditions exist of 500 psi or less. Polysulfone absorbs a modest amount of water (0.85 percent at equilibrium in boiling water). This is accompanied by very little dimensional change, approximately 0.1 percent.

The polymer is not attacked by water through chemical reaction (hydrolysis). Furthermore, it is resistant to mineral acid and salt solutions as well as many oils and alcohols. It is attached, however, by polar organic solvents such as ketones, chlorinated hydrocarbons, and aromatic hydrocarbons. Typical applications include hospital trays and dishes, medical and surgical instruments, and medical electrical and electronic components.

Polyvinyl Chlorides (PVC)

Polyvinyl chlorides are the most commonly used materials identified as vinyls. The term vinyl covers a broad range of materials. In general, vinyls are tough, have high inherent strength, abrasion resistance, and exceptional resistance to water and chemicals. In addition, they are among the few thermoplastics that are self-extinguishing, primarily because of their chlorine constituents.

Vinyls exhibit excellent resistance to weak acids, strong mineral acids, weak and strong alkalies, aliphatic hydrocarbons, and mineral, animal and vegetable oils. Solvents in which vinyls will dissolve include acetone, methyl ethyl ketone, diisobutyl ketone, cyclohexanone, tetrahydrofuran, toluene, xylene, and dimethyl dormamide.

The parent polymer is hard and horn-like, but through the use of additives it may be modified to provide varying flexibilities from tough and rigid to soft and pliable. Copolymers greatly extend the property range. PVC resins can be compounded to give any degree of flexibility and other desired end properties through the use of such additives as plasticizers, stabilizers, lubricants, and fillers.

In some instances, vinyls may present difficulties in hospital applications. The basic problem is that any plastics compound that is normally formulated with various additives may react with solutions that come in contact with it.

In fairness to vinyls, it should be pointed out that such a possibility is not restricted to vinyls since very few resins are used in their virgin state. Formulated products delivered to the surgeon may thus be complex, and obviously may very significantly from supplier to supplier, and from a given supplier, from time to time. Quality control procedures can be set up to meet specification requirements.

Typical application included for rigid PVC: tubing, soap dishes, laboratory equipment, transparent and opaque containers, pipe, film, and sheeting; for flexible PVC: tubing (medical, food, enema, drainage, endotracheal), blood collection and administration sets, stopclocks, surgical drapes, aprons, disposable gloves, pillow and mattress covers, diapers, film, sheeting and balloon-type splints. For medical and surgical applications, the vinyl polymers are supplied as foams, rods, tubes, sheets, films, filaments, and fabrics, and when further reshaping is required, this is normally accomplished mechanically.

A major surgical use is as tubing available in medical grades. PVC has been widely used for blood transfusion tubing in England since the 1950's. This was its first medical application, and it replaced glass and rubber tubing. Its transparency enabled cleanliness to be checked and liquid flow to be observed. [12]

PVC administration sets are supplied in pre-sterilized disposable packs and as a result the incidence of thrombophlebitis following transfusions has diminished. From these beginnings has come acceptance of flexible PVC moldings and extrusions for a wide variety of surgical and treatment uses.

There has been one problem, however. Flexible PVC compounds can contain up to 40 percent plasticizer and, while the chosen material is very carefully selected for its high purity and low toxicity, it can be extracted from PVC by contact with some fatty substances such as blood or the digestive system. Where contact times are short there is no difficulty but for a number of applications in which PVC may be in contact with a patient's system for longer periods, extraction of plasticizer is much less acceptable.

Stiffening of PVC due to plasticizer being extracted may cause patients considerable discomfort when a feeding or wound drainage tube is removed after prolonged use. Blood stored in PVC bags or flowing through PVC tubes for long periods will also extract plasticizer. While that most commonly used, DEHP, has been shown to be of low toxicity, it is naturally desirable to avoid any extra burden on a patient's system. This is obviously more important for those needing regular hemodialysis or blood transfusions.

BIP Vinyls of Turner & Newall Group, England, has been investigating this problem since 1975 in cooperation with the Department of Health and Social Security (DHSS). Development work at Aycliffe had been aimed at perfecting extraction-resistant PVC medical compounds which can be used safely in long-term contact with blood and human tissue. A five-year development program was started to perfect a new PVC compound.

Development of these new medical compounds involved a whole series of compounding and extrusion trials with a wide range of plasticisers. Besides satisfying toxicological tests a medical extrusion compound must be easily processed into tubing with high clarity and water-white color. Such an appearance is closely associated with cleanliness in this kind of application. In addition the product must obviously meet high physical standards as regards tensile strength, flexibility, and creep.

Materials meeting these criteria were then subjected to extraction tests using food and blood simulants in which samples of pressed sheet were immersed for long periods. Following this, physical properties were checked and analysis carried out to determine the degree of extraction.

In addition, samples were subjected to steam sterilization and sophisticated analytical technics were used to check whether plasticiser was extracted during autoclaving.

After full consultation with the DHSS, a wide range of toxicological tests were carried out on materials selected from the trials at Aycliffe and in addition a number of BIP customers commissioned their own toxicity testing at independent research houses in the United Kingdom and on the Continent.

As a result of all this development and research a new "Beetle" compound, VN 782, has been cleared by the DHSS for use in feeding and wound drainage tubing and also for blood contact applications. It also has been approved for use in feeding tubes in Denmark. Production started in 1980.

Silicones

Of the thermoset resins, silicones polysiloxanes are the most important as far as hospitals are concerned. They are unique among plastics in that they are semi-organic polymers (organopolysiloxanes) with a quartz-like structure. Those that are of major interest to hospitals are rubbers. The behavior of silicones at higher temperatures is one of the primary advantages of silicone rubber.

The silicones, are characterized by a backbone consisting of repeated silicon and oxygen atoms. Each silicon has two alkyl or aryl substituents, in the case of the medical grade silicones and the best known commercial elastomers, both are CH_3 groups and the polymer is thus known as polydimethylsiloxane.

Polymerization is accomplished by an acid-catalyzed ring-opening technique. The process may be carried to the gum stage and then continued on rubber processing equipment with the use of suitable fillers and peroxide catalysts to produce high-molecular weight, crosslinked, heat-cured elastomers. Cure-in-place materials (RTV, room temperature vulcanizing) rubber formulations are produced from suitable blends of the cyclic and linear species with stannous octoate as catalyst, the cured properties regulated by the parent oils, with overall properties generally inferior to those obtained with heat cures and crosslinking agents.

While the strength of all rubber materials diminished with increasing temperatures, the relative change in the properties of silicones is much less. In fact, above 390F, silicone rubber is the toughest of all rubbers. Equally impressive is the long-term retention of properties at elevated temperatures. Also, they are relatively unaffected by moisture, ozone, and many chemicals, and are not corrosive toward other materials. In addition, they possess unusual surface properties such as the ability to prevent other materials from adhering and they are among the most inert of all plastics.

Many silicone rubber compounds are available. There are two major types of silicone rubbers used for medical purposes: the heat vulcanizing type and the room temperature vulcanizing, or RTV type. In the main, the heat vulcanizing types are stronger and have greater tear strength. They are the material of choice where heat can be tolerated. When heat cannot be tolerated, RTV silicone rubbers are used.

Silicone resins are also employed in medical applications. For instance, silicone surface coating protect tissues from reactive foreign materials. Other products include a silicone antifoam defoams blood in heart-lung machines. Silicones (in fluid form) also are used to siliconize surfaces, rendering them non-wetable and non-adherent. In this regard, it should be noted that siliconized rubber is an organic rubber with a thin surface coat of silicone, while silicone rubber is an entity in itself.

Typical applications include catheters, drainage tubes, tubing for heart-lung machines, intestinal decompression tubes, intravenous tubing, heart valves, urethral valves, plastic surgery (rebuilding noses, cheek bones, jaw lines, breasts, ears), tubing for hydrocephalus, reinforcement of cranial aneurysms, implantable cardiac pacemakers, urinary drains, artificial bile ducts, esophageal prostheses, tracheal prostheses, laminates, retinal detachment surgery, housings, and foams.

Silicone rubber elastomers have been investigated as prosthetic ureters, esophaguses, bile ducts, blood vessels, tracheas, penises, testicles, mandibles, bladders, breasts, muscles, outer ears, and wrist and finger joints. They have been used as leaflets and balls/lenses/discs in artificial heart valves, and for post enucleation implants and as obturators for various applications. Most successful of the applications involve tissue augmentaton, including special breast prostheses, burr hole covers, chin, nose, and orbital implants, etc.

They have been used successfully for: a number of implantable drainage tracts, including lacrymal, glaucoma, and endolymphatic ducts and middle ear vents and for ventriculo-peritoneal shunts; used clinically as urethral, dura matter, and pericardial patches, for cushioning prosthetic heart valves and dentures; investigated as prosthetic ureter valves and used as valves for hydrocephalic shunts; used as interposition membranes to prevent adhesions after surgical procedures involving oviducts, middle ears, bones and joints; used as cornneal splints and water barriers and for scleral buckles; used as oxygenating membranes in heart lung machines, as coatings for sutures, as cuffs for tracheotomy tubes, as vascular occluders, blood compatible coatings, blood pump diaphragms, pacemaker encapsulants, and as microcapsules; and widely used for the construction of drains, catheters, and tubing, such as in the continuous anesthetic units, coronary artery cannulae, mushroom catheters, surgical sucker cannulae, thoracic drains and tracheotomy tubes.

Polyurethanes (PUR)

The polyurethanes have provided the medical industry with an important, viable plastics. Like the polyvinyl chlorides, there are many different formulations providing a broad range of properties. Chemical clean/pure grades are available.

Two basic types of polyurethanes have been used in surgical applications: the thermoplastic spandex types, which are complicated copolymers offering good elastic strengths and high orders of tissue compatibility; and the thermoset types, which is encountered as prefabricated or cure-in-place foams. Although the materials are grouped under the same generic heading, their properties are not too similar nor do their general commercial fields of application overlap.

Crosslinked materials have been investigated as bone glues, as sponges to promote adhesions, for mammary augmentation, as cavity liners, as dentures, as surgical sponges, and as dialysts membranes. The thermoplastic materials have been suggested as sutures and are under investigation as vascular prostheses, dialysis membranes, and diaphragms for blood pumps.

Foam Plastics

Foamed plastics are expanded materials with a cellular structure. They may be flexible, rigid, or semi-rigid. Most liquid resins can be made into foams by introduction of a dispersed gas and subsequently cooling or curing of the expanded mass.

Among the resins most commonly used in the production of foams are: acrylonitrile-butadiene-styrene polymers, cellulose acetate, epoxies, isocyanates (used to make urethane foams), phenolics, polyethylenes, polystyrenes, silicones, ureas, and vinyl copolymers. Other type foams include those produced with synthetic and natural rubbers.

Combinations of properties varies according to the type of resins and the formulation. Not all plastics foams possess all properties in the desirable ratio. Those of most interest to hospitals are urethane and vinyl foams. The latter compete with foam rubber and urethane foam as cushioning and padding material. Among the advantages of vinyl foam over other types are good resiliency, chemical resistance, and nonflammability.

Urethane foams have many things in their favor. They do not have undesirable bounce-back, they do not mat, stiffen, or crumble after long use or aging, they are nonallergenic, they are odorless, and they are unaffected by dampness. Moreover, since they are chemically inert, urethane foams are not affected by common cleaning chemicals, water, body acids, spilled foods, or liquids.

It is important to know in advance what foam properties will be required for a particular application. As with other plastics or any material, it is not enough to be told that a material is a plastics foam with remarkable properties.

Plastics Standard Classification System

A universal classification system for plastics is being developed by the American Society for Testing and Materials (ASTM) that can be used by all industries in specifying both commercially available and special plastics resins. Any company that is presently engaged in the design and/or manufacture of plastics, or any company, group or individual entering the field has great built-in potential. it will provide a basis for medical polymers where special "medical" requirements can be added by the individual material users that supercede or supplement the basic properties (using "Suffixes"). [13]
The standard is being promulgated by ASTM. It is called D 4000 classification system. The purpose of D 4000 is to provide guidance to the designer in the selection of practical, commercially available plastics, and further to provide a method for specifying these materials by use of a simple "line callout" designation.

The classification system will be developed to permit the addition of descriptive values for future plastics without reorganization of the classification system and to facilitate the incorporation of future new methods of testing to keep pace with changing industrial requirements.

The overall proposed system is detailed in Tables 3 through 7. Each type and all variations of a material will be assigned a callout number. The first letters (Table 3) identify the broad generic family such as PA for polyamide (nylon). Table 4 lists the abbreviations in the current ASTM D 1600 standard.

Table 3

Standard Classification System for Plastics

1	2 SPECIFIC			3	4	5	6 CELL REQUIREMENTS					7
Broad generic type	**Type**	**Class**	**Grade**	**Filler**	**%Filler**	**Table**	**Tensile strength**	**Flex. mod.**	**Izod impact**	**HDT**	**TBD**	**Suffix**

1 Two or more letters identify the generic material based on ASTM D 1600.
2 Three numbers identify the specific chemical type, the modification or use class, and the grade by viscosity or level of modification. A Basic Property Table will provide property values.
3 One letter identifies filler type.
4 Two numbers indicate percent of filler.
5 One letter refers to a Cell Table listing of physical specifications and test methods.
6 Five numbers refer to the specific physical parameters listed in the Cell Table.
7 Suffix codes indicate special requirements based on the application and identifies special tests.

Table 4

ASTM D 1600 Standard Plastics Abbreviations

Term	Abbreviation	Term	Abbreviation
Cellulose propionate	CP	Polyethylene terephtalate	PETP
Chorinated poly(vinyl chloride)	CPVC	Poly(methyl-α-chloroacrylate)	PMCA
Cresoi-formaldehyde	CF	Poly(methyl methacrylate)	PMMA
		Polyoxymethylene, polyacetal	POM
Diallyl phthalate	PDAP	Polypropylene	PP
		Polystyrene	PS
Epoxy, epoxide	EP	Polytetrafluoroethylene	PTFE
Ethyl cellulose	EC	Polyurethane	PUR
		Poly(vinyl acetate)	PVAC
Melamine-formaldehyde	MF	Poly(vinyl alcohol)	PVAL
		Poly(vinyl butyral)	PVB
Perfluoro(ethylene-propylene)	FEP	Poly(vinyl chloride)	PVC
copolymer		Poly(vinyl chloride-acetate)	PVCA
Phenol-formaldehyde	PF	Poly(vinyl fluoride)	PVF
Poly(acrylic acid)	PAA	Poly(vinyl formal)	PVFM
Polyacrylontirle	PAN		
Polyamide (nylon)	PA	Silicone plastics	SI
Polybutadiene-acrylonitirle	PBAN	Styrene-acrylonitrile	SAN
Polybutadiend-styrene	PBS	Styrene-butadiene	SB
Polycarbonate	PC	Styrene-rubber plastics	SRP
Poly(dially phthalate)	PDAP		
Polyethylene	PE	Urea-formaldehyde	UF

The next three digits further identify the material by specific *type, class,* and *grade*. Type identifies the material chemically, Class indicates modification or use, and Grade gives viscosity/flow or level of modification. A *Basic Property Table* will be prepared for each generic material. These tables will show the range of specifications by type, class, and grade of commercially available plastics. A callout such as PA 122 identifies a heat stabilized nylon 6/6 with medium viscosity as shown in the example of Table 5.

Table 5

Basic Property Table

Type	Class	Grade									
Description	***Description**	****Description**	**Relative Viscosity D 7B9 min**	**Melting point D 789°C**	**Specific gravity D 792**	**Flexural modulus D 790 MPa min.**	**Tensile strength D 638 MPa min**	**Elong. (ult.) D 638 / min.**	**Izod impact (notched) D 256 J/m min.**	**Heat defl. temp. D 648 455 kPa °C min.**	**1820 kPa °C min.**
6:6 Nylon	1 GP	1 LV	35	250-260	1.13-1.15	2600	76	10	40	180	65
		2 MV	45	250-260	1.13-1.15	2600	76	50	50	180	65
		3 HV	60	250-260	1.13-1.15	2600	76	50	50	180	65
		4 E	120	250-260	1.13-1.15	2600	76	50	50	180	65
		5 BM	300	250-260	1.13-1.15	2600	76	50	50	180	65
		0 Other									
	2 HS	1 LV	35	250-260	1.13-1.15	2600	76	10	40	180	65
		2 MV	45	250-260	1.13-1.15	2600	76	40	50	180	65
		3 HV	60	250-260	1.13-1.15	2600	76	40	50	180	65
		4 E	120	250-260	1.13-1.15	2600	76	40	50	180	65
		5 BM	300	250-260	1.13-1.15	2600	76	40	50	180	65
		0 Other									
	3 N	1 LV	35	250-260	1.13-1.15	2800	90	5	40	185	70
		2 MV	45	250-260	1.13-1,15	2800	90	5	40	185	70
		3 HV	60	250-260	1.13-1.15	2800	90	5	40	185	70
		4 E	120	250-260	1.13-1.15	2800	90	5	40	185	70
		5 BM	300	250-260	1.13-1.15	2800	90	5	40	185	70
		0 Other									
	4 IM	1 MI	–	250-260	1.09-1.11	1700	58	55	150	145	50
		2 HI	–	250-260	1.09-1.11	1500	48	50	800	145	55
		0 Other									
	5 IMHS	1 MI	–	250-260	1.09-1.11	1700	58	55	130	145	50
		0 Other									
	6 WS	1 MV	45	250-260	1.14-1.16	2700	80	20	40	180	65
		0 Other									
	0 O(s)	0 Other									
2 6 Nylon	1 GP	1 LV	3C	210-225	1.12-1.14	2600	75	40	50	–	65
		2 MV	4C	210-225	1.12-1.14	2500	75	40	50	–	65
		3 HV	5C	210-225	1.12-1.14	2500	75	100	50	–	65

*GP = General Purpose; HS = Heat Stabilized; N= Nucleated; IM = Impact Modified; IMHS = Impact Modified Heat Stablized; WS = Weather Stabilized; O(s) = Other (stabilized)

**LV = Low Viscosity; MV = Medium Viscosity; HV = High Viscosity; E = Extrusion; BM = Blow Molding; MI = Medium Impact; HI = High Impact

If the material requirements are fulfilled in one of these basic tables then no addition to the callout is needed. However, if special or filled versions of the material are needed, a letter followed by two numbers is added to the callout. The letter identifies the filler or reinforcement (possibly G for glass, C for carbon, etc.) and the two numbers indicate the percentage by weight.

To this is added an alphabetic cell identification code followed by the cell column numbers which contain specific physical characteristics. Thus, (proposed Cell Table 6) illustrates graphically the cell suffix A65480. Proposed Cell Table A pertains to filled, high performance plastics. In the example, PA 122 G33 A65480, G 33 indicates 33 percent glass reinforcement. A65480 refers to Cell Table A in which 6 indicates a tensile strength of 165 MPa, 5 a flexural modulus of 7.57 GPa, 4 and Izod impact of 96.1 J/m, etc.

Table 6

Cell Table

CELL A	0	1	2	3	4	5	6	7	8	9
Tensile strength D-638 MPa (psi)		96.3 (14000)	110 (16000)	123.8 (180000)	137.5 (20000)	151.3 (22000)	165 (24000)	192.5 (28000)	206.3 (30000)	220 (32000)
Flexural modulus D-790 GPa (10^6 psi)	UNSPECIFIED	3.44 (0.5)	4.82 (0.7)	5.51 (0.8)	6.88 (1.0)	7.57 (1.1)	8.26 (1.2)	8.95 (1.3)	9.64 (1.4)	11.0 (1.6)
Izod impact (notched) D-256 J/m (ft-lb/in.)		42.7 (0.8)	53.4 (1.0)	85.4 (1.6)	96.1 (1.8)	106.8 (2.0)	117.4 (2.2)	128.1 (2.4)	138.8 (2.6)	149.5 (2.8)
Heat deflection temperature (264 psi) D-648°C (°F)		138 (280)	143 (290)	149 (300)	160 (320)	193 (380)	204 (400)	227 (440)	238 (460)	249 (480)
To be determined		XX	XX	XX	XX	XX	XX	XX	XX	XX

Cell tables will be developed based on filled compounds now available. As new compounds are made available, their suppliers will provide physical characteristics data for the tables. These tables have the capacity to list the specifications of all commercially available plastic materials. With this system it would be possible to request, by callout number, a product that is not available or even impossible to compound. However, this could be circumvented by an additional list of all commercially available materials by specification.

Table 7 is the identification of a resin by the D 4000 standard classification system for plastics. The complete callout PA 122 G33 A65480 HXX FXX identifies a heat stablized medium

Table 7

Identification of a Resin by Standard Classification System for Plastics

ASTM D 4000 PA122 G33 A65480 Hxx Fxx

Material (plastic)	Basic Material	Special Material Requirements	Special Material for Application

	Broad generic type	Specific type	Class	Grade	Filter type	% Filler	Cell table	Tensile strength	Flexural modulus	Izod Impact	Heat deflection temperature	TBD*	Suffix	Special test requirements	Suffix	Special test requirement
ASTM D4000	**PA**	**1**	**2**	**2**	**G**	**33**	**A**	**6**	**5**	**4**	**8**	**0**	**H**	**xx**	**F**	**xx**

*To be determined

viscosity nylon 6/6, 33 percent glass reinforced with specific performance characteristics, and special requirements of heat resistance and flammability. The XX's will later identify the special tests to be established by ASTM and also permit user to specify their own requirements.

The final numbers in the identification callout allow for special requirements of materials based on application. ASTM will list certain tests, such as oxidation stability, solvent resistance, dimensional stability, etc. There also will be the opportunity for the plastics designer/user to list their own test requirements, such as sterilization limits, blood compatability, etc.

Processing Plastics

Many fabricating processes are employed. Which process to use depends upon the nature and requirements of the raw materials, the properties wanted in the finished product, the cost of the process, speed, and the volume to be produced. Some processes can be used with many kinds of plastics; others are specialized. [14]

Recognize that the final actual properties of a processed plastics for medical application is directly related to how the plastics is processed. If process controls are not properly set up, followed, and continually rechecked to insure meeting part performance requirements, products could be improperly processed.

This quality control requirement on processing plastics for medical use is no different than plastics used in other markets where high performance demands exist such as packaging food, beverages, aircraft structures, etc. Also similar process controls are required with materials other than plastics if tight requirements exist.

The extrusion process accounts for 38 percent of the plastics consumed for medical applications, injection molding at 32 percent, foam molding at 13 percent, blow molding at 9 percent, and other processes at 8 percent. Practically all the plastics are processed by the methods described in Table 8.

In any particular technological sphere, appreciable advance in knowledge are hardly possible in the long run without related progress in other fields. Indeed, the incentive for further development is often provided by forces not subject to scientific laws.

In some branches of plastics technology, particularly the field of processing techniques and machine construction, it was originally found to be sufficient to adapt existing equipment, at that time devoted mainly to rubber processing. The new thermoplastics had a wider range of working temperatures and viscosities compared with rubber, but it soon recognized that they required individual treatment in process design because of their special processing characteristics and their wide application potential.

It eventually became clear that very little was really known about what was happening inside the familiar processing machines—whether in the gap of a roll mill or calendar, or in the flights of a ram or screw. Only with the beginning of a deeper understanding of process mechanisms and their underlying physical laws, made close cooperation between theorists and practical men, has processing technology and machinery design made any real progress.

The 1940's and 1950's were the most productive periods in the latest phase of injection and extrusion development which at last became a province of the scientific engineer rather than the craftsman. The many publications of recent years describing investigatons of the rheological and thermodynamic phenomena occurring injection and extrusion, with their considerable use of mathematics can be appreciated only by a limited circle of specialists.

In spite of what has been achieved so far, the industry really surmounted only the first hurdle of systematic development. The industry must not regard the present state of injection and

Table 8

Methods for Processing Plastics

Process	Description	Limitations
Blow Molding	An extruded parison tube of heated elastomer is positioned between two halves of an open split mold and expanded against the sides of the closed mold via air pressure. The mold is opened and the part ejected. Low tool and die costs, rapid production rates, and ability to mold fairly complex hollow shapes in one piece.	Limited to hollow or tubular parts; wall thickness and tolerances can be difficult to control.
Calendering	Dough-consistent elastomer mass is formed into a sheet of uniform thickness by passing it through and over a series of heated or cooled rolls. Calenders are also utilized to apply elastomer covering to the backs of other materials. Low cost, and sheet materials are virtually free of molded-in stresses.	Limited to sheet materials, and very thin films are not possible.
Casting	Stock is poured into a mold without pressure, cured, and taken from the mold. Relatively low mold cost, capability to form large parts with thick cross sections, good surface finish, and convenient to low volume production.	Limited to relatively simple shapes. Most elastomers are not suitable for this method. Except for cast tires, method becomes uneconomical at high volume production rates.
Coating	Process methods vary. Various elastomers widely used in coating of numerous materials. Roller coating similar to calendering process. Spread coating employs blade in front of roller to position resin on material. Coatings also applied via brushing, spraying, and dipping.	Economics dependent upon close tolerance control generally.
Compression Molding	Principally, polymerized thermoset compound, usually preformed, is positioned in a heated mold cavity; the mold is closed (heat and pressure are applied) and the material flows and fills the mold cavity. Heat completes polymerization and the part is ejected. Large bulky parts can be molded; and process is adaptable to rapid automation (racetrack techniques, etc.)	Extremely intricate parts containing undercuts, side draws, small holes, delicate inserts, etc., very close tolerances difficult to produce.
Encapsulation	Mixed compound is poured into open molds to surround and envelope components; cure may be at room temperature with heated postcure. Generally, encapsulation includes several processes such as potting, embedding, and conformal coating.	Low volume process subject to inherent limitations on materials which can lead to product defect caused by exotherm, curing, or molding conditions, low thermal conductivity, high thermal expansion and internal stresses.
Extrusion Molding	Widely used for continuous production of sheet, tube, and other profiles; also can be used in conjunction with blow molding. Elastomer compound is fed from a hopper to a screw and barrel where it is heated to plasticity and then forwarded, usually via a rotating screw, through a nozzle possessing the desired cross section configuration. Production lines require input and takeoff equipment that can be complex. Low tool cost, numerous complex profile shapes possible, very rapid production rates, can apply coatings or jacketing to core materials (such as wire).	Limited to sections of uniform cross section.

Process	Description	Limitations
Filament Winding	Excellent strength-to-weight here. Continuous, reinforced filaments are saturated with resin and machine wound onto mandrels having shape of desired finished part. Once winding is completed part and mandrel are cured; mandrel can then be removed. High strength reinforcements can be oriented precisely in direction where strength is required. Good uniformity of resin distribution in finished part; mainly circular objects such as pipes.	Limited to shapes of positive curvature; openings and holes can reduce strength if not properly designed into molding operations.
Injection Molding	Very widely utilized method. High automation of manufacturing is standard practice. Stock is fed from the hopper and conveyed forward towards the nozzle by a rotating screw. Elastomer is thoroughly and uniformily heated to plasticity in the cylinder at controlled temperature, then forced under pressure through the nozzle into sprues, runners, gates, and cavities of mold. The material is restrained from extruding out the nozzle orifice during plasticizing. As the melted material accumulates at the front of the screw, it forces the rotating screw rearwards (away from the nozzle). Screw rotation and rearward motion stops when a preset position-signal is reached and immediately the screw acts as a ram forcing material to the mold cavity. Final cure occurs in the mold rapidly; the mold is opened; and the part ejected. There is no waiting for the mold to heat the compound. This factor is the basic reason for its high production rates. Efficient preheating of the rubber, just below cure, occurs in the screw. High production runs, low labor costs high reproducibility of complex details, and excellent surface finish exists.	High initial tool and die costs; not economically practical for small runs.
Laminating	Material, usually in form of reinforcing cloth, paper, foil, metal, wood, glass fiber, plastic, etc., preimpregnated or coated with elastomer is molded under pressure into sheet, rod, tube, or other simple shape. Excellent dimensional stability of finished product; very economical in large production of parts.	High tool and die costs. Limited to simple shapes and cross section profiles.
Pultrusion	This process is similar to profile extrusion, however, it does not provide flexibility and uniformity of product control, and automation. Used for continuous production of simple shapes (rods, tubes, and angles) principally incorporating cotton, wire, and fiberglass (or other reinforcement). High output possible.	Close tolerance control requires diligence. Unidirectional strength usually the rule.
Rotational Molding	A predetermined amount of powered or liquid elastomer is poured into mold; mold is closed, heated, and rotated in the exis of two planes until contents have fused to inner walls of mold; mold is then opened and part is removed. Low mold cost, large hollow parts in one piece can be produced, and molded parts are essentially isotropic in nature.	Limited to hollow parts; production rates are usually slow.
Slush Molding	Powdered or liquid elastomer is poured into a mold to capacity; mold is closed and heated for a predetermined time in order to achieve	Limited to hollow parts production rates are very slow; and limited choice of materials that can be processed.

Process	Description	Limitations
	a specified buildup of partially cured material on mold walls; mold is opened and unpolymerized material is poured out; and semifused part is removed from mold and fully polymerized in oven. Low mold costs and economical for small production runs.	Limited to hollow parts production rates are very slow; and limited choice of materials that can be processed.
Thermoforming	Heat softened elastomer sheet is positioned over male or female mold; air is evacuated from between sheet and mold, forcing sheet to conform to contour of mold. Variations include vacuum snapback, plug assist, drape forming, etc. Tooling costs are generally low, large part production with thin sections possible and often comes out economical for limited part production.	Limited to parts of simple configuration, high scrap, and limited number of materials from which to choose.
Transfer Molding	Related to compression and injection molding processes. Elastomer molding compound is fed from hopper into a transfer chamber where it is then heated to plasticity; it is then fed by means of a plunger through sprues, runners, and gates into a closed mold where it cures; mold is opened and part is ejected. Good dimensional accuracy, rapid production rate, and very intricate parts can be produced.	High mold cost; high material loss in sprues and runners; and size of parts is somewhat limited.

extrusion design and technology as the last word in progress. On the contrary, the great possibilities in development—many of which are undoubtedly still dormant—must be recognized and opened up by close cooperation between theorists and technologists.

Subjects of primary interest are:

1. Processing pressures and temperatures
2. Flow rate of plastics
3. Shear rate of plastics
4. Melt viscosity of plastics
5. Elastic shear stresses of plastics
6. Internal stresses in part
7. Instrumentation for measuring temperature, pressure and flow viscosity of plastics during processing
8. Instrumentation to measure internal stresses in the finished part.
9. Tests for physical/mechanical/and other properties of the part
10. Polymer chemistry

The increased use of injection molding and extrusion is due to the development of the screw and, more recently, a combination of better understanding the basic factors involved in the cost advantages and market requirements. As an example, previous to the reciprocating screw, injection machines were very similar to the compression-transfer molding types. Those conditions allow the injection process to be controlled as readily as the older, long-established processes. A sufficient and accurate prediction of the temperature rise on injection is possible, and simple method of optimising operating conditions can be applied to produce quality controlled products at fast rates of production.

Injection Molding [14]

The term injection molding is an oversimplified description of a quite complicated process which is controllable within specified limits. Melted or plasticized plastic material is injected or forced into a mold where it is held until removed in a solid state, duplicating the cavity of the mold. (Figure 3) The mold may consist of a single cavity or a number of similar or dissimilar cavities, each connected to flow channels or "runners" which direct the flow of the melted plastic to the individual cavities. The process is one of the most economical methods for mass producing a single item. Three basic operations exist:

1. Raising the temperature of the plastic to a point where it will flow under pressure. This is usually done by simultaneously heating and masticating the granular solid until it forms a melt at an elevated and uniform temperature and viscosity. Today, this is accomplished in the cylinder of an injection molding machine equipped with a reciprocating screw. The latter provides the mechanical working required in conjunction with the heating of the material. This overall process is called plasticizing (or plastication) of the material.

2. Allowing the plastic to solidify in the mold, which the machine keeps closed. The liquid, molten plastic from the injection cylinder of the injection machine is transferred through various flow channels into the cavities of a mold where it is finally shaped into the desired object by the confines of the mold cavity. What makes this apparently simple operation complex are the limitations of the hydraulic circuitry used in the actuation of the injection plunger and the complicated flow paths involved in the filling of the mold.

3. Opening the mold to eject the plastic after keeping the material confined under pressure as the heat which was placed into the material to liquify, it is removed to solidify the plastic and freeze it permanently into the shape desired.

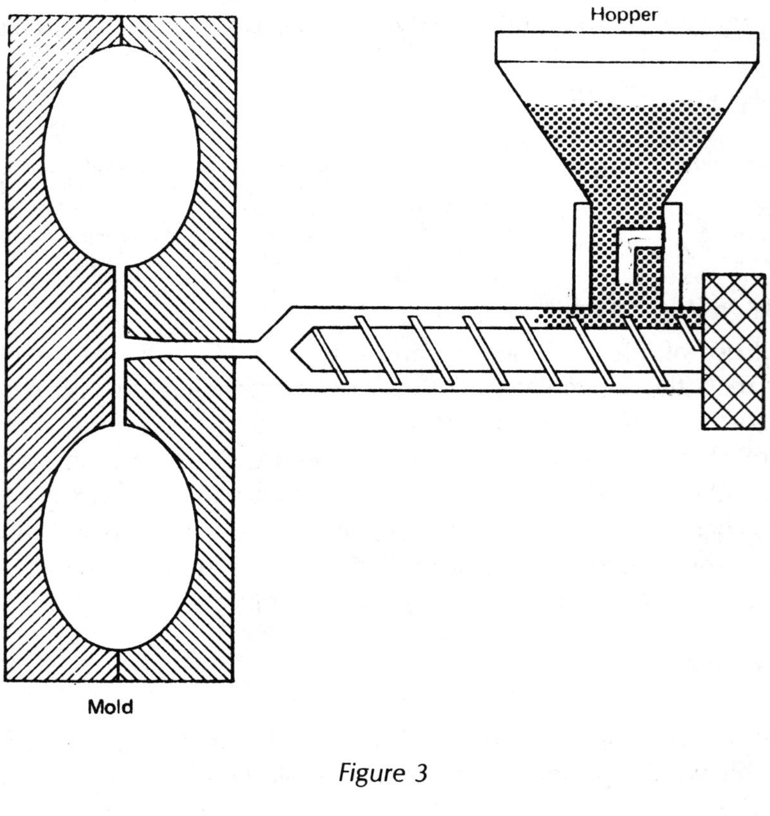

Figure 3

These three steps are the only operations in which the mechanical and thermal inputs of the injection equipment must be coordinated with the fundamental properties of the plastic being processed. These three operations also are the prime determinants of the productivity of the process since manufacturing speed will depend on how fast we can heat the plastic to molding temperature, how fast we can inject it, and how long it takes to cool the product in the mold.

The other operations in the injection process, such as clamping the mold, ejecting the part, feeding the machine, etc., are also important in the injection process. Their speed and effect on productivity will normally depend on factors other than the material being processed. They depend on factors such as hydraulics of the clamp system and design of the ejection system.

The basic machine is made up of the clamping end of a hydraulic machine; on the other end the injection unit of an inline reciprocating screw. The mold area is located in the center section. The empty space in the mold is filled with melted plastic under high pressure. The moving platen rides on steel bars call tie rods (or tie bars). The clamping force is generated by the hydraulic mechanism pushing against the moving platen and stretching the tie rods.

The part taken from the mold is, in most cases, a finished product ready to be packed and shipped or ready to be used as a part of an assembled unit. In contrast to metalforming, there is very little if any wasted material in injection molding. Most runners and sprues are reground and reused. By using hot runner molds, the sprue and runner system remain in a melted state in the mold and become part of the next finished part. The hot runners can be thought of as an extension of the plasticizing chamber. Usually, the part and mold can be designed so there is no subsequent machining required. If this is not possible for a certain design, conventional cutting tools can be used. Although some modifications of the cutting tip and periphery speeds are usually required to prevent a buildup of heat.

Materials having all shades of coloring can be purchased, or colorants can be preblended with clear pellets to obtain a desired color. Postformed coloring is eliminated and the color exists throughout the entire part.

Injection molding lends itself readily to automation in varying degrees, depending upon the ingenuity of the machine and mold designers, and the molder himself. The machine manufacturer can usually add components to the basic machine to implement any desired automatic arrangement. Molding cycles are relatively fast, and with new mold design developments constantly in progress, and centering around faster heat transfer within the mold, the molding cycle is continually being reduced.

Modern methods of material handling, both of the raw plastic and the finished product, are becoming more generally employed, further reducing costs of the finished part. Efficient use of leftover runners and sprues plays an important part in the overall economy of the molding plant, and increased attention is being given to this area. The reduction of raw material inventory is seriously considered today, and studies of production control methods are no longer uncommon, even by the small molder. All these economies are important in making plastic parts less expensive to manufacture and show plastics to be even more attractive to manufacturers dealing in all kinds of products.

The Injection Molding Systems

The basic components of an injection molding system which can be identified are: (1) blending, (2) drying, (3) hoppering, (4) metering, (5) plastication, (6) injection, (7) cooling, and (8) ejection. Plastic is usually purchased in pellet form and heated in the injection heating chamber until it reaches a viscous state in which it can be forced to flow into the mold cavities. Each plastic differs in its ability to flow under heat and pressure. For the best result, correct melting temperature, injection pressure and mold filling speed must be determined by trial for the particular plastic and mold used. Some molding conditions require that both the speed of injection and injection pressure vary during the filling process. A heat-sensitive plastic may be degraded if too fast a fill rate is used. Forcing the plastic through orifices at too high a velocity may increase the shear and temperature enough to cause overheating and burning.

However, thin-walled parts require a fast fill rate to prevent chilling of the plastic before the cavity has properly filled. Some molded parts carry both thin and thick sections, plus such interrupted flow patterns as are required to move around cored holes. Demanding requirements such as these require considerable versatility in the design of the injection unit. The programming of different injection speeds and pressures during the forward travel of the screw or plunger greatly aids in filling cavities properly. Programming or multi-stage injection is standard equipment on some machines.

The clamp of a machine must have sufficient locking force to resist the force of fluid plastic moving at high pressures from forcing apart the mold halves. (Figure 4) If the mating surfaces of the mold are forced apart, even a few thousandths/inch, fluid plastic will flow across the mating area or "flash." Amount of clamp force depends upon the projected area of the molded part; concern should also be given to a plastic's viscosity at the final fill stage. [15]

An experienced molder usually can judge the correct number of cavities to be used with his machines. The usual rule of thumb guide is to use 2 to 8 tons of available clamp/square inch of projected area (includes cavity and runner cross sectional areas). This guide can be used for parts having easy flow patterns and generous wall thicknesses, and which require medium injection pressures. Requirements for some molds and materials can be as high as 5 to 10 tons of clamp/square inch, but there is no exact method by which to predict requirements. Experience must be the real guide.

Plasticizing

The function of the injection molding machine heating cylinder is to thoroughly and uniformly convert (plasticize) the plastic feed material into a homogeneous heated plastic melt of controlled viscosity and then force it into the clamped mold where the end product is formed. Basically, the heating cylinder is a simple heat exchanger. Most cylinders have heavy steel walls with highly polished and hardened inner surfaces. For some purposes, the cylinder may be lined inside with a special corrosion-resistant material designed to resist the possible degradation products of thermally unstable resins.

It is important to note that only the cylinder temperature is directly controlled. The actual temperature of the plastic melt within the screw and as it is ejected from the nozzle can vary considerably, depending on the efficiency of the screw design and the method by which it is operated. Factors which affect the melt temperature include: the time the material remains in the cylinder; the internal surface heating area of the cylinder and screw per volume of material being heated; the thermal conductivity of both the cylinder and screw wall and the plastic material; the differential in temperature between the cylinder and the plastic; the wall thickness of the cylinder and of the stationary film (on the inner cylinder wall) of the plastic bein heated; and the amount of turbulence in the cylinder.

Since plastics, due to their molecular structure, have low thermal conductivities, it is difficult

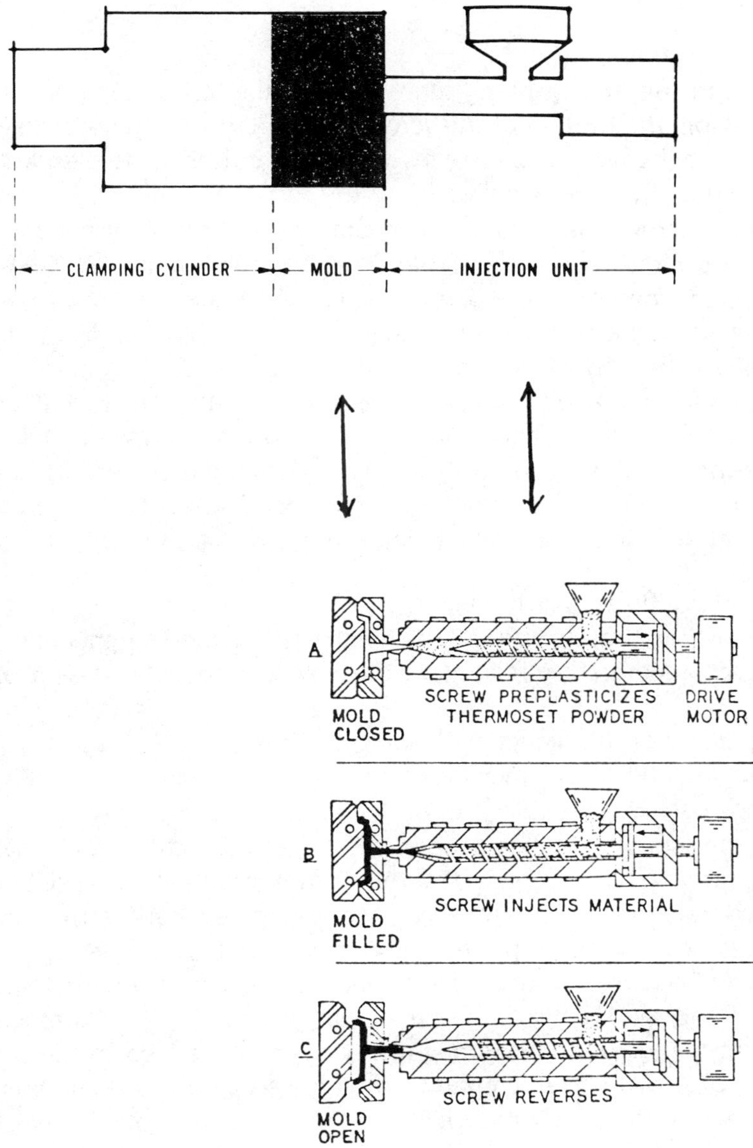

Figure 4

to transmit heat through them rapidly. In addition, plastic melts are very viscous, and it is difficult to create any turbulence or mixing action in them without the positive application of some form of mechanical agitation in the screw. The problem is further complicated by limitations on the length of time the plastic may be allowed to remain in the cylinder. In designing the screw, a balance must be maintained between the need to provide adequate time for proper heat exposure of material in the cylinder and the need to process maximum quantities of materials for most economical operation.

In general, the heat transfer problems have led injection screw designers to concentrate on making the screw more efficient heat transfer devices. As a result, the internal design and performance of these units varies considerably based on material to be processed.

Screw Design

The primary purpose for using a screw is to take advantage of its mixing action. Theoretically speaking, the motion of the screw should keep any difference in melt temperature to a minimum. It should also permit materials and colors to be blended better with the result that a more uniform melt is delivered to the mold.

The design of the screw is important for obtaining the desired mixing and melt properties as well as output rate and temperature tolerance on melt. Generally most machines use a single, constant-pitch, metering-type screw for handling the majority of plastic materials. A straight compression-type screw or metering screws with special tips (heads) are used to process heat-sensitive thermoplastics, etc.

The helix angle affects the conveying and the amount of mixing in the channel. Experience has shown that a helix which advances one turn per nominal screw diameter gives excellent results. This corresponds to an angle of 17.8° which has been universally adopted. The land width is 10% of the diameter. The radial flight clearance is the clearance between the screw flight and the barrel. It is specified considering the following effects:

1. Amount of leakage flow over the flights.
2. Temperature rise in the clearance. The heat is generated in shearing the plastic. The amount of heat generated is related to the screw speed, the design of screw and the material.
3. The scraping ability of the flights in cleaning the barrel.
4. The eccentricity of the screw and the barrel.
5. Manufacturing costs.

The length of the screw is the axial length of the flighted section. An important criterion of a screw design is the ratio of the length over the diameter of the barrel (L/D). Long screws with a 20:1 L/D are generally used. An advantage of a long screw can be that more of the shear heat is uniformly generated in the plastic without degradation. (Figure 5)

Basically, a screw has three sections: feed, melting (transition), and metering. The feed section which is at the back end of the screw can occupy from zero to 75% of the screw length. Its length essentially depends upon how much heat has to be added to the plastic in order to melt it. The pellet or powder are generally fed by gravity into this section and are conveyed some distance down the barrel, during which time they become soft. Heating is accomplished by both conduction and mechanical friction.

The melting (transition) section is the area where the softened plastic is transformed into a continuous melt. It can occupy anywhere from 5% to 50% of the screw length. This "compression" zone has to be sufficiently long to make sure that all of the plastic is melted. The straight compression-type screw is one having no feed or metering sections.

In the metering section, the plastic is smeared and sheared to give a melt having a uniform composition and temperature for delivery to the mold. As high shear action will tend to increase the melt's temperature, the length of the metering zone is dependent upon the resin's heat sensitivity and the amount of mixing required. For heat-sensitive materials, practically no metering zone can be tolerated. For other plastics, it averages out at about 20 to 25% of the total screw length. Both the feed and the metering sections have a constant cross section. However, the depth of the flight for the feed zone is greater than that in the metering zone. The screw's compression ratio can be determined by dividing the flight depth in the feed zone by that in the metering zone.

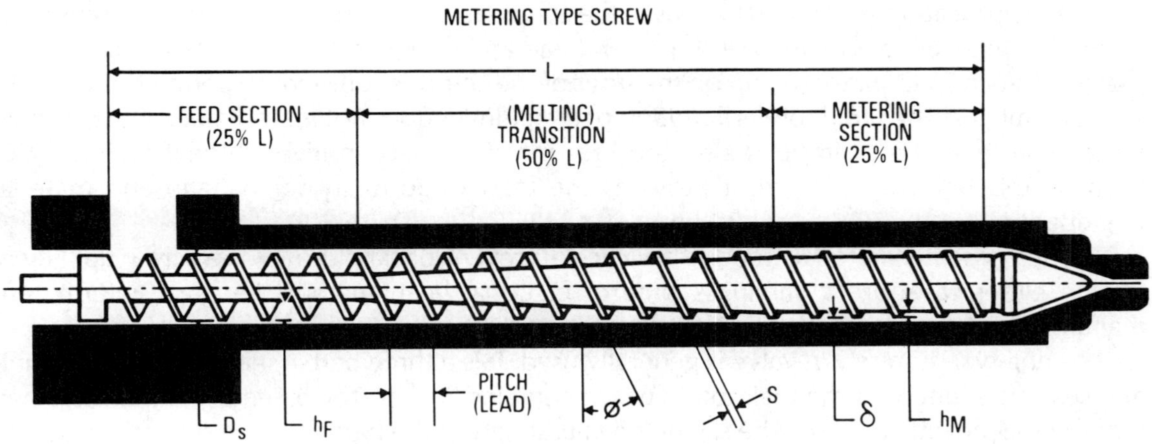

	D_S = diameter screw (nominal)		L = overall length
17.8°	ϕ = helix angle (one turn per screw diameter)	0.005	δ = flight clearance (radial)
0.250	s = land width	16:1 to 24.1	L/D = ratio of length to diameter
	h_F = flight depth (feed)	2.0 to 2.2	hF/hM = compression ratio
.22 minimum	h_M = flight depth (metering)		

Typical Screw Used in Injection Molding

Figure 5

At a fixed screw speed, the pitch, diameter, and depth of the channels determine output. A deep-channel screw is much more sensitive to pressure changes than a shallow channel. In the lower pressure range, a deep channel will mean more output; however, the reverse is true at high pressures. Shallower channels tend to give better mixing and flow patterns

The flow pattern in the screw flights changes with the back pressure. The flow of a particle in the flights with open discharge and in the blocked flow there is a similar circulatory motion between the flights, but no forward motion because the open end is closed. There is the greatest mixing when the flow is blocked. The importance of this flow concept is that it shows that the more blocked the flow, the better the mixing in the screw. The higher the pressure the greater the pressure flow and the lower the output. In injection molding, this pressure corresponds to the back pressure setting of the machine. This is the reason that color dispersion is improved and homogeneity increased by raising the back pressure. Often warpage and shrinkage problems can be overcome in this manner.

Developing Melt and Flow Control

The mechanism for melting starts after the plastics move from the hopper to the screw. Plastic touches the barrel to form a thin film of melted plastic on the barrel surface. The relative motion of the barrel and screw drag this melt which is picked up by the leading edge of the advancing flight of the screw. This flushes the polymer down in front of it, forming a pool which circulates. Heat is first conducted from the barrel through the film of plastic attached to it. Heat then enters the plastic by the shearing action, whose energy is derived from the turning of the screw. The width of the melted polymer increases as the width of the solid bed decreases. Melting is complete at the point where the width of the solid bed is zero.

The reciprocating screw machine uses the screw as a plunger. As the plunger comes forward, the material could flow past the screw head and back into the flights. For more viscous materials, such PVC, a tapered tip on the front of the screw is sufficient to permit the screw to act as a plunger. The rapid forward motion of the plunger does not let too much material flow back. Moreover, the plain tip is also good for molding heat-sensitive material such as PVC, because this type of screw front provides the least opportunity for hangup and material degradation.

The less viscous materials require a valve to prevent backflow over the screw tip. Screw tips, in either case, are a varying source of frictional heat, material hangups, intermittent malfunctioning, and potential high maintenance costs.

The ring-type non-return valve is generally used. It is a three part assembly. The check ring and seat are slipped on the main body which contains the tip. The assembly is then screwed into the reciprocating screw. The sliding ring fits snugly in the barrel. When the screw rotates, the force of the plastic pushes the ring toward the nozzle end and permits the plasticized material to flow under it through flutes or grooves on the main assembly. The screw slides back until the amount of material necessary for the shot is plasticized. On the forward or injection stroke, the ring slides toward the seat and seals the rear of the screw from the front so that material cannot leak by as the plunger comes forward.

Summary

As injection molding technology expands, requirements for precision injection molding machinery have followed suit. Profitable molding in today's highly technical and competitive world depends on precise clamping action coupled with both high plasticizing performance and reliability. This review has examined basic physical processes affecting the speed for productivity of an injection machine. These are the processes which must occur in any injection machine regardless of its specific design or of the refinements it contains in control systems or hydraulic circuitry.

Today, the actual injection machines which may be found on the market come in a myriad of sizes and designs. Because it is possible to combine a variety of different sizes of injection or plasticating systems with almost as many different sizes of clamp systems, there is almost no limit to the number of combinations available considering both the domestic and foreign sources of equipment. However, in every case, each machine must provide the necessary facilities to melt the plastic, inject it, and cool it.

Extrusion [14, 16]

When continuous profiles such as pipe, sheet, or profiles are required, a die of the desired shape is placed at the end of a heating chamber containing a feed screw that advances molding powder through the chamber where it becomes hot and soft and can be forced through the die. As the profile emerges it is cooled, as by an air blast or by immersion in a bath, carried away on a belt, and coiled or cut to suitable lengths. By varying the speed of the conveyor belt relative to the speed of extrusion, the profile can be drawn down to various sizes, but maintains the same proportions.

The most common and most versatile extruders in use today are of the single screw variety. In as many variations, the single screw extruder can convert a wide variety of raw thermoplastics into continuous melt streams which are then formed by dies into the desired shape for use or further manufacturing steps.

Every extruder includes these components: (Figure 6)

- barrel and feed section
- barrel heat input extraction mechanisms
- barrel (and die) temperature control systems
- screw
- gearbox and thrust bearing
- drive
- base

The screw is the heart of the extruder. Its design is the largest factor responsible for delivering fully melted, mixed polymer, at a uniform temperature—cross-bore and machine direction—and at a uniform output rate (usually judged by steady pressure level).

Today's standards for extruder output and extrudate quality are so highly advanced that no longer can one screw design be optimum for all materials and extrusion products.

Yet, every screw design is a compromise. Some of the factors which fight each other in this comprise are:

- More output at a lower temperature usually dictates a deeper screw: this yields poorer stability, less pressure pumping capability and less mixing or refinement of the polymer.
- More output usually dictates more speed (RPM), but this almost inevitably equates to a

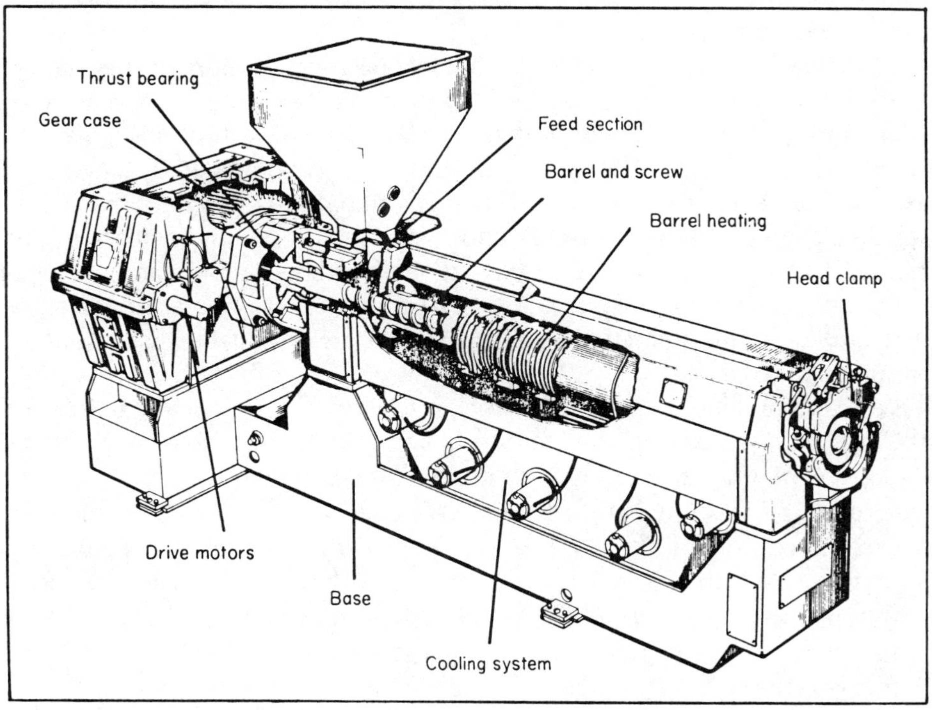

Figure 6

higher melt temperature, which often has adverse effects on both processability and finished pan properties.

• A longer screw yields greater output and melt homogenization, but usually raises melt temperature.

• While it is often desirable to remove excess melt heat in the metering section of the screw (through the barrel walls and heater/coolers), this tends to increase cross-bore temperature variation.

The common generic types of screws in use today are:

(A) *Basic Metering Screw* (Figure 7 (A)) Used extensively 20 years ago for the extrusion of most materials, this screw design is still utilized in the fiber industry and for the extrusion of PVC compounds.

It has the three zones common to all extrusion screws: a feed zone, a transition zone, and a metering or pumping zone.

The feed zone picks up the resin under the hopper and starts it into the externally heated barrel to begin polymer melting.

The transition zone compresses the material, eliminating air pockets and establishing a solid bed of unmelted pellets or powder with melt filling all voids. Much of the conversion of mechanical energy of the drive to heat occurs in this seciton, providing a major source of energy needed to melt the polymer.

The metering or pumping section of the screw generates the pressure needed to force the polymer through the die system. In the process, the rest of the polymer is melted and refined into a homogeneous mass.

(B) *Maddock (Union Carbide Corp.) Mixing Type Screw,* (Figure 7 (B)) This screw has become the workhorse of the polyethylene film industry. It refines the polymer through *one* close-clearance shear point to remove gels and fish-eyes, and yet yields a relatively high output of melt at a low stock temperature.

The UCC-Maddock section is usually located about 2-4 diameters to the rear of the tip of the screw to place it in an area of the barrel subject to the temperature control of heater/coolers and to provide some pumping capability beyond the mixing section.

(C) *Pin Mixing Screw* (Figure 7(C)) Heavily developed and optimized by Davis Standard, this screw's mixing action differs from the UCC-Maddock in that the multiple rows of pins break up the channel circulatory pattern repeatedly under low shear conditions, forcing it to re-establish itself in a random manner, rather than having one high shear mixing and homogenizing action. In the usual balance of output, rate degree of melt temperature uniformity, stock temperature, and pressure stability, the Davis-Standard Pin and the UCC-Maddock mixing screws are quite similar.

If there *is* a material difference, the Maddock screw may be marginally better at gel reduction, and the Pin Mixing screw may be marginally better in distributive mixing. The advantages of both mixing screws may also apply with increasing L/D ratios.

(D) *Compression Relief Mixing Screw* (Figure 7(D)) Used very successfully in longer (typically 34:1) extruders, the compression relief mixing screw has the feed, transition, and meter of the UCC and Pin Mixing Section, and offers deep channel low shear pumping, therefore, minimal stock temperature elevation. Further, this design tends to operate at a higher volumetric efficiency, as the first stage meter always pumps against a moderate (500-1500 PSI) pressure, not the usually higher (2500-6000 PSI) process head pressure

(E) *Vented Screw* (Figure 7(E)) The classical vented screw has feed transition, and metering sections in the first stage. This first meter dumps into the deep vent area which may be either

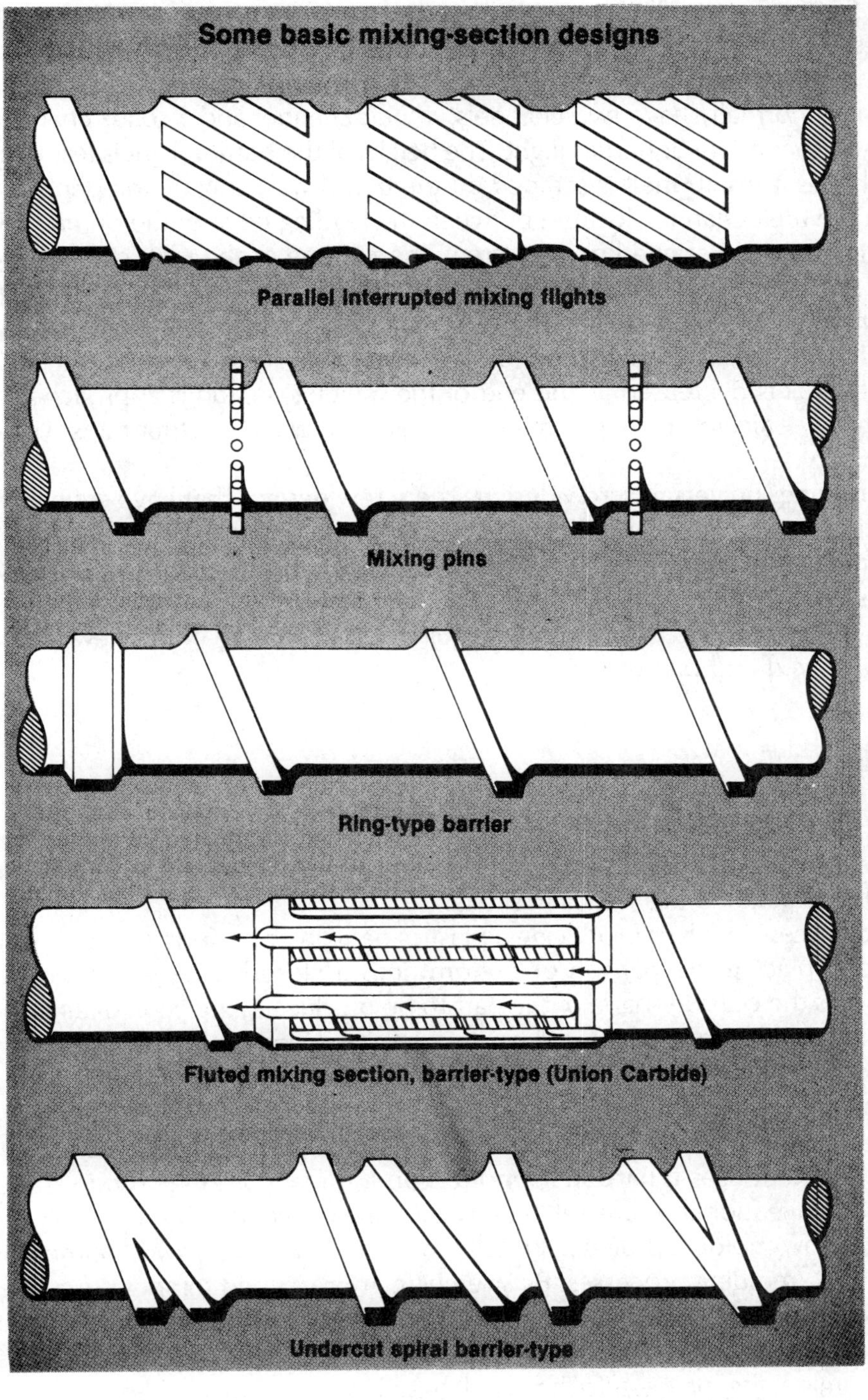

Figure 7

open to atmosphere or subjected to vacuum. Following the vent section is a recompression section, plus a second metering section, which pumps the polymer against the head or die pressure.

(F(*Barrier Screw* (Figure 7(F)) The melt separation or barrier type screw is available in many different designs, one or more of which may approach pressure optimum for your extrusion process.

These designs normally have two channels, a melt channel and a solids channel, which are separated by a secondary or barrier flight. The height of the barrier flight is less than that of the primary flight. As a result, melt is scraped off the barrel wall only by the primary flight and is collected in the melt channel, located between the leading edge of the primary flight and the barrier flight. In a well-designed barrier screw, the volume of the melt channel increases at a rate at least equal to the melting rate of the polymer which assures that no melt will collect in the solids channel. The increase in volume is accomplished either by deepening or widening the melt channel, or a combination of the two. In a reverse manner, the volume of the solids channel is decreased as the end of the melting section is approached. This design provides a highly efficient melting mechanism, resulting in high output rates with exceptional pressure stability.

There is no one "universal" screw design. The screw designs that have evolved as "best" for a particular industry or application are largely a function of compromises that application can accept in trading off output, melt temperature, mixing, and output uniformity while still meeting customer end product performance requirements. This evolutionary process will continue as resins, markets and property requirements change, and as new screw configurations are conceived and put into use.

Blow Molding [14]

Hollow plastics products such as squeeze bottles, milk bottles, fuel tanks, toys, oil containers, chemical tanks, furniture, electrical housing, etc. are blow molded. Different processes are used but the majority are basically similar.

The basic process involves producing a plastics parison or preform (tube, pipe, or test tube plastics shape), placing this parison or preform into a closed two-plate mold (cavity in the mold represents the outside shape of the part to be produced), injection of air into the heated parison to blow it out against the mold cavity, permit cooling of the expanded parison, opening the mold, and removing the rigid blow molded part.

Blow molding techniques can be divided into three major categories, namely, the extrusion blow molding process that principally uses an unsupported parison and injection blow molding process that uses a parison supported on a metal core pin. In turn these processes can be called conventional or unstretch-blow molding processes. The third major category is called stretch-blow molding process. Stretch-blow molding can start with either the extrusion or injection blow molding processes. By stretching at prescribed temperatures the properties of many plastics can be significantly improved providing cost/performance advantages.

These processes provide different advantages to produce all types of products so it is required to examine the process to be used based on product/performance requirements, materials (plastics) performance, and production quantity. As an example, the plastic bottle does more than hold the product. It combines safety, lightweight, design freedom, appealing colors, convenience, ease of dispensing, multi-decorating and low energy usage. Other factors to be examined in a blown container can be the desired shelf life, moisture barrier, oxygen barrier, drop strength, heat distortion, compatibility of plastic and product, top load, environmental stress cracking, clarity requirements, coloring of the plastic material, and cost.

When considering extrusion blow molding the advantages include high rate of production, low tooling cost, include blown handleware, wide selection of machine manufacturers, etc. Disadvantages are usually high scrap rate, recycling scrap, limited wall thickness control or material distribution, trimming can be accomplished in the mold for certain type molds or secondary trimming operations have to be included in the production lines, etc.

With injection blow molding, the major advantages include that no scrap or flash is molded, best wall thickness, and material distribution control, best surface finish of parts, low volume production quantities are economically feasible, etc. Disadvantages are high tooling cost, no handleware, based on the cost to produce large extruded blow molded parts the injection blow molded is limited to smaller sizes, etc. Advantages and disadvantages are similar for stretched injection blow molding. Major advantage is that cost/performance can be significant for certain size (and quantities) products such as the carbonated beverage bottle.

Important factors to consider when examining the blow molding process to be used usually start with part size, number to be manufactured, design/shape, and cost limitations.

Information is being presented to highlight past, present, and future developments in blow molding. The blow molding techniques to be reviewed have to take into consideration the melt process that occurs in the extruder or injection molding machine to produce the "ideal" parison or preform. So, in addition to analyzing the actual manufacturing process to be used in blow molding, it is extremely important to provide the properly designed machine to properly melt (and control the rheological/melt characteristic) of the parison or preform.

Blow molding of thermoplastics is now in its second century of operation. The first USA patent was filed May 22, 1880, published February 1, 1881 and issued to the Celluloid Manufacturing Company of New York. A fabricated cellulose nitrate tube was produced prior to heat/blowing. Later in history this tube was identified as a parison. A ram extruder was used to fabricate a tubular shaped sheet that was cemented along a scarf joint. Other methods to form the "parison" included the preparation of a high viscosity lacquer solution used to overcoat a mandrel. Vials and other containers were produced by these original concepts.

Major new developments occurred in blow molding during the 1920's and 1930's with the advent of extrudable cellulose acetate, ethyl cellulose, polystyrene, acrylic and most important, polyvinyl chloride. With the castable plastics, dip-coating of parisons became popular. Composite materials were used (similar to obtaining property/performance of our present coextrusion techniques) such as PVC adhesively bonded to pearlescent cellulose nitrate.

By the late 1930's, major new developments involved the use of controlled parison softening rate and relating the temperature profile to improving blow molding efficiencies. Prior technology involved basically the extrusion of a "pipe" that was positioned in ten to twenty blow molds operating in-line. Target was to provide sufficient heat to the pipe so that in-line bottles could be blown within certain time periods. With controlled parison temperature the present era of single and multiple blow molding started.

Multi-walled blow molded containers were produced during the late 1930's using double-walled tubes, stacked sheets or combinations of tube/sheet. Component adhesively assembled parts were produced; now the technique has been extended with the use of more thermoplastic solvent systems and sonic bonding. Rubber forming bags were used to produce blow molded double and single walled containers. This rubber bag technique started during the 1920's to produce single-wall blown parts. By the late 1930's, plants were producing different shaped pipes (different shaped water traps such as "S") by blowing PVC against a mold using a rubber coated spring; the spring would be positioned to provide the shape prior to blowing.

During the early 1940's, polystyrene extruded blow molded parts were very popular. Major commercial, large production parts were started during the 1950's using low density polyethylene to make squeeze bottles. By the early 1960's, work started in using high density polyethylene to produce extruded blow molded milk bottles . . . by the late 1970's, HDPE milk bottles reached a production in USA of over three billion bottles.

Since the 1940's, developments occurred in producing injection blow molded bottles and other containers. Developments of marketable, large production, did not occur until the 1970's with stretch-blow molding of 2-liter cabonated beverage bottles. Most of the original work started by Monsanto used acrylonitrile (AN), however production by others went to polyethylene terephthalate (PET). By 1980 over two billion PET carbonated bottles as Amoco Chemical, Continental Group, Hoover Universal, Imco, National Can, Owens-Illinois, Sewell Plastics, etc.

Extrusion Blow Molding

In extrusion blow molding, a parison is formed by an extruder. The plastic pellets are melted by heat which is transferred from the barrel and by the shearing action of the extruder screw as they pass through the extruder. The helical flights of the screw change configuration along its length from input to output ends to assure a uniformly homogeneous melt.

Turning continuously, the screw feeds the melt through the die-head as an endless parison or into an accumulator. Size of the part and the amount of material necessary to produce the part (shot size) dictate whether or not an accumulator offers an uninterrupted flow of plastic melt.

With the accumulator, flow of parison through the die is cyclic. The connecting channels between the extruder and the accumulator and within the accumulator itself, are designed rheologically to prevent restrictions which might impede the flow or cause the melt to hang up. Flow paths should have low resistance to melt flow to avoid placing unnecessary load on the extruder.

To ensure that the least heat history is developed during processing, the design of the accumulator should provide that the first material to enter the accumulator is the first to leave when the ram empties the chamber, and the chamber should be close to totally emptied on each stroke.

When the parison or tube exists the die and develops a preset length, a split cavity mold closes around the parison and pinches one end. Compressed air inflates the parison against the hollow blow mold surfaces which cool the inflated parison to the blow mold configuration. Upon contact with the cool mold wall, the plastic cools and sets the part shape. The mold opens, ejects the blown part, and closes around the parison to repeat the cycle.

Various techniques are used to introduce air into the parison. It may be accomplished through the extrusion die mandrel, through a blow pin over which the end of the parison has dropped, through blow heads applied to the mold, or through blowing needles which pierce the parison. The wall distribution and thickness of the blown part are usually controlled by parison programming, blow ratio, and the part configuration.

The mold clamping methods are hydraulic and/or toggle actuation. Sufficient daylight in the mold platen area is required to accommodate parison systems, unscrewing equipment, etc.

Clamping systems vary based on part configuration. Basically there exists, three types. The "L-shape" style has the parting line at an angle of 90° to the centerline of the extruder. The

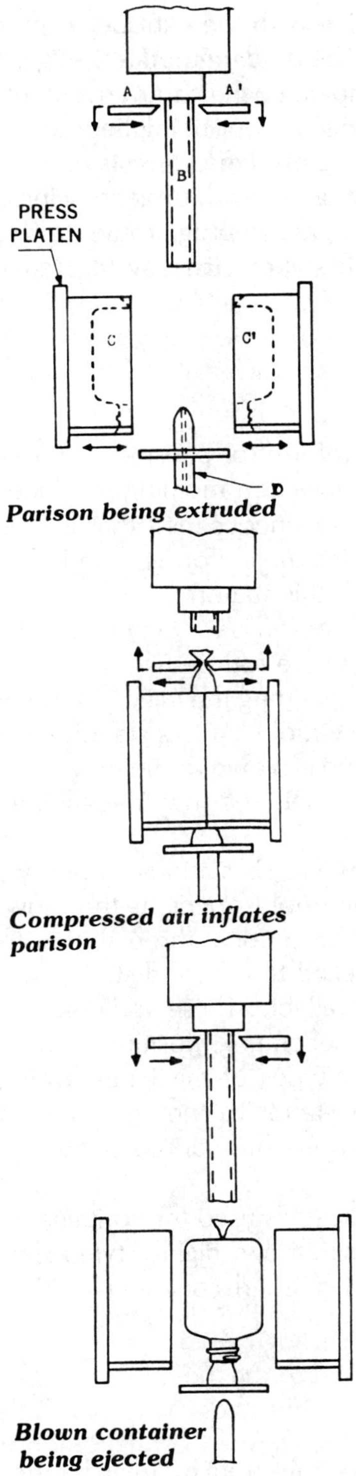
A
A'
B
PRESS PLATEN
C
C'
D
Parison being extruded
Compressed air inflates parison
Blown container being ejected

Figure 8

"T-shape" has the parting line in-line with the extruder centerline. Mold opening is perpendicular to the machine centerline. The third method is the "gantry" type. Extruder/die unit is arranged independently of the clamping unit. This arrangement permits the clamp to be positioned in either the "L" or "T" shape without being tied directly into the extruder.

The basic extrusion blow molding machine consists of an extruder, crosshead die (and accumulator), clamping arrangement, and mold. Variations include multiple extruders afor coextrusion of two or more materials, parison programmer to shape the parisons to match complex blown part shapes and multiple station clamp systems to improve output through the use of multiple molds.

Injection Blow Molding

In injection blow molding, a preform (or parison), is formed by a conventional injection molding machine plasticator. The injection molding machine injector provides an optimum plastics melt: with a uniformly homogeneous melt that is repeatable. This plastics melt is injected into the preform cavity forming the preform around the core rod. A completely finished injection molded neck is formed at this station.

In tool design the core rod and parison is very important. Each container to be blow molded has its own unique parison and core rod design.

The second stage consists of transferring the injection molded preform, either via the core rod, or the neck ring, into the blow mold. At this station compressed air enters through the core rod or seal ring and the preform is blown to the blow mold configuration. It is held in the cold blow mold until the material is set, and then the air is exhausted and the blown bottle ejected.

Machines are used with from two to six stations. In the two station machine, the finished container is ejected after the blow mold opens at the blow station by air pressure or by mechanical means. In the more conventional three station machine, the finished container stays with the core pin as it is indexed to the third station where ejection takes place. Four, five, and six station machines are available. These additional stations are used for further processing of the containers, such as decorating, positioning of blown parts, fillings, etc.

There have been several other types of machines available with different methods of transporting the core rods from one station to another. These include the shuttle, two position rotary, axial movement, and rotary with three or more stations used in conventional injection molding clamping units.

The injection blow molding process is used for containers that have very close tolerance threaded necks, wide mouth openings, and highly styled shapes. It features good materials distribution and the production of finished containers without the need for trimming and reaming.

Stretch Blow Molding

Since the late 1970's stretch-blow (injection) molding has become an important high speed, high production technique, largely due to the 2-liter carbonated beverage bottle that use PET resin. A variety of other bottling applications exist such as foods, cosmetics, etc. Stretched polypropylene (extrusion) blow molded bottles have been used since the early 1970's principally for packaging detergents.

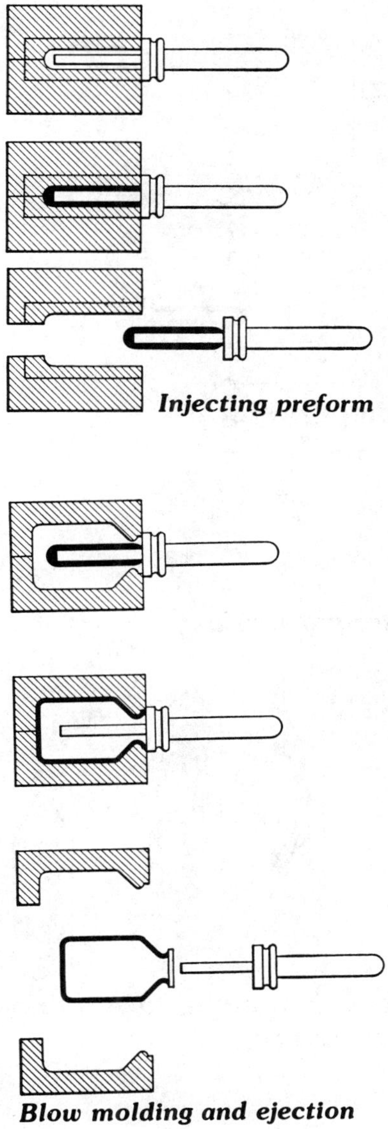

Figure 9

The stretch-blow process can give many resins improved physical and barrier properties. In biaxial orientation, bottles are stretched lengthwise by an external gripper, or by an interanl stretch rod, and then stretched radially by blow air to form the finished container against the mold walls. This process aligns the molecules along two planes providing additional strength, and even more important, better barrier properties than is possible without biaxial orientation. Other advantages include better clarity, increased impact strength, or toughness, and reduced creep. The actual increase is dependent on the ratio of blow up in each direction.

The carbonated beverage/soft drink bottles start with a tube or an injection molded preform. This preform is heated, stretched, and blown to its final shape. Due to the stretch and flow at a precise temperature, the molecules in the side wall become biaxially oriented,

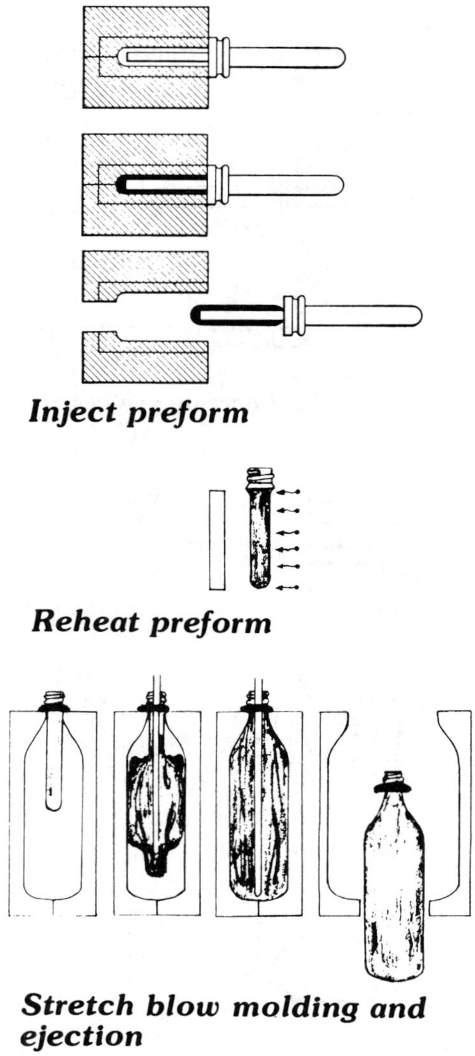

Figure 10

thus the term oriented. The top and bottom of these containers are not biaxially oriented, so these parts do not have the same physical properties as the side walls.

Ratios that are used to achieve the best properties in a PET bottle are 3.8 hoop by 2.8 axial. This will yield a bottle with hoop tensiles approximately 29,000 psi, and axials of 14,000 to 16,000 psi. Moisture barrier and CO_2 barrier are improved as a result of the process, also drop impact.

Stretch blow molding is possible for thermoplastic materials such as PET, PVC, polystyrene, acrylonitrile, polypropylene, and acetals. The amorphorous materials with a wide range of thermoplasticity are easier to stretch blow than the partially crystalline types. With the partially crystalline type (such as polypropylene), if the crystallizing is too rapid, the bottle is virtually destroyed.

Stretch-blow processing can be separated into two categories: in-line and two-stage. In-line processing is done on a single machine, while two stage processing requires either an extrusion or injection line to produce preforms, and a reheat-blow machine to make the finished bottles.

In the in-line an extruded or injection molded parison passes through conditioning stations which bring it to the proper orientation temperature. A rather tight temperature profile is held in the axial direction of the preform. Advantages of in-line systems are heat history is minimized (crucial for temperature-sensitive materials) and the preform can be programmed for optimum material distribution if it is maintained under continuous control.

With the two-stage, it uses extruded or injection molded preforms that have been cooled, and index them through an oven which reheats them to the proper orientation-blow temperature. (Temperature profile is held accurately in the axial direction of the preform.) Advantages of these processes can be that scrap production is minimized, improved thread finish, higher output rates, and the capability to stockpile preforms.

In-line injection stretch-blow systems, while offering more flexibility from material standpoint, do not give the degree of parison programming available in extrusion systems. An extruded parison can be heat stabilized, and then the parison is grabbed externally and pulled to give axial orientation while the bottle is blown radially. The process orients the entire bottle, including the thread area. Threads are then post-mold finished.

Extrusion processes also uses programed parisons and two sets of molds. The first mold is used to blow and temperature condition the preform, actually cool to orientation temperature, and the second mold uses an internal rod to stretch and blow the bottle.

When the two-stage, extrusion stretch-blow molding process is used, the preforms or parisons used are open-ended. They are reheated; then stretched by pulling one end while the other end is clamped in the blow mold. Minimum scrap is produced, and the compression molded threads provide a good neck finish. This system utilizes a conventional extrusion line and a reheat-blow machine whose oven contains quartz lamps to provide the proper temperature profile in order to obtain the proper container wall distribution.

The original designed two-stage machines have higher output rates than single-stage, while keeping scrap at a minimum. Preforms are injection molded on multicavity molds, including the thread finish, then cooled to ambient temperatures before going to the reheat-blow molding machine. Preforms are heated in a reflective radiant heat oven with provisions being made to shield preform thread areas.

After the oven heat exposure, preforms pass through an equilibration zone to allow the heat to disperse evenly through the preform wall. At the blow station, a center rod is inserted into the preform, stretching it axially, and to properly center the preform in the bottle mold. High-pressure air is then introduced to blow the preform to shape against the mold walls and give the bottle its radial orientation.

Based on the work conducted in stretch-blow molding, 2-liter containers of PVC, PET, and AN, average wall thicknesses of 0.012 to 0.015 inches have been used. Normal blow molding would use an average wall thickness of 0.018 to 0.022 inches, with no less than 0.009 to 0.010 inches in the thinnest point. The latter is used in either stretch blown or standard blow molding. Material so thin even though it will not fracture, is just too thin to prevent dimpling.

Relationship of wall thickness to degree of orientation is important. Control of the bottle's wall thickness can be as important, if not more, as the amount of biaxaial orientation. Soft drink bottles are pressurized to about 60 psi so the side walls of 0.009 to 0.015-inch cannot collapse due to internal pressure. However, a product such as mouthwash does not have internal pressure, and thin walls with 0.009 to 0.015-inch would experience paneling or wall collapse due to permeation losses.

Materials

Practically any thermoplastics can be blow molded; particularly the commodity type plastics. Different properties can be obtained with the different available and useful plastics that are now used to blow mold different size and shaped products. Properties can include strength toughness, clarity, gas barriers, chemical resistance, heat resistance, color, and many others. Different combinations of properties can be achieved by combining two or more plastics. Parisons can be coextruded, coated, dipped, coinjected, etc. in order to provide the combinations of different properties available in different plastics. Stretch-blow molding also provides an important processing technique to provide improved properties and reduce the quantity of plastics to improve cost/performance characteristics.

Examples of properties that can be obtained with the different plastics are as follows: Clarity—crystal polystyrene, acrylonitrile, styrene acrylonitrile, polyvinyl chloride, stretched PET, polysulfone; Moisture Barrier—polypropylene, low density polyethylene, high density polyethylene, transparent nylon, polymethypentene; Oxygen Barrier-PET, polyvinyl chloride, polyacrylonitrile, polysulfone, transparent nylon; etc.

Extrusion blow molding represents the biggest outlet for blow molded containers with high density polyethylene being the major plastics used; about 80 percent of all plastics consumed. Recognize that there are different grades of HDPE; with increased density stiffness, strength, hardness, creep resistance, softening temperature, and gloss improves. However, toughness, stress crack resistance, and permeability decreases. It resists most acids and salts but is attacked by strong oxidizing agents.

Polyvinyl chloride (PVC) is the second largest resin used in poundage in the USA today. Due to its low oxygen transmission, water clear clarity and relative ease of processing, it has captured the hair care, toiletries, cosmetics, household chemical and edible oil markets. It is now being challenged by stretch blown polypropylene and stretch blown PET.

This brief review on the different plastics is used to emphasize the importance of using the correct plastics to meet specific requirements. The real test on any material is that it is blown, either unoriented or stretch-oriented. Unfortunately, in the past, many simulated "fast" tests to evaluate plastic bottle performance have had "bad" records. But recognize that there are "fast" tests that have been developed to simulate actual performance.

SUMMARY

Hollow plastics products are produced ranging in volume from parts of an ounce to thousands of gallons. They are used to contain liquids, pastes, powders, and other solid particles. Use also extends into many other applications such as housings for tools, electronic hardware, wheels, and other parts of toys, medical devices, platforms, building panels, etc. When only examining the market for bottles over fifteen billion thermoplastics bottles were produced during 1980.

Even though blow molding is considered a major production process in USA, markets for new, as well as expanding present markets, is rather unlimited.

Examples of these markets include medical devices, automobile gasoline tanks, small carbonated beverage bottles, food containers, etc. These markets are also expanding since more action is developing co-extruded or coinjection materials to improve cost/performance of containers.

REFERENCES

1. Rosato, D. V., *Polymers, Processes and Properties of Medical Plastics,* University of Lowell Medical Polymer 4th International Seminar, Waban, MA., Apr. 1982.

2. Medical Market at $3.1 Billion, *Plastic World,* Boston, Ma., Cahners Publ., pp. 11-12, Aug. 1981.

3. Schuller, H., Plastics in Medicine, *The BASF Review,* BASF Corp., Germany, Vol. (23), pp. 28-37, May 1973.

4. Szycher, M. and Robinson, W. J., *Synthetic Biomedical Polymers: Concepts and Applications,* Westport, CT., Technomic Publ., 1980.

5. *World Health Market Research,* Cleveland, OH., Predicasts Inc., 1981.

6. Rosato, D. V., Fallon, W. K. and Rosato, D. V., *Markets for Plastics* (Medical), New York, NY., Van Nostrand Reinhold Co., pp. 281-289, 1969.

7. Polymers Advance the Ancient Art of Dentistry, *Southern Research Institute Bulletin,* Vol. (32), No. 1, pp. 16-19, Winter 1979-1980.

8. U.S. Dept. of Commerce, Medical and Dental Instruments and Supplies 1981, Santa Monica, CA., *Medical Devices and Diagnostic Industry,* Vol. (3), No. 8, pp. 38-48, Aug. 1981.

9 Bandy, W. C., 1981 U.S. Industrial Outlook-Medical and Dental Instruments and Supplies, Washington, DC., International Trade Commission, U.S. Dept. of Commerce, 1981.

10. Lee, H. and Neville, K., *Handbook of Biomedical Plastics,* Pasadena, CA., Pasadena Technology Press, 1971.

11. Rosato, D. V. and Schwartz, R. T., *Environmental Effects on Polymeric Materials,* Vol. 1 Environments and Vol. 2 Materials, New York, NY., Interscience Publ., pp. 1-2216, 1968.

12. Perfecting Flexible PVC for Medical use is Five Years Well Spent, *BIP Plastics Review,* London, England , p. 3, Nov. 1980.

13. Rosato, D. V., New ASTM Materials Standard for Designers, 33rd Annual Tech. Conference, Reinforced Plastics/Composites Institute, SPI, New York, Section 7-E, pp. 3-4, 1978.

14. Rosato, D. V., Injection Molding-Extrusion-Blow Molding, Plastics Seminars, University of Lowell, Waban, MA., 1982.

15. Beck, R. D., *Plastic Product Design,* New York, NY, Van Nostrand Reinhold Co. 1980.

16. Lounsbury, D. C., and Wheeler, N. C., *Know Your Extruder,* Davis Standard, Pawcatuck, CT., 1981.

SUBJECT INDEX

AUTHOR INDEX